TEXTBOOK
of
ORGANIC CHEMISTRY
for
PHARMACY STUDENTS

[General Organic Chemistry, Drugs and Chemistry of Natural Products]

TEXTBOOK
of
ORGANIC CHEMISTRY
for
PHARMACY STUDENTS

[General Organic Chemistry, Drugs and Chemistry of Natural Products]

Dr K S Mukherjee MSc, PhD

Ex-Professor and Head, Department of Chemistry
Formerly Principal, Siksha Bhavana (Dean, Faculty of Science)
Visva-Bharati, Santiniketan, West Bengal, India

New Central Book Agency (P) Ltd

LONDON
HYDERABAD ERNAKULAM BHUBANESWAR
DELHI KOLKATA PUNE

NCBA

REGD OFFICE

8/1 Chintamoni Das Lane, Kolkata 700 009, India
email: ncbapvtltd@eth.net

OVERSEAS

NCBA (UK) Ltd, 149 Park Avenue North, Northampton, NN3 2HY, UK

EXPORT

NCBA Exports Pvt. Ltd, 212 Shahpur Jat, New Delhi 110 049
email: ncbaexp@ncbapvtltd.com

BRANCHES

208B Peacock Lane, Shahpur Jat
New Delhi 110 049
email: ncbadel@ncbapvtltd.com

Shop Nos. 3 & 4, Vinayak Towers
681/B Budhwar Peth, Appa Balwant Chowk
Pune 411 002
email: ncbapune@ncbapvtltd.com

House No. 3-1-315, 1st Floor
Nimboliadda, Kachiguda, **Hyderabad** 500 027
email: ncbahydb@ncbapvtltd.com

GSS Shopping Complex, 1st Floor
Opposite College Post Office, Convent Road
Ernakulam 682 035
email: ncbaernk@ncbapvtltd.com

Shop No. 15, Bharati Towers, Ground Floor
Forest Park, **Bhubaneswar** 751 001
email: ncbabub@ncbapvtltd.com

TEXTBOOK OF ORGANIC CHEMISTRY FOR PHARMACY STUDENTS

First Published: 2010
Reprinted: 2012

PUBLISHER AND TYPESETTER
New Central Book Agency (P) Ltd
8/1 Chintamoni Das Lane, Kolkata 700 009

PRINTER
New Central Book Agency (P) Ltd
Web-Offset Division, Dhulagarh, Sankrail, Howrah

COVER DESIGNER
Soumen Paul

COVER PRINTER
Liba Graphics, Kolkata

TECHNICAL EDITOR
Dipan Roy

PROJECT TEAM
Swapan Sarkar, Prabhat Jas

ISBN: 978-81-7381-620-8

Price: ₹ 350.00

Contents

PART II

CHEMISTRY OF NATURAL PRODUCTS

Preface

In recent years the concept regarding the profession and role of pharmacists in our society have undergone an explosive change. The nature as well as the scope of their profession have been expanded profusely. The aim of this profession has now been shifted more towards the patients rather than the drugs. As a result, curricula of pharmacy (B.Pharma/ M.Pharma) have been changed significantly. In this changed scenario, chemistry particularly Organic Chemistry—occupies a vital position. This is because all the drugs are Chemical Compounds which are primarily Organic in nature and the study of pharmaceutical Organic Chemistry involves the discussion on the synthesis, storage, activities, toxicities, metabolism and management of drugs. As such, students of pharmacy are required to have a clear basic concept of chemistry, specially Organic Chemistry.

With the above objective, the present manual, entitled **Textbook of Organic Chemistry for Pharmacy Students** [General Organic Chemistry, Drugs and Chemistry of Natural Products] has been written. It provides comprehensive— but in concise form— the fundamental aspects of Organic Chemistry and discussion on the Chemistry of Organic Compounds, drug molecules and natural products as per the syllabi of the Pharma courses prescribed by AICTE and various Indian universities.

In each chapter attempts have been made to present the subject matter into an affordable and student-friendly manner with acute focus on the applications of Organic Compounds in relation to drug molecules. At the end of each chapter a set of Model Questions have been provided to guide and help the students in understanding the subject. I am sure the book will be useful to the pharmacy students and teachers alike. In this context I would like to mention that for general Organic Chemistry several chapters of the author's book **Textbook on Organic Chemistry** (NCBA) have been suitably revised, rearranged, and rewritten to meet the needs of the students of pharmacy.

In preparing the manuscript I have consulted a large number of books by national and international authors. I am grateful to them. I sincerely acknowledge the valuable assistance and helpful suggestions received from my son Sri Bodhisattwa Mukhopadhyay, MSc, Sr. Executive, Fresenius Kabi Oncology Limited, Kalyani, Nadia, West Bengal.

I would like to record my profound regards to my elder brothers Sri Shibsankar Mukhopadhyay, retired Assistant Teacher, Ramkrishna Sikshapith, Tumbani, Birbhum, and Dr Durgasankar Mukhopadhyay, Former Head, Department of Bengali, Calcutta University, for their hearty affection and constant inspiration. I am thankful to Dr Madhab Kumar

Chattopadhyay, Scientist, CCMB, Hyderabad, India, and Sri Sukanta Chattopadhyay, M.Pharma, Jubilant Organosys Limited, Noida, India, for their helpful suggestions. I wish to place on record my grateful thanks to my wife, Gouri, for her constant inspiration during the preparation of the book.

My heartfelt thanks to the authorities and the production staff of New Central Book Agency (P) Limited, Kolkata, for publishing this book promptly.

I would welcome any constructive criticism and suggestions for the improvement of the book.

26 January 2010
Phuler Madhu
Simantapalli, Santiniketan

K S Mukherjee

Introduction

Pharmaceutical Organic Chemistry is concerned with the studies of chemistry of those Organic Chemicals which are either used directly as medicines or are associated with the medicines as the starting materials for their syntheses. It may be mentioned that practically almost all the medicinal compounds are organic in nature and belong to different classes like hydrocarbons and their halogenated derivatives, alcohols, ethers, carbonyls, carboxylic compounds, aromatic, heterocyclic compounds etc. It is, therefore, obvious that pharmaceutical organic chemistry must involve the studies of these compounds. Again, it is known that activity of any organic compound as medicine is largely controlled by its chemical characteristics. Naturally, every student of pharmaceutical chemistry must be aware of some of the fundamental principles including stereochemistry and mechanistic aspects of organic reactions which determine the chemical characteristics of organic molecules.

It may be remembered that nature is the biggest source of organic chemicals. The existence of biologically active chemicals in natural resources, particularly in plants, has been known since the inception of human civilisation. The plant products have immense contribution in pharmaceutical science either as direct drugs or as the intermediates for the development of variety of drugs. Again, the study of various reactions of organic chemicals isolated from plant sources constituted the beginning of organic chemistry and indeed during the whole period of nineteenth century, only these natural products were the main source of organic chemicals and provided an immense fund of fascinating problems of organic chemistry. The structure investigation of these phytochemicals has resulted in the recognition of a large variety of organic compounds with diverse skeleton pattern. These vast number of organic compounds having complex chemical structures often exhibit highly specific pharmacological activities and possess curative properties against various diseases and find frequent applications in modern medicines. Statistically nearly 50% of the total consumable drugs in the present market are still derived directly or indirectly from the plant kingdom. The epoch-making tranquilliser drug, reserpine, from the genus **Rauwolfia,** effective antileukaemic drugs, vinblastine, vincristine, vincoleuco-blastine from **Vinca rosea** (Periwinkle), lympathomimetic drug, ephedrine from the genus **Ephedra**, the anti-malaria drug, quinine from **Cinchona** species, highly effective analgesic, morphine from **Papaver somniferum**, antimorbid swelling drug of **Podophyllotoxin** group, antidysentric drug, emetine from **Ipecae** roots, anticoagulant dicoumarol from **Rutaceae** family and use of various plant species of the genus **Swertia** in the treatment diseases like mental disorders, liver disorder, maleria, tuberculosis, hyperglycemic activity as well as in the treatment of central and cardiovascular systems, potent anticancer drug paclitaxel (Taxol) from **Taxaceae** family are only a few of the life saving potent drugs from natural sources on which entire human community is largely dependant. Again, rutin, a very well-known glycoside, originally derived from **Ruta graveolens** is now extensively used in the treatment of capillary fragility and after effects of exposure to atomic radiations. Recent view reveals that more than two dozens of phytochemicals have already been found to have antitumar activity and about forty per cent of the new drugs approved during the period between 1983 to 1994 are derived from plant sources. It is amazing to note that a few drugs such as angiotensin covering agents enalapril, captopril, nonsteroidal anti-inflammatory drugs diclofenac, naproxen, bronchodialator drug, salbutamol derived from plant sources occupy the positions world's best selling pharmaceuticals.

It may be mentioned that the use of plant products is not restricted to drugs alone but is applicable in the field of agriculture and sericulture. The isolation of the gibberellin group of plant growth hormone and the conversion of diosgenin to α-ecdysone has given a new dimension in the chemistry of natural products. Once again, many phytochemicals have been found to possess pesticidal properties and in recent years, in many instances, plant products are being used in protecting the loss of crop-production from the attack of insects and parasites. It has been observed that the nematodes, one of the important groups of parasites, affect both the animal and plant kingdoms and cause about 1461.6 million tons of annual world crop losses. These parasites were found to be highly resistant to the most of the pesticides synthesised so far. Moreover, the synthetic pesticides available in the market are highly costly often phytotoxic and cause environmental pollution. On the other hand, plant products have not only been found to be effective pesticides but are cheap, non-phytotoxic, non-pollutant, susceptible to bio-degradation and they do not leave any harmful residues in crops and soil.

Besides these material aspects, as mentioned before, chemical studies of plant products have unearthed a large volume of problems with tremendous academic interest. The solution of these problems in many instances have afforded the stimulus for the theories that are now fundamental to organic chemistry. Thus, the descriptions of non-classical carbocation and the theories of stereochemistry, including conformational analysis have firm foundation in natural product chemistry. Further, the structure of plant products, particularly complex molecules, have provided a challenging source of synthetic objectives. Again easy transformation of some of the phytochemicals to physiologically active hormone such as conversion of holaphylline, a steriodal alkamine of **Holarrhena floribonda**, to progesterone which can be transformed to cortisone through simple chemical orientations has stimulated active interest in the scientific research on plant products among the large number of chemists, clinicians and physiologists. It is, therefore, felt pertinent that the students of pharmacy should be acquainted with some preliminary ideas regarding the natural products. As such a few chapters comprising of the sources, chemistry and uses of some important groups of natural products have been incorporated in this text.

PART I

General Organic Chemistry

and

Drugs

CHAPTER ONE

Basic Concepts

Organic Chemistry is the chemistry of the compounds of carbon. Carbon possesses an unique character which primarily originates from its position in the periodic table. In order to understand the uniqueness in the character of carbon it is felt pertinent to present in this chapter a general discussion on some fundamental concepts.

1.1 Atomic Orbitals

Carbon atom has six electrons surrounding its nucleus. These six electrons according to Bohr theory are assumed to be arranged in different orbitals of varying energy. The precise definition of actual orbitals has, however, been emerged from the wave mechanical concept in conjunction with Heisenberg indeterminacy principle. According to these modern concepts, electrons are not fully particle in nature but they are sufficiently dynamic wave in character. So they do not stay still in a single position and what can be predicted is the relative probabilities of finding an electron at different positions from the nucleus. Consequently, classical concepts of orbitals have been replaced by three dimensional orbitals and these three dimensional nature of the orbitals can represent the shape and size of the space around the nucleus which can indicate the highest probability of finding a particular electron. According to *Pauli exclusion principle* an orbital can accommodate only two electrons having opposite spin. Again, *Hunds rule* states that the degenerate orbitals (orbitals having same energy) are half-filled before any of the orbitals are filled up by two electrons.

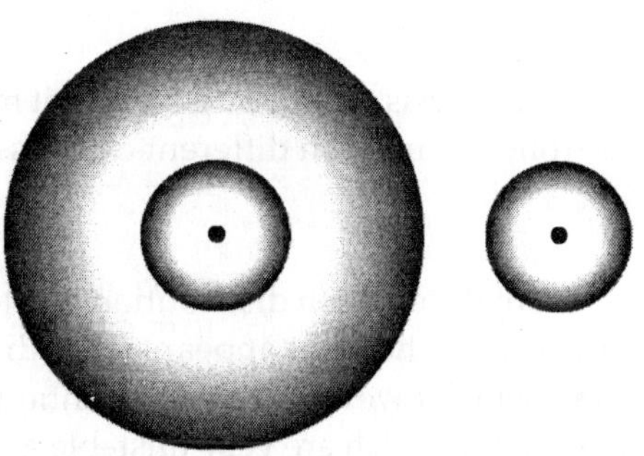

Fig. 1.1

The *Aufbau* process for periodic table is primarily based on these two rules. Wave mechanical analysis reveals that both 1*s*- and 2*s*-orbitals are spherically symmetrical but 1*s*-orbital is likely to be found closer to nucleus, having low energy and is more strongly held than an electron in a 2*s*-orbital. Two consecutive orbitals are separated by a space known as *nodal* *surface* where the probability of finding electrons is zero. A 1*s*-orbital thus has no node but 2*s* has a nodal surface as shown in the figure (Fig. 1.1).

According to wave mechanics, there should be three *p*-orbitals all having same energy and shape and these three *p*-orbitals are mutually perpendicular to each other along *x*-, *y*- and *z*-axes and are accordingly designated as $2p_x$, $2p_y$ and $2p_z$, respectively. These *p*-orbitals are dumb-bell shaped, two lobes of which touch each other at a point. This point has zero probability of finding electron and is known as nodal plane. These orbitals are pictured in the following figure (1.2):

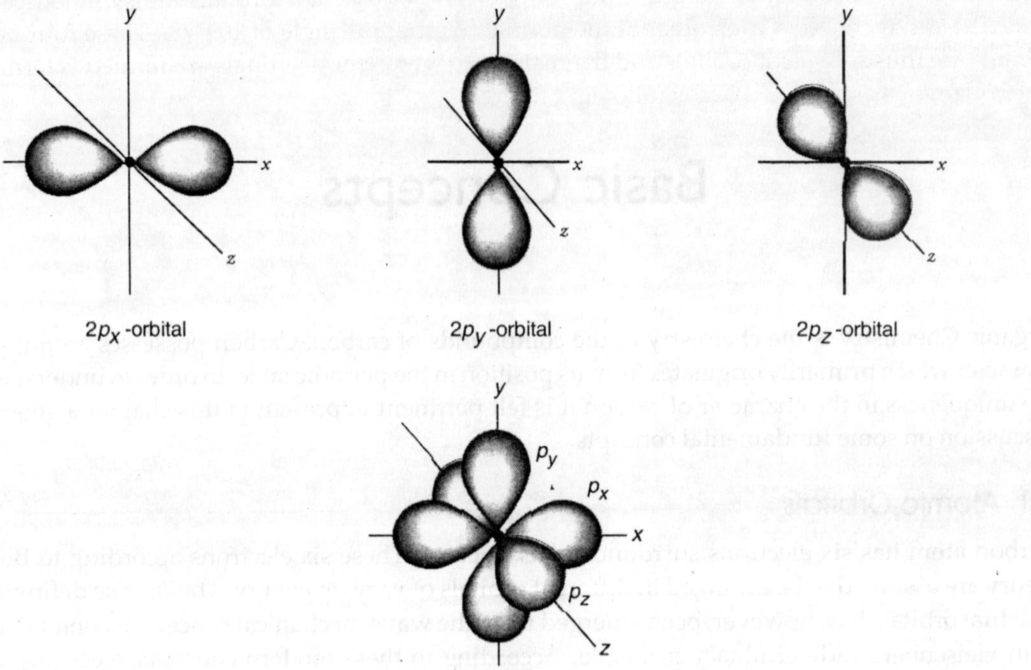

Fig. 1.2

On the basis of above discussion it may be concluded that the ground state distribution of six electrons of carbon in different orbitals may be written as:

$$1s^2 2s^2 2p_x^1 2p_y^1 2p_z^0$$

From the electron distribution written above it is evident that carbon has only two unpaired electrons and hence it appears to be divalent in nature but in actual practice carbon is always tetravalent. However, it may be mentioned in this connection that there are a few divalent carbon compounds which are very unstable and highly reactive. These are designated as *carbenes*.

It has been suggested that during any chemical reaction carbon atom can easily assume excited state by the dissociation of $2s^2$ electrons followed by the promotion of one of the dissociated electrons to the vacant $2p_z$ orbital without any additional requirement of energy because the energy required for dissociation of $2s^2$ electrons is much less than the energy produced during these two additional bond formation. As a result, carbon acquires such a configuration which has four unpaired electrons. Consequently it can form four rather than two bonds with other atoms or groups and so carbon can manifest its normal tetravalency having distribution of six electrons as:

$$1s^2\ 2s^1\ 2p_x{}^1\ 2p_y{}^1\ 2p_z{}^1$$

1.2 Hybridisation

1.2.1 sp^3-hybridisation

From the electron distribution given above it appears that tetravalent carbon should have two different types of valencies—one type due to three 2*p*-orbitals and the other one arising out of 2*s*-orbital. But in actual practice all the four valencies of carbon are equal and identical. This is only possible if all these four orbitals are intimately mixed together and divided in such a way that four equal and identical orbitals are formed. These four new orbitals are symmetrically disposed and inclined to each other at the normal tetrahedral angle of 109°28′. These four new orbitals are thus *sp^3-hybrid* orbitals and the manner in which these orbitals are formed is termed as *Hybridisation* as depicted in the following figures:

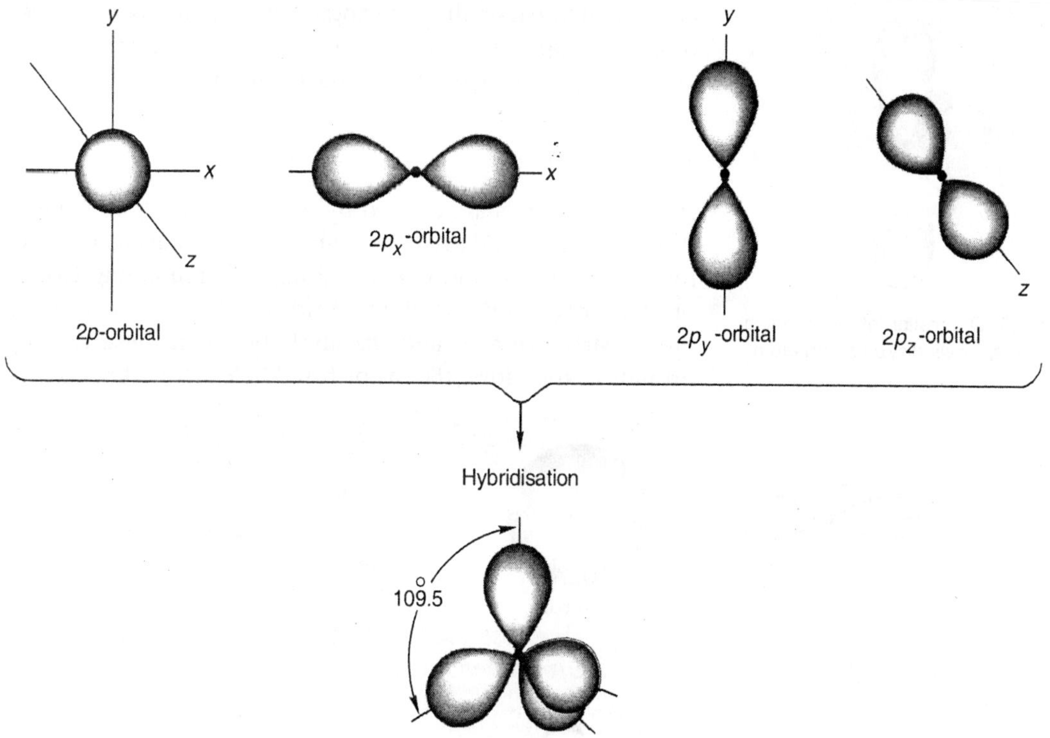

Four sp^3 atomic orbitals for one carbon
(small back lobes of orbitals omitted)

Fig. 1.3

1.2.2 sp^2 and sp-hybridisation

Two more hybrid orbitals are observed viz., sp^2- and *sp*-orbitals in the case of carbon atom.

1.2.3 sp^2-hybrid Orbitals

In this process of hybridisation one 2*s*- and two 2*p*-orbitals are mixed together to form three new equal and identical orbitals termed as sp^2 -orbitals as these hybrid orbitals are composed of one *s*- and two *p*-orbitals. Each of these three hybrid orbitals has one third *s*-character and two third *p*-character. The third $2p_z$-orbital is left unhybridised. The shape of sp^2-hybrid orbital may be depicted in the figure as under (Fig. 1.4):

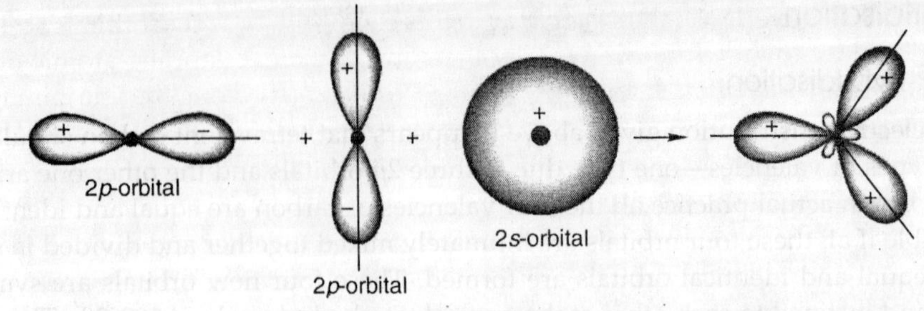

Fig. 1.4 : Shape and orientation of sp^2 A.O.s.

The three sp^2-orbitals lie in the same plane having a common axis passing through the nucleus and oriented trigonally. The angle between any two of these orbitals is 120°. The unhybridised *p*-orbital is oriented along an axis perpendicular to the plane of sp^2-orbitals as shown in the figure (Fig. 1.5).

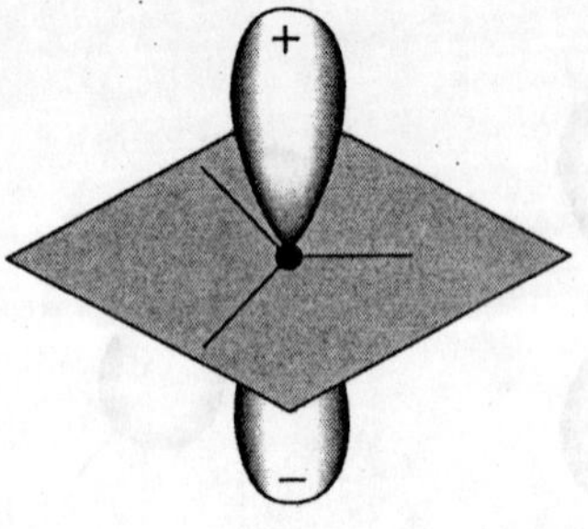

Fig. 1.5: Orientation of the p_z orbital of an sp^2 hybridised carbon atom

1.2.4 *sp*-hybrid Orbitals

sp-hybrid orbitals are formed by mixing 2s- and only one of three *p*-orbitals and are designated as *sp*-orbitals as they are formed by one s- and one *p*-orbitals. The remaining two *p*-orbitals are (p_y and p_z) left unhybridised. Two hybrid orbitals are linearly oriented and the angle between these two *sp*-orbitals is, therefore, 180° as pictured below (Fig. 1.6):

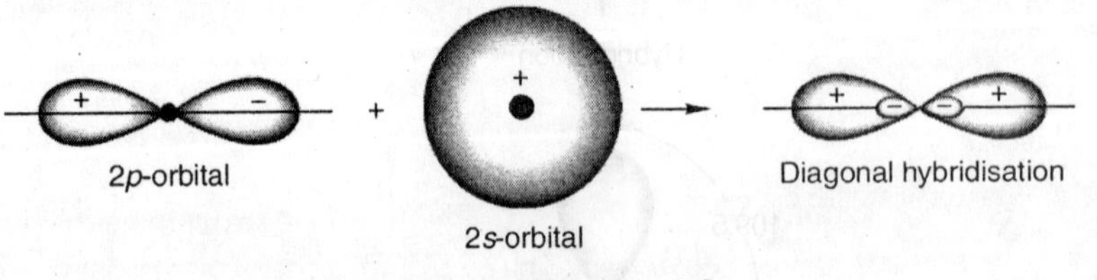

Shape and orientation of sp A.O.s.

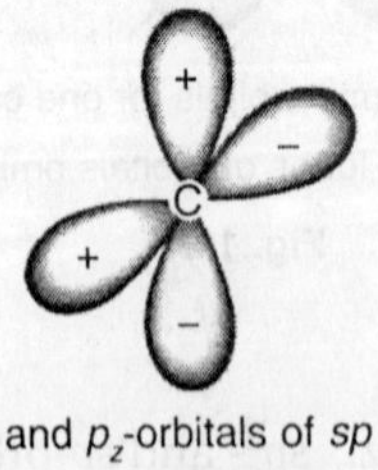

Orientation of p_y- and p_z-orbitals of *sp* hybridised carbon atom

Fig. 1.6

1.3 Chemical Bond Formation in Carbon•

According to *Molecular Orbital theory* a bond is formed between two atomic orbitals when they overlap each other—greater the overlapping, more stronger is the bond so formed.

When two atomic orbitals approach each other to overlap, there may be formation of two different new orbitals known as *Molecular Orbitals*—one such molecular orbital is formed when two atomic orbitals overlap in the *same phase*. In this condition these two orbitals add together to form a molecular orbital with lower energy than any of the overlapping atomic orbitals. This molecular orbital has a region of relatively high electron density along the line joining the nuclei of two participating atoms or in other words, the electrons in this molecular orbital is said to be localised. This higher electron density can easily attract the two positively charged nuclei and keep them together. For this reason this molecular orbital is known as *bonding molecular orbital*.

The other molecular orbital is formed when the atomic orbitals are *out of phase* during their overlapping. In this stage, atomic orbitals will tend to cancel each other so that there is a nodal plane where the probability of finding the electron is zero. This molecular orbital is of higher energy, i.e., less stable and has decreased electron density between the two nuclei and so the two positively charged nuclei are not eclipsed each other. Consequently two participating atomic orbitals repel each other and hence this orbital is termed as *antibonding molecular orbital*.

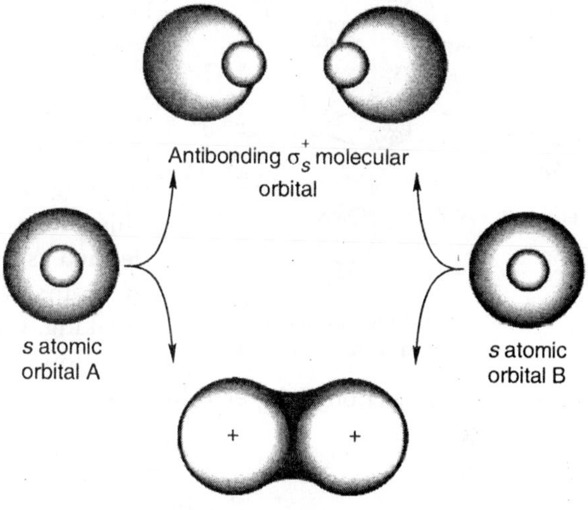

Fig. 1.7

Thus from the overlapping of two atomic orbitals two molecular orbitals are formed. In fact, this is a general phenomenon—whenever there are over-lapping of *n* number of atomic orbitals, the molecule so formed will have *n* number of molecular orbitals—half of which would be bonding in nature while remaining half of the orbitals would be antibonding in character. The above process of bond formation is portrayed in the figure above (Fig. 1.7).

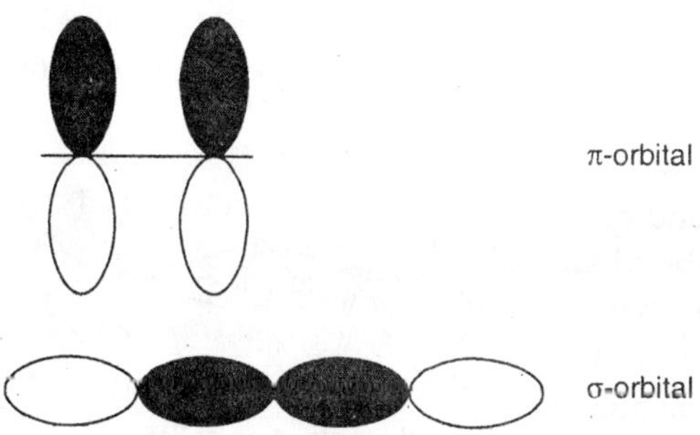

Fig. 1.8

1.4 Sigma (σ) and pi (π) Bonds

Overlapping of atomic orbitals leads to the formation of two types of covalent bonds—one is sigma (σ) and the other is pi (π) bonds, and the localised electrons of the corresponding covalent bonds are known as σ- and π-electrons, respectively. σ-bonds are formed when the overlapping of any two atomic orbitals takes place co-axially but when two *p*-orbitals overlap perpendicularly (sidewise) along the inter-nuclear axis, the bonds so formed are called π-bonds. It may be mentioned that the molecular orbital of σ-bond is known as σ-orbital and that of π-bond is called π-orbital.

1.4.1 Carbon-hydrogen Single Bond

During the combination with hydrogen, the four sp^3-hybrid atomic orbitals of carbon atom overlap co-axially with 1*s* atomic orbitals of four hydrogen atoms to form four strong and identical s-sp^3 hybrid σ-bonds making a normal tetrahedral angle of 109°28′ with each other. The orbital overlaps of four C—H bonds in methane are depicted in the figure (Fig. 1.9).

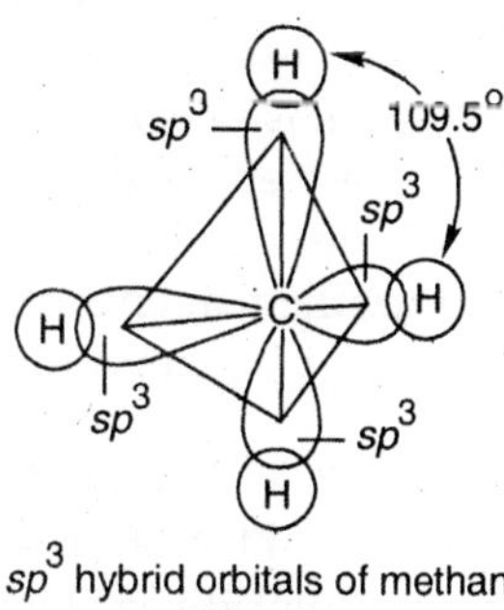

sp^3 hybrid orbitals of methane

Fig. 1.9

1.4.2 Carbon-Carbon Single Bond

Formation of carbon-carbon single bond as in ethane involves the co-axial overlapping of two sp^3-atomic orbitals—one from each carbon atom. The bond thus formed between the two carbon atoms is a strong σ-bond having bond length 1.54 Å. The bond is symmetrical about the inter-nuclear axis and is free to rotate along this axis.

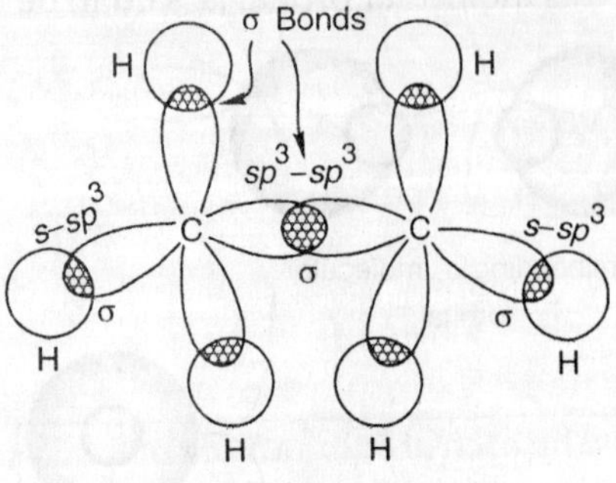

Orbital structure of Ethane

Fig. 1.10

This free rotation is significant in the sense that organic molecule can have infinite number of structures due to different spatial arrangements of hydrogen atoms on two bonding carbon atoms arising out of this free rotation. This phenomenon is known as *conformation* which is defined as the different arrangements of the same group of atoms which are interconvertible without bond breaking. Out of all the structures two extreme species are known as eclipsed and staggered forms as expressed by Newman projection. Staggered form is stable and is termed as preferred conformation.

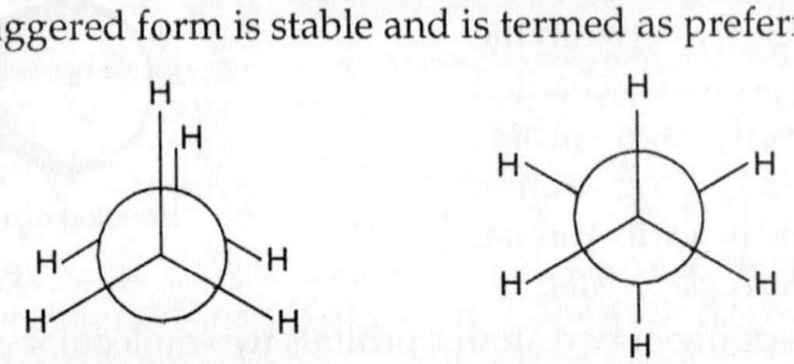

Eclipsed form Staggered form

Fig. 1.11

1.4.3 Carbon-Carbon Double Bond

Ethylene contains a double bond between two carbon atoms. In this carbon-carbon double bond each carbon atom is bonded with three other atoms—two of hydrogen and one of carbon. In between carbon atoms there are two bonds, one is σ formed by the linear (co-axial) overlap of two sp^2-hybrid orbitals one from each carbon and other is a π-bond formed by the parallel overlap of two unhybridised $2p_z$-orbitals—one from each carbon atom which are perpendicular to the plane of sp^2-orbitals. As the carbon atoms in π-bond are more tightly held, it has shorter (1.32Å) bond length than σ-bond and has restricted rotation. It is obvious that the overlap of two $2p_z$-orbitals will be maximum when two carbon atoms and four hydrogen atoms are exactly coplanar because it is in this position p_z-orbitals are exactly parallel to each other and hence maximum overlapping occurs. An important aspect of π-bonds is that there is no electron density between two participating nuclei. The electron cloud is concentrated above and below the plane of the bond. As the electron clouds in π-bond are less tightly held by the nuclei than the electron clouds in σ-bond, they readily take part in chemical reactions particularly with electrophilic reagents like halogens. Two hydrogen atoms in each carbon atom in ethylene are connected by σ-bond formed by co-axial $s—sp^2$ overlap as shown in figure (Fig. 1.12).

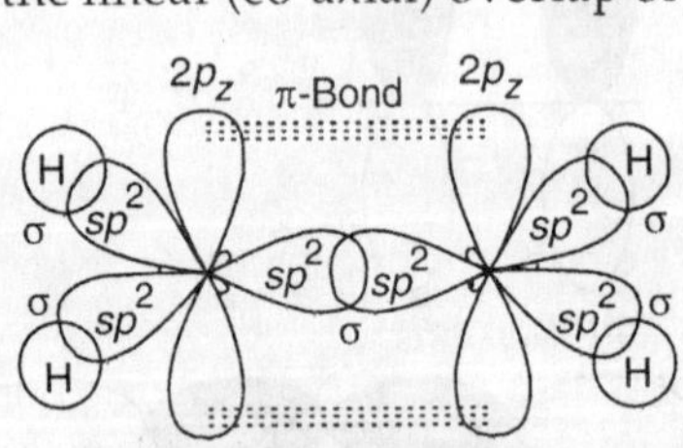

Orbital structure of Ethylene

Fig. 1.12

1.4.4 Carbon-Carbon Tripple Bond

The first member of carbon-carbon tripple bonded compound is acetylene in which carbon atoms are in *sp*-hybridised state. Out of three bonds between two carbon atoms one is σ-bond formed by the co-axial overlap of two *sp*-orbitals—one from each carbon and other two are π-bonds which involve the overlapping of $2p_y$- and $2p_z$-orbitals on each carbon which are mutually perpendicular to the σ-bond. Carbon-hydrogen bond in acetylene is due to *s-sp*-overlap which is at an angle of 180° to carbon-carbon σ-bond. This gives the molecule a linear shape with carbon-carbon bond length 1.20Å which is shorter than that in ethylene. The orbital picture of acetylene is shown (Fig. 1.13).

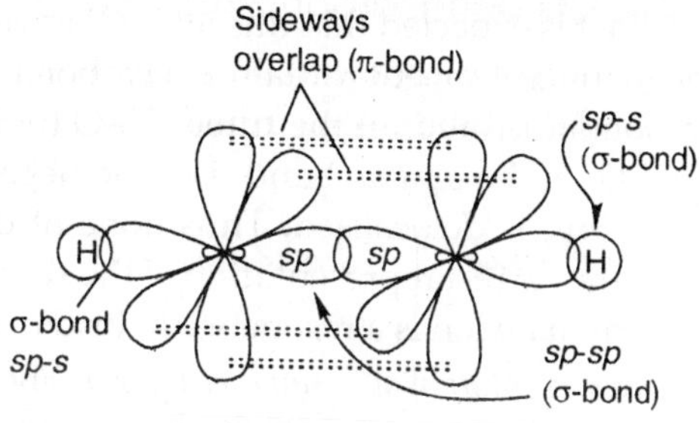

Orbital picture of acetylene

Fig. 1.13

PROBLEM 1.1

Indicate the type of bond and kinds of bonding orbitals used by each of carbon atom of the following molecules.

(a) $CH_2 = CH_2$, (b) $CH_3—CH_3$, (c) $HC = C—CH = CH—CH_3$

1.5 Bond Dissociation Energy

It is known that when atoms combine each other to form a bond a certain amount of energy is released as a result of which the energy of the molecule becomes less than that of constituent atoms. This amount of energy which is released during the bond formation is termed as *bond energy* (E), or heat of formation of bond. On the other hand, energy required to break a covalent bond is known as *dissociation energy* (D) which reflects the strength of the bond. It may be mentioned that the bond formation energy and bond dissociation energy are more or less equal in magnitude but opposite in sign.

$$H + H \rightarrow H - H, \Delta H° = -104.2 \text{ kcal/mole (Bond formation energy)}$$

$$H - H \rightarrow H + H, \Delta H° = 104.2 \text{ kcal/mole (Bond dissociation energy)}$$

Bond dissociation energy has an implication on chemical reaction as we know that chemical reaction involves the process of bond breakage and bond formation.

1.6 Resonance

The concept of resonance was first introduced by Heisenberg in 1920 and was generalised by Pauling in 1930. It has been observed that there are a large number of compounds, all the properties of which cannot be explained on the basis of a single structure. To explain different properties, different structures are to be assumed. These structures have no real existence. They are purely hypothetical and are interconvertible by the movement of electron pair only but the positions of atomic nuclei remain unchanged. The actual structure of the molecule is the average of all these hypothetical srructures, i.e., the structure of the molecule is a hybrid of all these hypothetical structures. This hybrid structure is usually known as *resonance hybrid* or delocalised structure and the different interconvertible hypothetical structures are termed as resonating, canonical or contributing structures. Let us consider carbonate ion for an example. It can be represented by three Lewis structures (I—III), all of which suggest that this ion has one double bond and two single bonds in between carbon and oxygen atoms.

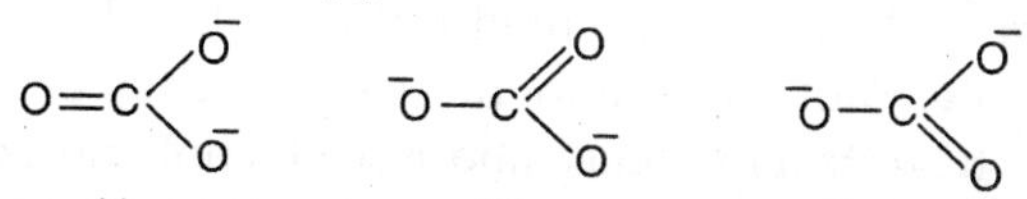

(I) (II) (III)

So it is expected that this ion will have two different carbon-oxygen bond lengths. But bond length measurement reveals that carbonate ion is completely symmetrical with a trigonal central carbon atom, and all the three C—O bonds are of equal length which is in between that of a double -and a single -bond, i.e., the negative charge is not localised to any one of the oxygen atoms but is delocalised. Thus none of the Lewis structure actually represents the carbonate ion—the correct representation of the structure of this ion is the average of these three structures. So carbonate ion is a resonance hybrid of the above three structures.

Representation of resonance hybrid: The resonance hybrid is represented by connecting all the contributing structures by double headed arrow. Thus

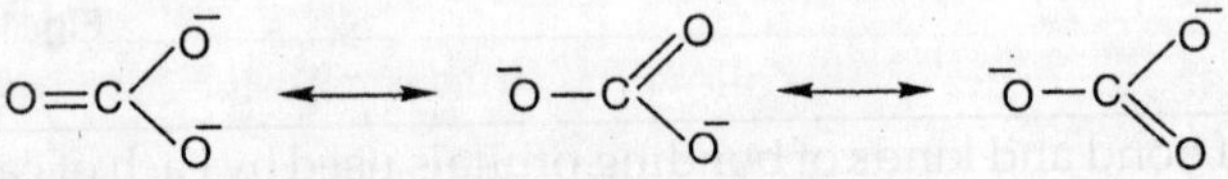

(I) (II) (III)

Conditions for resonance: The chief conditions for resonance are:

i. Resonance are observed only in π-bonded compounds.
ii. Different structures must be interconvertible.
iii. Each structure must have nearly the same internal energy.
iv. Position of nucleus of each atom in different structures must be the same.
v. All atoms involved in resonance must be more or less on the same plane.
vi. The number of unpaired electrons in each structure must be the same.

Effect of resonance: The effects offered by resonance may be enlisted as below:

i. The bond length becomes different, usually shorter than that of any contributing structure. Thus, benzene molecule which can be represented by two Kekule structures (IV) and (V) should have two different bond lengths, i.e., three C = C π-bonds with bond length 1.34 Å and three C—C σ-bonds having 1.54 Å bond distance. But X-ray analysis reveals that it has only one bond length of 1.39 Å. This is possible if benzene molecule exists in resonance hybrid of IV and V.

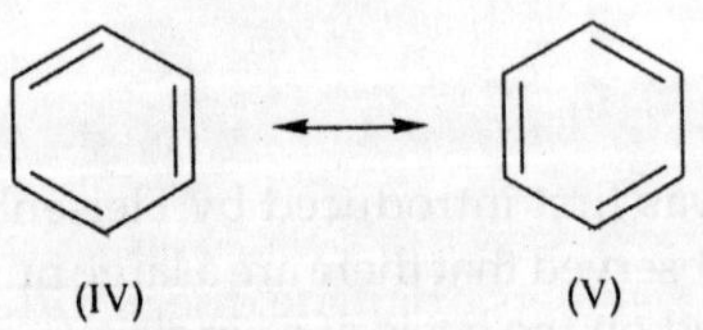

(IV) (V)

ii. Resonance increases the stability of the molecule. Thus heat of hydrogenation of benzene calculated on the basis of any one of the contributing structure (IV and V) is expected to be approximately 85.50 kcal/mole but the observed value is only 49.50 kcal/mole. The difference between calculated and observed heat of hydrogenation is known as *resonance or delocalisation energy* and it has been observed that higher the value of resonance energy more will be the stability of the molecule.

iii. An interesting effect offered by resonance is that observed dipole moment may be different from the calculated value.

Resonance vs. tautomerism: It may be pointed out that the phenomena of resonance and tautomerism are not the same. Tautomerism involves equilibrium between the structures, and different tautomeric forms have real existence and in fact, enol and keto forms of ethyl aceto-acetate have been isolated.

Another important aspect in which tautomerism differs from resonance is that in tautomerism no additional stabilisation of the molecule occurs.

Tautomerism also differs from resonance in the fact that in resonance only π-electrons are involved, σ-electrons remain intact while in tautomerism both π - and σ-frameworks are directly involved.

Lastly it may be mentioned that resonance effect should not be confused with mesomeric effect. Mesomeric effect is a case of permanent polarisation involving similar mechanism of electrons transfer as in electromeric effect but in resonance no such permanent polarisation occurs.

PROBLEM 1.2

Write all the resonance forms of the following molecules:

(i) CH_3—NO_2, (ii) $CH_2 = CHCH = CH_2$, (iii) 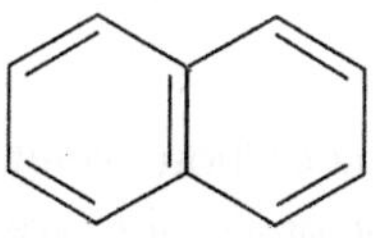

1.7 Isomerism

In organic chemistry it is frequently observed that a single molecular formula represents two or more compounds. These compounds differ from each other in physical and chemical properties and are known as *isomers* or *isomerides*. This phenomenon of real existence of two or more compounds having same molecular formula is termed as *isomerism*. The phenomenon of isomerism has been explained by assuming that the atoms or groups in a molecule are arranged in a definite manner and the difference in physical and chemical properties among the isomers is due to different modes of arrangement of atoms or groups in each isomer and so isomers differ in their structures. Again, carbon atom is tetrahedral in nature, so the spatial disposition of four groups towards four corners of tetrahedron may be different in different isomers. Thus, phenomenon of isomerism has been classified into two categories:

(a) Structural isomerism
(b) Stereo isomerism.

1.7.1 Structural Isomerism

In this isomerism, different isomers originate due to difference in the arrangements of atoms or groups within the molecule, i.e., if two or more compounds differ in their structural formulae, they are said to be structural isomers and the phenomenon is known as *structural isomerism*. There are different types of structural isomers as listed below:

(a) Chain isomerism
(b) Position isomerism
(c) Functional isomerism
(d) Metamerism
(e) Tautomerism.

1.7.1.1 Chain Isomerism

This type of isomerism arises from the difference in the carbon skeleton. Following examples may be cited:

(a) *n*-Butane and isobutane

$CH_3-CH_2-CH_2-CH_3$

n-Butane

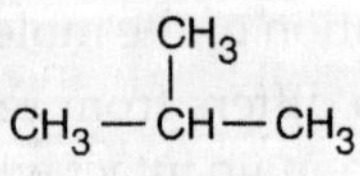

Isobutane

(b) Iso, Neo and *n*-Pentane

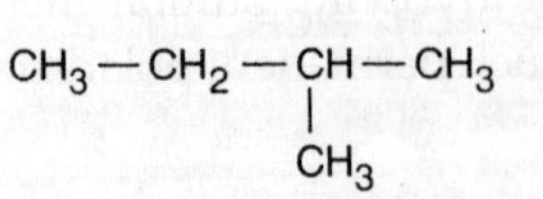

Isopentane

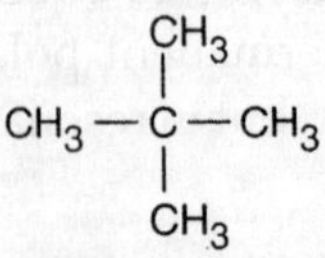

Neo-pentane

$CH_3-CH_2-CH_2-CH_2-CH_3$

n-Pentane

1.7.1.2 Position Isomerism

These isomers have the same carbon skeleton but differ in the position occupied by functional group. Examples of this type of isomers are:

(a) 1-Propanol and 2-Propanol

$CH_3-CH_2-CH_2-OH$

1-Propanol or *n*-propanol

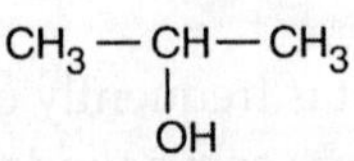

2-Propanol or isopropanol

(b) 1-Butene and 2-Butene

$CH_3-CH_2-CH=CH_2$

1-Butene

$CH_3-CH=CH-CH_3$

2-Butene

(c) *o* -, *p* - and *m* - dichloro benzene

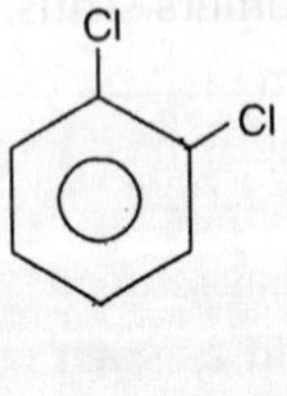

ortho-dichloro benzene

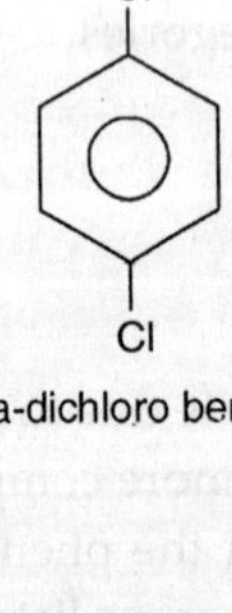

para-dichloro benzene

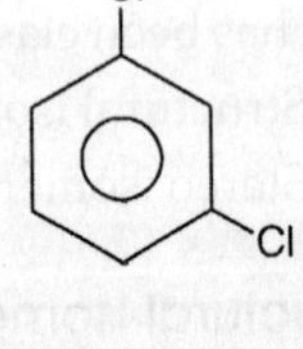

meta-dichloro benzene

1.7.1.3 Functional Isomerism

Isomers having same molecular formula but have different functional groups are known as functional isomerism.

- **Examples:**

(a) Dimethyl ether and ethyl alcohol

CH_3-O-CH_3

Dimethyl ether

CH_3-CH_2-OH

Ethyl alcohol

(b) Acetone and propionaldehyde

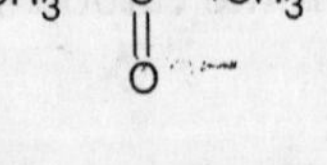

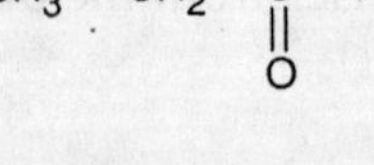

1.7.1.4 Metamerism

This is a special type of isomerism in which different isomers differ in the distribution of carbon atoms around a central atom.

- **Example:**

(a) Methyl propyl ether and diethyl ether

$$C_2H_5-O-C_2H_5 \qquad\qquad CH_3-O-CH_2-CH_2-CH_3$$

Diethyl ether   Methyl propyl ether

(b) Diethyl ketone and methyl propyl ketone.

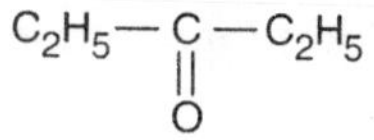

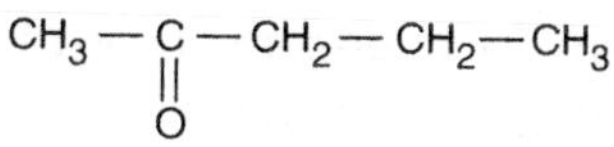

Problem 1.3

Indentify the nature of isomerism of the following pairs

(a) 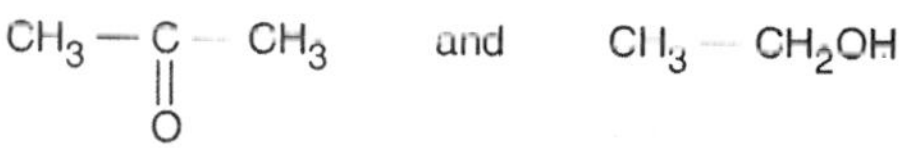

(b) $C_2H_5-O-C_2H_5 + CH_3-O-CH_2-CH_2-CH_3$

(c) 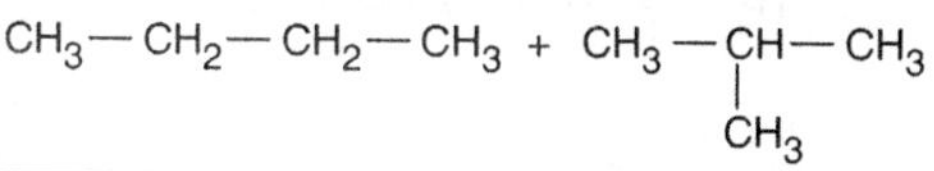

1.7.1.5 Tautomerism

It is an unique class of structural isomerism and to some extent different from other types of isomerism. It differs from the other isomerism in the fact that the isomers in this phenomenon are not static, they are dynamic in nature and are interconvertible. In fact, they exist in dynamic equilibrium with each other. According to modern approach tautomerism is due to the existence of two or more readily interconvertible forms which differ only in their electron distribution and in the position of mobile group. The different structures are termed as *tautomers*.

The mobile group concerned, may be a cation or any anion and as such tautomerism has been classified mainly as (i) *cationotropy* which involves the shifting of cations and (ii) *anionotropy* in which transfer of anions is observed. In overwhelming majority of cationotropy mobile group is a proton and that is why cationotropy is sometimes termed as *prototropy*. Highly illustrated examples of prototropic tautomerism are ethyl aceto-acetate and aliphatic nitro compounds while allylic compounds constitute the examples of anionotropy.

(a) Prototropy

i. 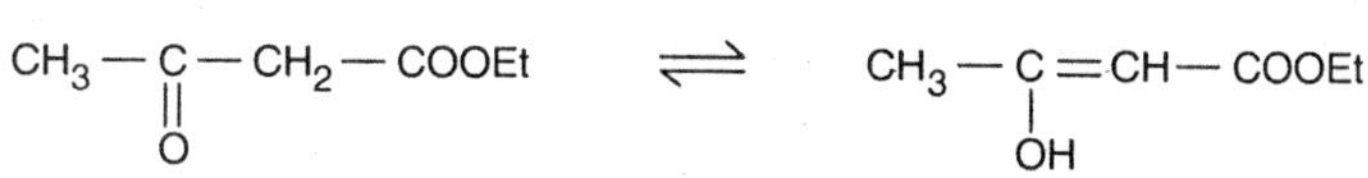

Keto form   Enol form

ii. 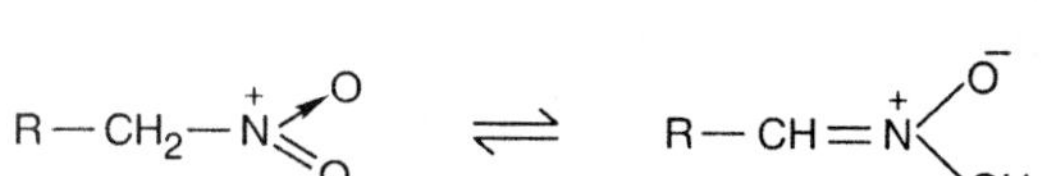

Pseudo acid form   Acid form

(b) Anionotropy

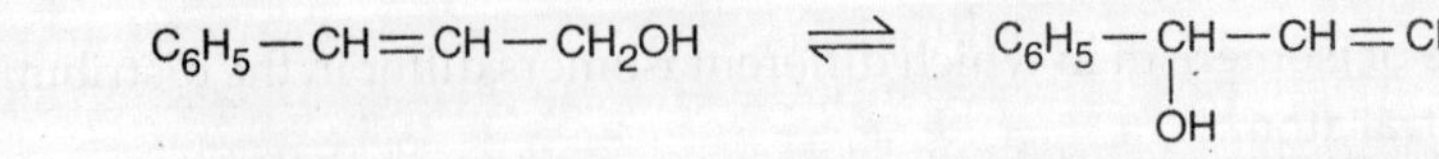

Cinnamoyl alcohol α-Phenyl allyl alcohol

Among the large number of tautomeric systems, keto-enol tautomerism is extremely common and has been widely studied. It has been observed that the inter conversion of both the forms may occur either by a stepwise or by a concerted mechanism. In the stepwise path, abstraction of proton from one atom takes place in the first step and redistribution of electrons followed by the addition of the proton abstracted in the first step to other atom occurs in the second step. In concerted mechanism abstraction and addition of proton proceed simultaneously. When a base is used as catalyst, stepwise inter-conversion becomes predominant while concerted mechanism is operative in acid catalysed transformation.

i. Stepwise path

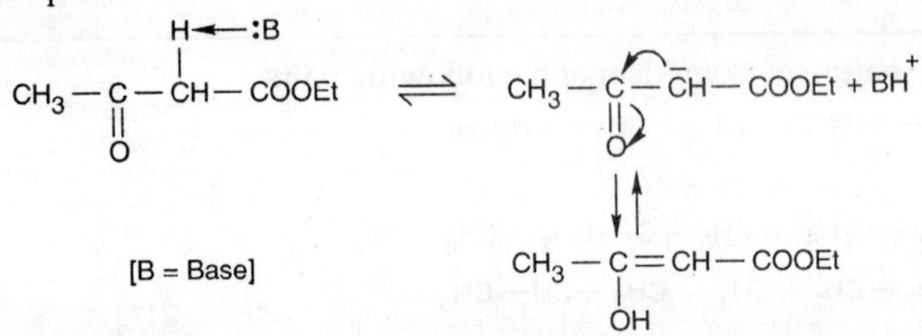

[B = Base]

ii. Concerted path

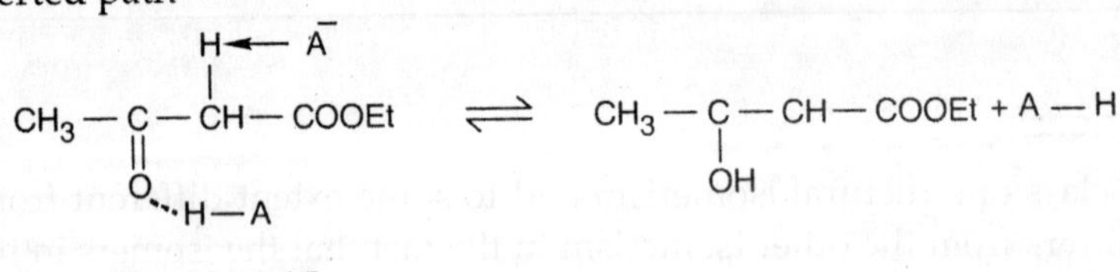

[A—H = Acid]

In general, keto form of keto-enol tautomerism predominates. But in certain cases where enol form can be stabilised, equilibrium may have substantial amount of enol content. Thus enol content of acetone is practically negligible but in acetyl acetone enol content is much higher than expected. This is due to the stabilisation of enol by H-bond formation.

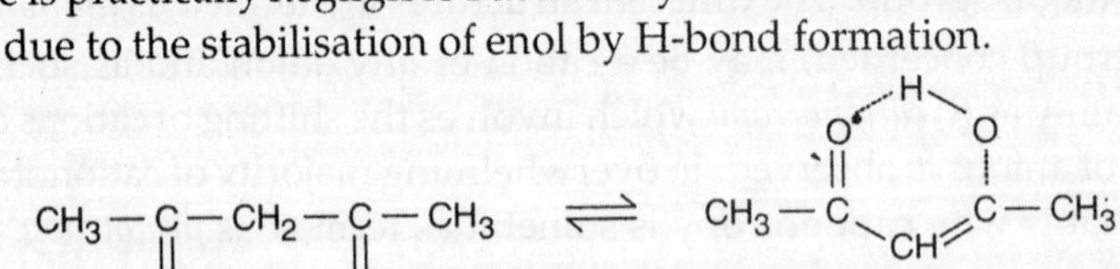

Keto form Enol form

Resonance may shift the keto-enol equilibrium by the stabilisation of the enol. For example phenol exists essentially cent per cent in enol form due to stabilisation.

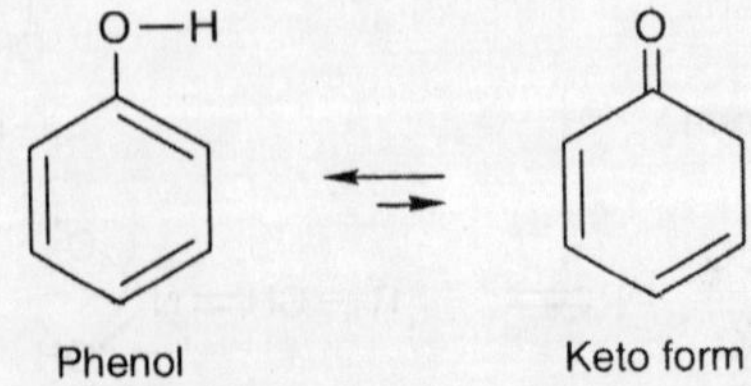

Phenol (Enol form) Keto form

It may be mentioned that tautomerism and resonance are not the same phenomenon. The major difference between these two is that the different structures in resonance hybrid are hypothetical but in tautomerism different tautomers have real existence and in suitable cases may be isolated and characterised as in ethyl aceto-acetate.

PROBLEM 1.4

How would you differentiate tautomerism from resonance?

1.8 Hydrogen Bond

The attraction of a hydrogen atom in a molecule by an electronegative atom results in the formation of a weak bond known as hydrogen bond. It is weaker than covalent bond with bond formation energy ranging from 2-10 kcal/mole. Both hydrogen and electronegative atoms may be in the same or in the different molecule. When both these atoms are present in the same molecule, the H-bond so formed is termed as *intramolecular hydrogen bond*, but when these atoms are from different molecules *intermolecular hydrogen bond* is formed. Hydrogen bond is represented by dotted line as depicted in Fig. 1.14.

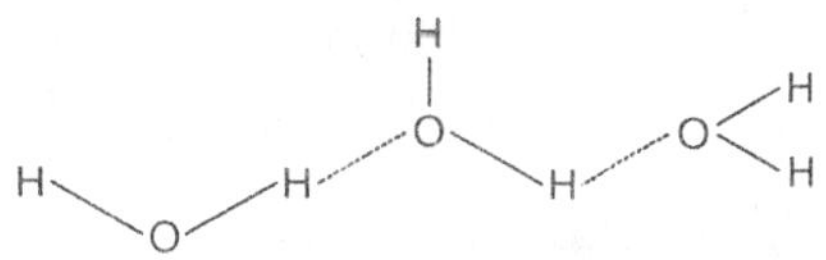

Intermolecular H bond in water molecules

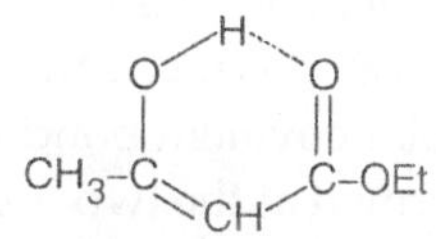

Enol of aceto acetic ester (Intramolecular H-bond)

Fig. 1.14

Generally compounds such as alcohols carboxylic acids, phenols, ammonia, water, hydrogen fluoride, etc. exhibit hydrogen bond formation ability. It has been established that different kinds of electrostatic forces are responsible for hydrogen bond formation. Different spectroscopic techniques specially IR and NMR are highly useful in detecting the existence of hydrogen bond. Hydrogen bond has significant influence on the behaviour of molecules. Essentially all the physical properties specially melting point, boiling point, solubility, heat of dilution and stability of molecules are prominently affected by hydrogen bonding.

PROBLEM 1.5

Explain

(a) Alcohols have higher boiling point than alkane of comparable molecular weight.

(b) Ethers are less soluble in water than alcohols.

1.9 Electronegativity

Electronegativity of an atom is defined as the intrinsic power of an atom to attract electrons towards itself. In general, it may be suggested that the tendency of an atom to attract electrons residing in the valency shell depends upon the magnitude of the positive charge on the nucleus of the atom—greater the magnitude of the positive charge on the nucleus—greater is the attraction for the negatively charged electrons and hence greater is the electronegativity. Again, more closer the valence electrons to the positive charge on the nucleus more will be attraction for electrons and hence more will be the electronegativity. Thus electronegativity depends upon the distance between the valence electron and nucleus—shorter this distance, i.e., smaller the atom greater will be the electronegativity. Again, attraction for electrons will be more for those atoms which have nearly filled orbital.

It has been observed that in the periodic arrangement of elements (periodic table) electronegativity increases from left to right and decreases downward in a vertical column. Thus fluorine is the most electronegative and caesium is the most electropositive elements. A number of attempts have been made to set up a quantitative table for electronegativity of which, prepared by Pauling is most acceptable and popular. He compiled a scale from thermochemical data. The most common elements with which the organic chemists are mainly concerned are carbon, hydrogen, nitrogen, oxygen, sulphur, phosphorus and halogens. These elements have different degrees of electronegativities and this accounts for the polarisation in the bond between two atoms. The values of electronegativities of these elements as deduced by Pauling are as follows:

Flourine	4.00	Iodine	2.50
Oxygen	3.50	Sulphur	2.50
Nitrogen	3.00	Carbon	2.50
Chlorine	3.00	Hydrogen	2.10
Bromine	2.80	Phosphorous	2.10

1.10 Dipole Moment

When a covalent bond is formed between two atoms having different electronegativities electron cloud in the bond is more attracted towards the atom with greater electronegativity, as a result of which a polar covalent bond is generated and a partial positive (δ^+) and a partial negative (δ^-) ends are formed at the two bonding atoms, i.e., the molecule becomes a dipole and hence it must have a dipole moment value.

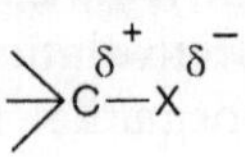

Thus it may be concluded that dipole moment is a molecular property which arises due to separation of charges. The dipole moment of a molecule is indicated by the symbol μ and is expressed in Debye units (D). It is defined as the product of multiplication of charge (*e*) in electrostatic units (esu) and distance (*d*) in centimetres (cm) between the bonding atoms, i.e.,

$$\mu = e.d$$

Dipole moment is an additive quantity, the total moment of the molecule is the vector sum of the individual bond moments and depends on the direction of the polarity of the polar bond. So it is highly rational that a molecule having polar bonds may be non-polar in nature. This situation arises when the symmetry of the molecule is such that the bond moments of individual bonds neutralise each other. Thus ethylene molecule although has a polar π-bond yet its net dipole moment is nil. This is because polarisation can occur on either side due to the symmetry of the molecule.

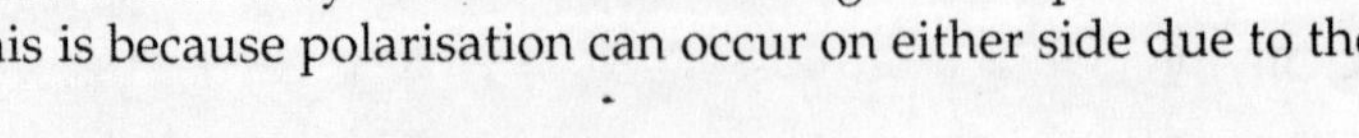

Similar is the case with *trans*-1, 2-dichloroethene.

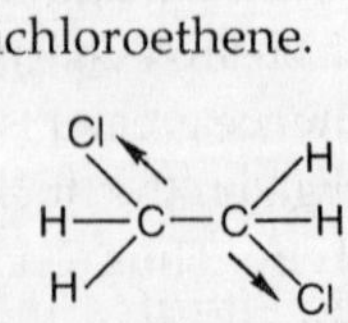

This type of molecule having polar bonds but without having any dipole moment is termed as *centro symmetric molecule.*

Dipole moment largely influences the properties of the molecule. This is because the polarity of the bonds depends upon dipole moment, and the reactivity of molecules in turn is mainly dependent upon polarity of the bond.

PROBLEM 1.6

Explain

(a) Both FCl and ICl have similar dipole moment but in one chlorine is positive and in other it is the negative end.

(b) CO_2 has no dipole moment but SO_2 has a net dipole moment.

(c) *cis*-1, 2-dimethyl ethylene has dipole moment but its *trans* isomer has no dipole moment.

1.11 Reactivity of Chemical Compounds

Reactivity of chemical compounds is reflected by their chemical reactions. Again, chemical reaction is always associated with the breakage and formation of bonds. Further, breakage of the bonds depends upon the electron availability surrounding the particular bond undergoing chemical reaction with a particular reagent. So it is felt pertinent to discuss factors which control the availability of electrons surrounding the bonds. There are a large number of factors of which some of the most important are discussed in sequel:

1.11.1 Inductive Effect

When a covalent bond is formed between two dissimilar atoms, bonding electron pair of σ-bond is attracted more towards the more electronegative atom as a result of which more electronegative atom becomes slightly negatively charged and less electronegative atom gains a slight positive charge as indicated below:

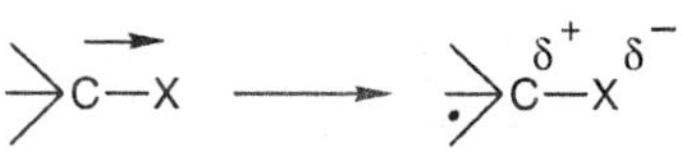

This effect is known as inductive effect. It is a permanent effect for polarisation of the molecule in the ground state. If the carbon atom bonded to electronegative atom is connected to a chain of further carbon atoms, this effect can be transmitted but its influence gradually decreases, i.e., the influence of this effect is maximum at C_1 and decreases slowly as the chain increases. Generally the influence of this effect is perceptible up to C_4-position after which the influence is practically nil.

$$C_4—C_3—C_2—C_1 \longrightarrow X$$

As mentioned earlier it is a permanent state of the molecule and is manifested in the form of dipole moment. It persists whether a reagent exists or not. But during the chemical reaction in presence of any reagent it increases to such an extent that a transition state for the reaction is formed. This enhanced inductive effect is designated as *inductomeric effect*. Inductomeric effect is a temporary effect and exists so long as the reagent is present. As soon as the reagent is withdrawn this effect ceases to operate and the molecule reverts to the ground state.

1.11.2 Mesomeric and Electromeric Effects

Mesomeric effect is observed in π-bonded compounds. It occurs due to the redistribution of π-electrons in between the atoms forming the π-bond. If the π-bond is present between a carbon and a more electronegative atom, π-electron density becomes higher at more electronegative atom. It is a case of permanent polarisation of π-bond. Thus,

$$>C=O \longleftrightarrow >\overset{\delta+}{C}-\overset{\delta-}{O}$$

In presence of any reagent, mesomeric effect is temporarily increased by the demand of the reagent. This temporary increase is due to complete transfer of π-electrons from less electronegative to more electronegative atom so that reaction can take place through formation of a transition state. Such temporary and increased mesomeric effect is brought into play by the demand of the reagent and is commonly termed as *electromeric effect*. i.e.,

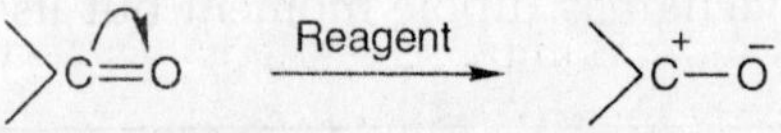

Electromeric effect is a case of complete polarisation of π-bond with the formation of positive charge centre at one end and negative charge centre at the other end of the π-bond.

1.12 Acids and Bases

According to definition proposed by Arrhenius, acids are compounds which yield hydrogen ions, H^+ in solution while bases are those compounds which can form hydroxyl ions, $\overline{OH}$. But these definations cannot be accepted as general, only applicable in aqueous solution. As a result, a large number of theories regarding acids and bases have been put forward.

According to Lowry and Bronsted theory, an acid is a substance that can donate a proton and any compound which can accept the proton is a base. This theory is also known as protonic concept of acids and base. The most important aspect of this concept is that a compound may be inherently acid or base but it can do so only in contact with other, i.e., acid-base reaction must proceed simultaneously or in other words, a substance can be regarded as an acid only when it can react with a base and vice versa, and this acid-base reaction is always an equilibrium reaction.

Thus,

$$A-H + B \rightleftharpoons \bar{A} + \overset{+}{B}H$$

A—H	B	$\bar{A}$	$\overset{+}{B}H$
Acid	Base	Conjugate base of the acid A—H	Conjugate acid of the base B

Further, this theory also proposes that acid and base terms are relative, and strength of an acid depends upon two factors, viz., (i) tendency of the acid to give its proton and (ii) stability of the conjugate base formed. Similar is the case with a base, i.e., tendency to accept a proton and the stability of the conjugate acid formed. Thus,

$$H_2SO_4 + H_2O \rightleftharpoons H\bar{S}O_4 + \overset{+}{H_3}O$$

H_2SO_4	H_2O	$H\bar{S}O_4$	$\overset{+}{H_3}O$
Acid	Base	Conjugate base	Conjugate acid

$$NH_3 + H_2O \rightleftharpoons \overset{+}{N}H_4 + \overline{OH}$$

NH_3	H_2O	$\overset{+}{N}H_4$	$\overline{OH}$
Base	Acid	Conjugate acid	Conjugate base

$$HCl + NH_3 \rightleftharpoons \overset{+}{N}H_4 + \bar{Cl}$$

HCl	NH_3	$\overset{+}{N}H_4$	$\bar{Cl}$
Acid	Base	Conjugate acid	Conjugate base

Again, we know that both HNO_3 and HF in general are acids but when they react with each other, one behaves as an acid while the other one as a base.

$$\underset{\text{Base}}{HNO_3} + \underset{\text{Acid}}{HF} \rightleftharpoons H_2\overset{+}{NO_3} + \bar{F}$$

It may be mentioned that although this protonic concept is well accepted, yet has a severe limitation. It is only applicable to those compounds which have protons. But there are a large number of compounds which can behave as acids but they have no proton.

So a more generalised theory has been provided by Lewis who defined acids as molecules or ions which can accept electrons, and bases are those which can donate electrons. Accordingly, this generalised definition of acid-base strength depends upon (i) electron availability, i.e., more electron deficient a compound more will be its tendency to be acidic, and more electron rich a compound more will be its basic strength (ii) stability of the corresponding conjugate ions. Thus Lewis acids include such compounds as boron trifluoride (BF_g), aluminium chloride ($AlCl_3$), tintetrachloride ($SnCl_4$), Zinc chloride, etc. Similarly Lewis bases are compounds having lone pair of electrons like hydroxide, amine, etc. It may further be mentined that protonic (Lowry and Bronsted) and electronic concepts are complimentary to each other—protonic concept is applicable only in the case of donation and acceptance of proton while electronic concept involves donation and acceptance of electron—in fact, proton donars (acids) are electron deficient (electron acceptors) while proton acceptors (bases) are electron rich (electron donors).

1.13 Reagents, Reaction and Mechanism

1.13.1 Reagent

Mentioned earlier that organic molecules manifest their chemical activities through chemical reactions which are always associated with the breakage and formation of one or more bonds. It has been observed that in the process of breakage and formation of bonds, presence of at least two substances is essential—one is known as *Substrate* while the other is called *Reagent*. When the reactions involve one organic and another inorganic substances, organic substance is usually termed as *Substrate* and the inorganic component is designated as *Reagent*. Thus,

i. 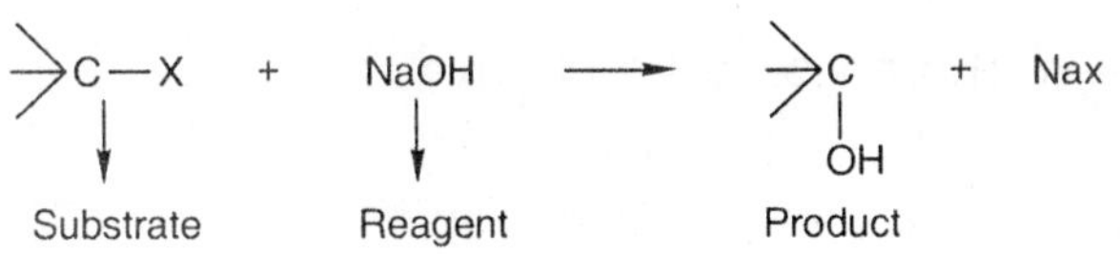

ii. 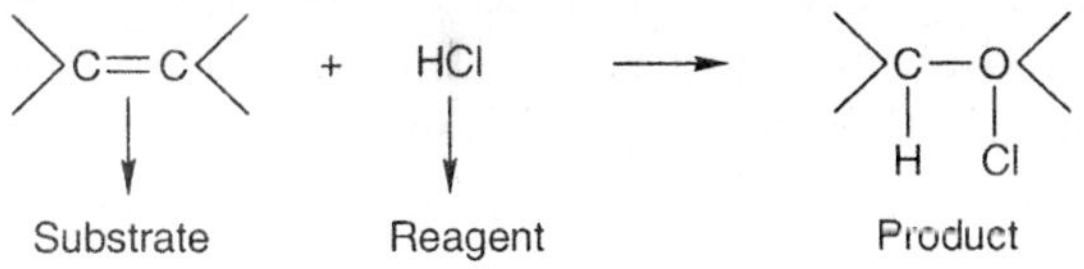

It may be mentioned that in the case of reactions where both the substances are organic in nature the choice is arbitrary.

1.13.2 Classification of Reagents

When the reactions (i) and (ii) mentioned above are properly explained, it appears that the reagent in the reaction (i) does not react as such, but its active species $\overline{O}H$ plays the major role as reagent. This active species functions as electron donor. i.e.,

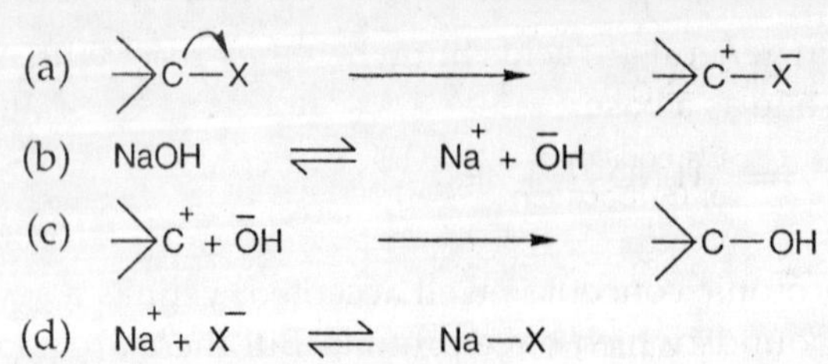

Similarly in reaction (ii),

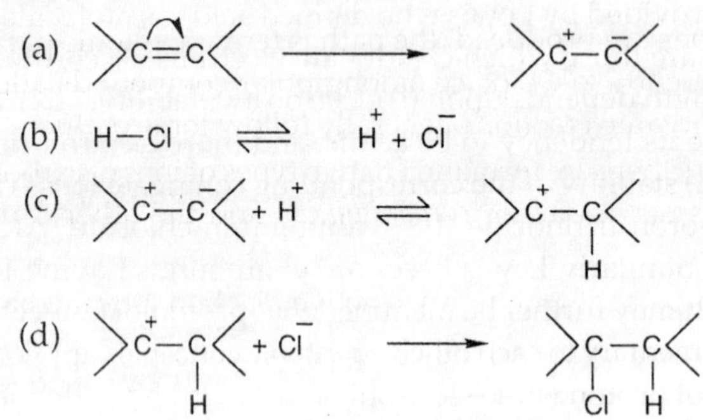

The active part of the reagent is H^+ which acts as electron acceptor.

Thus reagents may be classified into two categories—

1. Electron donor commonly designated as *Nucleophilic reagents* or *Nucleophiles.*
2. Electron acceptor usually known as *Electrophilic reagents* or *Electrophiles.*

It may be mentioned that electrophiles and acids are not identical although both are electron acceptors. Similar is the case with nucleophiles and bases though both act as electron donor. Acid base reactions always involve equilibrium state but reaction between electrophile and nucleophile may or may not form equilibrium state.

1.13.3 Some Common Electrophiles and Nucleophiles

Electrophiles: Cl^+, Br^+, I^+, $-NO_2$, $>\overset{+}{C}<$, $>C{=}O$, $R-\underset{\underset{O}{\|}}{C}-Cl$, H_2SO_4, HNO_3, HCl, $AlCl_3$, BF_3, etc.

Nucleophiles: $\overline{O}H$, $\overline{Cl}$, $\overline{Br}$, $\overline{I}$, $\overline{CN}$, $>\overline{C}<$, H_2O, R— OH, $\overline{O}$— R, NH_3, etc.

1.13.4 Reaction and Mechanism

It has already been mentioned that chemical reaction is a process of a chemical change which is always associated with the breakage and formation of bonds. This process of breakage and formation of bonds in chemical reaction is initiated by two different paths:

1. Homolytic cleavage: In this process of breakage, bonding electron pair is equally shared by both the bonding atoms.

The products formed are *Free Radicals.* As free radicals have an unpaired electron they are highly active. For this reason reactions occurring through free radical path is very rapid and is catalysed by heat, light and peroxides or by any source of oxygen.

2. Heterolytic Fission: In this fission electron pair in bonding orbital may be transferred to any one of the bonding atoms with the formation of ions.

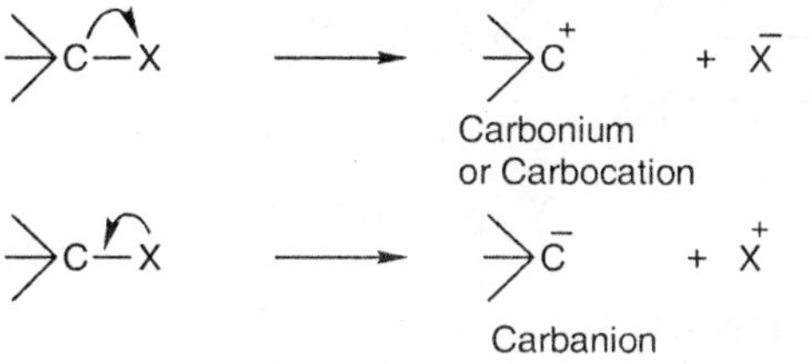

[Arrow indicates flow of electrons]

Since in this process of bond cleavage ions are produced, the path is termed as ionic path of the reaction. This type of bond fission frequently takes place among polar compounds and in polar solvents. Overwhelming majority of organic reactions generally follow ionic paths.

As seen above, in this bond fission process there are formation of two types of ions of carbon—one is positively charged carbon known as *carbocation* or *carbonium ion* and the other carbon bearing negative charge termed as *carbanion*.

Carbocation or carbonium ion: They are important and highly reactive reaction intermediates. They readily combine with nucleophiles such as $\bar{C}l$, $\bar{B}r$, $\bar{C}N$, $\bar{O}H$, etc., i.e.,

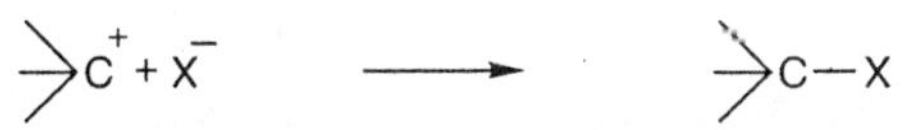

The stability of carbocations depends on the number and nature of substituents on carbon atom. Electron releasing substituents like alkyl groups increase the stability of carbocation and obviously more the number of alkyl group substituents on carbon greater is the stability of carbocation. Depending on the number of alkyl substituents carbocations may be primary or 1°, ccondary or 2° and tertiary or 3° in nature. These cations are planar having three α-bonds in the same plane with an angle of 120° as shwon below.

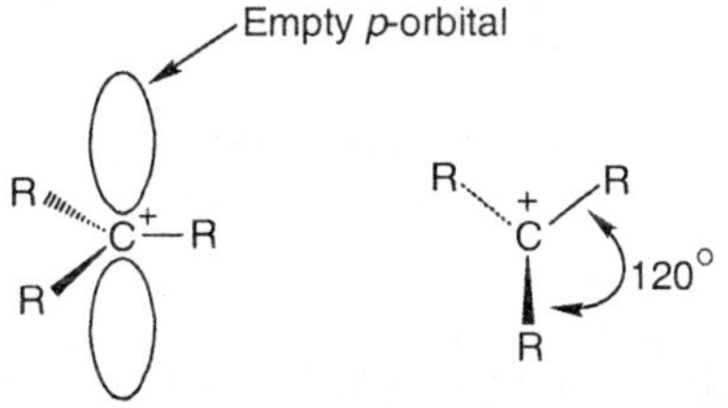

(Carbocation)

Carbanions: Organic anion bearing negative charge on carbon atom are known as *carbanions*. They have pyramidal structure.

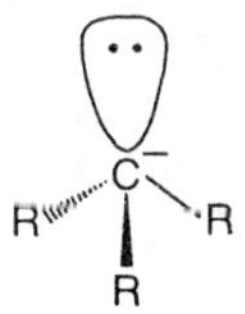

Carbanion

They are less stable than carbocations; however, electron withdrawing substituents can stabilise these anions. Thus,

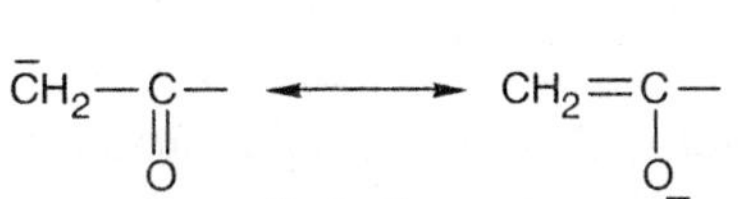

Carbanion

PROBLEM 1.7

> Arrange the following carbocations in order of increasing stability.
>
> i. $CH_3-\overset{+}{C}H$ (with CH_3 below), (ii) $(CH_3)_3\overset{+}{C}$, (iii) $\overset{+}{C}H_3$, (iv) $CH_3-\overset{+}{C}H_2$

1.13.4.1 Mechanism

Mechanism of chemical reactions is usually defined as the step by step detail description of paths by which reactants are converted into products. But the detail study of stepwise change occurring in each and individual substrate is not only an up-hill task but also practically impossible. Fortunately, survey on the vast number of organic reactions reveals certain similarities among the reactions. Consequently organic reactions have been classified into a few groups—each group has been found to have some common criteria. Main classes of organic reactions recognised are:

1. Substitution Reactions
2. Elimination Reactions
3. Addition Reactions
4. Rearrangement Reactions
5. Pericyclic Reactions.

1.13.4.2 Substitution Reactions

Substitution reactions are those in which an atom or a group of atoms connected to a carbon atom is directly replaced by another atom or a group of atoms. Thus,

$$>C-X + \underset{\text{(Incoming group)}}{Y} \longrightarrow >C-Y + \underset{\text{(Outgoing group)}}{X}$$

The incoming group may be either an electrophile, nucleophile or a free radical. Therefore, substitution reactions have been divided into three categories.

(a) Electrophilic substitution Reactions
(b) Nucleophilic substitution Reactions
(c) Radical substitution Reactions.

Of these classes of substitution reactions free radical substitution reactions are not so common, and electrophilic substitutions are of frequent occurrence in aromatic compounds (**vide Chapter Fourteen**) while nucleophilic substitution are primarily observed in saturated aliphatic compounds.

1.13.4.2.1 Nucleophilic Substitution Reactions

In nucleophilic substitution reactions, a nucleophile attacks the attacking centre forming the product by replacing a group attached to the attacking centre as nucleophile, i.e.,

$$>C-X + \bar{Y} \longrightarrow >C-Y + \bar{X}$$

$\bar{Y}$ ↓ (obtained from the reagent)

1.13.4.2.1.1 Mechanism of Nucleophilic Substitution Reaction

Mechanistically this reaction can occur through two distinct paths.

(a) *Stepwise path*

Step I: Slow removal of leaving group from reaction centre under the influence of the reagent.

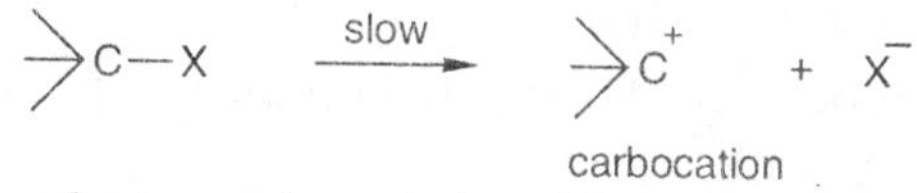

Step II: Rapid attack by the incoming nucleophile at carbocation.

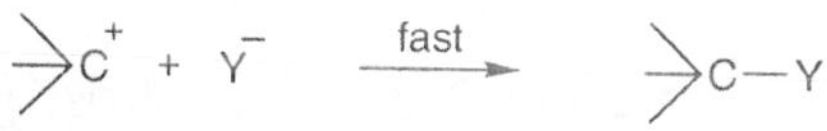

(b) *Simultaneous* or *concerted path*

In this path, attack by incoming nucleophile and removal of outgoing nucleophile take place simultaneously.

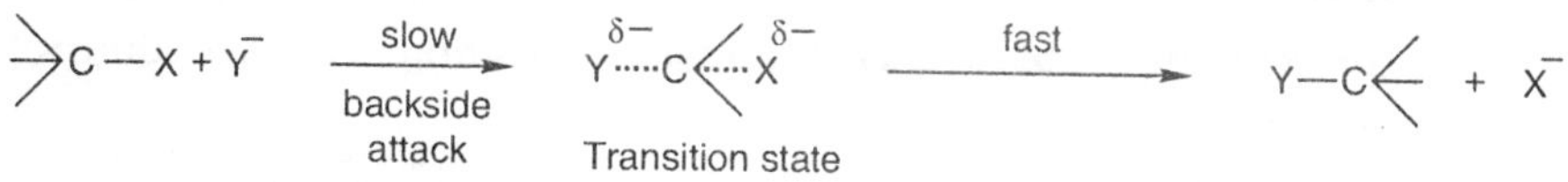

A scrutiny of above two paths suggests that in stepwise path, step I, i.e., the formation of carbocation is the slowest path and in this path only one molecular species—the substrate is involved. So from the view point of chemical kinetics it is unimolecular nucleophilic substitution reaction abbreviated as S_{N1} . But in the simultaneous path, formation of transition state—the slowest path involves both the substrate and the attacking nucleophile. So kinetically this path is bimolecular in nature and is known as bimolecular nucleophilic substitution reaction usually expressed as S_{N2}.

1.13.4.2.1.2 Factors Governing S_{N1} and S_{N2} Path

Whether a particular nucleophilic substitution takes place through S_{N1} or S_{N2} path depends upon some factors like the structures of the substrate, nature of the solvent, nature of incoming and out going nucleophiles, etc. as discussed below:

(a) **Structure of the Substrate:** From the mechanistic path it is evident that any substitution reaction must proceed either through S_{N1}or S_{N2} path. In the case of S_{N1} path there must be formation of carbocation. So it is reasonable to conclude that any structure which can favour the formation of stable carbocation will favour S_{N1} path. This condition is considered to be primry factor which controls the S_{N1} path because the formation of carbocation is an endothermic reaction. It has been observed that in endothermic reaction there must be a close similarity between the product and the transition state. In S_{N1} path the formation of carbocation may be regarded as the product of the 1st step of the reaction. Since carbocation is ionic in character its transition state must be ionic in nature which is actually found to be the fact, i.e.,

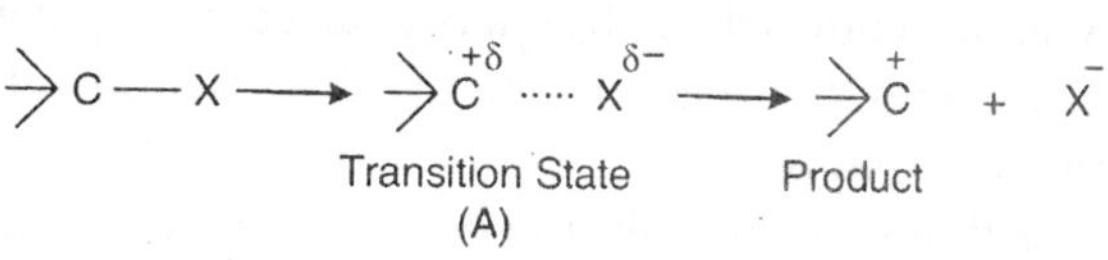

Thus it is obvious that any factor which stabilise carbocation will stabilise the transition state (A). Again, greater the stability of (A) more is the probability of formation of carbocation because the stable transition state will reduce the energy of activation for the formation of carbocation, and so the path will be S_{N1}.

A few examples may be cited in favour of the above concludion

i. In the series, $CH_3—X$, $R—CH_2—X$, $R_2CH—X$, $R_3C—X$
I, II, III, IV

the order of probability of SN¹ path becomes

IV > III > II > I

because the order of stability of carbocation is

$$R_3\overset{+}{C} > R_2\overset{+}{C}H > R—\overset{+}{C}H_2 > \overset{+}{C}H_3$$

on the contrary, the probability of S_{N^2} path becomes higher with the lesser stability of carbocation.

ii. The presence of double bond in the adjacent position may have some role in stabilising the carbocation.

Thus, $R—CH=CH—CH_2—X \longrightarrow R—CH=CH—\overset{+}{C}H_2 \longleftrightarrow R—\overset{+}{C}H—CH=CH_2$

iii. In some cases steric factors may play important role in the substitution. Thus the hydrolysis of neopentyl halide is extremely slow. This is because if it undergoes hydrolysis the path should be either S_{N^1} or S_{N^2}. As there is formation of I⁰ carbocation which is very unstable S_{N^1} path is not favoured. Again, backside attack by the incoming nucleophile is not possible due to the crowded nature of the central carbon atom. So SN² is not also favoured. Thus,

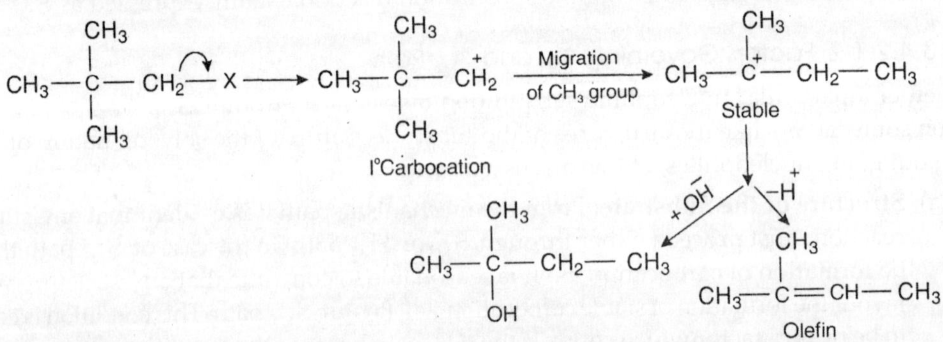

As shown above if the reaction occurs at all, the product will be rearranged.

(b) **Role of solvent:** In SN reactions a C—X bond must undergo cleavage. Naturally, question arises, where from the energy required for bond cleavage is supplied? In the case of S_{N^2} path along with the breakage of the bond there is also formation of the bond occurs. It is known that during bond formation energy is accumulated. So in S_{N^2} path the energy needed for bond breakage comes from the energy stored during the formation of the bond. But in the case of S_{N^1} path, there is no such bond formation before the cleavage of the bond. In this situation most of the energy required for bond cleavage is supplied by solvent. It has been suggested that solvent molecule particularly polar and protic can easily form H-bond with nucleophilic part of the substrate. Ss a result energy develops and hence favours the bond cleavage. Thus,

$$>C—X \xrightarrow[\text{Polar protic solvent}]{H—A} >C—X \cdots H—A \rightleftharpoons >\overset{+}{C} + \overset{-}{X}\cdots N—A$$

(H-bond formation) (Stabilised)

The nucleophilic group is stabilised by H-bond formation so the probability of reverse reaction becomes high and hence formation of carbocation (S_{N1} path) is enhanced. Since S_{N2} is a path of non-ionisation the polarity of the solvent has no direct role. However, it has been observed that the rate of S_{N2} path is decreased, if polar particularly protic is used in place of non-polar solvents.

(c) **Nature of the leaving group:** Substitution reaction requires the cleavage of C—X bond. The cleavage of the C—X bond depends upon the nature of the leaving nucleophilic group (X). Greater the electron demand of this nucleophilic group (X) more will be the tendency of C—X bond to undergo eleavage, or in other words, less the electron density at the leaving group (X) more is its tendency to leave the reaction centre and so more is the probability of SN reaction. It is, therefore, concluded that the electron density at the leaving group (X) is the deciding factor for determining the activity of the group as leaving nucleophile. Again, electron density is related to the basicity. Thus, less the basicity of the leaving group (X), more is the probability of SN reaction to occur. Thus, in the halide series the order of SN reaction is

$$\bar{I} > \bar{Br} > \bar{Cl} > \bar{F}, \text{ because the order of basicity stands as } \bar{F} > \bar{Cl} > \bar{Br} > \bar{I}$$

(d) **Nature of the attacking nucleophile:** The incoming group in SN reaction attacks as nucleophile. So it is logical to assume that greater the nucleophilicity of the group more is its activity as attacking nucleophile and hence more is the probability of SN reaction. In the halide series the order of activity as incoming nucleophilies is

$$\bar{I} > \bar{Br} > \bar{Cl} > \bar{F}, \text{ because they have same order of nucleophilicity.}$$

1.13.4.2.1.3 Stereochemical Implications of SN Reactions

As revealed from mechanistic path, SN reaction may proceed either through S_{N1} or S_{N2} path. In S_{N1} path, substitution occurs via the formation of carbocation. Carbocation is planar in character and so the incoming nucleophile may attack the reaction centre from either side. So the nature of the product should be racemic if the reaction centre is chiral, i.e.,

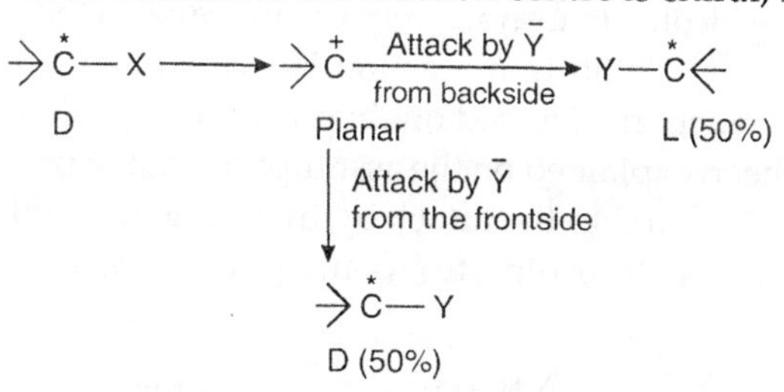

It may be mentioned that although there is probability of formation of racemic product but in most of the cases inverted product predominates.

When the substitution reaction takes place through S_{N2} path, the product is always inverted because in this path incoming nucleophile attacks the reaction centre from the backside of the leaving nucleophile. Thus,

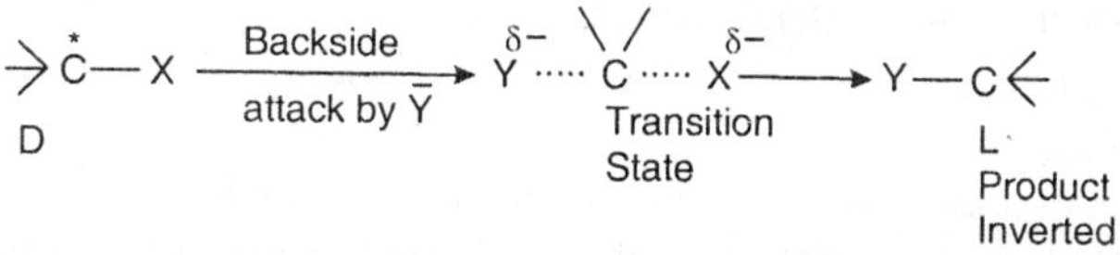

Thus S_{N2} reaction may be looked upon as stereospecific and stereoselective.

1.13.4.2.1.3.1 Retention in Configuration

Under normal situation path of substitution is either S_{N^1} or S_{N^2} and as shown above there is no probability of formation of product with retention in configuration. However, under certain conditions, configuration of the substrate may be retained in the product. Two such situations may be mentioned below.

(a) **Attack by specific incoming nucleophile**

It has been observed replacement of certain groups by some specific reagents, the configuration of the starting compound may be retained in the product. The most highly illustrated example of such reaction is the replacement of hydroxyl function by chlorine by the use of thionyl chloride, $SOCl_2$. Thus,

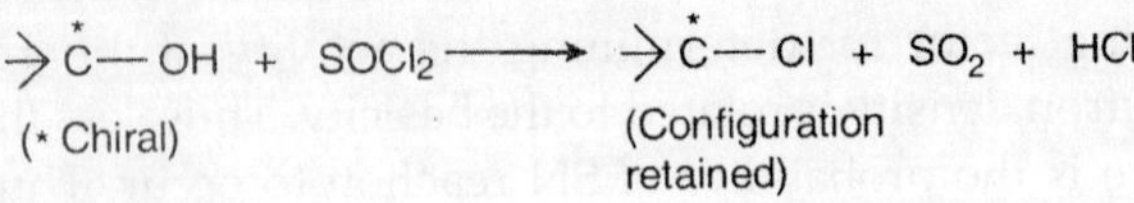

The retention of configuration in this reaction has been explained on the basis of formation of an intermediate chlorosulphite. This intermediate forms a cyclic transition state as shown below.

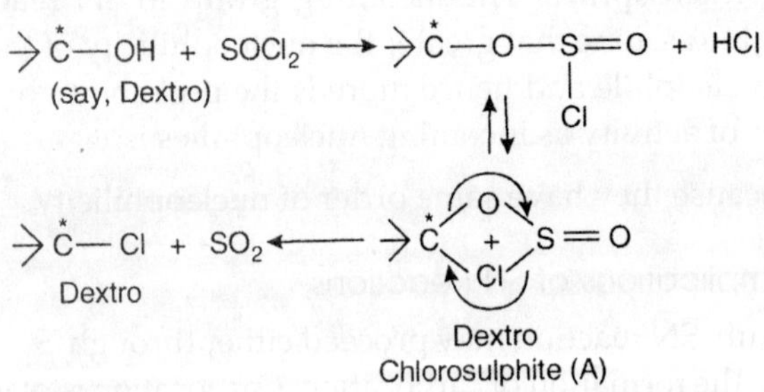

Since chlorine attacks chiral carbon (*) atom from the same direction at which C—O bond is attached, configuration of the starting alcohol (substrate) remains the same in the product, chloride. This mechanistic path of nucleophilic substitution reaction is termed as internal nucleophilic substitution (S_{Ni}). However, if the reaction is carried out in presence of pyridine as catalyst, the configuration is inverted. This has been explained on the assumption that in presence of pyridine that path of substitution becomes S_{N^2} due to the attack by free Cl^- generated by the action of HCl produced during the formation of chlorosulphite (A) and pyridine which is a base.

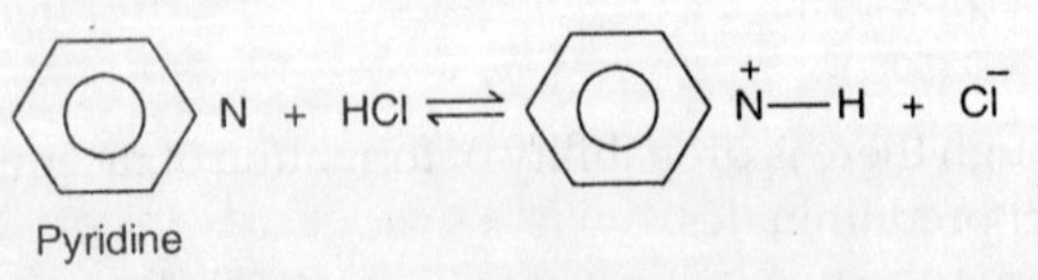

This free Cl^- ion attacks chlorosulphite (A) from the opposite direction of C—O bond and hence configuration is inverted.

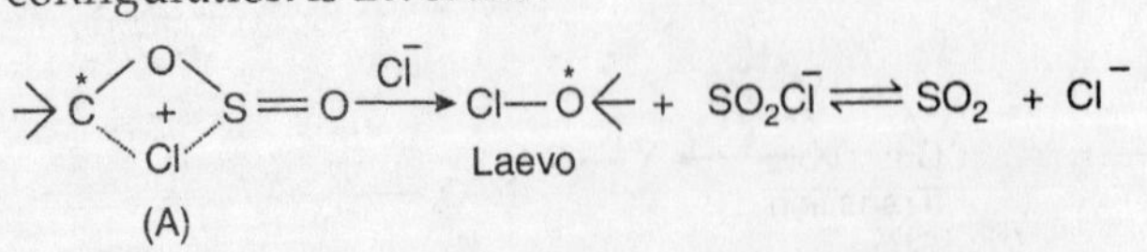

It may be mentioned that in presence of pyridine, there are two nucleophiles—one is uncharged internal chlorine and the other is negatively charged free external Cl^- ion which is better nucleophile and so free Cl^- attacks the transition state as shown.

(b) Neighbouring group participation

Sometime neighbouring group present in the substrate may participate in SN reaction in such a way that the rate of the reaction and the configuration of the product may be unexpectedly affected. During such participation of neighbouring group, reaction in general, occurs through S_{N2} path but instead of inversion, retention in configuration takes place. This is explained by assuming that the reaction proceeds in two different stages. In first stage, the leaving nucleophile is eliminated by the backside attack of the neighbouring group (first S_{N2}; first inversion) with the formation of an intermediate. In the second stage, external nucleophile attacks that reaction centre in the intermediate from the backside (2nd S_{N2}, 2nd inversion) forming the final product which retains the configuration of the substrate, Thus,

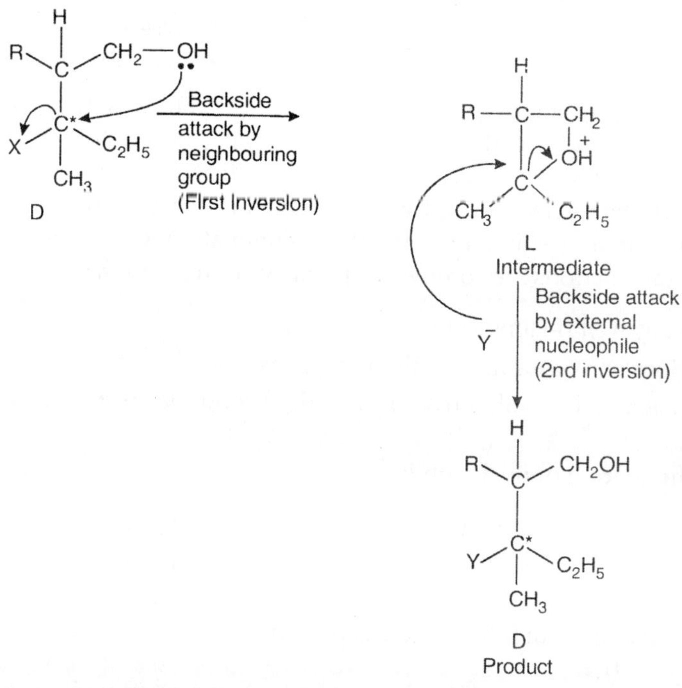

Mention may be made in this connection that the neighbouring group which participates in the reaction should be electron donor in nature such as having lone pair of electrons and should be present either at γ or δ position with respect to reaction centre.

1.13.4.2.1.4 Single Electron Transfer Mechanism of SN (SET)

It has been observed that in some cases the substitution reactions may take place in such a way that the path may be looked upon as an ionic as well as radical in character. Generally, this type of mechanistic path is observed when the reaction is S_{NI}. If the Carbocation that is formed is highly stable (high half-life period) can take up one electron from the ionic species of the incoming nucleophile. As a result, there are formation of radicals as shown below:

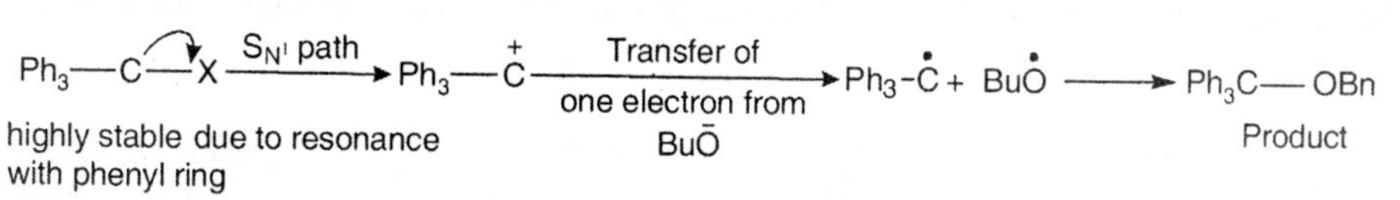

As there is transfer of single electron from the attacking reagent (butoxide ion) before the formation of the product, the path of SN is termed as single electron transfer mechanism (SET mechanism).

1.13.4.3 Elimination Reactions

Elimination reactions are those in which two species—one electrophile and another nucleophile are eliminated from the substrate as a neutral molecule with the formation of an alkenes. The electrophile eliminated is, in most of the cases, a proton. Thus,

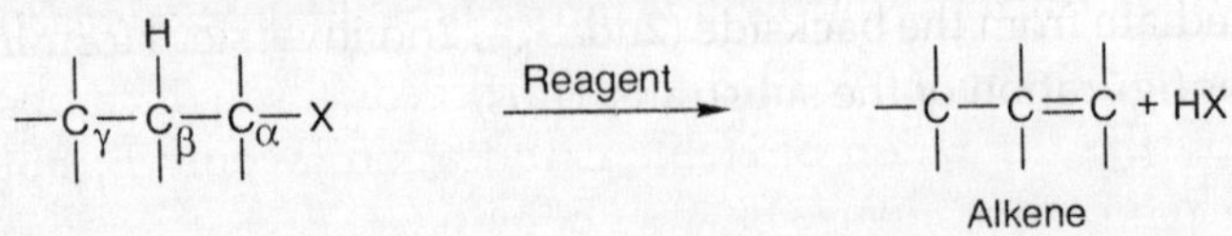

[X is any nucleophile]

Elimination reactions generally prefer basic reagents as catalysts. However, in some cases they can occur in acidic catalysts. It may be pointed out that as the formation of alkene is the essential condition of elimination reaction, presence of hydrogen atom at the β-carbon atom (the carbon atom at which the nucleophilic group is attached is designated as α) is a must. For this reason common elimination reactions are termed as β-elimination reaction and most of the studies regarding elimination reactions are confined to β-elimination reactions.

1.13.4.3.1 Mechanism of β-Elimination Reactions

β-elimination reactions can occur in two different paths.

(a) *Stepwise path*: In this path β-hydrogen and nucleophile are eliminated in two separate steps.

Step I: Elimination of nucleophile

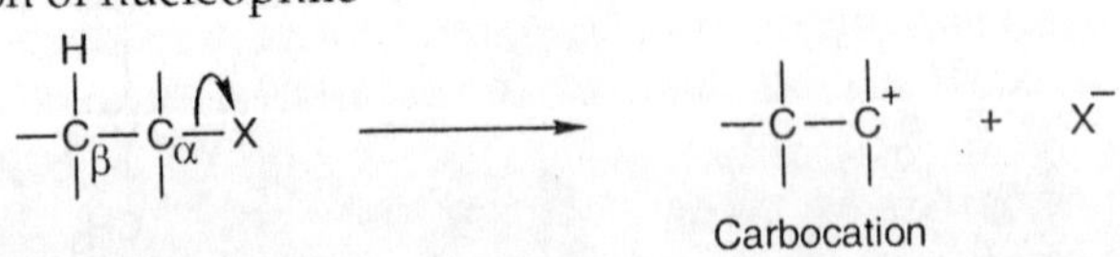

Step II: Elimination of β-hydrogen as proton

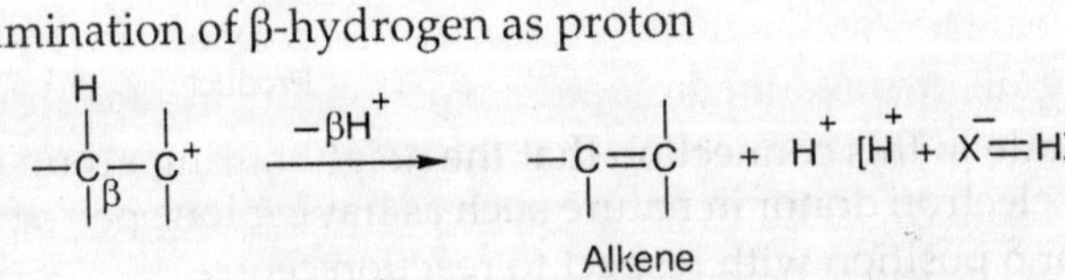

Like nucleophilic substitution and on the ground of chemical kinetics stepwise path is unimolecular in nature and is indicated by E_1. The simple example of E_1 is the dehydration of ethyl alcohol to ethylene.

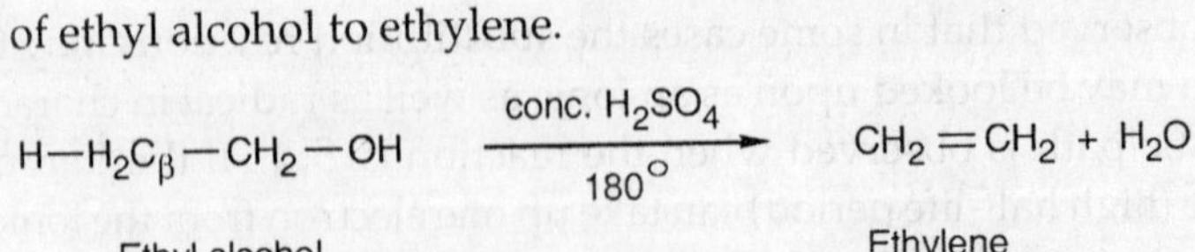

(b) *Simultaneous path*: In this process both β-hydrogen and nucleophile are eliminated at the same time, i.e.,

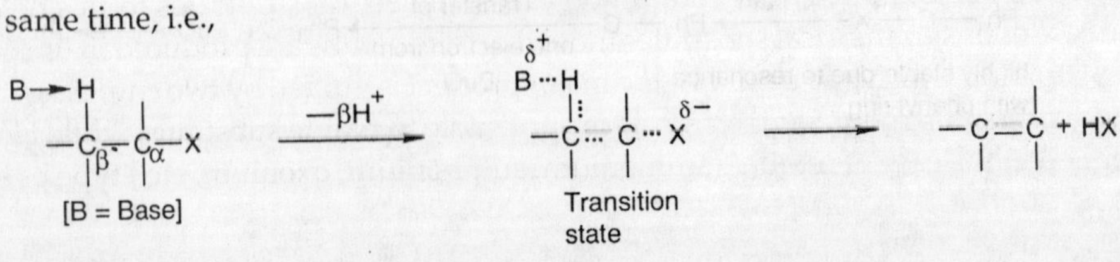

Simultaneous path is similarly E_2 reaction. Hofmann exhaustive methylation followed by the treatment with alkali constitutes the very common example of E_2.

$$\underset{\text{Ethyl amine}}{CH_3-CH_2-NH_2} \xrightarrow[\text{Excess}]{CH_3I} CH_3-CH_2-\overset{+}{N}(CH_3)_3\ \bar{I} \xrightarrow[\text{Heat}]{\text{Alkali}} \underset{\text{Ethylene}}{CH_2=CH_2} + N(CH_3)_3 + HI$$

1.13.4.3.2 Factors Controlling Elimination Reactions

Following are usually the factors which guide the path of elimination reaction.

(a) **Structure of the substrate:** As E_1 reaction proceeds through carbocation any structure which favours the formation of stable carbocation favours E_1 but not E_2 path. Thus substritution at α-carbon always favours E_1 path.

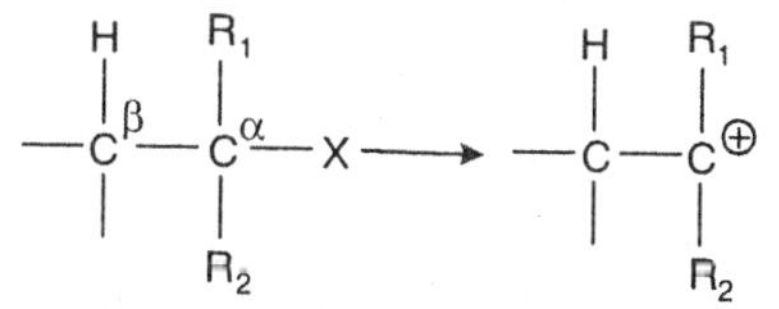

(Stable C^+)

But if the substituents are present at β-position, it may create steric hindrance to H atom. So the β-H atom may not be readily eliminated. Again, the presence of electron releasing group at β-position reduces the acidity of β-H atom as a result of which its elimination may be difficult. On the other hand, electron withdrawing group if present at β-position increases the acidity of β-H atom and so elimination reaction is favoured.

(b) **Nature of base:** Since in elimination reaction β-H atom is eliminated as proton, basic reagent normally catalyses elimination reaction. But in E_1 path as the base does not directly participate in the reaction, increase in the strength of basic catalyst does not change the rate of E_1. In the case of E_2, however, base being a direct participant the increase in the base strength favours E_2 path.

(c) **Nature of the leaving nucleophilic group:** Generally poor leaving nuclerphilic groups like OH, OR, etc, do not favour elimination reaction. But in such situation acidic catalyst if used elimination reaction may take place smoothly. The most common example cited in this context is the dehydration of alcohol to olefin in presence of concentrated mineral acid. The path ($-O-\underset{\underset{O}{\|}}{C}-R$), if present, elimination through E_1 path takes place favourably. Presence of moderate leaving group like halogens usually favours E_2 path.

(d) **Nature of the solvent:** Polar solvents favour E_1 path while E_2 path of elimination is favoured by non-polar slovents.

1.13.4.3.3 Orientation of Double Bonds in the Olefin Formed

It may be pointed out in this connection that symmetrical substrates form single alkene. But in the case of unsymmetrical substrates more than one olefins are produced in unequal amounts. In this situation which one would be the major product is guided by two empirical rules—Saytzeff's and Hofmann's rules. Saytzeff's rule is applicable to halide substrates while Hofmann's rule is applied in the case of 'oniun' (ammonium, sulphonium, oxonium, etc.) type os substrates.

According to Saytzeff's rule most highly substituted olefin becomes the major product while Hofmann's rule states that the least substituted alkene will be the major product. Thus,

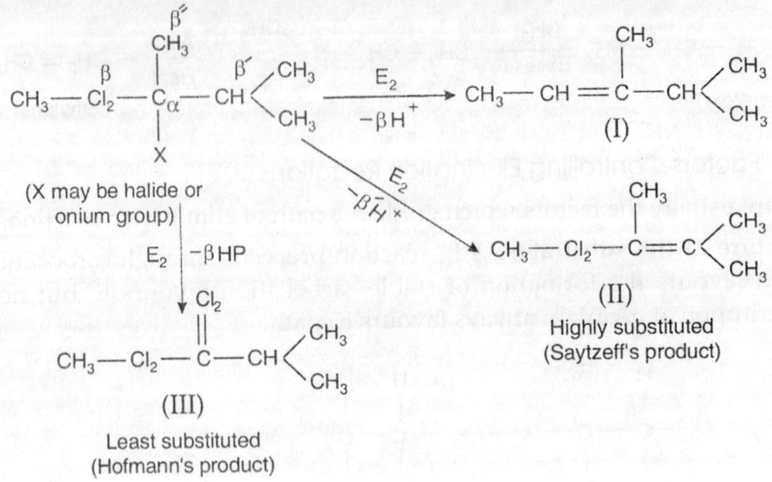

The justification of those two emperical rules may be explained on the basis of following factors:

i. Relative stabilities of different alkenes formed
ii. Relative acidity of different β-H atoms
iii. Relative case of elimination of different β-H atoms.

The hightly substituted alkene is the most stable due to hyper conjugation. As stablest product becomes the major product according to Saytzeff's rule, it is in accordance with the essential requirement of the reaction and so Saytzeff's rule although emperical is justified.

But in the case of Hofmann's elimination the two factors become the deciding factors. The onium group is bulky and so it can create enough steric hindrance to β-H. Again, substitution, preferably alkyl substitution, at β-position reduces the acidity of β-H. So β-H having least substituents is more acidic and so will be more readily eliminated with the formation of least substituted alkene.

Thus in the case of formation of Saytzeff's product thermodynamic (stability) factor plays the important role while steric factor and acidity of β—H become the key-factors for the formation of Hofmann's product.

1.13.4.3.4 Stereochemical Requirement of Elimination Reactions

The stereochemical requirement for elimination may be deduced from the consideration of structures of transition states of E_2 and E_1 paths. E_2 path proceeds through the following transition state.

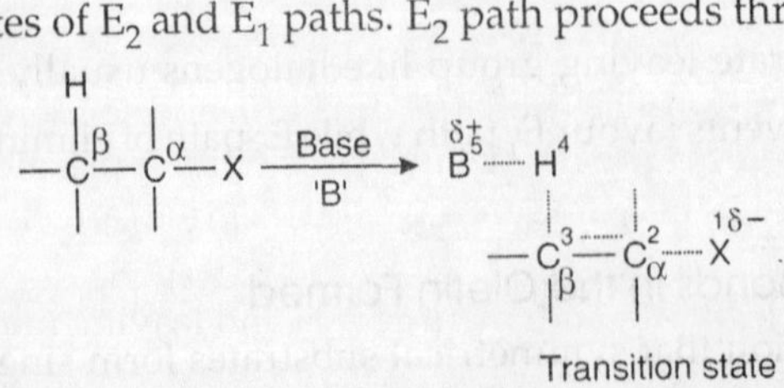

Transition state for E_2 path

From the structure of transition state it is seen that the bonding electron at β-position is being gradually delocalised towards the vacant orbital at α-position generated by the departure of the leaving nucleophile (X) to form π-bond in between α and β carbon atoms. It is known that the essential condition required for the formation of π-bond is the planarity of the overlapping orbitals.

So it is ligical to conclude that as E_2 path is a concerted one, all the five centres (1→5) including the base must be in the same plane in the transition state, i.e., all these five centres are coplanar (periplanar). This periplanarity is to be maintained throughout the reaction for smooth occurrence of elimination reaction.

This periplanarity may be developed in two ways:

(a) When β-H and the leaving nucleophile are trans (anti) to each other as shown below:

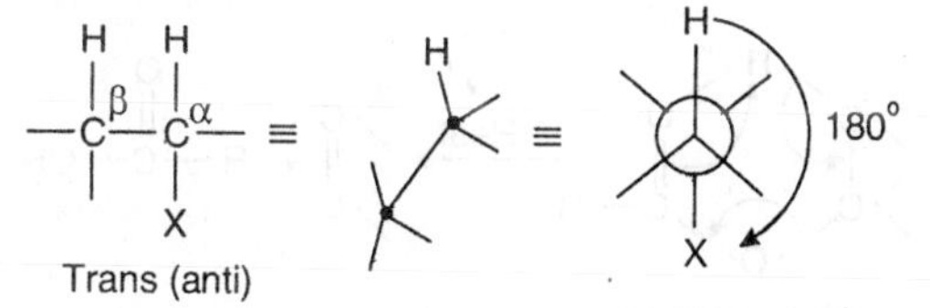

Trans (anti)

In this orientation the dihedral angle between β-H and the departing group is 180°

(b) β-H and the leaving nucleophile are *cis* (syn) to each other, i.e.,

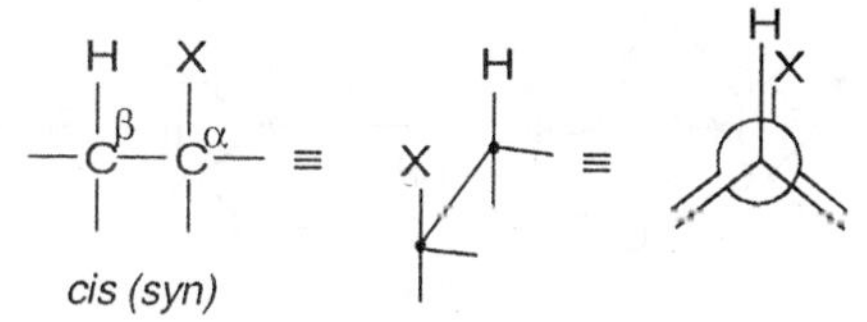

cis (syn)

The dihedral angle in this **cis** arrangement of β-H and leaving nuclerphile is virtually zero degree.

Out of these two arrangements *syn* arrangement is less stable because in this arrangement C_β–H electron pair and $\overline{X}$ are in the same direction and so there is probability of repulsion between these two species. This repulsive force decreases the stability of transition state. But in the anti arrangement probability of operation of such repulsive force is much less and so the stability of the transition state is not hampered. Again, in *syn* arrangement as both β-H and departing nuclerphile are in the same direction some amount of steric hindrance may be created while possibility of such hindrance is much less in *anti*-arrangement. So for E_2 path *anti (trans)* periplanarity is the most favourable condition.

Similar conclusion may be drawn in the case of E_1 elimination. In E_1 path, reaction proceeds through carbocation as transition state.

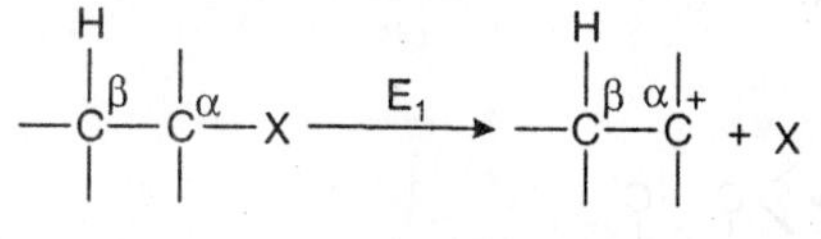

In this path after the formation of carbocation β-H is eliminated as H^+ leaving its bonding electron pair at β-postion.

Now is *syn* arrangement, the β-H and $\overline{X}$ are in the same direction and so there is possibility of generating a repulsive force while in *anti*-arrangement such possibility is practically nil. Thus in the case of *syn*-arrangement reaction may be hampered while in *anti*-arrangement elimination may occur smoothly.

It is, therefore, evident that in E_1 path *anti*-arrangement of β-H and leaving nucleophilic group is the favoured situation.

Thus in general, for any elimination (E_1 or E_2) *anti (trans)* periplanarity is the desired condition. That is why it is stated that common elimination reaction is the anti (trans) elimination reaction. It may be mentioned that elimination reaction particularly E_2 elimination is stereospectic and stereoselective in nature.

1.13.4.3.4.1 *Cis* (*syn*) Elimination

Although *trans* (*anti*) elimination is the common elimination reaction yet in some cases elimination reactions may occur in *cis* (*syn*) manner. Such elimination reactions do not require any catalyst but normally takes place under pyrolytic (thermal) condition. For this reason *cis*-elimination reactions are sometimes termed as pyrolytic elimination reactions. The most common examples of *cis*-elimination reactions are the pyrolysis of esters, xanthates and tertiary amine oxides. Thus,

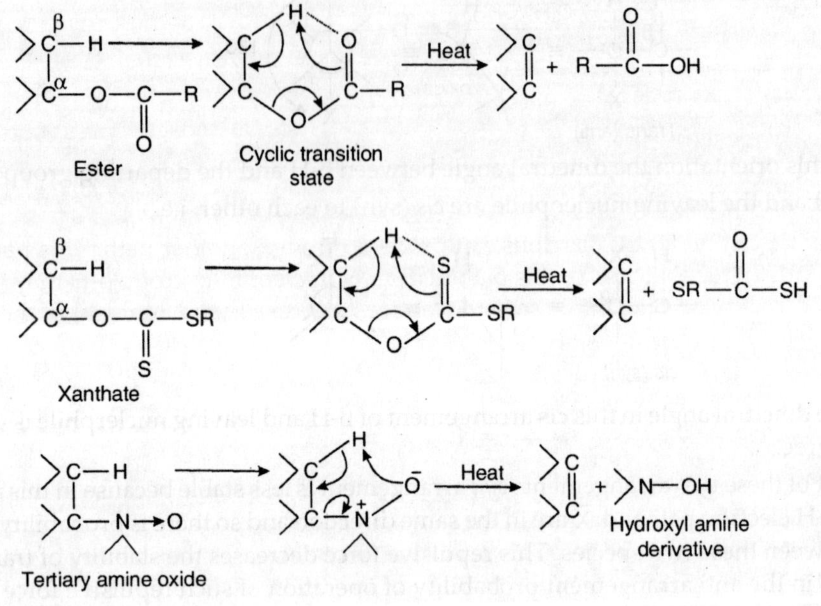

The pyrolysis of esters and xanthates have been studied by **Tschugaev** and accordingly known as **Tschugaev** elimination while Cope investigated the pryolytic elimination of tertiary amine oxide and so it is known as **Cope's elimination**.

1.13.4.3.5 α-Elimination Reaction

In some cases elimination reactions may occur when both H atom and departing nucleophile are eliminated from the same carbon atom.

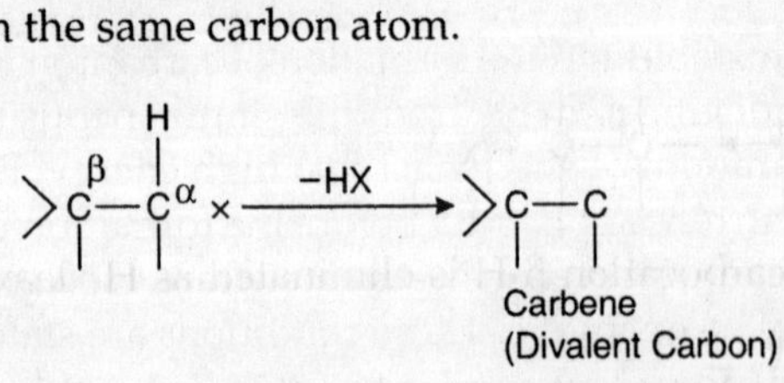

Carbon in Carbene is divalent in nature. This means there are two non-bonded electrons on carbon atom. These two non-bonded electrons may be distributed in two ways—(i) both the electrons may exist in one *p*-orbital leaving another *p*-orbital vacant. This state is SP^2-hybridised state (ii) each of the two electrons may be present in each *p*-orbital creating *SP* state of hybridisation. So it is logical to assume that the chemical activity of carbene is very much similar to π-bonded species. In this respect carbene may be looked upon as an olefinic compound, the formation of which is one of the most essential condtion for elimination and hence α-elimination may be regarded as an elimination reaction. But due to high instability of carbene, α-elimination reaction is very rare. The most illustrated example is the hydrolysis of chloroform with alkali. Thus,

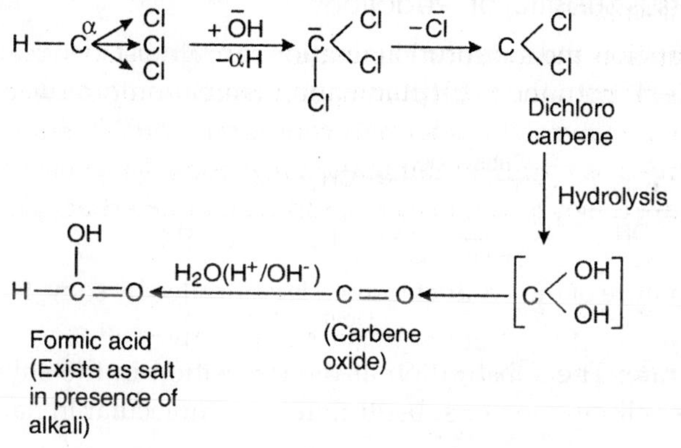

1.13.4.3.6 E_1 CB Elimination

Mechanistically elimination reactions can proceed through another path. This path like E_1 is a stepwise path. In the first step of this path instead of nucleophilic group β-H may be eliminated forming a carbanion which in the second step forms alkene by the removal of the nucleophilic group as depicted below:

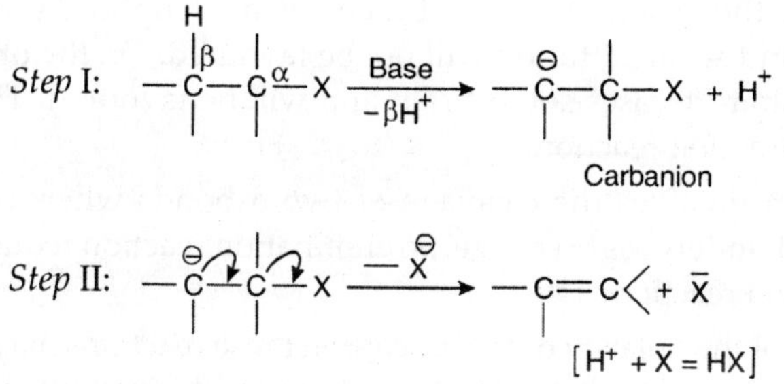

This path like E_1 is unimolecular and the carbanion formed may be regarded as the conjugate base of the substrate. So this mechanistic path is known as unimolecular elimination reaction occurring through conjugate base abbreviated as E_1 CB.

1.13.4.3.6.1 Validity of E_1 CB

It is known that the carbanion is very unstable and the formation of carbanion is reversible. As a result this path becomes kineticully indistinguishable from the simultaneous (E_2) path. Again, formation of carbanion requires high amount of energy. At that high energy, E_2 path can easily take place. So there is possibility of occurrence of E_2 path before the formation of carbanion. For this reason carbanion pathway for elimination reaction is extremely rare. However, under certain conditions this path of elimination may be operative. These conditions are stated below:

i. Presence of highly acidic β-H atom.
ii. Highly electron withdrawing nucleophilic group and
iii. In presence of strong base.

A few examples of E_1 CB may be cited in this connections:

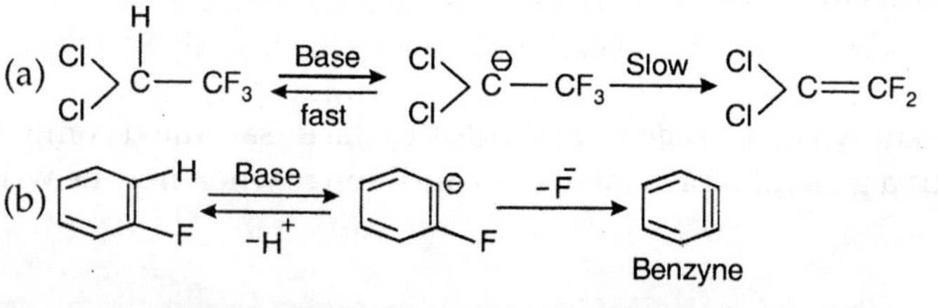

1.13.4.3.7 Elimination Versus Substitution Reactions

The conditions of both elimination and substitution reactions are almost identical. So it is expected that in a substrate having β-H, both the substituion and elimination products may be formed. Thus,

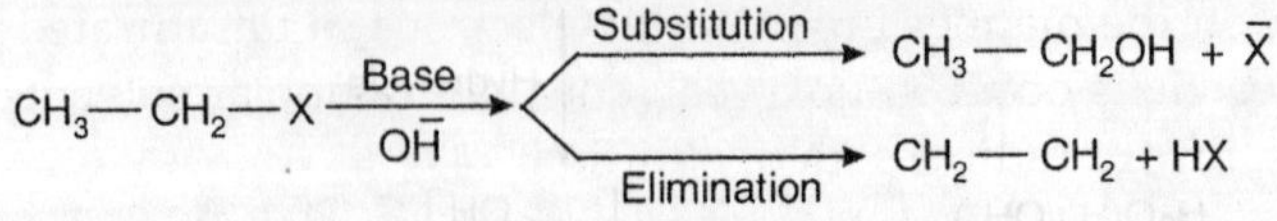

Under this situation the nature of the product formed is controlled by some factors as discussed below:

1. **Nature of the substrate:** The substitution at the α-position in the substrate makes the reaction path whether elimination or substitution is unimolecular in nature, i.e.,

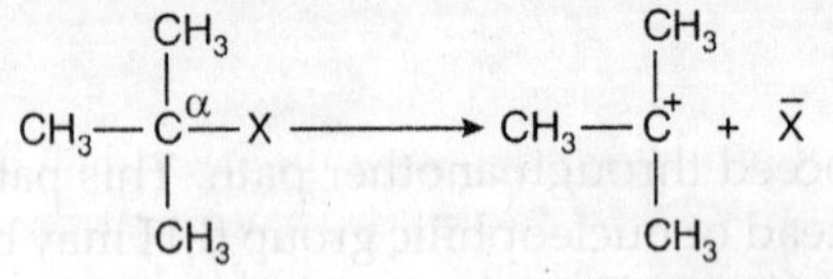

Transition state

In the structure of transition state it is evident that it is strained due to overcrowding. So it will have its tendency to release the strain. The attachment of nucleophilic group (substituion) increases the strain and so substitution will not be favoured. On the other hand, elimination of a hydrogen atom releases some strain and will be favoured. Thus such type of substrate favours elimination reaction.

2. **Temperature:** Elimination reaction involves the cleavage of two δ-bonds whereas in substitution reaction only one bond undergoes breakage. So elimination reaction requires higher temperature than substitution reaction.

3. **Polarity of the base:** The influence of the polarity of the base upon these reactions may be explained on the basis of consideration of transition states of bimolecular path of these two reactions.

(a) Transition state of $S_{N}2$

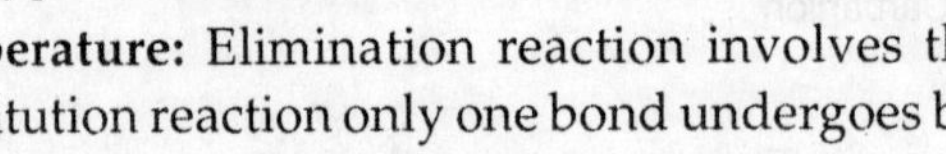

(b) Transition state of E_2

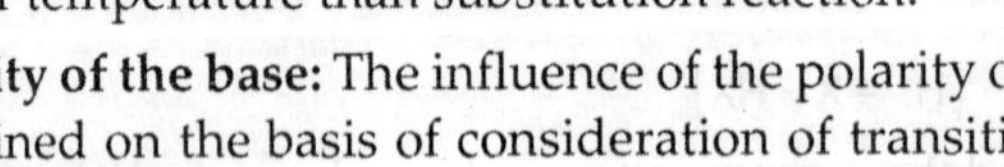

From these two transition states it is seen that the basic strength (polarity) is distributed over three centres in substitution while the strength of the same base in the case of elimination is spread over five centres. So the basic strength required per unit centre in elimination reaction is less than that of substitution reaction. So more polar solvent favours substitution while elimination reaction takes place in less polar solvent.

1.13.4.4 Addition Reactions

In addition reaction a compound known as *addendenum* is added to the unsaturated compound to form a saturated molecule. Thus a general representation of addition reaction may be written as:

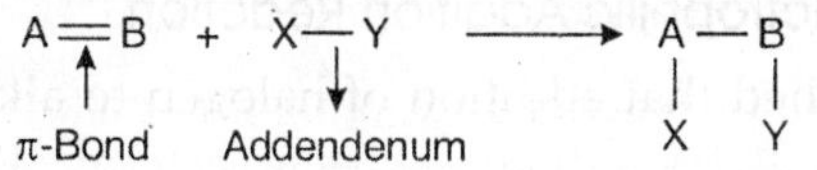

Addition reactions occur in organic compounds having multiple bonds. This reaction may be ionic or radical depending on the manner in which the electrons in unsaturated (π)-bond are polarised. Ionic addition reactions occur in polar solvents, but nonpolar solvents and oxygen source primarily peroxides, favour radical path of addition.

Ionic addition reactions may be electrophilic or nucleophilic in nature. Electrophilic additions are generally observed in C — C multiple bonds such a alkenes and alkynes while nucleophilic addition reactions commonly occur in compounds with multiple bonds between carbon and a hetero atom, such as $>C{=}O$, $>C{=}N{-}H$, etc.

1.13.4.4.1 Electrophilic Addition Reactions

In this type of addition reaction positive part of the addendenum initially attaks the π-bond of the unsaturated compound forming a σ-bond at one end and a carbocation at the other end in the first step, and in the second step negative part of the addendenum combines with carbocation formed.

Step I: / *Step* II:

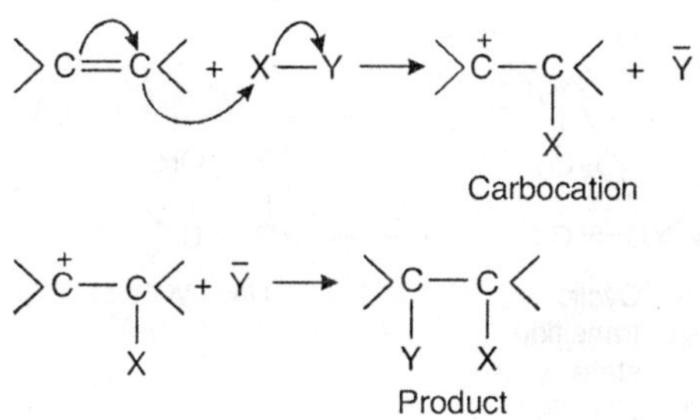

In the case of addition reactions of unsymmetrical alkenes or alkynes which part of the addendenum will combine with which end of unsaturation is guided by an empirical rule known as ***Markownikoff's rule***. The rule states that the negative part of the addendenum combines with highly substituted carbon atom, i.e.,

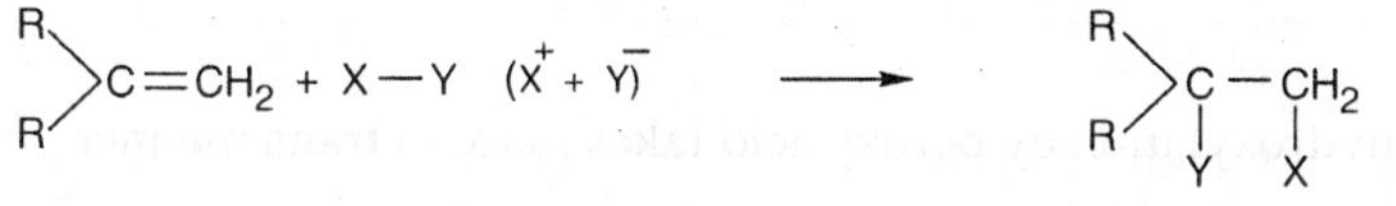

It may be emphasised that although Markownikoff's rule is empirical yet it is applicable in most of the cases with a few exceptions. Thus, in presence of peroxides addition occurs in reverse direction. This deviation from Markownikoff's rule has been explained on the basis of the fact that in presence of peroxide addition path is a radical one.

$$H{-}O{-}O{-}H \longrightarrow 2\dot{O}H$$

$$\dot{O}H + H{-}Br \longrightarrow \dot{Br} + H_2O$$

$$R{-}CH{=}CH_2 + \dot{Br} \longrightarrow \underset{2^{o}\text{ radical, stable}}{R{-}\dot{C}H{-}CH_2{-}Br} \quad \text{or} \quad \underset{(1^{o}\text{ radical less stable})}{(R{-}\underset{|}{\overset{Br}{C}}H{-}\dot{C}H_2}$$

$$R{-}\dot{C}H{-}CH_2{-}Br + HBr \longrightarrow R{-}CH_2{-}CH_2{-}Br + \dot{Br}$$

1.13.4.4.1.1 Some Typical Examples of Electrophilic Addition Reaction

(a) *Addition of halogen:* It has been established that addition of halogen to alkene proceeds through a cyclic intermediate.

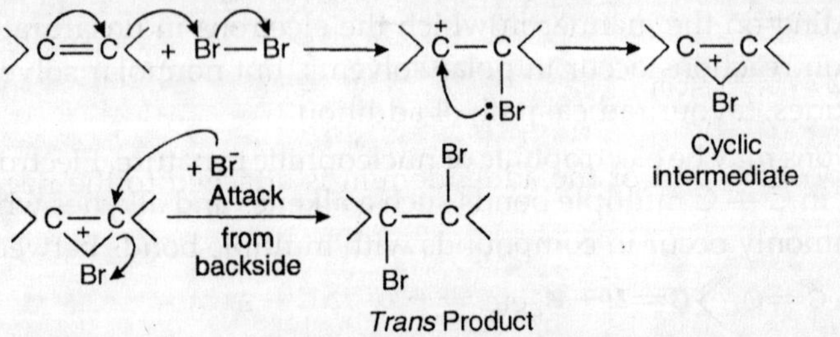

This *anti* addition has been found to be stereoselective.

(b) *Hydroxylation:* Hydroxylation of alkene may be carried out by different reagents such as $KMnO_4$, OSO_4 and peroxy acid. All these hydroxylations are stereoselective. In the case of $KMnO_4$ and OSO_4 addition occurs in *syn* manner with the formation of *syn* (*cis*) diol.

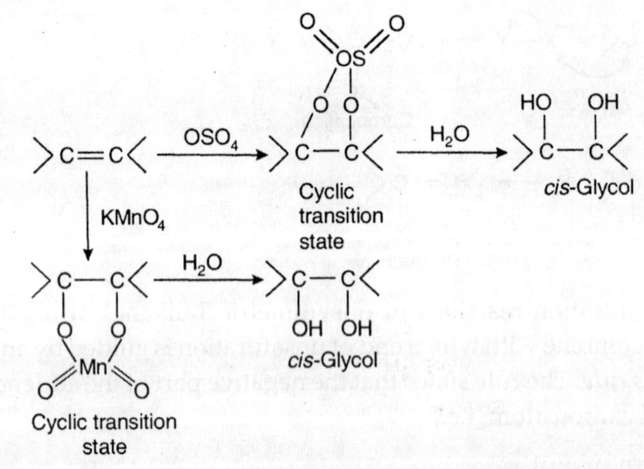

However, hydroxylation by peroxy acid takes place in **trans** manner.

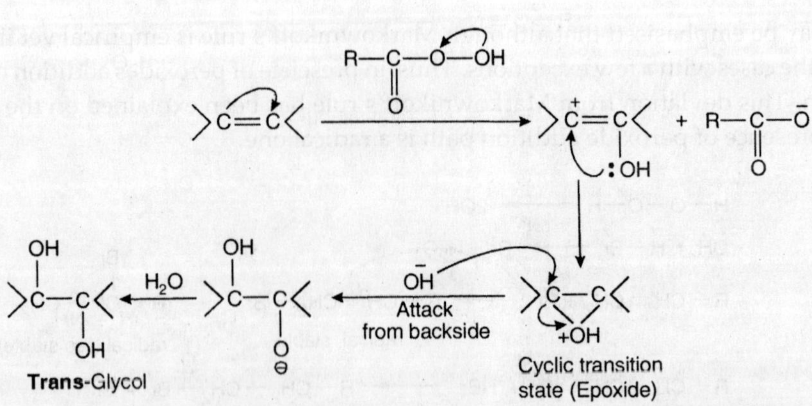

1.13.4.4.2 Nucleophilic Addition Reactions

This type of addition reaction takes place in a stepwise manner. In the first step negative of the addendenum combines with carbon atom to which hetero atom is connected by multiple bond.

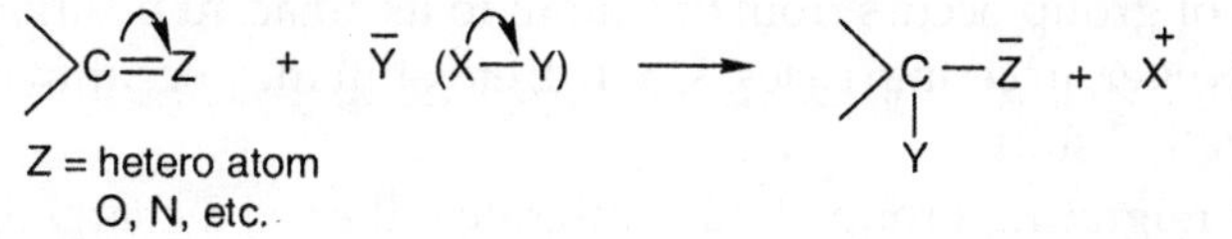

In the next step's positive part of the addendenum is attached to the negatively charged hetero atom.

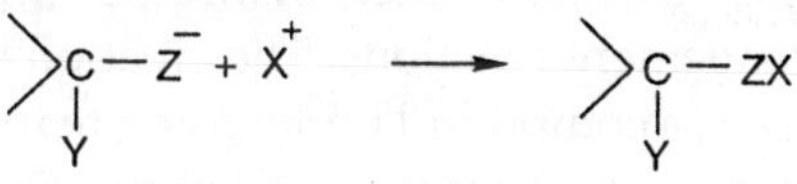

Some common examples of nucleophilic addition reactions are:

(a) Addition in carbonyl compounds.

(i)
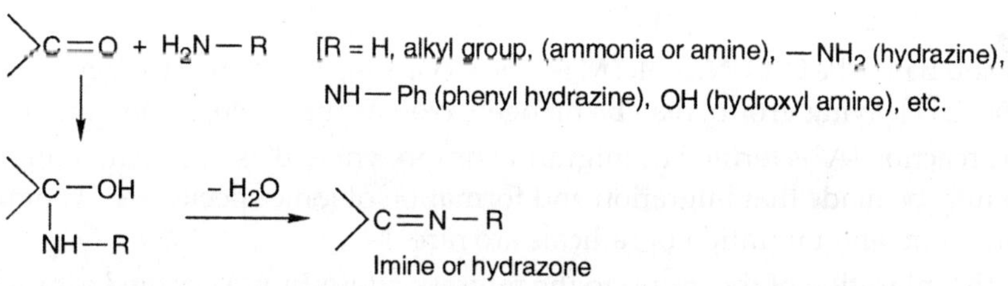

(ii)
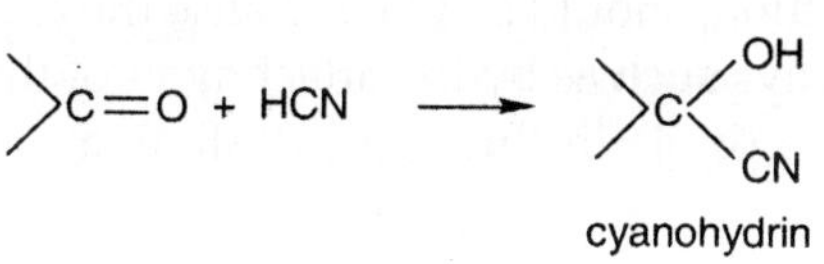

(iii)
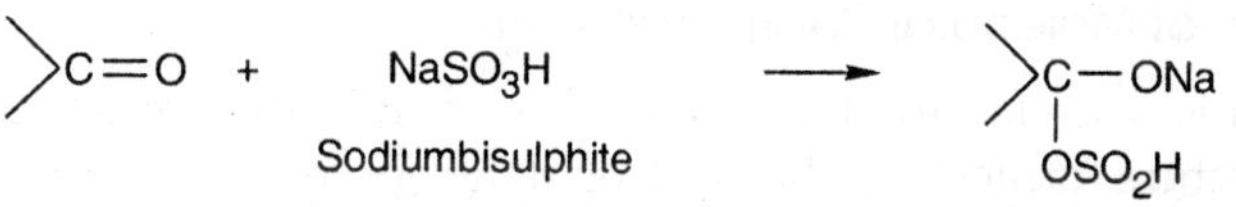

(b) Hydrolysis of nitriles.

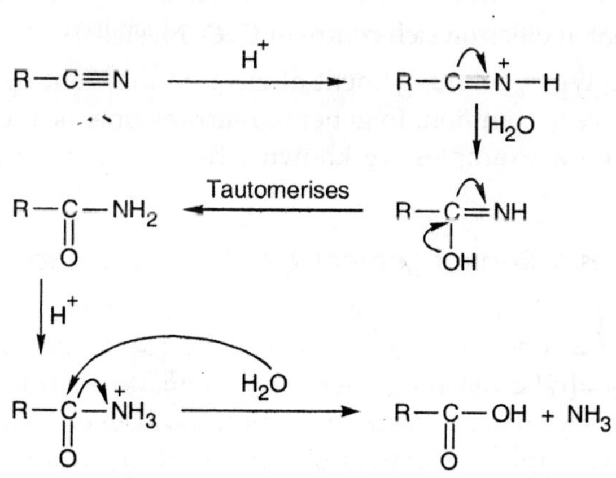

1.13.4.5 Rearrangement Reactions

As name suggests, these are special type of reactions. In this type of reactions an atom or a group of atoms migrates from one atom to another within the molecule or the carbon skeleton is modified. Normally migration of group occurs from one atom to its adjacent position, i.e., commonly 1, 2 shift takes place. However, in certain cases, 1, 3; 1, 4; etc. shift may occur which may be explained in terms of successive 1, 2 shifts.

It is obvious that migrating group should migrate either as a charged species (ion) or as a radical. Further, it is natural that the migrating group should migrate to ionic or radical centre depending upon its nature. Thus it is evident that in order to have a rearrangement reaction, a charged (ionic) or radical centre must be created before the migration starts and this is the prerequisite of molecular rearrangement reactions. The creation of desired centres can only be done by the removal of a group, i.e., a compound undergoing rearrangement reaction must have a leaving group. Thus, a general picture of rearrangement reaction may be shown as under,

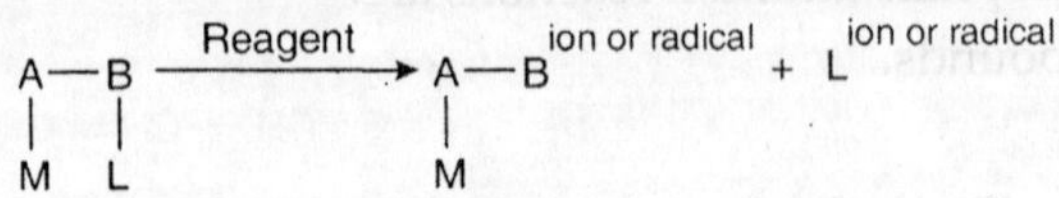

where A and B may be C, O, N, S, etc. M is any alkyl, aryl, or halogen, oxygen, nitrogen containing group and L is leaving group, may be halogen, oxygen, nitrogen, S containing group.

In this reaction 'A' is termed as migration origin while 'B' is designated migration terminus. Mention may be made that migration and formation of ionic species are of common occurrence while formation and migration of radicals are rare.

After the migration of the group to the migration terminus a charged centre is created at the migration origin. So the final step of the reaction, should be to neutralise the charged migration origin which may be achieved by various ways such as by the attachment of the leaving group (L) or attacking reagent or by the formation of olefin through the elimination of β-H, if it is available.

1.13.4.5.1 Classification of Molecular Rearrangement

The molecular rearrangement is classified on the basis of nature of charged centre formed at migration terminus. The centre formed may be electron deficient (positively charged) or electron rich (negatively charged). Thus rearrangement reactions may be classified under two headings.

(a) Rearrangement at electron deficient centre which may be C, N, O, etc.

(b) Rearrangement at electron rich centre of C, O, N, etc.

Out of these two types, rearrangement at electron deficient centre particularly at electron deficient carbon are very common. In general, rearrangements at electron deficient carbon are acid catalysed but a few examples are known where rearrangements proceed in presence of basic catalysts.

1.13.4.5.2 Examples of Rearrangement Reactions at Electron Deficient Centres

Most common examples of molecular rearrangement occurring at electron deficient carbon are (i) rearrangement of alcohol (ii) pinacol-pinacolone rearrangement, (iii) benzil-benzilic acid rearrangement, (iv) allylic rearrangement, (v) Demjanov-Tiffinu rearrangement, (vi) Wolf rearrangement while Hofman bromamide reaction and Baeyer-Villiger oxidation constitute two widely illustrated examples of rearrangement at electron deficient nitrogen and oxygen respectively. A short resume on these rearrangements is furnished in the sequel.

1.13.4.5.2.1 Molecular Rearrangement at Electron Deficient Carbon

In general, these rearrangements occur in presence of acidic catalyst. However, in certain cases bases may be used as catalyst.

i. *Rearrangement of alcohol:*

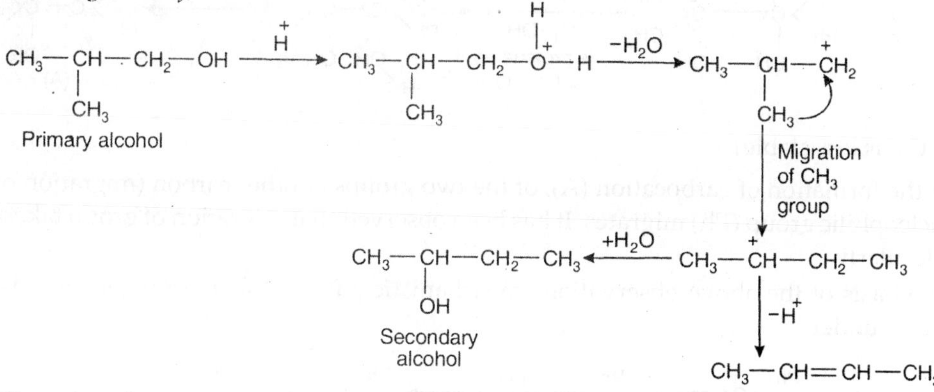

The migrating group in this rearrangement migrates as nucleophile. So if there are more than one migrating group at the migration origin, more nuclecophilic group, generally, migrates. Similar type of rearrangement may occur with olefin and halides.

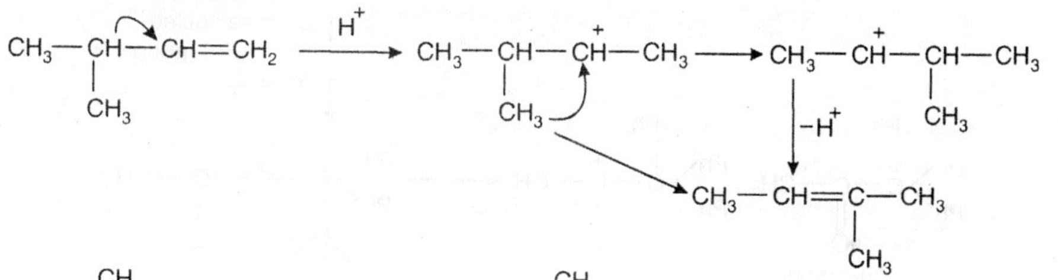

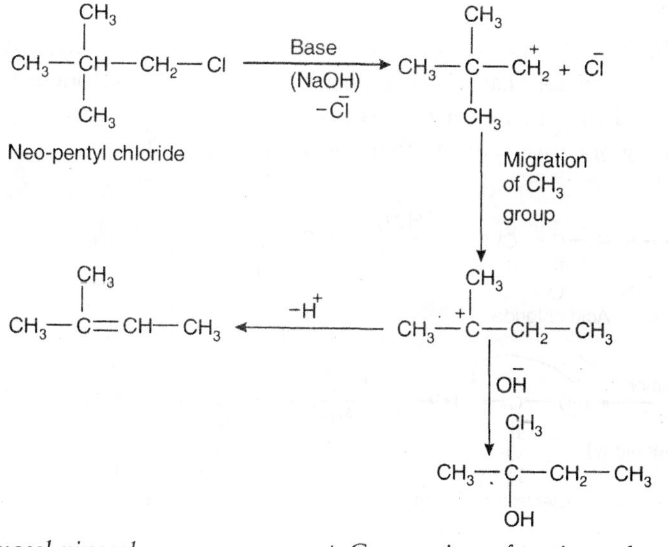

ii. *Pinacol-pinacolone rearrangement:* Conversion of tertiary glycol to a ketone, pinacolone in presence of acid as catalyst is known as pinacol-pinacolone rearrangement.

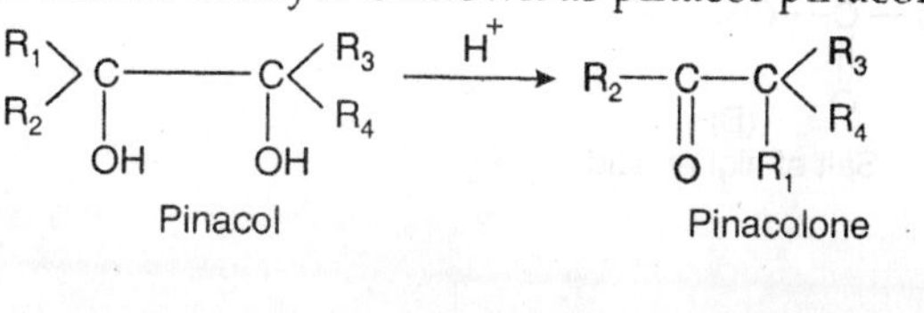

Mechanism: Out of two OH groups only one is protonated. Normally that hydroxyl group is protonated from which relatively stabler carbocation is formed.

Thus,

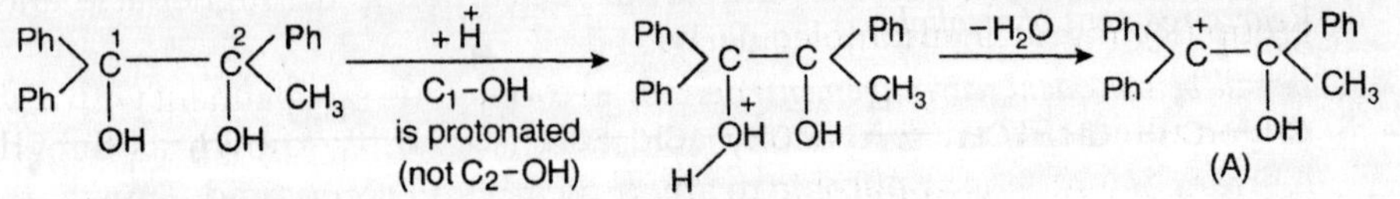

(NB: C_2^+ is less stable).

After the formation of carbocation (A), of the two groups at other carbon (migration origin) more nucleophilic group (Ph) migrates. It has been observed that migration of group takes place intramolecularly.

On the basis of the above observations meachanistic path of this rearrangement has been proposed as under.

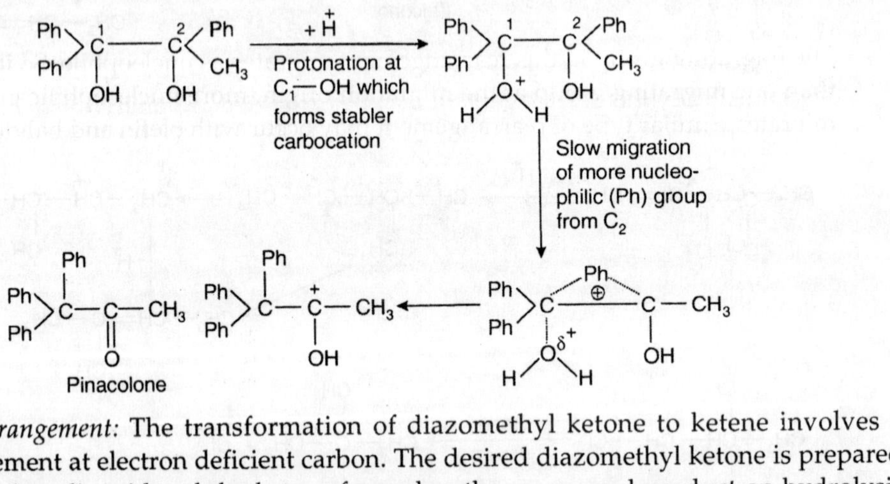

iii. *Wolf-rearrangement:* The transformation of diazomethyl ketone to ketene involves a rearrangement at electron deficient carbon. The desired diazomethyl ketone is prepared from a carboxylic acid and the ketene formed as the rearranged product on hydrolysis yields another acid having one more carbon than the starting acid. Thus,

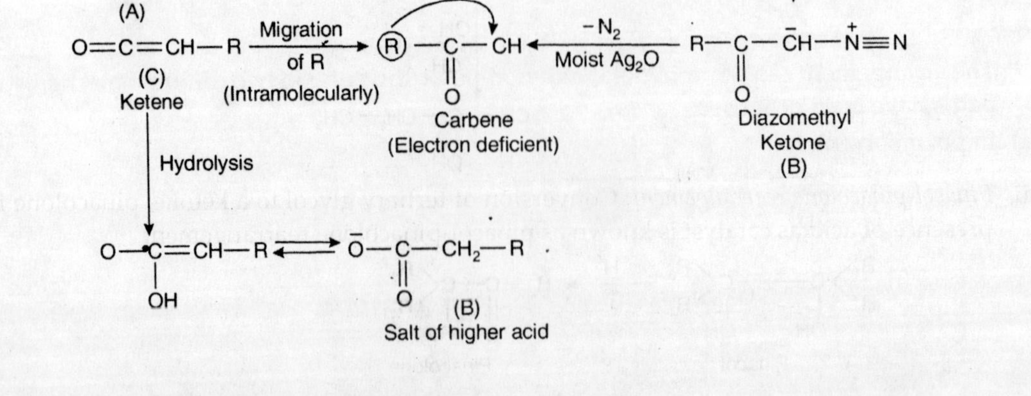

The whole process of conversion of (A) to the higher homologue (D) is known as **Arndt-Eistart synthesis.**

In the conversion of diazomethyl ketone (B) to ketene (C) the carbonyl carbon of diazomethyl ketone becomes the carboxylic carbon in the higher acid and the migrating group (R) migrates intramolecularly.

iv. *Benzil-benzilic acid rearrangement:* Benzil, an α-diketone on treatment with a base is converted to benzilic acid, an α-hydroxy acid and is usually known as benzil-benzilic acid rearrangement. It is applicable to any α-dicarbonyl compound. Thus,

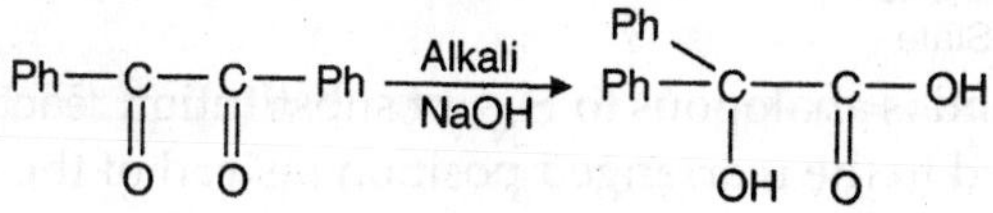

Benzil — Benzilic acid

In general,

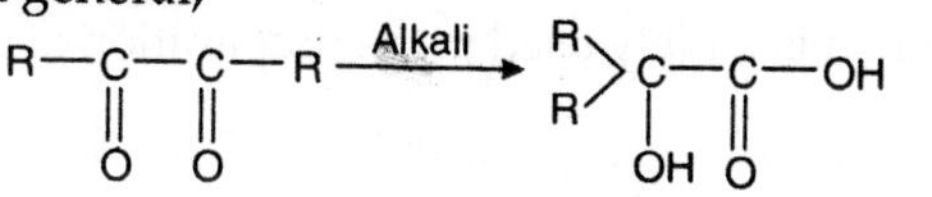

α-Diketone — α-Hydroxy acid

Mechanistically this rearrangement may be expressed as under:

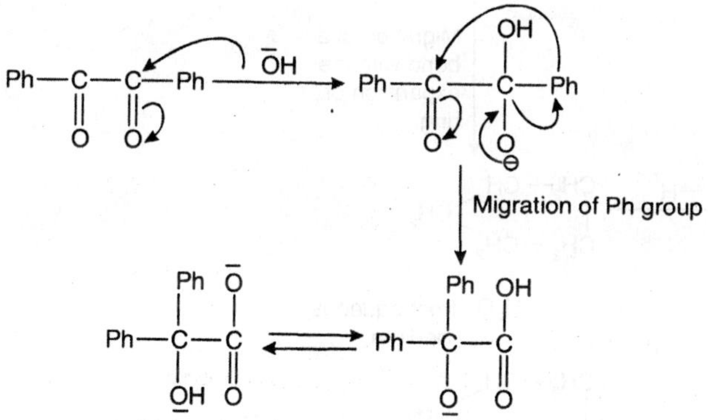

v. *Allylic rearrangement:* It is a rearrangement in which a group is migrated from an allylic position to another carbon atom under the reaction condition. The most well illustrated example is the conversion of α-phenyl allyl alcohol to cinnamoyl alcohol.

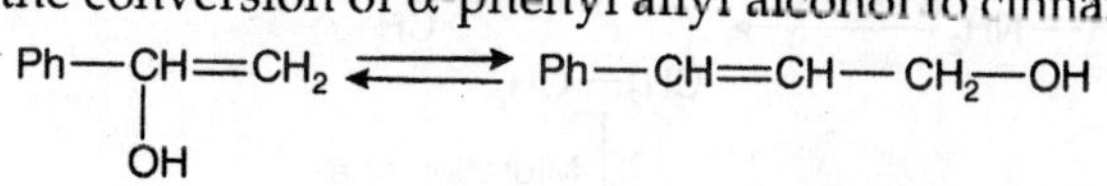

α-Phenylallyl alcohol — Cinnamoyl alcohol

The arrangement can occur in polar and non-polar solvents. So two different mechanistic paths have been proposed.

(a) In polar solvent:

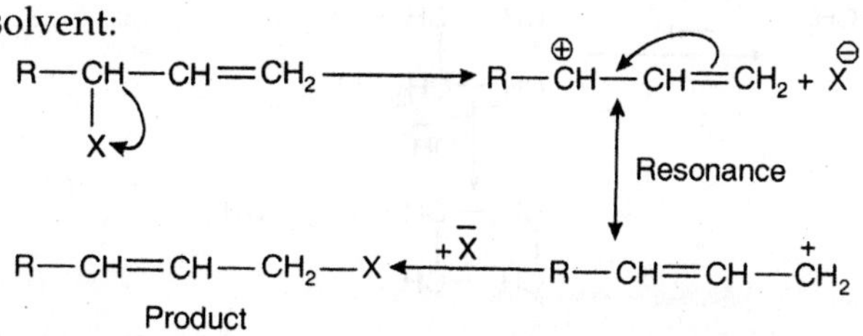

This path is analogous to S_{N^1} path but the product formed is not a normal substitution as the nucleophilic group ($\bar{X}$) is attached to rearranged position. So this path is termed as $S_{N^{1'}}$.

(b) In non-polar solvent: In non-polar solvent rearrangement takes place through a cyclic transition state.

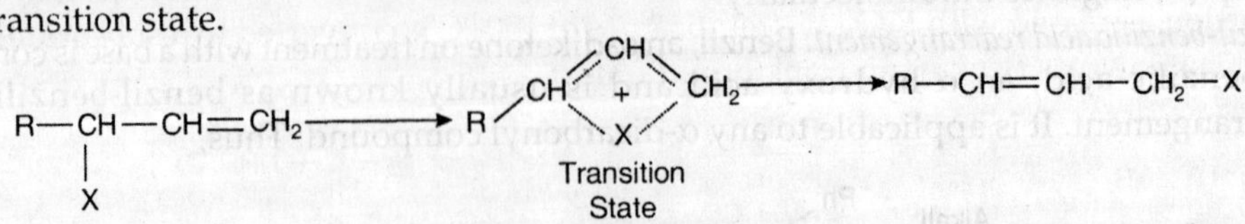

This path is intramolecular in nature and is analogous to S_{N^2} of substitution reaction but the leaving nucleophilic group attached to the rearranged position instead of the normal position and hence is indicated by $S_{N^{2'}}$.

vi. *Demjanov-Tiffinu rearrangement:* In this rearrangement carbon cation is generated from primary amino group through diazotisation. It is widely used in the preparation of alicyclic compound.

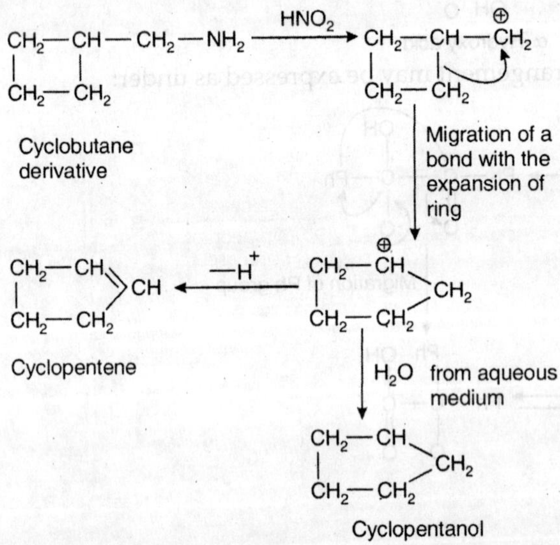

If primary amino group is attached to the ring carbon atom, contraction of ring occurs.

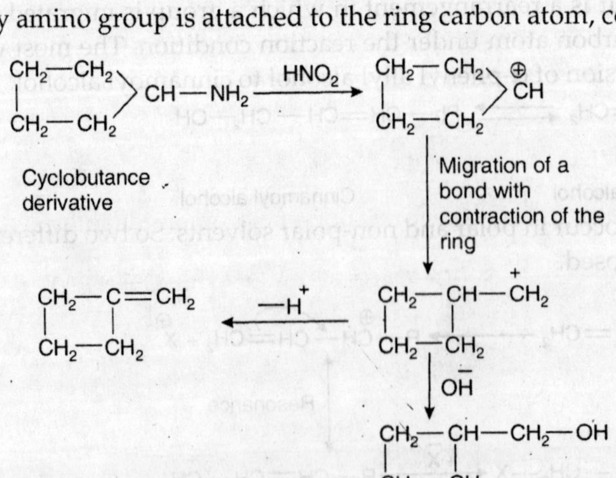

1.13.4.5.2.2 Rearrangement at Electron Deficient Nitrogen

Two most common examples of rearrangement occurring at electron deficient nitrogen are Beckmann transformation and Hofmann bromamide reaction.

i. *Beckmann transformation:* Oxime of carbonyl compound preferably ketoxime when in ether solution is treated with P_2O_5 at a temprature of 100 °C is converted to a substituted amide and is known as Beckmann transformation.

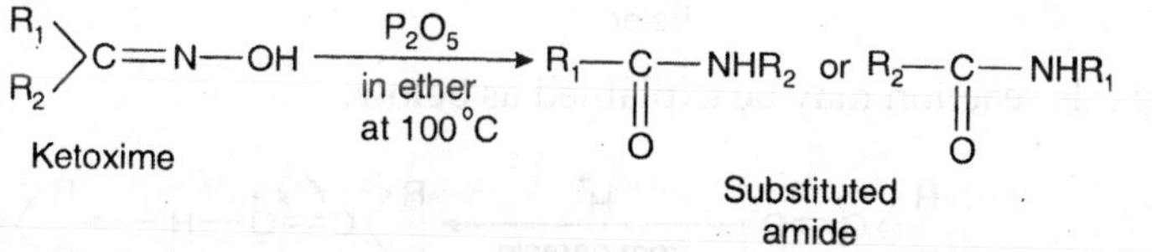

The characteristic features of this rearrangement are as under:

1. Migration of group occurs intramolecularly.
2. The group which is *trans* to oxime hydroxyl always migrates.
3. The oxygen of amide carbonyl oxygen comes from water during decomposition of the intermediate complex.
4. Along with substituted amide there is always formation of cyanide.

On the basis of above observations following mechanism has been suggested for Beckmann rearrangement.

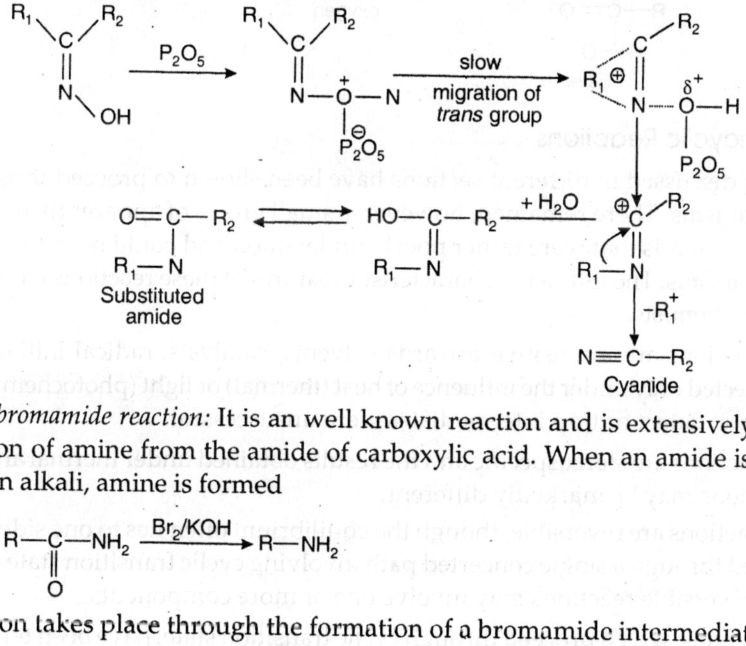

ii. *Hofmann bromamide reaction:* It is an well known reaction and is extensively used for the preparation of amine from the amide of carboxylic acid. When an amide is treated with bromine in alkali, amine is formed

The reaction takes place through the formation of a bromamide intermediate.

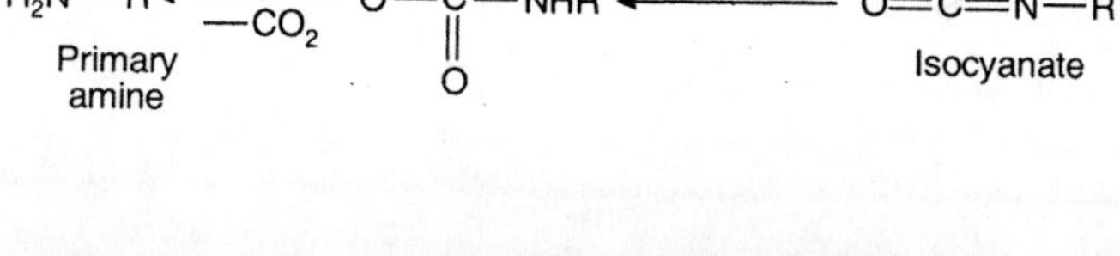

1.13.4.5.2.3 Rearrangement at Electron Deficient Oxygen

The only best known example is Baeyer-Villiger oxidation. In this reaction a ketone is oxidised with peracid when ester of a carboxylic acid is formed.

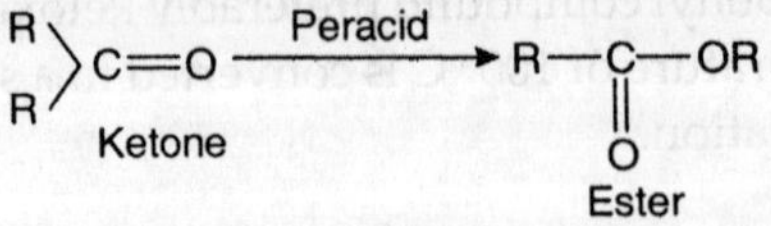

Mechanistically this reaction may be explained as below:

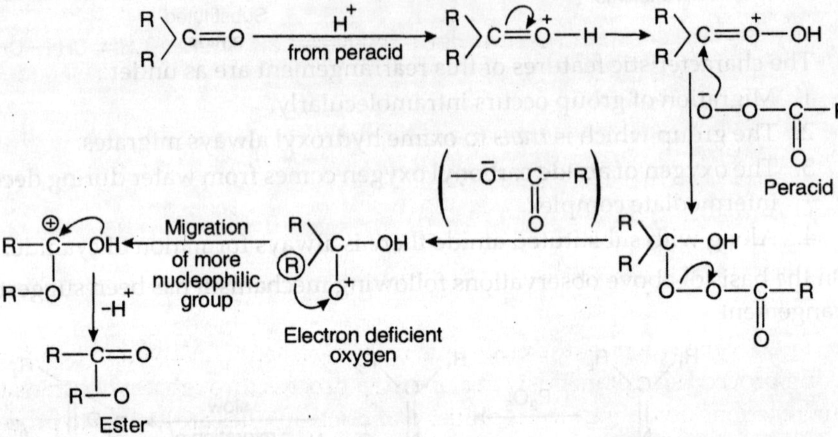

1.13.4.6 Pericyclic Reactions

The reactions discussed in different sections have been shown to proceed through ionic or free radical mechanisms. There remained, however, a small group of apparently unrelated reactions of olefinic compounds that were rather poorly understood and could not be explained by either of these mechanisms. The following characteristic features of these reactions were of great concern to the organic chemists.

i. The reactions are insensitive towards solvents, catalysts, radical initiators or inhibitors and effected only under the influence of heat (thermal) or light (photochemical). All attempts to isolate, detect or trap intermediates were unsuccessful.
ii. The reactions are stereospecific and the results obtained under thermal and photochemical conditions may be markedly different.
iii. The reactions are reversible, though the equilibrium often lies to one side or the other, and proceed through a single concerted path involving cyclic transition state and either side of these reversible reactions may involve one or more components.

These reactions, which proceed through cyclic transition state, have been termed as pericyclic reactions and these pericyclic reactions generally undergo reversible cyclisation and ring opening in most of the cases. The classical and widely illustrated examples of these reactions are shown below:

1 (a) 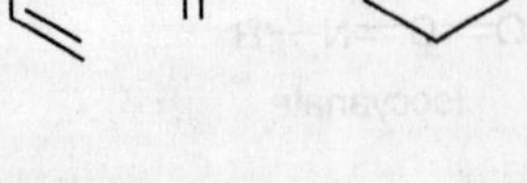

(b) 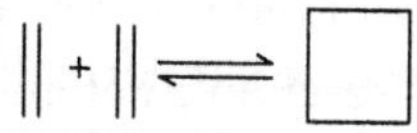

2. (a) 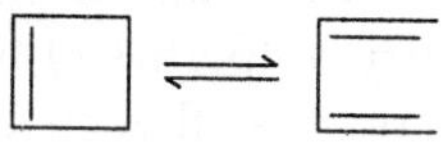

(b) 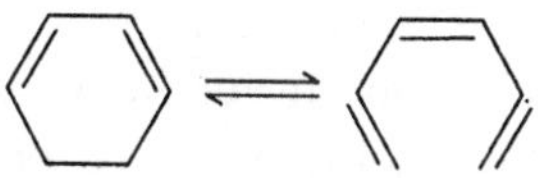

3. (a) $R-CH_2-CH=CH_2 \xrightleftharpoons{1,\,3\ \text{shift}} CH_2=CH-CH_2-R$

(b) 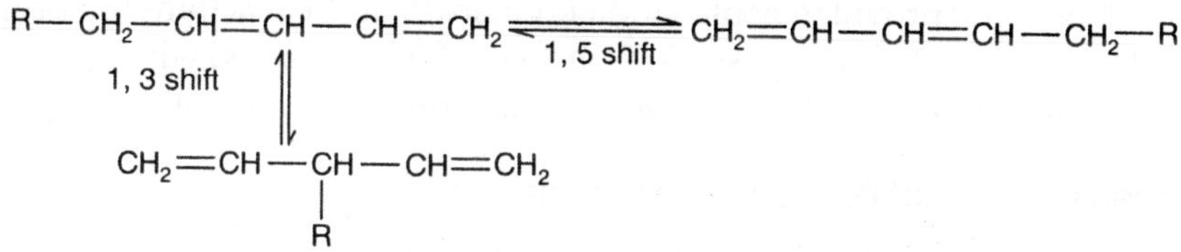

4. 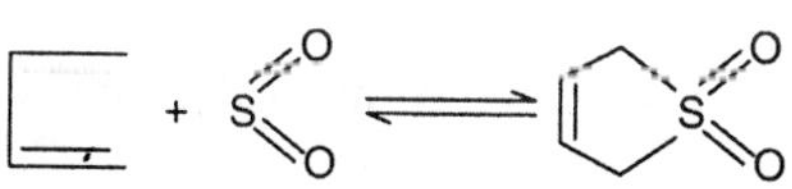

In a pericyclic reaction, the electronic rearrangements involved in bond-making and bond-breaking proceed simultaneously in a one-step process through a cyclic transition state. Though certain reactions involving electrophilies and nucleophilies are known to proceed through cyclic transition states and some rearrangements may even take place in a concerted manner but these reactions do not fulfil all the criteria of pericyclic reactions and, therefore, there is no scope for confusion.

1.13.4.6.1 Classification of Pericyclic Reactions

On the basis of differences in the overall nature of the reaction and the number of participating molecules as well as from the number of sigma (σ) bonds formed or broken, five subsclasses of pericyclic reaction are recognized. These are

1. *Cycloaddition:* It is an adduct-forming pericyclic reaction ($X + Y \rightarrow X - Y$). In this reaction, one side of reversible process has more than one pi (π) bonded molecule, which undergo cyclisation forming two new sigma (σ) bonds. [Examples 1 (a) and 1(b)].
2. *Electrocyclic Reactions:* These are reversible ring closure-ring opening pericyclic reactions with the formation of a new σ or π bond. Only a single molecule lies on either side of the reversible process. [Examples 2(a) and 2(b)].
3. *Sigmatropic Rearrangements:* Molecular rearrangements in which a σ bonded atom or group, flanked by one or more π-electron systems, shifts to a new location with a corresponding recorganization of π-bonds are sigmatropic rearrangements. [Examples 3(a) and 3(b)]
4. *Cheletropic Reaction:* Addition of a single species to an olefin giving rise to a cyclic compound is known as cheletropic reaction (Example 4).
5. *Group Transfer Reaction.*

1.13.4.6.2 Central Theme of Pericyclic Reactions

A careful scrutiny of classical examples of pericyclic reactions reveals that in these reactions, there is a smooth interconversion pi (π) and sigma (σ) bonds. It has been established that such facile interconversion is only possible when the activation energy of the reaction is very low. Again, for a reaction to have low activation energy there must be some similarity between the involved molecular orbitals of the participating molecules, that is, similarity in symmetry properties of their molecular orbitals. It is known that if symmetry properties of the involved molecular orbitals of the reactants and products are conserved in a reaction, the activation energy of the reaction becomes very low and in such a situation the reaction becomes synchronous. The energy necessary for formation and cleavage of the bond is largely derived from the cleavage and formation of the bond and only a small amount of energy becomes necessary to initiate the reaction. The conservation of symmetry of molecular orbitals, the central theme of pericyclic reactions, was advanced by Woodward and Hoffmann, a revolutionary theory in organic chemistry, which not only provided explanation for many of these reactions but predicted many reactions which were considered impossible. The theory also explained why some reactions can be effected under the influence of heat and some others under the influence of light.

1.13.4.6.3 Interpretation of Pericyclic Reactions

Since the initiation of investigation by Woodward and Hoffmann for the application of orbital symmetry analyses to pericyclic reactions, three main approaches have so far been developed and these are (i) Correlation diagram method (ii) Frontier orbital method and (iii) Mobius-Hückel method.

Historically, the first approach was due to Woodward and Hoffmann according to which the symmetry properties of the involved molecular orbitals of the reactants and products are correlated in a diagram, Known as **correlation diagram.** On the basis of such correlation diagram, a set of rules, known as **selection rules**, were formulated for different pericyclic reactions. According to these rules, reaction paths of some concerted reactions were described as **symmetry-allowed**, while some others as **symmetry-forbidden**.

The Second approach and perhaps the most popular approach is the **Frontier molecular orbital** (FMO) approach, developed by Woodward and Fukui and and this is poularly known as **Homo-Lumo** method. According to this approach, the symmetry properties of only **Highest energy occupied molecular orbital** (HOMO) and **lowest energy unoccupied molecular orbital** (LUMO) are the guiding factors for the interpretation of these concerted reactions.

The thrid approach was developed by Mobius and Hückel and popularised by H. Zimmermann and H.J.S. Dewar. The idea behind this method is that a pericyclic reaction that proceeds through a cyclic transition state with aromatic characteristics is energetically favourable and thus allowed. This is known as **Mobius-Hückel method**.

1.13.4.6.4 Electrocyclic Reactions

In electrocyclic reaction a conjugated open chain polyene undergoes reversible ring opening and ring closing reaction or in other words in electrocyclic reaction a conjugated polyene forms a cycloalkene and in reverse reaction a cycloalkene yields a conjugated polyene. In these reactions during cyclistion a new sigma bond is formed between the terminals of the linear conjugated polyene and the net change that occurs in the open chain conjugated polyene is the loss of two π-electrons with the formation of a σ (sigma) bond and in the reverse reaction, a σ-bond is converted to a π-bond with the concomitant ring opening. So, the electrocyclic reaction may be expressed as:

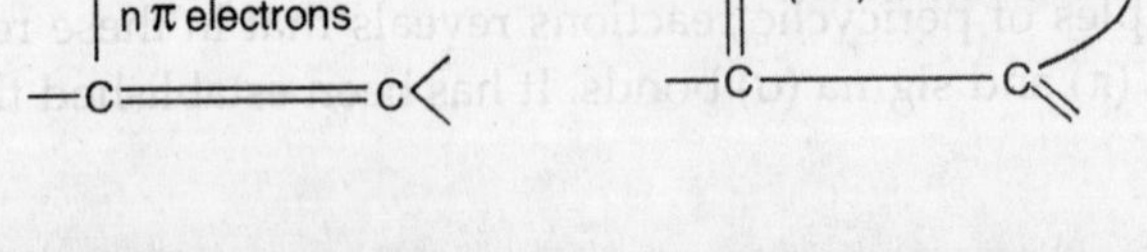

1.13.4.6.5 Classification of Electrocyclic Reactions

Depending upon the of number of π electrons present in open chain partner, electrocyclic reactions have been classified into two groups:

(a) Electrocyclic reactions involving conjugated linear polyenes containing (4n + 2) π electrons where n may be 0, 1, 2, 3 .... n

(b) Electrocyclic reactions of conjugated linear polyene system having 4nπ electrons where n may be 1, 2, 3 .... n

Some typical examples of the above two groups of electrocyclic reaction are as noted below:

(a) (4n + 2) π electron system (n, may be 0, 1, 2, 3, ... n)

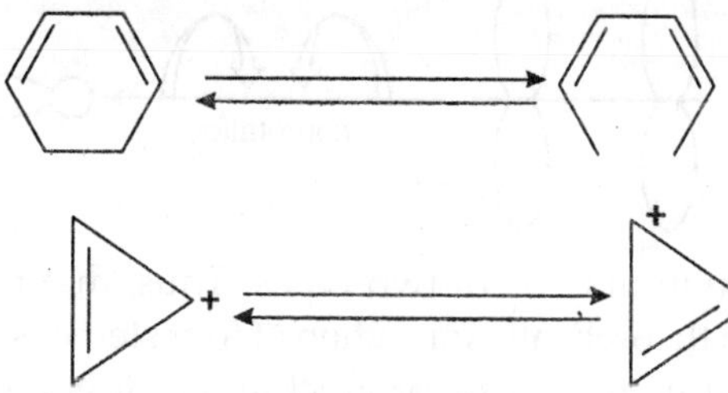

(b) 4 n π electron system (n, may be 1, 2, 3 .... n)

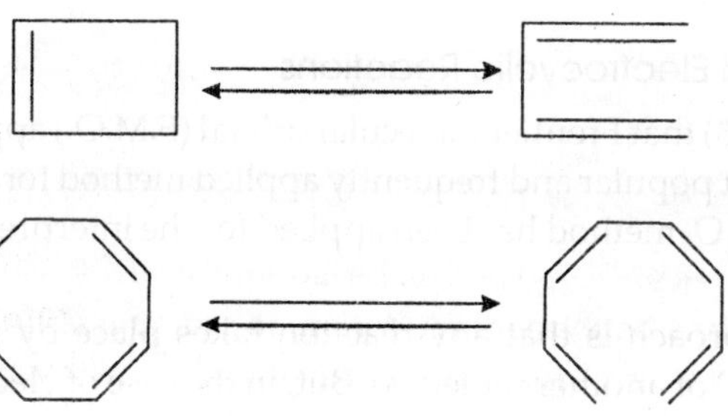

1.13.4.6.6 Explanation of Electrocyclic Reactions

A careful scrutiny of organic molecules undergoing electrocyclic reactions clearly suggests that these reactions involve the conversion of a C—C pai bond into a C—C sigma bond and vice versa. Although C—C sigma bond formation generally takes place by the overlapping of sp^3 orbitals yet due to greater contribution of *p*-orbital in this hybridization, for simplicity, the importance of only *p*-orbital in these reactions has been given more importance. Again, as pointed out earlier, in electrocyclic reaction there is an interconversion of π & σ bonds, the perquisite or pre-condition of the reaction is the rotation of the atomic orbitals of the involved M.O. by 90°, because the mode of overlapping of atomic orbitals for π and π bond formation are different, π bond formation requires parallel overlapping of *p*-orbitals while σ bond formation is possible if co-axial overlapping of *p*-orbitals takes place as depicted below:

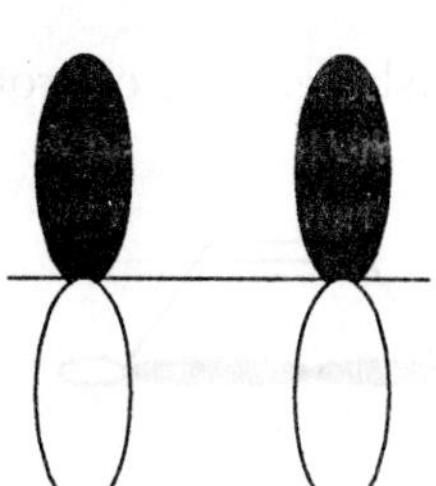

π-orbital

Further, as a consequence of rotation of atomic orbitals by 90°, two more basic aspects which come up for considerations are: (i) rotation of atomic orbitals by 90° is always associated with the rotation by 90° of the atoms or groups connected to these orbitals. and (ii) rotation of both the atomic orbitals of the M.O. may be in the same direction (both clockwise or both anti clockwise)-termed as *conrotation* or the rotation of both the atomic orbitals may be in the opposite direction (one in clockwise and other in anti clockwise) designated as *disrotation* as indicated in the figure below:

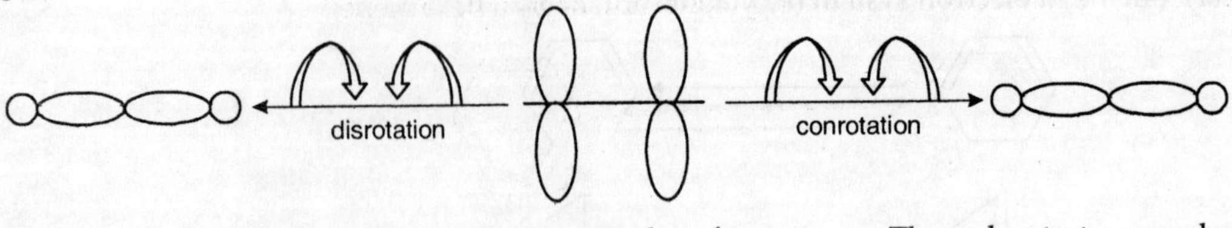

Once again, conrotation and disrotation may be of two types. Thus, due to two modes of conrotation and two modes of disrotation theoretically formation of four stereo isomeric products are possible, out of which only one will be the major product and that is the beauty of this reaction.

1.13.4.6.7 F.M.O. Approach and Electrocyclic Reactions

As mentioned (vide section 1.13.4.6.3) that Frontier molecular orbital (F.M.O.) approach developed by Woodward and Fukūi is the most popular and frequently applied method for the interpretation of pericyclic reactions. As such F.M.O. method has been applied for the interpretation of different type of pericyclic reactions.

The basic theme of F.M.O. approach is that any reaction takes place by the interaction of HOMO of one molecule and LUMO of another molecule. But, in the case of electrocyclic reaction as only one molecule reversibly undergoes ring opening and ring closing, only the HOMO is regarded as the controlling factor. It has been observed that if HOMO of the open chain partner under the reaction conditions has C_2-axis of symmetry, reaction will proceed in conrotatory manner. On the other hand, if this HOMO has m (plane/mirror plane) symmetry, reaction will occur in disrotatory manner.

Now in the case of $4n\pi$ electron system (butadiene & cyclobutene) under thermal condition, the HOMO of the open chain partner is ψ_2 (bonding M.O with highest energy). This ψ_2 has C_2 symmetry. Therefore, under thermal condition butadience—cyclobutene interconvertion will occur in conrotatory way, the same conclusion has been drawn from correlation diagram. In photochemical condition the HOMO will be the first excited state. Thus, such HOMO of open chain partner is ψ_3 here (n – 1) is even, so its symmetry is plane of symmetry (mirror plane). So, under this condition the path of the reaction will be disrotatory. The above statement may be explained on the basis of orbital picture of HOMO.

In Thermal condition HOMO of Butadiene is ψ_2, it obviously requires conrotation as shown in figure (1.15).

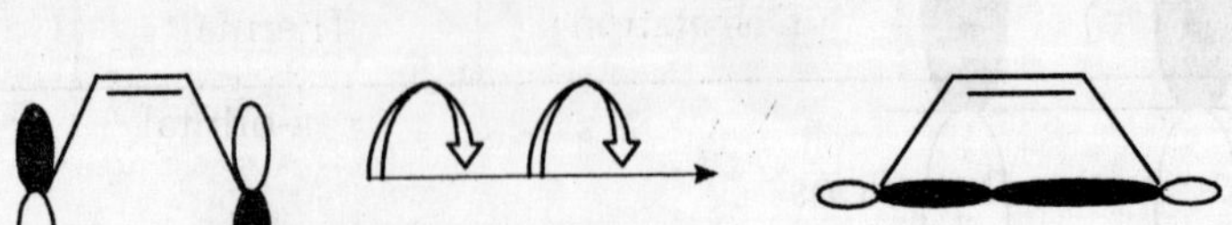

Fig. 1.15

Under photochemical condition first excited of butadiene is ψ_3, its orbital picture reveals that bond formation is only possible through disrotation.

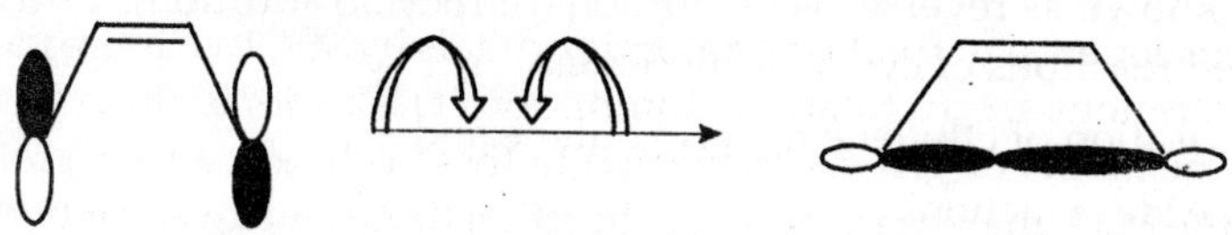

Fig. 1.16

In the case of (4n + 2) π electron system, similar explanation may be given. The most classical example is the interconversion of of cyclohexadiene into hexatriene:

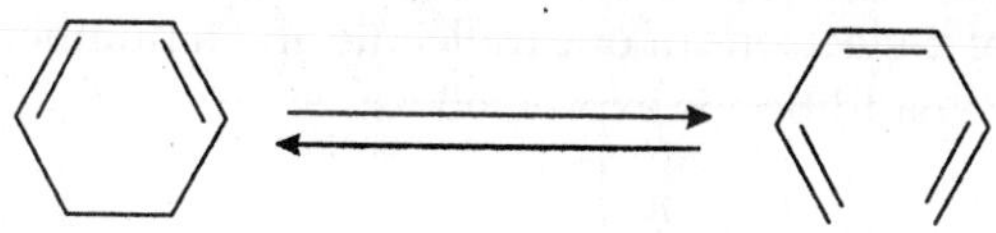

(i) (ii)

Under thermal condition HOMO of hexatriene is ψ_3 (bonding MO with highest energy). Here (n – 1) is even, so it will have plane of symmetry, so the path of reaction will be disrotation. Again in photochemical condition HOMO of hexatriene is ψ_4 (first excited state), as (n – 1) is odd, it will have C_2-symmetry so reaction will occur in conrotatory manner. Orbital pictures (Fig. 1.17) of HOMO's, ψ_3 & ψ_4 of above two states are in complete agreement with this view.

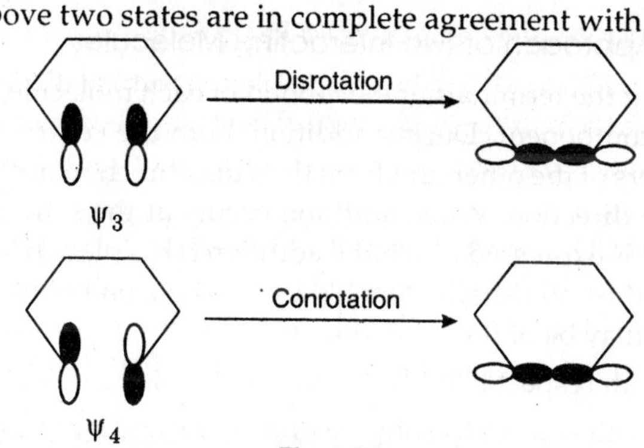

Fig. 1.17

1.13.4.6.8 Selection Rules for Electrocyclic Reactions

Woodward and Hoffmann proposed a set of selection rules for electrocyclic reactions as tabulated below:

No of π-electron	Mode of rotation	Condition	Remarks
4nπ electrons (n = 1, 2, 3 ... n)	Conrotation Disrotation	Thermal Photochemical	Allowed Allowed
(4n + 2) π electrons (n = o, 1, 2, 3 ... n)	Conrotation Disrotation	Photochemical Thermal	Allowed Allowed

1.13.4.6.9 Cycloaddition Reactions

It is a special type of pericyclic reaction in which two π-bonded compounds undergo reversible addition reaction with the formation of a cyclic compound. In such reaction addition takes place at the terminals of the π-bonds with the formation of two σ-bonds along with generation of a cyclic compound. The reverse reaction is the opening of the cyclic compound with the formation of two π-bonds is known as reverse cycloaddition (retrocyclo addition). Two most classical and extensively studied reactions of cycloaddition are:

i. Dimerisation of ethylene to cyclo butane and

ii. Diels Alder reaction.

1.13.4.6.10 Classification of Cycloaddition Reactions

Cycloaddition reactions have been classified with respect to two aspects (i) number of π-electron involved in each of the participating molecule. (ii) mode of approach of two π-bonded compounds during addition. When *m* number of π-electrons of one molecule and *n* number of π-electrons of other molecule are involved, the cycloaddition is expressed as:

$$\pi^m + \pi^n$$

and the reaction is called (m + n) cycloaddition reactions. The total number of π-electrons of both the molecules, (m + n), may be represented either by the general expression, 4qπ or by (4q + 2)π, where q may be 1, 2, ... or 0, 1, 2, ... n, consequently cycloaddition reactions have been grouped into two categories: (i) cyclo addition of 4qπ electron system and (ii) the second type is the cyclo-addition reactions of (4q + 2)π electron system.

1.13.4.6.11 Mode of Approach of Two Interacting Molecules

As addition takes place at the terminals of the π-bond of each molecule, the reaction must occur at two centres of each component. During addition, both the centres of one component may combine at the two centers of the other unit from the same direction or the combination may take place from the opposite direction. When addition occurs at the same direction it is known as suprafacial addition and is expressed as s, but if addition takes place from opposite direction it is termed as antarafacial addition usually denoted by, a. Thus, on the basis of mode of approach, cycloaddition reactions may be of the following types:

i. Suprafacial with respect to both the units expressed as (s-s)

ii. Antarafacial with respect to both the units indicated by (a-a) and

iii. Suprafacial with respect to one and antarafacial with respect to another represented by (s-a).

The above approach may be pictorically (Fig. 1.18) represented as:

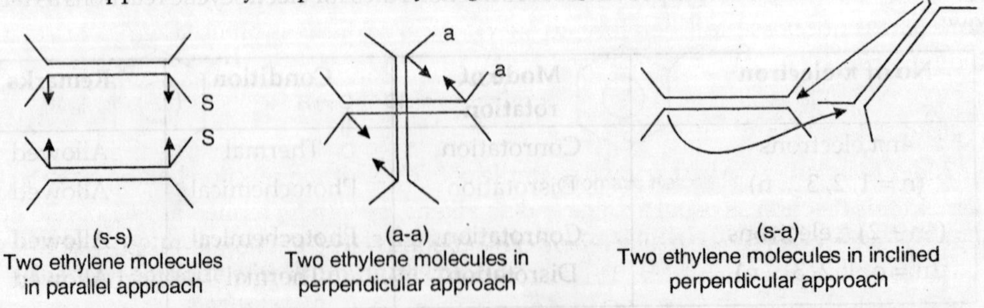

Fig. 1.18

From the above pictorial representation it is evident that in the case of (s-s) mode of combination parallel approach of two interacting units occurs, but in the case of (a-a) or (s-a) mode of combinations perpendicular approach of two units is observed.

Among these three modes of addition (a-a) is very rare and (s-s) approach is extremely common. Taking into account of both two aspects of classifications, cycloaddition reactions are generally expressed as:

$$\text{(i) } \pi_s^m + \pi_s^n; \quad \text{(ii) } \pi_s^m + \pi_a^n; \quad \text{(iii) } \pi_a^m + \pi_a^n$$

The most common and widely investigated cycloaddition is $\pi_5^4 + \pi_5^2$ category.

1.13.4.6.12 Explanation of $\pi_s^4 + \pi_s^2$ Cycloaddition in the Light of F.M.O.

Cycloaddition may precisely be interpreted in the light of F.M.O. approach. According to F.M.O. concept HOMO of one component and LUMO of another are involved in chemical reaction. In this particular reaction either HOMO of butadiene and LUMO of ethylenic component will interact each other or LUMO of butadiene and HOMO of alkene will participate. But as butadiene component is relatively more electron rich it will act as electron donor i.e., HOMO of diene system will preferably interact with the LUMO of alkene. Thus ψ_2, the HOMO of diene component under thermal condition will interact with ψ_2, the LUMO of alkene under the same condition. As the signs of lobes at 1, 4 positions of HOMO of diene component under thermal condition will interact with ψ_2, the LUMO of alkene under the same condition. As the signs of lobes at 1, 4 positions of HOMO of diene component match with the signs of lobes at 1, 2 positions of LUMO of alkene, the addition under thermal condition is a symmetry allowed process. Similar conclusion may be drawn by considering the LUMO of diene and HOMO of alkene.

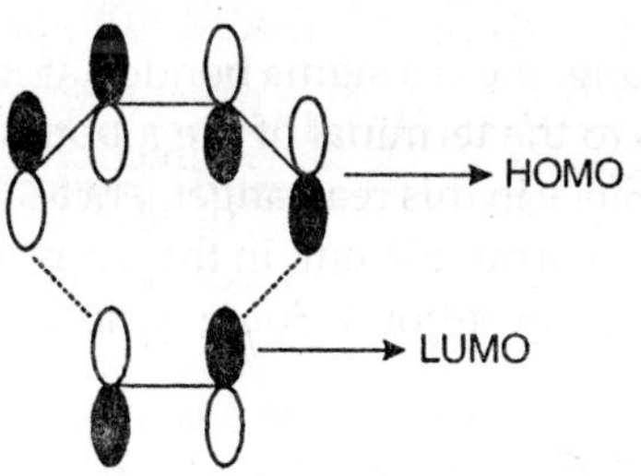

Fig. 1.19a

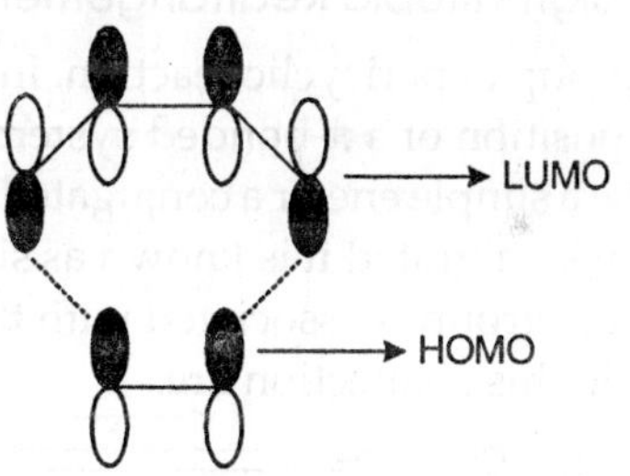

Fig. 1.19b

Again, in photo chemical condition HOMO of diene is ψ_3 and LUMO of alkene is ψ_2. These two orbitals will be the interacting entities. Inspection of orbital pictures clearly indicates that there is no matching of lobes of same sign in the both the directions and the formation of cyclohexene is not possible. Therefore, $\pi_s^4 + \pi_s^2$ cyclo addition is photo chemically a symmetry forbidden process.

1.13.4.6.13 Diels Alder Reaction

Diels Alder reaction is the best known example of cycloaddition reaction belonging to $\pi_s^4 + \pi_s^2$ system. In this reaction as usual a diene and an alkene, generally, termed as dienophile undergo addition reaction to form cyclohexene derivative and this reaction is of immence synthetic importance in organic chemistry. This reaction has several characteristic features all of which can precisely be explained by F.M.O. treatment.

1. Theoretically HOMO of either diene or dienophile may interact with LUMO of alkene or diene. But, in actual practice smooth reaction occurs if HOMO of diene & LUMO of alkene interacts, this is because in such situation energy difference between HOMO and LUMO is small and so overlapping of these two orbitals takes place smoothly.

2. It has been observed that the presence of electron releasing group in diene and electron withdrawing group in dienophile makes the reaction very facile. This is in conformity with the F.M.O. concept. The presence of electron releasing group in diene will increase the energy of HOMO while the presence of electron withdrawing substituent in dieneophile will decrease the energy of the LUMO. As a result energetically HOMO & LUMO will be closer and so overlapping of these two M.O's will be very facile.
3. In some cases Diels Alder reaction may takes place unhampered if electron releasing group is present in dienophile and electron withdrawing group is associated with diene. This situtation is termed as *reverse or inverse electron demand* in Diels-Alder reaction. According to F.M.O. treatment, presence of electron releasing group in dienophile will increase its electron density and hence it will behave as electron donor. So its HOMO not its LUMO will participate in the reaction. Similarly, presence of electron withdrawing group in diene will decrease its electron density and so it will act electron acceptor and hence its LUMO will be the active participant in this reaction because, in this particular situation, HOMO of dienophile & LUMO of diene are energetically closer.
4. It has been observed that in some cases Diels Alder reaction is catalysed by Lewis acid. This phenomenon is not contrary from F.M.O. view point. The Lewis acidic catalyst forms a complex with dienophile. As a result, the dienophile behaves as if it has an electron withdrawing group. So the energy of its LUMO will be lowered to some extent and hence, energetically it will be more closer to HOMO of diene. Therefore reaction will be favoured.

1.13.4.6.14 Sigmatropic Rearrangement

It is another group of pericyclic reaction. In this rearrangement a sigma bonded atom or a group at the allylic position of a π-bonded system migrates to the terminal of the π-bond. The π-bond system may be a simple ene or a conjugated polyene. Since in this rearrangement a sigma bonded group or atom is migrated it is known as sigmatropic rearrangement. In this rearrangement the migration of the group is associated with the shifting of the π-bond. Some typical examples that may be cited in this connection are:

i. $R{-}CH_2{-}CH{=}CH_2 \rightleftharpoons CH_2{=}CH{-}CH_2{-}R$

ii. 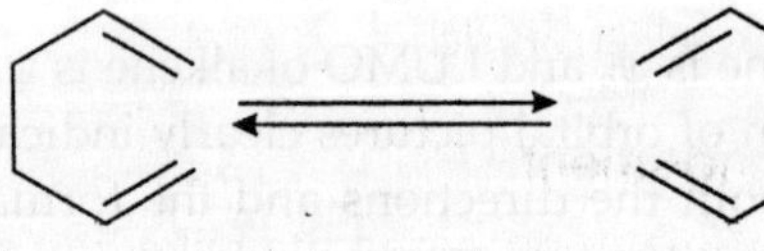

1.13.4.6.15 Classification of Sigmatropic Rearrangement

Classification of sigmatropic rearrangement is based on two aspects.

(a) Nature of migration
(b) Stereochemical course of the reaction.

(a) Nature of the migration means the range of transfer i.e., from what position the allylic group (the group at allylic position) migrates to what position of the π-bonded system. Normally, the σ-bonded group has two sides which are indicated by I, I and the position of π-framework to which the group is migrated is indicated as J. In some cases only one side may migrate to a particular position say j of the π-framework and other end may be connected to migrating group as in example (i) or the nature of the migrating group may be such (like H atom) that there is no question of migration of both ends. This type of migration is expressed as (I, j) shift sigmatropic rearrangement. In some cases both the sides of the migrating group may migrate to the different positions of the π-framework, one side may migrate to position, say, i, while other end may be connected to position, say, j of the π-framework. Such type of rearrangement is termed as (i, j) shift sigmatropic rearrangement as in example (ii) Actual classification of sigmatropic rearrangement is based on the summation of (I + j) or (i + j). The nature of the summation may be such that these rearrangements has been grouped into two categories.

i. (I + j) or (i + j) may be expressed as 4n system and
ii. (I + j) or, (i + j) may be represented as (4n + 2) system where, n = 1, 2, 3 ... etc. in-both the cases.

(b) *Stereochemical aspects:* As regards to stereochemical aspect, the σ-bonded migrating group may migrate from the same direction of the π-bonded terminal or it may migrate from the opposite direction of the π-bonded terminal. When migration occurs from the same direction it is termed as suprafacial while transfer of σ-bonded group from the opposite direction of π-bonded terminals is known as antarafacial rearrangement.

1.13.4.6.16 Interpretation of Sigmatropic Rearrangement

Although this rearrangements is intramolecular in nature yet no correlation diagram can be drawn because the starting compound. is not symmetrical, so the maintenance of symmetry through out the course of reaction does not arise. But the cyclic transition state that is involved has symmetry properties. Consequently, these rearrangements may be explained in terms of F.M.O. method based on the symmetry nature of HOMO of the reacting system. For these purpose it has been imagined that in the initial stage, the σ-bonded group undergoes homolytic cleavage with the formation of two radicals namely one σ-radical and other one is π-radical. It is these two radicals which ultimately interact to form a rearranged product.

It may be pointed out that as the reaction is concerted, the migrating group never becomes detached from the migration origin. So, the migrating group maintains the bonding character both at the origin and at the terminus. In order to maintain such bonding character at both the centers, HOMO of both the radicals (σ, π) must involve in the formation of the rearrangement product. However, out of two HOMO's, HOMO of π-radical system plays the most important role in predicting the course of the reaction as it is more electron rich.

1.13.4.6.17 Selection Rules of Sigmatropic Rearrangement

On the basis of the above argument Woodward & Hoffmann proposed the following selection rules for sigmatropic rearrangement.

i. For 4n system of sigmatropic rearrangement thermally allowed rearrangement is antara facial while photo chemically allowed rearrangement is suprafacial.
ii. For (4n + 2) system, just the reverse of the 4n system occurs. These two rules may be tabulated as:

System	Allowed	Forbidden
4n	i. Thermal (antara)	i. Thermal (supra)
	ii. Photochemical (supra)	ii. Photo (antara)
(4n + 2)	i. Thermal (supra)	i. Thermal (antara)
	ii. Photochemical (antara)	ii. Photo (antara)

1.13.4.6.18 [1, j]-Shift Sigmatropic Rearrangement

In this type of shift the most common migrating group is H atom. However in some cases other groups like alkyl, aryl, oxygen, nitrogen or sulphur containing group may act as migrating groups. The basic difference between the mode of migration of H atom and other group is that since H has only 1s-electron, it will always use (+) lobe for overlapping. On the other hand, the group having other atom has *p*-orbital and so can use either (+) or (–) sign lobe for overlapping. Therefore, in the case of H, simple suprafacial or antarafacial migration will occur but in the case of other groups along with suprafacial and antarafacial migration retention or inversion in configuration of the migrating group will be associated. It has been observed that if the migration is supra facial with respect to allylic radical as well as migrating group, configuration is retained but when the migration is antarafacial with respect to both, inversion in configuration occurs. The most common (1, j)-shifts that are frequently observed belong to [1, 3].

i. **[1, 3]-shift:** The frequently encountered example of 1, 3-shift is the allylic rearrangement.

$$R—CH_2—CH=CH_2 \rightleftharpoons CH_2=CH—CH_2—R$$

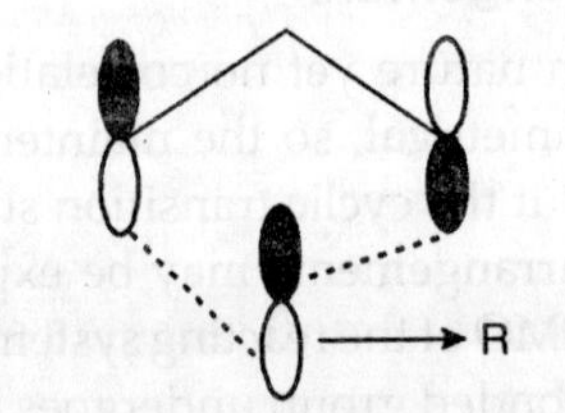

Fig. 1.20a

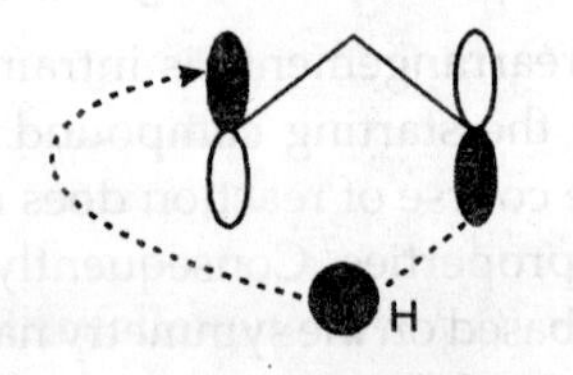

Fig. 1.20b

The HOMO of allylic radical under thermal condition, is ψ_2. From the orbital picture (Fig. 1.20a) it is seen that it has C_2 symmetry. So in *antara* facial migration inversion in configuration of the migrating group will occur. But if R=H, it will use (+) lobe and so bonding interaction is only possible if antara facial migration (Fig. 1.20b) takes place but such antara facial shift for H is geometrically impossible which arises from the fact that a rigid three carbon atom chain is too short to allow H atom to transfer from top to bottom. That is why [1, 3] H-shift under thermal condition is extremly rare. For this reason the triene (A) does not isomerise to toluene (B) under thermal condition.

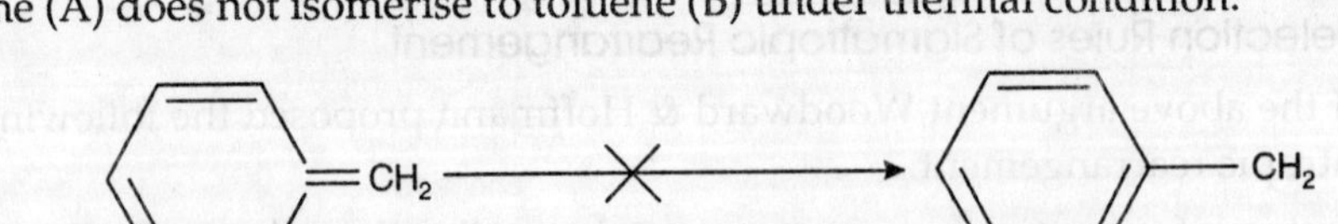

(A) (B)

But photo chemical migration is possible because under this condition HOMO is ψ_3 which has m-symmetry and hence suprafacial migration can occur.

1.13.4.6.19 [i, J]-Shift Sigmatropic Rearrangement

Cope rearrangements is the most common and highly illustrated example of [i, J] shift sigmatropic rearrangement.

Cope rearrangement: It is [3, 3] shift sigmatropic rearrangement. It involves six Carbon atoms with two double bonds forming two separate allylic systems as indicated.

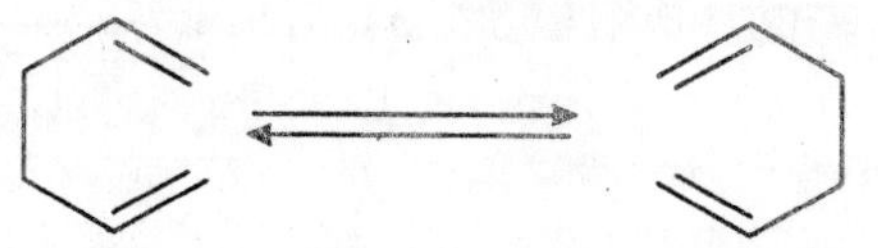

Explanation: Since in this rearrangement six carbon atoms are involved, it has been assumed that cyclic transition state of this rearrangement bears a close similarity with cyclohexane. Hence this transition state may exist either in chair form or in boat form of conformation as shown below (Fig. 1.21).

Out of these two forms of transition states, chair form is preferable as it is stabler than the boat form. The experimental evidence has also been obtained in favour of chair conformation.

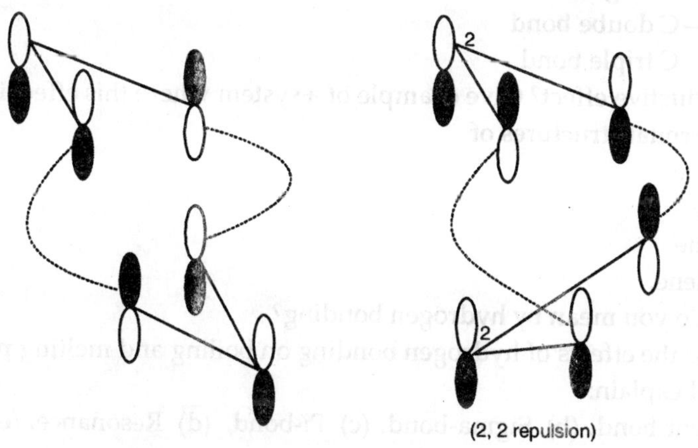

Fig. 1.21

Model Questions

1. Describe homolytic and heterolytic fission of a covalent bond. How carbonium ions, carbanions and free radicals are formed?
2. (a) Write note on inductive effect.
   (b) What is the difference between inductive and mesomeric effect?
3. Write notes on
   (a) Carbonium ions
   (b) Carbanions
   (c) Free radicals
   (d) Electromeric effect.
4. (a) What are electrophiles?
   (b) What are nucleophiles?
5. (a) What are different types of organic reactions?
   (b) What is the essential difference between a free radical reaction and an ionic reaction?
6. (a) What are carbocations? Describe their characteristics, stability and structures.
   (b) What are carbanions? Discuss their formation, stability and structures.

7. Wrire notes on
   (a) Bond dissociation energy
   (b) Hydrogen bond
   (c) Resonance
   (d) Dipole moment
   (e) Electronegativity
   (f) Inductive effect.
8. (a) How will you establish that carbon is tetravalent?
   (b) How the equivalency of all the four valencies of carbon has been explained?
   (c) Draw the orbital picture of
      (i) C–C single bond
      (ii) C–C doube bond
      (iii) C–C triple bond.
9. What is inductive effect? Give example of a system where this effect is operative?
10. Draw the orbital structures of
    (a) Methane
    (b) Ethane
    (c) Ethylene
    (d) Acetylene.
11. (a) What do you mean by hydrogen bonding?
    (b) Discuss the effects of hydrogen bonding on boiling and melting points.
12. Define and explain:
    (a) Covalent bond, (b) Sigma-bond, (c) Pi-bond, (d) Resonance, (e) sp^3-, sp^2 - and *sp*-orbitals.
13. Give the bond length, and bond angles in
    (a) ethylene and, (b) acetylene.
14. Write notes on
    (a) Nucleophilic substitution reaction
    (b) Elimination reaction
    (c) Addition reaction.
15. (a) Comment on the hybridisation state and geometry of carbanions
    (b) Arrange the following carbocations in order of increasing stability and give reason thereof:

$$CH_3-\overset{+}{C}H-CH_3,\ CH_2{=}CH-\overset{+}{C}H_2,\ CH_3-CH_2-\overset{+}{C}H_2,$$

    (c) Name the fragments in the homolytic and heterolytic cleavage in ethane C–C bond.
    (d) Define the terms inductive effect and electromeric effect.
    (f) Indicate the state of hybridisation of reactive carbon of carbocation, carbanion and free-radical.
16. What do you mean by pericyclic reactions? What is its central theme? How it differs from S_{N^2} and E_2 reactions.
17. Write notes one
    (a) Different approaches for the unterpretation of pericyclic reaction.
    (b) Electrocyclic reaction
    (c) Cycloaddition reaction
    (d) Sigmatropic rearrangement.

CHAPTER TWO

Classification and Nomenclature of Organic Compounds

2.1 Classification

Carbon atom has a unique character of forming covalent bond with elements like H, N, O, halogens, S, etc. Similarly, it can form bonds with other carbon atoms as well without any limit. Again, carbon atom during combination with other carbon atoms as well as with other atoms can form single, double or triple bonds involving different types of hybridisations. Due to this unusual and distinctive characteristic carbon atom forms a vast number of organic compounds of varied nature. The study of individual species of this class of innumerable compounds is practically impossible. In order to systematise the study of organic compounds, this group of vast number has been primarily classified into two categories, viz.

i. *Open chain compounds*: These compounds are usually known as aliphatic or fatty compounds. They are also known as acyclic compounds. Earlier, compounds of this category were obtained from fats and hence the name *"aliphatic"*. In this class of compounds the open chain may be *straight (normal)* and *branched* in nature. Thus,

$$CH_3-CH_2-CH_2-CH_2-CH_3$$

Pentane

Straight chain or normal

$$CH_3-CH_2-\underset{\displaystyle CH_3}{\underset{|}{CH}}-CH_3$$

Isopentane
(Branched)

ii. *Cyclic compounds*: Carbon compounds with closed chains are termed as cyclic compounds. Cyclic compounds have been found to be of two types—(i) homocyclic containing same atoms generally carbon atoms and (ii) heterocyclic compounds containing other atoms such as N, O, S beside carbon atom in the ring formation. Again, cyclic compounds both homo - and heterocyclic have been found to form a special class of compounds which contain single and double bond at alternate positions. This special class of cyclic compounds are known as *aromatic* compounds.

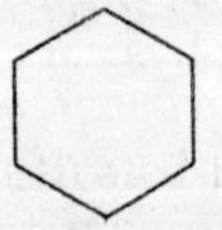

Cyclohexane
(Homocyclic)

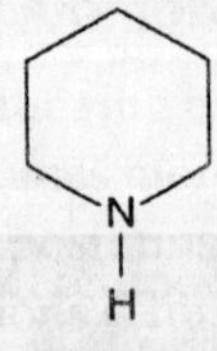

Piperidine
(Heterocyclic)

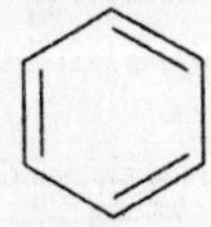

Benzene

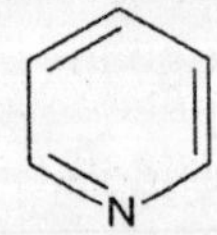

Pyridine

Aromatic

Once again, in order to study the organic compounds in a more systematic and useful manner, each of these categories of compounds has been divided into different classes on the basis of type of *functional groups* present in the compounds. A *functional group* is the chemically reactive part of the molecule and an organic compound owes to it the characteristic chemical properties. So the functional group may be defined as the atom or a group of atoms which determines the class structure as well as chemical characteristics of a particular family of organic compounds. Thus carbonyl group (>C=O) is the functional group of a family of compounds known as carbonyl compounds. Similarly, carboxylic group (— COOH) is the functional group of carboxylic compounds. Some of the most common functional groups and the corresponding classes of compounds are enlisted below:

Functional group	**Names of class of compounds**
Hydroxyl (— OH)	Hydroxy compounds, alcohols, phenols
Carbonyl ($>C=O$)	Carbonyl compounds, (aldehydes, ketones)
Carboxyl (— COOH)	Carboxylic acids
Ether (— O —)	Ethers
Ester (— COOR)	Esters
Amino (— NH_2)	Amines
Amido (— $CONH_2$)	Amides
Nitro (— NO_2)	Nitro compounds

In addition to above functional groups there are a series of important and very common univalent groups. These groups are formed by the removal of the hydrogen atom from hydrocarbon (compounds containing only carbon and hydrogen atoms). These groups are known as *alkyl or aryl groups*. The name of each individual group is obtained by changing the suffix 'ane' of corresponding hydrocarbon by -yl. Thus,

Hydrocarbon	**Alkyl**
Methane (CH_4)	Methyl (CH_3 —)
Ethane (C_2H_6)	Ethyl (C_2H_5 —)
n-Propane ($CH_3 — CH_2 — CH_3$)	*n*-porpyl ($CH_3 — CH_2 — CH_2$ —)
Benzene (C_6H_6)	Aryl or phenyl (C_6H_5 —)

In this connection it is necessary to mention the name of a series called *homologous series*. it is a series of compounds of the same family in which any two consecutive members differ only by a methylene (CH_2) group. Thus methane (CH_4), ethane ($CH_3 — CH_3$), *n*-propane ($CH_3 — CH_2 — CH_3$), *n*-butane ($CH_3 — CH_2 — CH_2 — CH_3$) belong to a homologous series because each member of this series differ from its immediate member by CH_2. Each individual member is in general known as homologue. Members of homologous series have similar chemical properties which mainly originate from the functional group but they differ in physical properties.

2.2 Nomenclature of Organic Compounds

There are several methods for naming organic compounds of which following two are most important.

2.2.1 Trivial Name

In this system name of the compound is derived from the source from which the compound has been first obtained or from the characteristic property of the compound. Thus, formic acid was first obtained from *formica,* the latin name of red ants, and name of glucose was derived from Greek word 'glukos' meaning sweet. This trivial name is also known as *common name.* Trivial or common names of a few compounds are tabulated below:

Formula	Name
CH_4	Methane
CH_3-CH_3	Ethane
$CH_3-CH_2-CH_3$	Propane
$CH_3-(CH_2)_2-CH_3$	Butane
$CH_3-(CH_2)_3-CH_3$	Pentane
$CH_3-(CH_2)_4-CH_3$	Hexane
$CH_2=CH_2$	Ethylene
$CH_3-CH=CH_2$	Propylene
$CH_3-CH_2-CH=CH_2$	Butylene
CH_3-OH	Methyl alcohol
CH_3-CH_2-OH	Ethyl alcohol
$CH_3-CH_2-CH_2-OH$	Propyl alcohol
$HC\equiv CH$	Acetylene
CH_3-Cl	Methyl chloride
$CH_3-CH_2-O-CH_2-CH_3$	Diethyl ether
$HCHO$	Formaldehyde
CH_3-CHO	Acetaldehyde
$CH_3-\underset{\underset{O}{\Vert}}{C}-CH_3$	Acetone
$H-COOH$	Formic acid
CH_3-COOH	Acetic acid
$H-\underset{\underset{O}{\Vert}}{C}-NH_2$	Formamide
$CH_3-\underset{\underset{O}{\Vert}}{C}-NH_2$	Acetamide

CH_3-NH_2	Methylamine
$CH_3-CH_2-NH_2$	Ethylamine
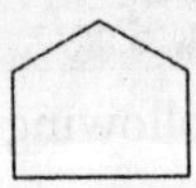	Cyclopentane
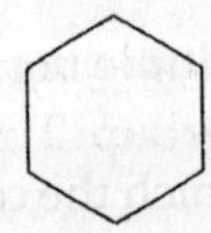	Cyclohexane
CH_3COOCH_3	Methyl acetate
$CH_3COOC_2H_5$	Ethyl acetate

2.2.2 Systematic Naming of Organic Compounds

The magnitude of numbers of organic compounds is so vast that it is not possible to remember the common names of all the organic compounds. So it was felt that a systematic nomenclature of organic compounds is urgently essential. The system proposed by *International Union of Pure and Applied Chemistry* abbreviated as IUPAC is that desired method of systematically naming the organic compounds. In IUPAC system of nomenclature, organic compounds are named as derivatives of open chain normal hydrocarbons. There are certain rules for guiding the naming of organic compounds. These rules may be enunciated as below:

1. In the first step the longest possible chain of carbon atoms containing the main functional group and also as many as carbon -carbon multiple bonds is chosen. The name of this longest chain is derived from the name of the corresponding hydrocarbon. Thus,

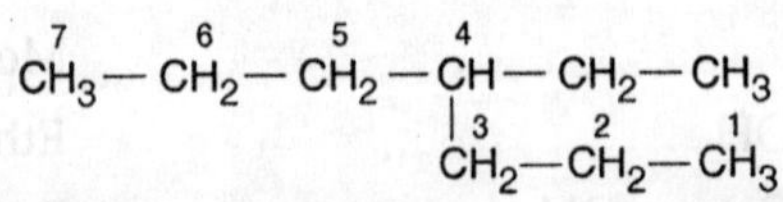

contains seven carbon atoms in longest chain and this hydrocarbon is named as the derivative of heptane.

2. (a) The location of the substituents is indicated by number.

   (b) During numbering, the carbon chain is numbered from that end which is nearest to the substituent.

   (c) If the same substituents occur more than once, prefixes di, tri, tetra, etc. are used. For example,

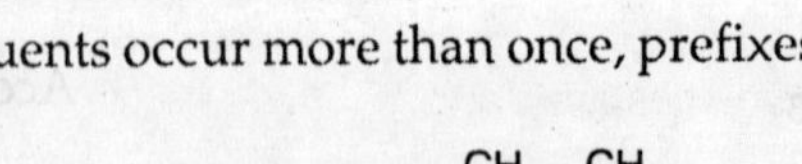

2, 3-dimethyl hexane

   (d) But if two or more substituents located are different the lower number is assigned to that group which is alphabetically first, i.e.,

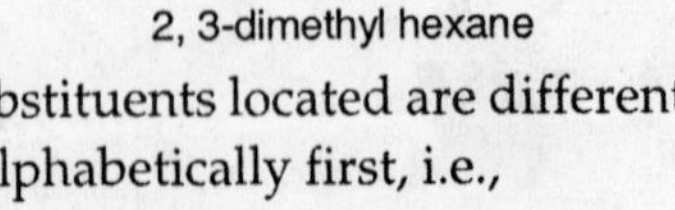

2-Ethyl-4-methyl pentane

(e) During naming the compounds, the substituents are placed in alphabetical order. For example,

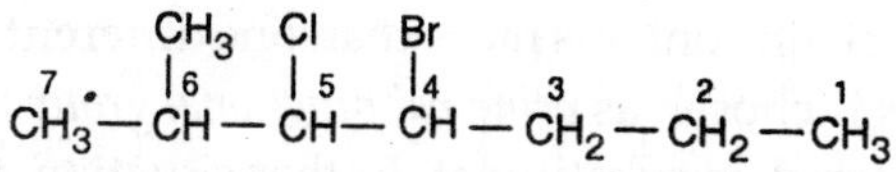

4-Bromo-5-chloro-6-methyl heptane

3. (a) When a compound contains a functional group including multiple bonds and other substituents, the lowest number is assigned to the functional group. Thus,

(i) 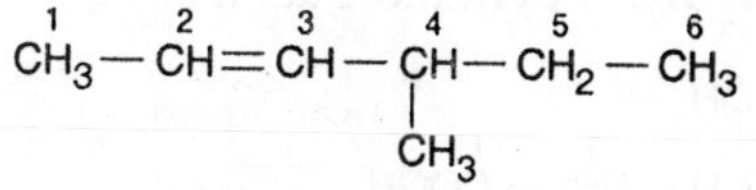

4-Methyl-pent-2-ene

(ii) 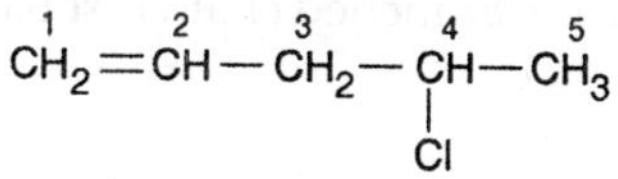

4-chloro-pent-I-ene

In this connection it must be remembered that in the case of compound having only one functional group, the name of the compound is obtained by adding a *suffix* to the name of hydrocarbon of longest possible chain replacing 'e' of - 'ane'. Suffixes of common functional groups are tabulated below:

Functional group	Suffix
Alcohol (– OH)	– ol
Carbonyl (>C=O)	– one
Aldehyde (H>C=O)	– al
Carboxylic (– COOH)	– oic
Esters (– COOR)	– oate
Alkene (>C=C<)	– ene
Alkyne (—C≡C—)	– yne

For example, 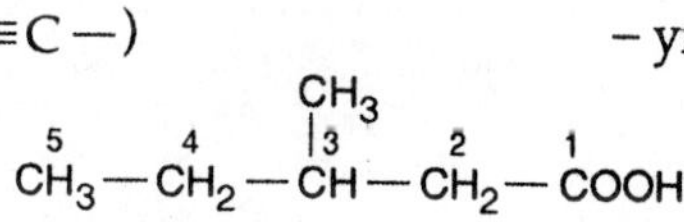

3-Methyl pentanoic acid

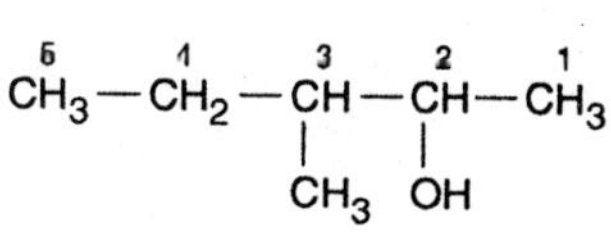

3-Methyl-pentan-2-ol

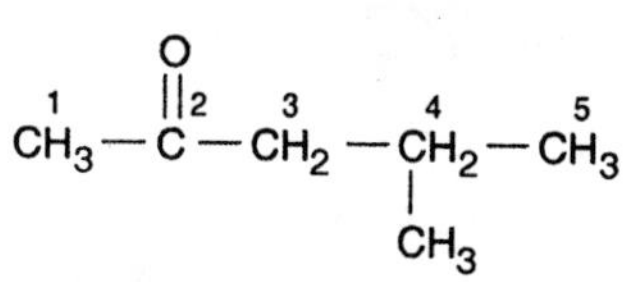

4-Methyl-pentan-2-one

In the case of compound containing aldehyde, and carboxylic groups, the numbering of the parent chain starts from the carbon atom of those functional groups.

(b) When the longest chain contains more than one different functional groups, one of the functional groups is chosen as *principal functional group* and the remaining functional groups are considered as substituent. In that situation, the priority of the functional groups is of the following order:

carboxylic acid> ester > aldehyde > ketone > alcohol > – ene > – yne.

An example cited in this connection is 3-hydroxy pentanoic acid.

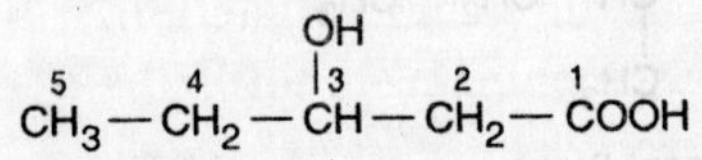

If the branched-chain contains functional groups, the branched chain is separately numbered. Thus,

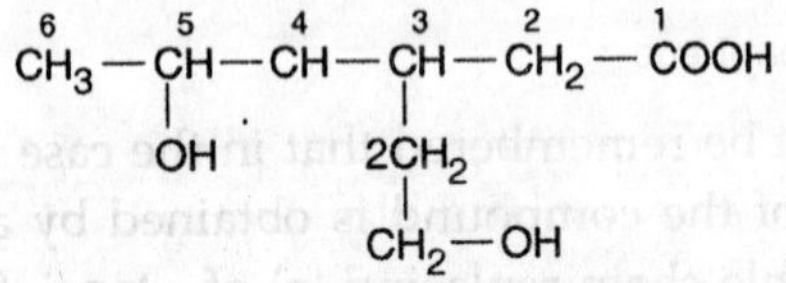

5-Hydroxy-3-(1-hydroxy ethyl)-hexanoic acid

Model Questions

1. Write IUPAC names of the following:

(a) HC≡C–CH$_2$–CH=CH$_2$

(b) 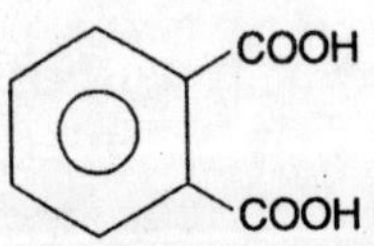

(c) 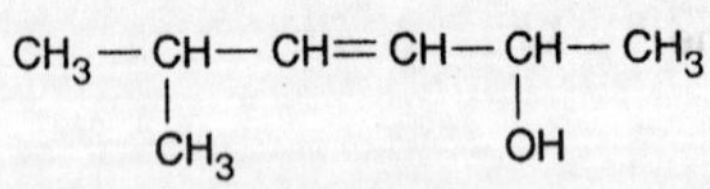

(d) 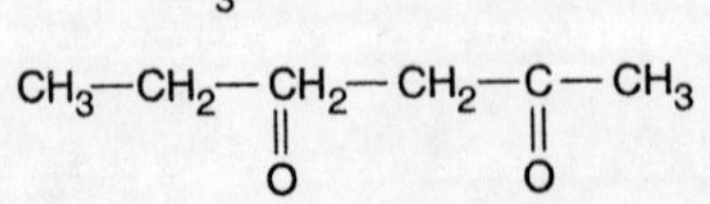

(e) 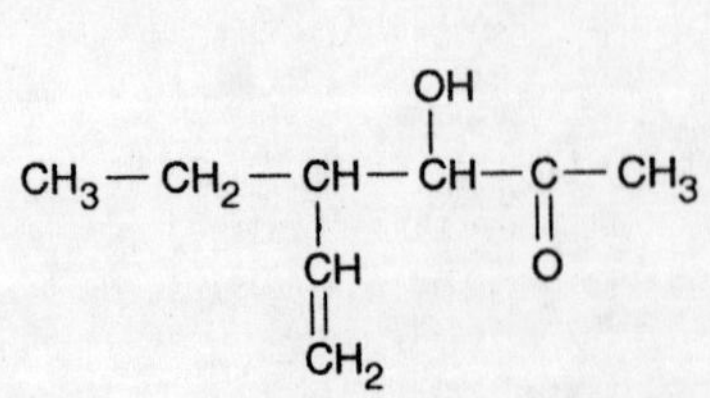

(f) 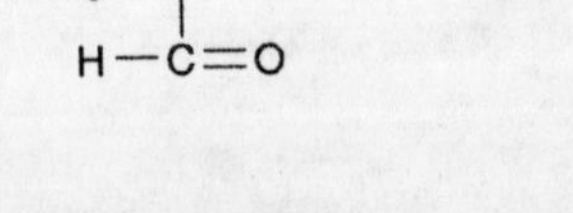

(g) 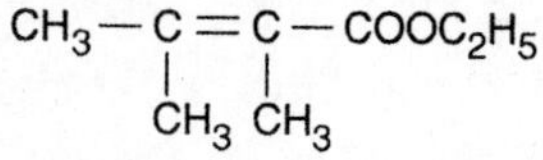

(h) 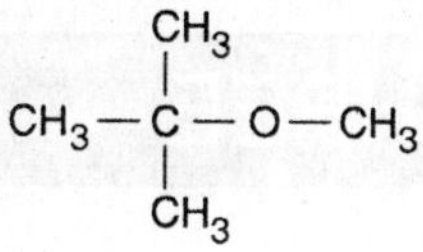

(i) $(CH_3)_2—CH—CH_3—CH_3—COCl$

(j) $CH_2{=}CH—CH_2—CH_2—CONH_2$

2. Write structural formulae of the following:
   (a) 2-Ethyl-but-1-ene
   (b) 2-Ethoxy chloroethane
   (c) 2, 4-Dimethyl-3-ethyl hexane-2-ol
   (d) 2-chloro-5-methyl hexanal
   (e) 2,2, 4-Trimethylheptane
   (f) 1, 5–Heptadiene
3. (a) What do you understand by the term functional group? Name the five important functional groups.
   (b) Write notes on homologous series.

CHAPTER THREE

Stereoisomerism

3.1 Introduction

Carbon compounds are covalently bonded and it is known that covalent bond is directional in nature. This means each group or atom connected by covalent bond must have specific direction obviously in space. So the different groups attached to covalent bond in a particular structure may be arranged in several ways in its three dimensional structure (space) giving rise to a class of isomers known as *stereoisomers* and the phenomenon is termed as *stereoisomerism*. In other words, stereoisomerism is exhibited by compounds having the same structure but differing in molecular configuration, called stereoisomers, and the phenomenon is known as *stereoisomerism*. The molecular configuration means the three dimensional arrangement of atoms and groups (i.e., spatial arrangement) in a molecule. The difference in molecular configurations, i.e., three dimensional arrangements of groups and atoms may originate mainly due to three specific causes, viz., restricted rotation around a bond, difference in light absorption propety of different stereoisomers and rotation around a σ-bond. Consequently stereoisomerism has been classified into three categoires:

(a) Geometrical isomerism

(b) Optical isomerism

(c) Conformation.

3.2 Geometrical Isomerism

Geometrical isomerism arises from the restricted rotation around a double bond in acylic compounds and a single bond in cyclic compounds.

According to *Molecular Orbital theory* each carbon atom of the double bond has three sp^2 hybridised orbitals and the remaining one is *p*-orbital. The σ-bond between the two carbon atoms is formed by the overlap of sp^2 hybrid orbitals, and the π-bomd is formed by the overlap of *p*-orbitals in parallel direction. Such overlap of *p*-orbitals requires the existence of both the carbon atoms involved in π-bond formation in the same plane. In order to maintain such planarity, rotation around the σ-bond must be restricted or in other words, the presence of π-bond locks the molecule at a particular position. So the two carbon atoms of the double bond and the four groups, two in each carbon lie in the same plane and their positions are fixed in space. As a result, geometrical isomerism originates. This type of isomerism takes place in such type of compounds in which each of the doubly bonded carbon atom is attached to two different atoms or groups, and different geometrical isomers arise due to difference in the relative spatial arrangements of groups around C=C bond.

In cyclic compounds rotation about C—C single bond forming a ring is restricted because rotation would prevent the formation of the ring. However, for exhibiting geometrical isomerism, there must be at least two substituents on two differtent ring carbon atoms.

Groups around the bond with restricted rotation, either double bond or single bond in certain cyclic compounds, can be arranged spatially to give two types of isomers—one isomer in which two similar groups are on the same side of the bond (double bond or single bond in cyclic compound) is known as *cis*-isomer, while in other isomer, two similar groups exist in opposite direction and is called *trans*-isomer. For this reason geometrical isomerism is also known as *cis-trans* isomerism. Geometrical isomerism is also exhibited by compounds having C = N, N = N bonds.

Geometrical isomers have different physical and chemical properties. It has been observed that *trans*-isomers are more stable than *cis*-isomers. This is due to the less steric repulsion of groups in *trans*-isomer than in *cis*-isomer. Since *cis*-isomer is less stable it can be converted to trans-isomer. Thus maleic acid can be easily converted into fumaric acid by simple heating.

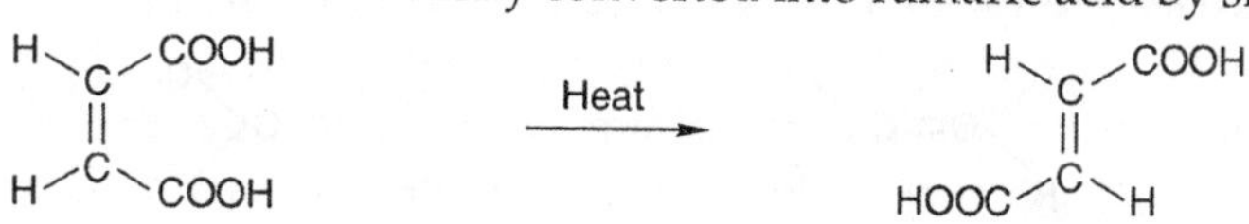

Maleic acid (*cis*-isomer) Fumaric acid (*trans*-isomer)

The configuration of geometrical isomer can be determined by some standard methods. One group of methods is based on some physical properties. It has been observed that *cis*-isomer has greater dipole moment, higher boiling point and lower melting point compared to *trans*-isomer. So determination of these physical properties settles the configuration of the isomer. In suitable cases from the formation of cyclic compounds, configuration of the isomer may be determined. Thus, maleic acid readily forms anhydride at 150 °C while fumaric acid fails to form anhydride at such temperature.

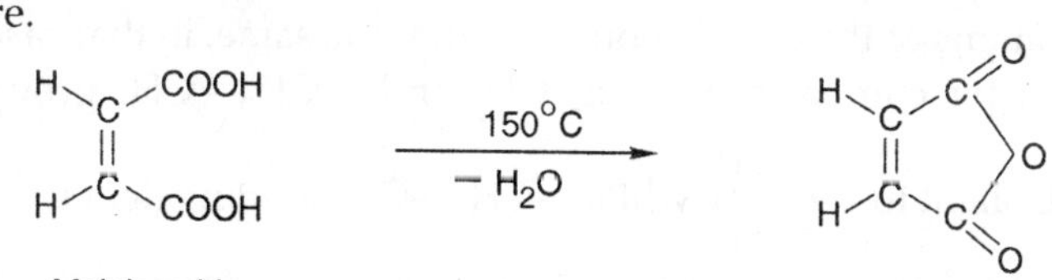

Maleic acid Anhydride

Sometimes spectroscopic measurements like IR and NMR are used to distinguish between cis and *trans*-isomers.

PROBLEM 3.1

How maleic and fumaric acids can be distinguished?

3.2.1 E and Z System of Nomenclature

The *cis* and *trans* designation of the isomers can successfully be used for compounds in which two carbon atoms of the double bond have similar groups or atoms. But when there are different atoms or groups attached to carbon atoms of the double bond it is very difficult to assign *cis* or *trans configuration*. Let us consider an arbitrary compound in which different groups are attached to two carbon atoms of the double bond:

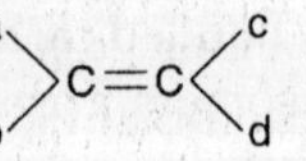

In this configuration existence of similar groups in the same or opposite direction does not arise and designation of isomers as *cis* and *trans* is not possible. To overcome this difficulty, a more general system for designating the configuration of geometric isomers has been adopted. This system has been developed by Cahn, Ingold and Prelog and is known as E (from German word *entgegen* meaning across or opposite) and Z (derived from German word *zusammen* meaning together) system. This system is based on the priority of the attached group. The atoms and groups connected to each carbon atom of the double bond are assigned first and second priority. Priority of groups on each carbon atom of the double bond is compared with each other. If the higher priority atoms or groups are on the same direction of the double bond the configuration is designated as Z and if the atoms or groups of higher priority are on the opposite side of the double bond the configuration is termed as E.

The priorities of atoms or groups are determined on the basis of atomic numbers or atomic weights of the atoms directly connected to carbon atoms of the double bond. Higher priority is given to atoms of higher atomic number. Thus in the halogen series, order of priority is I>Br>Cl>F. Thus (a) is Z- and (b) is E-isomer,

(a) Z-isomer (b) E-isomer

When a doubly or triply bonded atom is present it is regarded as equivalent to two or three such atoms. $-C{\equiv}C-$ group is considered as if carbon has three single bonds to carbon. Thus,

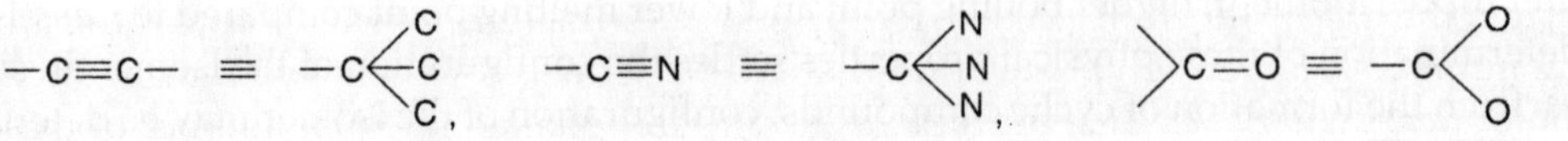

If the priorities of any two groups calculated on the basis of atomic number of atoms directly connected to carbon atoms of the double bond becomes the same, in that case next atoms in the group are considered for comparison. Thus, CH_3 and —CH_2—CH_3 groups. Here —CH_3 is considered to be equivalent to $-C\begin{matrix}H\\-H\\H\end{matrix}$, while —$CH_2$—$CH_3$ is equivalent to $-C\begin{matrix}H\\-C\\H\end{matrix}$. So the sum of atomic numbers of three H atoms and C atom (3 + 6) is 9 for methyl while for —CH_2—CH_3 the sum of atomic numbers is 2 + 6 + 6 = 14. Thus, ethyl group gets priority over methyl.

3.3 Optical Isomerism

Optical isomerism arises from the optical activity of chemical compounds. It has been observed that when chemical compounds placed in the beam of polarised light, can rotate the plane of polarised light either to left or to right. Such compounds are called optically active and those compounds which cannot rotate the plane of polarised light are optically inactive.

The optically active compound which rotates the plane of polarised light to right is said to be *Dextrorotatory* and is indicated by (+) sign. The compound which rotates the plane of polarised light to the left is designated as *Laevorotatory*, expressed by (–) sign. Originally these optical isomers were indicated by the prefix d for dextro and l for laevorotatory. Thus compounds having the same molecular formula which rotate the plane of polarised light in different directions—right or left—are called *Optical Isomers* and the phenomenon is known as *Optical Isomerism*.

It may be mentioned in this connection that light is an electromagnetic radiation and is a wave phenomenon. It consists of two component forces, electrical and magnetic, which acting perpendicular to each other propagates through vibration. At any point of propagation these two component forces are acting in all possible directions. Hence the picture of ordinary light may be indicated as shown in Fig. 3.1. When it is passed through a Nicol prism (made of calcite, $CaCO_3$), placed in a polarimeter all the electrical components vibrate within one plane, while all the magnetic components vibrate in other plane. Thus the two components of light are allowed to propagate in two different planes perpendicular to each other. Such light is known as *polarised light* and the plane through which this polarised light popagates is known as *plane of polarised light*. Polarised light has been found to be circular in character and its plane of polarisation is continuously rotating across the plane of propagation. Another characteristic of circularly polarised light is that each of the components, electrical and magnetic, made up of two parts—one is right circularly polarised part and the other is left circularly polarised part. At ordinary condition of polarised light, i.e., in absence of any medium each of these components propagates in the resultant directions. The two resultants, one for electrical components and the other for magnetic components are mutually perpendicular to each other. It has been assumed that when such polarised light is passed through a solution of a compound it is the electrical component of the polarised light primarily interacts with the molecule since molecule may be looked upon as an assembly of electrons. So the left and right circularly polarised electrical components polarise the total number of molecules present in a gram mole of the compound. This is a case of random polarisation. As a result of such random polarisation, the total number of molecules (N_0, Avogadro number) is polarised into two sets—one due to right and the other due to left circularly polarised electrical components. If both the sets contain equal number of molecules, plane of resultant of electrical component will remain unchanged. So no optical activity will be observed. But if the sets contain unequal number of molecules, plane of resultant changes causing development of net rotation and so optical activity originates. Thus it may be concluded that the *optical activity or inactivity is not the property of individual molecule, rather it is due to average of random polarisation*.

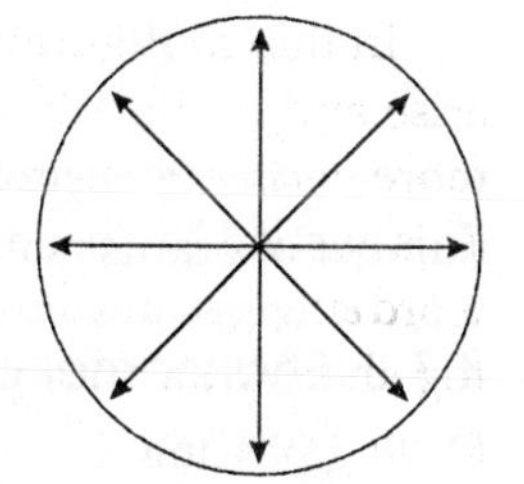

Ordinary light

Fig. 3.1

3.3.1 Optical Rotation and Its Measurement

The instrument by which the optical rotation is measured is called *Polarimeter*. It consists of a light source, two nicol prisms, a sample tube in between nicol prisms. Schematic representation of a polarimeter is as given below in Fig. 3.2:

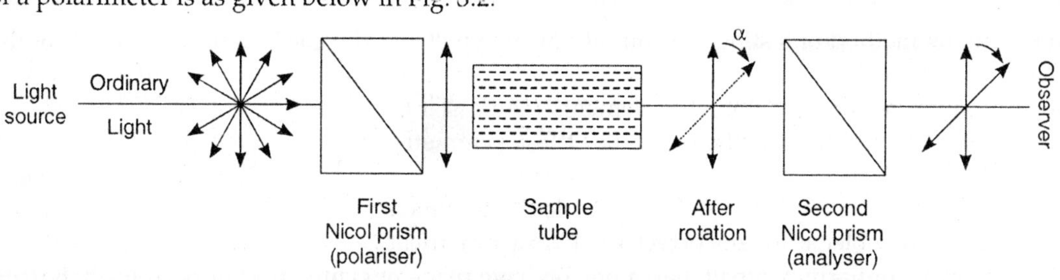

Fig. 3.2

3.3.2 Specific Rotation

Specific rotation is defined as the angle of rotation of plane polarised light produced by a solution of length 10 centimetres and unit of concentration (g/ml) for the given wavelength of light at a given temperature. It also depends upon the nature of the solvent used. It is expressed as $[\alpha]_D^t$ and is a constant quantity, characteristic of a particular substance. It is given by the expression,

$$[\alpha]_D^t = \frac{100 \times \alpha}{l \times C},$$

where α is the observed rotation in degrees, l is the length of the tube in decimetres, C is the number of grams per 100 ml of the solution and D is the sodium D-line and t is the temperature.

3.3.3 Enantiomer and Enantiomerism

During passing through polarised light it has been observed that the total number of molecules are polarised into two sets. Again, both the sets contain the same molecules; hence one set may be regarded as the image of other set. When both the sets contain different number of molecules, then one set (say object) is not superimposable with its image, i.e., the other set. In such a situation, rotation of plane polarised light occurs and the substance is said to be optically active. These stereoisomers, which are non-superimposable with each other, are known as *enantiomers*, and the phenomenon is referred to as *enantiomerism*.

Enantiomers are also called optical isomers or optical antipode. Enantiomerism or non-superimposibility of mirror images arises due to *chiral* or *dissymmetric* nature of the molecule. A molecule is said to be chiral if it has no plane of symmetry and is non-superimposable on its mirror image as is seen in the in Fig. 3.3.

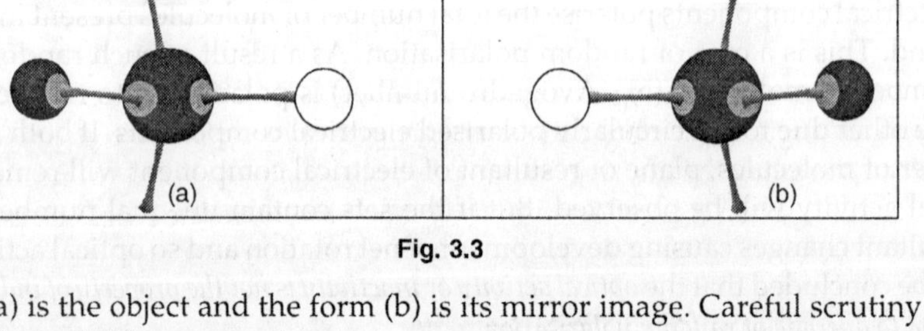

Fig. 3.3

The form (a) is the object and the form (b) is its mirror image. Careful scrutiny reveals that the two forms (a) and (b) are enantiomer to each other and are optically active. It is, therefore, concluded that the *chirality* is the fundamental and essential requirement for enantiomerism or optical isomerism. Our hands, shoes, socks, etc. are dissymmetric or chiral objects, while ball is a symmetric object.

3.3.4 Symmetry Elements

The ultimate method of testing the chirality or dissymetry is the construction of models of the object and its mirror image, and determination of their non-superimposability. However, determination of certain symmetry elements may assist in recognising dissymmetry in the molecule. These symmetry elements are:

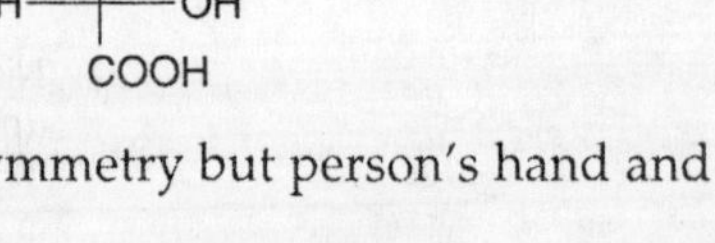

i. *Plane of Symmetry*: It is defined as the plane which divides a molecule or any object into two symmetrical halves. Similarly, football, hat, a person have plane of symmetry but person's hand and gloves do not have plane of symmetry. It has been observed that a molecule or an object which does not contain any plane of symmetry is usually chiral or dissymmetric.

ii. *Centre of Symmetry*: A centre of symmetry is a point in the centre of a molecule or an object such that any straight line drawn through this point encounters identical parts of the object or molecule on either side of the centre. This element of symmetry is usually present in ring system.

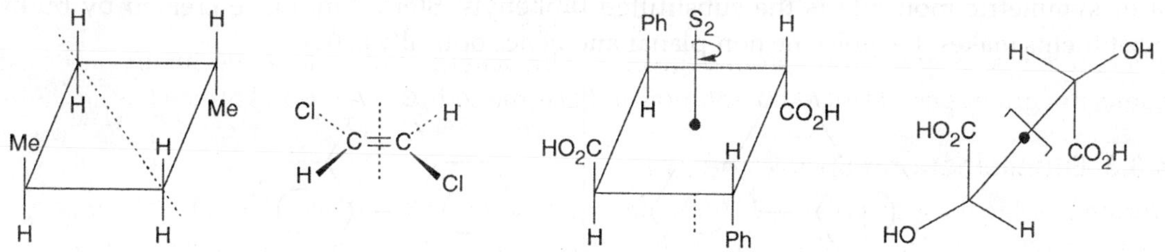

iii. *Alternating Axis of Symmetry*: This symmetry element is to some extent rare. A molecule is said to have *n*-fold axis of symmetry only when it is rotated through an angle of $360°/n$ about this axis (alternating axis) followed by reflection in a plane perpendicular to the axis, generates the orginal molecule.

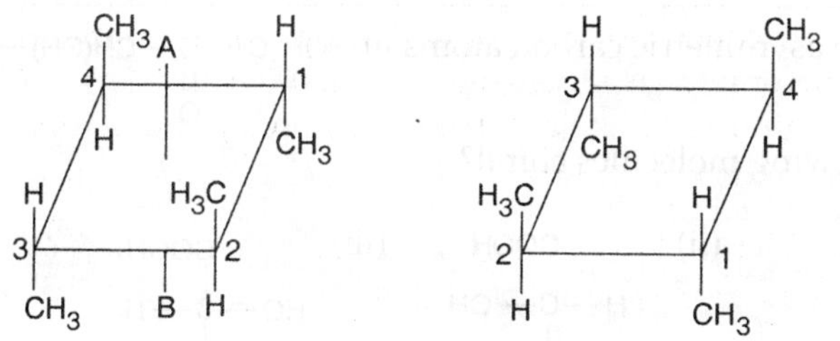

(a) (b)

Thus the above molecule (a) has four-fold axis of symmetry. This is because when form (a) is rotated through an angle of 90° about the axis AB passing through the centre of the ring and is perpendicular to the plane of the ring, the form (b) is obtained. Form (a) becomes the mirror image of the form (b) when it is reflected in the plane parallel to the ring, i.e., perpendicular to the axis AB.

3.3.5 Essential Condition for Optical Activity

Absence of all the elements of symmetry makes a molecule or an object completely non-symmetrical which is usually termed as asymmetry. Asymmetric object will definitely have non-superimposable image and hence will show optical activity. For this reason compounds containing asymmetric carbon (carbon atom having four different groups directly attached to it) exhibit optical activity. But sometimes there are deviations. For example, in tartaric acid different groups may be so arranged that an isomeric form known as mesoform may be developed. This form of tartaric acid has two asymmetric carbon, yet it fails to exhibit any optical activity because it has a plane of symmetry.

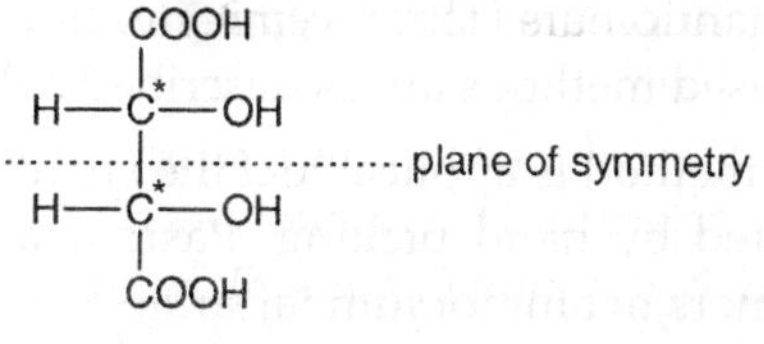

Again, an allene derivative,

$$R-CH=C=CH-R$$

has no asymmetric carbon, still it can show optical activity. This is because the molecule is overall dissymmetric or chiral in nature. A dissymmetric or chiral molecule or an object is that which lacks the plane of symmetry. From the above it is thus concluded that *it is the dissymmetry* or chirality (stereogenicity) *not the asymmetry is the essential criterion for optical activity.* Another class of dissymmetric molecule is the substituted biphenyls. Steric hindrance created by bulky substituents makes the molecule non-planar and hence optically active.

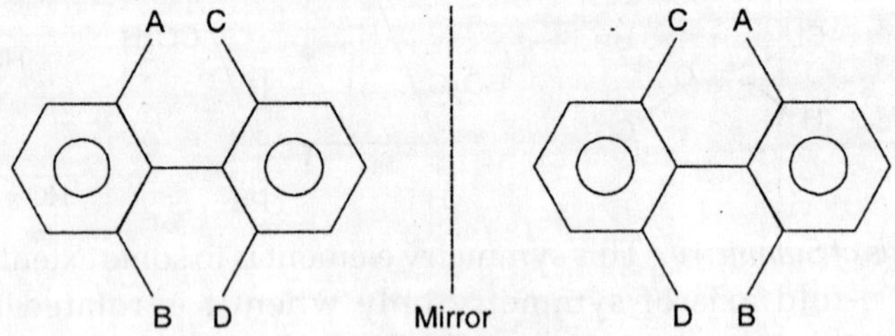

substituted biphenyl

PROBLEM 3.2

1. Circle all the asymmetric carbon atoms in $HOH_2C-C(=O)-CH(OH)-C(=O)-CH_2OH$

2. Are the following molecules chiral?

(i) 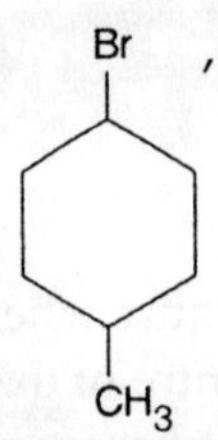

(ii) 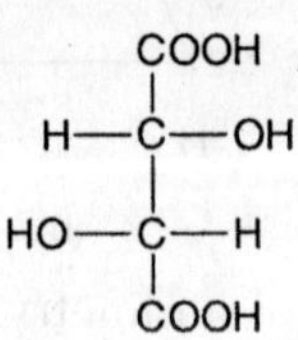

(iii) 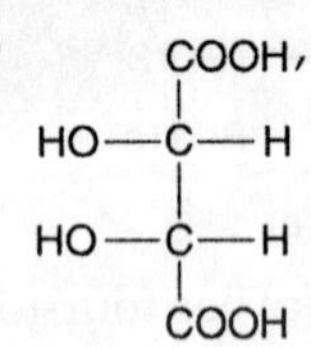

(iv) 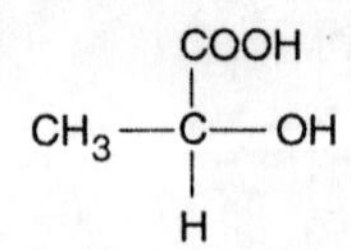

3.3.6 Racemic Modification

It has been observed that in the case of large number of dissymmetric molecules no optical activity is observed. This is because such molecules are constituted of equal numbers of dextro rotatory (+) and laevorotatory (–) molecules so that the average rotation is zero. Such a mixture of equal number of enantiomers is called *Racemic Modification* denoted by the prefix (±).

3.3.6.1 Resolution of Racemic Modification

If and when necessary the two enantiomers of racemic modification may be separated by suitable methods. Since the enantiomers have identical physical and chemical properties except towards optically active reagents, they cannot be separated by normal processes like chromatography, fractional distillation and fractional crystallisation. So some special procedures are to be adopted. This process of separation of enantiomers from racemic modification is known as *Resolution.* A few important and frequently used methods are as described below:

(a) *Mechanical Method*: This method is applicable if the enantiomers are crystaline in nature. The crystals are separated by hand picking. Pasteur adopted this technique for the separation of optical isomers of ammonium tartarate.

(b) *Chemical Method*: This is the most general method. In this method racemic mixture is converted to a pair of non-identical derivatives by the treatment with optically active reagent. These derivatives differ in their physical properties and can be separated by physical means. This method is highly suitable for the resolution of carboxylic acids and amines.

For example, racemic mixture of tartaric acid is treated with a base (–) cinchonidine when two non-identical salts— (+) tartarate of (–) cinchonidine and (–) tartarate of (–) cinchonidine are formed. These two salts appreciably differ in solubility and are separated during fractional crystallisation. After the separation each salt is decomposed with sulphuric acid to get pure (+) and (–) tartaric acids.

(±)Tartaric acid + (–) Cinchonidine

↓

(+)Tartarate – (–) Cinchonidine and (–) Tartarate – (–) Cinchonidine
(Mixture of salts)

↓ Fractional crystallisation

Pure (+) (–) salt	Pure (–) (–) salt
↓ H^+	↓ H^-
Pure (+) tartaric acid	Pure (–) tartaric acid

(c) *Enzymatic Method*: Certain enzymes when allowed to grow in dilute solution of racemic mixture preferentially consumes one enantiomer leaving other untouched. Thus when a racemic mixture of ammonium tartarate is treated with the mould, *penicillium glaucum*, only the dextro form is consumed leaving laevo form practically intact. This method suffers from the drawback that one of the enantiomers is destroyed.

3.3.6.2 Racemisation

Racemisation is a process of converting one of the pure enantiomer into racemic modification. Thus when dextro form of tartaric acid is heated with alkali at 175 °C it is converted into inactive racemic modification. There are various methods for racemisation. One of the general methods is the thermal process. This process involves temporary breakage of one of the four bonds of chiral centre and recombination of the broken bond in either side yielding racemic mixture.

3.3.7 Number of Stereoisomers

How many stereoisomers are possible for a molecule depends upon the number of chiral centres present in the concerned molecule. Thus lactic acid has only one asymmetric atom in its molecule. It can exist in three forms of which two are optically active and the other is optically inactive.

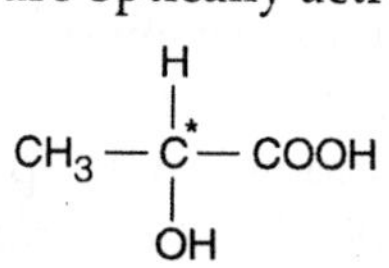

Lactic acid ($\overset{*}{C}$ is asymmetric)

Out of two optically active forms one is dextro rotatory and rotates the plane of polarised light in the right-hand direction and the other is laevorotatory and rotates the plane of polarised light in the left-hand direction. These two forms are mirror images to each other.

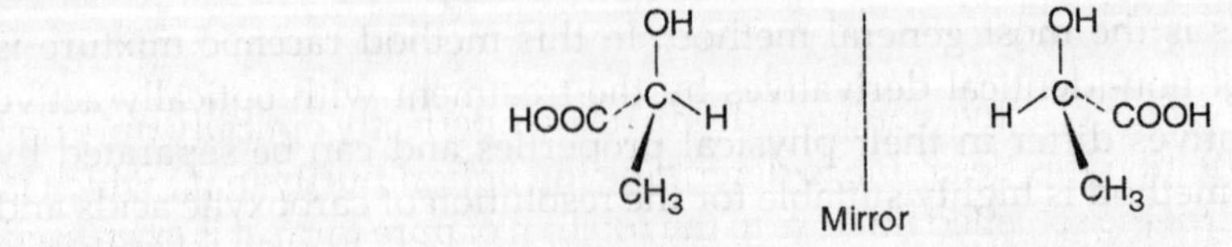

(+) Lactic acid (–) Lactic acid

The third one is equimolar mixture of above two forms known as racemic mixture and is optically inactive, i.e., (±) lactic acid. Racemic form may be regarded as *externally compensated form*. Tartaric acid contains two asymmetric carbon atoms—each one is attached to H, OH, COOH and CH (OH) COOH groups, i.e., in tartaric acid two asymmetric carbon atoms are silmilar.

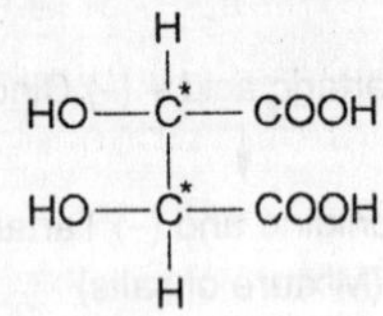

Tartaric acid

The groups on the two asymmetric carbon atoms may be spatially arranged in four different ways as indicated below:

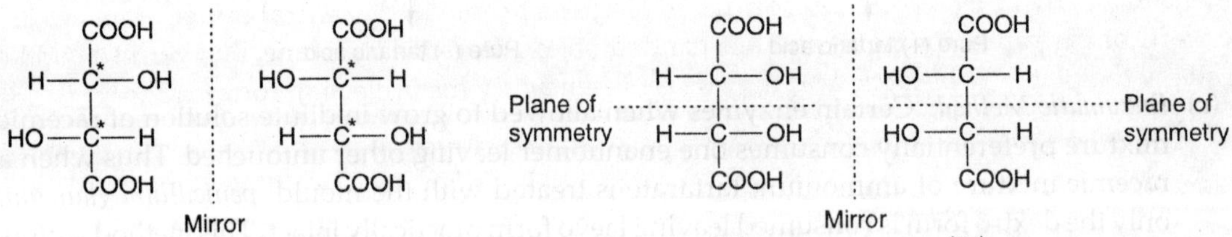

(I) (II) (III) (IV)

Optically active Optically inactive

The structures (I) and (II) are non-superimposable and so are optically active. They are enantiomers to each other. But structures (III) and (IV) have a plane of symmetry which bisects the molecule into two equal and identical halves. So the optical activity of one half is exactly cancelled by other half. As a result the net rotation exhibited by the compounds becomes zero and so both of them are optically inactive. Their optical inactivity is due to internal compensation. Such forms are known as *mesoform*. Both (III) and (IV) are identical and constitute only one mesoform. It cannot be resolved. Over and above, of these three forms, there exists a *racemic form* which is equimolar mixture of two enantiomers (I) and (II), which can be resolved into two active forms. Therefore, altogether, tartaric acid having two chiral centres has four stereoisomers — dextro (+), laevo (–), meso and racemic forms.

From the above it may be concluded that a compound having *n* number of chiral centres has 2^n stereoisomers. In this connection it may be mentioned that the structures (I) & (III), (I) & (IV), (II) & (III) and (II) & (IV) are neither enantiomers nor superimposable. This type of stereoisomers are called *diastereoisomers* or *diastereomers*. Thus diastereomers may be defined as stereoisomers which are not mirror image to each other.

Diastereoisomers are similar but not identical in properties. They have different physical properties and can be separated by suitable means. Diastereoisomers may or may not be optically active.

3.3.8 Optical Purity

In some cases it is found that optically active compounds are neither perfectly optically pure nor racemic mixtures. In such situation it is desirable to determine the optical purity (o.p.) which is defined as the ratio of rotation of the so-called mixture to the rotation of pure form. It is expressed as:

$$\text{o.p.} = \frac{\text{observed rotation of the sample}}{\text{optical rotation of pure sample}} \times 100.$$

Optical purity also indicates the amount of the excess in percentage of the predominant enantiomer. Thus the value of o.p. = + 15% means that (+) form is 15% excess of (–) form and the remaining 85% is optically inactive and racemic. In other words, (15 + 85/2) = 57.5% is (+) form and 44.5% is (–) form. This relative amount of enantiomer is termed as *enantiomeric excess (e.e.)*.

Problem 3.3

What does it imply if a mixture has an enantiomeric excess 30%?

3.3.9 Projection Formula for Representation of Enantiomers

Initially Fischer proposed a projection formula for representing tetrahedral carbon atom as a two dimensional structure on paper. According to Fischer's proposal, the central carbon atom lies on the plane of the paper, the right- and left-handed bonds lie above the plane, and vertical bonds lie below the plane. Thus lactic acid may be represented by the projection formula as—

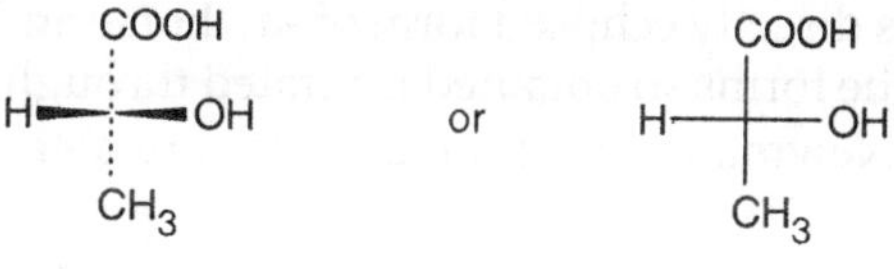

It may be mentioned that the most important functional group is placed at the top, and the main chain of carbon atoms in the molecule should be represented along the vertical line. If necessary, projection formula may be rotated by 180° because such rotation does not produce any change in the structure but cannot be rotated either by 90° or 270°.

Interchange of two pairs of substituents in one Fischer projection will create another identical structure. Thus,

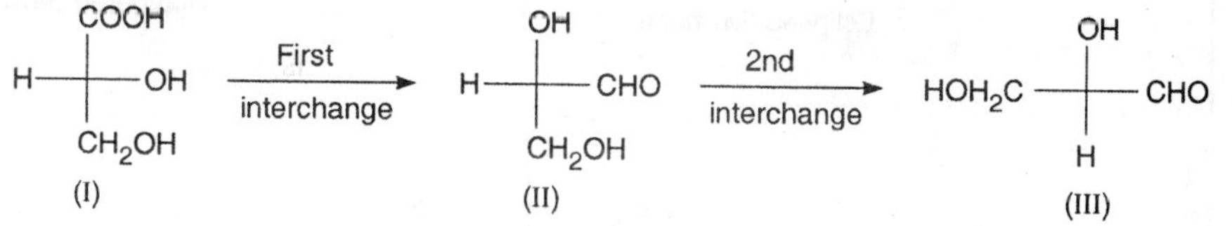

(I) (II) (III)

Structures (I) and (III) are same, but (I) and (II) or (II) and (III) are not the same. This means two changes are to be made.

Fischer projection formula is not sufficiently adequate for representing compounds containing more than one asymmetric carbon atoms. In such cases '*Sawhorse*' and Newman projection formula are very convenient and useful representation. In the Sawhorse representation, the molecule is shown in three dimensions. The bond between two asymmetric atoms is diagonally written and bulky groups are oriented far away from each other. Thus, the Sawhorse representation of erythrose may be shown as in Fig. 3.4.

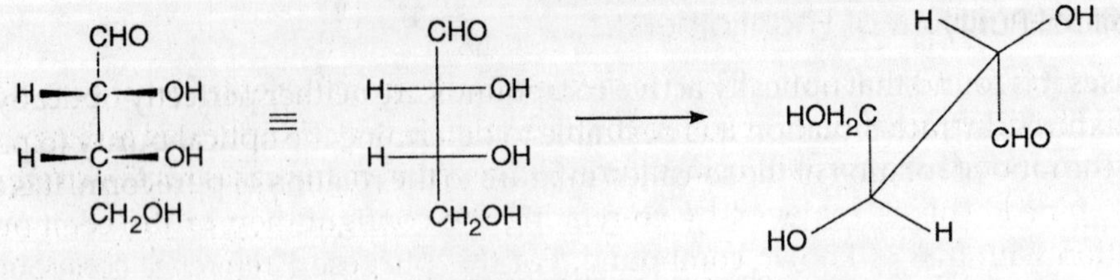

Fig. 3.4

In Newman projection formula, the molecule is viewed from front to back in the direction of the bond between chiral carbon atoms which are represented by two superimposable circles. The groups and bonds associated with chiral carbon are projected into a vertical plane. The representation of erythrose in Newman formula thus stands as in Fig. 3.4:

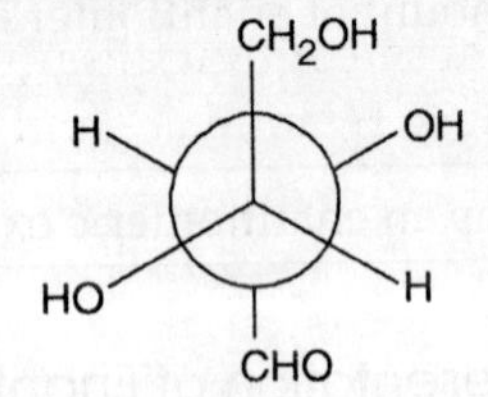

Erythrose

Fig. 3.5

Fischer, Sawhorse and Newman projection formulae are interconvertible as shown below in Fig. 3.6. The bottom carbon atom in Fischer projection formula is written at the front, and top atom is placed at the side while other groups are placed in the front and in the rear as in Fischer projection formula. This gives directly eclipsed form of sawhorse and Newman projection. In the next step the front carbon of the forms so obtained is rotated through 180° around the C—C bond when normal sawhorse and Newman projection formulae are obtained. Thus,

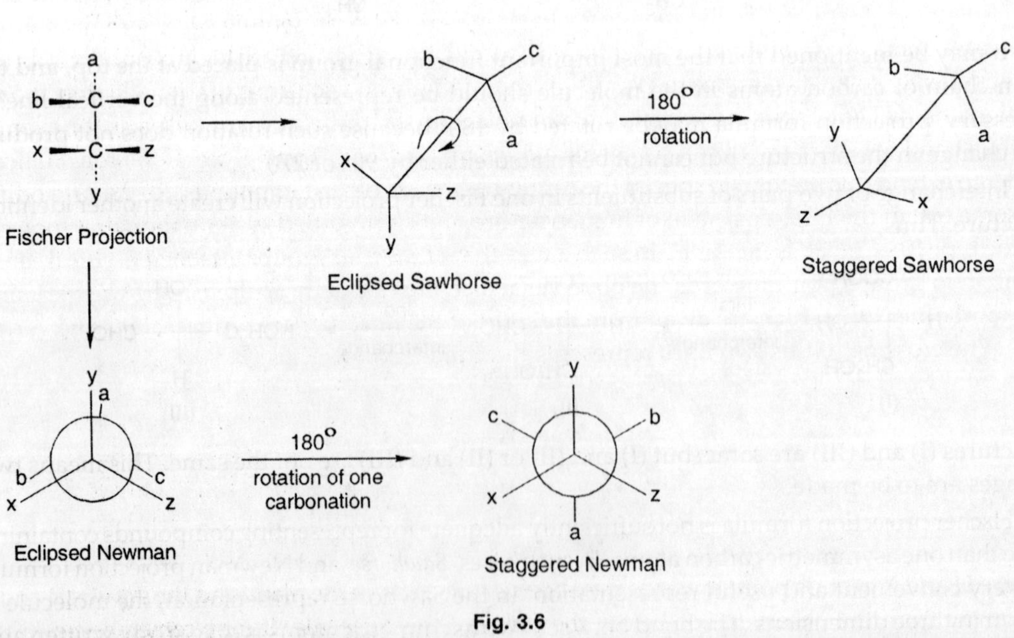

Fig. 3.6

Similarly, by reversing the above procedure sawhorse and Newman projection formulae can be converted to Fischer projection formula.

3.3.10 Nomenclature of Enantiomers

The *absolute configuration* of a compound is defined as the spatial orientation of groups relative to each other. The determination of absolute configuration is very complicated and is possible only when the compounds are crystalline in nature. However, in many cases *relative configuration* has been determined. This is achieved by co-relating the configuration of the compound under consideration with that of known compound. For this purpose a reference compound is to be used. An widely used such compound is glyceraldehyde. This compound has one asymmetric carbon and can exist in dextro (+) and laevo (–) forms and their configurations are known. In (+) forms, the OH group is attached to the chiral carbon atom in the right-hand direction and its configuration is indicated by D (+). Similarly, in (–) forms the said OH group is present in left-hand direction and its configuration is represented by the symbol L (–). The configuration of the compound that could be derived from D (+)-glyceraldehyde is regarded as the member of D-family. Similarly, the compound whose configuration can be correlated with that of L (–) glyceraldehyde is considered to belong to L-family. D- and L- glyceraldehyde have the following configurations:

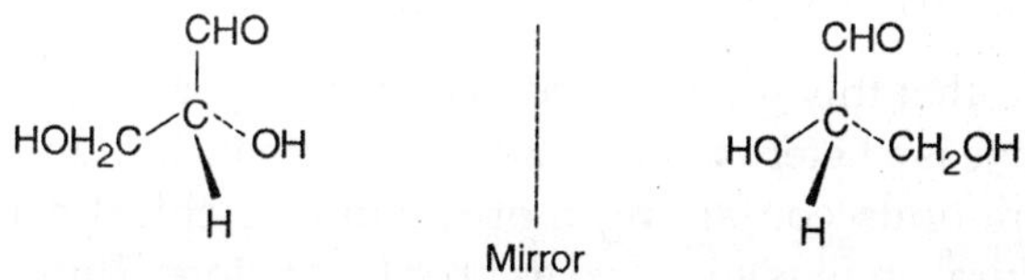

D (+) Glyceraldehyde L (–) Glyceraldehyde

In this connection it may be mentioned that D, L and d, l are not identical. Capital letters indicate configuration only but small letters indicates rotation, d for rotation in the right, while l for rotation in the left.

The above system of nomenclature was introduced by Emil Fischer during his studies on carbohydrate chemistry and is the most oldest method of representing the configuration of a molecule. It may be mentioned that although most of the sugars and analogous compounds may be genetically correlated either to D or L- glyceraldehyde and so configurationally they may be designated as D or L but this system fails to work satisfactorily in many cases as for example both (+) and (–) - lactic acid can be chemically correlated with same glyceraldehyde. Hence in order to extend this method to specify the configurations of other compounds, Rosanoff modified to some extent the Fischer system of nomenclature. In this modified system, the chiral molecule of the type R—CHXR′ is imagined in such a way that of the four groups attached to chiral carbon atom, two groups point towards the observer which are normally written along the horizontal line and other two which are away from the sight of the observer are written along the vertical line. The crossing of this two lines represents the chiral carbon. Thus,

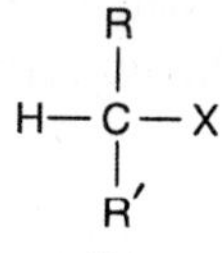

(A)

Fig. 3.7

where H and X groups point towards the observer , i.e., above the plane and the groups R and R′ are away from the observer, i.e., below the plane of the molecule. It may remembered in this connection that the longest chain (here R—C—R′) of carbon atoms should be represented along the vertical line and the most highly oxidisable carbon is to be on the top. In such representation, if the group X is on the right, the molecule is termed as D and the molecule is called as L when X is on the left. On this basis D (–) lactic acid may be represented as

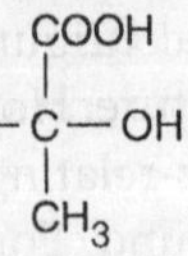

D (–) lactic acid

As mentioned earlier that the rotation by 90° or 270° changes the configuration of the molecule and the interchange of the positions of any two groups leads to inversion in configuration but two consecutive interchanges in the positions of the groups neutralise the effect. Thus,

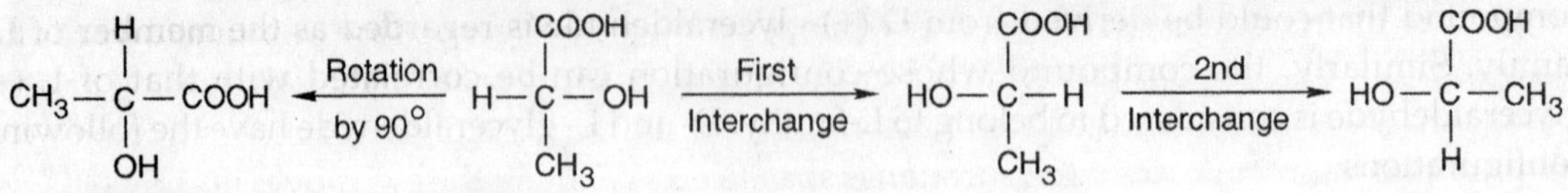

L (+) lactic acid D (–) lactic acid L (+) lactic acid D (–) lactic acid

It has been observed that this system of nomenclature operates successfully when X in the expression [Fig. 3.7] above is a hetero atom or any hetero atomic group and may be extended for nomenclature of compounds containing more than one chiral carbon atoms where the configuration of each chiral atom is specified as D or L as before. Thus,

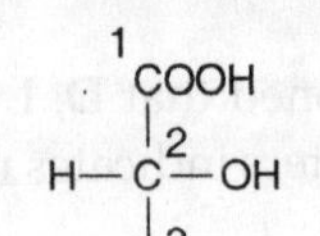

2D-Hydroxy-3D-methyl-
3L-hydroxy-pentanoic acid

The system is also applicable to compounds having chiral carbon in the ring.

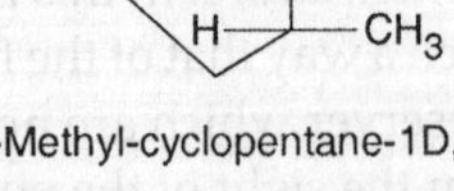

3D-Methyl-cyclopentane-1D, 2D-diol

However, this system of nomenclature is not free from drawbacks. It can only be applied usefully to those molecules which can be projected in a fashion comparable to glyceraldehyde. Thus, this system cannot be applied to 1-phenyl butyric acid as it cannot be written in Fischer-projection.

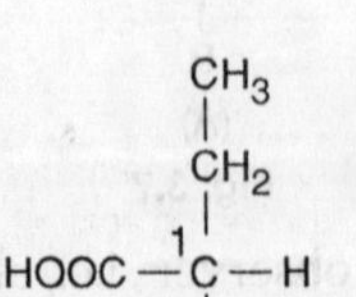

1-phenyl buityric acid

3.3.10.1 R and S Nomenclature

In order to avoid any confusion an independent system has been developed by Cahn, Ingold and Prelog based on actual three dimensional formula to indicate the configuration without any reference to glyceraldehyde. This independent system of nomenclature is known as R and S system of nomenclature where R stands for *rectus* meaning right and S for *sinister* which means left. It is also known as Cahn, Ingold and Prelog (CIP) system. It may be mentioned that like D and L, R and S are spatial descriptors and have nothing to do with the signs of rotations.

This method of nomenclature distinctly consists of two different steps. Step-I involves the assignment of groups attached to chiral centre a sequence of priority determined by following a set of sequence rules (discussed below) and in the step II, (application of chirality rule) the arrangement of groups is visualised in such a way that the atom or group of lowest priority is directed away from the sight of observer while remaining three groups are pointing towards the observer. Now on viewing at these three remaining groups in the order of their decreasing priority from the side remote from the lowest priority group if eye of the observer moves in clockwise (right-handed) direction, the configuration is specificed as *R* and if the eye moves in anticlockwise (left-handed) direction the configuration is S. This is known as the *chirality rule*. The method of specifying the configuration as R and S may be illustrated by the following example. Let us assume a compound x, a, b, c, and d where x is the chiral carbon atom and a, b, c and d are four groups. According to sequence rule, their priority in the decreasing order is a > b > c > d. i.e., *d* is the lowest priority group and *a* has the highest priority.

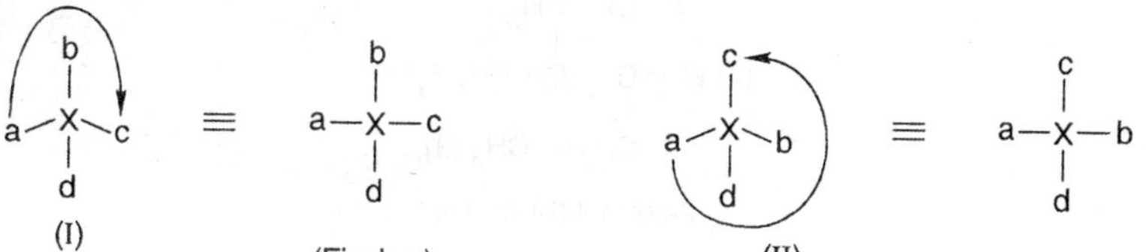

(I) (R) (Fischer) (II) (S) (Fischer)

Thus, (I) has R configuration while S configuration is assigned to (II).

3.3.10.1.1 Sequence Rules

In order to determine the sequence of priority of groups attached to chiral carbon there are some sequence rules as depicted below:

Sequence rule 1: The sequence of priority of four groups attached to chiral carbon atom is determined on the basis of atomic number of the atom of the groups directly attached to the chiral centre. The atom of higher atomic number gets higher priority. For example, in chloroiodomethane sulphonic acid, the priority sequence is I > Cl > SO_3H > H

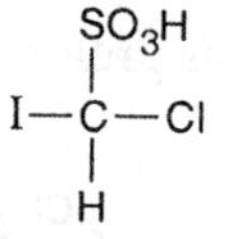

Chloroiodomethane sulphonic acid

Sequence rule 2: In the situation when the atoms attached to chiral carbon are the same, their respective states of substitution are also considered. Thus, the priority sequence of the following groups may be written as:

—CH_2OH > —CH_2—CH_3 > —CH_3. This is because the sum of atomic numbers in CH_3 is 12 + 3 = 15, in —CH_2—CH_3 is 12 + 2 + 12 = 26 and in CH_2OH is 12 + 2 + 16 = 30.

Following examples may be cited for the elaboration of the above rule.

In 2-butanol, atoms of two groups, —CH_3 and —CH_2—CH_3 directly attached to chiral centre are carbon. In order to decide the priority between these two groups atomic number of other atoms connected to these atoms (carbon) are to be considered. In CH_3, three H atoms are connected. Hence total atomic number becomes 12 + 1 + 1 + 1 = 15. In —CH_2—CH_3 group, there is one carbon and two H atoms attached (–C(H)(H)–C), so its total atomic number stands as 12 + 1 + 1 +12 = 26. Thus, ethyl group gets priority over methyl. Thus, the sequence of priority of different groups in 1-butanol is OH > CH_2—CH_3> —CH_3> H.

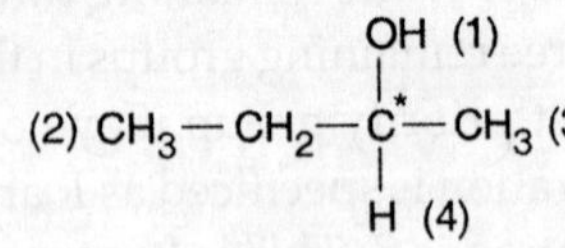

2-Butanol

Similarly, in 2-methyl-3-pentanol, priority sequence of four groups stands as

OH > $CH(CH_3)_2$ > CH—CH_3 > H

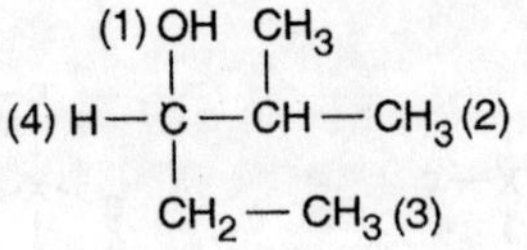

2-Methyl-3-pentanol

Sequence rule 3: Doubly or triply bonded atoms are considered to be duplicated or triplicated at both the ends of multiple bonds. Thus,

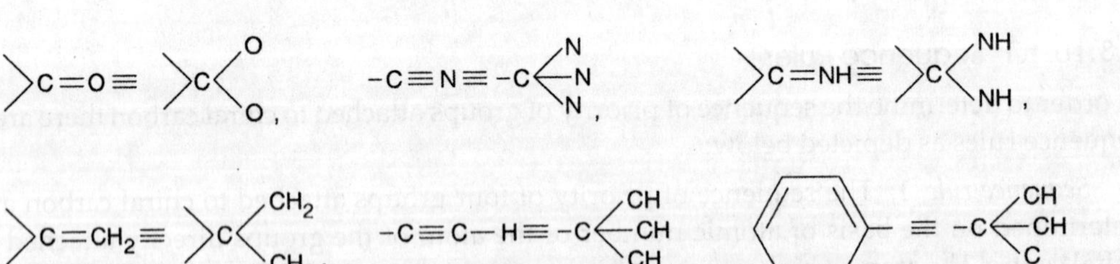

It may be mentioned that $>C=CH_2$ has preference over $>C(CH_3)_2$. Similar is the case with

–C≡C—H which has higher priority than –$C(CH_3)_3$.

By applying the above sequence rules priority of some common substituents stands as under:

$-I > -Br > -Cl > -SO_2R > -SR > -SH > -F > -O-\overset{\overset{O}{\|}}{C}-R > -OR > -OH >$

$-NO_2 > -NHCOR > -NR_2 > -NHR > -NH_2 > -SR > -CCl_3 >$

$-\underset{\underset{O}{\|}}{C}-Cl > -COOR > -COOH > -CONH_2 > -CHO > -CH_2OH >$

$-C_2H_5 > -CR_3 > -CHR_2 > -CH_2R > -CH_3 > -H$

3.3.10.1.2 Configuration on the Basis of Projection Formula

Fischer projection formula has been found to be suitable for designating the configuration of the molecule without constructing the model. In order to determine whether the eye of the observer moves clockwise or anticlockwise always the group or ligand of lowest priority must be at the bottom on the Fischer projection formula. But in fact, lowest priority goups may or may not always be at the bottom of the Fischer projection formula. So in assigning the configuration following situations may arise.

(a) *The group of lowest priority is at the bottom of the projection formula*: This is the simplest situation. In this case eye is rotated in the order of decreasing priorities and to observe whether eye rotates in clockwise or anticlockwise manner. Thus,

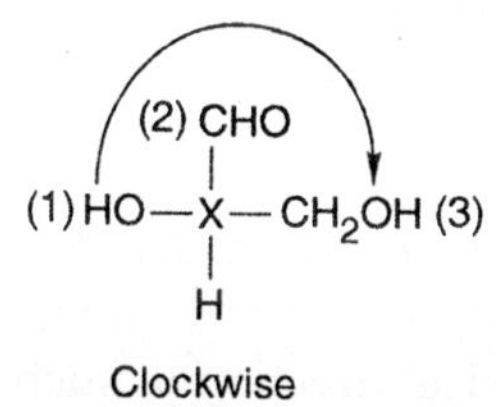

Clockwise

R-Glyceraldehyde

(b) *The lowest priority group is at the left-hand side*: In this situation, keeping the position of group or ligand at the top of the vertical end, the positions of other groups are changed in the anticlockwise direction so that lowest priority group becomes at the bottom and next the direction in the order of decreasing priorities is found out. Thus,

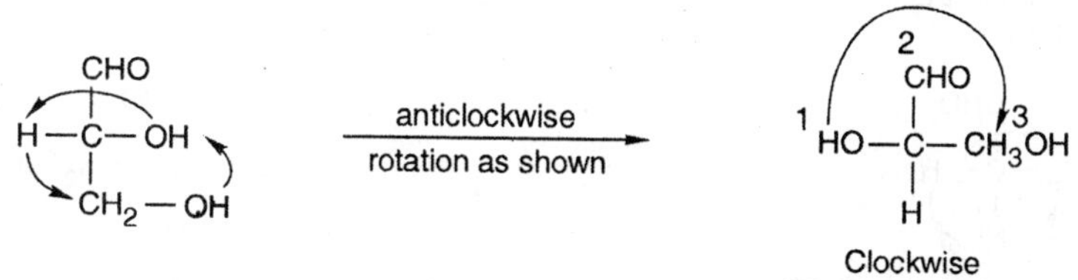

Clockwise

(R)-Glyceraldehyde

Similarly, other examples that may be cited in this connection are as discussed below.

i. 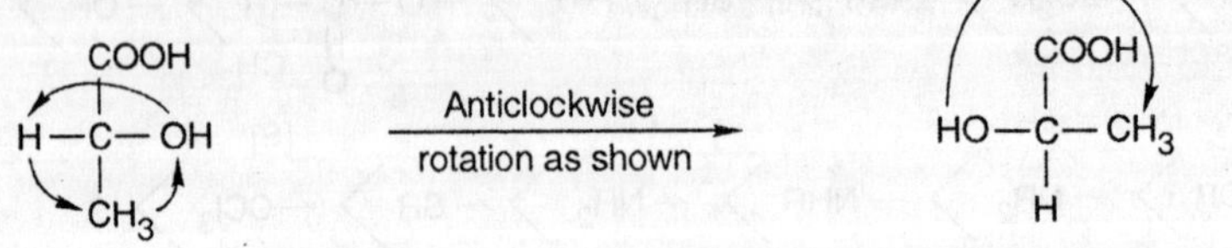

(R)-lactic acid

ii. 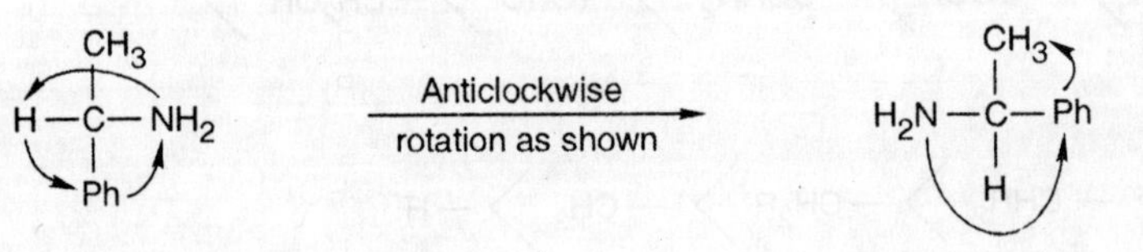

S-α-phenyl alanine

iii. 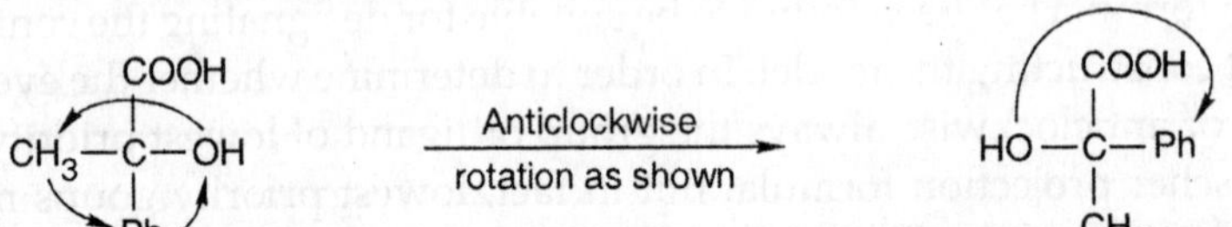

Lowest priority group is CH_3

R-Atrolactic acid

iv. 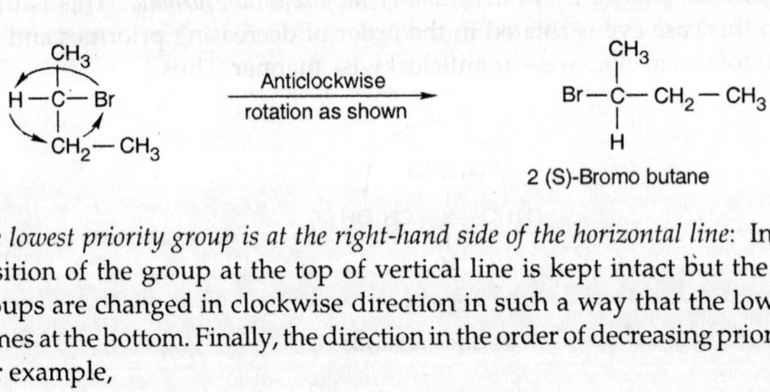

2 (S)-Bromo butane

(c) *The lowest priority group is at the right-hand side of the horizontal line*: In this situation, the position of the group at the top of vertical line is kept intact but the positions of other groups are changed in clockwise direction in such a way that the lowest priority group comes at the bottom. Finally, the direction in the order of decreasing priorities is determined. For example,

i. 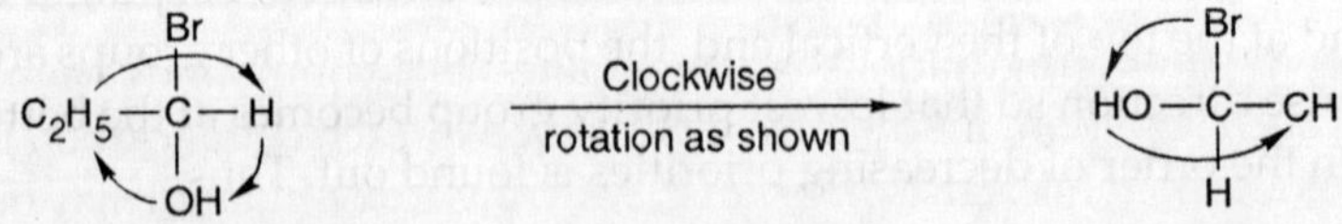

Lowest priority atom is H

[S]

ii. 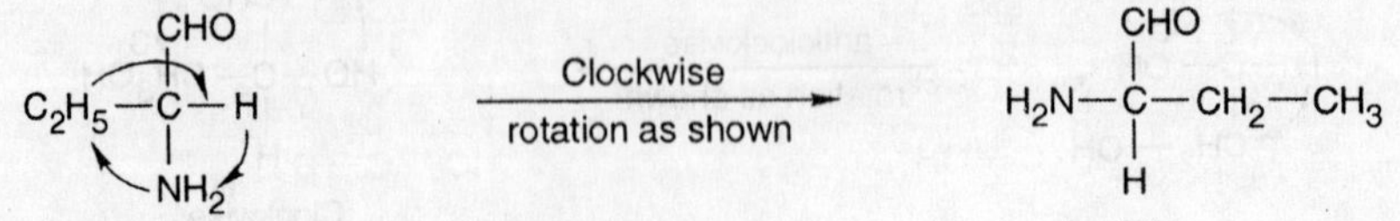

Lowest priority atom is H

[R]

iii. 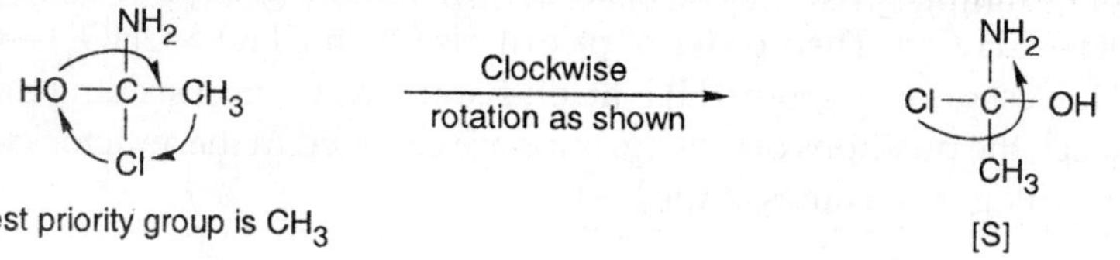

Lowest priority group is CH_3

iv. 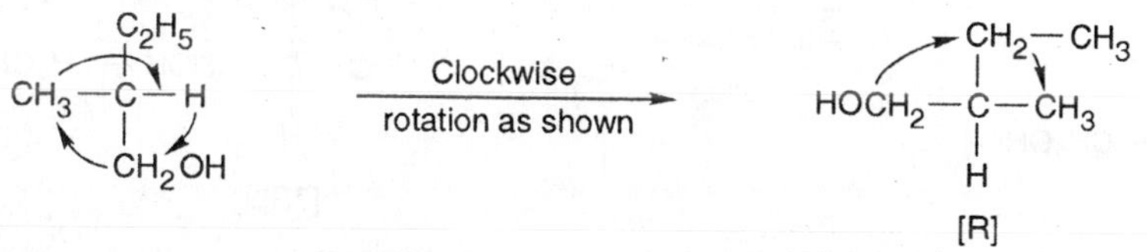

v. 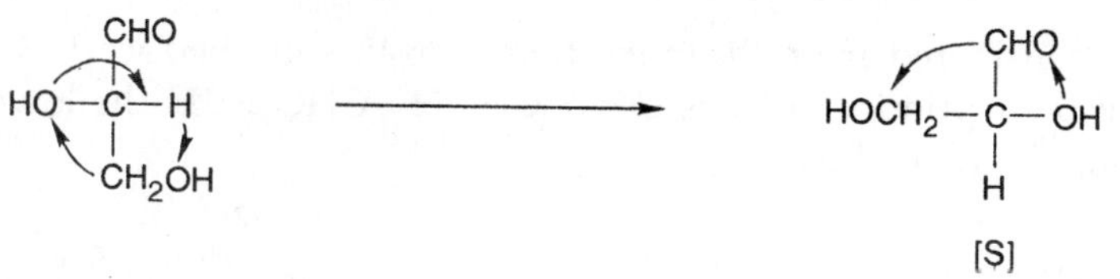

(d) *The lowest priority group is at the top of the vertical line*: In this case the molecule is rotated by 180° so that the lowest priority group takes the bottom position of the vertical line. This is normally done by reversing the positions of all the groups. This is followed by determination of direction in the order of decreasing priorities. Thus,

i. 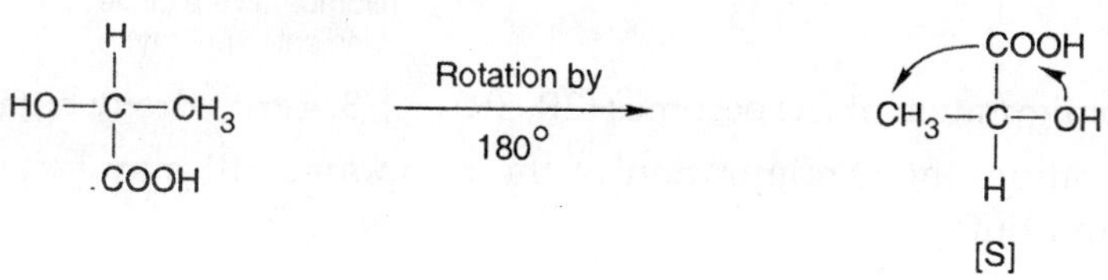

ii. 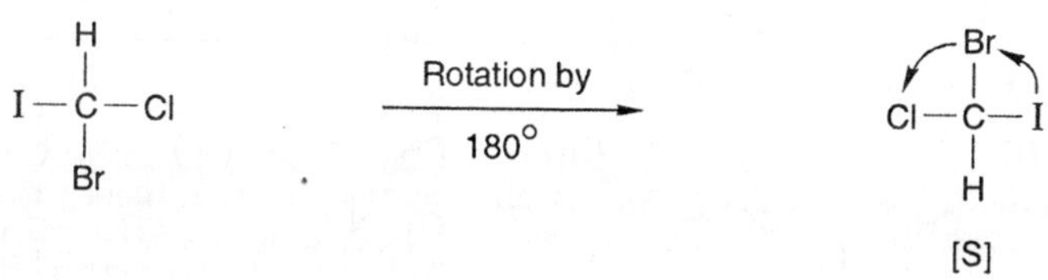

3.3.10.1.3 Configuration of Compounds Containing More than one Chiral Centres

This system of specifying the configurations is also applicable to compounds having more than one chiral carbon. In such situation, firstly the configuration of each chiral carbon is settled and then a symbol R or S is attached to each. Isomers of 2, 3, 4-trihydroxy-butanol may be cited in this connection as an example. Thus,

(A) (B)

In both the compounds C_2 and C_3 are chiral. In (A), the four groups attached to C_2 are CHO, OH, H and CHOH—CH_2OH. Their order of priority is OH > CHO > CHOH—CH_2OH > H. In chiral carbon (C_2) lowest priority group (H) is at left-hand direction. So keeping the group (ligand) CHO at the top intact, the positions of other groups are changed in the anticlockwise direction so that the lowest priority group comes at the bottom.

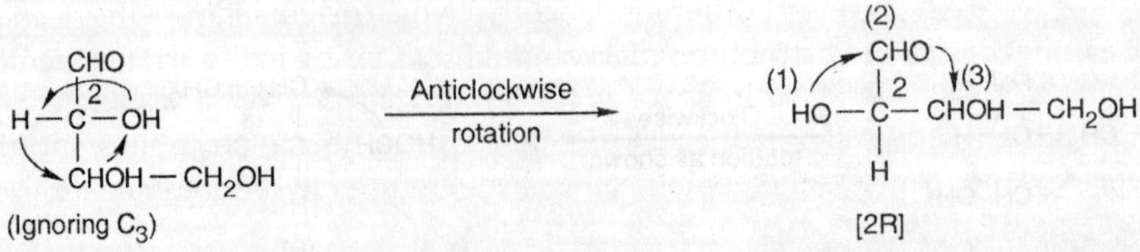

(Number in the circle indicates priority)

Similarly, C_3 may be considered. Here, the four different groups attached are, H, OH, CH_2OH and CHOH—CHO and their priority order is OH > CHOH—CHO > H. The lowest priority group (H) is at left-hand direction. Thus,

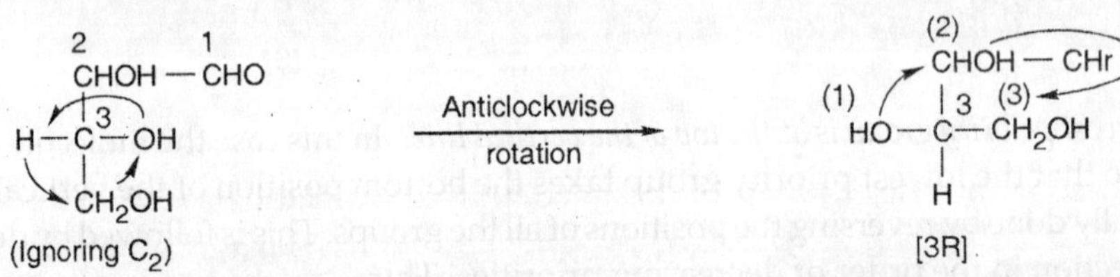

(Number in the circle indicates priority)

Thus, the overall configuration of (A) becomes (2R, 3R)— 2, 3, 4-trihydroxy butanol.

By similar consideration, the configuration of the compound (B) may be specified as (2S, 3S)—2, 3, 4-trihydroxy butanol.

PROBLEM 3.4

Assign R and S configurations to the following:

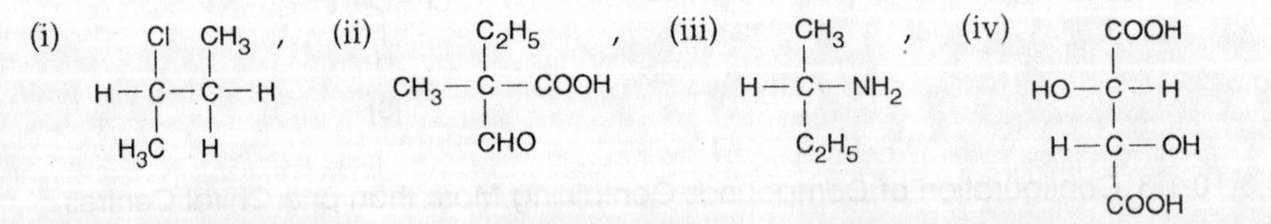

3.4 Conformational Isomerism

Conformations or conformational or rotational isomers or simply conformers originates from the different arrangements of atoms or groups in space by the rotation of carbon-carbon single bond. Conformers are interconvertible by rotation around carbon-carbon single bond. The different conformers obtained from particular configuration differ in energy content and hence in stability. In non-rigid systems, isolation of all the conformers is practically impossible. It has been observed that a difference of al least 20 kcal/mole energy barrier between any two conformers is required for their existence at ordinary condition. The conformer with lowest energy content is relatively stable and is generally known as *preferred conformation*. An analysis of energy changes that a molecule involves due to rotation of groups or atoms around a single bond is termed as *conformational analysis*.

In this context it must be remembered that the terms conformation and configuration are not the terms of the same phenomenon but they differ from each other. As mentioned before conformation is a phenomenon of different arrangements of atoms or groups in a molecule in space resulting in the generation of different structures which originate from the *rotation around a single bond* while the different structures of a compound differing in the arrangement of atoms or groups *around a particular atom* in space is known as *configuration*. The different forms of conformation are termed as stagged, eclipsed, gauche or skew conformations and the terms enantiomers, diasteroisomers and geometrical isomers are used to differentiate different types of configurations.

The phenomenon of conformation is exhibited by variety of compounds like alkanes, cycloalkanes and other compounds having single bonds in rigid system.

3.4.1 Conformation of Ethane

Ethane is the simplest molecule having a carbon-carbon single bond. So it is expected that it should exhibit the phenomenon of conformation. In ethane (CH_3—CH_3) two carbon atoms are connected by a single bond and each carbon atom is attached with three hydrogen atoms. A large number of conformers of ethane may be originated by the rotation of one of the carbon atoms about the carbon-carbon bond keeping other carbon stationary. It may, however, be mentioned that the rotation about a carbon-carbon single bond is not quite free, there is an energy barrier of about 3 kcal/mole. This amount of energy required to rotate ethane molecule around carbon-carbon bond is called *torsional energy*.

Out of infinite number of conformers, two extreme cases are staggered and eclipsed forms. In staggered from H atoms of two carbons are far apart while in eclipsed conformation H atoms of one carbon are just behind those of the front carbon. These two forms are converted into each other by rotation of one of the carbon atoms against other through 60°. The other possible conformations in between these two extreme conformers are known as *skew* or *gauche* conformations.

3.4.2 Representation of Conformations

To represent conformations normally two types of three dimensional formulae, viz, Sawhorse and Newman projections are used.

In *Sawhorse representation*, the C—C bond is viewed sideways. This bond is drawn diagonally and is slightly longer. The lower left-hand carbon is considered as front carbon and the upper right-hand carbon is taken as back carbon. The staggered and eclipsed conformations of ethane may be represented by the Sawhorse projection as depicted below:

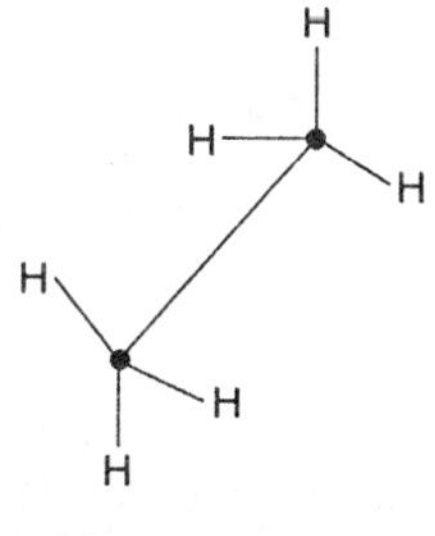

Staggered conformation (s)

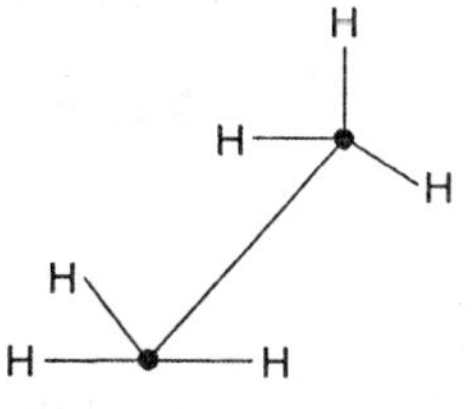

Eclipsed conformation (e)

In *Newman projection* formula, the carbon-carbon bond lies along the line of vision and cannot be seen. The carbon nearer to the vision is represented by a point and other three bonds attached to it are shown by three lines at an angle of 120° to each other. The other carbon atom which is away from the sight is represented by a circle and the three bonds of this carbon are shown by a shorter lines and are at an angle of 120° to one another. Newman projection formulae for staggered and eclipsed conformations of ethane may be indicated in Fig. 3.8 as below.

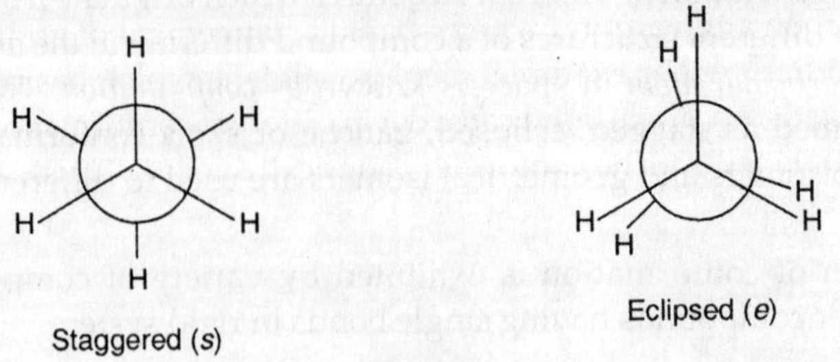

Fig. 3.8

The potential energy of the molecule in general is minimum for staggered conformation and it increases with rotation and becomes maximum at the eclipsed conformation. Most of the molecules of a compound naturally exist in the most stable staggered conformation. The potential energy changes during rotation about carbon-carbon single bond in ethane may be shown in Fig. 3.9 as below.

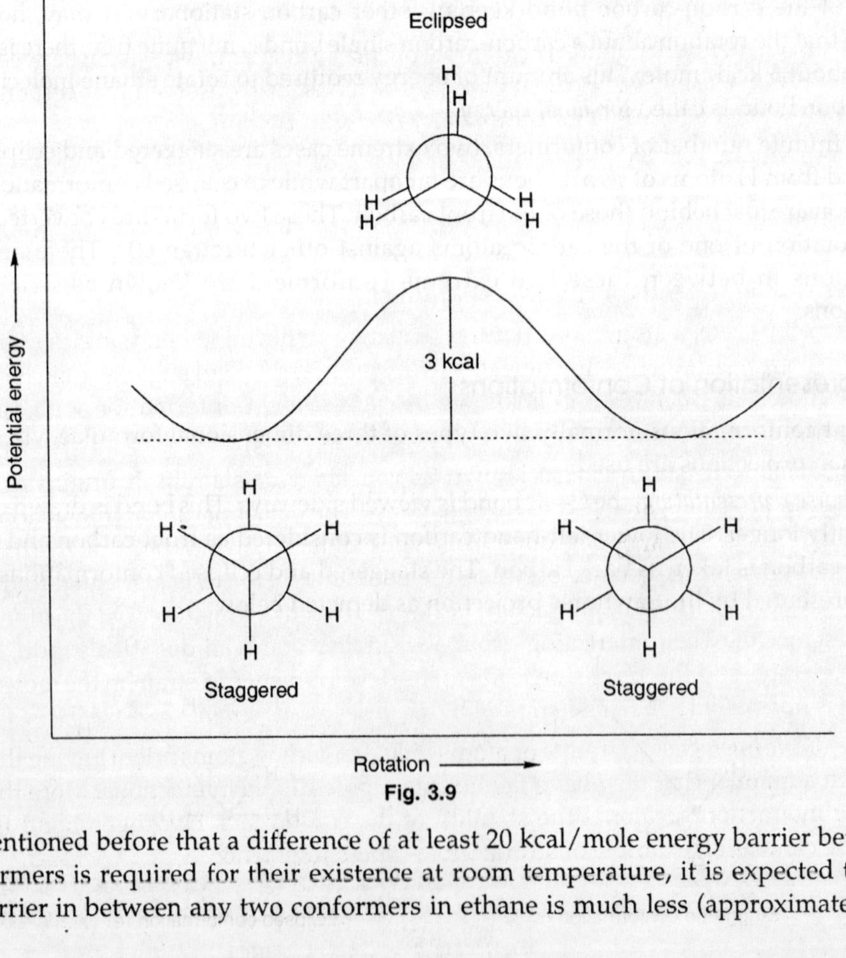

Fig. 3.9

As mentioned before that a difference of at least 20 kcal/mole energy barrier between any two conformers is required for their existence at room temperature, it is expected that as the energy barrier in between any two conformers in ethane is much less (approximately 3 kcal/

mole) than the required energy, the different conformers of ethane may not exist at all and in fact, different conformers of ethane are readily interconvertible and as such ethane exists in only one conformation, i.e., in staggered conformation.

It is noteworthy that since conformational isomers differ from each other only in their arrangement of atoms or groups in space, they, can also be looked upon as stereoisomers. Like stereoisomers of any kind a pair of conformers may or may not be the mirror images of each other provided the carbon atom around which spatial arrangement of groups or atoms is being considered is chiral in nature. For example, dichloro stilbene which has two chiral carbons C_1 and C_2 that are connected by a single bond can exist in different conformation. Its staggered form is optically inactive while the gauche conformer is optically active. Thus,

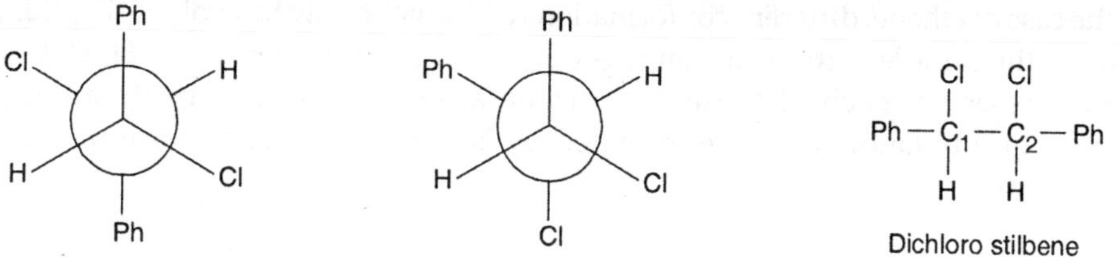

(Staggered) Inactive

(Gauche) Active

Dichloro stilbene

3.4.3 Factors Controlling the Relative Stability of Conformations

It has already been mentioned that 20 kcal/mole of energy barrier must exist in between any two conformers for their existence at ordinary condition. It has been observed that certain factors as mentioned below are responsible for the stability of conformations.

1. *Torsional Strain*: It is known that the rotation about a C—C single bond is not completely free. There exists a potential energy barrier which restricts the free rotations. This energy barrier is known as torsional energy and according to Pitzer it originates due to a strain usually termed as *torsional strain*. More the torsional strain, more is the torsional energy barrier and higher is the stability of conformers.
2. *Angle Strain*: Every atom has a natural tendency to have the bond angles matching the bonding orbitals. If there is any deviation from the normal bond angle, a strain is developed in the molecule. Such a strain is known as *angle strain*. Conformation with appreciable angle strain are less stable.
3. *Steric Strain*: This strain is also known as van der Waals strain. It originates from the interaction of groups attached to carbon atoms. The actual nature of interaction depends upon the size and polarity of groups. This type of interaction may be attractive or repulsive in nature. When the distance between the interacting groups is just equal to the sum of their van der Waals radii, interaction becomes attractive in nature. On the other hand, if the distance between interacting groups is smaller than van der Waals radii, repulsive force operates and this repulsion leads to the development of a strain in the molecule. This strain is normally termed as *steric strain* or *van der Waals strain*.
4. *Dipole-dipole Interaction*: Groups or atoms linked to carbon atoms orient among themselves in such a manner that they have favourable dipole-dipole interactions. More the dipole-dipole interaction greater is the stability of the conformers. Hydrogen bond formation may be cited as an example of strong diple-dipole interaction.

3.4.4 Conformation of *n*-Butane

Structurally *n*-butane ($\overset{1}{C}H_3-\overset{2}{C}H_2-\overset{3}{C}H_2-\overset{4}{C}H_3$) may be looked upon as a derivative of ethane ($H-CH_2-CH_2-H$), in which one hydrogen atom of each carbon has been replaced by a methyl group. So it is expected that the conformational analysis of *n*-butane may be elaborated similarly. But as one hydrogen atom of each carbon has been replaced by a slightly bulkier (methyl) group, the factors particularly torsional and of steric strains may have some influence on the stability of the conformation. In fact, it has been found to be so. The energy barrier has been observed to be slightly higher than in ethane. Due to this higher energy barrier several conformers of *n*-butane are possible.

As in the case of ethane, different conformations of n-butane may be evolved. For this purpose, the rotation of the middle carbon-carbon (C_2—C_3) bond is considered while H, H, CH_3 are the substituents present at each of these two carbon atoms. On such consideration probable conformations of *n*-butane may be represented by Newman Projection formulae as depicted below in Fig. 3.10.

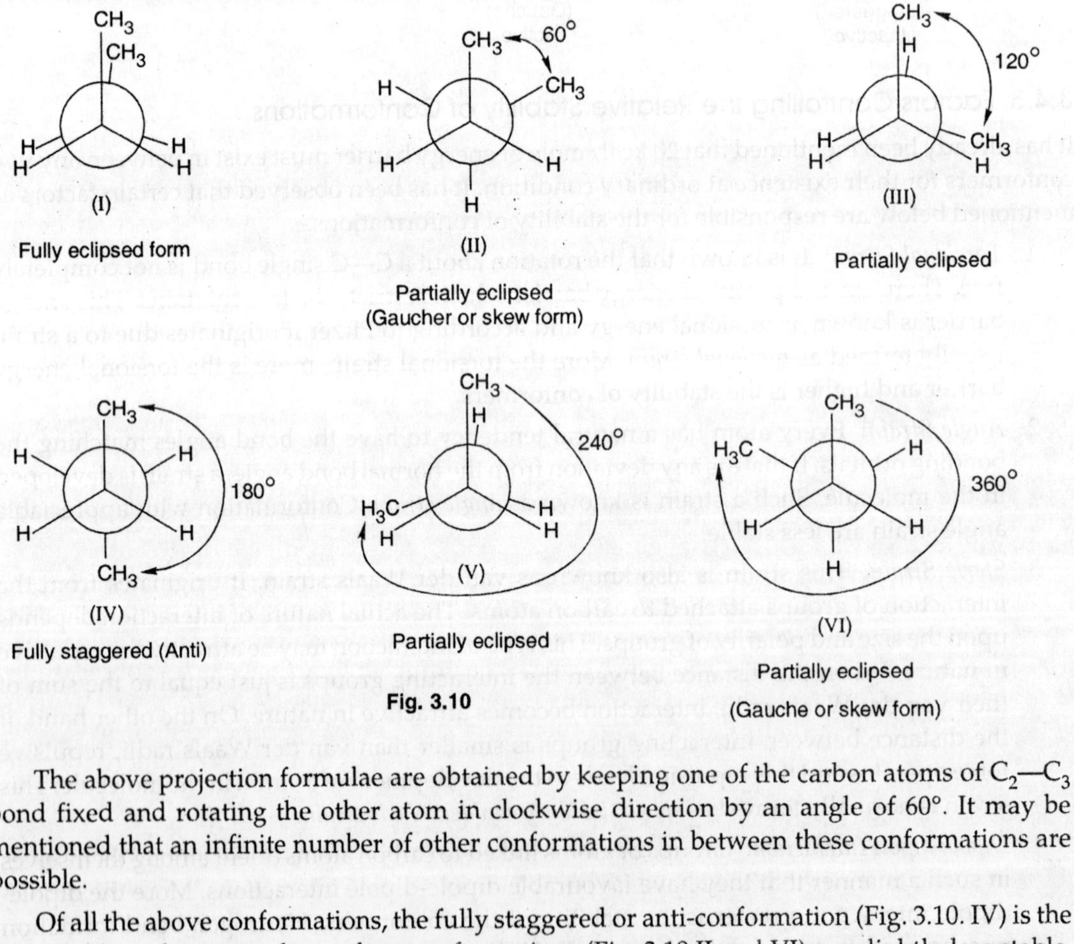

Fig. 3.10

The above projection formulae are obtained by keeping one of the carbon atoms of C_2—C_3 bond fixed and rotating the other atom in clockwise direction by an angle of 60°. It may be mentioned that an infinite number of other conformations in between these conformations are possible.

Of all the above conformations, the fully staggered or anti-conformation (Fig. 3.10. IV) is the most stable and two gauche or skew conformations (Fig. 3.10.II and VI) are slightly less stable. The eclipsed form (Fig. 3.10.I) is least stable while two partially eclipsed forms (Fig. 3.10.III and V) is slightly more stable than (Fig. 3.10.I). The energy difference between the most stable form

(Fig. 3.10.IV) and least stable conformation (Fig. 10.I) is about 6.8 kcal/mole while the difference between anti (most stable) form (Fig. 3.10.IV) and gauche forms (Fig. 3.10. II and VI) is about 0.8 kcal/mole. So it is expected and in fact, at ordinary condition *n*-butane predominantly exists in anti form along with some gauche forms. The potential energy changes during the rotation of C_2—C_3 bond in *n*-butane may be shown in Fig. 3.11 by the following graph.

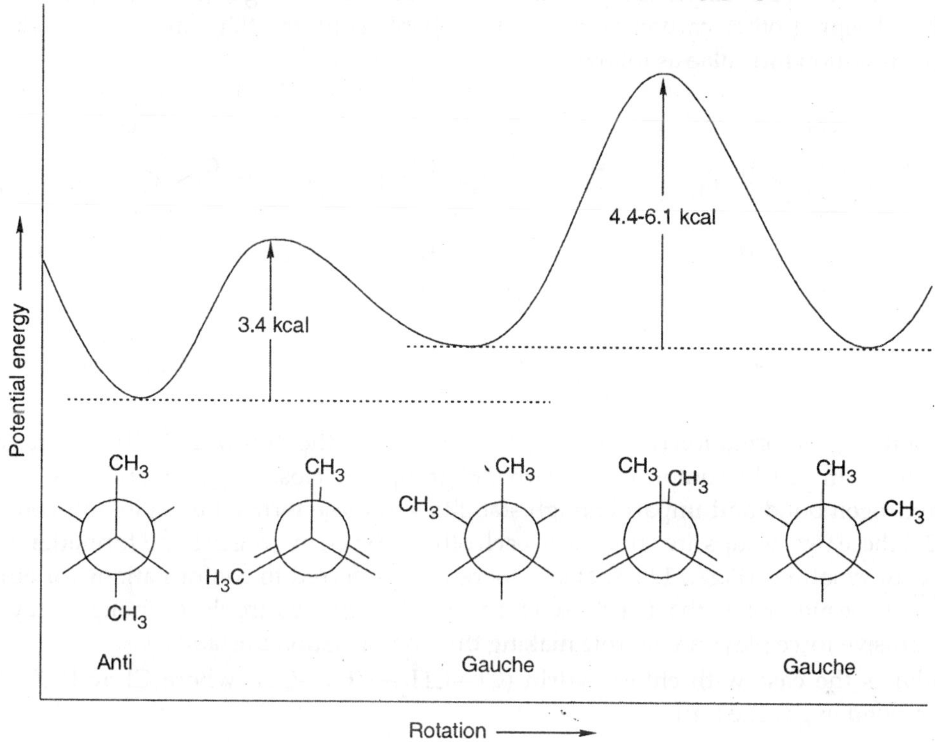

Fig. 3.11

3.4.5 Butane Gauche Interaction

As mentioned that in the case of butane, gauche forms are slightly less stable than the fully staggered form. This is due to the fact that in gauche forms probable interacting groups are close together as a result of which there may be interaction between them. The origin of this interaction may be due to different factors like angle strain, van der Waals strain, dipole-dipole interactions etc. These interactions change the energy content of the gauche forms—the energy may either be raised or may be diminished. So difference in stabilities between the fully staggered and gauche forms occur. This type of interaction due to which difference in stability originates in gauche forms is known as *gauche interactions*. Since occurrence of such interaction was first observed in the case of gauche forms of butane, it is usually termed as *butane gauche interaction*. The gauche interaction plays an important role in conformational analysis. Generally, torsional strain in gauche form is minimum, so gauche interaction has been assumed to originate from non-bonded interaction between two gauche groups which are sufficiently close and hence van der Waals strain develops. It may be mentioned that in acyclic and cyclic compounds conformational energy which is defined as the difference in energy between the most stable form and less stable gauche conformer, originates from gauche interaction.

3.4.6 Conformation of Some Alkane Derivatives

A few examples of conformations of alkane derivatives may be cited in this connection which provide interesting gauche interactions originating from different factors.

3.4.6.1 Conformations of Ethylene Glycol (HO—CH_2—CH_2—OH)

Ethylene glycol, like butane may be considered as a derivative of ethane in which one hydrogen of each carbon has been substituted by a hydroxyl group. So its conformation may be handled in the similar manner as in the case of ethane and butane.

The different forms of ethylene glycol may be evolved by rotating one of the carbon atoms of C—C bond keeping other carbon atom fixed. Probable conformations may be expressed by Newman projection formulae as follows:

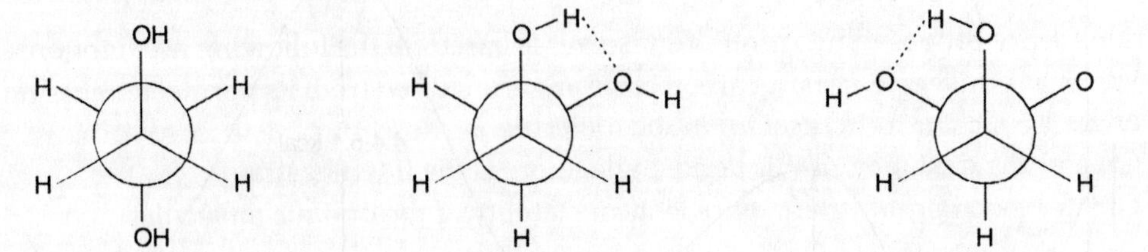

(a) Fully Staggered form (b) Gauche form (c) Gauche form

Fig. 3.12

Out of these, conformation (Fig. 3.12a) is staggered and other two (Fig. 3.12b & c) are gauche conformations. In gauche conformations two OH groups are closer together and they can form strong hydrogen bond and impart enough stabilities to these forms. But as in anti-conformer (Fig. 3.12a) these two groups are opposite to each other no such hydrogen bond formation occurs. Gauche conformations (Fig. 3.12b & c) are, therefore, preferred to conformations for ethylene glycol. It may be mentioned that in eclipsed form although groups are closer enough but van der Waals repulsive force plays a vital role making this conformation unstable.

Similar is the case with chlorohydrin (Cl—CH_2—CH_2—OH) where Cl and OH forms hydrogen bond in gauche form.

3.4.6.2 Conformations of 2, 3-Dimethyl Butane [CH_3—CH(CH_3)—CH(CH_3)—CH_3]

2, 3-dimethyl butane provides an interesting example of existence of bond angle strain. It exists in three different conformations as shown below in Fig. 3.13.

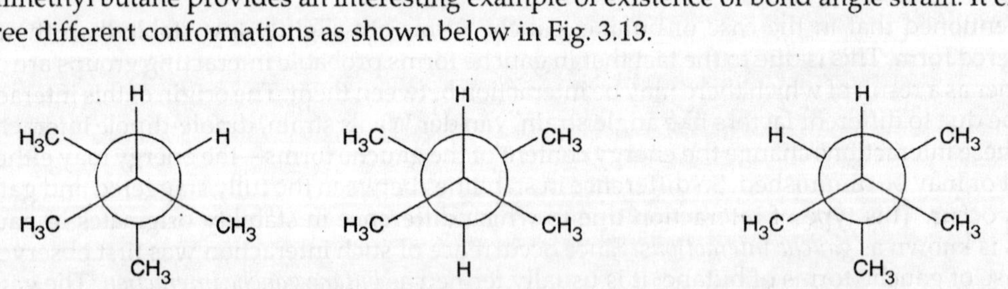

(a) Gauche form (b) Anti form or Fully staggered form (c) Gauche form

Fig. 3.13

From IR and NMR spectral measurements it has been established that at ordinary condition all the three conformations are present in equal proportion and the total concentration of gauche form is twice that of antiform. The conformational energy is, therefore, zero.

However, monomethyl butane preferably exists in antiform.

3.5 Baeyer's Strain Theory

For a long time it is an amazing experience to the chemists that smaller ring compounds are highly reactive and undergo ready ring opening reactions, and immense difficulty is faced in synthesising higher cyclic compounds. This observation prompted Baeyer to propose his theory known as **Baeyer's strain theory** in order to explain the high reactivity and instability of smaller ring compounds.

3.5.1 Assumption of Baeyer's Strain Theory

The strain theory proposed by Adolf Von Baeyer is based on the following assumptions:

i. When in a molecule carbon-carbon bond angle is shifted from its normal tetrahedral bond angle 109°28′, a strain is set up in the molecule.
ii. Greater the deviation of this bond angle, more is the internal strain.
iii. Greater the internal strain, more is the instability of the organic molecules.
iv. All the carbon atoms in cycloalkanes are coplanar.

Baeyer calculated the internal strain of different cycloalkanes and suggested that the rings smaller or larger than cyclopentane or cyclohexane are unstable and it is due to this instability smaller ring compounds readily undergo ring opening reactions while great difficulty arises to prepare the higher members of cycloalkanes.

However, Coulson and his associates on the basis of wave mechanical calculations observed that the high reactivity of small ring compounds is not due to ring as envisaged by Baeyer but due to incomplete overlapping of atomic orbitals during the formation of carbon-carbon bonds in cyclic compounds and so they challenged the validity of Baeyer's strain theory.

3.5.2 Theory of Strainless Ring (Conformation)

Under these circumstances *Sachse* and *Mohr* advanced their theory of *strainless ring*. According to their opinion, in cyclopropane and in its higher homologues the carbon atoms may not lie in the same plane as assumed by Baeyer but may assume strainless puckered configurations. In fact, it has been possible to prepare two models for cyclohexane ring system, the most common and significant member of alicyclic family, both of which are free from ring strain. These two models are chair and boat forms as shown below in Fig. 3.14.

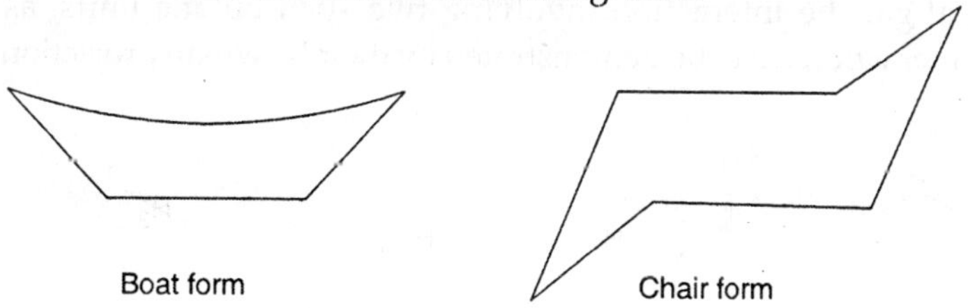

Boat form   Chair form

Fig. 3.14

Electron diffraction and thermodynamic considerations convincingly support the view that the chair form is the most stable form and at room temperature cyclohexane entirely exists in the *chair conformation*.

The chair conformation of cyclohexane possesses six-fold axis of symmetry which divides twelve carbon-hydrogen (C—H) bonds into two types. Six C—H bonds are parallel to the axis and are designated as *axial* bonds indicated by the symbol '*a*' while other six C—H bonds are directed upward at an angle of 109.5° to the axis and are known as *equatorial bonds* expressed by the symbol '*e*'. It may further be mentioned that cyclohexane ring is quite flexible, as a result of which one chair form may flip into another chair form. So bonds which are axial in one form become equatorial in other and viceversa. The energy barrier to this flipping is very small, it is approximately 10 kcal / mole. In the case of unsubstituted cyclohexane two forms are perfectly equivalent and indistinguishable as shown in Fig. 3.15.

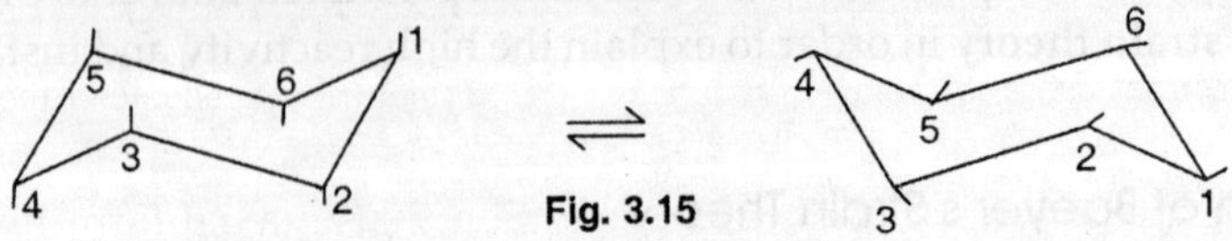

Fig. 3.15

Thus, the study of cycloalkanes marked the beginning of the study of a new concept—conformational analysis of stereochemistry.

3.5.2.1 Conformational Analyses of Substituted Cyclohexanes

Although, two forms of unsubstituted cyclohexane are perfectly equivalent and indistinguishable, but the situation is completely different in the case of substituted cyclohexanes. This is because in substituted cyclohexane, the substituent(s) can occupy either axial or equatorial positions and so different non equivalent conformations may originate. The different situations that may arise may be considered under following headings:

3.5.2.1.1 Conformations of Mono Substituted Cyclohexane

In mono substituted cyclohexane like methyl cyclohexane, the substituent-methyl group may be either at axial or at equatorial positions and exists in two non-equivalent diastereomeric conformations, one with methyl group in equatorial position and the other with methyl group in axial positions. These two forms exist in equilibrium as shown below in Fig. 3.16.

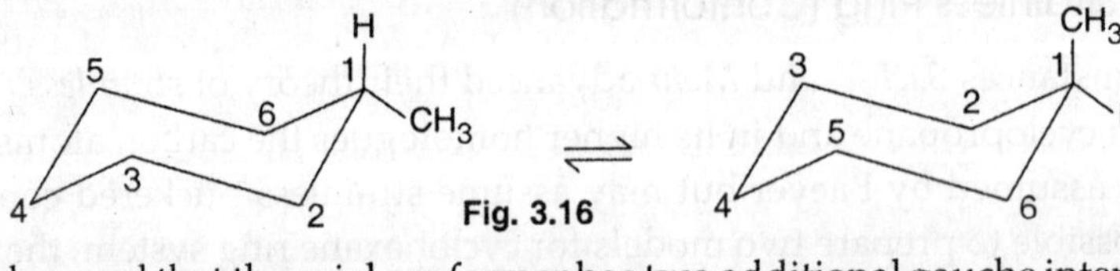

Fig. 3.16

It has been observed that the axial conformer has two additional gauche interactions involving $CH_3—C_1—C_2—C_3$ and $CH_3—C_1—C_6—C_5$ butane units while the equatorial conformation is free from any additional gauche interaction involving two such butane units, as they have anti-orientation. These interactions may be demonstrated by their Newman projection formulae drawn below (Fig. 3.17).

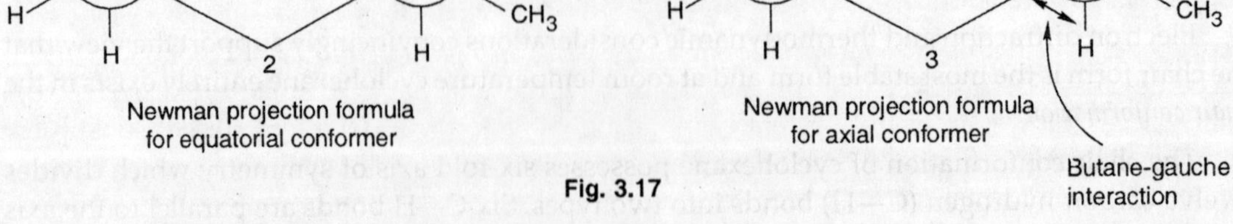

Fig. 3.17

The overall interactions of both the axial and equatorial conformers may be evident from the scrutiny of their structures as shown below in Fig. 3.18.

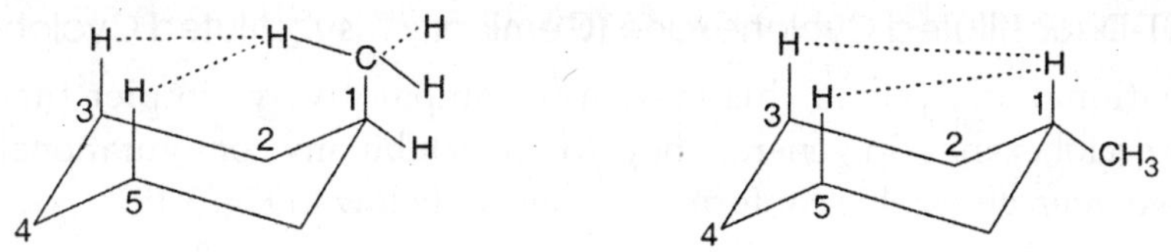

Conformer with axial methyl Conformer with equatorial methyl

Fig. 3.18

It is seen from the above structural representation that in axial form two axial hydrogen atoms on C_3 and C_5 are very close to axial methyl hydrogen. As a result there is a repulsive interaction due to over crowding in this conformer. On the otherhand, in equatorial form axial C_3—H and C_5—H are to some extent far apart from equatorial-methyl hydrogen. So there is less repulsive interaction.

Based on this observation it has been shown that the chair conformation with methyl group in equatorial position is stabler than its axial counterpart and in equilibrium equatorial conformer has predominant contribution (90%). It may be mentioned in this connection that when the substituent larger than methyl group is present, the predominancy of equatorial conformation is raised to 100%. This is due to the fact that in the case of large substituent, flipping of the ring is prevented. These interactions of axial atoms or groups at 1 and 3 or 5-positions are known as 1, 3-*diaxial interaction*. It has been observed that due to this 1, 3-diaxial interaction very large group like tert-butyl always occupies equatorial position in its preferred form and is often called *anchoring group*.

In many cases a large energy difference between the axial and equatorial conformers is observed. The energy difference [conformational free energies (– 4G° values)] of some common substituents are tabulated below.

Group	Conformational free energy (– 4G°) kcal/mole	Group	Conformational free energy (– 4G°) kcal/mole
$—CH_3$	1.74	—Cl	0.50
$—C_2H_5$	1.75	—F	0.25
$—CH(CH_3)_2$	2.15	OH	0.92
$—C(CH_3)_3$	4.85	$—NH_2$	1.40
$—C_6H_5$	2.75	$—OCH_3$	0.75
—I	0.45	—OAC	0.72
—Br	0.48	—OTS	0.52

3.5.2.1.2 Conformations of Disubstituted Cyclohexanes

The general principle of conformational analysis as applied in the case of mono-substituted cyclohexane is also applicable for the conformational analysis of disubstituted cyclohexane derivatives. However, in this system two additional factors viz., (i) interaction of substituents among themselves sterically or in other way and (ii) existence of disubstituted system in two or more diastereo forms, each of which can have two or more conformers, may be involved. So in order to have an insight into conformational aspects of disubstituted cyclohexanes these two additional factors are to be considered. As a result conformational analysis of this system may be to some extent complicated.

3.5.2.1.3 1,1-Disubstituted Cyclohexane (Geminally Disubstituted Cyclohexanes)

The conformational analysis of this system is comparatively simpler than that of other disubstituted cyclohexanes. In general, they do not exhibit any configurational isomerism but can exist in two interconvertible conformers as shown below in Fig. 3.19.

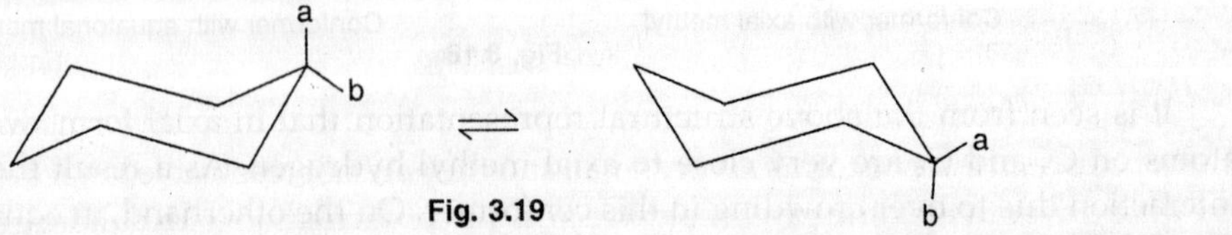

Fig. 3.19

When the two substituents a and b are the same as in 1, 1,— dimethyl cyclohexane two conformers are identical but when a and b are different two conformers are diastereomers and are present in unequal amount in the equilibrium. In general, the conformer with bulkier substituent at the equatorial position predominantes. However, other factors like steric interaction may interfere.

3.5.2.1.4 Other Disubstituted Cyclohexanes

Non-geminally disubstituted cyclohexanes can exist in three isomeric forms, e.g., 1, 2; 1, 3 and 1, 4 —isomers and each isomer can structurally be *cis* or *trans*. The different situations that may arise are tabulated below.

Compound	Isomer	
	cis	*trans*
1, 2-Disubstituted cyclohexane	ae or ea	ee or aa
1, 3-Disubstituted cyclohexane	ee or aa	ae or ea
1, 4-Disubstituted cyclohexane	ae or ea	ee or aa

a = axial, e = equatorial

3.5.2.1.4.1 1, 2-Disubstituted Cyclohexane

From the above table it is evident that *trans* 1, 2-disubstituted cyclohexane can exist in two conformations. In one, both the substituents are in axial position and in other, both the groups are equatorially oriented. Thus,

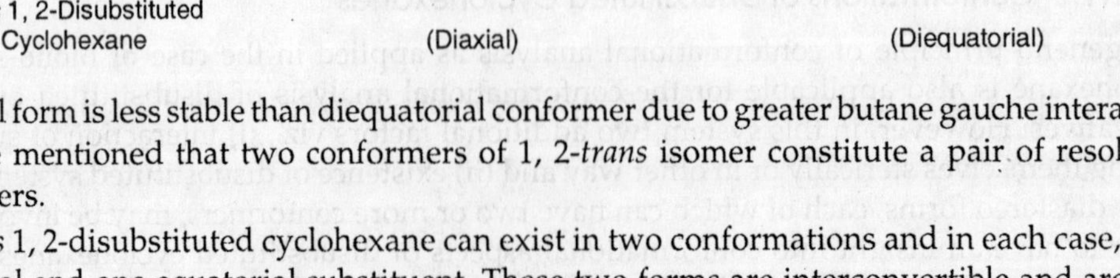

trans 1, 2-Disubstituted Cyclohexane (Diaxial) (Diequatorial)

Diaxial form is less stable than diequatorial conformer due to greater butane gauche interaction. It may be mentioned that two conformers of 1, 2-*trans* isomer constitute a pair of resolvable enantiomers.

The *cis* 1, 2-disubstituted cyclohexane can exist in two conformations and in each case, there is one axial and one equatorial substituent. These two forms are interconvertible and are non-super imposable mirror images of each other.

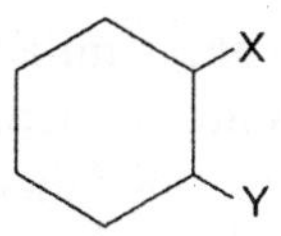

cis-1, 2-Disubstituted Cyclohexane

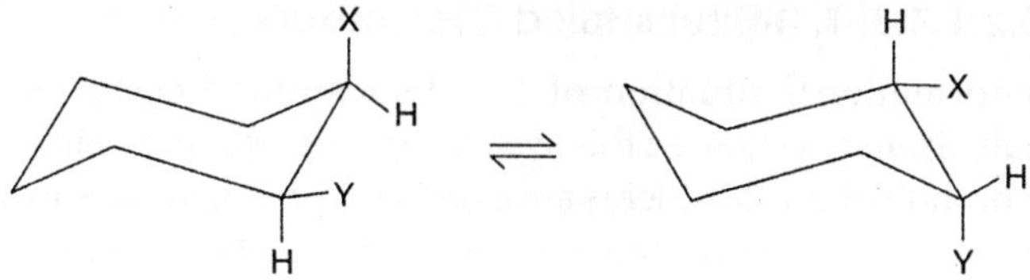

Axial-equatorial

Equatorial-axial

When both the groups are identical, as in the case of 1, 2-dimethyl cyclohexane, the energy barrier between the two forms is very small and they are not resolvable but if the two substituents are different both the forms are resolvable and the conformation with bulkier group in equatorial position predominates.

3.5.2.1.4.2 1, 3-Disubstituted Cyclohexane

The situation is entirely reverse in the case of 1, 3-disubstituted cyclohexanes. As seen from the above table, in this system *cis*-isomer can assume either diaxial or diequatorial conformation while *trans*-isomer is axial-equatorially (a, e) or equatorial-axially (e, a) oriented. As usual, the diaxial conformation of *cis*-isomer is less favourable than its diequatorial conformation due to gauche interaction involving severe steric overcrowding by two axial substituents while no such gauche interaction is present in diequatorial conformation. So the diequatorial conformation is the preferred conformation for *cis*-1, 3-disubstituted cyclohexanes. On the other hand, *trans*-isomer (a, e or e, a) suffers from gauche interaction and is less stable than *cis*-isomer. Thus, unlike 1, 2-disubstituted system, the *cis*-1, 3-system is more stable than 1, 3-trans isomer. When the two groups are different, both *cis*- and *trans*-isomers are resolvable, *cis*-isomer obviously exists in diequatorial conformation and the *trans*-isomer in equatorial-axial conformation with bulkier substituent in equatorial position. But if the two groups are identical as in the case of 1, 3-dimethyl cyclohexane, they cannot be resolved and so they are *meso*.

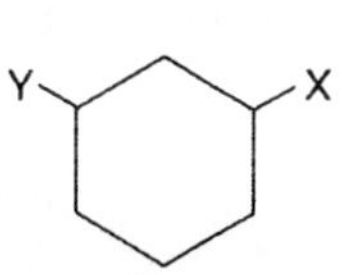

cis-1, 3-Disubstituted Cyclohexane

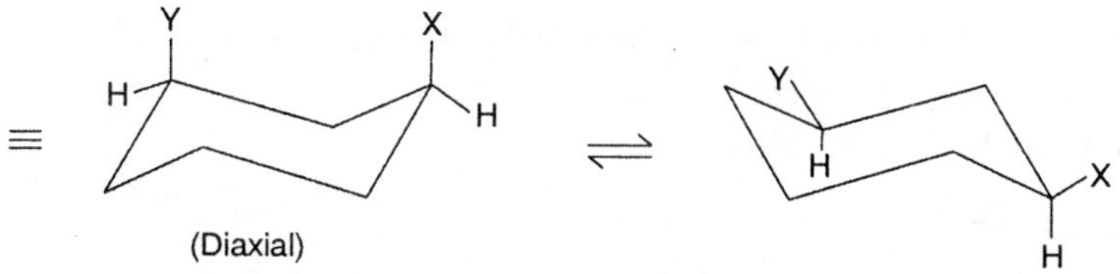

(Diaxial)

(Diequatorial)

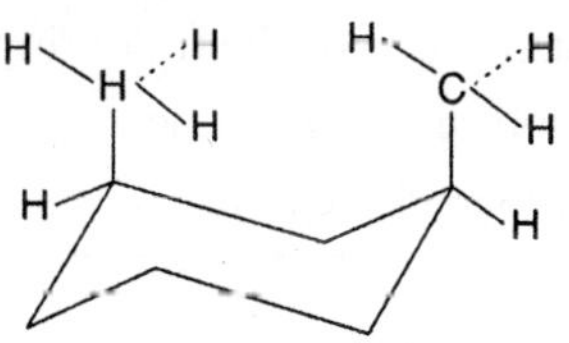

Steric interference of diaxial conformer of 1, 3-dimethyl cyclohexane

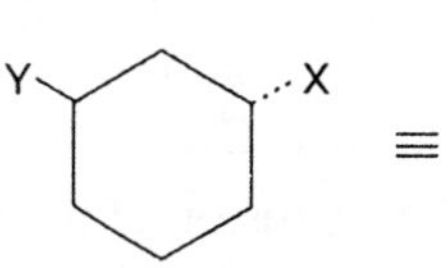

trans -1, 3-Disubstituted

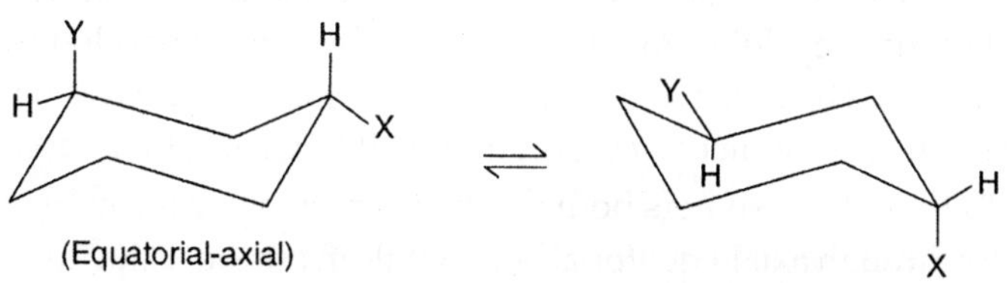

(Equatorial-axial)

(Axial-Equatorial)

3.5.2.1.4.3 1, 4-Disubstituted Cyclohexane

Conformational situation of 1, 4-disubstituted cyclohexane system is very similar to 1, 2-disubstituted system. In this system *trans*-isomer exists in two non-equivalent conformations — in one, both the substituents are axial while in other, they are equatorial. As expected diequatorial conformation is more stable and is present in 99% at equilibrium. The *trans*-isomer is also more stable than *cis*-isomer which exists in two identical axial-equatorial (a, e) or equatorial-axial (a, e) conformations. When both the substituents are different, the 1, 4-*trans*-isomer preferably exists in diequatorial conformation but *cis*-isomer exists predominantly in equatorial-axial conformer with the larger group at equatorial position. It may be mentioned that when both the substituents are identical, these two stereoisomers are achiral as they possess a plane of symmetry.

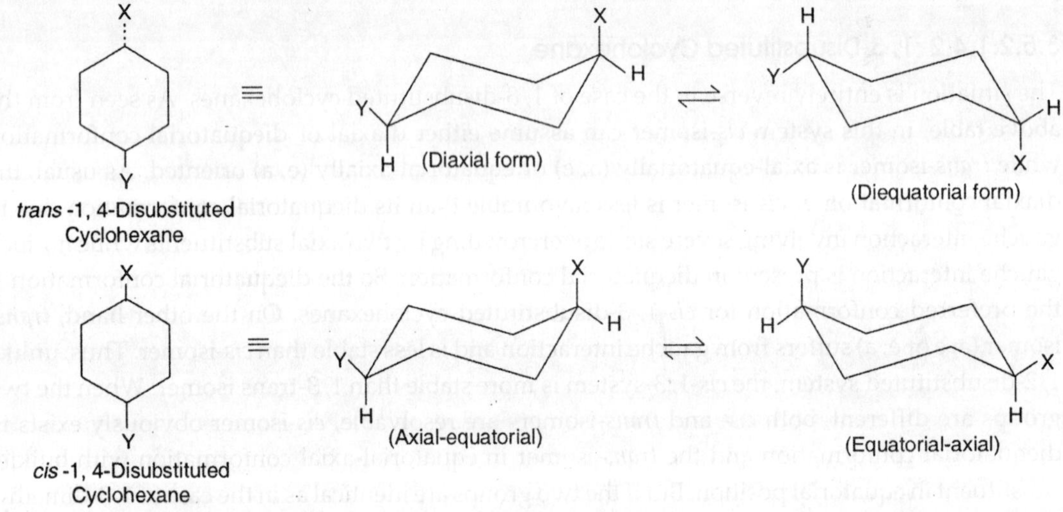

In conclusion it may be mentioned that although the views discussed above for the disubstituted cyclohexane system is valid in most of the cases but in some instances discrepancy may arise due to interference of some factors like dipole-dipole interaction, hydrogen bond formation, high steric effect, etc.

PROBLEM 3.5

1. Predict which form of methyl cyclohexane predominates at equilibrium.
2. Draw the preferred conformations of the following:
   (a) *trans*-1-*tert*-butyl-2-2methyl cyclohexane.
   (b) *cis*-1-methyl-3-*iso*-propyl cyclohexane.

3.5.2.2 Conformational Analysis of Fused Ring System (Decalin)

Decalin is a very commonly encountered organic compound. It may be looked upon as a 1, 2-disubstituted cyclohexane derivative. In decalin two cyclohexane rings are fused together at 1, 2-positions. The fusion of two cyclohexane may be in *cis* or in *trans* manner and so it can exist in two geometric isomers—*cis*-decalin (bp 195 °C) and *trans*-decalin (bp 184 °C).

In these two isomers both the rings are in chair form. In *cis*-isomer, fusion of the two rings occurs through axial-equatorial bond while in *trans*-decalin, fusion of the rings involves equatorial-

equatorial bonds. In *trans*-decalin there is no additional gauche-butane interaction whereas in *cis*-decalin there are three such additional interactions involving C_1—C_9—C_8—C_7, C_1—C_9—C_{10}—C_5 and C_3—C_4—C_{10}—C_5 butane units. So *cis*-decalin is less stable than *trans*- isomer. Since ring juncture of *cis*-decalin involves axial-equatorial bonds it has one equatorial and one axial angular hydrogen. This imparts this isomer a higher degree of flexibility. But as the ring fusion in *trans*-decalin takes place through two equatorial bonds it has two angular hydrogen in axial conformation. This makes the structure of *trans*-decalin rigid. For this reason *cis*-decalin can be readily converted to *trans*-isomer on heating but it is impossible to convert *trans*-decalin into its *cis* counterpart.

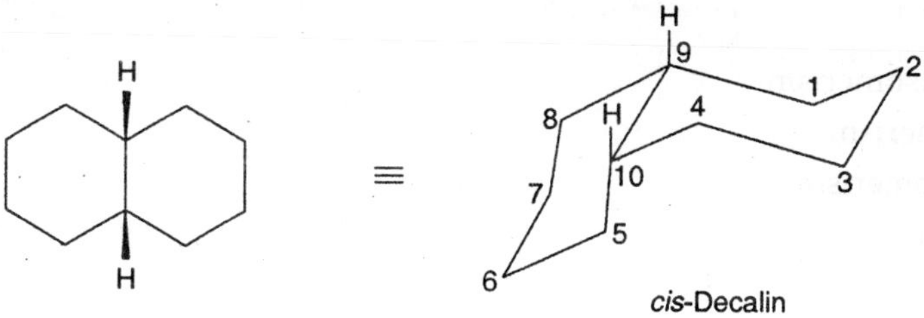

cis-Decalin

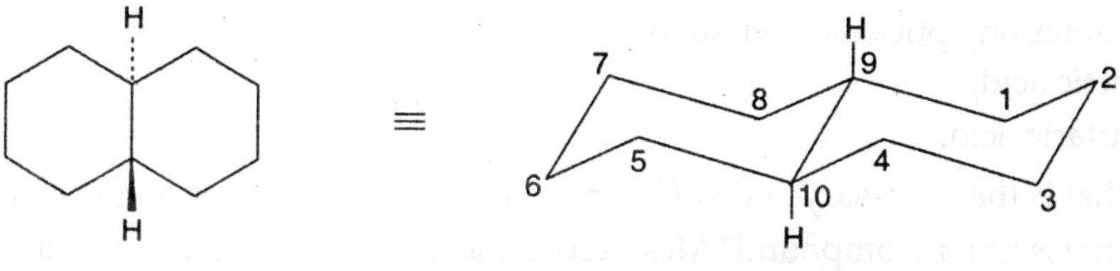

trans-Decalin

PROBLEM 3.6

Draw the conformational structures of chlorohydrin and monomethyl butane.

Model Questions

1. What is stereoisomerism? What are different kinds of stereoisomerism?
2. What is meant by the following:
   (a) Plane polarised light,
   (b) Optical activity,
   (c) Specific rotation of an optically active substance,
   (d) Enantiomerism,
   (e) Fischer's projection formula,
   (f) Racemic modification.
3. (a) What is the essential condition of optical activity of a substance?
   (b) Prove that presence or absence of a chiral carbon in a molecule is not the necessary and sufficient criterion for the existence of optical activity.
4. (a) Explain giving example the phenomenon of racemisation.
   (b) How will you distinguish Meso and Racemic forms?

5. Describe various methods for resolution of racemic mixtures.
6. What is asymmetric synthesis?
7. What is meant by geometrical isomerism? Show that hindered rotation around a carbon-carbon double bond gives rise to geometrical isomerism.
8. (a) What are the conditions to be fulfilled for exhibiting geometrical isomerism by a compound?
   (b) How will you determine the configuration of a geometrical isomer?
9. Explain clearly E and Z designations of geometrical isomers.
10. Write notes on
    (a) Structural Isomerism
    (b) Chain Isomerism
    (c) Position Isomerism
    (d) Metamerism
    (e) Enantiomers
    (f) Diastereomers
    (g) Racemisation.
11. Write notes on optical isomerism of
    (a) Lactic acid,
    (b) Tartaric acid.
12. (a) What is the necessary and sufficient condition for a compound to be optically active?
    (b) What is a *meso* compound? Meso-tartaric acid is optically inactive due to the presence of plane of symmetry within the molecule-how far this statement is correct?
    (c) Explain the term optical purity.
13. (a) What are geometrical isomers? How do they differ from optical isomers? Explain with example.
    (b) Discuss the chirality of tartatic acid in terms of symmetry elements.
    (c) What is the optical purity of a sample isolated from a reaction having an obs = 6°, if $[\alpha]_D = +12°$?
14. (a) What do you mean to say by "enantiomeric excess"?
    (b) How do the terms 'asymmetric' and 'disymmetric' differ?
    (c) "Plane of symmetry and centre of symmetry both may be regarded as the special case of alternating symmetry."— Justify the statement.
    (d) What do you mean by the terms "enantiomers" and "diastereoisomers"? How do they differ?
15. Assign R and S configuration to the following:

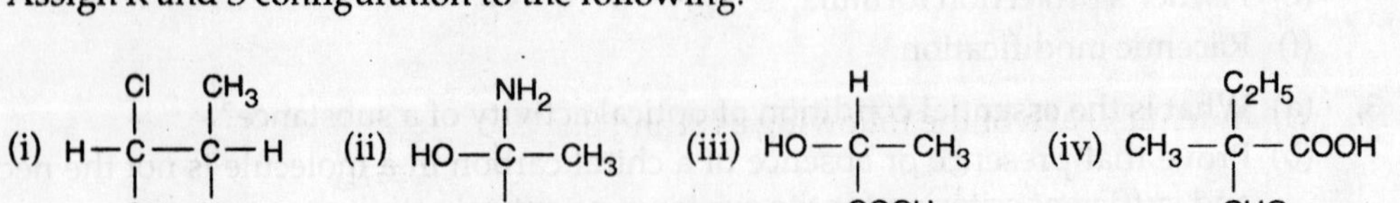

(v) 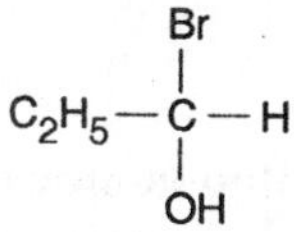 (vi) 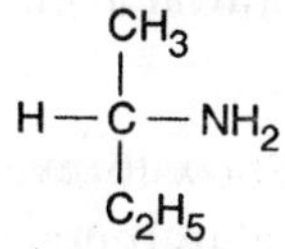 (vii) 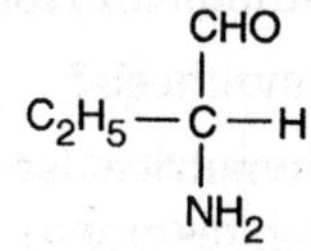 (viii) 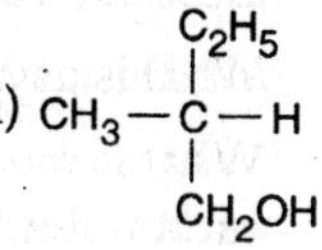

(ix) 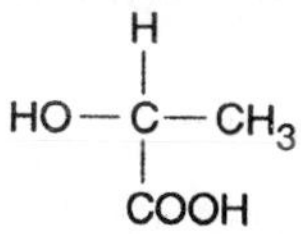 (x) 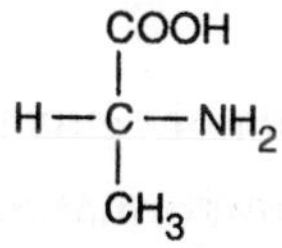 (xi) 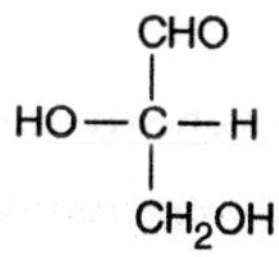 (xii) 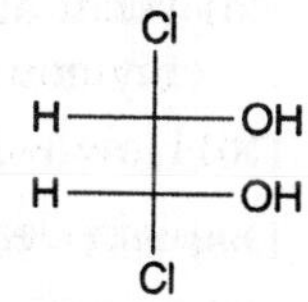

(xiii) 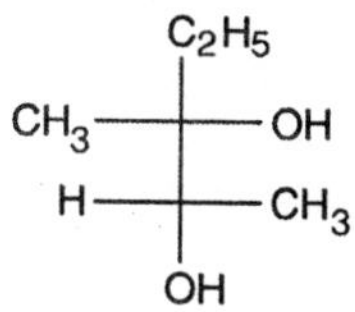 (xiv) 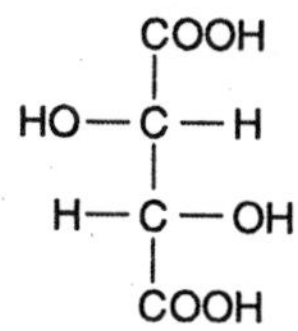 (xv) 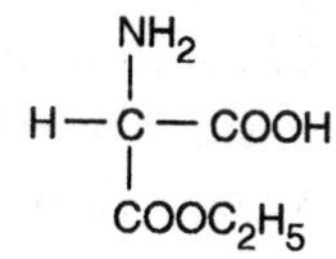

(xvi) 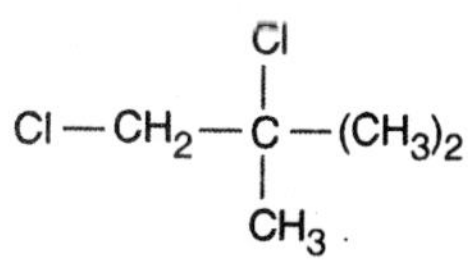 (xvii) 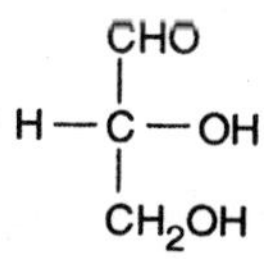 (xviii) 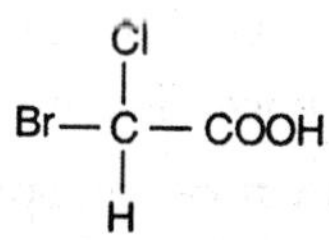

(xix) 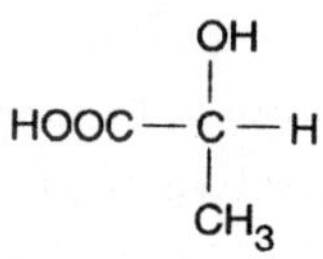 (xx) 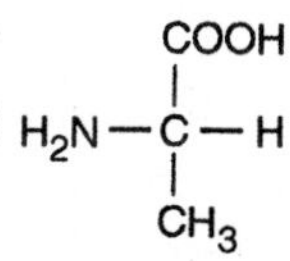 (xxi) 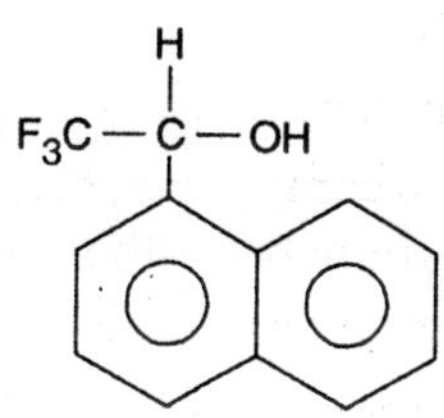 (xxii) 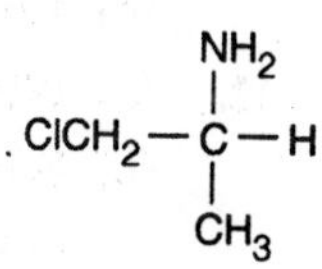

16. Write down the Fischer projection forms of the following compounds:

i. (2R, 3R)-Butane dioic acid.
ii. (3S, 4R)-3-chloro-4-4methyl hexane.
iii. (R)-3, 4-dimethyl-pent-1-ene
iv. (2R, 3R)-2, 3-dihydroxy-1, 4-butane dioic acid
v. (2R, 3R, 4S)-2, 3, 4-trihydroxy glutaric acid

17. Assign E/Z configurations to each of the following alkenes:

(i) 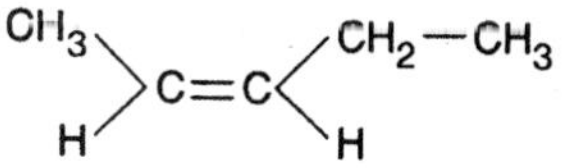 (ii) 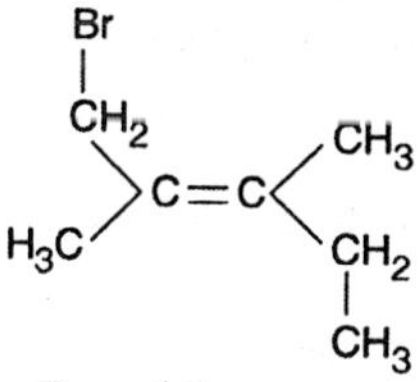

18. (i) Indentify each of the following as R and S:

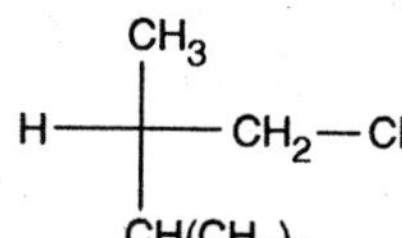 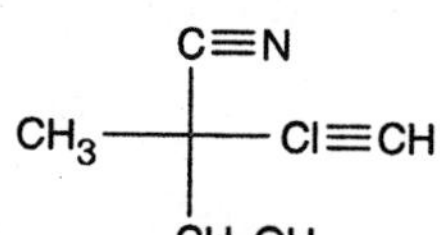

(ii) What is the simplest alkane that is optically active?

(iii) Designate 2-Butanol in R, S nomenclature.

19. What is butane-gauche interaction? Draw the conformation 2-methyl butane for rotation about C_2—C_3 bond in Newman projection formula and compare their relative stabilities.

20. What do you mean by conformational analysis? Draw the qualitative enrrgy profile diagram for ethylene glycol.

21. Discuss Newman and Sawhorse representations of ethane.

22. Discuss factors affecting relative stability of conformations.

23. Discuss the conformation of stilbene dichloride.

24. Explain the conformation of butane.

CHAPTER FOUR

Hydrocarbons (Alkanes and Cycloalkanes)

As the name implies this class of organic compounds contain only carbon and hydrogen atoms in their molecule. There is no conventional functional groups in this type of compounds. Based on their structures and reactivity hydrocarbons have been classified into two main categories- *aliphatic hydrocarbons* and *aromatic hydrocarbons*.

Aliphatic hydrocarbons are further subdivided into four major groups — alkane, alkene, alkyne and their cyclic analogs — alicyclic or cyclic aliphatic. Thus,

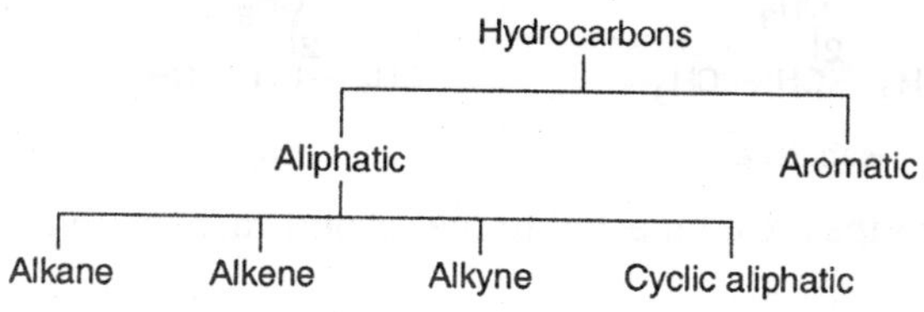

Alkanes are hydrocarbons in which all the bonds are single bonds, alkenes contain carbon-carbon double bond(s), alkynes possess carbon-carbon tripple bond(s) while cyclic aliphatic hydrocarbons may or may not contain any double or tripple bond but they are cyclic in nature.

Aromatic hydrocarbons are different in properties from aliphatic hydrocarbons. They are cyclic unsaturated (double bonded) compounds having unusual properties. They are also known as *arenes*.

Various principles of organic chemistry can be developed in a systematic manner by examining different hydrocarbons separately in the order of alkane, alkene, alkyne, alicyclic and arenes and as such these different classes of hydrocarbons have been discussed in the order mentioned above in different chapters.

4.1 Alkanes

Alkanes are the simple aliphatic organic hydrocarbons. They are expressed by the general formula, C_nH_{2n+2}, where n is any integer, 1, 2, 3, 4, etc. Carbons in these hydrocarbons are connected to each other by single covalent bond and hydrogen atoms involved are also bonded by covalent bonds. As there is no π-bond in their structures, they are fully saturated by hydrogen atoms. For this reason they are also known as *Saturated Hydrocarbons.* Since in alkanes strong carbons-carbon and carbon-hydrogen bonds are involved they display stability towards variety of reagents, i.e., they are chemically inert. That is why they are also known as *paraffins* meaning less affinity towards reagents.

Alkanes enjoy special importance due to the fact that they are the major constituents of petrol, kerosene oil, diesel oil and lubricants and numerous commodities in common use in our day-to-day life.

4.1.1 Nomenclature of Alkanes

First four members of alkanes are known by their trivial names, methane, CH_4, ethane, C_2H_6, propane, C_3H_8 and butane, C_4H_{10} but for the higher members names are derived from Greek numerals to indicate the number of carbon atoms in the molecule. To the prefix of such numerals suffix-*'ane'* is added. Thus, pentane has five carbon atoms, hexane six, heptane seven and so on. In trivial system of nomenclature, a prefix *n* is used for straight chain hydrocarbon, *n* stands for normal.

$CH_3-CH_2-CH_3$	$CH_3-CH_2-CH_2-CH_3$	$CH_3-CH_2-CH_2-CH_2-CH_3$
n-propane or normal propane	*n*-butane or normal butane	*n*-pentane or normal pentane

But in the case of branched chain alkane, prefix *'iso'* and *'neo'* are used. When only one methyl group is attached to second carbon of the straight chain, it is known as *'iso'*. For example,

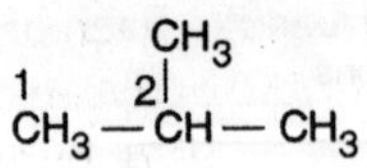

isobutane

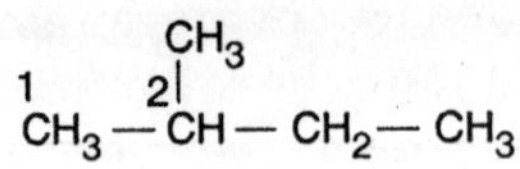

isopentane

But if two methyl groups are connected to the second carbon atom, the prefix *'neo'* is used. Thus,

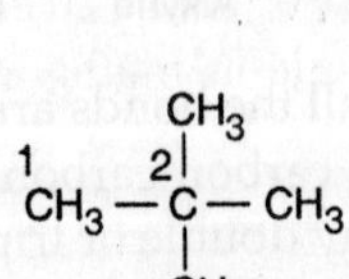

Neopentane

In trivial system carbom atoms have been classified as *primary, secondary, tertiary,* and *quaternary.*

i. When a carbon atom is attached to only one or no other carbon atom, it is known as *primary carbon* or 1° carbon.
ii. When a carbon atom is connected to two other carbon atoms, it is *secondary carbon* or 2° carbon.
iii. If a carbon atom is connected to three other carbon atoms, it is called *tertiary carbon* or 3° carbon.
iv. A carbon atom with four carbons attached to it is known as *quaternary carbon* denoted by 4°.

A single example may be cited to elaborate the above four types of carbon atoms.

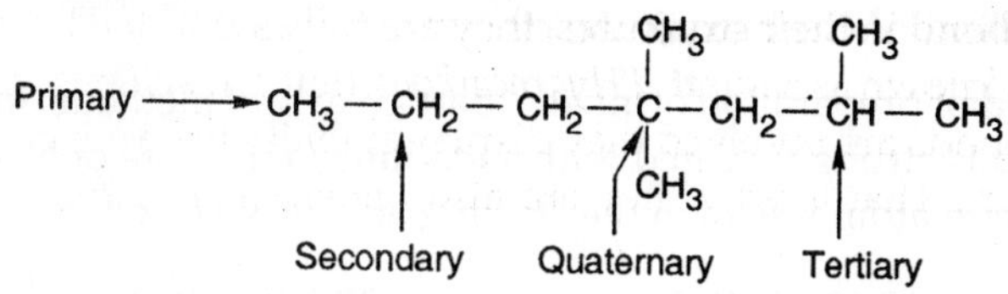

However, alkanes are systematically named following IUPAC system of nomenclature as discussed in chapter **three**. For example,

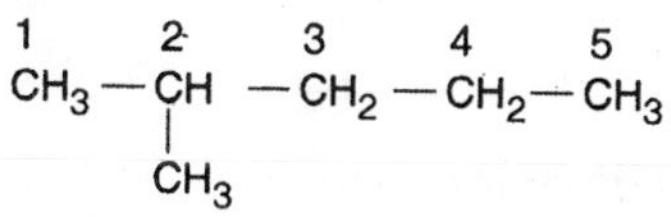

2-Methyl pentane

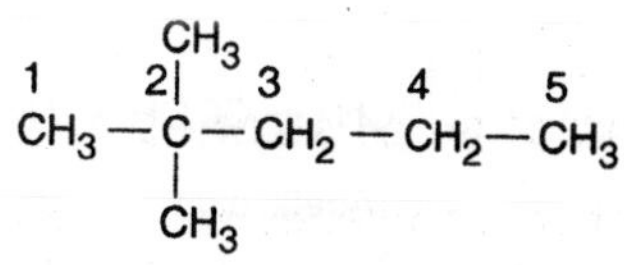

2, 2-Dimethyl pentane

4.1.2 Methane

The first and simplest member of alkane group of hydrocarbons is methane. Its molecular formula is CH_4. The study of this alkane in detail will allow us to have a clear picture regarding the various aspects of alkane family because most of the characteritics of methane are applicable to other members of alkane family with minor modifications. We, therefore, confine our discussion on this member with some additional points applicable to other members.

4.1.2.1 Structure of Methane

Methane has one carbon and four hydrogen atoms in its molecule. Each of these four hydrogen atoms are bonded to carbon atom by covalent bond. The bonding between carbon and hydrogen involves overlapping of sp^3-hybrid orbitals of carbon and *s*-orbitals of hydrogen atom.

All the four C—H bonds are σ in nature. The configuation of ground state is a perfect tetrahedron and the four hydrogen atoms are located at the four corners of this tetrahedron. Since in this tetrahedral arrangement most effective overlapping of orbitals is possible, the σ-bond formed is very strong. The bond angle in methane is 109.28° and C—H bond length is 1.09Å (Fig. 4.1).

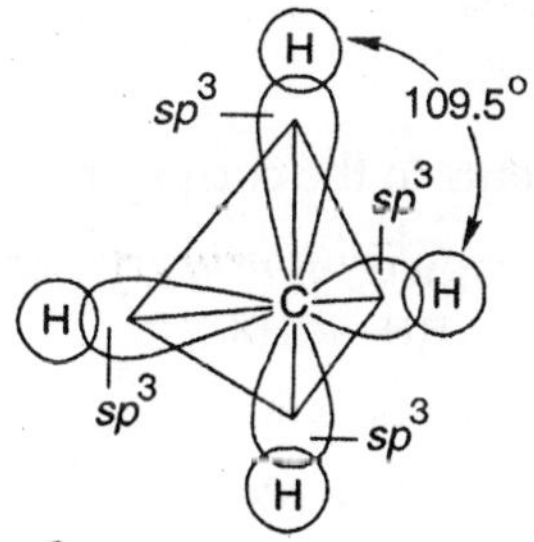

sp^3 hybrid orbitals of methane

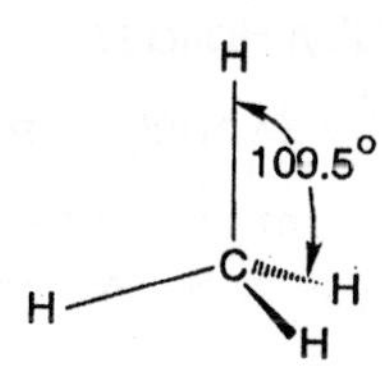

Methane molecule

Structure of Methane

Fig. 4.1

4.1.3 General Methods of Preparation of Alkanes

Some of the most common methods of preparation of alkanes are discussed in the sequel.

4.1.3.1 Decarboxylation of Carboxylic Acids

It is a laboratory method of preparation of alkane, particularly of methane. In this method sodium salt of a carboxylic acid is strongly heated with soda lime (a mixture of NaOH and CaO), when alkane having one carbon atom less than the starting acid is obtained.

$$R{-}COOH + NaOH \longrightarrow R{-}COONa + H_2O$$

$$R{-}COONa \xrightarrow[\text{Heat}]{\text{Soda lime}} R{-}H + Na_2CO_3$$

$$\underset{\text{Acetic acid}}{CH_3{-}COOH} + NaOH \longrightarrow \underset{\text{Na-acetate}}{CH_3{-}COONa} + H_2O$$

$$CH_3COONa \xrightarrow[\text{Heat}]{\text{Soda lime}} CH_4 + Na_2CO_3$$

Since in this process a molecule of CO_2 is eliminated it is known as decarboxylation process.

Mechanistically dcarboxylation takes place as

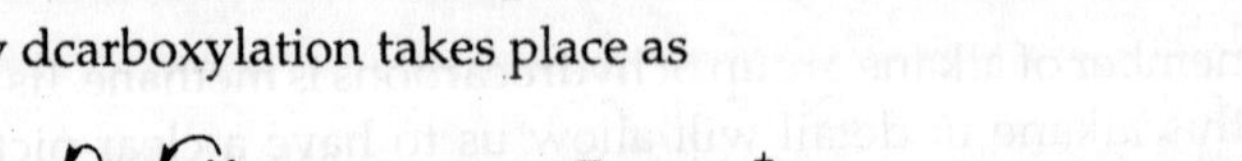

From above path it is evident that decarboxylation is due to flow of electron-pair from oxygen of carboxylic OH to carbon. So if the density of electrons on oxygen of OH is increased, rate of decarboxylation will be high. Metallic salt of any acid can readily ionise forming carboxylate anion having higher electron density and hence decarboxylation takes place rapidly.

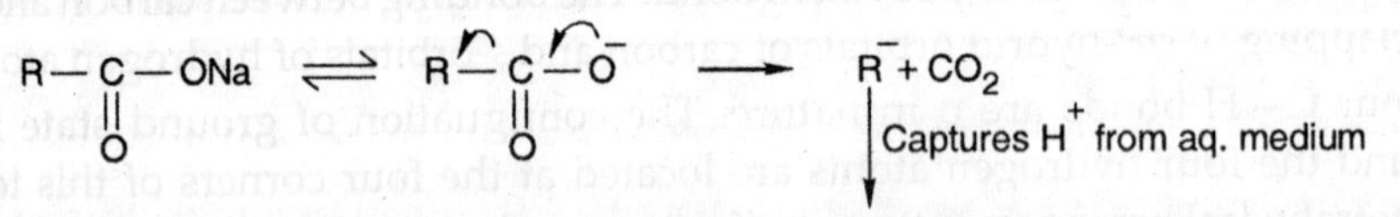

For this reason salt of an acid decarboxylates more rapidly than free acid and hence in this method salts but not the free acids are used.

4.1.3.2 Reduction of Alkyl Halides

Alkyl halide is reduced by a variety of reducing agents to the corresponding hydrocarbon.

$$R{-}X \xrightarrow[\text{agent}]{\text{Reducing}} RH + HX$$

$$CH_3{-}X \xrightarrow[\text{agent}]{\text{Reducing}} CH_4 + HX$$

Reducing agents commonly used are zinc and acetic acid, zinc-copper couple and alcohol, magnesium amalgam and water, etc. In the case of reduction of alkyl iodide mixture of HI and red phosporus are used.

$$CH_3{-}CH_2{-}CH_2{-}I \xrightarrow{\text{HI, P}} CH_3{-}CH_2{-}CH_3 + I_2$$

4.1.3.3 Decomposition of Grignard Reagent

In this method, a Grignard reagent is prepared in the first step by reaction of an alkyl halide with magnesium metal in dry ether.

$$R-X + Mg \xrightarrow{\text{dry ether}} \underset{\text{Grignard reagent}}{R-MgX}$$

In the next step, Grignard reagent is decomposed with water to form alkane.

$$R-MgX + H_2O \longrightarrow R-H + Mg(OH)X$$

$$CH_3-Br + Mg \xrightarrow[\text{ether}]{\text{dry}} CH_3MgBr$$

$$CH_3MgBr \xrightarrow{H_2O} CH_4 + Mg\langle{}^{OH}_{X}$$

4.1.3.4 Kolbe's Electrolytic Process

In Kolbe's process alkanes are obtained when concentrated solution of sodium or potassium salts of fatty acids are electrolysed.

$$2R-COONa \xrightarrow{\text{Electrolysis}} R-R + 2CO_2 + 2NaOH + H_2\uparrow$$

The process is regarded as a free radical reaction. Sodium salt ionises to yield carboxylate anion which loses an electron at the anode to form carboxylate radical. This radical rapidly loses CO_2 to generate an alkane radical. Two such alkane radicals combine each other to form a hydrocarbon.

$$R-COONa \rightleftharpoons RCO\bar{O} + \overset{+}{Na}$$

$$RCO\bar{O} \xrightarrow{-e} R-CO\dot{O} \xrightarrow{-CO_2} \dot{R} + CO_2$$

$$\dot{R} + \dot{R} \longrightarrow R-R \quad \text{[at anode]}$$

$$2\overset{+}{Na} + 2e \longrightarrow 2\dot{Na} + H_2O \longrightarrow 2NaOH + H_2\uparrow \text{[at cathode]}$$

From the above path it is evident that methane cannot be prepared by this process. This method is applicable for the preparation of alkanes containing at least two carbon atoms.

4.1.3.5 Wurtz Reaction

This reaction involves the reaction between two molecules of alkyl halides in presence of metallic sodium in dry ether.

$$2R-X + 2Na \xrightarrow{\text{dry ether}} R-R + 2NaX$$

Two different mechanisms have been suggested—one involves free radical path while the second one conceives the existence of sodium alkyl intermediate.

$$R-X + Na \longrightarrow \dot{R} + NaBr$$

$$\dot{R} + \dot{R} \longrightarrow R-R$$

Or

$$R-X + 2Na \longrightarrow \overset{-}{R}\overset{+}{Na} + NaX$$

Sodium Alkyl

$$\overset{-}{R}\overset{+}{Na} + R-X \longrightarrow R-R + NaX$$

Comments: (i) This process is applicable for the synthesis of alkanes containing more than two carbon atoms. (ii) When interaction between two different alkyl halides takes place, mixtures of alkanes are obtained. Separation of individual alkane is extremely difficult due to their little difference in physical properties.

$$R-X + R'-X + 2Na \xrightarrow{\text{dry ether}} R-R + R'-R' + R-R' + 2NaX$$

4.1.3.6 Corey-House Synthesis

This synthesis involves the use of an important organometallic compound lithium dialkyl-cuprates. In this method an alkyl halide and lithium dialkyl cuprate are allowed to react to give higher hydrocarbon.

$$R'-X + (R)_2CuLi \longrightarrow R-R' + RCu + LiX$$

The key step of mechanism appears to be nucleophilic attack to alkyl halide by negatively charged copper.

$$(R)_2CuLi \rightleftharpoons R_2\overset{-}{Cu} + \overset{+}{Li}$$

$$(R)_2-\overset{-}{Cu} + R'-X \longrightarrow \left[R_2-Cu-R'\right]^{+}X \longrightarrow R-R' + RCu + \overset{-}{X}$$

This is a very good method and can be used for the preparation of straight chain, branched chain, symmetrical and unsymmetrical hydrocarbons. To get reasonably better yield both alkyl halide and alkyl groups in dialkyl cuprate should be primary to avoid steric hindrance that may be created by secondary and tertiary alkyl groups.

4.1.4 Properties of Alkanes

4.1.4.1 Isomerism

As there is a great possibility of arranging carbon atoms in different manners in higher members (containing more than three carbon atoms) of alkane family this class of hydrocarbons constitutes an widely illustrated example of *structural, particularly* of *chain isomerism*. Number of isomers increases with the increase in carbon atoms in alkanes. For example,

i. $CH_3-CH_2-CH_2-CH_3$ $CH_3-\underset{}{CH}(CH_3)-CH_3$

n-Butane   isobutane or 2-methyl propane

ii. $CH_3-CH_2-CH_2-CH_2-CH_3$

n-pentane

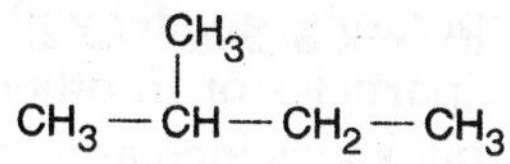

2-methyl butane
or
isobutane

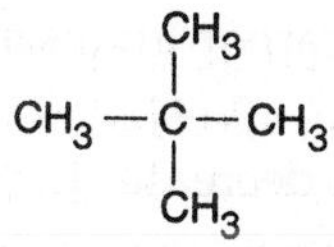

neopentane (2, 2-dimethyl propane)

iii. $CH_3-CH_2-CH_2-CH_2-CH_2-CH_3$

n-hexane

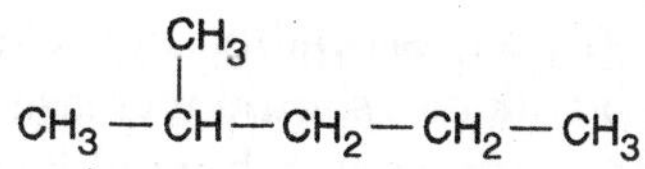

2-methyl pentane

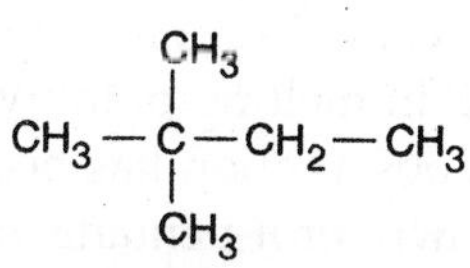

neohexane
or
(2, 2-dimethyl butane)

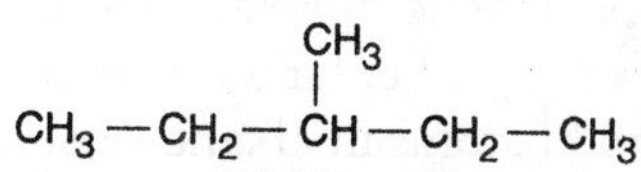

3-methyl pentane

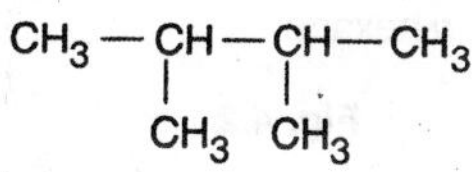

2, 3-methyl butane

4.1.4.2 Physical Characteristics of Alkanes

The first four members—methane, ethane, propane and butane are gaseous in nature at room temperature. Alkanes from C_5—C_{16} are colourless liquids while members from C_{16} onwards are waxy solids. Since there is no polar bond in alkanes, they are insoluble in polar solvents like water but are soluble in nonpolar solvents such as carbon tetrachloride.

4.1.4.2.1 Boiling Point

It has been observed that boiling point of liquid alkanes increases with the increase in carbon atoms; increase of each CH_2 group corresponds to an approximate increase of 25-30 °C in the boiling points. Thus *n*-pentane and, *n*-hexane boil respectively at 36.10 °C and 68.7 °C while the boiling point of *n*-heptane is 98.40 °C. The branching in the chain has the reverse effect, i.e., boiling point decreases with greater number of branching in isomeric alkanes. Such observations may be explained on the basis of association of molecular particles. It is known that a chemical compound whether it is in gaseous, liquid or in solid state, it tends to remain as associated particles. The association of particles in the molecule originates from the cohesive forces operating among the particles. More the cohesive forces, more will be the association. Cohesive forces arise from van der Waals forces. With gradual decrease in cohesive forces nature of compound changes from solid to gas through liquid, i.e., solid → liquid → gas. Again, during boiling, a liquid changes from liquid to gas. For this change energy is required to break the association. It is obvious that more the cohesive forces operating, greater will be the association and hence more energy will be required to dissociate the particles or in other words, liquid will boil at higher temperature. Increase in carbon atoms in alkanes increases the cohesive forces. So higher energy is needed to dissociate molecular particles and hence to change from liquid to gaseous state. That is why a sharp rise in boiling points is observed as one goes on increasing the carbon atoms in the chain of normal alkanes.

But increase of branching makes molecule more compact which decreases the surface area. It is known that cohesive forces decrease with the decrease in surface area. So less energy is required to change from liquid to gas, i.e., liquid boils at lower temperature.

4.1.4.2.2 Melting Point

As there is greater association of molecular particles in solid state it is expected that melting points of solid alkanes should increase with increase in carbon atoms in the chain. In fact, there is increase in melting points but unlike the change in boiling point no regularity in the change in the melting point has been observed either in normal or in branched chain alkanes. However, in some cases, such irregularities can be justified on the basis of crystal structure. Thus as we move up from *n*-pentane to *n*-hexane there is an increase of 35 °C in melting point whereas moving from *n*-hexane to *n*-heptane the increase is only 4 °C. This observation has been explained as follows: carbon atoms in alkane exist in zig-zag form as shown for *n*-pentane, *n*-hexane and *n*-heptane in Fig. 4.2.

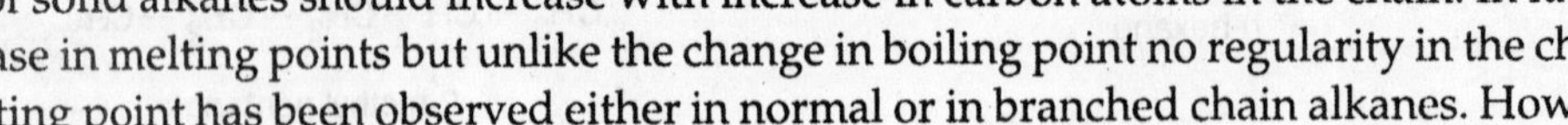

n-pentane *n*-hexane *n*-heptane

Fig. 4.2

From above zig-zag structure it is seen that in *n*-hexane terminal methyl groups are in opposite directions. This arrangement permits the chain to fit very closely in crystal structure as a result of which overall packing arrangement of the chain becomes very compact. Due to this very compact packing arrangement association of molecular particles becomes very strong and so requires more energy for dissociation and hence it melts at higher temperature. But in *n*-pentane and *n*-heptane terminal methyl groups are in the same directions and so the association of molecular particles in these compounds is not so strong due to less compact packing arrangement of the chain. So these alkanes melt at low temperature.

4.1.4.3 Chemical Properties

It was pointed out during the discussion of the structure of methane that in alkanes all bonds are covalent in nature and are very strong. Due to this fact alkanes are chemically very inert and indifferent towards chemical reagents. However, under drastic conditions they can undergo certain chemical reactions as described below:

1. *Halogenation*: In this reaction hydrogen atoms of alkanes are replaced by halogen atoms. Methane on treatment with chlorine in presence of diffused sunlight or on heating at a high temperature of 250 °C-400 °C forms monochloro methane.

$$CH_4 + Cl_2 \xrightarrow[\text{250–450°C or sunlight}]{\text{Heat at}} \underset{\text{Methyl Chloride}}{CH_3Cl} + HCl$$

If excess chlorine is present, reaction continues further, and step by step all the hydrogen atoms are replaced.

$$CH_3-Cl + Cl_2 \longrightarrow \underset{\text{Dichloromethane}}{CH_2Cl_2} + HCl$$

$$CH_2Cl_2 + Cl_2 \longrightarrow \underset{\substack{\text{Trichloromethane} \\ \text{(chloroform)}}}{CHCl_3} + HCl$$

$$CHCl_3 + Cl_2 \longrightarrow \underset{\substack{\text{Tetrachloromethane} \\ \text{or} \\ \text{Carbon Tetrachloride}}}{CCl_4} + HCl$$

Bromine reacts similarly but less rapidly while direct iodination is not possible because the reaction is reversible.

$$CH_4 + I_2 \rightleftharpoons CH_3I + HI$$

If, however, in presence of oxidising agent which reacts with HI, stops the reverse reaction, so direct iodination may occur.

$$5HI + HIO_3 \longrightarrow 3I_2 + 3H_2O$$

The order of reactivity among halogens is $Cl_2 > Br_2 > I_2$. Ethane and higher alkanes react in similar fashion and all the possible products are formed. Numbers of isomers to be formed depend upon the nature of replaceable hydrogen atoms (primary, secondary and tertiary).

$$\underset{n\text{-propane}}{CH_3-CH_2-CH_3} + Cl_2 \longrightarrow \underset{n\text{-propyl chloride}}{CH_3-CH_2-CH_2-Cl} + \underset{\text{Isopropyl chloride}}{CH_3-\overset{\overset{\large Cl}{|}}{C}H-CH_3}$$

Similarly, isopentane will form three isomeric monochloro derivatives as there are three types of replaceable hydrogen atoms—primary, secondary and tertiary. Mechanistically halogenation takes place in radical path as indicated below:

Step I: $Cl-Cl \xrightarrow[\text{or Heat}]{\text{Light}} \dot{Cl} + \dot{Cl}$

Step II: $CH_3-H + \dot{Cl} \longrightarrow \dot{C}H_3 + HCl$

Step III: $\dot{C}H_3 + Cl-Cl \longrightarrow CH_3-Cl + \dot{Cl}$

Steps I and II are repeated till the termination of the chain by the combination of any two free radicals occurs.

$$\dot{C}H_3 + \dot{Cl} \longrightarrow \underset{\text{Methyl Chloride}}{CH_3-Cl}$$

$$\dot{C}H_3 + \dot{C}H_3 \longrightarrow CH_3-CH_3$$

$$\dot{Cl} + \dot{Cl} \longrightarrow Cl_2$$

Before the termination of chain, reaction can take place in other way also if excess of chlorine is present to form other products.

$$\underset{\text{Methyl Chloride}}{Cl-CH_2-H} + \dot{C}l \longrightarrow \underset{\text{Chromethyl radical}}{\dot{C}H_2Cl} + H-Cl$$

$$\dot{C}H_2-Cl + Cl-Cl \longrightarrow CH_2Cl_2 + \dot{C}l$$

In similar way chloroform and carbon tetrachloride may be formed.

2. *Sulphonation*: When alkanes are treated with fuming sulphuric acid one hydrogen atom of alkanes is replaced by sulphonic acid group ($-SO_3H$). This process of replacement of a hydrogen atom by $-SO_3H$ is known as sulphonation process.

$$R-H + (HO)_2S(=O)=O \longrightarrow R-S(=O)(=O)-OH + H_2O$$

The order of replacement of hydrogen atom from alkane is tertiary > secondary > primary.

3. *Nitration*: This involves the replacement of a hydrogen atom from alkane by nitro ($-NO_2$) group on treatment with fuming nitric acid at a very high temperature.

$$R-H + HO-N(\rightarrow O)=O \longrightarrow R-N(\rightarrow O)=O + H_2O$$

4. *Oxidation*: When alkanes are burnt in presence of excess of oxygen, carbon dioxide and water are formed. This process is known as combustion.

$$CH_4 + 2O_2 \longrightarrow CO_2 + 2H_2O$$

It is an exothermic reaction and a large amount of heat is evolved. For this reason, alkanes are used as fuels in the form of kerosene oil, gasoline, LPG, etc.

But when alkanes are heated in limited supply of oxygen or air at high pressure and in presence of suitable catalyst, alcohols, aldehydes or fatty acids are obtained.

$$2CH_4 + O_2 \xrightarrow[\text{Cu}]{250\,°C,\ 100\ \text{atmos}} 2CH_3OH$$

$$2CH_4 + O_2 \xrightarrow[Mo_2O_3]{400\,°C,\ 200\ \text{atmos}} HCHO + H_2O$$

5. *Cracking or Pyrolysis*: Higher alkane molecules are decomposed into a number of simpler molecules by the action of heat. This thermal process of decomposition is called pyrolysis or cracking. This process involves the breakage of C—C and C—H bonds and takes place generally at a temperature of 600 °C-800 °C. For example,

$$\underset{\text{Ethane}}{CH_3-CH_3} \xrightarrow{\Delta} \underset{\text{Ethylene}}{CH_2=CH_2} + \underset{\text{Methane}}{CH_4} + H_2$$

$$CH_3-CH_2-CH_2-CH_3 \longrightarrow CH_3-CH_2-CH=CH_2 + CH_3-CH=CH_2 + CH_2-CH_2 + CH_3-CH_3 + CH_4 + H_2$$

Petrolium industry uses this cracking process to convert higher hydrocarbons into smaller hydrocarbons which are useful fuels.

4.1.5 Uses of Alkanes

Alkanes are primarily used as fuel and lubricating oils. Alkanes are also used for the preparation of nitro-paraffins.

4.2 Alicyclic Hydrocarbons (Cycloalkane)

Alicyclic hydrocarbons are also known as cycloalkanes. In fact, these are alkanes containing rings of carbon atoms only and in general, chemistry of alicyclic hydrocarbons is essentially the chemistry of alkanes. Cycloalkanes are represented by the general formula, C_nH_{2n}. The cyclic nature of these compounds confers on them some special properties which are considered to be the beginning of the study of some important concepts of chemistry. One of such concepts is the conformational analysis of the stereochemical aspects of organic molecules. The cyclic nature can impart variety of effects such as shape of the molecules, change of steric restrictions, stability of the molecules, etc., which have created a stir among the organic chemists for over the years.

It may be mentioned in this connection that the stability of alicyclic compounds has been explained by Baeyer and coulson (vide 3.5.2, p. 91).

4.2.1 Classification of Cycloalkanes

Cycloalkanes may be classified into following categories:

(a) *Monocyclic Compounds*: Cycloalkanes containing only one ring system are categorised as monocyclic compounds; for example,

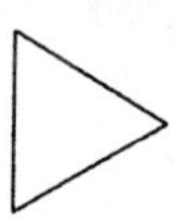

Cyclopropane

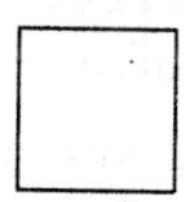

Cyclobutane

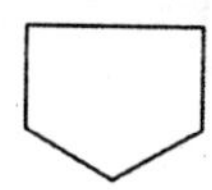

Cyclopentane

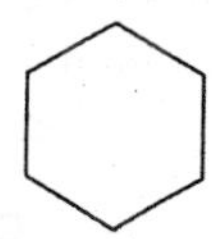

Cyclohexane

(b) *Polycyclic Compounds*: Compounds having two or more than two rings and whose rings share one or more common atoms are called polycyclic compounds. The polycyclic compounds may further be divided into the following groups:

i. *Spirocyclic Compounds*: A polycyclic compound containing rings with one common carbon atom is called *spirocyclic* compound.

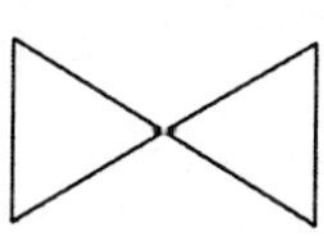

Spiro [2, 2] pentane

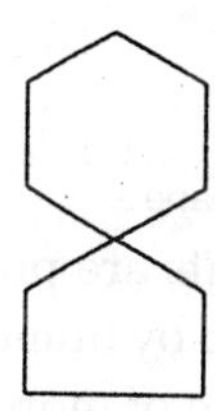

Spiro [5, 4] nonane

ii. *Condensed Polycyclic Compounds*: Polycyclic compounds in which rings are fused with two *adjacent* carbon atoms are called condensed polycyclic compounds.

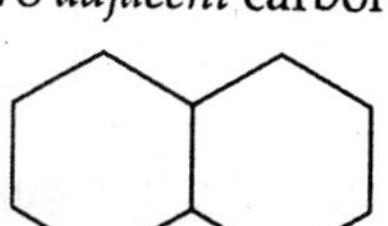

Decation

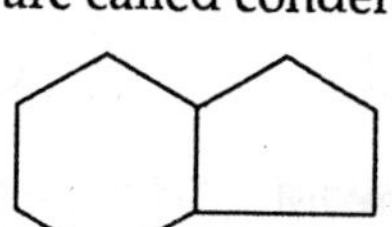

Hydrindane

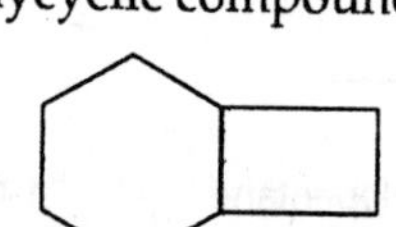

Bicyclo [4, 2, 0] octane

iii. *Bridged Polycyclic Compounds*: When two rings are fused through *non-adjacent carbon* atoms, and the rings have two or more common atoms, a bridged ring system originates and the corresponding compounds are called *bridged polycyclic compounds*.

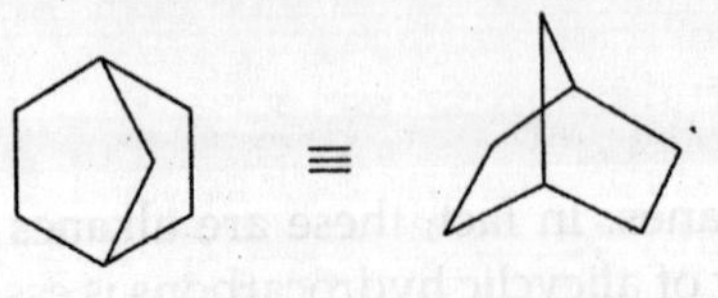

Bicyclo [2, 2, 1]-heptane

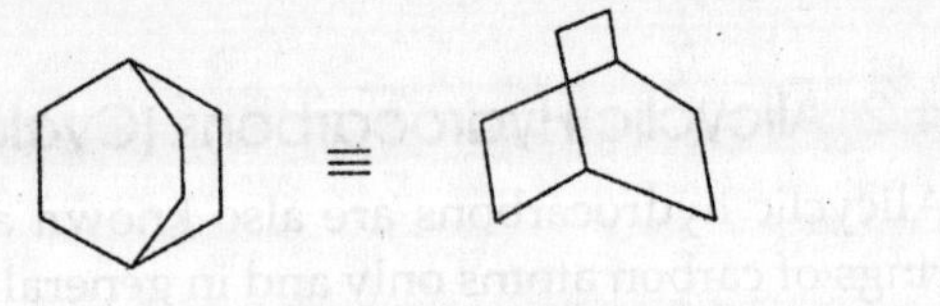

Bicyclo [2, 2, 2]-octane

iv. *Simple Polycyclic Compounds*: There are some polycyclic compounds which are joined by a carbon-carbon single bond.

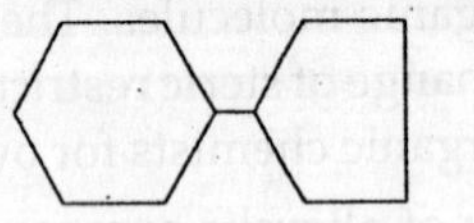

Cyclo-hexane-Cyclopentane

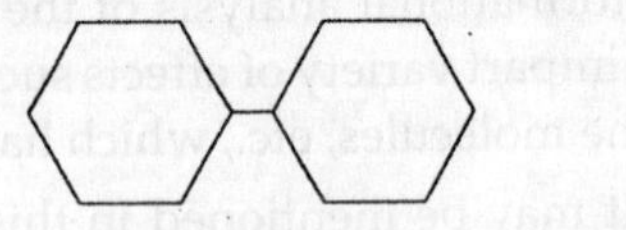

Dicyclo-hexane

v. *Polycyclic Compounds with Strange Shapes*: There are some polycyclic compounds which have strange and wonderful shapes.

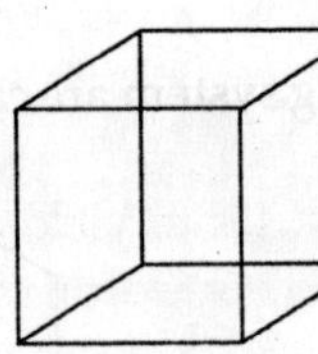

Cubane

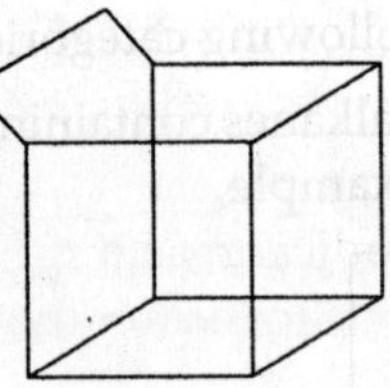

Basketane

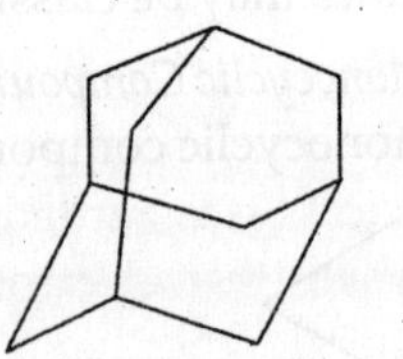

Adamantane

4.2.2. Nomenclature of Cycloalkanes

Alicyclic hydrocarbons or cycloalkanes are named by putting a prefix *cyclo* to the name of the corresponding open chain hydrocarbon having the same number of carbon atoms as the ring. Thus,

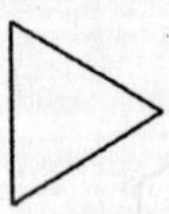

Cyclopropane

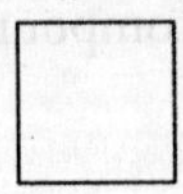

Cyclobutane

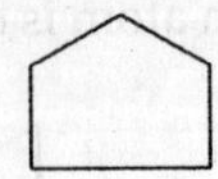

Cyclopentane

But when substituents are present in the ring, alkyls or other groups, the positions of the substituents are indicated by numbers in the ring. When single substituent is present, its position is always 1 but in the case of more than one substituents, they are named in alphabetical order. Thus,

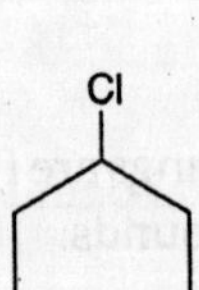

1-Chloro cyclopentane or chloro cyclopentane

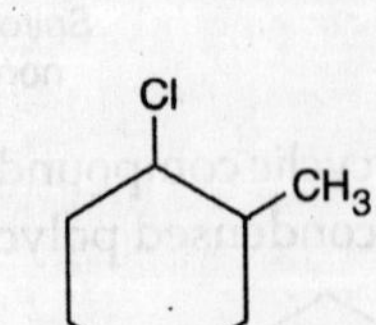

1-Chloro-2-methyl cyclohexane

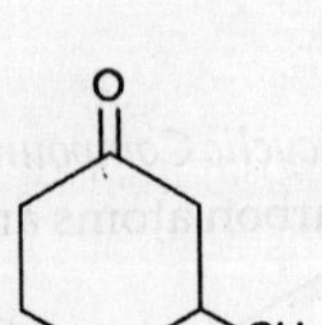

3-Methyl-cyclohexanone

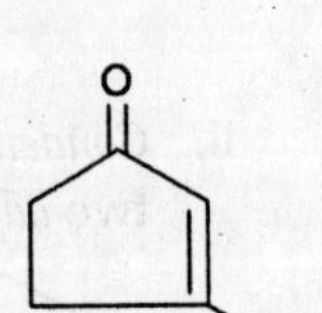

3-Methyl-cyclopent-2-enone

Polycyclic compounds are named according to the nature of the combination of the rings. Spirocyclic compounds are named by adding prefix *spiro* with name of parent hydrocarbon, the name of which is obtained by counting the total number of carbon atoms present in the compound. The number of carbon atoms on each side of the common atom is indicated in the bracket. Thus,

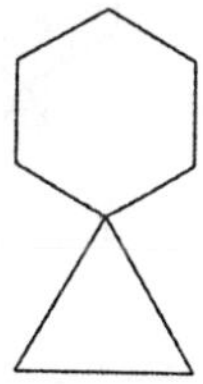

Spiro [5, 2] heptane

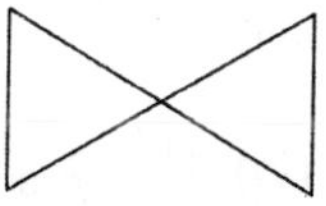

Spiro [2, 2] pentane

In the case of condensed ring system, the prefix *bicyclo* is used with the name of parent hydrocarbon and the number of carbon atoms on each side of the two common atoms are indicated by number in the bracket. Since in condensed system, there is no bridging, hence number of carbon atoms in the bridge in this system is always zero. Thus,

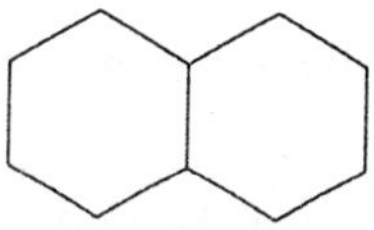

Bicyclo [4, 4, 0] docane

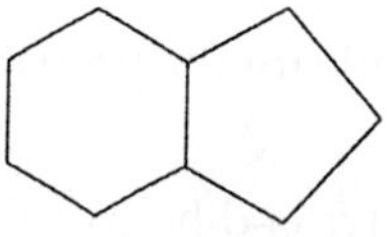

Bicyclo [4, 3, 0] nonane

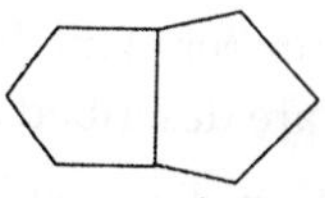

Bicyclo [2, 2, 1] octane

Similarly, bridged ring systems are named but in this case since there is a bridge, number of carbon atoms involved in the bridge must be indicated.

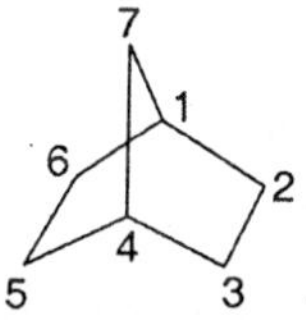

Bicyclo [2, 2, 1]-heptane

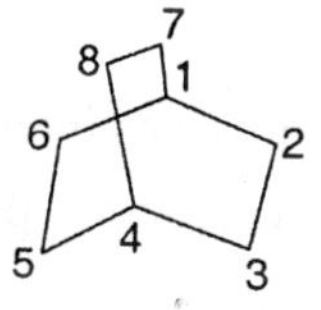

Bicyclo [2, 2, 2]-octane

When the different rings are joined by carbon-carbon single bond, naming is done by using the names of different ring systems.

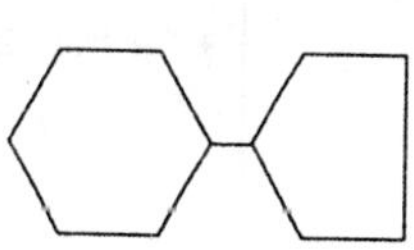

Cyclo-hexane-Cyclopentane

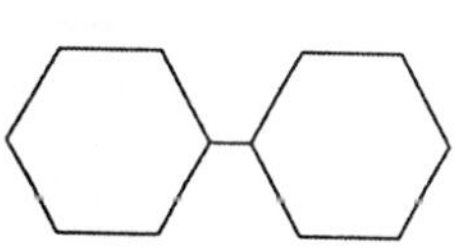

Dicyclo-hexane

Polycyclic compounds having strange shape are named on the basis of their shape as exemplified earlier.

PROBLEM 4.1

Suggest the names of the following:

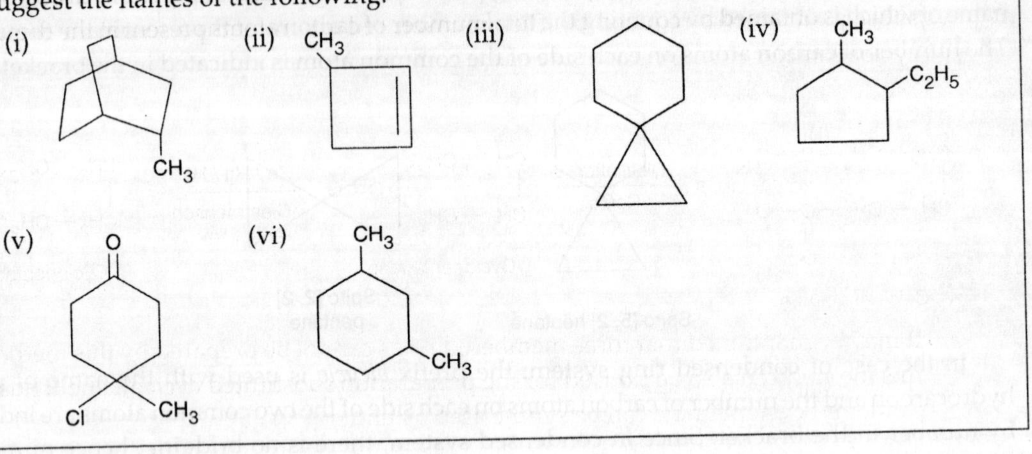

4.2.3 Preparation of Cycloalkanes

A large number of methods are available for the preparation of cycloalkanes. Some of the typical methods are described below.

1. *Wurtz Reaction*: In this method α, ω-dihalo derivatives of alkanes are treated with metallic sodium or zinc when corresponding cycloalkanes are obtained. Thus,

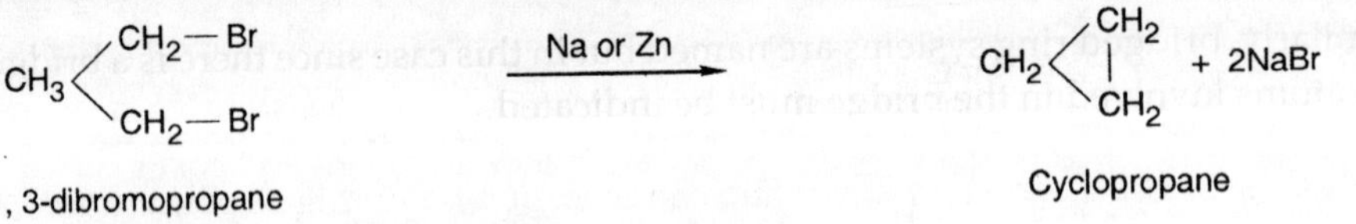

This reaction is known as *Internal Wurtz Reaction*.

Mechanistically the reaction proceeds as under:

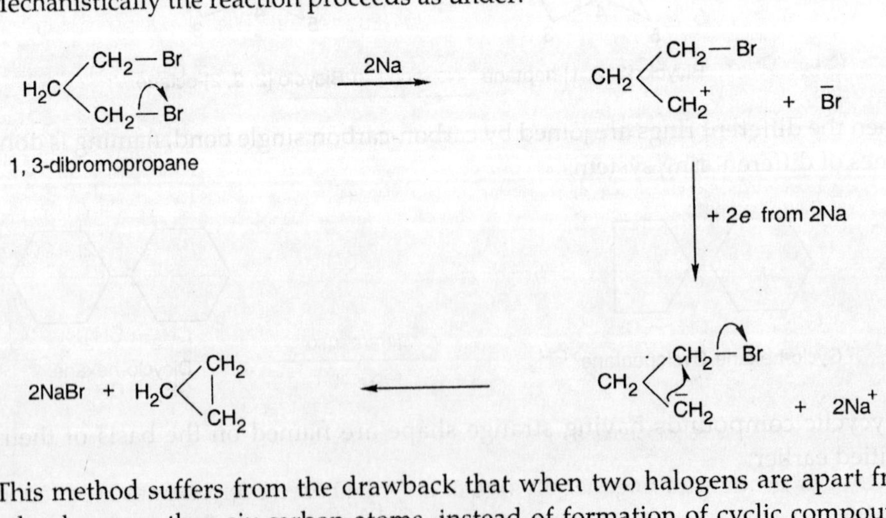

This method suffers from the drawback that when two halogens are apart from each other by more than six carbon atoms, instead of formation of cyclic compound, open chain hydrocarbons are formed by normal Wurtz reaction.

2. *Distillation of Salts of Dibasic Acid*: This method involves the distillation of calcium or barium salt of a dicarboxylic acid. In the initial stage a ketone is formed which in the subsequent step is reduced by Clemmenson reduction method to obtain the desired cycloalkane.

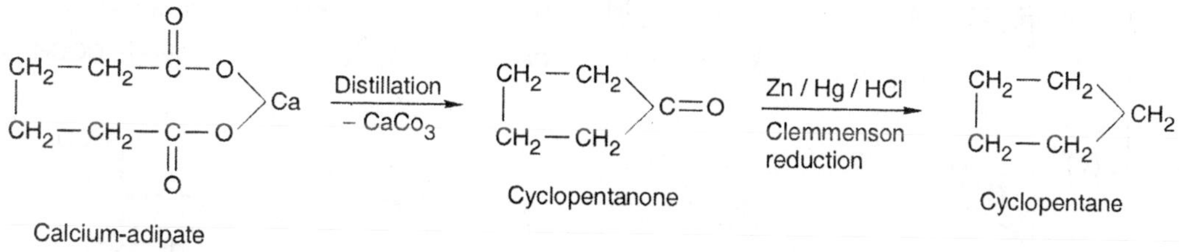

It may be mentioned that three membered rings cannot be prepared by this method. But this method can also be utilised for the preparation substituted cycloalkane. Thus, ethyl or methyl cyclopentane can be synthesised as under:

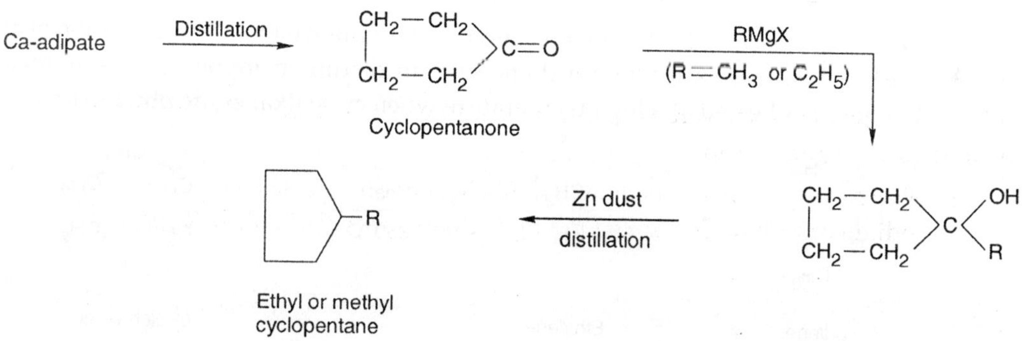

3. *Dickmann Condensation*: Dickmann condensation is nothing but the intramolecular claisen condensation. In this reaction, esters, or ester and ketone in presence of basic reagent such as alkoxide, undergo intramolecular aldol condensation to form cycloalkanes.

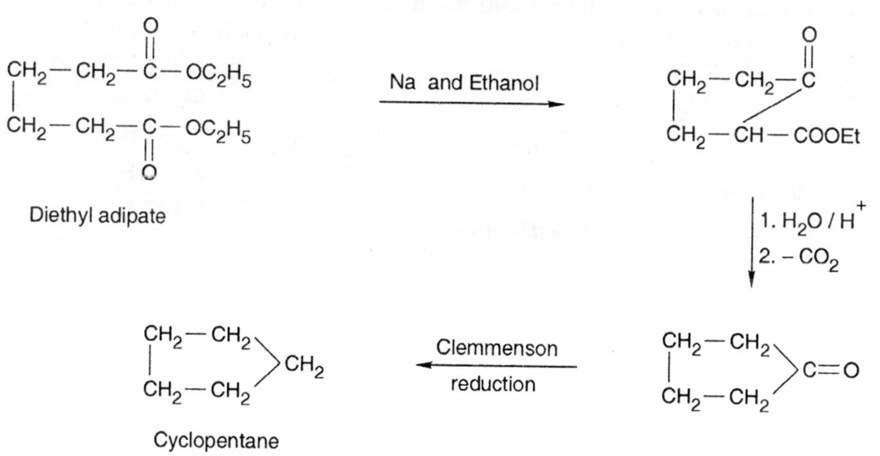

By this condensation generally five or six membered cycloalkanes are prepared.

4. *Thorpe-Zeigler Reaction*: In this method a dinitrile is treated with $LiN(C_2H_5)_2$ in benzene or in toluene. A cyclic imino compound is formed in the initial stage which on hydrolysis

yields a cyclic ketone. Ketone may be reduced by clemmenson reduction to get the desired cycloalkanes.

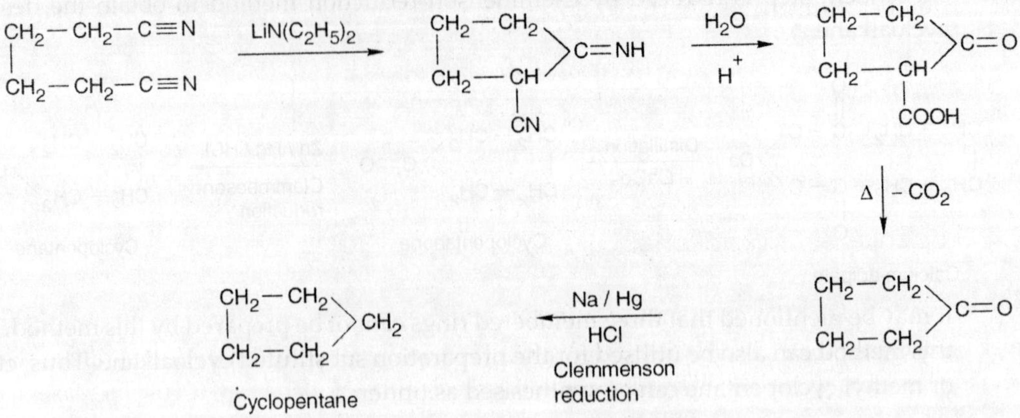

5. *Diels-Alder Reaction*: Diels-Alder reaction can be employed for the preparation of alicyclic compounds. In this reaction a diene and an olefinic compound usually termed as dienophile is heated at a high temperature when cycloalkanes are obtained.

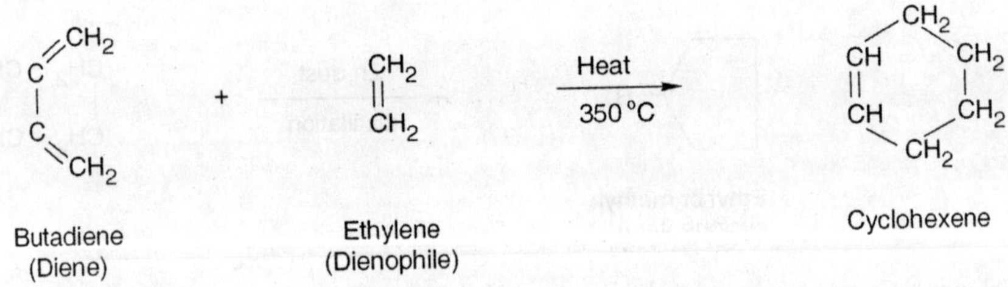

Diels-Alder reaction is a special type of reaction known as pericyclic reaction which is neither ionic nor radical in nature but can be explained in terms of orbital symmetry.

6. *Perkin's Method*: This is a very old method. This method involves the reaction between malonic ester and ω-dihalide in presence of alkoxide as basic catalyst.

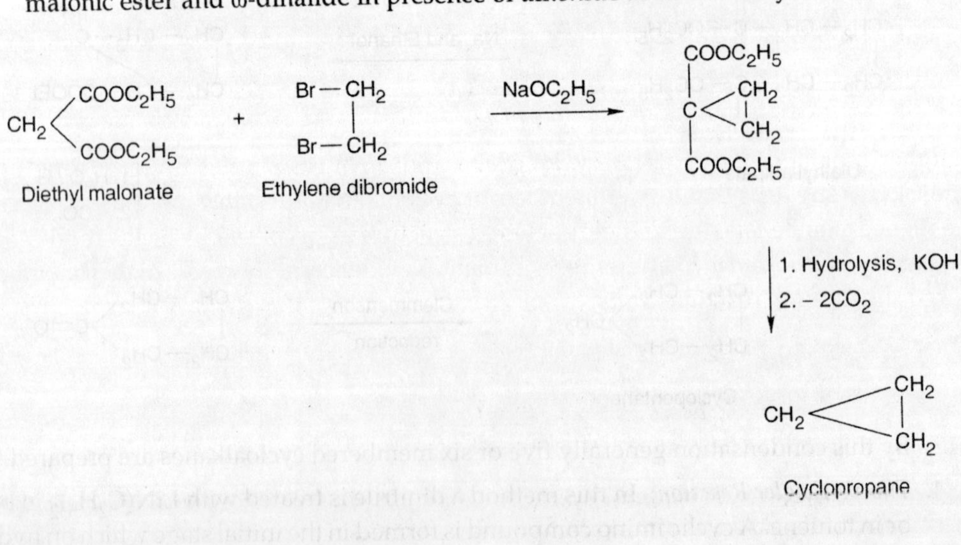

7. *Reduction of Aromatic Compounds*: Aromatic compounds can afford cyclohexane and its derivatives on reduction. The reduction is carried out in presence of nickel as catalyst at a temperature of 250-275 °C.

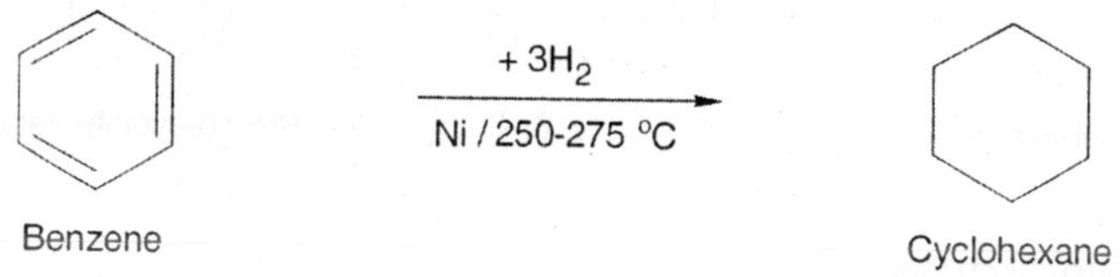

4.2.4 Properties of Cycloalkanes

4.2.4.1 Physical Properties

Lower members, viz., cyclopropane and cyclobutane are gases at ordinary temperature while others are liquid in character. The boiling points of cycloalkanes increase with the increase in the size of the ring and are higher than the corresponding open chain alkanes.

4.2.4.2 Chemical Properties

Lower members are very unstable and readily undergo ring opening reactions.

(i) 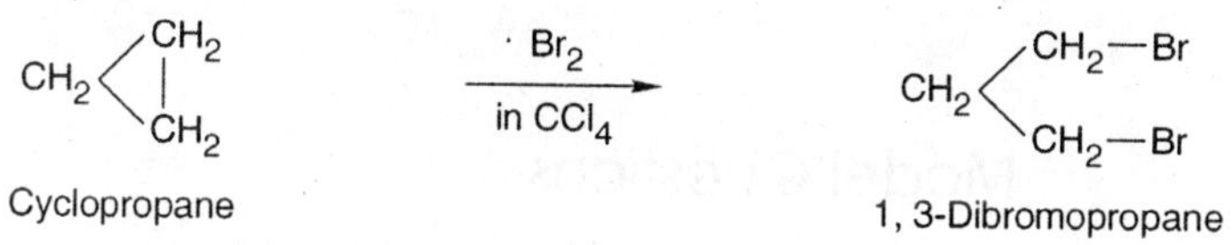

(ii) 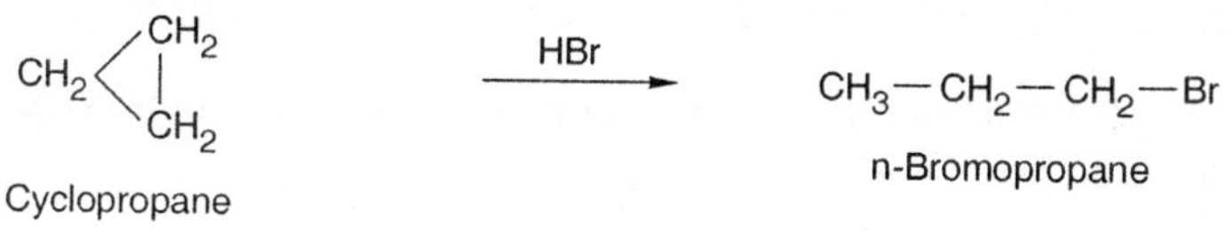

However, in presence of UV-light they can undergo substitution reaction.

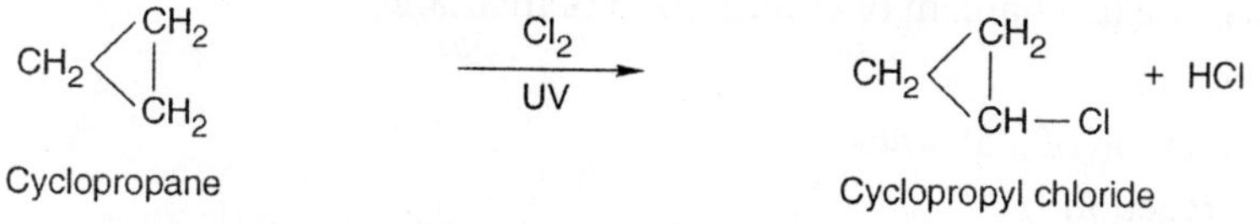

Higher members particularly cyclohexane and onwards do not undergo ring opening reactions. This suggests that higher members of cycloalkanes are stable molecules. The stability of the higher members is due to their puckered structure as proposed by Sachse and Mohr and subsequently supported by different experimental evidences. However, higher members can undergo substitution reaction. Thus,

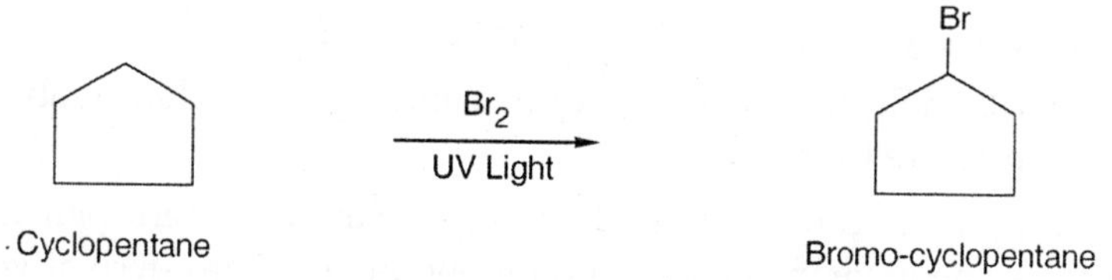

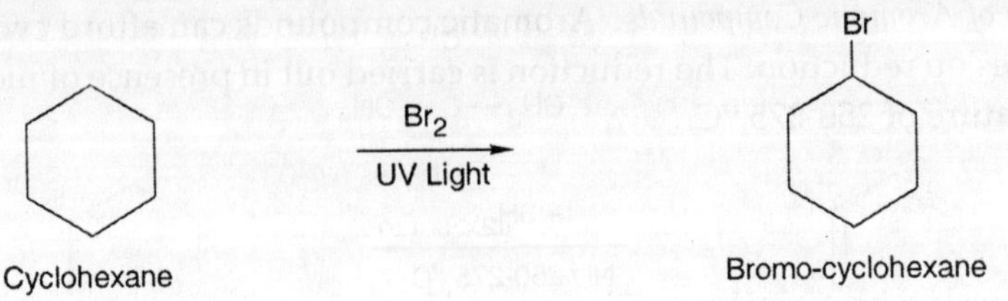

4.2.4.3 Uses of Cycloalkanes

Cycloalkanes are used for variety of purposes. Cyclohexane is frequently used as a solvent while a few other members of this family find extensive applications as medicines. Cyclopropane itself is a potent anaesthetic, and cyclohexanol derivative (cyclomethycaine Sulpahte) is an effective topical anaesthetic in thermal and chemical burns. Some cyclopentene derivatives of fatty acids occurring in nature are important in medicines particularly in the treatment of congestive heart failure, hepatic cirrhosis, leprosy, tuberculosis and in the nephritic stage of glomeru nephrits. Some natural products such as steriods and terpenes are cycloalkanes and used as important pharmaceuticals. γ-Isomer of hexachloro cyclohexane is extensively used as a powerful insecticide.

Model Questions

1. What are alkanes? How are they prepared? Discuss some characteristic properties of alkanes.
2. (a) Write the structural formula of *n*-pentane, isopentane and neopentane. Which of these has the highest boiling point and why?
   (b) Discuss the variation of m.p. in alkanes.
   (c) Explain the mechanism of halogenation of alkane.
   (d) Discuss the mechanism of chlorination of methane.
3. Write notes on:
   (a) Halogenation of a alkanes.
   (b) Wurtz reaction.
   (c) Kolbe's electrolytic process.
   (d) Korey-House Synthesis.
4. What happens when
   (a) Ethyl chloride is treated with sodium metal.
   (b) Methane is treated with iodine in presence of an oxidising agent, HIO_4.
   (c) Ethane is treated with concentrated nitric acid at 450 °C.
5. (a) An alkane with molecular weight 72 formed only one monochloro substitution product. Suggest a structure for the alkane.

   Hints: Mol. wt. indicates that its mf is C_5H_{12}. So three isomeric pentanes are possible. Out of these, neopentane can form only one monochloro derivative because it has only one type of hydrogen, i.e., primary.

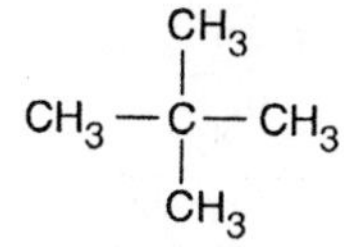

Neopentane

(b) Give the structure of pentane that would be expected to produce the largest number of isomeric monochloro derivatives.

Hints: Out of three isomeric pentane, isopentane has the largest number of variety of replaceable hydrogen (three different types) and so this isomer will form the largest number of isomeric monochloro derivatives.

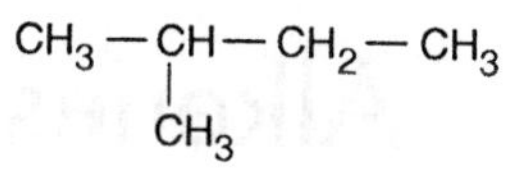

Isopentane

6. What are alicyclic compounds? How are they classified? Give some general methods of preparation of these compounds.
7. Write notes on:
   (a) Axial and equatorial bonds
   (b) Dickmann reaction
   (c) Baeyer's Strain theory
   (d) Conformation of cyclohexane.
8. How will you prepare
   (a) Cyclopentane from ethyl adipate
   (b) Ethyl cyclopentane
   (c) Methyl cyclopentane.
9. Explain
   (a) Why cyclohexane is more stable than cyclopropane
   (b) The statbility of cycloalkanes.
10. How will you distinguish
    (a) Cyclohexane and cyclohexene
    (b) Cyclopentane and cyclopentene
    Hints: Cyclohexene and Cyclopentene decolourise (i) bromine in CCl_4 and (ii) dilute $KMNO_4$

CHAPTER FIVE

Alkenes

Alkenes are unsaturated hydrocarbons containing one double bond. They are expressed by the general formula C_nH_{2n}, where n is any integer, 1, 2, 3, ... They are also known as olefins meaning oily liquid, because lower members are found to form oily products with halogens and halogen acids. Alkenes are very significant organic compounds because they are one of the major products of cracking of petroleum and also serve as intermediates for the synthesis of large variety of compounds having biochemical importance.

In accordance with the general formula, C_nH_{2n}, the first member should have been methylene, CH_2. But methylene is very unstable and does not exist in stable form. Consequently, the alkene family begins with two carbon atoms containing member, ethylene, C_2H_4. Structurally this simple and most common member is represented as below:

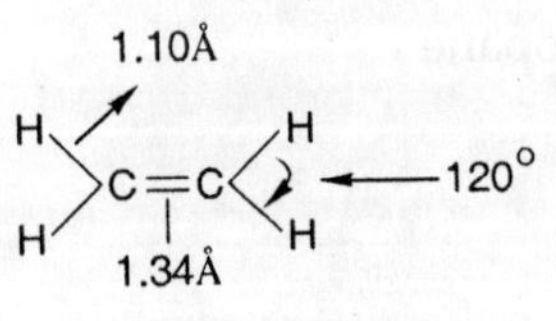

Structural formula of ethylene

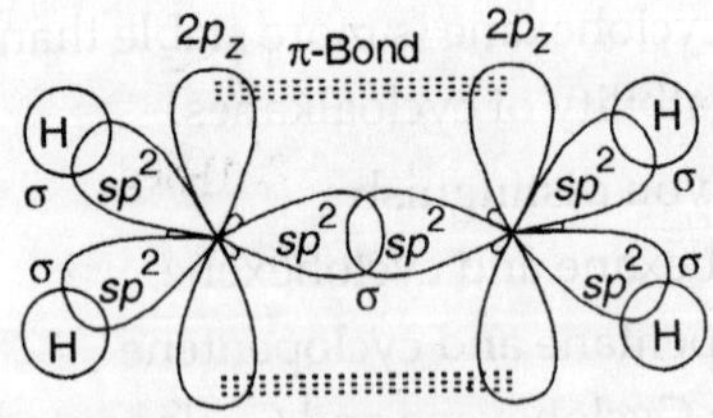

Molecular orbital structure of ethylene

Two carbon atoms in ethylene are connected by a σ-bond formed by overlapping one sp^2-hybrid orbital of each and by a π-bond which is formed by the parallel overlapping $2p$-orbital of each carbon atom. Thus the double bond between the carbon atoms consists of one σ -and one π-bond. Four hydrogen atoms are connected by σ-bonds formed by the overlapping of sp^2-orbitals of carbons and s-orbital of hydrogen.

5.1 Nomenclature

Lower members are known by names derived from the corresponding *alkane* by replacing the suffix -'ane' by -'ylene'. Thus,

Ethylene (C_2H_4)
(Ethane $\longrightarrow$ Eth + ylene $\longrightarrow$ Ethylene)

Propylene (C_3H_6)
(Propane $\longrightarrow$ Prop + ylene $\longrightarrow$ Propylene)

However, higher members are named according to IUPAC system of nomenclature as discussed in chapter **three** . The position of the double bond is indicated by number remembering that both the carbon atoms of the double bond are given the lowest possible numbers. Thus,

$$\overset{1}{C}H_2{=}\overset{2}{C}H{-}\overset{3}{C}H_2{-}\overset{4}{C}H_2{-}\overset{5}{C}H_3$$

1-Pentene or Pent-1-ene

$$\overset{1}{C}H_3{-}\underset{}{\overset{\overset{CH_3}{|}}{\overset{2}{C}}}H{=}\overset{3}{C}H{-}\overset{4}{C}H_2{-}\overset{5}{C}H_3$$

2-Methyl-2-pentene
or
2-Methyl pent-2-ene

5.2 Preparation of Alkenes

Most of the common methods of preparation of alkenes follow the path of elimination reactions. For examples,

(a) *Dehydration of alcohols*: As the name of the process implies this method involves the elimination of one molecule of water from alcohol. The simplest member, ethylene is prepared by heating ethyl alcohol at a temperature of 180 °C in presence of concentrated sulphuric acid.

$$CH_3-CH_2-OH \xrightarrow[180\,^{\circ}C]{\text{conc. } H_2SO_4} CH_2{=}CH_2 + H_2O$$

This is the laboratory method of preparation of ethylene. Sometimes alcohol vapours are passed over alumina, Al_2O_3, at about 350 °C of temperature.

Mechanistically dehydration occurs in stepwise manner. It is an unimolecular elimination reaction.

Step I: $CH_3-CH_2-O-H \overset{\overset{+}{H}}{\rightleftharpoons} CH_3-CH_2-\underset{\underset{H}{|}}{\overset{+}{O}}-H \xrightarrow[\text{slow}]{-H_2O} CH_3-\overset{+}{C}H_2$

Intermediate carbocation

Step II: $\underset{\underset{H}{|}}{C}H_2-\overset{+}{C}H_2 \xrightarrow[\text{fast}]{\overset{+}{H}} CH_2{=}CH_2 + \overset{+}{H}$

Comments: (i) Dehydration proceeds smoothly in the case of tertiary (3°) alcohol. For this reason tertiary alcohols undergo dehydration under milder condition while primary alcohols require to some extent drastic condition for dehydration. The reason for smooth dehydration of tertiary alcohol is that the intermediate carbocation formed is more stable and so its formation is favoured and again as this carbocation is strained due to steric reasons, it can readily eliminate a proton (H^+) to form alkene.

(ii) Sometimes rearranged alkene is formed instead of expected one.

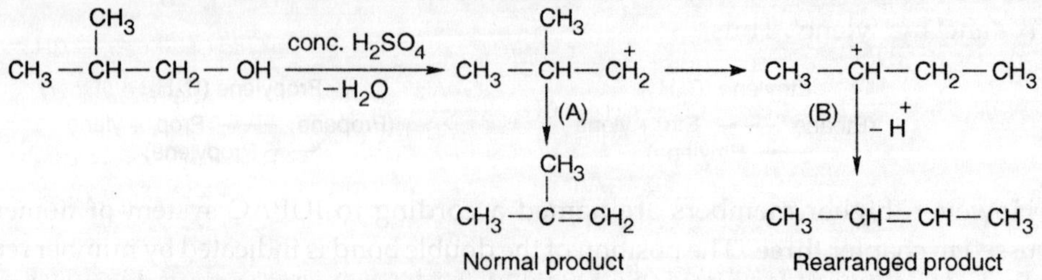

This is due to the fact that the intermediate carbocation (A) formed is primary (1°) and is unstable but the migration of a methyl group from adjacent carbon generates a 2° carbocation (B) which is relatively stable.

(iii) In some cases more than one alkenes may be formed.

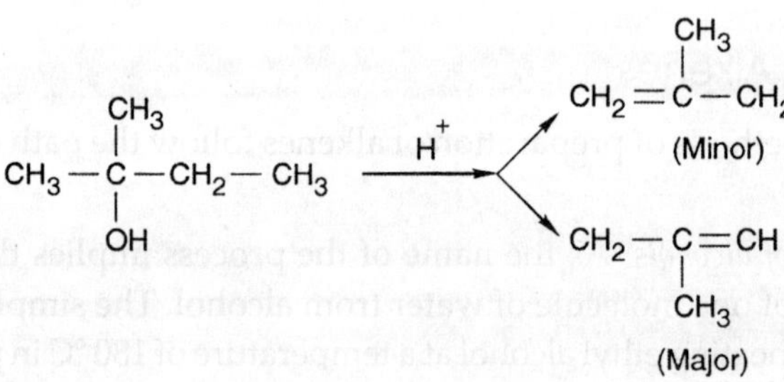

In this situation highly substituted alkene (substituted at the both ends of double bond) becomes the major product because such alkene is more stable. This guiding rule is known as *Saytzeff's rule* which was initially in use in the case of formation of alkene from dehydrohalogenation of alkyl halides.

(b) *Dehydrohalogenation of Alkyl halides*: Alkyl halides on treatment with alcoholic potassium hydroxide or any base eliminate a molecule of hydrogen halide with the formation of alkenes. It is also a case of elimination reaction.

$$CH_3-CH_2-X \xrightarrow[KOH]{Alcoholic} CH_2=CH_2 + HX$$

In this elimination reaction halide anion ($\bar{X}$) and the adjacent proton are removed simultaneously as HX as indicated below:

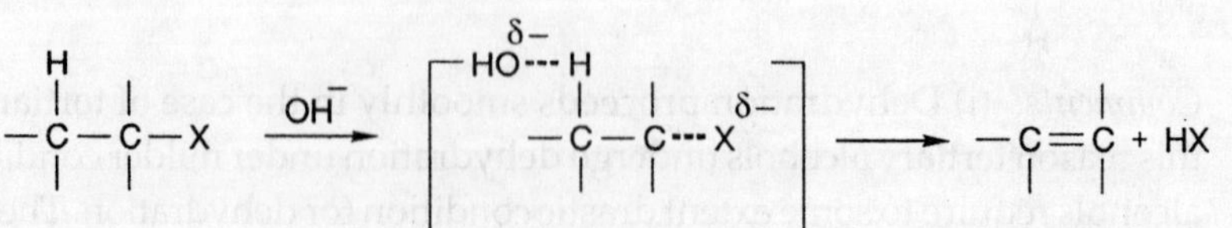

This mechanistic path is bimolecular in nature as both the basic catalyst and the substrate are directly involved. This path is indicated by E_2. In the case of unsymmetrical alkyl halide more than one products may be formed and according to Saytzeff's rule highly substituted alkene becomes the major product. For example,

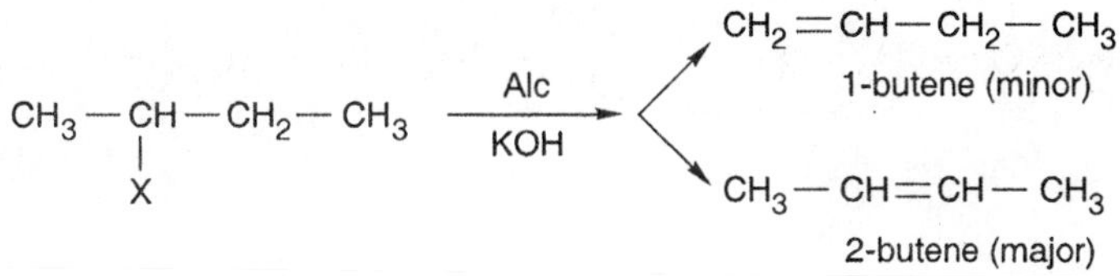

The order of reactivity of alkyl halides is tertiary > secondary > primary.

In the case of some secondary and tertiary halides hydrogen and halogen atoms may be removed in a stepwise manner.

Step I:

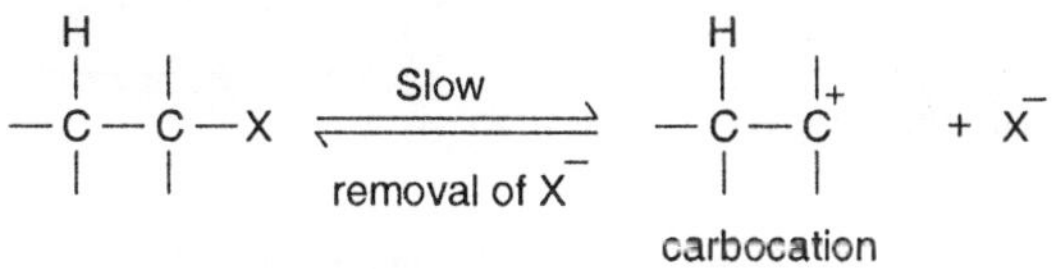

Step II:

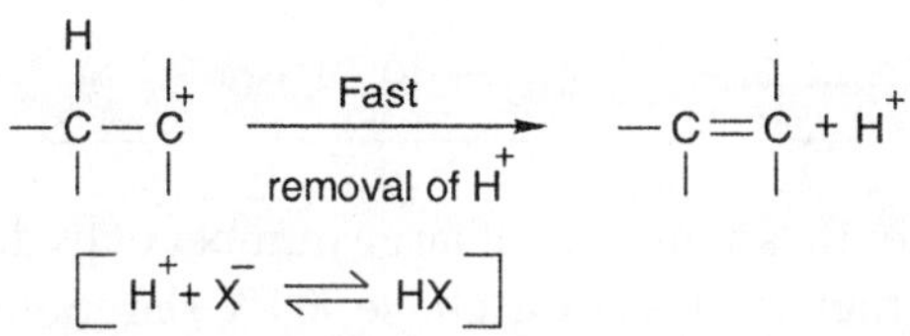

As in the case of dehydration of alcohol, in certain alkyl halides rearrangement can occur forming rearranged alkene. For example,

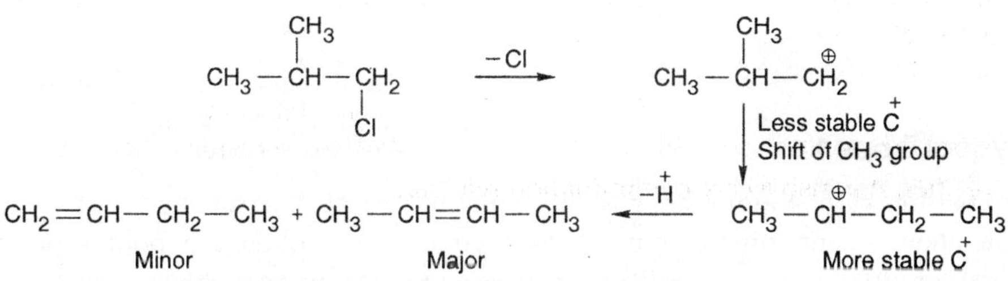

(c) *Dehalogenation of Vicinal dihalides* (1:2 *dihalo alkane*): When reactive metals like zinc in acetic acid are allowed to react with vicinal dihalides alkenes are formed.

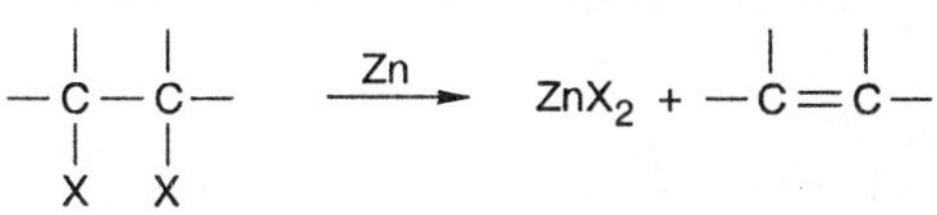

For example,

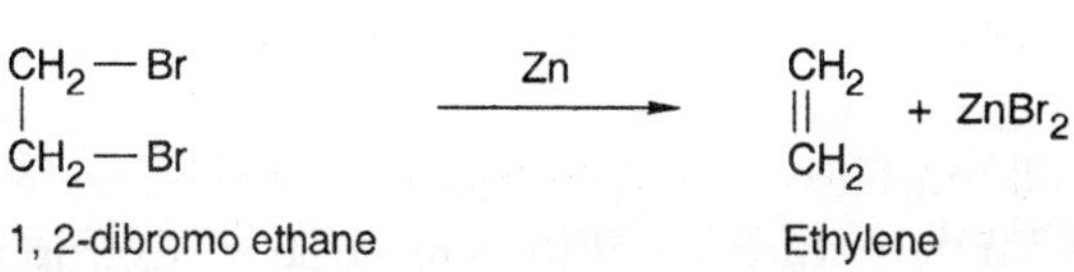

Metallic Zn acts as nucleophile and reaction takes place through bimolecular path (E_2), i.e.,

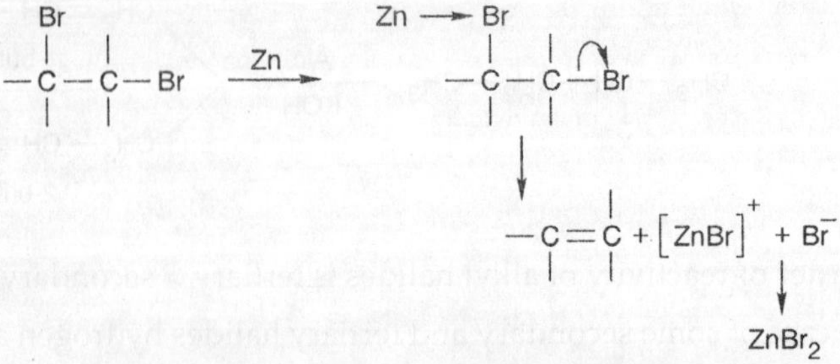

PROBLEM 5.1

Suggest probable mechanism of the following reaction:

(a) $CH_3-CH_2-CH_2-OH \xrightarrow[200\,^\circ C]{\text{Conc. } H_2SO_4} CH_3-CH=CH_2 + H_2O$

(b) $CH_3-CH_2-Cl \xrightarrow{\text{Alcoholic KOH}} CH_2=CH_2 + HCl$

(d) *Cracking of Petroleum*: Petroleum is a mixture of large number of hydrocarbons. When petroleum is heated at a very high temperature (above 500 °C) large amount of mixtures of alkenes and alkanes are obtained.

$$CH_3-CH_2-CH_2-CH_3 \xrightarrow[600\,^\circ C]{\text{Heat}} CH_2=CH-CH_3 + CH_4 + CH_3-CH_3 + CH_2=CH_2$$

5.3 Properties of Alkenes

5.3.1 Physical Properties

Alkenes up to three carbon atoms are gaseous in nature and alkenes having C_4—C_{15} atoms are liquid while alkenes containing carbon atoms beyond 15 are solids. The boiling point of the liquid alkenes gradually increases with the increase in molecular weight as is observed in the case of alkanes and such increase can be explained on the basis of cohesive forces operating between the molecular particles. Like alkanes, melting points of solid alkenes also increase in an irregular manner. Presence of π-bond in alkene restricts the rotation of carbon-carbon single bond as a result of which alkenes exhibit geometrical isomerism (vide chapter-**four**).

5.3.2 Chemical Properties

Presence of π-bond makes the alkenes very active towards chemical reagents. Due to the less stability of π-bond than σ-bond, alkenes have the tendency to be converted to stable alkane derivatives. For this reason, the most interesting class of chemical reactions of alkenes is the addition reaction around π-bond. Further, as the electrons in π-bond are less firmly held in alkenes, they are readily available. So the nature of addition reaction is electrophilic, i.e., the addition to π-bond is initiated by the electrophilic part of the addendenum (reagent). So the general path of addition reaction in alkenes may be depicted as below:

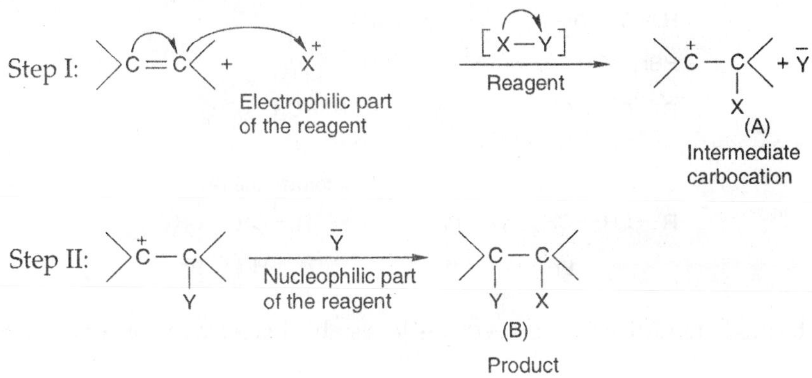

5.3.2.1 Direction of Addition Reaction

An obvious question arises at which carbon atom of the double bond electrophilic part of the addendenum (reagent) attacks? In symmetrical olefins (both ends of double bond contain identical substituents) and in the case of symmetrical addendenum (as for example, hydrogen and halogen molecules) this question is immaterial. But when both the olefins and addendenum are unsymmetrical, this is a significant issue. In this addition, there is an empirical rule proposed by Russian chemist *Markownikoff* which is popularly known as *Markownikoff's rule*. This rule states, during the addition of unsymmetrical addendenum to unsymmetrical alkene it is the negative part of the addendenum which is attached to the highly substituted (electron releasing substituent) carbon atom of the double bond. Thus,

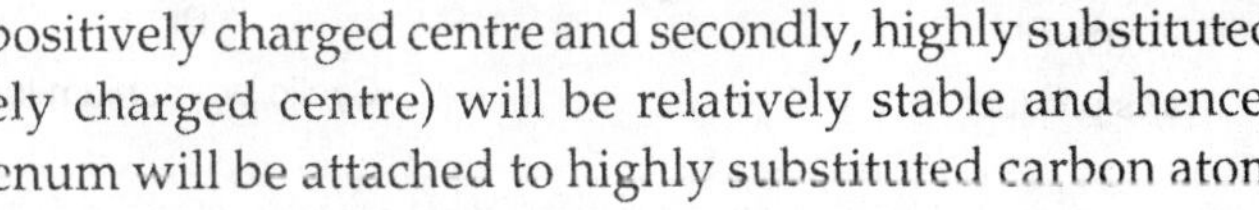

Although Markownikoff's rule is empirical, it has enough justification. Firstly, the substituents are electron releasing, electron will flow from more electron rich carbon (containing more substituents) to less electron rich carbon (containing lesser number of substituents) making highly substituted carbon positively charged centre and secondly, highly substituted intermediate carbocation (A) (positively charged centre) will be relatively stable and hence negatively charged portion of addendenum will be attached to highly substituted carbon atom.

5.3.2.2 Deviation of Markownikoff's Rule

M.S. Kharasch, an American chemist, observed that in presence of peroxide or any oxygen source addition occurs in the reverse way of Markownikoff. For example,

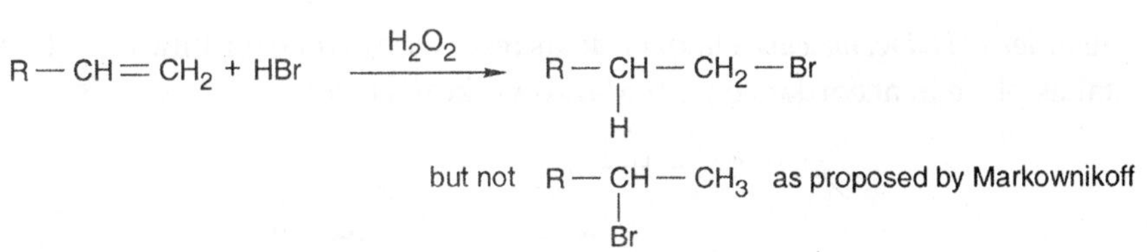

This anomaly has been explained by the observation that in presence of peroxide, the path of addition is free radical not ionic as shown below:

$$H{-}O{-}O{-}H \longrightarrow 2\dot{O}H$$

$$HBr + \dot{O}H \longrightarrow \dot{Br} + H_2O$$

$$R{-}CH{=}CH_2 + \dot{Br} \longrightarrow R{-}\dot{C}H{-}CH_2Br$$

Intermediate (A)

$$R{-}\dot{C}H{-}CH_2Br + H{-}Br \longrightarrow R{-}CH_2{-}CH_2Br$$

Alternative intermediate radical $R{-}CH(Br){-}\dot{C}H_2$ is less stable because the order of stability of free radical is tertiary>secondary>primary and so the addition takes place in the direction opposite to that proposed by Markownikoff. This effect is known as *Peroxide effect* or *anti-Markownikoff rule.*

5.3.2.3 A Few Common Addition Reactions

Some of the most common addition reactions undergone by alkenes are discussed below:

(a) *Addition of Halogens*: Addition of halogens to alkenes follows the general path discussed above but a noticeable observation which has been recorded is that the two halogen atoms in the reaction product (B) remain in opposite directions, i.e., *trans* to each other. Formation of *trans* dihalo product has been explained by assuming the formation of cyclic halonium ion before the attack by nucleophilic halogen. As for example,

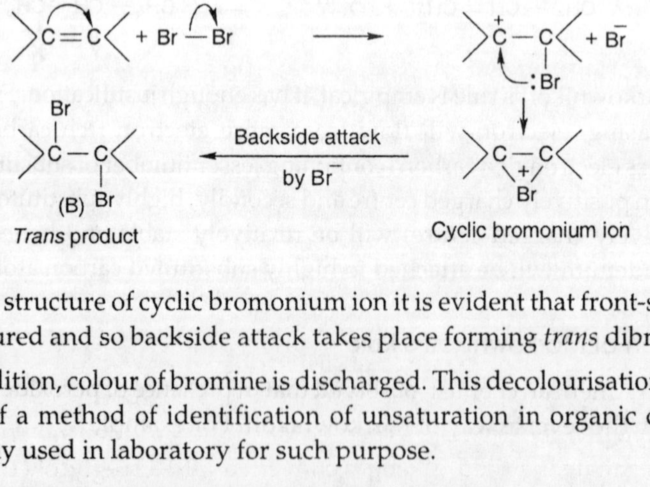

From the structure of cyclic bromonium ion it is evident that front-side attack by Br^- is not favoured and so backside attack takes place forming *trans* dibromo compound.

After addition, colour of bromine is discharged. This decolourisation of bromine forms a basis of a method of identification of unsaturation in organic compounds and is frequently used in laboratory for such purpose.

(b) *Addition of Halogen Acids*: Halogen acids react with alkene forming alkyl halide. Addition takes place in accordance with Markownikoff's rule.

(c) *Addition of halogens in presence of water*: Olefins on treatment with halogen in presence of water forms halohydrin.

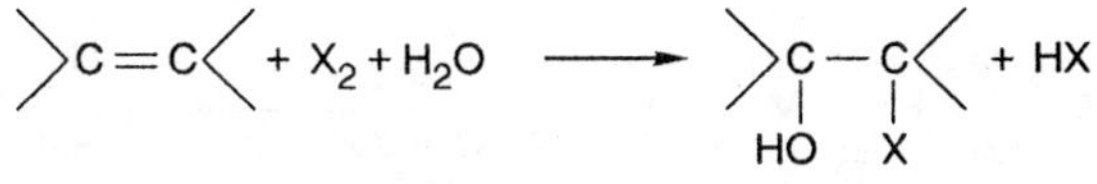

Halohydrin

Mechanism of this addition is similar to that mentioned in general pathway. In the first step electrophilic halogen adds to form halonium ion which is attacked by water from the backside in the second step.

Step I:

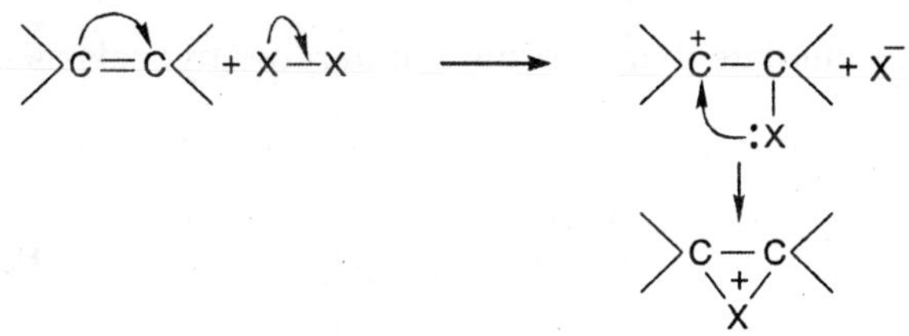

Step II:

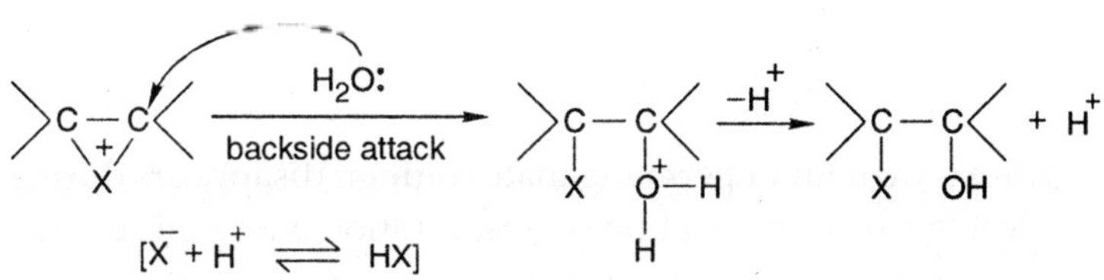

(d) *Hydration of olefins (Addition of water)*: Addition of acidulated water to olefins yields alcohol. Normally 65-75% H_2SO_4 is used. Path of addition follows Markownikoff's rule.

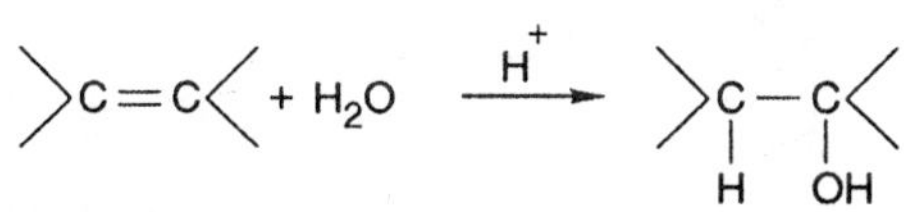

Alcohol

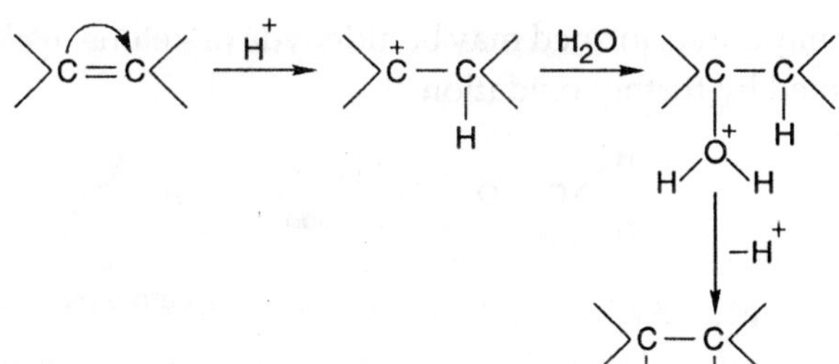

(e) *Hydroxylation by $KMnO_4$*: When cold, dilute and neutral solution of potassium permanganate is added, alkene is converted into a *cis*-glycol (1:2 *cis* diol). Potassium permanganate solution is decolourised and a brown suspension of MnO_2 appears.

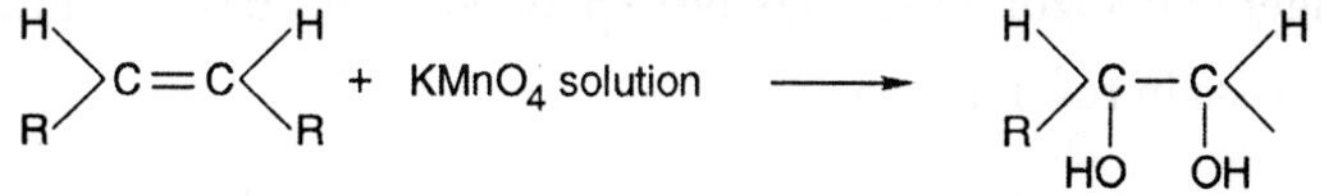

cis-Glycol

This reaction has been interpreted as discussed below:

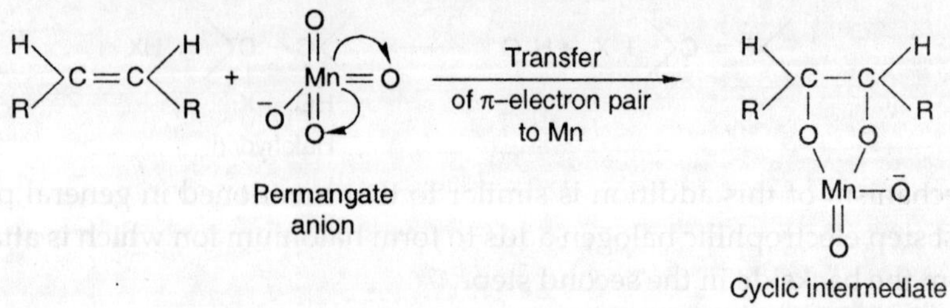

The cyclic intermediate that is formed undergoes hydrolysis in the next step to form *cis*-glycol.

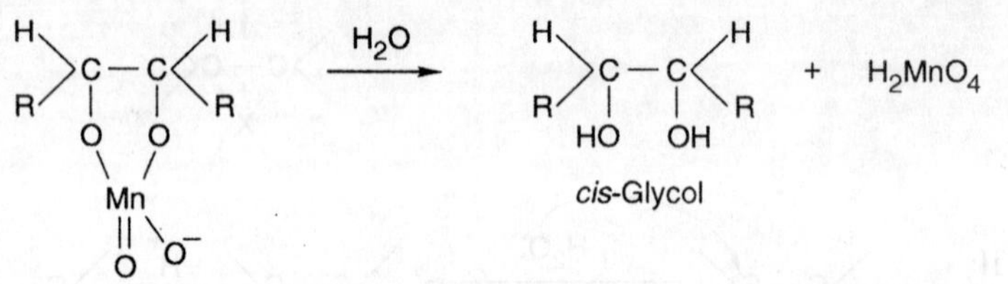

Since the colour of permanganate solution disappears during the reaction, it is used as a test for the identification of unsaturation in organic compounds.

When hot permangate solution is used, the glycol formed undergoes carbon-carbon bond cleavage forming carbonyl and carboxylic compounds depending upon the nature of substituents present on double bonded carbon atoms.

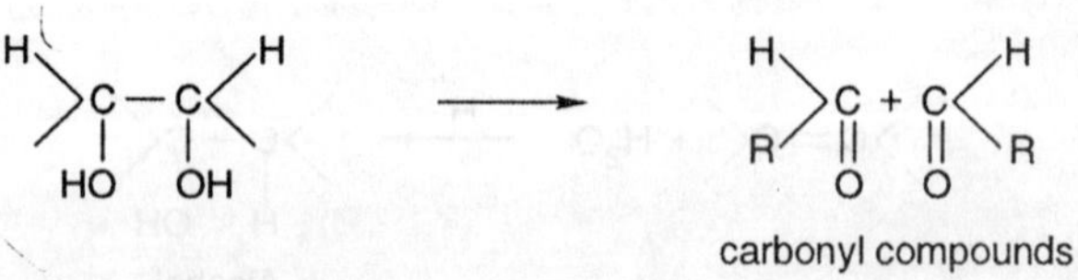

Carbonyl compounds formed may be aldehyde or ketone. If aldehyde, carboxylic acid may be formed by further oxidation.

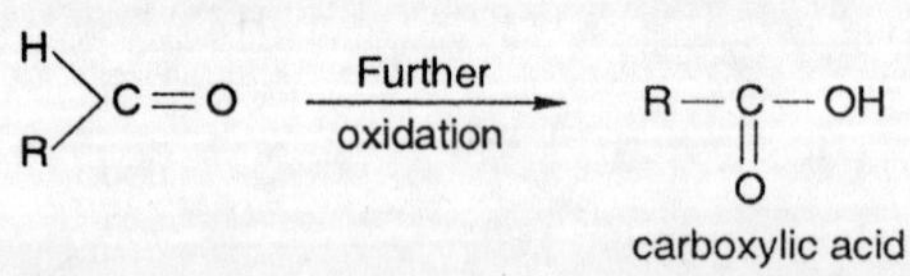

(f) *Addition of ozone (ozonolysis)*: The reaction of ozone (O_3) with alkene is very interesting. When ozone is passed through alkene in an inert solvent at room temperature, addition of ozone to alkene takes place forming a very unstable compound known as mole ozonide or primary ozonide. This unstable compound is readily converted to another addition product usually termed as *iso-ozonide* or simply ozonide undergoing rearrangement. Ozonolysis may be explained as discussed below:

Ozone exists in resonance as

$$C=\overset{+}{O}-\overset{-}{O} \longleftrightarrow \overset{-}{O}-\overset{+}{O}=O \longleftrightarrow \overset{-}{O}-O-\overset{+}{O}$$

when ozone is added reaction takes place as under:

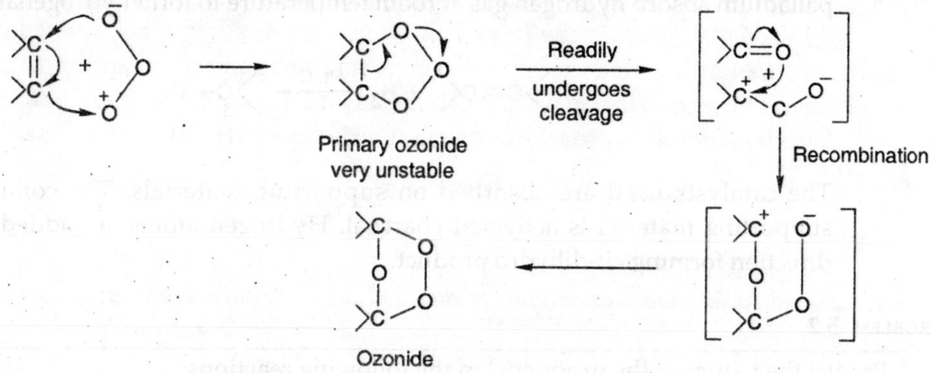

Ozonide formed is not so stable that it could be isolated. They can be readily reduced to carbonyl compounds by the use of mild reducing agent like Zn/H_2O.

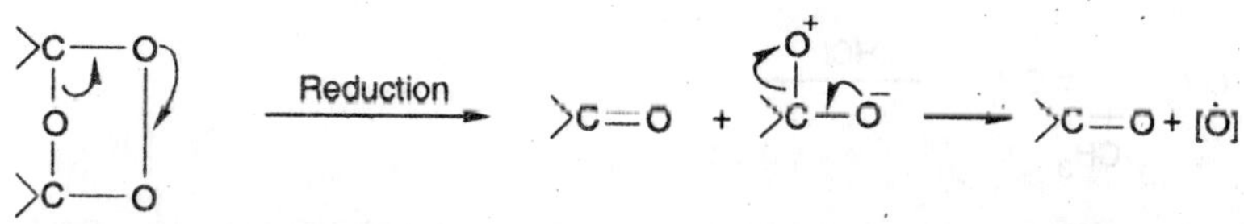

The whole process of formation of ozonides and their cleavage to yield carbonyl compounds in known as *ozonolysis*.

The process of ozonolysis is a very good method for the determination of the position of double bond in alkene. For example,

$$\overset{1}{CH_3}-\overset{2}{CH}=\overset{3}{CH}-\overset{4}{CH_3} \xrightarrow[\text{Ozonolysis}]{O_3} 2CH_3-CHO$$

$$\overset{1}{CH_3}=\overset{2}{CH}-\overset{3}{CH_2}-\overset{4}{CH_3} \xrightarrow[\text{Ozonolysis}]{O_3} \begin{matrix}H\\H\end{matrix}\!\!>C=O + CH_3-CH_2-CHO$$

Thus, from the identification of carbonyl compounds location of the double bond can be easily settled.

(g) *Epoxidation*: When alkene is treated with peracid or H_2O_2, epoxide is formed.

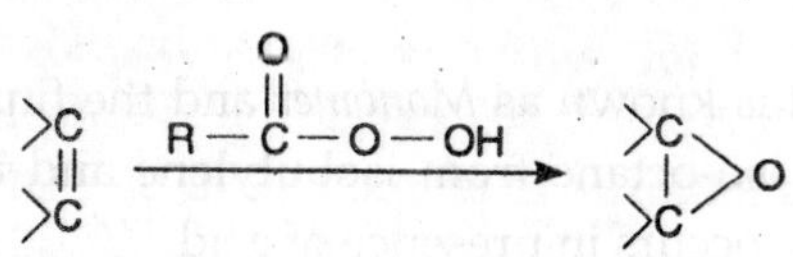

The addition is stereospecific *cis*-addition.

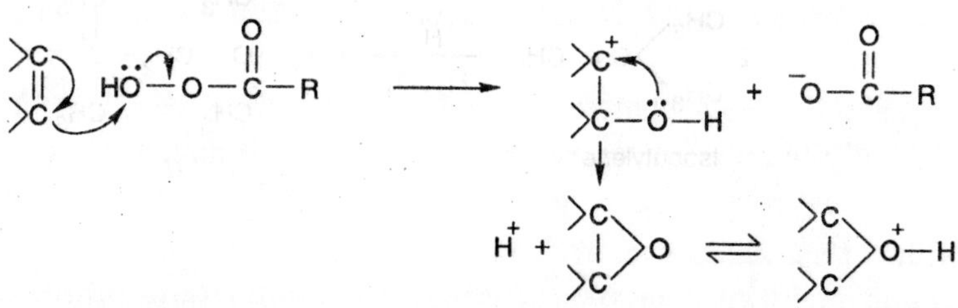

(h) *Catalytic Hydrogenation*: Alkenes in presence of metallic catalysts such as platinum or palladium absorb hydrogen gas at room temperature to form hydrogenated product.

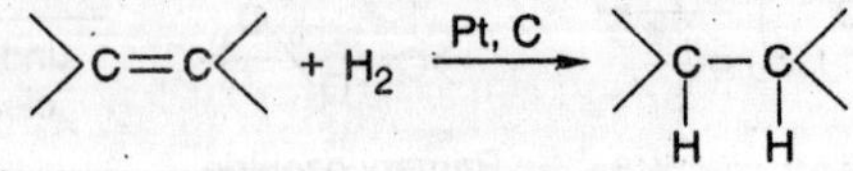

The catalysts used are absorbed on supporting materials. The commonly used supporting material is activated charcoal. Hydrogen atoms are added from same direction forming *cis*-dihydro product.

PROBLEM 5.2

Predict the nature of the product(s) in the following reactions:

(a) $CH_3-CH=CH_2 \xrightarrow{O_3}$

(b) $CH_3-\underset{CH_3}{\underset{|}{C}}=CH_2 \xrightarrow{HCl}$

(c) $CH_3-CH=CH_2 \xrightarrow[\text{Peracid}]{HCl}$

5.3.2.4 Polymerisation of Alkenes

Alkenes at high pressure and temperature in presence of traces of oxygen readily undergo polymerisation reaction. Polymerisation reaction is a process of formation of a large molecule from small molecules. Thus, when ethylene is heated at high temperature and pressure in presence of traces of oxygen, it undergoes polymerisation forming the product known as polythene.

$$\underset{\text{(Monomer)}}{\underset{\text{Ethylene}}{n\,CH_2=CH_2}} \xrightarrow[\text{Traces of oxygen}]{\text{High temperature and pressure}} \underset{\text{(Polymer)}}{\underset{\text{Polythene}}{(-CH_2-CH_2-)_n}}$$

The starting material is known as *Monomer* and the final product is called *Polymer*. In this connection formation of iso-octane from isobutylene and isobutane may be mentioned. This polymerisation, however, occurs in presence of acid.

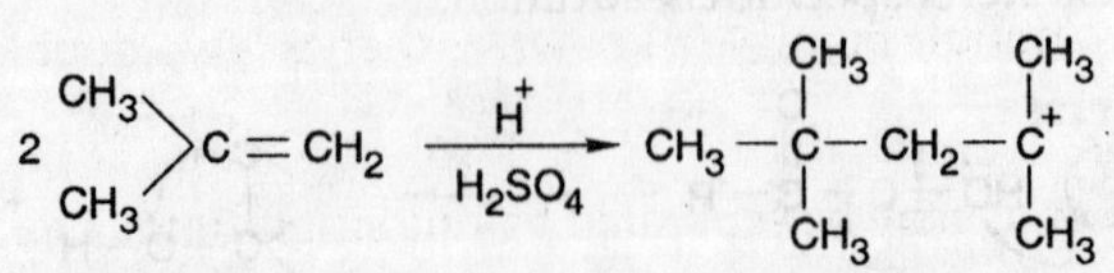

Isobutylene (A)

The intermediate (A) loses a proton to form the dimer of isobutylene or can abstract a hydride ion from isobutane.

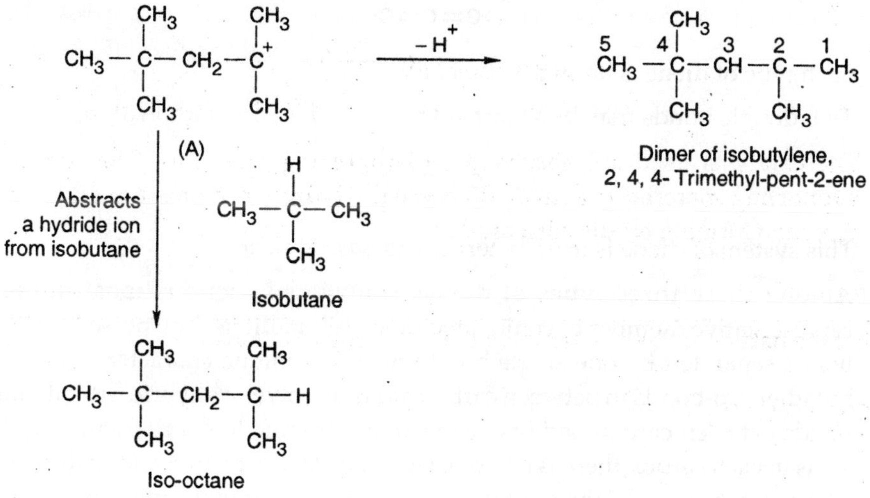

This conversion of isobutylene to iso-octane by the addition of isobutane is of industrial importance for the production of high grade motor fuels.

Again, addition of isobutylene is repeated to generate polyisobutylene, i.e.,

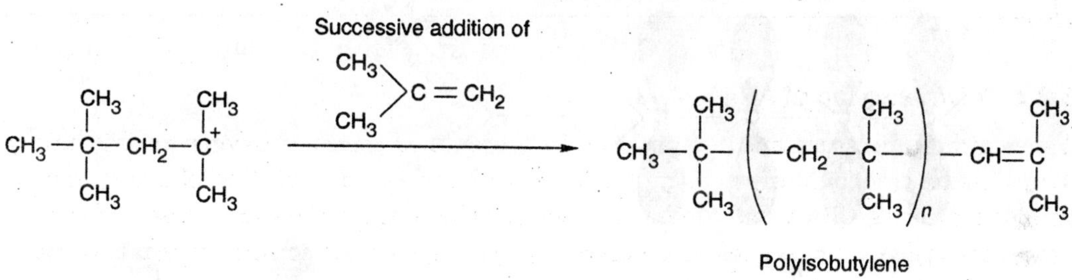

PROBLEM 5.3

From which alkenes the following compounds may be prepared?

(a) $CH_3-CH(OH)-CH_3$ (b) $CH_3-CH_2-CH_2-OH$

5.4 Dienes

Alkenes that contain two double bonds are known as dienes. Two double bonds may be present in three different manners:

i. Two double bonds may be separated by one single bond, i.e.,

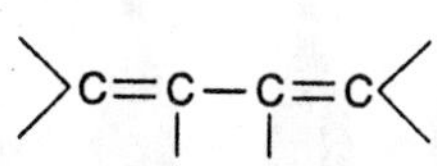

This type of diene is called *conjugated diene.*

ii. Both the double bonds may be present in two consecutive carbon atoms like the type shown below:

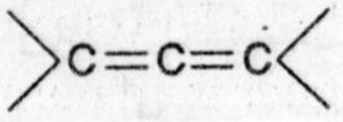

Such type of diene is known as *cumulative* diene.

iii. Two double bonds may be separated by more than one carbon atom.

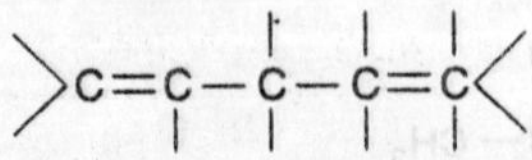

This system of diene is usually termed as *isolated diene.*

Among these three types of dienes conjugated diene is most important. The representative member of conjugated diene is butadiene. The presence of two double bonds separated by one single bond imparts a unique character of these dienes. In butadiene, σ-bonds in between carbon atoms involve sp^2-hybrid orbitals and covalent bonds between carbon and hydrogen atoms are due to overlapping of sp^2-s orbitals. Thus in each carbon there is one free *p*-orbital. All the carbon and hydrogen atoms are in the same plane and the π-orbitals are perpendicular to the plane of σ-bonds. Four *p*-orbitals, one in each carbon atom, can overlap each other in two different ways and so can form resonating structures.

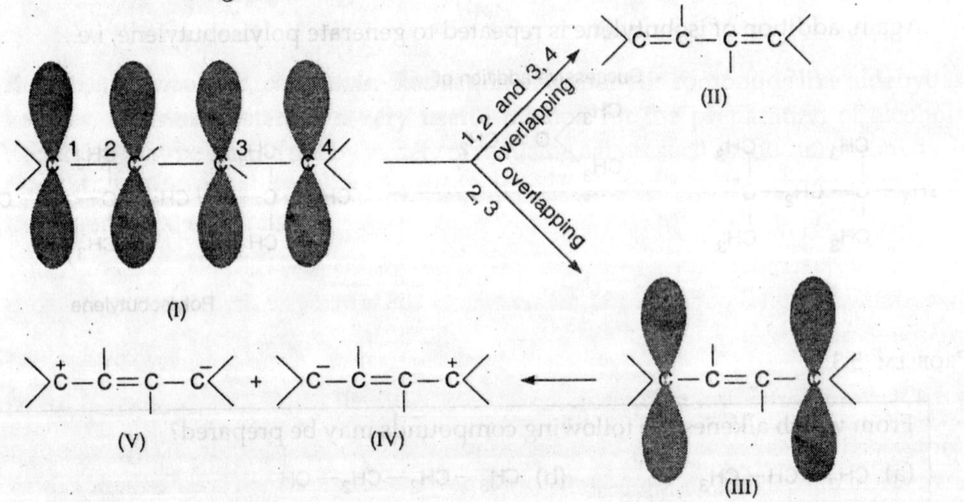

Since electrons are dynamic, electrons in *p*-orbitals at C_1 and C_2 in (II), may move in either directions resulting the structures (IV) and (V). All these structures are inter-convertible and hypothetical, and hence the actual structure of butadiene is the average of all these five structures which is nothing but delocalised structures (VI) or in other words, butadiene exists in resonance hybrid.

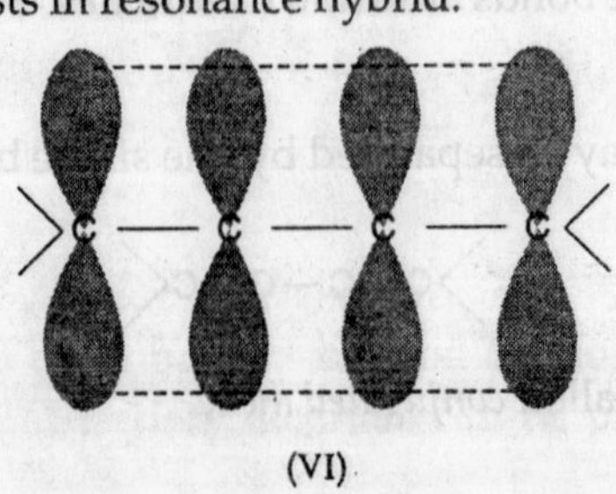

(VI)

Resonance structure of butadiene has been supported by bond length measurement. The C—C single bond length is 1.47Å (normal C—C single length 1.51Å) and that of C—C double bond is 1.36Å higher than normal double bond length (1.32Å).

Butadiene is a gas at room temperature. It may be prepared by a variety of methods of which the most common is the dehydration of a diol.

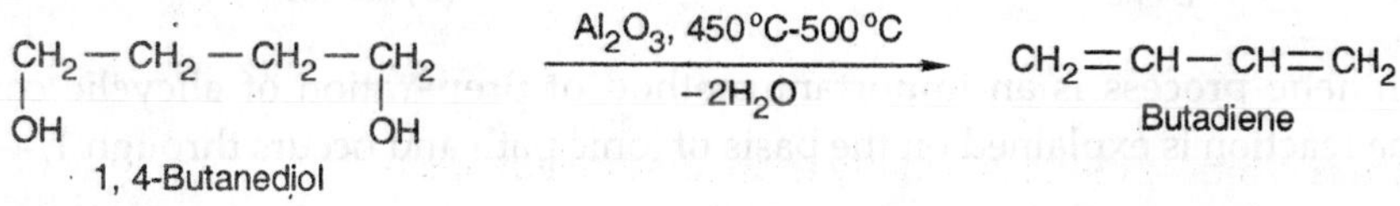

5.4.1 Reactions of Butadiene

The most important class of reactions undergone by butadiene or any conjugated diene is the addition reactions. Addition reaction of butadiene is to some extent unusual. The addition takes place either at 1, 2- or at 1, 4-positions.

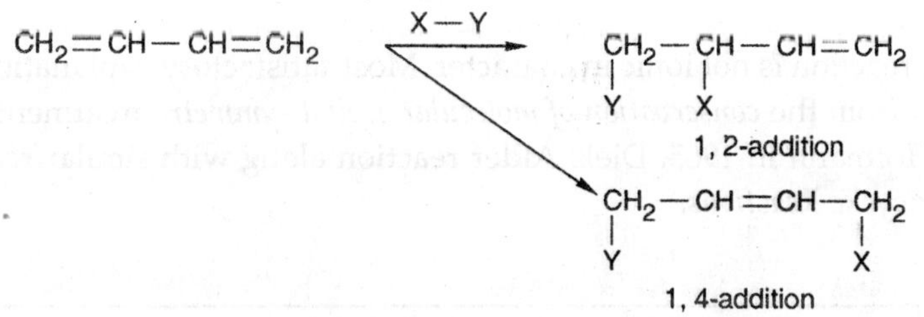

The formation of above products can be easily explained on the basis of resonance structure as discussed above. It has been observed that at low temperature 1, 2-addition predominates while at high temperature 1, 4-product becomes the major. Different addendenum (reagents) that commonly take part in addition reaction with butadiene are halogens, halogen acids and hydrogen molecules.

5.4.1.1 Polymerisation of Dienes

Conjugated diene particularly butadiene undergoes polymerisation in presence of peroxide or any radical initiator. Thus, butadiene forms polybutadiene which is a synthetic rubber known as *Buna Rubber*.

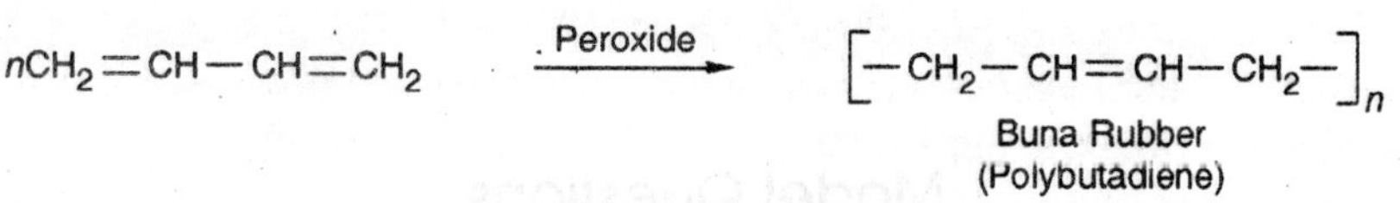

Polymerisation is assumed to take place through 1, 4-addition.

5.4.1.2 Diels-Alder Reaction

Butadiene or any conjugated diene serves a very good diene in Diels-Alder reaction for the synthesis of cycloalkenes. The reaction occurs between a diene and an alkene generally termed as dienophile at high temperature in non-polar solvents to form a cyclic compound known as adduct.

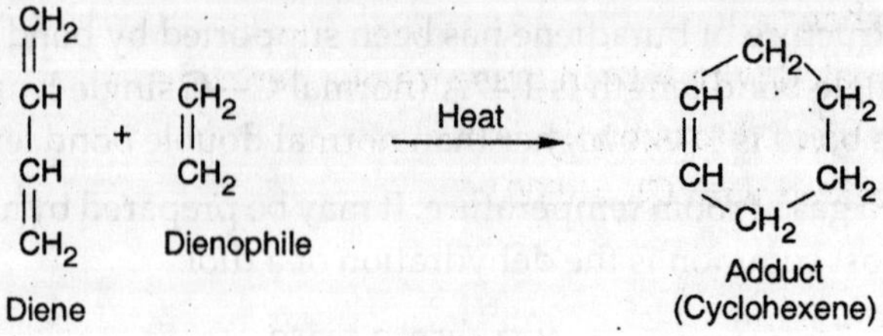

This synthetic process is an important method of preparation of alicyclic compounds. Normally the reaction is explained on the basis of ionic path and occurs through 1, 4-addition.

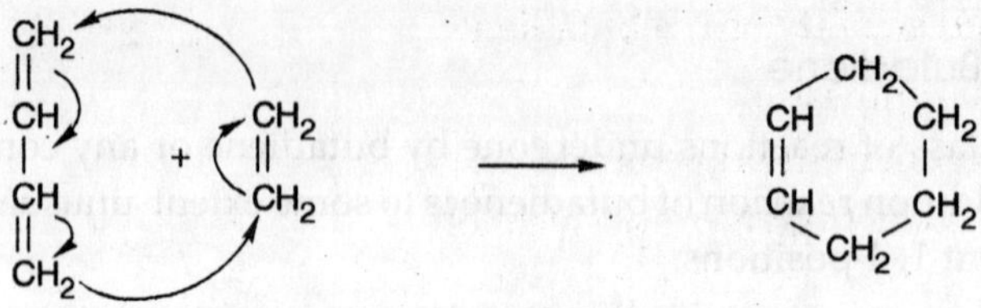

However, the reaction is not ionic in character. Most satisfactory explanation of the reaction has been obtained from the *conservation of molecular orbital symmetry* treatment as proposed by Woodward and Hofmann in 1965. Diels-Alder reaction along with similar reactions has been categorised as *Pericyclic Reactions.*

PROBLEM 5.4

(a) Write the resonating structure of butadiene.

(b) Suggest the product(s) of the following reaction:

$$CH_2{=}CH-CH{=}CH_2 + Br_2 \longrightarrow$$

5.5 Uses of Alkenes

Alkenes are used (a) in large quantities as raw materials in chemical industries for the preparation of many useful products such as polymer (PVC, polythene, polystyrene etc), glycols, dioxine, etc, (b) ethylene is used to hasten the ripening of fruits like citrus, tomatoes, (c) ethylene in the form of oxy-ethylene flame for cutting welding, (d) ethylene and its tri and tetra chloro-ethylene are effective anthelmintic anti-filarial agent frequently used against hookworms and intestinal flukes.

Model Questions

1. Describe the preparation of alkene by dehydration of alcohol giving the mechanism of the reaction.
2. What is dehydrohalogenation of alkyl halides? How can we obtain alkenes by this method? Expalin the mechanism of dehydrohalogenation.
3. Write the structural formulae and IUPAC names for iosmeric alkenes having molecular formula, C_5H_{10}.

4. What happens when
   (a) Propene is treated with HBr in presence of a peroxide.
   (b) Propene is subjected to ozonolysis.
   (c) Propene is treated with Cl_2 at 500 °C.
5. Write notes on
   (a) Markownikoff's rule.
   (b) Peroxide effect
   (c) Ozonolysis
   (d) Diels-Alder reaction
   (e) Structure and stability of 1, 3-butadiene.
6. How would you synthesise
   (a) *n*-Propyl alcohol from propene and
   (b) Isopropyl alcohol from *n*-propyl alcohol?

   Hints: $n\text{-Propyl alcohol} \xrightarrow[\text{conc. } H_2SO_4]{-H_2O} \text{Propene} \xrightarrow{H_2O / \overset{+}{H}} \text{Isopropyl alcohol}$

   (c) *n*-propyl bromide from isopropyl bromide.

   Hints: $\text{Isopropyl bromide} \xrightarrow{-HBr} \text{propene} \xrightarrow[H_2O_2]{HBr} n\text{-Propyl bromide}$

   (d) 1, 3-butadiene from 1-butene.
7. How would you distinguish between.
   (a) 1-hexene and *n*-hexane.
   (b) Propane and propene
   (c) 1, 3-butadiene and *n*-butane.
8. What happens when 1, 3-butadiene is treated with HBr in CCl_4?
9. (a) How would you obtain alkenes by reduction of alkynes?
   (b) Describe the mechanism of addition of bromine to ethene.
   (c) Name and explain the mechanism of addition of an unsymmetrical molecule over an unsaturated double bond.

   Hints: Markownikoff's rule and anti-Markownikoff's rule.

   (d) What is meant by anti-Markownikoff's addition. Give its mechanism.
   (e) Explain why peroxide effect or anti-Markownikoff's rule (or Kharasch effect) is observed in the addition of HBr and not in HI or HCl addition?

   Hints: H—Cl bond is stronger than H—Br and so cannot be easily cleaved in presence of peroxide to form free radical and hence addition of HCl to alkene is not possible. H—I bond although weaker than HBr yet addition to alkene is not possible because iodine radical formed readily combines to form iodine molecule and so does not add to alkene.
10. On reductive ozonolysis an unsaturated hydrocarbon gave the following:
    (i) Ethane diol, (ii) Propanone, (iii) Ethanol.
    Write the structural formula of the hydrocarbon and write IUPAC name.

Hints:

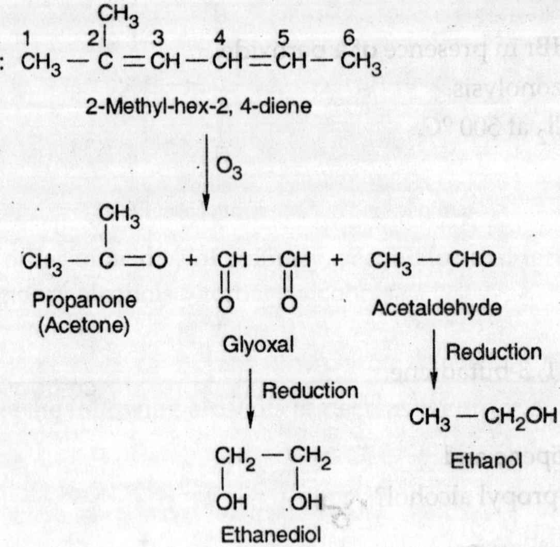
2-Methyl-hex-2, 4-diene
O_3
Propanone
(Acetone)
Glyoxal
Acetaldehyde
Reduction
Reduction
Ethanol
Ethanediol

CHAPTER SIX

Alkynes

Alkynes are a special type of unsaturated aliphatic hydrocarbons. The special characteristic of this group of hydrocarbons is the presence of a *tripple* bond in between two carbon atoms. They are expressed by the general molecular formula, C_nH_{2n-2}. The first and most important member of the series is acetylene, H—C≡C—H. This member is so important and highly representative alkyne that the class as a whole is referred to as *acetylenes* and the corresponding triple bond is termed as *acetylenic* bond. The simple structural representation of this hydrocarbon is

H—C≡C—H
Acetylene

The carbon atoms in acetylene is in *sp*-hybridised state. Two carbon atoms are connected by one σ-bond and two π-bonds. The σ-bond is formed by the co-axial overlapping of *sp*-orbital of each carbon atom. The C—H σ-bond is due to co-axial overlap of *sp*-orbital of carbon and *s*-orbital of hydrogen atom. Since the *sp*-orbitals of each carbon atom exists in a straight line and bond formation occurs by co-axial overlapping of these orbitals, two carbon and two hydrogen atoms of acetylene lie in the same straight line. As a result, acetylene becomes a *linear* molecule. In each carbon atom, there are two unused *p*-orbitals which are mutually perpendicular to each other and are also perpendicular to plane containing two carbon and two hydrogen atoms. These two *p* orbitals of each carbon atom overlap in the parallel direction with two *p*-orbitals of other carbon atom forming two π-bonds. Such type of overlapping gives rise to a cylindrical shape which is co-axially symmetrical.

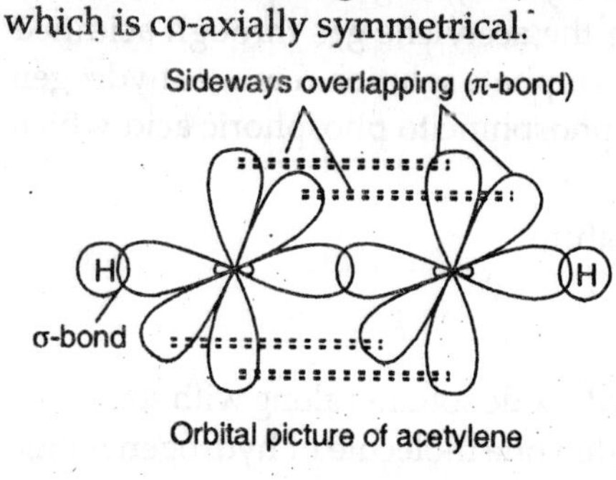

Orbital picture of acetylene

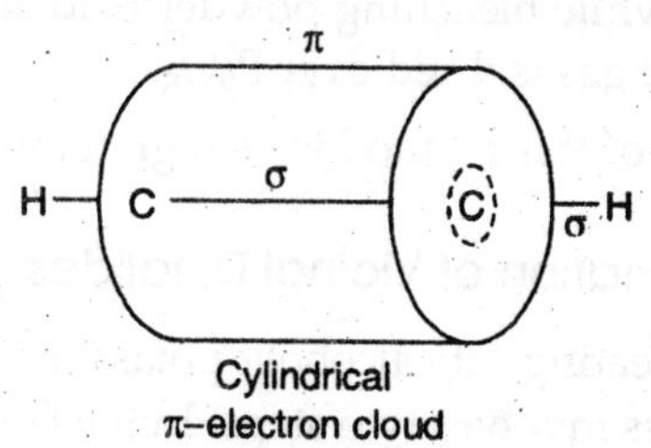

Cylindrical
π–electron cloud

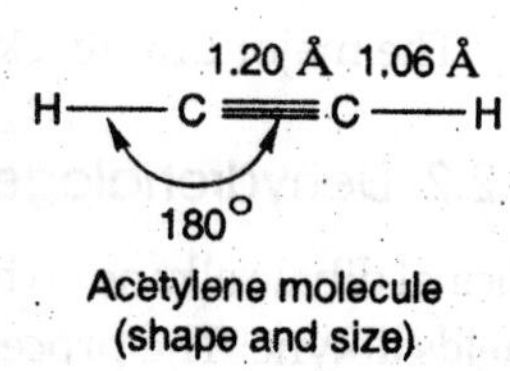

Acetylene molecule
(shape and size)

Thus, in acetylene, triple bond in between two carbon atoms consists of one *sp-sp* σ-bond and two π-bonds. The carbon-carbon bond distance is 1.20Å and C—C—H bond angle is 180°.

6.1 Nomenclature of Alkynes

Alkynes are normally named by applying general rules of IUPAC system of nomenclature. In IUPAC system, the suffix *-ane* of alkane is changed to *-yne* and the position of the triple bond is indicated by the number. Sometimes they are also named as derivatives of acetylene. A few examples that may be cited are as below:

$$\overset{1}{CH_3}-\overset{2}{C}\equiv\overset{3}{C}-\overset{4}{CH_3}$$

2-Butyne (But-2-yne)
or
Dimethyl acetylene

$$\overset{1}{CH_3}-\overset{2}{CH_2}-\overset{3}{C}\equiv\overset{4}{C}-\overset{5}{CH_3}$$

3-Pentyne (Pent-3-yne)
or
Ethyl methyl acetylene

$$\overset{6}{CH_3}-\underset{\displaystyle CH_3}{\overset{5}{CH}}-\overset{4}{CH_2}-\overset{3}{CH_2}-\overset{2}{C}\equiv\overset{1}{CH_3}$$

5-Methyl -1-hexyne (5-Methyl-hex-1-yne)
Or
(2-Methyl)-Butyl acetylene

6.2 Methods of Preparation of Alkynes

6.2.1 From Calcium Carbide

The first and most common member, acetylene, is prepared in the laboratory by the hydrolysis of calcium carbide. Calcium carbide is readily obtained by heating a mixture of limestone and coke at 2000 °C in an electric furnace.

$$CaCO_3 \xrightarrow{\text{Heat}} CaO + CO_2$$

$$CaO + 3C \longrightarrow \underset{\text{Calcium Carbide}}{CaC_2} + CO$$

$$CaC_2 + 2H_2O \longrightarrow H-C\equiv C-H + Ca(OH)_2$$

Acetylene so obtained is not pure. It contains small quantity of hydrogen sulphide, ammonia and phosphine. These impurities are removed by passing the acetylene gas through acidified solution of copper sulphate and bleaching powder. Copper sulphate solution removes hydrogen sulphide and ammonia while bleaching powder oxidises phosphine to phosphoric acid which remains in the water. The gas is dried over P_2O_5.

The major drawback of this method is its high temperature.

6.2.2 Dehydrohalogenation of Vicinal Dihalides

Vicinal dihalo alkane on heating with alcoholic potassium hydroxide solution along with sodamide yields alkyne. The process involves two steps. In the first step one molecule of hydrogen halide is eliminated with the formation of mono halo alkene.

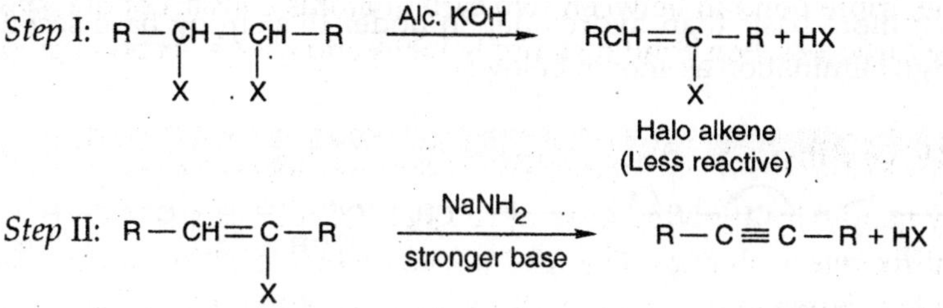

In some cases particularly for the preparation of I-alkynes other than propyne only $NaNH_2$ is used. This is because of the fact that in alcoholic KOH isomerisation of 1-alkyne to 2-alkyne may occur.

6.2.3 Dehalogenation of Tetrahalides

It is also a general method for the preparation of alkynes. In this method vapours of 1, 1, 2, 2-tetrahalides are passed over heated zinc powder when halogens are removed as zinc halide and alkynes are formed.

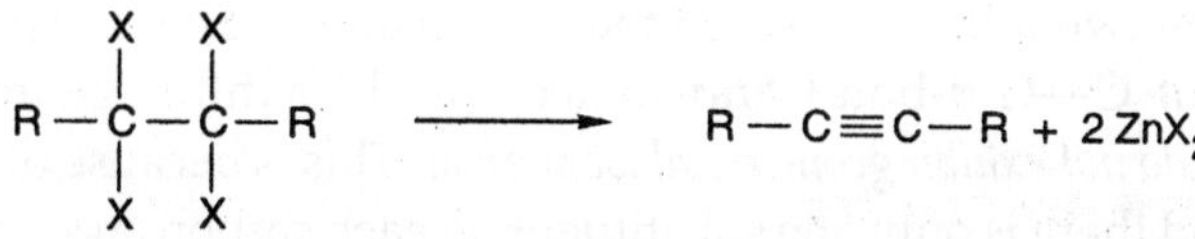

Although the method appears to be a general one but it is not of much importance because the required tetrahalides are usually prepared from alkynes by the addition of halogens.

6.2.4 Alkylation of Acetylene

It is a very good method of preparation of higher alkynes from lower alkynes. This synthetic process comprises of two separate reactions. In the first step, acetylene or any alkyne having terminal hydrogen is converted to its salt by treatment with sodamide.

$$R-C\equiv C-H + NaNH_2 \longrightarrow \underset{\text{Sodium salt of alkyne}}{R-C\equiv CNa} + NH_3$$

In the second step, an alkylhalide preferably primary alkylhalide is allowed to react with sodium salt of alkyne. Salt of alkyne acts as nucleophile and it replaces halide ion from alkylhalide and forms a new carbon-carbon bond.

$$R-C\equiv CNa + R-X \longrightarrow R-C\equiv C-R + NaX$$

$$\underset{\text{Acetylene}}{H-C\equiv CH} + NaNH_2 \longrightarrow H-C\equiv CNa \xrightarrow{CH_3-CH_2-Br} \underset{\text{1-Butyne}}{HC\equiv C-CH_2-CH_3}$$

Thus, it is a case of nucleophilic substitution occurring through SN^2 path.

The reaction is usually carried in liquid ammonia; however, other solvents like ether and tetrahydrofuran may be used.

The most significant drawback of this method is that it proceeds smoothly with good yield, only in the case of primary alkylhalides. The reason for this limitation is that salt of alkyne is a very strong base, even more basic than hydroxide. So under this strong base secondary and tertiary halides undergo elimination as shown below:

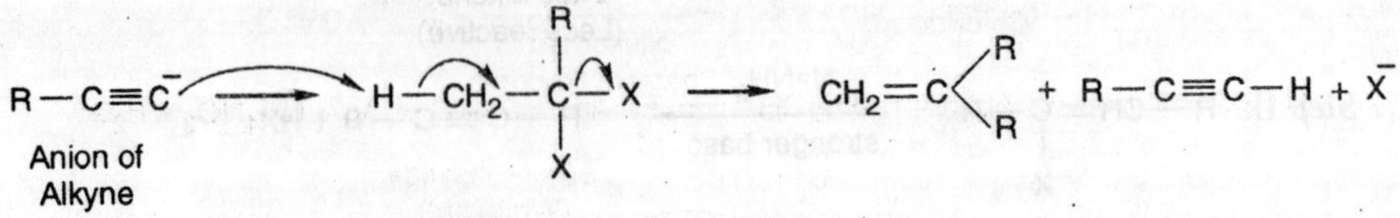

6.3 Properties of Alkynes

Lower members (C_1—C_3) are gases, alkyne containing C_4—C_{10} are liquids while others are solids. The boiling points and melting points of alkynes regularly increase with increase in molecular weights. Alkynes have slightly higher boiling points than corresponding alkanes and alkenes. This is due to the fact that since alkynes are linear in nature successive molecules in crystal require more space, as a result of which surface area is increased. So it will require more energy to pass from liquid to gaseous state.

In alkynes, there are two π-bonds betwen the carbon atoms. So it is expected that they may restrict the rotation of C—C σ-bond and hence should exhibit geometrical isomerism. Unfortunately alkynes *do not exhibit geometrical isomerism*. This is because of the fact that alkynes are linear molecules and there is only one substituent on each carbon atom. In such molecule the steric hindrance is not so high to produce appreciable restriction in rotation and no geometrical isomerism is observed in alkynes.

6.3.1 Chemical Properties of Alkynes

Acidity: Acetylene itself and terminal alkynes ($R-C\equiv C-H$) are acidic in nature. The acidity originates from the fact that in such alkynes hydrogen atom is connected to a *sp*-hybridised carbon atom. In this orbital *s*-character is appreciably predominant. Electrons in *s*-orbital is closer to the nucleus. This means electrion pair of C—H bond in acetylene and terminal alkynes is more towards carbon nucleus. This makes C—H bond to some extent less stronger and so H atom can be easily abstracted with the formation of conjugate base.

$$H-C\equiv C-H \xrightarrow[B]{\text{Base}} \underset{\text{Conjugate Base}}{H-C\equiv \bar{C}} + \overset{+}{B}H$$

Therefore, acetylene and terminal alkynes are acidic in nature and can act as nucleophlic. The acidic nature of such alkynes are manifested from the following reactions:

i. Acetylene and terminal alkynes on treatment with $NaNH_2$ in liquid ammonia form salts.

$$H-C\equiv C-H + NaNH_2 \xrightarrow[NH_3]{\text{liq.}} \underset{\text{Sodium Acetylide}}{H-C\equiv \bar{C}\overset{+}{Na}}$$

$$R-C\equiv C-H + NaNH_2 \xrightarrow[NH_3]{\text{liq}} \underset{\text{Sodium Alkylide}}{R-C\equiv \bar{C}\overset{+}{Na}}$$

ii. Acetylene and terminal alkynes also form salts with silver and copper ions.

$$\mathrm{H{-}C{\equiv}C{-}H} + \underset{\text{Cuprous Chloride}}{\mathrm{Cu_2Cl_2}} + \mathrm{NH_4OH} \longrightarrow \underset{\text{Copper-acetylide (Red ppt)}}{\mathrm{Cu{-}C{\equiv}C{-}Cu}} + \mathrm{NH_4Cl} + \mathrm{2H_2O}$$

$$\mathrm{H{-}C{\equiv}C{-}H} + \mathrm{AgNO_3} + \mathrm{NH_4OH} \longrightarrow \underset{\text{Silver-acetylide (White ppt)}}{\mathrm{Ag{-}C{\equiv}C{-}Ag}} + \mathrm{NH_4NO_3} + \mathrm{H_2O}$$

These acetylides are insoluble in water and have characteristic colours. For this reason, formation of these acetylides are used for identification of acetylenic bond and to *differentiate alkynes from alkenes.* It may be mentioned, with excess of $NaNH_2$ acetylene may form disodium salt $\mathrm{Na{-}C{\equiv}C{-}Na}$.

iii. Acetylene or terminal alkyne can function as nucleophile.

$$\mathrm{CH{\equiv}CH} + \mathrm{NaNH_2} \longrightarrow \mathrm{CH{\equiv}\overset{-}{C}} + \mathrm{CH_3{-}X} \longrightarrow \underset{\text{Propyne}}{\mathrm{CH{\equiv}C{-}CH_3}}$$

PROBLEM 6.1

(a) Explain why acetylenic proton is acidic?

(b) Predict the product:

$$\mathrm{R{-}C{\equiv}C{-}H} + \mathrm{NaNH_2} \xrightarrow[\mathrm{NH_3}]{\text{Liq.}}$$

6.3.2 Other Chemical Properties of Alkynes

Chemical activities of acetylene and alkynes in general originate from the two π-bonds present in these compounds. Since these hydrocarbons are rich in electrons major reactions are of electrophilic addition reactions. However, although there are two π-bonds in these compounds, they are less reactive than alkenes. The less activity of alkynes towards electrophilic reagent than alkenes may be interpreted from their molecular orbital structures.

The carbon atoms in alkynes are in *sp*-hybridised state but in alkenes they are in sp^2-hybridised state. This means *s*-character of orbital in alkynes is higher than that of alkenes. We know that more the *s*-character of an orbital, more tightly the electrons of that orbital are held by the nucleus. Therefore, π-electrons in alkynes are more strongly held by carbon atoms in alkynes. Consequently, they are less readily available for the attack by electrophilic reagent.

Again, π-electrons in alkynes assume a co-axially symmetrical cylindrical shape having a large volume. So electron density per unit volume becomes low. This makes less availability of π-electrons in alkynes for electrophiles. But in alkenes no such decrease in π-electron density occurs. For these reasons alkynes are less reactive towards electrophilic reagents than alkenes. The most common addition reactions that are found to occur frequently in alkynes are mentioned in the sequel.

(a) *Hydrogenation of Alkynes*: Hydrogenation of alkynes takes place in presence of catalysts like finely divided platinum, palladium, nickel, etc. Two molar equivalents of hydrogen are added to the triple bond and alkanes are formed.

$$CH{\equiv}CH + 2H_2 \xrightarrow{Pt} \underset{\text{Ethane}}{CH_3-CH_3}$$

$$R-C{\equiv}C-R + 2H_2 \xrightarrow{Pt} \underset{\text{Alkane}}{R-CH_2-CH_2-R}$$

Hydrogenation takes place in two stages. In the first stage one molar equivalent of hydrogen is added to form alkene which in the second stage adds one mole equivalent of hydrogen more to yield alkane.

Stage I: $H-C{\equiv}C-H + H_2 \xrightarrow{Pt} \underset{\text{Ethylene}}{CH_2{=}CH_2}$

$$R-C{\equiv}C-R + H_2 \xrightarrow{P} \underset{\text{Alkene}}{R-CH{=}CH-R}$$

Stage II: $CH_2{=}CH_2 + H_2 \xrightarrow{Pt} \underset{\text{Ethane}}{CH_3-CH_3}$

$$R-CH{=}CH-R + H_2 \xrightarrow{Pt} \underset{\text{Alkane}}{R-CH_2-CH_2-R}$$

If partial hydrogenation occurs alkene may be formed and in actual practice that has been found to be so. A special type of catalyst known as *Lindlar Catalyst* which is a combination of palladium on calcium carbonate with lead acetate and quinoline has been developed for this purpose. Lead acetate and quinoline deactivate the catalyst making it a poor catalyst for hydrogenation of alkene, but it remains sufficiently active for hydrogenation of alkyne to alkene.

$$H-C{\equiv}C-H + H_2 \xrightarrow[\text{2. lead acetate and quinoline}]{\text{1. Pd/CaCO}_3} CH_2{=}CH_2$$

$$R-C{\equiv}C-R + H_2 \xrightarrow[\text{2. lead acetate and quinoline}]{\text{1. Pd/CaCO}_3} R-CH{=}CH-R$$

This partial hydrogenation of alkynes by the use of Lindar catalyst finds a useful method of synthesis of alkene.

(b) *Addition of Halogen Acids*: Addition of halogen acid to alkynes also takes place in two stages.

$$H-C{\equiv}C-H + HX \longrightarrow \underset{\text{Vinyl halide}}{H-\underset{H}{C}{=}\underset{X}{C}-H}$$

$$R-C{\equiv}C-R + HX \longrightarrow R-\underset{H}{C}{=}\underset{X}{C}-H$$

If another molecule of HX is added,

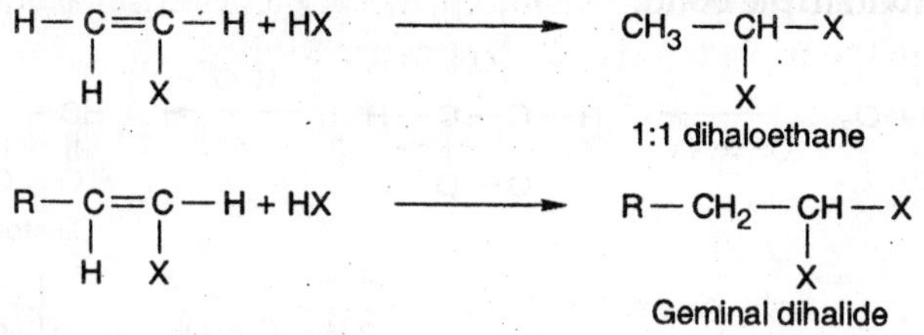

In the case of unsymmetrical alkynes addition follows Markownikoff's rule.

(c) *Addition of Halogens*: Addition of halogens to alkynes is also a two-step reaction forming dihalo and tetra-halo alkanes.

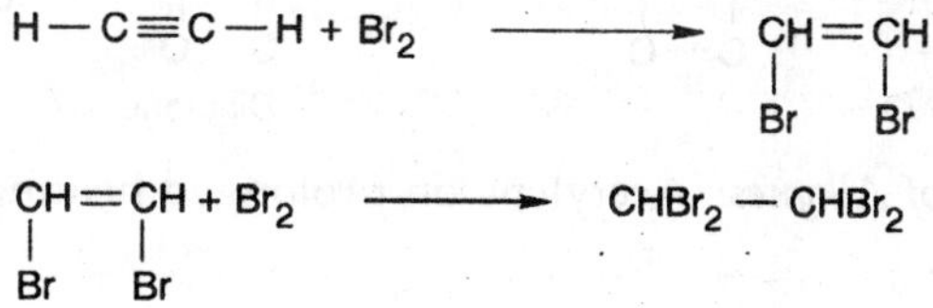

(d) *Addition of Water (Hydration)*: Acetylenes and alkynes on treatment with water in presence of sulphuric acid and mercuric sulphate as catalyst form carbonyl compounds (aldehyde or ketone).

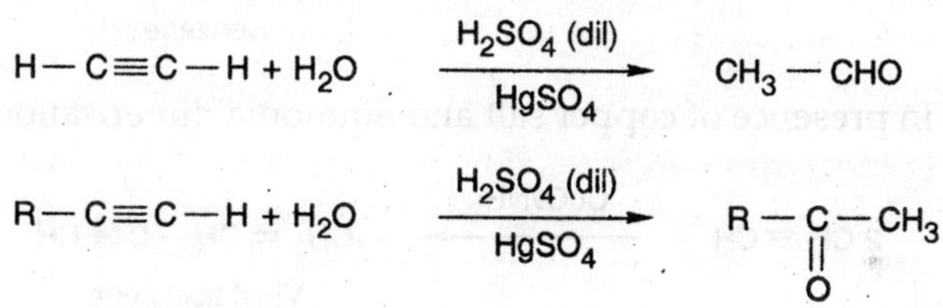

Addition of water takes place in accordance to Markownikoff's rule.

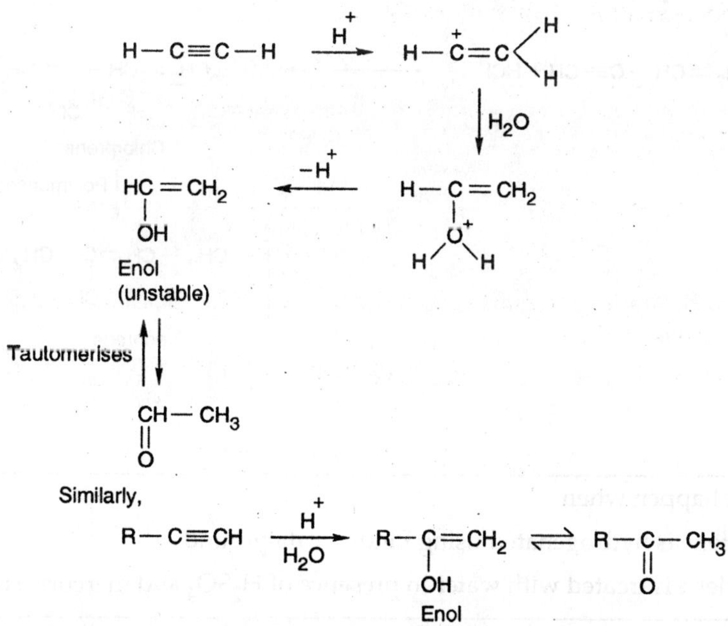

(e) *Ozonolysis of Alkyne*: Ozonolysis of alkynes forms carboxylic acids by the cleavage of carbon-carbon triple bond.

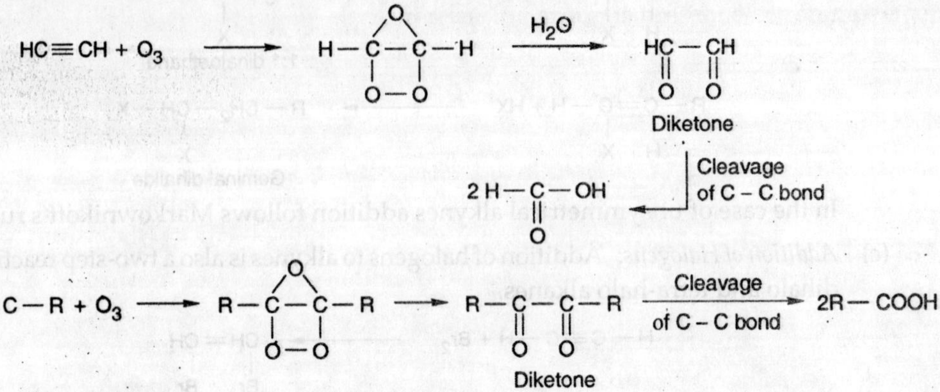

(f) *Polymerisation of Alkynes*: Acetylene on prolonged heating at temperature of 500 °C forms benzene.

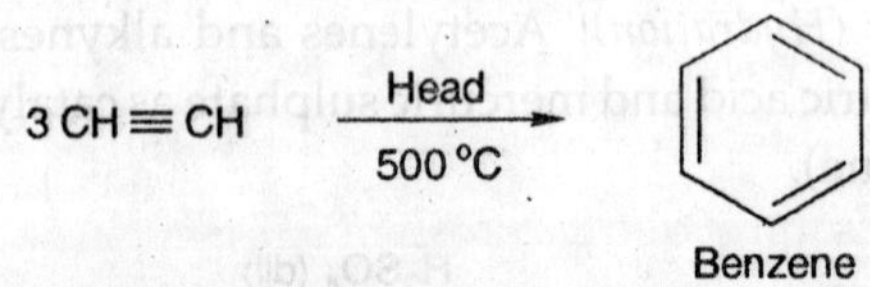

Benzene

However, in presence of copper salt and ammonia dimerisation takes place.

$$2\,CH{\equiv}CH \xrightarrow{CuCl/NH_3} CH_2{=}CH{-}C{\equiv}CH$$

Vinyl acetylene

Vinyl acetylene is an intermediate for the synthesis of synthetic rubber, *Neoprene*.

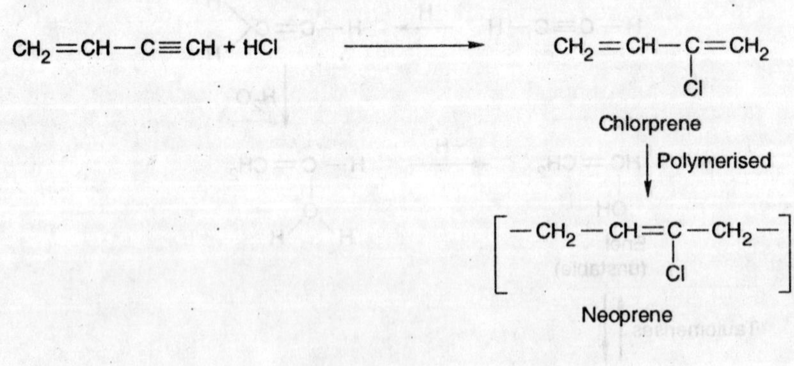

PROBLEM 6.2

What will happen when

(a) Acetylene is hydrogenated using Lindlar catalyst and

(b) Acetylene is treated with water in presence of H_2SO_4 and mercuric sulphate?

6.4 Uses of Alkynes

Acetylene on burning with oxygen produces an intensely hot flame which is used for cutting and welding of metals. Acrylonitrile prepared by the addition of HCN to acetylene in presence of $CuCl/NH_4Cl$ catalyst [($CH \equiv CH + HCN \xrightarrow{CuCl/NH_4Cl} CH_2 = CH - CN$) (acrylonitrile)] is a raw material for synthetic fibre *Orlon* and *Acrylon*.

Accetylene is also used for the preparation of other useful materials such as vinyl chloride which is used in plastics (PVC) etc, vinylacetate used in paints, adhesives, plastics, etc., tri- and per-chloroethrylenes used as an important dry cleaning solvent, methohexital sodium, an important general anaesthetic and an effective sedative, ethinamate, etc.

Model Questions

1. What are alkynes? How are they prepared?
2. Explain: (i) Alkynes are less reactive than alkene towards electrophilic addition.
   (ii) Alkynes undergo nucleophilic as well as electrophilic.
   (iii) Actylenic protons are acidic in nature.
3. How acctylene is prepared industrially?
4. What happens when
   (a) Calcium carbide is treated with water?
   (b) Acetylene is passed through red hot iron tube?
   (c) Acetylene is passed through ammoniacal silver nitrate solution?
   (d) Acetylene is passed through ammoniacal cuprous chloride solution?
   (e) Acetylene is passed through dilute sulphuric acid in the presence of mercuric sulphate?
5. How will you distinguish
   (a) Acetylene and ethylene?
   (b) 1-Butyne and 2-Butyne?
6. How will you synthesise
   (a) Acetaldehyde from acetylene?
   (b) Acetylene from ethylene?
   (c) 1-Butyne from acetylene?
   (d) Acetone from propene?
   (e) Neoprene from acetylene?

CHAPTER SEVEN

Aliphatic Halogen Compounds

Aliphatic halogen compounds are primarily halogen derivatives of aliphatic hydrocarbons formed by replacing their hydrogen atoms. Among them halogen derivatives of saturated hydrocarbons (alkanes) are important. They are classified into following groups:

i. *Monohalogen Compounds*: These compounds contain one halogen atom in their molecule. Common members are methyl chloride, ethyl chloride, propyl chloride, etc. These are most important class of aliphatic halogen compounds and are generally known as *alkylhalides* and are expressed by the general formula, $C_nH_{2n+1}X$ or R—X, where R is any alkyl group and X represents a halogen atom such as Cl, Br, I, F. Alkylhalides may be primary, secondary and tertiary in nature depending upon the nature of alkyl group (see chapter **two**) to which the halogen atom is attached.

ii. *Dihalogen Compounds:* These halogen compounds contain two halogen atoms. For example, methylene dichloride (CH_2Cl_2), dichloro ethane (CH_3—$CHCl_2$).

iii. *Trihalogen Compounds*: Compounds like chloroform, $CHCl_3$, iodoform CHI_3 which contain three halogen atoms in the molecule are known as trihalogen compounds.

iv. *Tetrahalogen Compounds*: There are four halogen atoms in the molecule; as for example, carbon tetra, chloride (CCl_4).

7.1 Alkylhalides (Monohalogen Compounds)

Alkylhalides constitute one of the most important intermediates in the synthesis of organic compounds. This is due to ability of alkylhalides to undergo a wide variety of chemical reactions. They are used as eco-friendly insecticides.

7.1.1 Nomenclature of Alkylhalides

There are two ways by which alkylhalides may be named.

i. *Popular System*: In this method alkylhalides are named according to the name of alkyl group to which halogen atom is attached. Thus, methyl chloride, ethyl chloride, propyl chloride, butyl chloride, etc.

ii. *IUPAC System*: According to this system, alkylhalides are named as *haloalkane* and the position of halogen atom in the longest chain is indicated by number following the general rules:

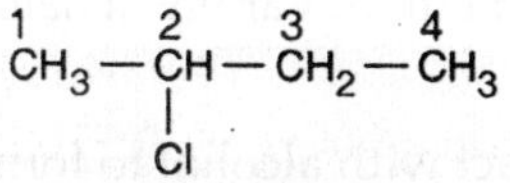

2-Chlorobutane

$$CH_3-CH_2-CH_2-CH_2-CH_2-Br$$

1-Bromo pentane

The highly illustrated member of this family is methyl halides. However, they are not typical members but ethylhalides may be looked upon as typical member because variety of chemical activities exhibited by alkylhalides can be illustrated taking ethylhalides as examples.

7.1.2 Structure of Alkylhalides

The first and most popular member methylhalide (CH_3X) has three H atoms and one halogen atom attached with carbon atom. Carbon atom as usual is in sp^3-hybridised state and halogen atom has half-filled *p*-orbital in its valence shell. Each of the three C—H bonds is formed by the co-axial overlap of sp^3 orbital of carbon and *s*-orbital of hydrogen forming σ-bond and C—X bond is due to co-axial overlap of sp^3-orbital of carbon and half-filled *p*-orbital of halogen giving rise to another σ-bond. Overall shape of the halide is tetrahedral.

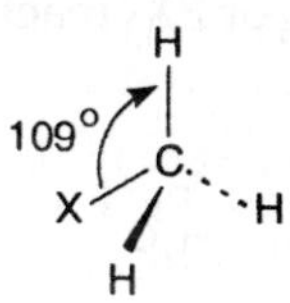

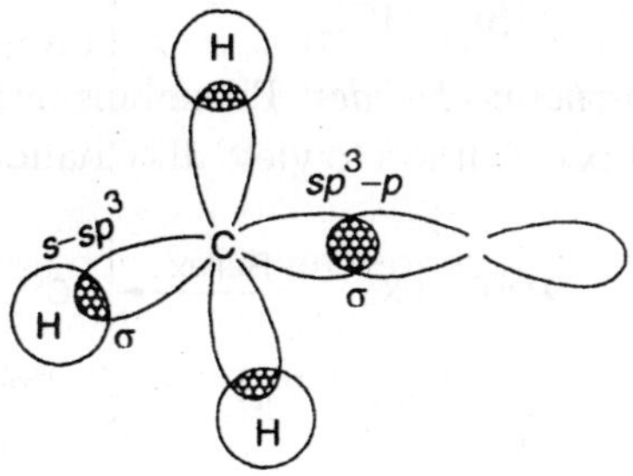

Orbital structure of Methylhalide

PROBLEM 7.1

> How many structures are possible for a compound whose molecular formula is C_4H_9Br. Name all these according to IUPAC system.

7.1.3 Preparation of Alkylhalides

Alkylhalides are normally prepared in the laboratory by the following general methods:

(a) *Halogenation of Alkanes*: In presence of UV-light or any oxygen source, halogens, particularly chlorine and bromine, replace hydrogen atom to form alkylhalides.

$$CH_4 + X_2 \xrightarrow[\text{light}]{\text{uv}} CH_3X + HX$$

$$R-H + X_2 \xrightarrow[\text{light}]{\text{uv}} R-X + HX$$

This method is used in industry, but it is not suitable for laboratory preparation. Because along with alkylhalide always there is formation of polyhalides and so complication regarding the separation arises, i.e.,

$$CH_3-X \xrightarrow[uv]{Cl_2} CH_2Cl_2 \xrightarrow[uv\ light]{Cl_2} CHCl_3 \xrightarrow[uv\ light]{Cl_2} CCl_4$$

(b) *Replacement of Alcoholic Hydroxyl Group:* Preparation of alkylhalides by the replacement of hydroxyl group of alcohol is a very common method. Variety of halogen compounds may be used.

i. *Halogen Acids:* Halogen acids readily react with alcohol to form alkylhalides.

$$\underset{\text{Methyl alcohol}}{CH_3OH} + HX \longrightarrow \underset{\text{Methyl halide}}{CH_3X} + H_2O$$

$$R-OH + HX \longrightarrow \underset{\text{Alkylhalide}}{R-X} + H_2O$$

HBr and HI react with alcohols directly but HCl requires the presence of a catalyst like $ZnCl_2$ and better yield is obtained when dry HCl is used.

$$CH_3-CH_2-OH + HCl\ (dry) \xrightarrow{ZnCl_2} \underset{\text{Ethyl halide}}{CH_3-CH_2-X}$$

The order of reactivity of primary, secondary and tertiary alcohols is tertiary alcohol > secondary alcohol > primary alcohol and that of halogen acids is HI > HBr > HCl.

ii. *Phosphorous Halides:* Phosphorous halides PX_5 or PX_3 react with alcohols under reflux condition to yield alkylhalides.

$$CH_3-OH + PX_5 \xrightarrow{Reflux} CH_3-X + POX_3 + H_2O$$

$$CH_3-\underset{|\atop OH}{CH}-CH_2-CH_3 + PX_5 \xrightarrow{Reflux} CH_3-\underset{|\atop X}{CH}-CH_2-CH_3 + POX_3 + H_2O$$

Phosphorous bromide and iodides are prepared *in situ* by adding red phosphorous to corresponding halogen.

$$2P + 3Br_2 \longrightarrow 2PBr_3$$

$$2P + 3I_2 \longrightarrow 2PI_3$$

iii. *Thionyl Chloride:* Thionyl chloride ($SOCl_2$) is an important halogen containing reagent which can readily replace alcoholic hydroxyl group by chlorine.

$$CH_3-OH + SOCl_2 \longrightarrow CH_3-Cl + SO_2 + HCl$$

$$R-OH + SOCl_2 \longrightarrow R-Cl + SO_2 + HCl$$

(c) *Addition of Halogen Acids to Alkene:* When halogen acids are allowed to react with alkene, corresponding alkylhalides are formed. This process is followed in industry as a commercial method for the preparation of alkylhalides.

$$\underset{\text{Ethylene}}{CH_2=CH_2} + HX \longrightarrow \underset{\text{Ethyl halide}}{CH_3-CH_2-X}$$

7.1.4 Properties of Alkylhalides

7.1.4.1 Physical Properties of Alkylhalides

Methylhalides are gases but alkylhalides containing carbon atoms up to 16 are liquids, and beyond C_{16} are solids. Alkylhalides are insoluble in water although they contain polar C—X bond. This is due to the fact that the difference of electronegativity between halogen and hydrogen is negligible and so H-bond formation between the molecules of alkylhalides and water is not possible. The boiling points of alkylhalides for a given halogen atom increases with the increase in the size of alkyl groups, and for a given alkyl group, boiling point increases with the increase in atomic weight of halogen, i.e., the order of boiling points is RI > RBr > RCl > RF for a given alkyl group.

Boiling points of some alkylhalides (in °C)

Alkyl group	I	Br	Cl	F
CH_3—	42.5	4	– 24	– 78
CH_3—CH_2—	72.5	38	12.5	– 38

7.1.4.2 Chemical Properties of Alkylhalides

The most significant and widely discussed property of alkylhalides is their *nucleophilic substitution reaction*. In this substitution reaction halogen atom can be replaced by a variety of nucleophilic reagents with the formation of various products. Thus,

i. *Action of aqueous Potassium Hydroxide*

$$R-X + KOH\ (\text{aqueous solution}) \longrightarrow \underset{\text{Alcohol}}{R-OH} + KX$$

$$\underset{\text{Ethyl Bromide}}{CH_3-CH_2-Br} + Aq.\ KOH \longrightarrow \underset{\text{Ethyl Alcohol}}{CH_3-CH_2-OH} + KBr$$

ii. *Reaction with Alkoxide*

$$R-X + \underset{\substack{\text{Sodium}\\\text{Ethoxide}}}{C_2H_5ONa} \longrightarrow \underset{\text{Ether}}{C_2H_5-O-R} + NaX$$

$$CH_3-X + C_2H_5ONa \longrightarrow \underset{\text{Ethylmethyl Ether}}{C_2H_5-O-CH_3} + NaX$$

This is the well known method for the synthesis of ether termed as *Williamson Synthesis*.

iii. *Reaction with Sodium Cyanide*

$$R-X + NaCN \longrightarrow \underset{\text{Alkyl Cyanide}}{R-CN} + NaX$$

$$CH_3-X + NaCN \longrightarrow \underset{\text{Methyl Cyanide}}{CH_3-CN} + NaX$$

$$\underset{\text{Ethyl Bromide}}{CH_3-CH_2-Br} + NaCN \longrightarrow \underset{\text{Ethyl Cyanide}}{CH_3-CH_2-CN} + NaBr$$

iv. *Reaction with Ammonia*

$$R-X + NH_3 \longrightarrow \underset{\text{Alkyl Amine}}{R-NH_2} + HX$$

$$CH_3-X + NH_3 \longrightarrow \underset{\text{Methyl Amine}}{CH_3-NH_2} + HX$$

$$CH_3-CH_2-X + NH_3 \longrightarrow \underset{\text{Ethyl Amine}}{CH_3-CH_2-NH_2} + HX$$

v. *Reaction with Acetylide*

$$R-X + \underset{\text{Sodium Acetylide}}{HC\equiv \overset{-}{C}\overset{+}{Na}} \longrightarrow \underset{\text{Alkyne}}{HC\equiv C-R} + NaX$$

vi. *Reaction with Silver Nitrite*

$$R-X + AgNO_2 \longrightarrow \underset{\text{Nitroparaffin}}{R-NO_2} + AgX$$

$$CH_3-X + AgNO_2 \longrightarrow \underset{\text{Nitromethane}}{CH_3-NO_2} + AgX$$

vii. *Reaction with Salts of Carboxylic Acids*

$$R-X + R'-COONa \longrightarrow \underset{\text{Ester}}{ROCOR'} + NaX$$

$$\underset{\text{Ethyl Bromide}}{CH_3-CH_2-Br} + CH_3COONa \longrightarrow \underset{\text{Ethyl Acetate}}{CH_3COOCH_2CH_3} + NaBr$$

All the above reactions (i-vii) are nucleophilic substitution (SN) reaction and can proceed either by S_{N^1} or S_{N^2} depending upon the conditions of the reaction and nature of alkyl group of the alkyl halide (see chapter **two**). In general, the order of activity of alkylhalides for S_{N^2} path is:

Primary Alkylhalide > Secondary Alkylhalide > Tertiary Alkylhalide and in the case of S_{N^1} the order is reverse.

Problem 7.2

Suggest the order of the following alkylhalides for SN^2 hydrolysis:

$$CH_3-CH_2-Cl, \quad CH_3-\underset{\displaystyle CH_3}{\underset{|}{CH}}-Cl, \quad CH_3-\underset{\displaystyle CH_3}{\underset{|}{\overset{\displaystyle CH_3}{\overset{|}{C}}}}-Cl$$

viii. Another interesting type of reactions undergone by alkylhalides is the *Elimination Reactions.* The most important reaction is the dehydro halogenation of alkylhalides. In this reaction a molecule of hydrogen halide is eliminated and the product is commonly an alkene. For the smooth elimination of hydrogen halide molecule followed by the formation of alkene, halogen and hydrogen atoms must be situated at consecutive carbon atoms or in other words, alkylhalides to undergo elimination reaction there must be a hydrogen atom at the β-position (carbon atom at which halogen is attached is considered to be α). Methylhalide does not have β-hydrogen atom and hence cannot undergo elimination reaction. On the other hand, ethylhalide has β-hydrogen atom.

$$\overset{\beta}{H-CH_2}-\overset{\alpha}{CH_2}-X$$

So it can undergo elimination reaction. That is why ethylhalide, not methylhalide, is regarded as a typical and representative member of alkylhalides (Ethylhalide can also undergo all other reactions of alkylhalide).

The elimination reaction of alkylhalides smoothly takes place in presence of alcoholic potassium hydroxide solution under reflux. Thus,

$$\underset{\text{Ethyl halide}}{H-CH_2-CH_2-X} \xrightarrow[\text{Heat}]{\text{Alc. KOH}} \underset{\text{Ethylene}}{CH_2=CH_2} + HX$$

The path of elimination may be either E_1 or E_2. Which one will actually be the path that is governed by some factors and in the case of unsymmetrical alkylhalide product formation is controlled by Saytzeff's rule and normally highly substituted alkene alkene becomes the major product (see chapter **one**).

PROBLEM 7.3

Suggest the possible products and indicate which one is the major product.

$$CH_3-\underset{\substack{|\\X}}{CH}-CH_2-CH_3 \xrightarrow[\text{Heat}]{\text{Alc. KOH}}$$

Other type of Reactions of Alkylhalides

i. *Formation of Grignard Reagent*: Alkylhalide in dry ethereal solution reacts with dry magnesium ribbon to form Grignard compound.

$$R-X + Mg \xrightarrow{\text{dry ether}} \underset{\text{Grignard compound}}{RMgX}$$

$$CH_3-I + Mg \xrightarrow{\text{dry ether}} \underset{\text{Grignard compound}}{RMgI}$$

Grignard reagent has immense applications in synthetic organic chemistry for the preparations of variety of compounds.

ii. *Formation of Other Organometallic Compound*: Other metals like Li and Zn can react with alkylhalides to form alkyl metal compounds which are also used in the synthesis of organic compounds.

$$C_2H_5Br + 2\,Li \xrightarrow{\text{dry ether}} C_2H_5Li + LiBr$$

$$R-X + 2\,Li \xrightarrow{\text{dry ether}} RLi + LiX$$

iii. *Wurtz Reaction*: Alkylhalides participate in Wurtz reaction for the preparation of alkane. The reaction occurs in presence of metallic sodium under reflux condition in an appropriate solvent.

$$2R-X + 2Na \xrightarrow[\text{Reflux}]{\text{Solvent}} R-R + 2NaX$$

$$\underset{\text{Ethyl Bromide}}{2CH_3-CH_2-Br} + 2Na \xrightarrow[\text{Reflux}]{\text{Solvent}} \underset{n\text{-Butane}}{CH_3-CH_2-CH_2-CH_3}$$

iv. *Friedel-Crafts Reaction*: Friedel-Crafts reaction is a process of preparation of alkyl derivatives of aromatic hydrocarbons in presence of anhydrous aluminium chloride. Alkylhalides in this reaction serves as the source of alkyl group.

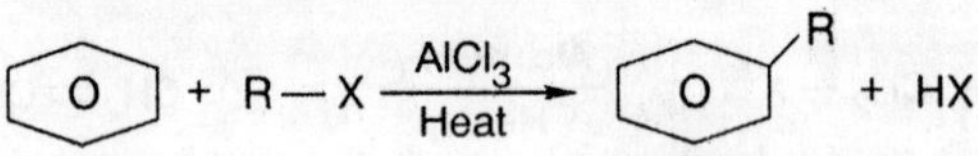

Benrenl

Alkyl derivative benrenl

7.2 Haloethanes

Monohalogen drivatives of ethane are termed as haloethanes. These members are ethyl chloride, ethyl bromide and ethyliodide. Ethyl chloride is commonly prepared by the following methods:

i. By the action of hydrogen chloride gas on ethyl alcohol in presence of anhydrons zinc chloride:

$$C_2H_5OH + HCl \xrightarrow{ZnCl_2} \underset{\text{Ethyl Chloride}}{C_2H_5Cl} + H_2O$$

ii. By the addition of hydrogen chloride to ethylene in presence of aluminium chloride:

$$\underset{\text{Ethylene}}{C_2H_4} + HCl \xrightarrow{AlCl_3} C_2H_5Cl$$

Ethyl chloride exhibits the common properties of alkylhalide.

Ethyl bromide is prepared in large scale by passing a mixture of ethylene and hydrogen bromide through a suspension of aluminium bromide at low temperature:

$$\underset{\text{Ethylene}}{CH_2=CH_2} + HBr \xrightarrow{AlBr_3} \underset{\text{Ethylbromide}}{C_2H_5Br}$$

In the laboratory it is conveniently prepared by distilling a mixture of KBr, C_2H_5OH and conc. H_2SO_4.

$$KBr + H_2SO_4 \longrightarrow KHSO_4 + HBr$$

$$C_2H_5OH + HBr \longrightarrow C_2H_5Br + H_2O$$

Like ethyl chloride it shows the common properties of alkylhalides.

Ethyliodide is normally prepared by warming a mixture of ethyl alcohol, red phosphorous and iodine

$$2P + 3I_2HC_2H_5OH \longrightarrow \underset{\text{Ethyl iodide}}{6C_2H_5I} + 2H_3PO_4$$

7.3 Dihalogen Derivatives of Alkanes

Two types of dihalogen derivatives of alkanes are known, viz,

(a) Gem-dihalide—in which both the halogen atoms are attahed to the same carbon atom. Most common members of this group are methylene chloride CH_2Cl_2 and 1, 1-dichloroethane, CH_3—$CHCl_2$. They are prepared by the following methods:

i. By the addition of halogen acid to alkynes:

$$HC{\equiv}CH + HCl \longrightarrow CH_3{-}CCl_2$$

Acetylene → 1, 1-Dichloroethane

ii. By direct halogenation of alkanes:

$$CH_4 + Cl_2 \xrightarrow[\text{light}]{\text{UV}} CH_2Cl_2$$

Methylene chloride

(b) *Vic Dihalides*: In this type of dihalides, two halogen atoms are attached to two consecutive carbon atoms. Most important member is ethylene dibromide Br—CH_2—CH_2—Br.It may be prepared by the following methods:

i. When hydrogen halides or phosphorous halides react with glycol, 1, 2-dihalo compound is formed.

$$CH_2OH{-}CH_2OH + HBr \longrightarrow CH_2Br{-}CH_2Br$$

Ethylene glycol → 1, 2-Dibromo ethylene

ii Ethylene on treatment with halogen forms 1, 2-dihalo derivative.

$$CH_2{=}CH_2 + Br_2 \longrightarrow CH_2Br{-}CH_2Br$$

Properties: Dihalo alkanes are liquids and insoluble in water. Chemically they are much similar to mono halogen derivative and undergo substitution and elimination reactions. Thus,

i. $$CH_2Cl_2 + KOH \xrightarrow[\text{Heat}]{H_2O} CH_2(OH)_2 \xrightarrow{-H_2O} H{-}C(H){=}O$$

Methylene chloride → Formaldehyde

$$Cl{-}CH_2{-}CH_2{-}Cl + KOH \xrightarrow[\text{Heat}]{H_2O} CH_2OH{-}CH_2OH + 2KCl$$

Ethylene dichloride → Ethylene glycol

ii. $$Cl{-}CH_2{-}CH_2{-}Cl \xrightarrow[\text{Heat}]{\text{Alc. KOH}} CH_2{=}CH_2 + 2KCl + H_2O$$

Ethylene

7.4 Trihalo Alkanes

In this class of halides all the three halogen atoms are attached to the same carbon atom. Most of common members of this family are chloroform, $CHCl_3$; Iodoform, CHI_3; and trichloro ethylene, C_2HCl_3.

7.4.1 Chloroform ($CHCl_3$)

Chloroform is prepared in the laboratory by the reaction of bleaching powder and ethyl alcohol. Bleaching powder, $Ca(OCl)_2$ is taken in a flask and a paste is made with water. To it ethyl alcohol is added and distilled. It is purified by redistillation and dried over anhydrous $CaCl_2$. The reaction taking place may be depicted as below:

$$Ca(OCl)_2 + H_2O \rightleftharpoons Ca(OH)_2 + Cl_2$$

$$\underset{\text{Ethylalcohol}}{CH_3-CH_2OH} + Cl_2 \xrightarrow[\text{[O]}]{Ca(OH)_2} \underset{\text{Acetaldehyde}}{CH_3CHO} + HCl$$

$$CH_3-CHO + 3Cl_2 \xrightarrow[\text{reaction in presence of } Ca(OH)_2]{\text{Haloform}} CCl_3CHO + 3HCl$$

$$CCl_3-CHO \xrightarrow{\text{Hydrolysis}} \underset{\text{Chloroform}}{CHCl_3} + \underset{\text{Ca-formates}}{Ca(O-\overset{\displaystyle O}{\overset{\|}{C}}-H)_2}$$

In place of ethyl alcohol acetone may be used. Procedure in this case is similar and the reaction occurring is known as haloform reaction, i.e.,

$$\underset{\text{Acetone}}{CH_3-\underset{\underset{\displaystyle O}{\|}}{C}-CH_3} + 3Cl_2 \longrightarrow CCl_3-\underset{\underset{\displaystyle O}{\|}}{C}-CH_3$$

$$CCl_3-\underset{\underset{\displaystyle O}{\|}}{C}-CH_3 \xrightarrow[\text{Hydrolysis}]{Ca(OH)_2} CHCl_3 + \underset{\text{Ca-acetate}}{(CH_3-COO)_2Ca}$$

7.4.1.1 Properties of Chloroform

Chloroform is a colourless liquid with a pleasant smell. It is used as solvent and also as anaesthetic. Some important reactions of chloroform are noted below:

(a) *Hydrolysis*: On hydrolysis with aqueous alkali it forms formic acid.

$$CHCl_3 + NaOH \xrightarrow{\text{Heat}} \underset{\text{Na-formate}}{H-COONa} + H_2O + NaCl$$

(b) *Reaction with primary amine*: Chloroform when heated with primary amine in presence of alcoholic alkali obnoxious smelling isocyanide is formed.

$$R-NH_2 + CHCl_3 \xrightarrow[\text{KOH}]{\text{Alcoholic}} \underset{\text{Isocyanide}}{R-N\overset{\rightarrow}{\equiv}C} + 3KCl + 3H_2O$$

Formation of isocyanide may be explained as

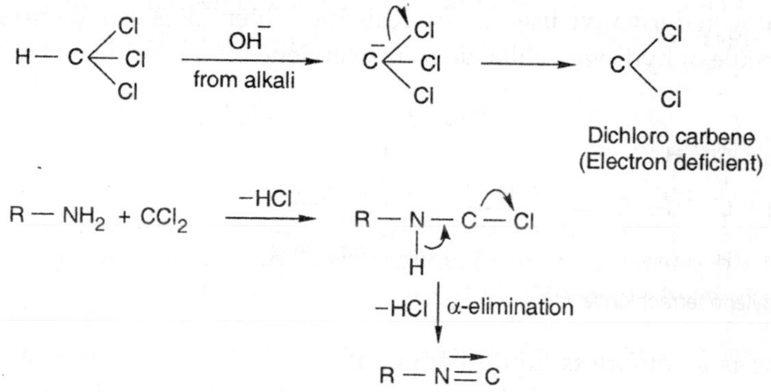

This reaction is employed as a test for detecting primary amine known as *carbylamine test*.

(c) *Nitration*: Chloroform on nitration with HNO_3 forms nitrochloroform known as *chloropicrin* used as pesticide.

$$H-CCl_3 + HNO_3 \longrightarrow Cl_3-C-NO_2 + H_2O$$

Chloropicrin

(d) *Reimer-Tiemann Reaction*: Chloroform is one of the reactants in Reimer-Tiemann reaction which is a general reaction for the preparation of aromatic hydroxy aldehydes. Thus,

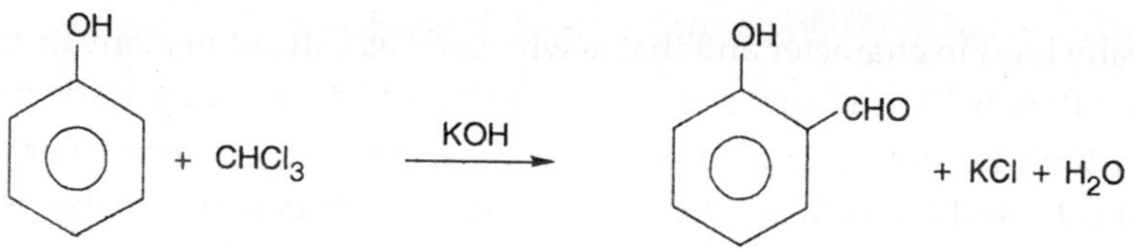

Phenol Salicyldehyde

It is an electrophilic substitution reaction to aromatic ring and chloroform acts as the source of electrophile by forming dichloro carbene in presence of alkali.

7.4.2 Iodoform (CHI_3)

It is a yellow crystalline solid. It is prepared in the laboratory by the action of iodine on acetone or ethyl alcohol following the similar procedure as in the case of chloroform. The reaction in this particular case is termed as *iodoform* reaction. This reaction is applicable to compounds having ketomethyl ($CH_3-\underset{\underset{O}{||}}{C}-$) group or those compounds which may be readily converted to ketomethyl compounds under the reaction condition. For this reason iodoform reaction is used for the detection of ketomethyl ($CH_3-\underset{\underset{O}{||}}{C}-$) group or for identifying those compounds which are readily transformed into ketomethyl compound under the reaction condition, such as ethyl alcohol, isopropyl alcohol, etc. Iodoform is used *as antiseptic*.

7.5 Trichloroethylene (C_2HCl_3)

It is an important halogen derivative used as fire-resisting solvent. It is usually prepared by the removal of one molecule of hydrogen chloride from acetylene tetrachloride with alkali.

Ethyliodide

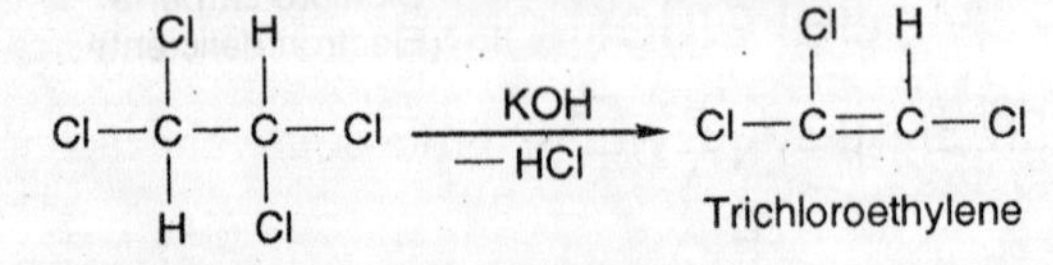

Acetylene tetrachloride → Trichloroethylene

Trichloroethylene is a colourless liquid boiling at 88 °C. It is relatively stable than other polyhalogenated derivatives of saturated hydrocarbons. The stability of this molecule retards loss of second molecule of hydrogen chloride and permits the reaction to stop at this stage.

As stated, it is extensively used as a fire-extinguishing solvent.

7.6 Polyhalogen Derivative: Carbon Tetrachloride (CCl_4)

Carbon tetrachloride is the most important member of alkylhalide having four chlorine atoms attached to the same carbon atom. It is a colourless liquid and insoluble in water. It is prepared from methane as indicated below:

$$CH_4 + 4Cl_2 \xrightarrow[400\,^\circ C]{Heat} CCl_4 + 4HCl$$

It is chemically inert in character and that is why used as solvent in many organic reactions. It is highly non-inflammable and so it is *used as fire extinguisher* under the trade name *Pyrene.*

On reaction with hydrofluoric acid in presence of catalyst, antimony pentafluoride, the product formed is *Freon*-12, which is extensively used as a refrigerant and also as propellant in aerosol sprays.

$$2HF + CCl_4 \xrightarrow{SbF_5} \underset{\text{Dichloro-difluoro carbon (Freon-12)}}{CCl_2F_2} + 2HCl$$

7.7 Uses of Alkylhalides

Some of the important uses of alkylhalides are as mentioned below:

i. Some alkylhalides, viz., chloroform, ethylchloride, fluothane (2-Bromo-2-Chloro-1, I, I-trifluoro ethane) are potent anaesthetics.

ii. Bromoform is used for whooping cough and iodoform is used as an antiseptic.

iii. Carbon tetrachloride is an anti-hookworm drugs. It is also used as an insecticide and as a good fire extinguisher under the name *pyrene.*

iv. Chloretone, a condensation product between chloroform and acetone, is used as a hypnotic drug.

v. Nitrochloroform known as *chloropicrin* is a powerful insecticide.

vi. Dichlorodifluromethane is used as refrigerant under the name *Freon.*

vii. Chloroform and carbon tetrachloride are imporant solvents.
viii. Ethyl chloride is used in the preparation of tetraethyl lead.
ix. All the haloethanes are used as ethylating agent.

Model Questions

1. What are alkylhalides? How are they prepared? Give some characteristic reactions of alkylhalides.
2. Give the laboratory methods of preparation of
   (a) Ethylbromide
   (b) Iodoform
   (c) Chloroform.
3. What happens when
   (a) Ethyl alcohol is treated with bleaching powder?
   (b) *n*-propyl bromide is treated with alcoholic KOH?
   (c) Chloroform is treated with ethyl amine in presence of KOH?
4. How will you synthesise
   (a) isopropyl bromides from *n*-propyl bromide?
   (b) *n*-propyl bromide from isopropyl bromide?
   (c) Propionic acid from ethyl bromide?

Hints: (a)

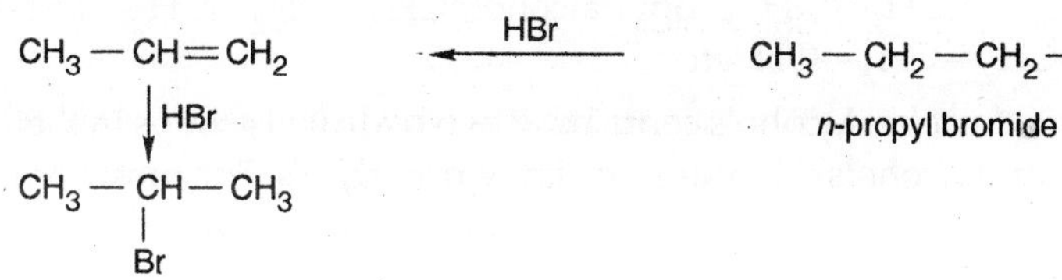

(b)

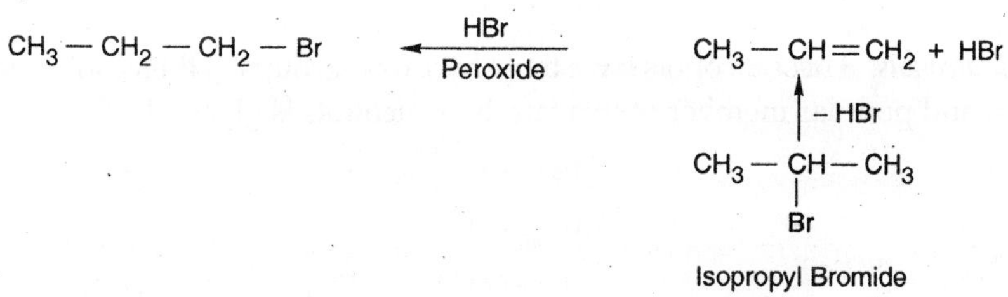

(c)

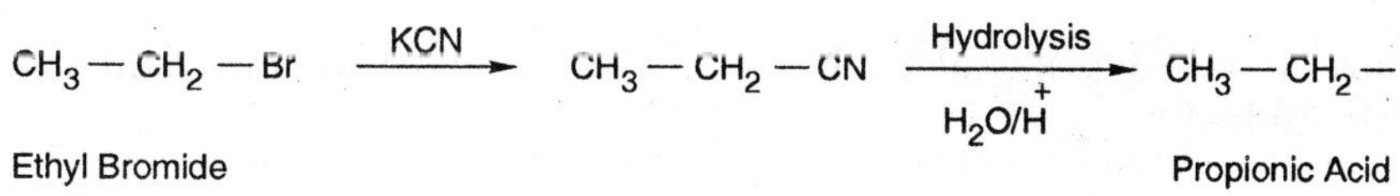

5. Discuss the preparation and uses of
   (a) Chloroform
   (b) Freon-12
   (c) Iodoform
   (d) Carbon tetrachloride.

CHAPTER EIGHT

Alcohols

Alcohols are the hydroxy derivatives of aliphatic hydrocarbons. They may contain one or more hydroxyl (OH) groups in their molecule and hence are classified as:

i. *Monohydric alcohols*: These alcohols contain only one hydroxyl (OH) group in their molecules. They may be expressed by a general formula, C_nH_{2n+1} OH or R—OH. Some of the common members of this group of alcohols are methyl alcohol, CH_3-OH, ethyl alcohol, CH_3CH_2—OH, propyl alcohol, CH_3—CH_2—CH_2—OH, butyl alcohol, CH_3—CH_2—CH_2—CH_2—OH, etc.

ii. *Dihydric alcohols*: Alcohols containing two hydroxyl groups in their molecules are known as dihydric alcohols. They are also known as *glycols*. The most common glycol is ethylene glycol:

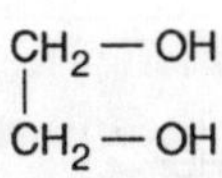

iii. *Trihydric alcohols*: These alcohols have three hydroxyl groups in their molecule. The most common and popular member of this family of alcohols is glycerol:

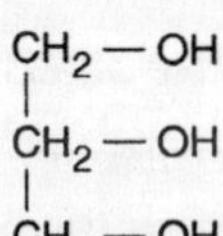

glycerol

Among all these types of alcohols, monohydric alcohols are important and have been widely studied.

8.1 Monohydric Alcohols

Monohydric alcohols, R—OH have been classified into three groups depending upon the nature of alkyl (R) group to which the OH function is attached.

(a) *Primary alcohols*: Primary alcohols are those in which hydroxyl group is connected to primary carbon atom. Thus,

$CH_3—OH$,
Methyl alcohol

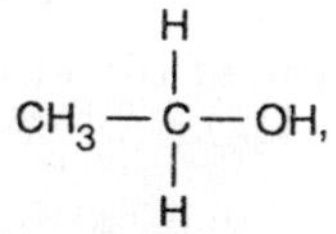
Ethyl alcohol

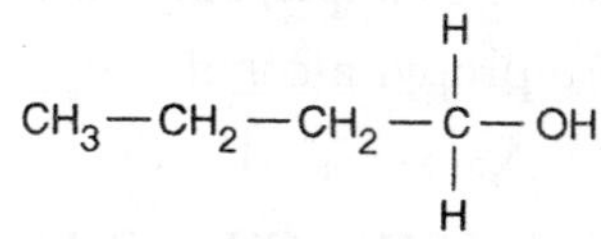
Propyl alcohol

or, in other words, alcohols having —CH_2—OH grouping are primary alcohols.

(b) *Secondary alcohols*: In these monohydric alcohols hydroxyl function is attached to secondary carbon, i.e., monohydric alcohols containing — CHOH functionality are secondary alcohols. Common members are, *iso*-propyl alcohol, 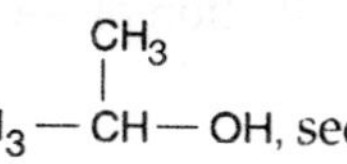, secondary butyl alcohol, 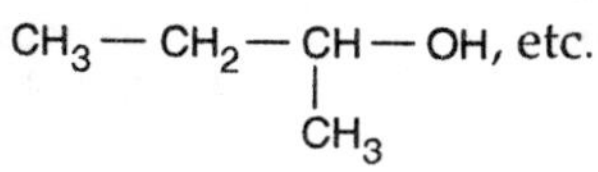, etc.

(c) *Tertiary alcohols*: In tertiary alcohols, hydroxyl group is connected to tertiary carbon, i.e., 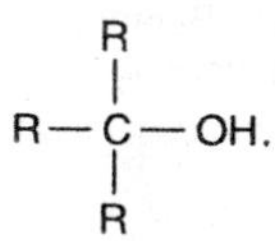. Highly illustrated example of this category of alcohol is *tert*-butyl alcohol,

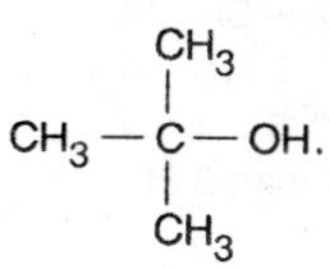.

PROBLEM 8.1

Write the structural formulae of the isomeric alcohols possible with the molecular formula, $C_4H_{10}O$ and classify them as primary, secondary or tertiary.

8.1.1 Nomenclature of Alcohols

There are three systems for the nomenclature of alcohols.

1. *Common System*: Lower members of alcohol family are named by adding the word *alcohol* after the name of alkyl group to which the hydroxyl group is attached. Thus,

$CH_3—OH$
Methyl alcohol

$CH_3—CH_2—OH$
Ethyl alcohol

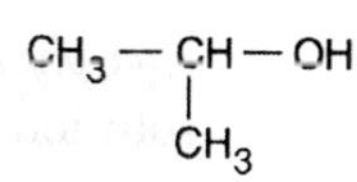
Isopropyl alcohol

$CH_3—CH_2—CH_2—OH$
n-propyl alcohol

$CH_3—CH_2—CH_2—CH_2—OH$
n-butyl alcohol

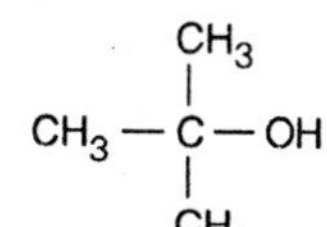
tert-butyl alcohol

ii. *Carbinol System*: According to this system, all alcohols are named as the derivatives of carbinol, the first member of which is carbinol, i.e., methyl alcohol. The other members as for example, ethyl alcohol, $CH_3—CH_2—OH$ is named as methyl carbinol. Similarly, *iso*-propyl alcohol, $CH_3-CH(CH_3)-OH$ is called dimethyl carbinol and *n*-propyl alcohol, $CH_3—CH_2—CH_2—OH$ is ethyl carbinol.

This system of nomenclature for alcohols is not popular and is rarely used.

iii. *IUPAC System*: In this system the longest chain containing the hydroxyl function is selected as the parent alkane and the suffix *-ol* is added in place of 'e' of alkane. The position of —OH group is indicated by the number. Thus,

CH_3-OH
Methanol

CH_3-CH_2-OH
Ethanol

$CH_3-CH_2-CH_2-OH$
n-propanol or
Propan-1-ol (1-Propanol)

$CH_3-CH(OH)-CH_3$
Propan-2-ol (2-Propanol)
(Isopropyl alcohol)

$CH_3-CH_2-CH_2-CH_2-OH$
Butan-1-ol (1-Butanol)
(*n*-Butyl alcohol)

$CH_3-CH_2-CH(OH)-CH_3$
Butan-2-ol (2-Butanol)
(Sec-Butyl alcohol)

$CH_3-C(OH)(CH_3)-CH_3$
2-methyl-Propan-2-0l
or
2-methyl-2-propanol
(Tert-butyl alcohol)

PROBLEM 8.2

Give the carbinol and IUPAC name of the following alcohols:

1. $CH_3-CH(CH_3)-CH_2-OH$
2. $CH_3-CH(CH_3)-CH_2-CH_2-OH$

8.1.2 General Methods of Preparation of Alcohols

Some of the most common methods of preparation of alcohols are summarised below:

1. *Hydrolysis of alkylhalides*: Alkylhalides on hydrolysis with sodium or potassium hydroxide solution form alcohols.

$$\underset{\text{Alkylhalide}}{R-X} + NaOH \longrightarrow R-OH + NaX$$

$$\underset{\text{Methyl chloride}}{CH_3-Cl} + NaOH \longrightarrow CH_3-OH + NaCl$$

Hydrolysis may also be carried out with moist silver oxide.

2.(a) *Fermentation of carbohydrates* (Commercial method of preparation of ethanol): This is the oldest method of preparation of alcohols, particularly ethyl alcohol and this is still in use for the industrial preparation of beer, brandy and wine. Starch is the starting material which is normally obtained from the *grain*, i.e., wheat or barley. Grains are mashed with hot water and then warmed with germinated barley, usually known as malt, for nearly an hour. The enzyme *diastase* present in malt hydrolyses starch into maltose.

$$\underset{\text{Starch}}{(C_6H_{10}O_5)_n} + \frac{n}{2} H_2O \xrightarrow{\text{diastase}} \underset{\text{Maltose}}{\frac{n}{2} C_{12}H_{22}O_{11}}$$

Maltose is fermented with yeast for 2-3 days when the enzyme *maltase* present in yeast converts maltose into glucose and another enzyme, zymase which is also present in yeast converts glucose into ethanol.

$$C_{12}H_{22}O_{11} \xrightarrow[+H_2O]{\text{maltase}} \underset{\text{Glucose}}{2C_6H_{12}O_6}$$

$$C_6H_{12}O_6 \xrightarrow{\text{Zymase}} \underset{\text{Ethanol}}{2C_2H_5OH} + 2CO_2$$

In the similar way, cane sugar can form ethanol by enzymatic hydrolysis.

$$\underset{\text{Cane sugar}}{C_{12}H_{22}O_{11}} + H_2O \xrightarrow{\text{invertase}} \underset{\text{Glucose}}{C_6H_{12}O_6} + \underset{\text{Fructose}}{C_6H_{12}O_6}$$

$$C_6H_{12}O_6 \xrightarrow{\text{Zymase}} \underset{\text{Ethanol}}{2C_2H_5OH} + 2CO_2$$

i. *Absolute Alcohol*: Ethyl alcohol prepared is not 100 per cent pure. It contains 5% water. However, this small amount of water can be removed by distilling ethanol obtained. Ethanol obtained is mixed with appropriate quantity of benzene and is subjected to fractional distillation. The first fraction which contains all the water is rejected and the remaining fraction is anhydrous ethanol and is distilled at 78 °C. This is *absolute alcohol*. Sometimes absolute alcohol is prepared by passing the vapours of ordinary alcohol through a dehydrating agent like calcium oxide.

   Absolute alcohol so obtained is toxic in nature due to the presence of traces of benzene. This absolute alcohol is termed as 200 *proof*. A *proof spirit* is a solution of alcohol in water containing half of its volume of absolute alcohol. Mixture of 50 ml absolute alcohol and 54 ml of water is 100 ml of 100 proof spirit. Since during mixing of absolute alcohol with water, contraction in volume occurs slight excess of water than absolute alcohol is to be mixed. Industrial alcohol containing 95% alcohol is known as *rectified spirit*.

ii. *Denatured Alcohol* (Methylated spirit) : It is a commercial alcohol, which is denatured by adding some poisonous chemicals like methyl alcohol and pyridine to it. It is duty free.

iii. *Determination of Alcohol in Pharmaceutical Preparations:* To estimate the quantity of alcohol in pharmaceutical preparations *alcoholometry* is applied. In this method 100 ml of pharmaceutical preparation is diluted with distilled water and distilled. Distillation is continued till 100 ml of distillate is collected in a measuring flask. Specific gravity of the distillate is determined and the percentage of alcohol is read against this value of specific gravity from ready reference table.

Normally percentage of alcohol is expressed in terms of proof spirit. Proof-spirit is aqueous ethyl alcohol containing 57.10% by volume of ethyl alcohol. The sample is referred to as over-proof or under-proof according as it is stronger or weaker than proof-spirit. A 20° under-proof sample means that the 100 volumes of sample contain as much alcohol as 80 volumes of proof spirit. Similarly, 20° over-proof sameple is one whose 100 volumes contain as much alcohol as 120 volumes of proof-spirit.

(b) *Commercial Method of Preparation of Methanol*: Methanol, another member of alcohol, is however, industrially manufactured by the destructive distillation of wood. For this reason methanol is also known as *Wood alcohol*. Dried wood on heating at a high temperature of 360 °C in absence of oxygen furnishes a liquid product known as *pyroligneous acid*. It contains methanol, acetone and acetic acid. This liquid product is subjected to fractional distillation and the vapours are passed through hot milk of lime when acetic acid is separated out as calcium acetate and the remaining vapour is condensed to liquid and further subjected to fractional distillation for separation of acetone, b.p. 56 °C and methanol, b.p. 65 °C. This is the oldest method for the preparation of methanol. Nowadays methanol is manufactured by more *sophisticated method* from *water-gas*. Water-gas is prepared by passing steam on hot-cake and the water-gas so obtained is mixed with half its volume of hydrogen gas and is passed over a mixed catalyst containing oxides of copper, zinc and chromium at a pressure of 200 atmosphere and temperature of 300 °C.

$$CO + 2H_2 \longrightarrow CH_3OH$$

This method is very useful with the yield of nearly 100 per cent and of 99% purity.

3. *Preparation of alcohols from alkenes*: Alcohols are prepared from alkenes adopting various procedures, a few of which are discussed as under:

(a) *Hydration of alkenes*: Alkenes on hydration in presence of mineral acid as catalyst readily form alcohols.

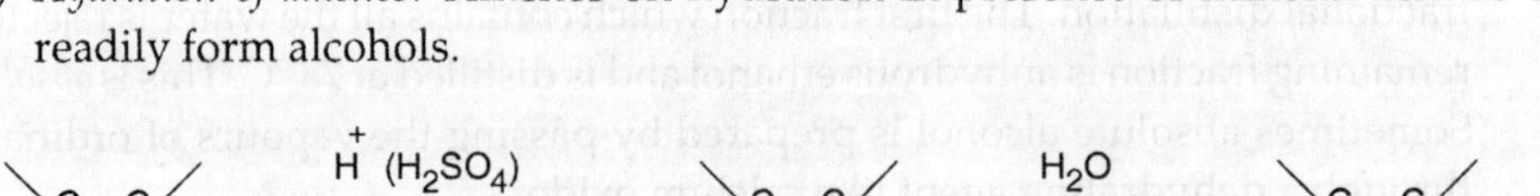

Alcohol

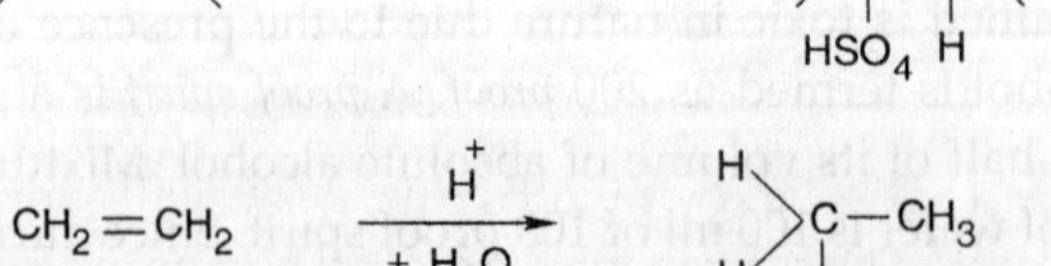

Ethyl alcohol

(b) *Oxymercuration-demercuration of alkenes*: This is an important method for the preparation of alcohols. The process involves two steps. In the first step alkene is allowed to react with mercuric acetate in tetrahydrofuran (THF) and water mixture when hydroxy alkyl mercury compound is formed. This process is termed as *oxymercuration*. In the second step mercuric acetate is replaced by reduction with sodium borohydride. This is known as *demercuration*. Both oxymercuration and demercuration take place smoothly at room temperature and the hydroxy alkyl mercury compound formed in the first step is not usually isolated and the reduction by sodium borohydride is carried out *in situ*. Thus,

$$R-CH=CH_2 \xrightarrow[\text{THF, } H_2O \text{ (Oxymercuration)}]{Hg(OAC)_2} R-\underset{OH}{\underset{|}{CH}}-CH_2Hg(OAC)$$

$$R-\underset{OH}{\underset{|}{CH}}-CH_2Hg(OAC) \xrightarrow[\text{Demercuration}]{NaBH_4} R-\underset{OH}{\underset{|}{CH}}-CH_3 + Hg$$

The process is a case of addition reaction to alkene and proceeds following Markownikoff's rule. In the first step, electrophilic attack takes place by $H\overset{+}{g}OAC$ followed by nucleophilic attack by water forming hydroxy alkyl mercury compound.

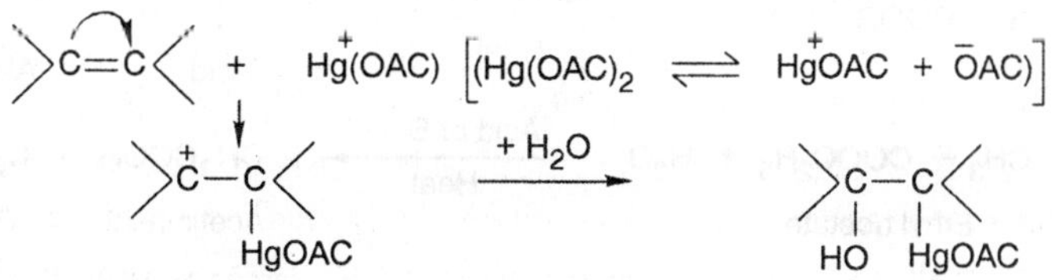

In the second step hydride ion ($\bar{H}$) replaces HgOAC group, i.e.,

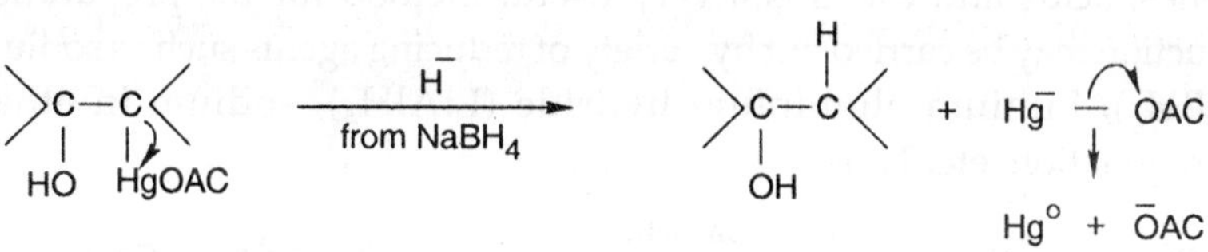

(c) *Hydroboration-oxidation of Alkenes*: Alkenes on reaction with diborane B_2H_6 readily forms tri-alkyl boranes which on oxidation with hydrogen peroxide in alkaline medium yields alcohols. This addition follows *anti*-Markownikoff's rule.

$$R-CH=CH_2 \xrightarrow{B_2H_6} \underset{\text{Trialkyl borane}}{(R-CH_2-CH_2)_3B}$$

$$(R-CH_2-CH_2)_3B \xrightarrow{H_2O_2,\ \bar{O}H} R-CH_2-CH_2-OH$$

Since this reaction takes place via anti-Markownikoff's rule, it is usually applied for the preparation of only *primary alcohols*. The conversion of tri alkyl borane to alcohol may be explained as shown below:

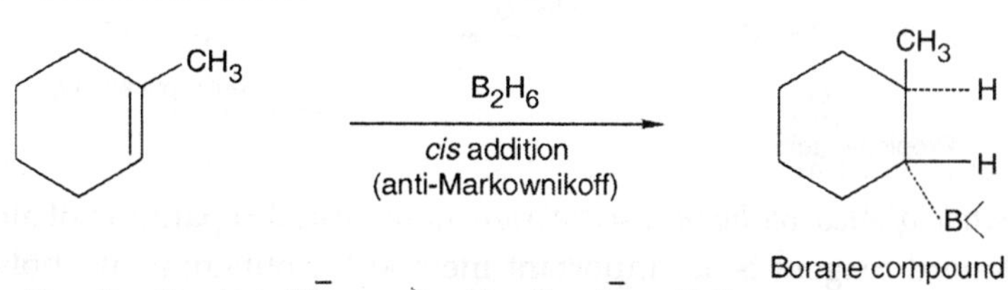

$$H-O-O-H + \bar{O}H \rightleftharpoons H-O-\bar{O} + H_2O$$

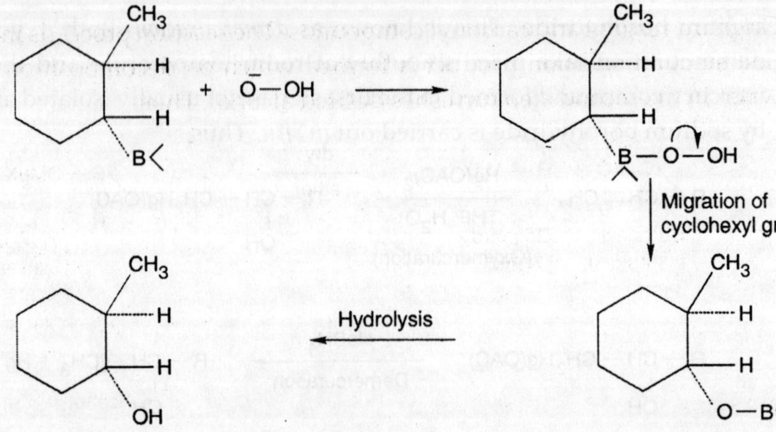

4. *Hydrolysis of Esters*: Preparation of alcohols by the base or acid catalysed hydrolysis of ester is a very common process.

$$\underset{}{R-COOR'} + H_2O \xrightarrow[\text{Heat}]{\text{Acid or Base}} \underset{\text{Acid}}{R-COOH} + \underset{\text{Alcohol}}{R'-OH}$$

$$\underset{\text{Ethyl acetate}}{CH_3-COOC_2H_5} + H_2O \xrightarrow[\text{Heat}]{\text{Acid or Base}} \underset{\text{Acetic acid}}{CH_3COOH} + \underset{\text{Ethyl alcohol}}{C_2H_5OH}$$

5. *Reduction of carbonylic compounds*: Reduction of carbonylic compouds like aldehydes, ketones, acids and esters is a very useful method for the preparation of alcohols. Reduction may be carried out by variety of reducing agents such as sodium borohydride ($NaBH_4$), Lithium aluminium hydride ($LiAlH_4$), sodium in ethanol, catalytic hydrogenation, etc. Thus,

$$\underset{\text{Acetaldehyde}}{CH_3-\underset{\underset{O}{\|}}{C}-H} \xrightarrow[\text{Ni or Pt}]{\text{Cat. [H]}} \underset{\text{Ethyl alcohol}}{CH_3-CH_2-OH}$$

$$\underset{\text{Acetone}}{CH_3-\underset{\underset{O}{\|}}{C}-CH_3} \xrightarrow{NaBH_4} \underset{\text{Isopropyl alcohol}}{CH_3-\underset{\underset{OH}{|}}{CH}-CH_3}$$

$$\underset{\text{Ethyl acetate}}{CH_3-\underset{\underset{O}{\|}}{C}-OC_2H_5} \xrightarrow{\text{Na / Ethanol}} \underset{\text{Ethyl alcohol}}{2CH_3-CH_2-OH}$$

$$\underset{\text{Propionic acid}}{CH_3-CH_2-\underset{\underset{O}{\|}}{C}-OH} \xrightarrow{LiAlH_4} \underset{n\text{-Propyl alcohol}}{CH_3-CH_2-CH_2-OH}$$

6. *Preparation of Alcohols by the use of Grignard reagent*: Preparation of alcohols by the use of Grignard reagent is an important method for obtaining alcohols in good yields. Primary, secondary and tertiary alcohols can be prepared by the action between

Grignard reagent and carbonyl compounds. The reaction proceeds in two steps. In the first step, an addition product is formed which on decomposition with acidulated water in the second step furnishes desired alcohol. Thus,

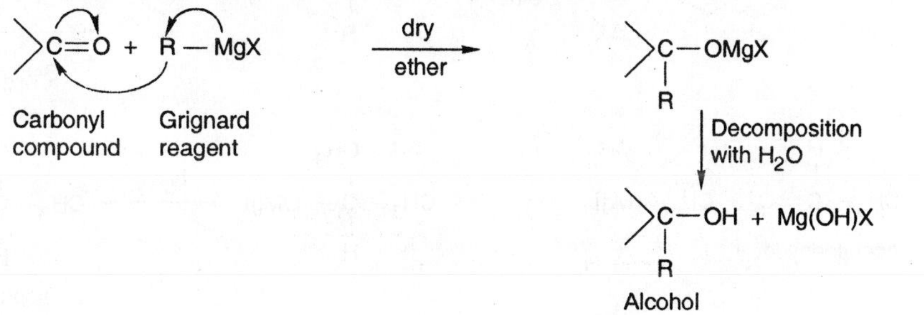

i. In order to prepare primary alcohol, reaction is to be carried out in between formaldehyde and Grignard reagent.

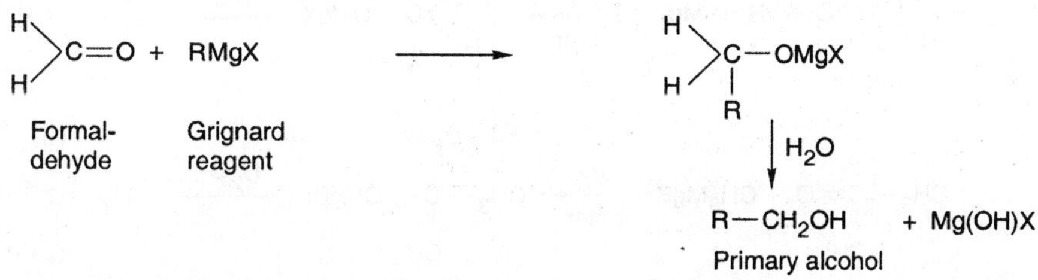

Suitably selecting the alkyl group (R) of Grignard reagent desired primary alcohol may be obtained. For example,

(a)

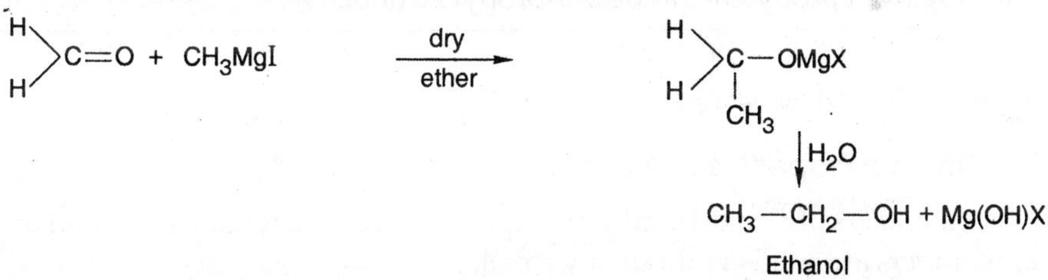

(b)

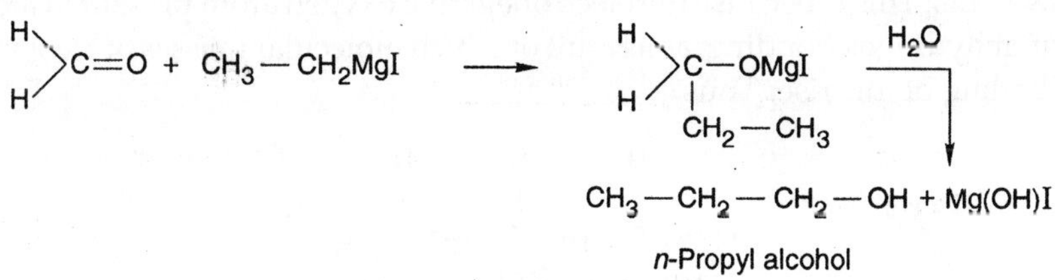

Primary alcohols may also be obtained by the reaction between ethylene oxide and Grignard reagent.

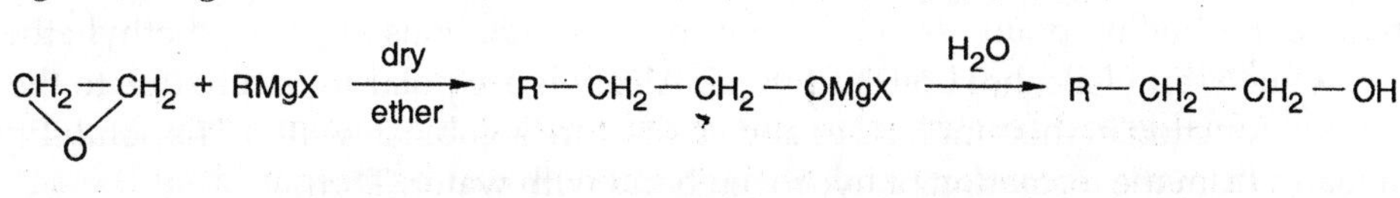

ii. Secondary alcohols are obtained when any aldehyde other than formaldehyde is used.

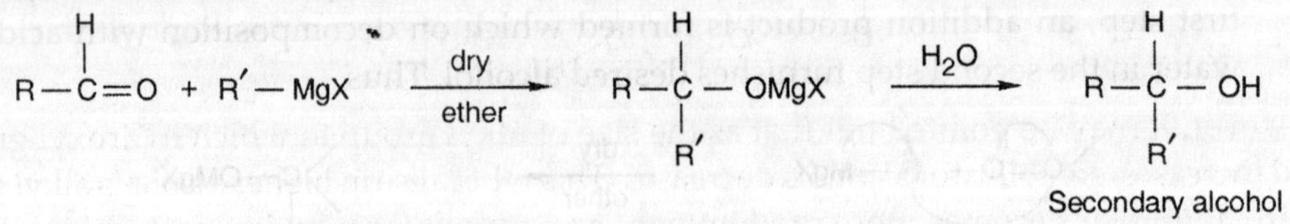

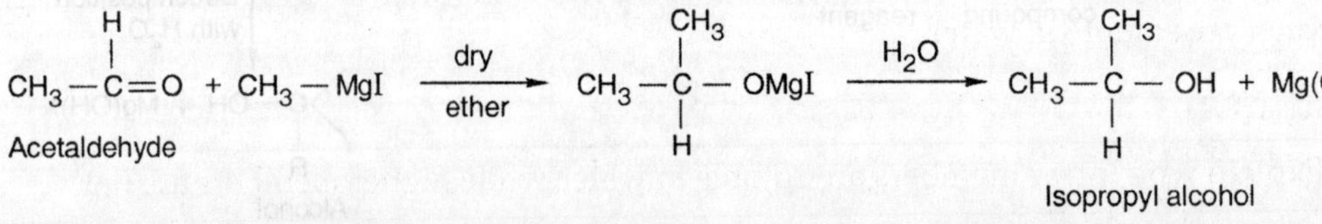

iii. Tertiary alcohols are obtained by the reaction between a ketone and Grignard reagent.

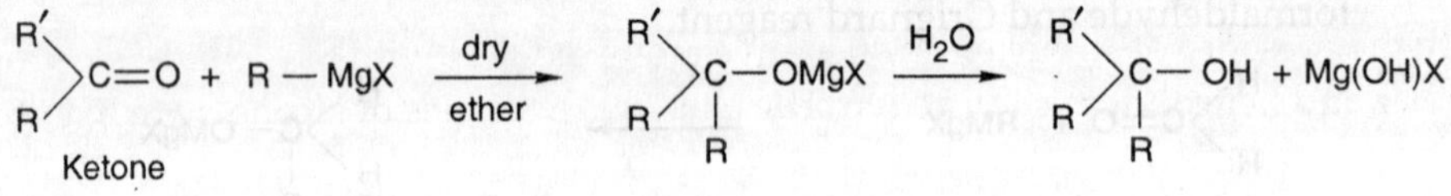

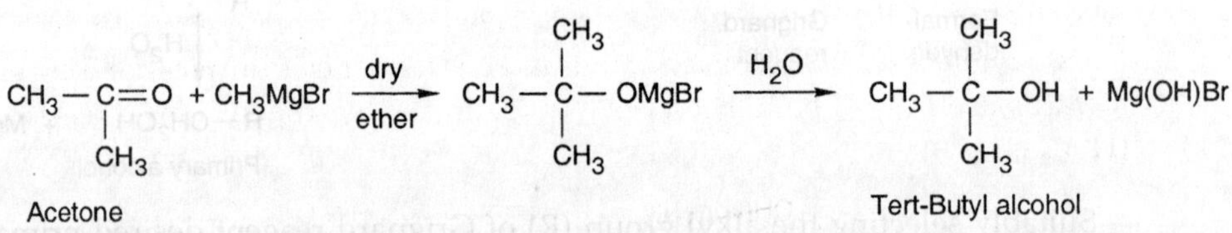

Problem 8.3

Starting from propylene prepare *n*-propyl alcohol.

8.1.3 Properties of Alcohols

8.1.3.1 Physical Properties of Alcohols

The lower members of alcohol family are liquids with characteristic smell and burning taste. The higher members are solids without any smell.

Alcohols have higher boiling points than ethers, alkanes and alkylhalides of comparable molecular weights. This is because the electronegative oxygen atom present in alcohols can form intermolecular hydrogen bonding, as a result of which molecular masses of alcohols are increased and hence boiling points rise. Thus,

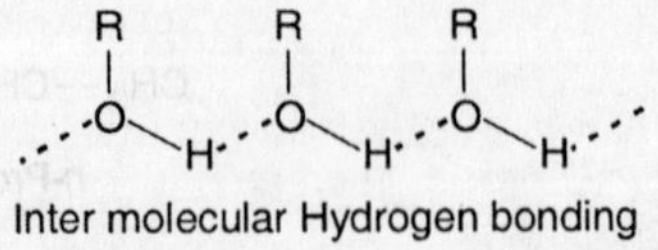

Inter molecular Hydrogen bonding

On the other hand, ethers, alkanes and alkylhalides cannot form such intermolecular hydrogen bonding. So there is no increase in molecular mass and hence boiling points do not rise. Thus, *n*-butane has boiling point —0.5 °C, isopropyl chloride boils at 47 °C, diethyl ether does so at 35 °C while *n*-butyl alcohol boils at 118 °C. Alcohols are polar in nature due to the presence of hydroxyl function in their molecules and so they are soluble in water. The solubility of alcohols originates from the formation of hydrogen bond with water. Thus,

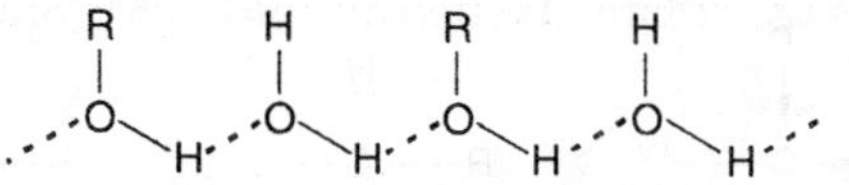

However, it may be pointed out that as the size of alkyl group to which hydroxyl group is attached increases, solubility of alcohols decreases. This is because in higher alcohols alkyl groups which are non-polar becomes more predominant and cannot form hydrogen bond, and hence solubility decrease. For this reason *n*-hexanol is insoluble in water whereas methnol, ethanol and propanol are soluble in water.

Problem 8.4

Explain why lower members are soluble in water while higher members are not.

8.1.3.2 Chemical Properties of Alcohols

Due to the presence of strong electronegative atom, oxygen, with lone pair of electrons, alcohols are polar and hence chemically active. The chemical activities of alcohols are manifested by the following reactions:

(a) *Acidity of Alcohols*: The acidity of alcohols originates from the polarity of O—H bond. Since oxygen is highly electronegative and has tendency to attract bonding electron pair towards itself O—H bond becomes weaker and so hydrogen atom is released as proton (H^+), i.e.,

$$R{-}O{-}H + \bar{O}H(\text{from NaOH}) \rightleftharpoons \underset{\substack{\text{Alkoxide ion}\\ \text{(conjugate base)}}}{R{-}\bar{O}} + H_2O$$

But since the oxygen atom of OH group of alcohol is attached to electron releasing alkyl group the release of proton from O—H bond is not so easy as expected. For this reason alcohols are weak acids, weaker than water. The acidic character of alcohols is exhibited by their reaction with active metals like sodium and potassium:

$$\underset{\text{Alcohol}}{2R{-}O{-}H} + 2Na \longrightarrow \underset{\substack{\text{Alkoxide}\\ \text{(conjugate base)}}}{2R{-}ONa} + H_2\uparrow$$

$$\underset{\text{Methanol}}{2CH_3OH} + 2Na \longrightarrow \underset{\text{Sodium methoxide}}{2CH_3ONa} + H_2\uparrow$$

$$\underset{\text{Ethanol}}{2C_2H_5OH} + 2Na \longrightarrow \underset{\text{Sodium ethoxide}}{2C_2H_5ONa} + H_2\uparrow$$

From the above discussion it is evident that acidic character of alcohols depends upon the release of proton from O—H bond. So it is obvious that the acidity of alcohols will be controlled by the ability of releasing electrons by the alkyl group to which the oxygen atom of O—H bond is attached—greater the ability of releasing electron, less will be the acidity. As the releasing of electrons by primary, secondary and tertiary alkyl groups is in the following order:

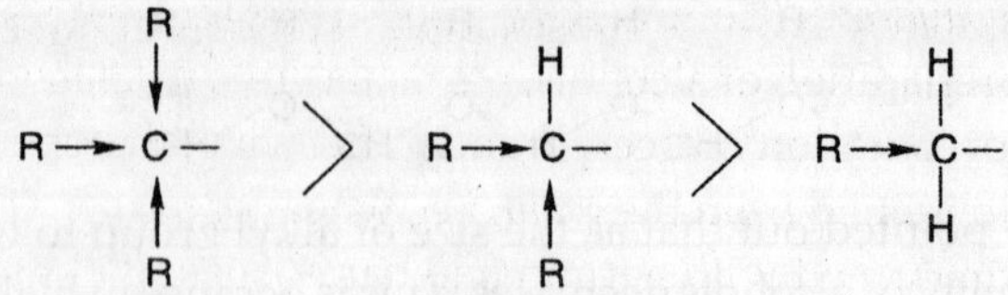

Tertiary alkyl group > Secondary alkyl group > Primary alkyl group

The order of acidity of primary, secondary and tertiary alcohols is primary alcohols > secondary alcohols > tertiary alcohols,

PROBLEM 8.5

Arrange the following alcohols in decreasing order of acidity:

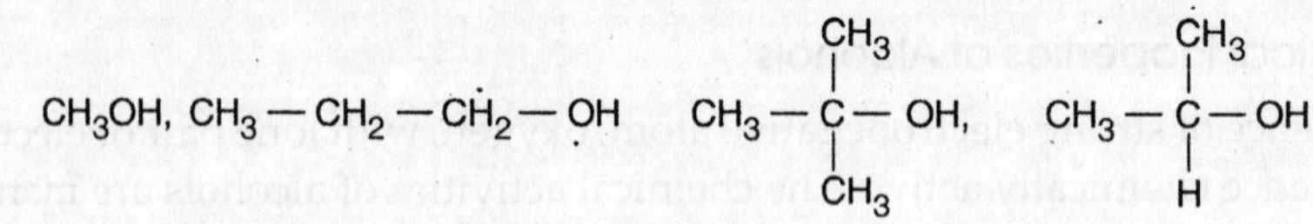

(b) *Reaction with Grignard Reagents*: Alcohols contain an active hydrogen atom. So they react with Grignard reagents to form hydrocarbon (Zerewittinoff active hydrogen determination).

$$R-OH \quad + \quad R'MgX \longrightarrow R'-H + Mg(OR)X$$

$$\underset{\text{Methanol}}{CH_3-OH} \quad + \quad \underset{\text{Ethyl magnesium iodide}}{C_2H_5MgI} \longrightarrow \underset{\text{Ethane}}{C_2H_6} \quad + \quad Mg(OCH_5)I$$

$$\underset{\text{Ethanol}}{C_2H_5-O-H} \quad + \quad \underset{\text{Methyl magnesium bromide}}{CH_3MgBr} \longrightarrow \underset{\text{Methane}}{CH_4} \quad + \quad Mg(OC_2H_5)Br$$

(c) *Dehydration of Alcohols*:

i. *Formation of alkene:* Alcohols when heated at a temperature of 180 °C in presence of concentrated sulphuric acid, one molecule of water is eliminated and there is formation of *alkenes*.

$$\underset{\text{Ethanol}}{CH_3-CH_2-OH} \xrightarrow[180\,°C]{\text{conc. } H_2SO_4} \underset{\text{Ethylene}}{CH_2=CH_2} + H_2O$$

Mechanistically dehydration proceeds via the formation of a *carbocation* as an intermediate. So it is reasonable to assume that more stable the carbocation, more easier becomes the dehydration. Hence the ease of dehydration of three types of alcohol is of the order: tertiary alcohols > secondary alcohols > primary alcohols.

ii. *Formation of ether*: On dehydration, alcohols can form ether. On heating alcohols at a lower temperature in presence of mineral acids ethers are formed.

$$\underset{\text{Alcohol}}{2R-O-H} \xrightarrow{H^+} \underset{\text{Ether}}{R-O-R} + H_2O$$

Formation of ether is a case of substitution reaction but not an elimination reaction and the path of reaction is SN^1

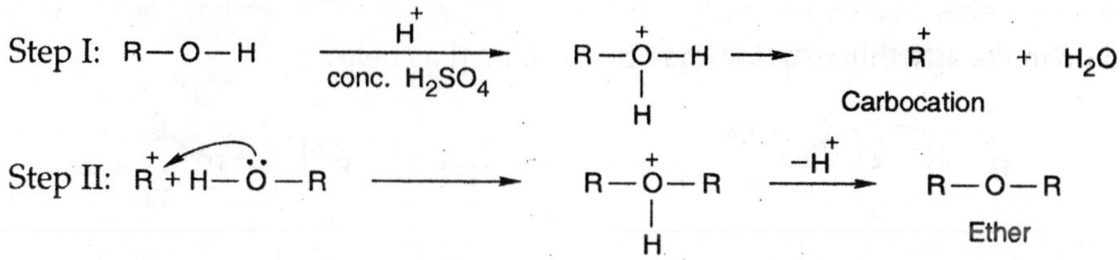

(d) *Dehydrogenation of Alcohols*: When the vapour alcohols are passed over copper at a very high temperature of 300 °C, primary, secondary and tertiary alcohols form different products.

i. Primary alcohols are dehydrogenated to aldehydes. .

$$\underset{n\text{-Propyl alcohol}}{CH_3-CH_2-CH_2-OH} \xrightarrow[300\,^\circ C]{Cu} \underset{\text{Propionaldehyde}}{CH_3-CH_2-CHO}$$

ii. Secondary alcohols form ketones. Thus,

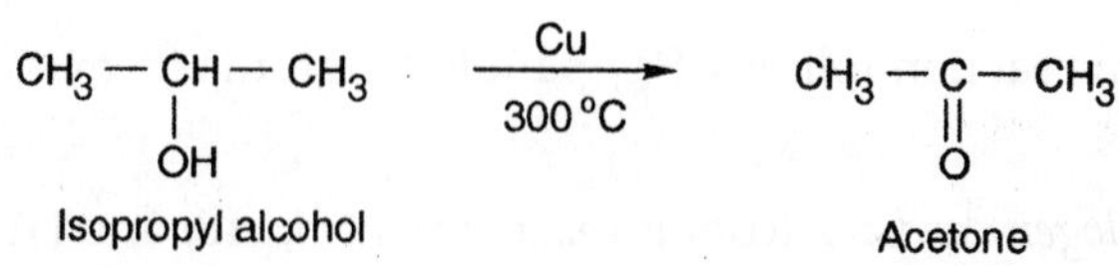

iii. Tertiary alcohols yield alkene.

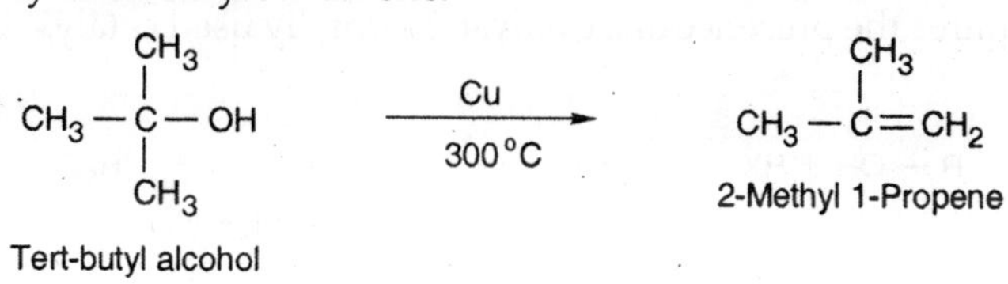

(e) *Formation of Alkylhalides by Alcohols*: Alcohols react with reagents like phosphorous pentachloride, phosphorous tribromide and thionyl chloride with the formation of alkyl-halides. Thus,

i. $R-OH + PCl_5 \longrightarrow \underset{\text{Alkyl chloride}}{R-Cl} + POCl_3 + HCl$

Reaction proceeds as under:

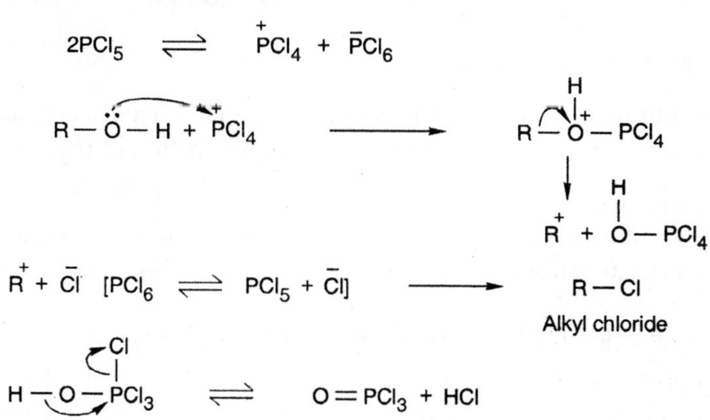

ii. $R-OH + PBr_3 \rightleftharpoons R-Br + H_3PO_3$

Alkyl bromide; Phosphorous acid

Mechanistically this reaction may be explained as below:

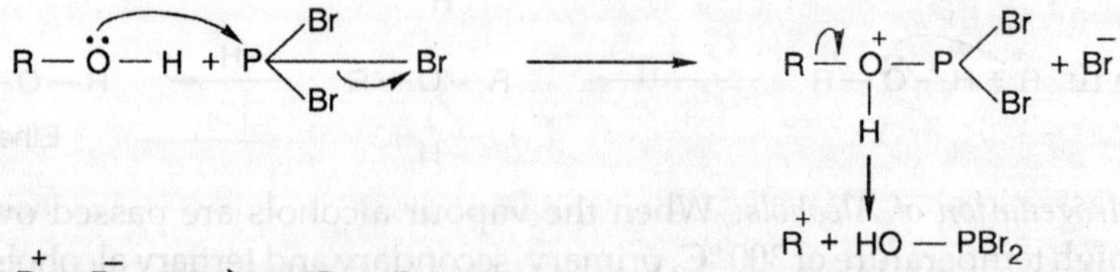

$\overset{+}{R} + \overset{-}{Br} \rightleftharpoons R-Br$

Alkyl bromide

$HO-PBr_2$ on hydrolysis forms $P(OH)_3$ or H_3PO_3

iii. $R-OH + SOCl_2 \rightleftharpoons R-Cl + SO_2 + HCl$

Thionyl chloride; Alkyl chloride

This substitution reaction follows S_{Ni} path through the formation of chlorosulphite as intermediate.

(f) *Reaction with Halogen Acids:* Alcohols react with HCl, HBr and HI to form corresponding alkylhalides and water. HBr and HI do not require any catalyst but reaction with HCl normally requires the presence of a catalyst. Normally used catalyst is anhydrons $ZnCl_2$. Thus,

$$R-OH + HX \longrightarrow \underset{\text{Alkylhalide}}{R-X} + H_2O$$

Reaction occurs through SN^1 path. In the first step a carbocation is formed which combines with halogen ion in the next step.

Step I: $R-O-H + \overset{+}{H}$ (from halogen acid) $\longrightarrow R-\overset{+}{O}-H \xrightarrow{-H_2O} \underset{\text{Carbocation}}{\overset{+}{R}}$

Step II: $\overset{+}{R} + \overset{-}{X} \longrightarrow R-X$

The order of reactivity of halogen acids is HI > HBr > HCl. This is because the order of nucleophilicity is $I^- > Br^- > Cl^-$. In general, among the different types of alcohols, the order of reactivity is tertiary alcohol > secondary alcohol > primary alcohol.

It may be mentioned in this connection that if an alcohol is heated with HI in presence of red phosphorous hydrocarbon is formed instead of alkylhalide, i.e.,

$$R-OH + 2HI \xrightarrow{\text{Heat}} RH + H_2O + I_2$$

(g) *Oxidation of Alcohols*: Alcohols on oxidation form different products. Exact nature of the product depends upon the nature of the alcohol and the conditions of the reaction. Commonly used oxidising agents are aqueous acidified or alkaline potassium permanganate, acidified potassium dichromate or nitric acid.

i. Primary alcohols on oxidation form aldehydes and carboxylic acids without any loss of carbon atom.

$$\underset{\text{Ethyl alcohol}}{CH_3-CH_2-OH} \xrightarrow{[O]} \underset{\text{Acetaldehyde}}{CH_3-CHO} \xrightarrow{[O]} \underset{\text{Acetic acid}}{CH_3COOH}$$

ii. Secondary alcohols on oxidation yield ketones having same number of carbon atoms but on further oxidation form carboxylic acids with lesser number of carbon atoms than the original alcohol. Thus,

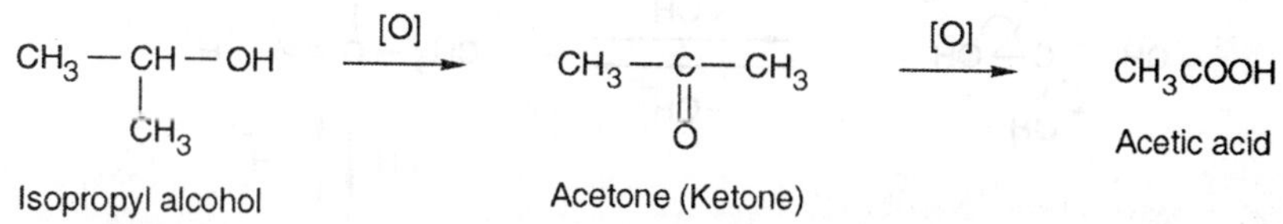

iii. Tertiary alcohols under normal condition fail to undergo oxidation. However, if drastic condition is applied, they can be oxidised to ketones and carboxylic acids, both containing lesser number of carbon atoms than the original alcohol, i.e.,

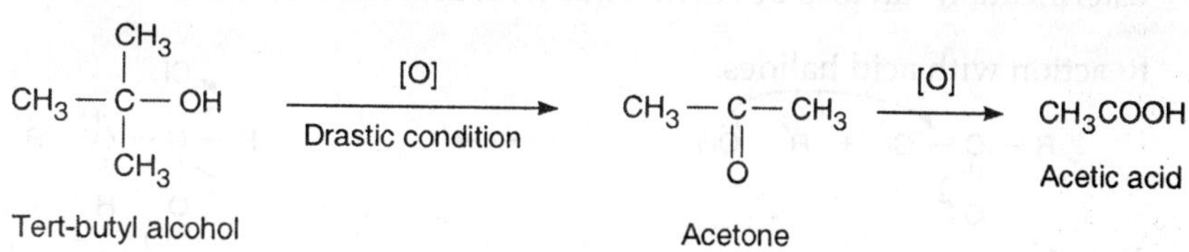

From the identification of the nature of products, three types of alcohols can be easily differentiated and in fact, oxidation is used for such purpose.

(h) *Esterification*: In presence of mineral acids preferably concentrated sulphuric acid as catalyst, alcohols react with carboxylic acids to form esters. The reaction is reversible in nature.

$$\underset{\text{Methanol}}{CH_3OH} + \underset{\text{Acetic acid}}{CH_3COOH} \overset{\overset{+}{H}}{\rightleftharpoons} \underset{\text{Methyl acetate}}{CH_3COOCH_3} + H_2O$$

Because of reversible nature of the reaction, excess amount of alcohol is used in order to get appreciable yield of ester.

Mechanism of esterification may be depicted as below:

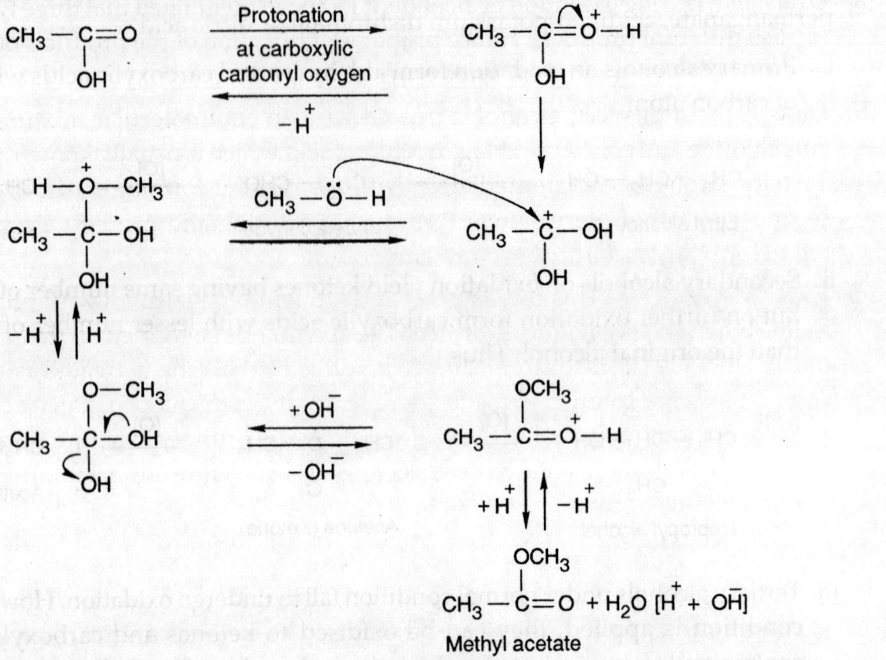

Esterification can also be carried out with acid halides and acid anhydrides. Thus,

i. Reaction with acid halides:

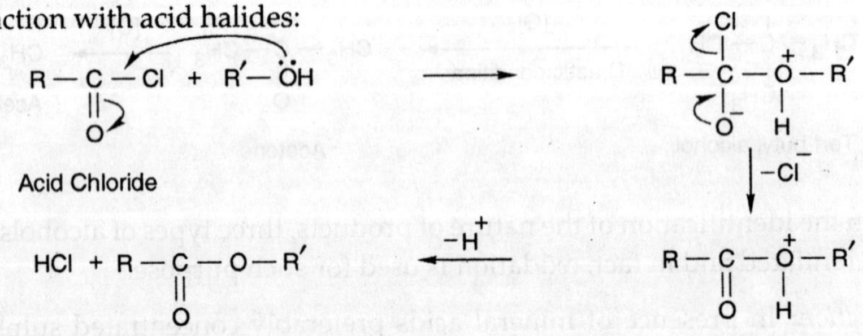

ii. Reaction with acid anhydride:

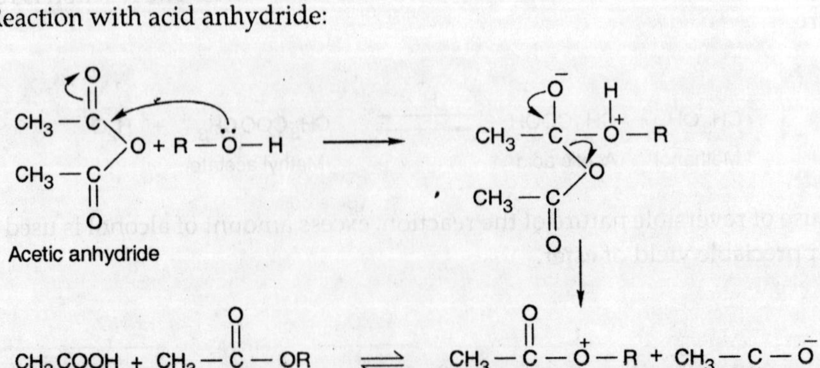

8.1.3.3 Distinction between Primary, Secondary and Tertiary Alcohols

Primary, secondary and tertiary alcohols may be distinguished by the following methods:

(a) *Oxidation*: During oxidation of alcohols it has been mentioned that three types of alcohols furnish different products. Hence proper identification of the products of oxidation will lead to the differentiation of three types of products.

(b) *Lucas Test*: In this test, alcohol is treated with an equimolecular mixture of anhydrous zinc chloride and concentrated hydrochloric acid which is usually known as *Lucas reagent*. Tertiary alcohols react immediately with the reagent forming a turbid solution while secondary alcohols very slowly form turbid solution and primary alcohols practically fail to form any turbidity at room temperature.

(c) *Victor Meyer's Test*: This test consists of treatment of an alcohol with phosphorous and iodine when an alkylhalide is formed. The alkylhalide so formed on treatment withsilver nitrite ($AgNO_2$) forms nitroalkane. When this nitroalkane is treated with nitrous acid solution and the solution is made alkaline, colour is developed. Development of blood red colouration suggests that the original alcohol is primary in nature, secondary alcohol gives blue colouration while tertiary alcohol fails to produce any colouration. The reactions occurring in the test are:

i. *Primary alcohol*

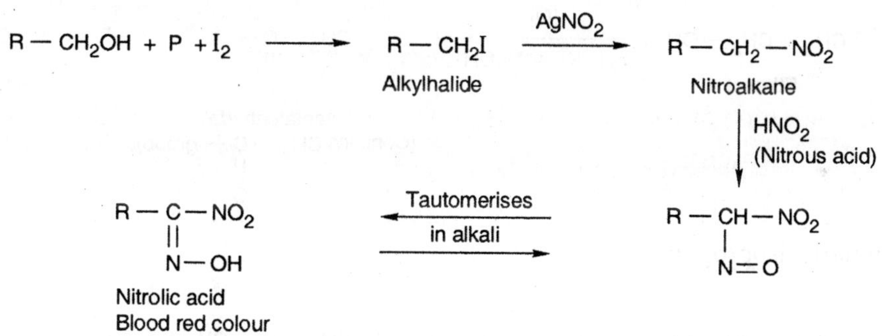

ii. *Secondary alcohol*

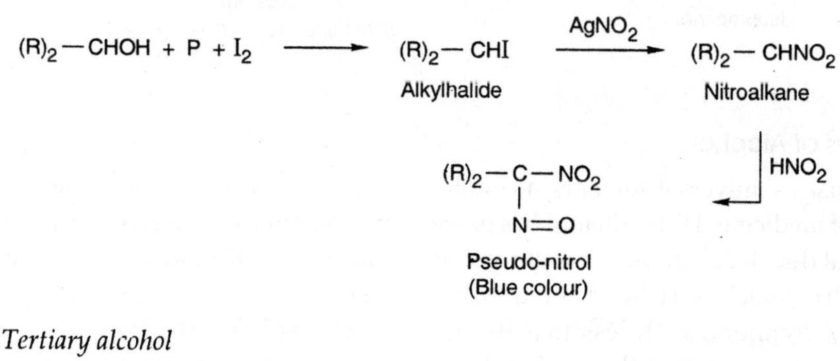

iii. *Tertiary alcohol*

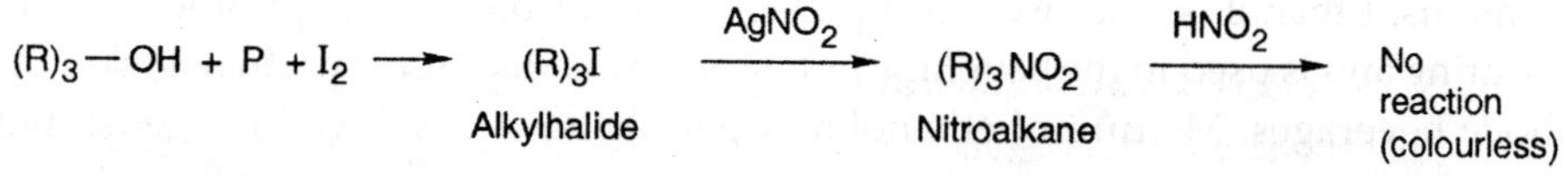

8.1.3.4 Qualitative Tests for Alcohols

Alcoholic hydroxyl function can be identified by the following tests:

i. Liberation of hydrogen gas by adding a small piece of sodium metal indicates the presence of hydroxyl group.

$$2R-OH + 2Na \longrightarrow R-ONa + H_2\uparrow$$

ii. Formation of ester (acetyl derivative) on treatment with acid chloride suggests the presence of OH function.

$$R-OH + CH_3COCl \longrightarrow CH_3-COOR + HCl\uparrow$$

iii. Certain type of alcohols, particularly those which can generate keto methyl group ($CH_3-\underset{\underset{O}{||}}{C}-$) during oxidation by mild oxidising agent, can be identified by *Iodoform test*.

In this test aqueous solution of alcohol is made alkaline with sodium hydroxide and to this alkaline solution iodine in potassium iodide solution is added and warmed on water bath. Formation of yellow precipitate of iodoform suggests the presence of alcoholic OH group. Ethanol and isopropanol respond to this test but methanol does not. Thus,

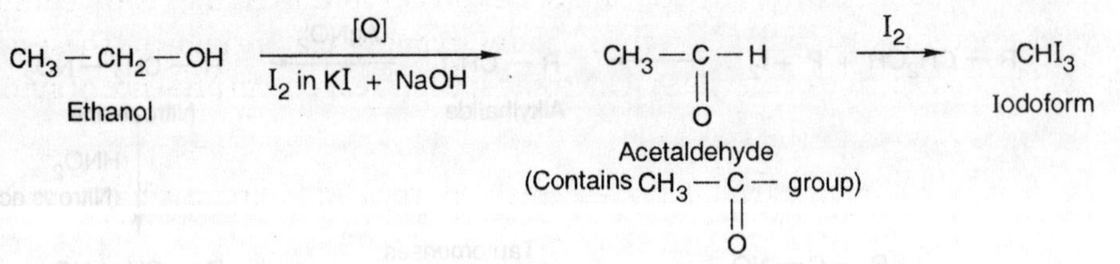

Similarly, isopropanol

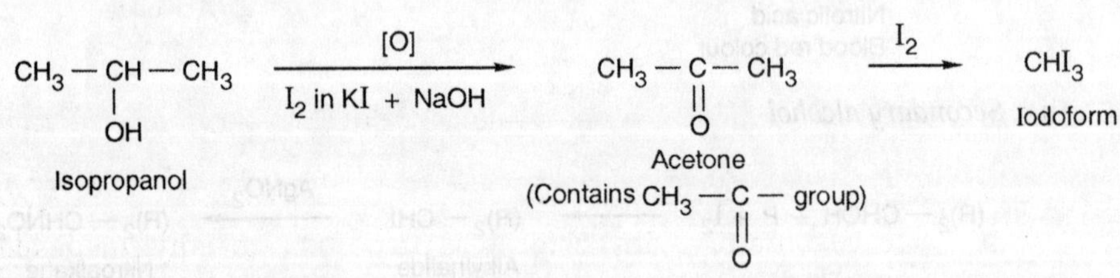

8.1.3.5 Uses of Alcohols

Besides the use as universal solvents, alcohols have immense utility in other fields, particularly in the field of medicine. Thus, ethanol has played a prominent role as a sedative and hypnotic for centuries. But due to development of chronic alcoholism its continuous use is avoided and other depressant drugs such as trichloro and tribromo ethanol have been favoured. Both of these drugs are powerful hypnotic with less toxicity. Further, ethanol and isopropanol are very good antiseptics and are freqeuntly used in hospitals as disinfectant for the skin and surgical instruments. Ethanol is also used as a preservative for biological specimen. Again, ethanol is intoxicating and is used in the beverage industry for making brandy, gin, whisky, rum and other alcoholic beverages. Mixture of ethanol and petroleum is employed for generation of power.

This is known as **power** *alcohol*. Methanol is used for denaturing industrial alcohols (methylated spirit) and in antifreeze composition of automobile and aeroplane radiators.

8.2 Unsaturated Alcohols

The most commonly known unsaturated alcohols are:

$CH_2{=}CH{-}OH$	$CH_2{=}CH{-}CH_2{-}OH$	$CH_3{-}CH{=}CH{-}CH_2OH$
Vinyl alcohol	Allyl alcohol	Crotyl alcohol

8.2.1 Vinyl Alcohol ($CH_2 = CH{-}OH$)

Vinyl alcohol is the simplest member of this group of alcohols. It may be regarded as the hydroxy derivative of ethylene. It has been found to be very unsatable and is rapidly converted to corresponding aldehyde, i.e.,

$$\underset{\text{Vinyl alcohol (unstable)}}{CH_2{=}CH{-}OH} \rightleftharpoons \underset{\text{Acetaldehyde (stable)}}{CH_3{-}\underset{\mid \atop H}{C}{=}O}$$

Due to instability, vinyl alcohol cannot be directly prepared and is practically unknown. However, some of its derivatives such as halides, cyanide, etc, are known. These derivatives are prepared by the reaction of acetylene with some specific reagents in presence of suitable catalysts.

(a) *Vinyl chloride*, $CH_2 = CH{-}Cl$

Preparation: Following methods are usually applied for the synthesis of vinyl chloride.

i. $$\underset{\text{Acetylene}}{H{-}C{\equiv}C{-}H} + HCl \xrightarrow{Hg^{2+}} \underset{\text{Vinyl chloride}}{CH_2{=}CH{-}Cl}$$

ii. $$\underset{\text{Calcium carbide}}{CaC_2} + HCl \xrightarrow{Hg^{2+}} CH_2{=}CH{-}Cl$$

iii. In the laboratory, vinyl chloride is prepared from ethylene dichloride.

$$\underset{\text{Ethylene dichloride}}{\underset{Cl}{CH_2}{-}\underset{Cl}{CH_2}} \xrightarrow[-\ HCl]{\text{Alcoholic KOH}} CH_2{=}CH{-}Cl + HCl$$

Above starting material is used in the industrial manufacture but instead of using alcoholic potassium hydroxide it is decomposed by heating at a temperature of 600-650 °C.

Properties: The halogen atom of vinyl halides is not reactive. They do not undergo usual reactions of alkyl halides and do not form Grignard reagents. But substituted vinyl halides can undergo Grignard reaction.

The exact reason for inactivity is not known but it is assumed that due to resonance halogen acquires double bond character and thereby strongly bound to carbon atom.

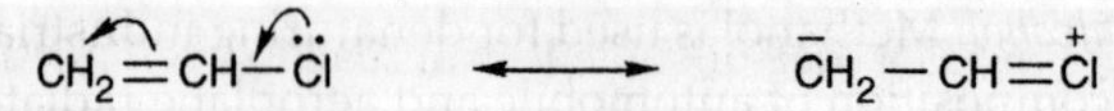

But when substituents specially electron releasing group is present electron movement occurs in the opposite direction.

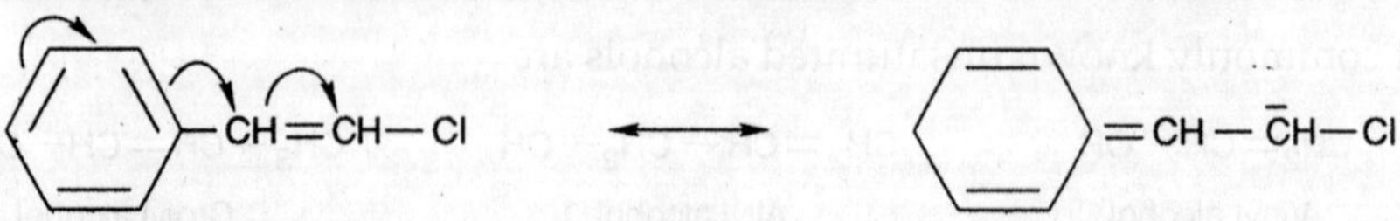

(b) *Vinyl cyanide*, $CH_2 = CH—CN$

It is prepared from acetylene as indicated below.

$$\underset{\text{Acetylene}}{H—C\equiv C—H} + HCN \xrightarrow[\text{Carbon}]{Ba(CN)_2} CH_2{=}CH—CN$$

Vinyl cyanide is industrially very important. It is used for the preparation of polymer, vinyon and vinyl acetate which are used in thermoplastic filter cloth. Vinyl cyanide is also used in the manufacture of synthetic rubber—buna-N-brand.

8.2.2 Allyl Alcohol, $CH_2 = CH—CH_2OH$ (Prop-2-en-1-ol)

It differs from vinyl alcohol in structure. The hydroxyl group is not attached to the doubly bonded carbon atom.

Preparation: Preparation of this unsaturated alcohol is carried out by the following methods:

i. $$\underset{\text{Allyl chloride}}{CH_2{=}CH—CH_2—Cl} \xrightarrow[\text{dilute NaOH}]{\text{Boiled with}} \underset{\text{Allyl alcohol}}{CH_2{=}CH—CH_2—OH} + NaCl$$

This method is followed for the commercial synthesis.

ii. It is also prepared by heating glycerine with formic acid or oxalic acid.

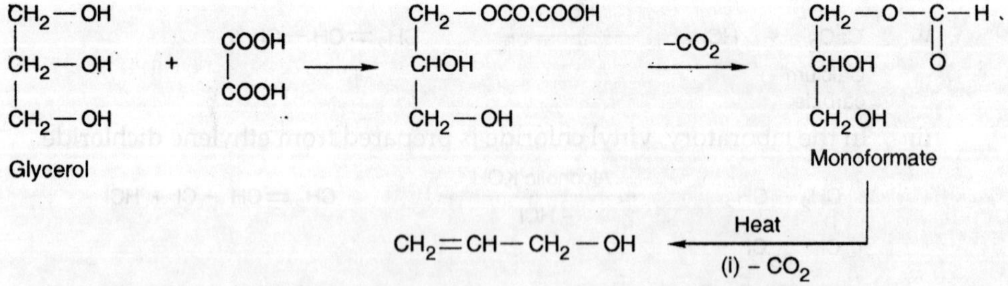

For better yield formic acid is used.

Properties:

Physical properties: It is a colourless liquid with pungent smell, soluble in water.

Chemical properties: Allyl alcohol exhibits the properties of both the unsaturation and alcohol as mentioned:

i. *Oxidation*: On oxidation with dilute alkaline permanganate solution it yields glycerol.

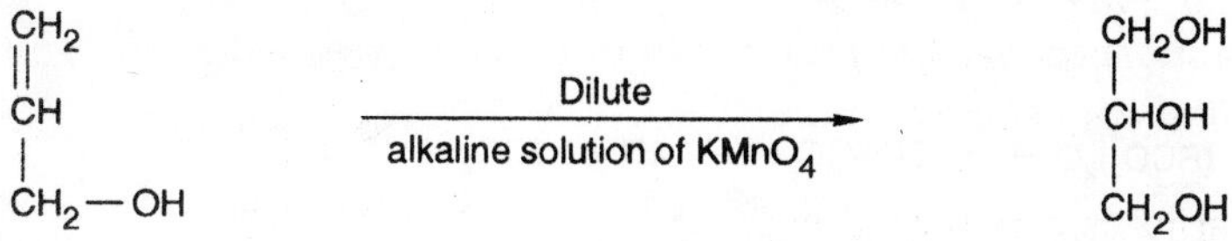

Allyl alcohol Glycerol

ii. *Addition of halogen acids*: Allyl alcohol undergoes addition reaction with halogen acids. Thus,

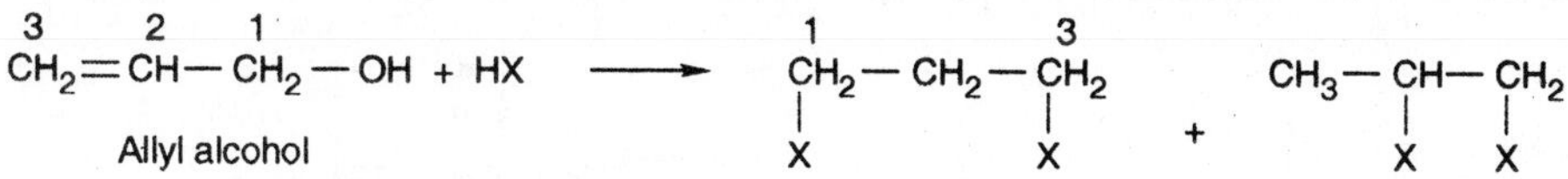

Allyl alcohol 1:3 1:2

It has been observed that in presence of peroxides, 1:3 product is predominant while in absence of peroxide or any oxygen source, 1:2 product is obtained in 90% yield but under normal condition both the products are obtained. Formation of these two products may be rationalised as:

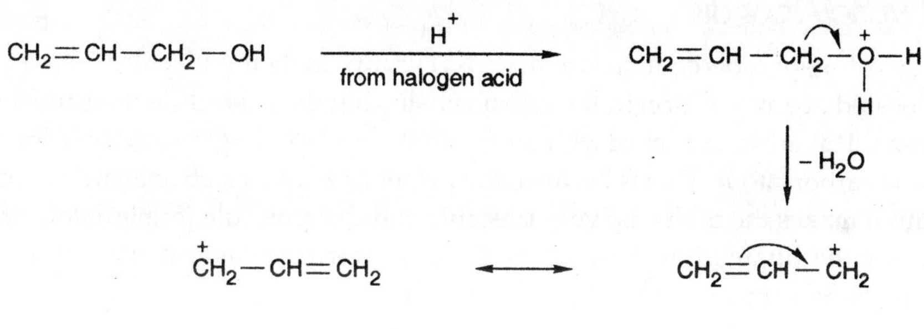

(II) (I)

Now,

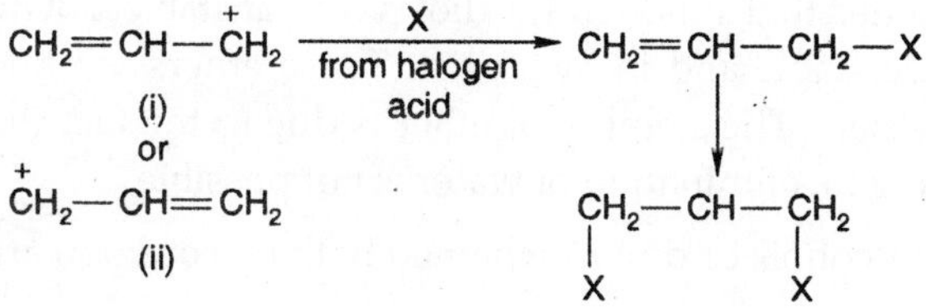

1, 3-product

Again,

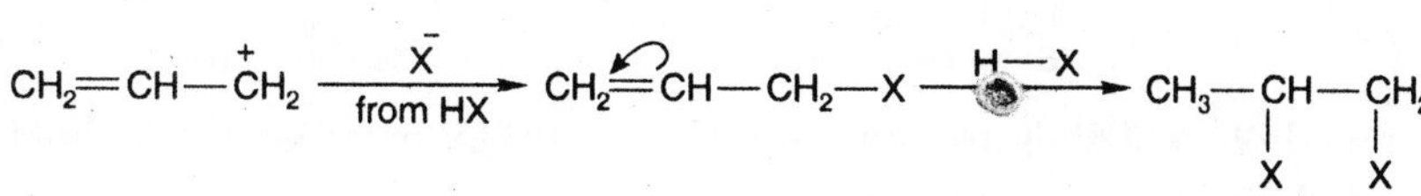

1, 2-product

In presence of peroxides the reaction path is radical in nature

$$(RCO_2)_2O \longrightarrow 2R\dot{C}OO \longrightarrow 2\dot{R} + 2CO_2$$

Peroxide

$$(RCO_2)_2O \longrightarrow 2R\dot{C}OO \longrightarrow 2\dot{R} + 2CO_2$$

$$\dot{R} + HX \longrightarrow R{-}H + \dot{X}$$

$$CH_2{=}CH{-}CH_2{-}OH \xrightarrow{HX} CH_2{=}CH{-}CH_2{-}X$$

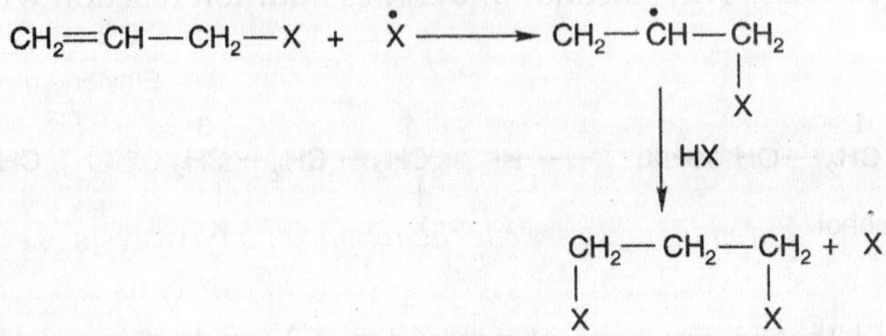

Allyl alcohol is used as a starting compound for the manufacture of allyl caproate which is used in perfumes.

8.3 Dihydric Alcohols

Dihydric alcohols or diols contain two hydroxyl groups in their molecules. These two OH groups may be located at any position in the carbon chains but they should not be attached to the same carbon atom. This is in accordance with the fact that two electronegative atoms cannot be connected at the same carbon atom. This is because the presence of two electronegative atoms at the same carbon atom makes the molecule very unstable and the molecule immediately undergoes bond cleavage wih the elimination of one of the electronegative atoms as neutral molecule. In the case of 1,1-diol, there is ready elimination of water, i.e.,

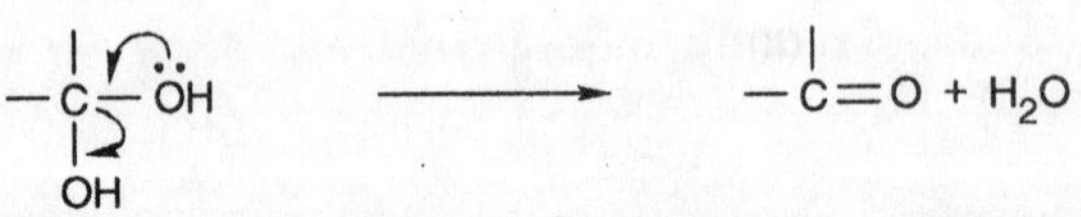

However, it may be mentioned that although 1, 1-diol is very unstable, but their corresponding ethers (mono- or diethers) are stable and in fact, exist. These ethers are known as *hemiacetal* (mono- ether) and acetal (diether). The stability of ether is due to the fact that as there is a no hydrogen atom bonded to oxygen, elimination of water is not possible.

Nomenclature: Dihydric alcohols or diols are named both by common and IUPAC system. Thus,

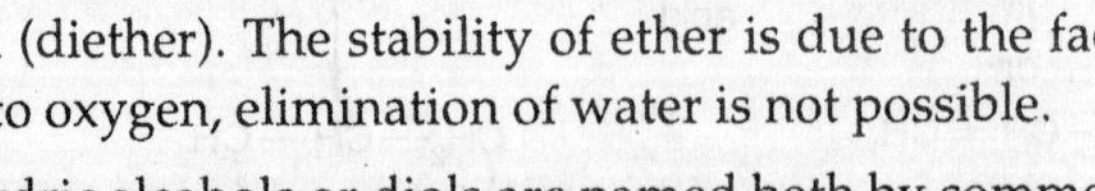

1, 2-Ethane diol (Ethylene glycol) 1, 2-Propane diol (Propylene glycol)

Among diols, 1, 2 diols are common. The important member of 1, 2-diol is *ethylene glycol* (1, 2-ethane diol) which is usually known as *glycol*.

8.3.1 Preparation of Ethylene Glycol

This diol is prepared by the following methods.

(a) *Hydroxylation*: Hydroxylation of ethylene is normally carried out by cold dilute alkaline solution of potassium permanganate. The reaction proceeds through cyclic intermediate (vide chapter **one**).

$$CH_2{=}CH_2 + H_2O \xrightarrow[\text{KmnO}_4\text{ solution}]{\text{alkaline}} \underset{OH}{CH_2}-\underset{OH}{CH_2}$$

Ethylene glycol
cis

Hydroxylation may also be carried with osmium tetroxide (OSO_4).

(b) *Hydrolysis of ethylene dibromide and ethylene chlorohydrin*: Hydrolysis of ethylene dibromide and ethylene chlorohydrin form ethylene glycol. Hydrolysis is carried out with the aqueous solution of sodium carbonate. Thus,

$$\begin{matrix} CH_2-Br \\ | \\ CH_2-Br \end{matrix} + H_2O \xrightarrow[\text{Aq.}]{Na_2CO_3} \begin{matrix} CH_2-OH \\ | \\ CH_2-OH \end{matrix} + 2NaBr + CO_2$$

Ethylene dibromide → Ethylene glycol

$$\begin{matrix} CH_2-OH \\ | \\ CH_2-Cl \end{matrix} + H_2O \xrightarrow[\text{Aq.}]{Na_2CO_3} \begin{matrix} CH_2-OH \\ | \\ CH_2-OH \end{matrix}$$

Ethylene chlorohydrin

(c) *Hydrolysis of epoxides*: Ethylene oxide on hydrolysis in presence of acid or base as catalyst forms ethylene glycol. Since ethylene oxide is a three membered ring compound it is highly unstable and can readily undergo hydrolysis.

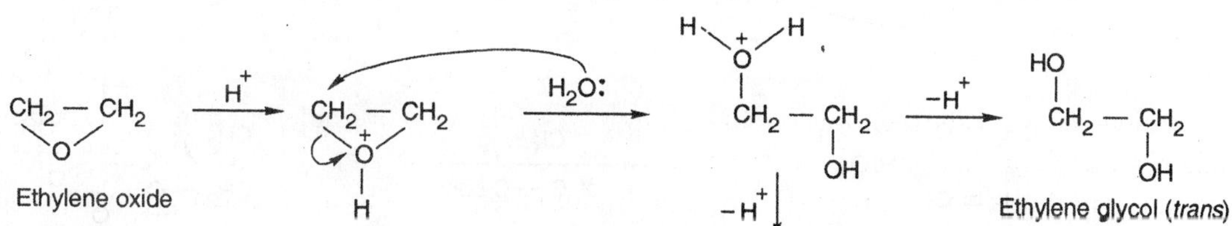

This reaction forms *trans* 1, 2-glycol but $KMnO_4$ or OSO_4 forms *cis* glycol.

8.3.2 Physical Properties of Ethylene Glycol

It is a colourless syrupy liquid. It has high boiling point (198 °C). The higher boiling point is due to the formation of strong intermolecular hydrogen bonding. Because of the formation of strong hydrogen bond it is highly soluble in water.

8.3.3 Chemical Reactions of Ethylene Glycol

Ethylene glycol undergoes all the chemical reactions of monohydric alcohols. However, reaction may be conducted in such a way that sometimes out of two one of the hydroxyl groups may undergo reaction. Some of the important reactions of ethylene glycol are discussed:

(a) 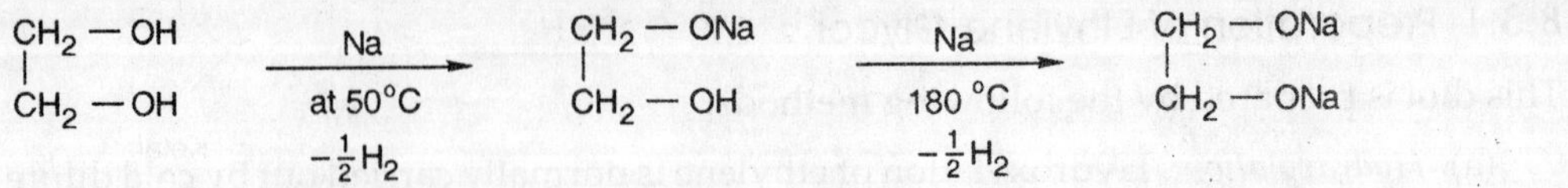

(b) 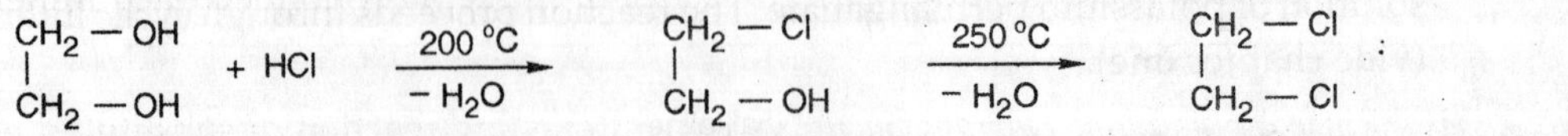

(c) Oxidation of ethylene glycol is an important reaction. Variety of products are formed under different experimental condition.

i. On oxidation with *nitric acid* ethylene glycol furnishes the following products:

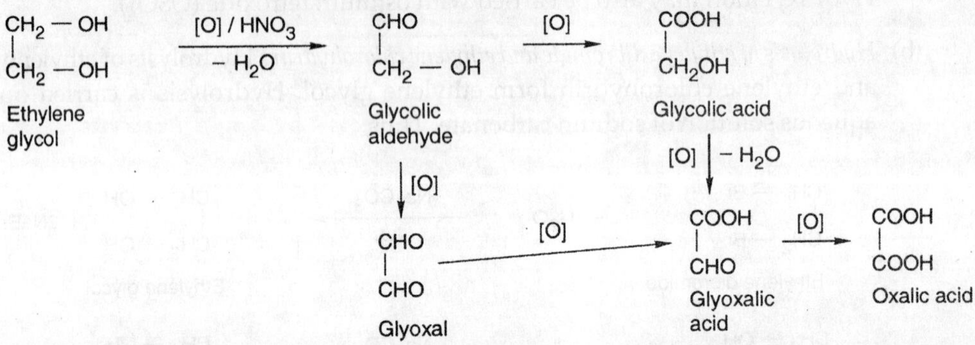

ii. If periodic acid (HIO_4) or lead tetra acetate, $Pb(OCOCH_3)_4$ is used as oxidising agent oxidative cleavage occurs forming different types of carbonyl compounds. Oxidation in both the cases takes through the formation of cyclic intermediate. Thus,

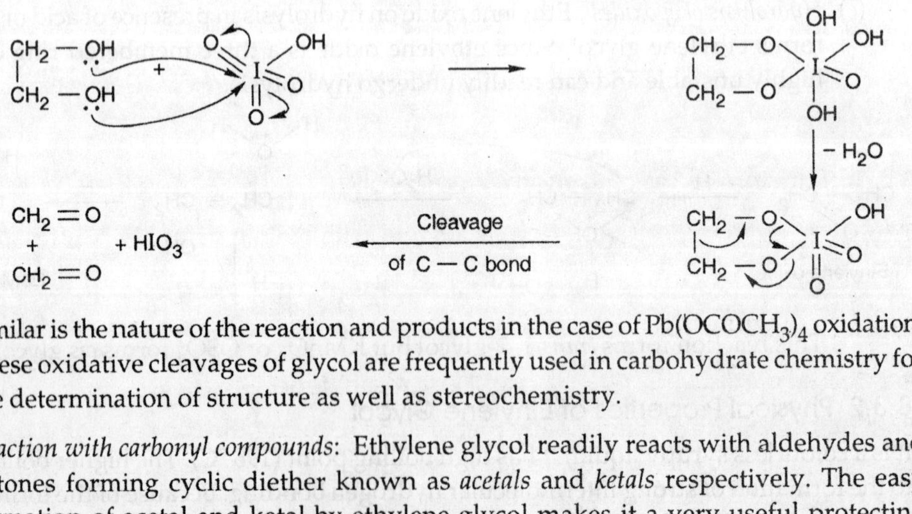

Similar is the nature of the reaction and products in the case of $Pb(OCOCH_3)_4$ oxidation. These oxidative cleavages of glycol are frequently used in carbohydrate chemistry for the determination of structure as well as stereochemistry.

iii. *Reaction with carbonyl compounds*: Ethylene glycol readily reacts with aldehydes and ketones forming cyclic diether known as *acetals* and *ketals* respectively. The easy formation of acetal and ketal by ethylene glycol makes it a very useful protecting agent for carbonyl compounds. Thus,

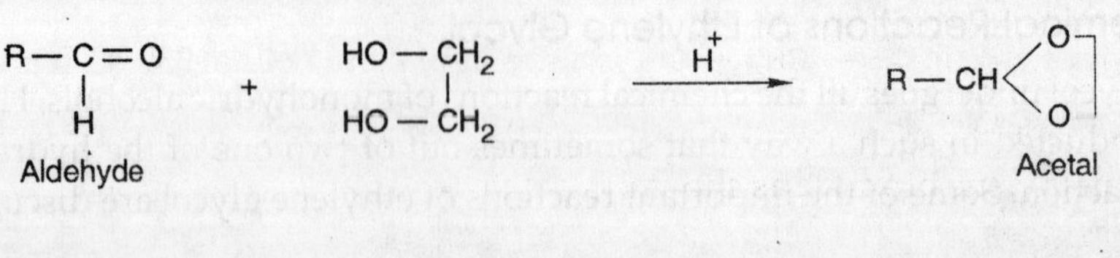

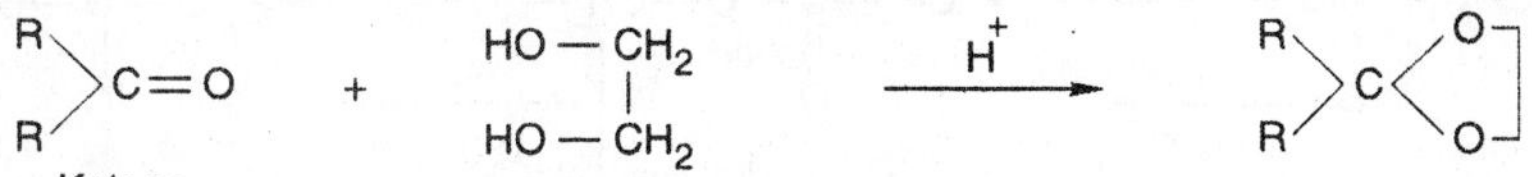

Ketone Ketal

The reaction occurs smoothly in presence of moderately connectrated mineral acid (HCl or H_2SO_4).

iv. *Pinacol-pinacolone rearrangement*: A very interesting reaction of substituted ethylene glycol is the pinacol-pinacolone rearrangement. Pinacol which is a tertiary glycol, in presence of mineral acid undergoes a skeletal rearrangement with the formation of a ketonic product termed as pinacolone, i.e.,

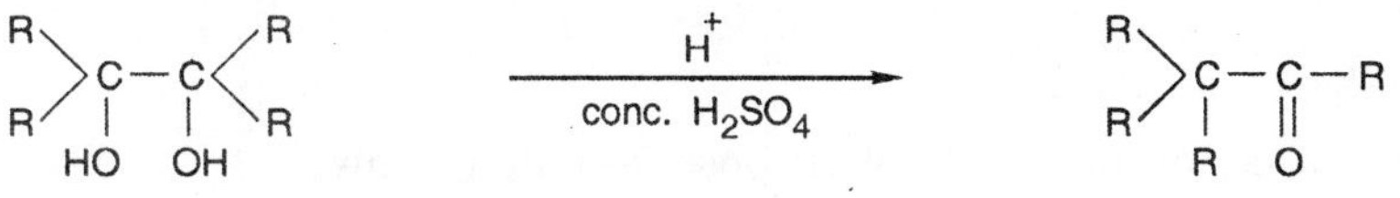

Pinacol Pinacolone

This rearrangement is known as pinacol-pinacolone rearrangement.
Mechanism of the reaction may be discussed as below:

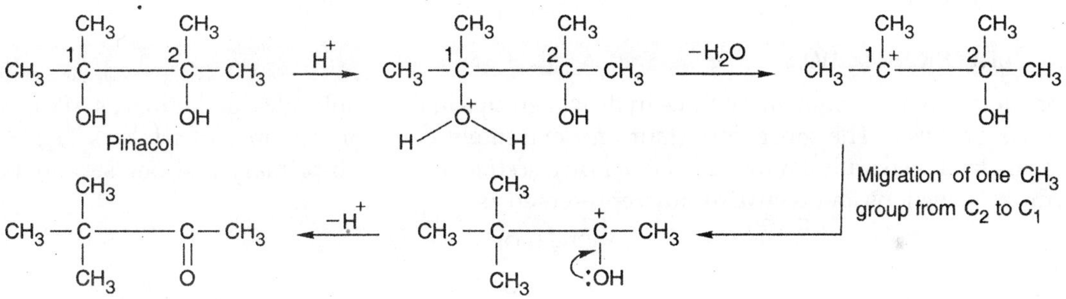

Pinacolone

8.4 Polymethylene Glycols

8.4.1 Propane-1, 3-diol (Trimethylene glycol)

Trimethylene glycol, $CH_2(OH)—CH_2—CH_2(OH)$ is a liquid with boiling point 214 °C. It is prepared by the hydrolysis of trimethylene bromide or by fermentation of glycerol by *Schizomycetes.*

8.4.2 Tetramethylene Glycol and Hexamethylene Glycol

Both these glycols are conveniently prepared by reducing the corresponding α, ω-dicarboxylic esters i.e., succinic and adipic esters respectively. Teramethylene glycol is prepared industrially by hydrogenating butynediol. It is used for preparing butadiene and tetrahydrofuran.

8.4.3 Pentamethylene Glycol

Pentamethylene glycol, $CH_2(OH)—(CH_2)_3—CH_2(OH)$ is also a liquid and boils at 239 °C. It is usually prepared from pentamethylene bromide as shown:

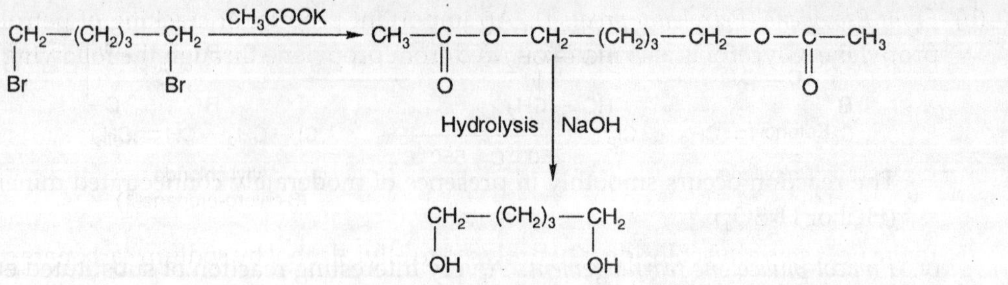

Pentamethylene Glycol

The polymethylene glycols can be readily converted into mono- and di-halogen derivatives by halogen acids. These halogen derivatives are useful reagents in organic synthesis.

8.4.4 Uses of Glycols

Ethylene glycol is used for the variety of purposes as noted below:

i. As a protecting agent for carbonyl group during the synthesis of organic compounds.
ii. In the manufacture of synthetic fibre, **Dacron** (Terylene)
iii. As antifreeze for automobile and coolant for aeroplane motors under the trade name **prestone.**

8.5 Trihydric Alcohols

Organic compounds containing three hydroxyl groups in their molecules are known as *trihydric alcohols* or *Triols*. The most important and extremely common member of triols is 1, 2, 3-propanetriol, generally known as *glycerol* or *glycerine*. It has two primary and one secondary hydroxyl functions and is structurally represented as:

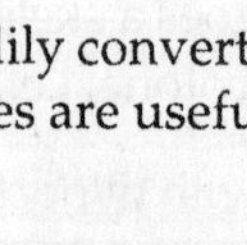

8.5.1 Preparation of Glycerol

Glycerol is normally prepared by the following methods:

(a) *From Fats*: The oldest and most important source of glycerol is natural fats and oils. Oils and fats are the triesters of long chain fatty acids primarily palmitic, stearic and oleic acids. These esters are known as *glycerides*. Glycerides on hydrolysis with sodium hydroxide form glycerol and salts of fatty acids. The process of hydrolysis is known as *saponification*. Originally saponification of fats and oils is carried out for the manufacture of soap, and glycerol is obtained as a by-product.

Glycerides are hydrolysed by boiling with sodium hydroxide solution when the fatty acids are precipitated as their sodium salt. This is filtered out and the filtrate usually known as *spent lye* contains glycerol. This spent lye is subjected to different processes of purification after which 90% pure glycerol is obtained. The reactions taking place are as under

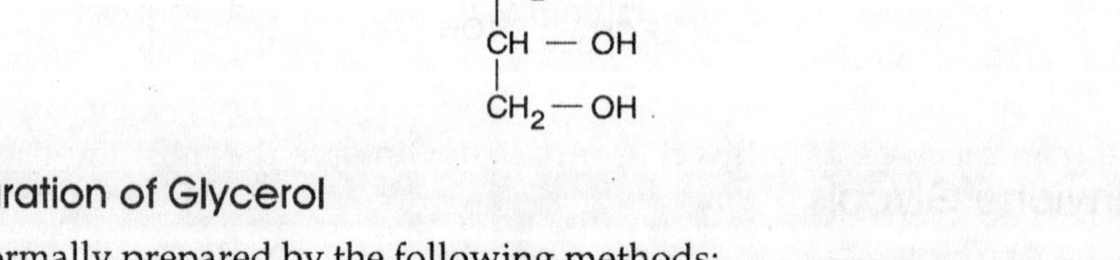

(b) *From Propylene (Petroleum product)*: An important product of cracking of petroleum is propylene. Glycerol is also manufactured from propylene through the following steps:

$$\underset{\text{Propylene}}{CH_3-CH=CH_2} + Cl_2 \xrightarrow[500\,°C - 550\,°C]{Cl_2} \underset{\substack{\text{Allyl chloride}\\ \text{(3-chloro-propane-1)}}}{Cl-CH_2-CH=CH_2}$$

In the next step allyl chloride is hydrolysed to allyl alcohol by sodium carbonate solution at a temperature of 150 °C.

$$Cl-CH_2-CH=CH_2 + H_2O \longrightarrow \underset{\text{Allyl alcohol}}{HO-CH_2-CH=CH_2}$$

Allyl alcohol thus formed is treated with hypochlorous acid (HOCl) to form chloro-hydrin.

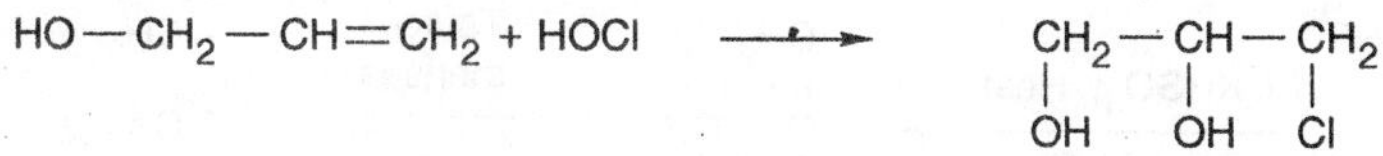

Glycerol-α-chlorohydrin

In the final step chlorohydrin is hydrolysed by sodium hydroxide solution when glycerol is obtained.

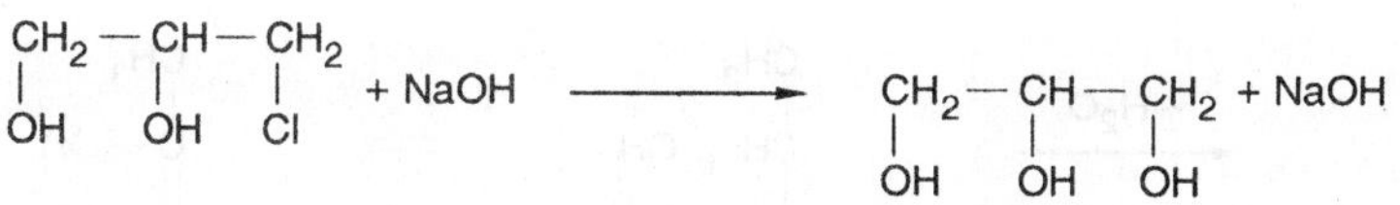

Glycerol

8.5.2 Properties of Glycerol

Glycerol is a colourless, viscous liquid with very high boiling point (300 °C). It is soluble in water. Its high boiling point and greater solubility in water is due to more hydrogen bond formation by three hydroxyl groups.

Glycerol has two primary and one secondary hydroxyl functions. Primary hydroxyl group is more reactive than secondary hydroxyl group. Following are the most important reactions exhibited by glycerol.

i. *Reaction with* HI: Glycerol on reaction with HI yields 2-iodopropane (isopropyl iodide):

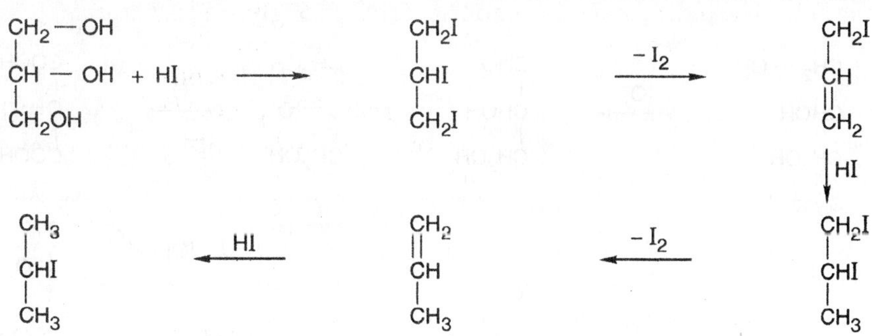

Isopropyl iodide Propylene

ii. *Reaction with Nitric acid*: Glycerol on nitration with the mixture of nitric acid and sulphuric acid below the room temperature furnishes glyceryl trinitrate, commonly known as *nitroglycerine*.

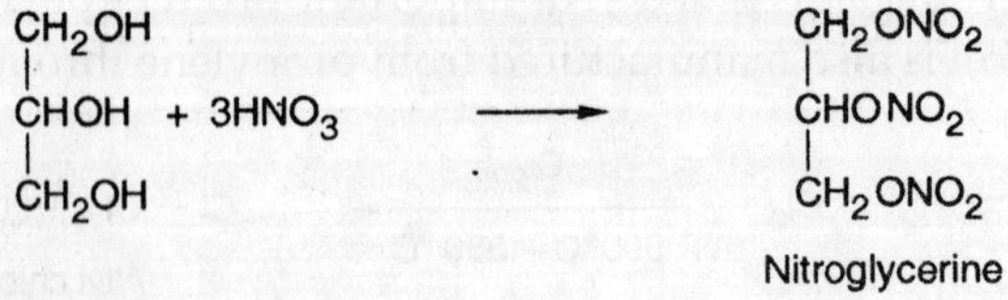

Nitroglycerine is a powerful explosive discovered by Alfred Nobel. That is why it is known as *Nobel's oil*.

Nitroglycerine when absorbed on kieselguhr, a special type of clay, dynamite is obtained. It is less powerful and so can be handled safely.

iii. *Dehydration of Glycerol*: Glycerol when heated with dehydrating agent preferably potassium hydrogen sulphate undergoes dehydration with the formation of acrolein.

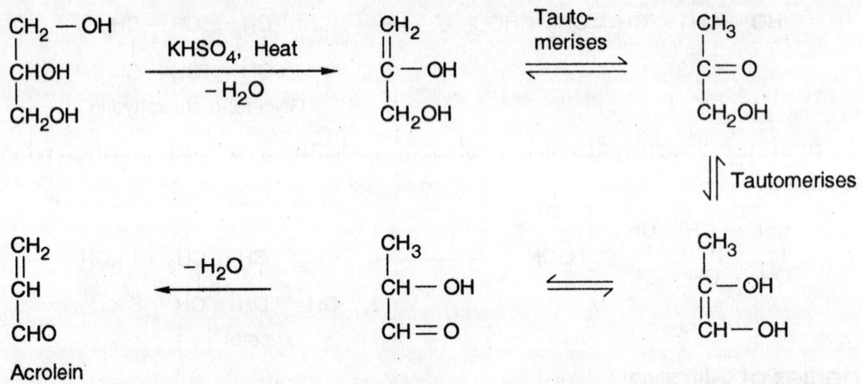

This reaction is utilised for the identification of glycerol and is known as *Acrolein Test*. Acrolein has pungent smell.

iv. *Oxidation of Glycerol*: Oxidation of glycerol is very interesting and a variety of products are obtained depending upon the nature of oxidising agent.

When mild oxidising agent is used, the products are glyceraldehyde and dihydroxy acetone, but on oxidation with strong oxidising agent glyceric acid, mesooxalic acid, oxalic acid and tartonic acid are formed.

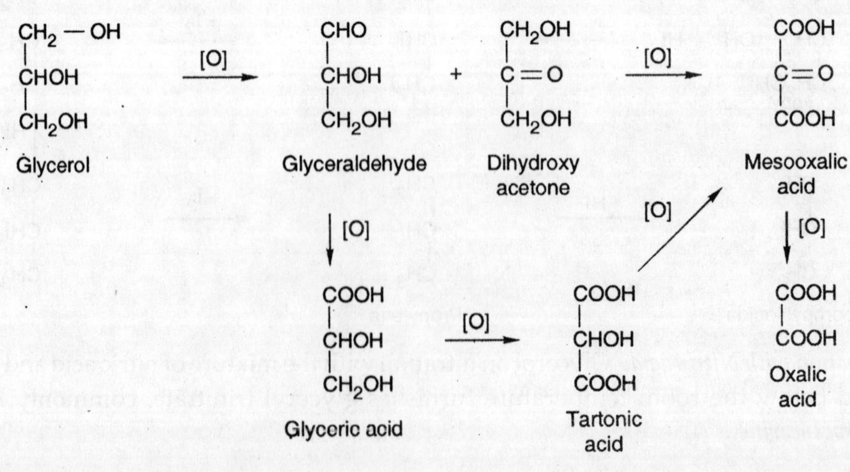

8.5.3 Uses of Glycerol

Glycerol is used in the manufacture of (i) cosmetics, (ii) nitroglycerine, which is an important chemical compound used for variety of purposes. It is used as a vasodilator applied in heart disease called angina pectoris.

It has action typical of nitrites but its action is developed slowly and is of longer duration. Its side effects are occassional throbbing headache and dizziness. It is also used as medicine in asthma.

It is also used in the preparation of explosives.

Model Questions

1. Write the structural formulae and give IUPAC names of all isomeric alcohols of the molecular formula, $C_4H_{10}O$.
2. How are alcohols prepared? Describe their important reactions.
3. How is methyl alcohol manufactured?
4. How is ethyl alcohol manufactured from starch or molasses?
5. How does ethyl alcohol reacts with (a) Na, (b) conc. $H_2SO_4/170$ °C, (c) PCl_5, (d) $K_2Cr_2O_7/H^+$?
6. What happens when propanol is treated with: (a) PCl_5, (b) $SOCl_2$, (c) Na, (d) conc. $H_2SO_4/$ 170 °C?
7. How do primary, secondary alcohols differ towards oxidation?
8. How will you distinguish primary, secondary and tertiary alcohols?
9. Explain: (i) Alcohols have higher boiling points than ether of comparable molecular weight.
   ii. n-Hexanol is insoluble in water.
   iii. Lower members of alcohols are soluble in water while higher members are not.
   iv. Bioling point of I-Propanol is lower than 1, 2-ethane diol.
   v. Alcohols are weak acids.
   vi. Alcohols have higher boiling points than alkyl halides or alkane of comparable molecular weight.
10. How will you convert the followings?
   (a) Isopropyl alcohol ⟶ Tert-butyl alcohol

   Hints: Isopropyl alcohol

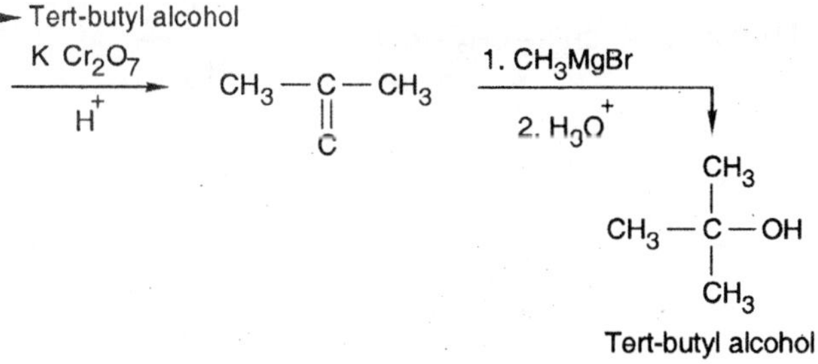

Tert-butyl alcohol

   (b) Isopropyl alcohol ⟶ *n*-propyl alcohol

Hints: 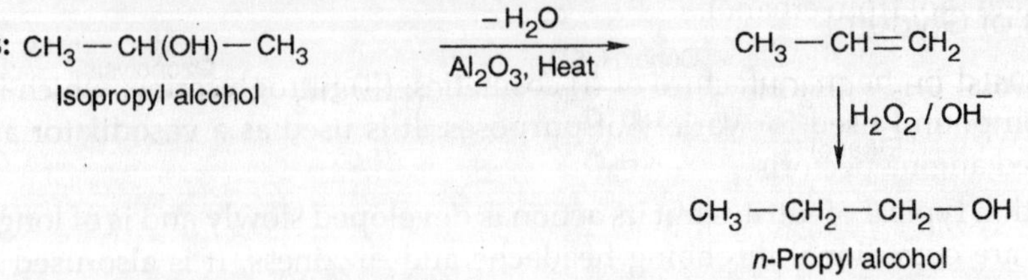

(c) Isobutyl alcohol ⟶ Tert-butyl alcohol

Hints: 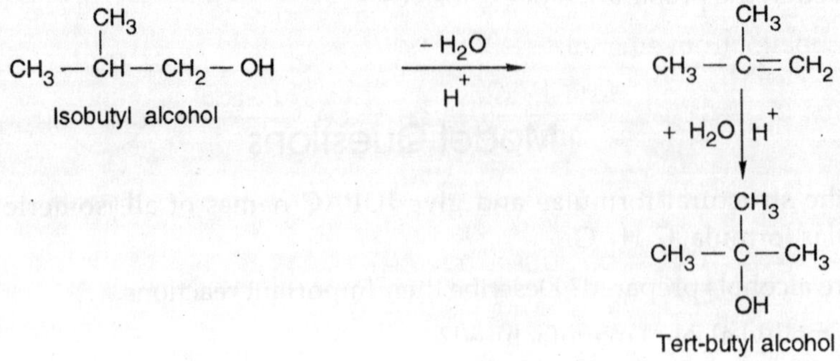

11. Identify the products:

$$\text{Isopropyl alcohol} \xrightarrow[H_2SO_4]{K_2Cr_2O_7} (A) \xrightarrow{CH_3MgBr} (B) \xrightarrow{Al_2O_3} (C)$$

Hints: (A) is acetone, (B) is 2-Methyl 2-propanol, (C) is 2-Methyl-propene

12. How will you synthesise the followings:

(a) *n*-propanol from methanol.

Hints: 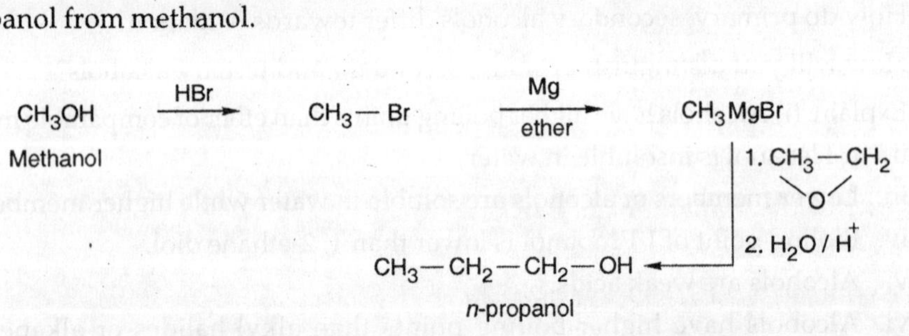

(b) Isopropyl alcohol from *n*-propyl alcohol.

Hints: 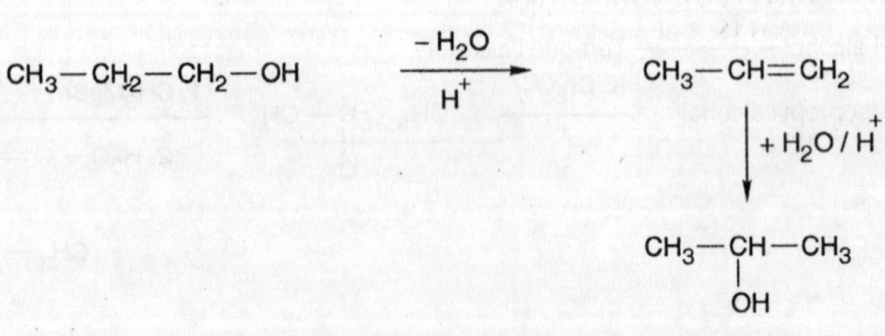

(c) Methanol from ethanol.

Hints:

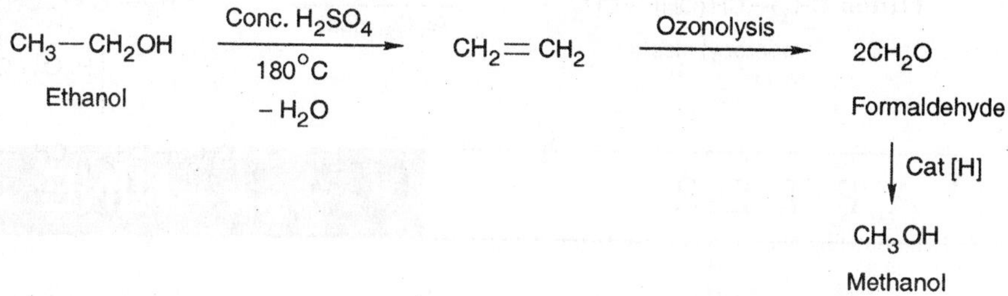

(d) *n*-propanol from ethanol.

Hints:

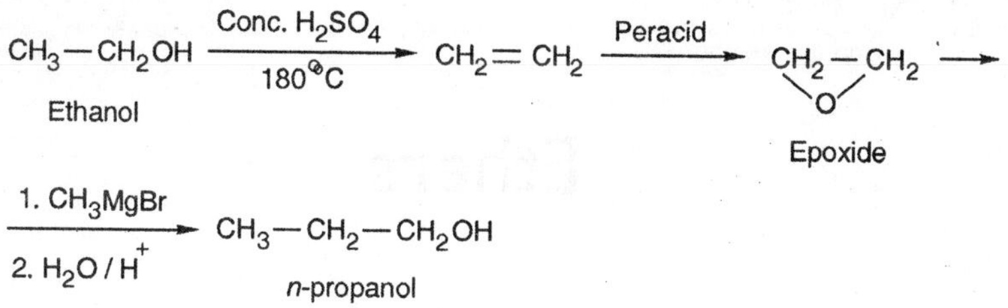

13. How will you distinguish the following?
    (a) Methyl alcohol and ethyl alcohol.
    (b) *n*-butyl alcohol and diethyl ether.

    Hints: (a) Ethyl alcohol responds to Iodoform test but methyl alcohol does not. (b) On treatment with metallic Na *n*-butyl alcohol liberates hydrogen but ether does not.

14. Write notes on
    (a) Methylated spirit
    (b) Absolute alcohol
    (c) Proof-spirit
    (d) Fermentation
    (e) Denaturated alcohol.
15. Describe the preparation of ethylene glycol.
16. Describe the properties of ethylene glycol.
17. Describe the preparation of glycerol.
18. How is glycerol obtained from pertroleum products?
19. Describe properties of glycerol.
20. How can you obtain Nobel's oil and 2-propenol from glycerol?

Hints:

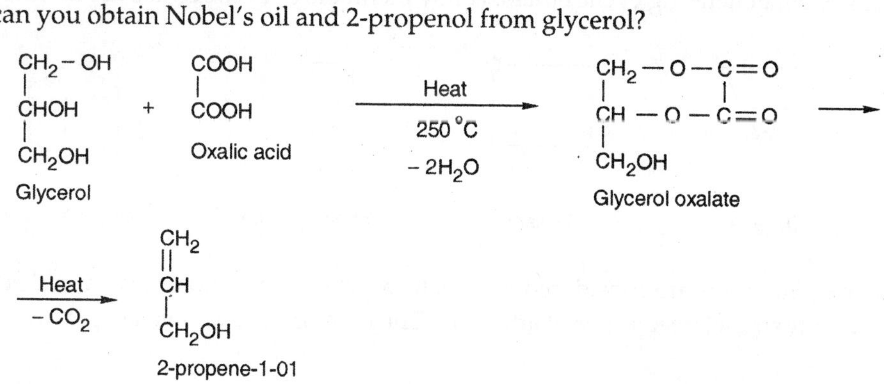

CHAPTER NINE

Ethers

Ethers are organic compounds in which both the valencies of oxygen atom are satisfied by the combination of two organic groups—alkyl or aryl. They are represented by the general structure.

$$R—O—R$$

From the above structural representation it is evident that ethers may be considered as the derivatives of water in which both the hydrogen atoms have been replaced by two organic groups. They may also be looked upon as the derivative of alcohol in which hydrogen atom has been substituted by any organic group.

Two R groups in the structure may be same or different. When both the groups are identical, ether is said to be *symmetrical*, but if the two groups are different *unsymmetrical* ether results. Some of the most common members of ether are stated below:

$CH_3—O—CH_3$	$C_2H_5—O—C_2H_5$	$C_2H_5—O—CH_3$
Dimethyl ether	Diethyl ether	Ethylmethyl ether

Among the ethers, highly illustrated and extensively studied ether is diethyl ether. It is so popular that simply ether means diethyl ether. Sometimes ether oxygen atom may be present in a cyclic system generating cyclic ethers. A few members of cyclic ethers are mentioned below:

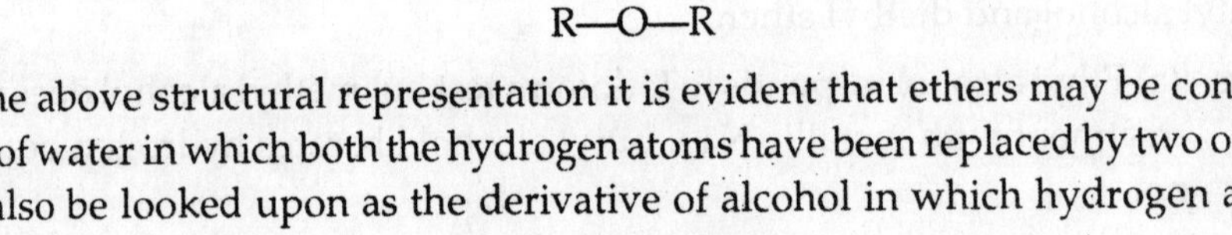

Oxirane   Oxetane   Tetrahydro furan   Tetrahydro pyran

Such cyclic ethers are considered to be heterocyclic compounds. However, three membered cyclic ether (oxirane) needs special attention. They are usually known as *epoxides*.

9.1 Structure and Bonding in Ethers

Since ethers are considered to be the derivatives of water there must be some similarity in shapes and structures between these two compounds. The oxygen atom in ethers is in sp^3 hybridised state and two C—O bonds are formed by the overlapping of sp^3—sp^3 orbitals. The unpaired electrons on oxygen is also in sp^3 hybrid orbitals. The C—O—C bond angle in ethers is 110° which is very close to tetrahedral angle (109° 28′) but it is bigger than H—O—H bond angle (105°) in water. This enhancement in bond angle is due to the steric hindrance created by organic groups associated with oxygen atom. It has been observed that more bulkier the organic groups, more increase will be in the bond angle. That is why in di-tert-butyl ether C—O—C bond angle is very high (132°).

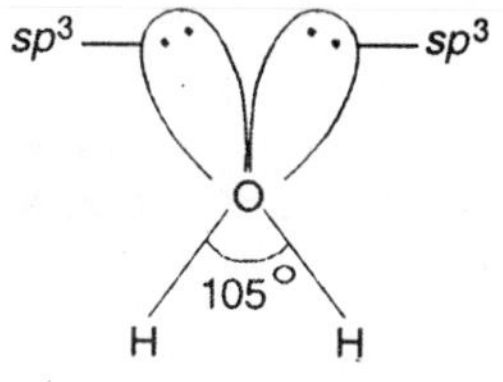

Orbital structure of water molecule

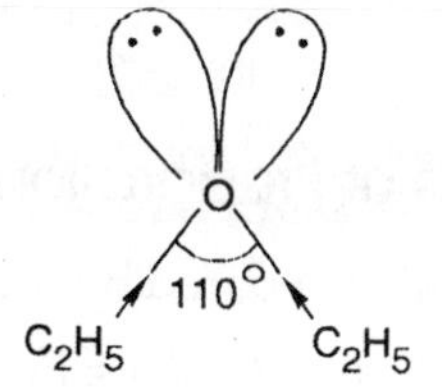

Orbital structure of diethyl ether

However, C—O bond distances in ethers (1.41Å) are somewhat shorter than C—C bond distance (1.53Å).

The value of C—O—C bond angle (110°) in ethers is much below 180°. This is a strong indication that the ethers are not linear molecules and so dipole moments of two C—O bonds do not cancel each other and hence ethers must have net dipole moment and in fact, it has been found to be so. The dipole moment for diethyl ether is 1.18D.

PROBLEM 9.1

Explain: C—O—C bond angle in diethyl ether is bigger than that in dimethyl ether.

9.2 Nomenclature of Ethers

There are two systems for naming ethers, viz.

Common system: In this system word 'ether' is added after the name of alkyl groups attached to oxygen atom. However, in the case of unsymmetrical ether, alkyl groups are written in alphabetical order as separate word while for symmetrical ether, the prefix *di* precedes the name of alkyl group.

In IUPAC system the ethers are named as the alkoxyl derivative of alkanes. Alkyl group having higher number of carbon atoms is taken as the parent hydrocarbon. Ethers are mainly named by common system, IUPAC system is rarely used. Thus,

Compound	Common name	IUPAC name
$CH_3—O—CH_3$	Dimethyl ether	Methoxy methane
$CH_3—O—C_2H_5$	Ethyl methyl ether	Methoxy ethane
$C_2H_5—O—C_2H_5$	Diethyl ether	Ethoxy ethane
$C_2H_5—O—CH_2—CH_2—CH_3$	Ethyl propyl ether	Ethoxy propane

In some cases particularly in the case of aromatic ethers, special names are used. For example,

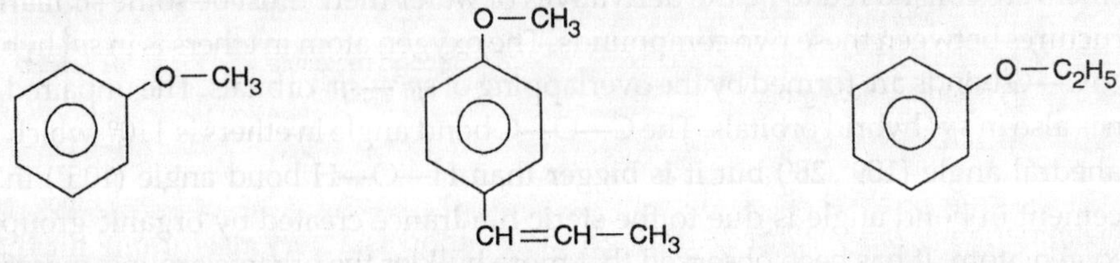

Anisole (Methyl phenyl ether) | Anethole [Methyl-(para propylene)-phenyl ether] | Phenetole (Ethyl phenyl ether)

9.3 Methods of Preparation of Ethers

Ethers are usually prepared by the following methods:

1. *Dehydration of Alcohols*: Formation of ethers by dehydration of alcohol is a very common and useful method. The dehydration of alcohol is carried out by heating excess of alcohols with concentrated sulphuric acid at a temperature of not more than 140 °C. Reaction taking place is

$$2R-OH \xrightarrow[140\,^{\circ}C]{\text{conc. } H_2SO_4} R-O-R + H_2O$$

Mechanistically the reaction is a nucleophilic substitution reaction. The reaction proceeds as:

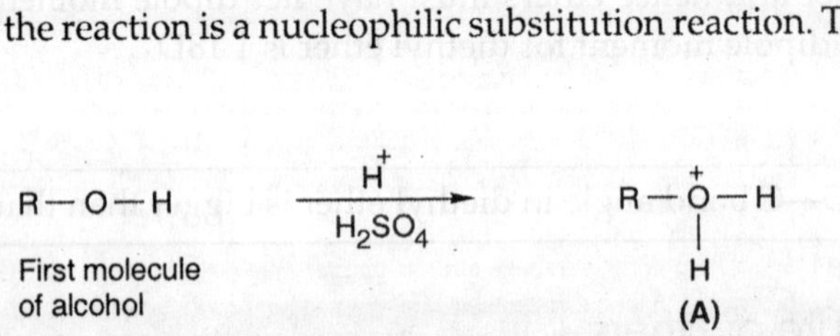

When R is primary alkyl group, as the carbocation to be formed by elimination of water from protonated alcohol (A) is unstable, the second molecule of alcohol attacks the protonated alcohol from the backside, i.e., through S_{N^2}

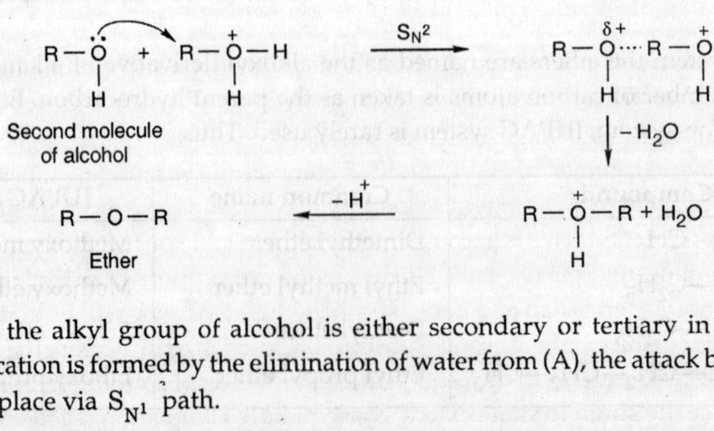

But if the alkyl group of alcohol is either secondary or tertiary in nature, the stable carbocation is formed by the elimination of water from (A), the attack by second molecule takes place via S_{N^1} path.

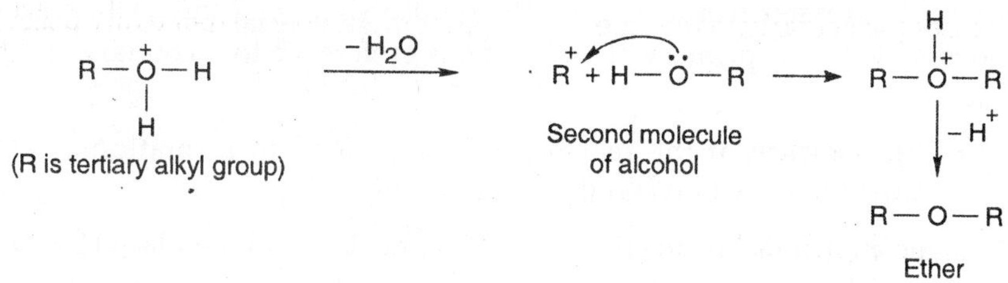

Limitation of this method: Although the method is a very useful one for the large scale production of ethers, yet it suffers from some severe drawbacks, viz.

i. Alcohols used should be primary in character, otherwise if secondary and tertiary alcohols are used dehydration may lead to the formation of alkenes as major products.

ii. Even in the case of primary alcohols there is always possibility of formation of alkenes. However, the formation of alkenes may be avoided by the rigorous control of temperature and using large excess of alcohol. The temperature must be kept below 140 °C. If the reaction temperature raises up to 180 °C and ratio of alcohol and concentrated sulphuric acid becomes 1:1, the major product will be alkenes.

iii. Unsymmetrical ethers cannot be prepared in appreciable yield by this method. This is because mixture of two different alcohols would lead to the formation of mixture of three different ethers which will involve complicated procedure of separation.

2. *Williamson's Synthesis*: Most probably this is the best method for the preparation of ethers in the laboratory. In this method alkyl halide is treated with an alkoxide.

$$\underset{\text{Alkyl halide}}{RX} + \underset{\text{Alkoxide}}{R'-O-Na} \longrightarrow R-O-R' + NaX$$

The reaction is a case of S_{N^2} type of nucleophilic substitution. Mechanistic path of the reaction may be depicted as under:

$$R'-O-Na \rightleftharpoons \underset{\text{Alkoxide ion}}{R'-\bar{O}}$$

Backside attack by alkoxide to alkyl halide:

$$R'-\bar{O} + R-X \longrightarrow R'-O-R + \bar{X}$$

By this method both symmetrical and unsymmetrical ethers can be synthesised successfully with very good yields.

Limitation of Williamson's Synthesis: Although the method is a successfull one yet it is not free from drawbacks. This method has following limitations:

i. Since alkoxides are strong bases, there is every possibility of occurrence of elimination reaction by their attack to alkyl halide as competiting reaction to substitution. Tertiary alkyl groups and to some extent secondary alkyl group have more tendency to undergo elimination reaction. This is because they can form stable carbocations and so the reaction path will follow *unimolecular path*. Further, as the carbocations from tertiary and secondary alkyl groups are crowded and hence strained, their tendency will be to reduce the strain. Attachment of nucleophilic group (substitution reaction) will increase the strain and hence will not be favourable. On the other hand, elimination of a proton (elimination reaction) will reduce the strain to some extent, consequently elimination reaction will favourably occur. For this reason in order to get better yield as well as to conduct the reaction smoothly, it is desirable to use primary alkyl halide in preference to secondary and tertiary alkyl halides.

ii. Higher temperature of the reaction may also lead to formation of alkene. Hence temperature of the reaction should be moderate.

iii. As halogen atom attached to aromatic ring cannot be readily replaced by the nucleophilic reagent, aryl halides cannot be used in this reaction. For the preparation of aromatic ethers, alkyl halides and phenoxide should be used.

PROBLEM 9.2

> **Select the preferred combination of alkyl halide and alkoxide or phenoxide for the preparation of following ethers by Williams's method: (i) Ethyl-tert-butyl ether (ii) Methyl phenyl ether (anisole) (iii) Isopropyl methyl ether.**

3. *The Reaction of Alcohols with Diazomethane*: Methyl ether may be prepared by the action between alcohol and diazomethane in presence of HBF_4. Thus,

$$R-O-H + CH_2N_2 \xrightarrow{HBF_4} \underset{\text{Methyl ether}}{R-O-CH_3} + N_2$$

Mechanistically this reaction takes place as

$$CH_2=\overset{+}{N}=\overset{-}{N} \longleftrightarrow \overset{-}{C}H_2-\overset{+}{N}\equiv N \longrightarrow \underset{\substack{\text{Carbene}\\ \text{(Electron deficient)}}}{CH_2} + N_2\uparrow$$

$$R-\ddot{O}-H + CH_2 \longrightarrow R-\underset{\underset{^{-}CH_2}{|}}{\overset{+}{O}}-H \rightleftharpoons R-O-CH_3$$

9.4 Properties of Ethers

9.4.1 Physical Properties

Only two members—dimethyl ether and ethyl methyl ether, are gases and rest of the members are colourless liquids with sweet smell. Lower members are highly inflammable.

The boiling points of ethers gradually increase with the increase in carbon atoms. It has been observed that ethers have lower boiling points than isomeric alcohols. This is because of the fact that oxygen atom of ethers is not connected to hydrogen atom and so they cannot form any intermolecular hydrogen bonding among themselves as a result of which boiling point does not increase. On the other hand, alcohols have hydrogen atom attached to alcoholic oxygen and hence can form intermolecular hydrogen bonding forming associated molecule; consequently their boiling points become high.

Ethers are soluble in water and in this respect they have comparable solubilities with isomeric alcohols. This is due to the fact that ether oxygen atom can form hydrogen bond with water, i.e.,

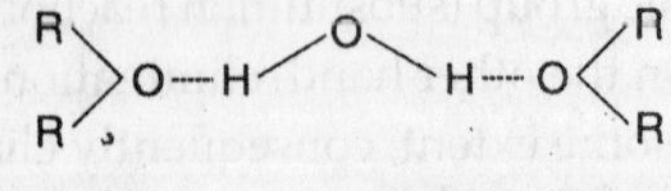

9.4.2 Chemical Properties

Ethers are chemically least reactive organic compounds. Because of this low reactivity in conjunction with their capability of dissolving a large number of organic compounds, specially nonpolar compounds, ethers are extensively used as solvents in organic reactions, but care should be taken because of their inflammable character. The presence of lone pair of electrons on sp^3-orbitals of oxygen atom in ethers, however, makes them to exhibit some chemical activities which are discussed below:

i. *Basic character*: Ethers exhibit *weak basic character* obviously due to the presence of lone pair of electrons on their oxygen atoms. The basic character is revealed from their formation of unstable oxonium salts on reaction with strong acids.

$$R-O-R \xrightleftharpoons{HX} \left[R-\overset{+}{\underset{|\atop H}{O}}-R\right]\overset{-}{X}$$

Dialkyl oxonium salt

In this connection it may be mentioned that basic character is also manifested from the reaction of ethers with Lewis acids. On reaction with boron triflouride, ethers form a very useful acidic catalyst—*boron triflouroetherate.*

$$R-\ddot{O}-R + BF_3 \longrightarrow R_2\overset{+}{O}-\overset{-}{B}F_3.$$

Borontriflouro etherate

ii. *Cleavage of ether linkage*: The presence of lone pair of electrons on oxygen atoms facilitates the cleavage of C—O bonds in ethers by halogen acids. When ethers are heated with halogen acids alkyl halides and alcohols are formed. However, if excess of halogen acids are used alcohol formed is converted to alkyl halides:

$$R-\ddot{O}-R + HX \longrightarrow \underset{\text{Alcohol}}{R-OH} + \underset{\text{Alkyl halide}}{RX}$$

$$R-OH \xrightarrow{\text{Excess HX}} RX + H_2O$$

iii. *Formation of peroxides*: Formation of peroxides is a dangerous property of ethers. Air oxidation of ethers yield peroxides. These peroxides are highly explosive in nature. Thus,

$$\underset{\text{Diethyl ether}}{C_2H_5-O-C_2H_5} \xrightarrow{O_2} CH_3-\underset{|\atop HOO}{CH}-O-CH_2-CH_3$$

1-Ethoxy ethyl-hydroperoxide

It may be mentioned in this connection that if ethers are briefly exposed to atmospheric oxygen, peroxides may be formed. For this reason extreme care must be taken before handling the old bottle of ethers.

iv. *Halogenation:* Ethers on treatment with halogens in presence of sunlight, halogen derivatives of ethers are formed.

$$C_2H_5-O-C_2H_5 \xrightarrow[h\nu]{Cl_2} C_2Cl_5-O-C_2Cl_5$$

Perchloro ethyl ether

Problem 9.3

Following ethers are allowed to react with excess of HBr with the following results. Identify the ether in each case:

i. one ether gives methyl bromide and ethyl bromide.

ii. second ether forms only methyl bromide.

9.5 Some Important Members

9.5.1 Diethyl Ether, $C_2H_5—O—C_2H_5$

The most important member of ether family is diethyl ether which is commonly known as "ether" or "solvent ether".

Preparation: It is prepared in the laboratory as well as on a commercial scale by heating a mixture of ethyl alcohol and concentrated sulphuric acid at 140 °C

i. $C_2H_5OH + H_2SO_4 \longrightarrow \underset{\text{Ethylhydrogen sulphate}}{C_2H_5HSO_4} + H_2O$

ii. $C_2H_5HSO_4 + C_2H_5OH \longrightarrow \underset{\text{Ethel}}{C_2H_5—O—C_2H_5} + H_2SO_4$

Preparation: It is a colourless highly volatile liquid boiling at 35 °C. It is fairty soluble in water but completely miscible with alcohol in all proportion. It is highly inflammable in nature and on mixing with oil it forms an explosive. This is its great disadvantage in its use as an industrial solvent. It exhibits characteristic reactions of ether.

9.5.1.1 Anaesthetic Ether

The ether obtained industrially is not so pure and safe for its use as anaesthetic. As such industrial ether so obtained is subjected to fractional distillation and the distillate is treated succesively with the solutions of sodium bisulphite and sodium carbonate. The ether, thus, obtained is washed with water, dried over solid anhydrous sodium hydroxide when sufficiently pure ether is obtained. This ether is now safe for use as anaesthetic and is known a **anaesthetic ether**.

9.5.1.2 Absolute Ether

In some reactions particularly in Grignard reactions, either should be free from traces of water and alcohol. This ether is known as **absolute ether**. This is prepared by the distillation of ordinary ether from concentrated sulphuric acid followed by its storage over metallic sodium.

9.5.2 Divinyl Ether (Vinethene)

Divinyl ether is prepared from ethylene chlorohydrin involving the following steps of reactions.

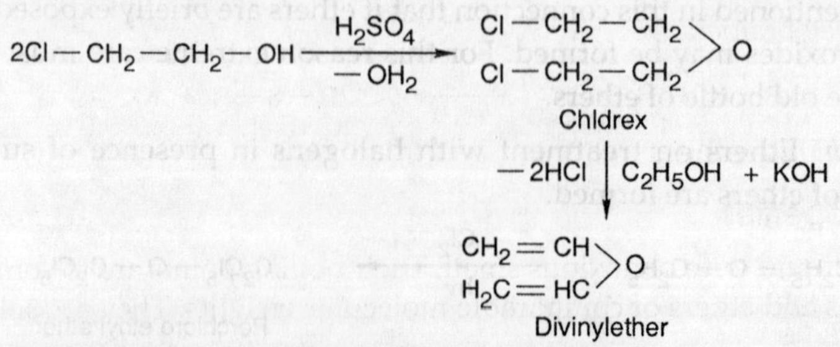

Divinyl ether is a highly inflammable liquid boiling at 39 °C.

9.6 Thio-ethers

Thio-ethers are derived from ethers by the replacement of oxygen atom by sulphur atom. They may also be derived from hydrogen sulphide by replacing two hydrogen atoms by alkyl groups and for this reason thio-ethers are also known as **alkyl sulphide**.

$R-O-R$	$R-S-R$
Ether	Thio-ethers
$H-S-H$	$R-S-R$
Hydrogen Sulphide	Alkyl Sulphide (Thio-ether)

In this thio-ether, the functional group is sulphide (—S—) in trivial system, their names are derived from the names of two organic groups attached to sulphur. The names of organic groups are added as prefix to the word sulphide.

CH_3-S-CH_3	$CH_3-S-CH_2-CH_3$
Dimethyl Sulphide	Ethyl methyl sulphide

In IUPAC system, RS-groups are alkyl thio-groups. Out of two organic groups thio-ethers are named according to the name of organic group containing long chain and the smaller organic group is considered as substituent .

CH_3-S-CH_3	$CH_3-S-CH_2-CH_3$
Mythyl Thio methane	Mythyl Thioethane
$CH_3-S-CH_2-CH_2-CH_3$	$CH_3-S-CH_2-CH_2-CH_2-CH_3$
Methyl Thiopropanre	Methyl Thiobutane

9.6.1 Preparation of Thio-ethers

(a) The most important method of preparation of thio-ethers is analogous to Williamson's ether synthesis involving nucleophilic substitution reaction. Primary alkyl halide is treated with alkyl thiolate ion.

$$R-X + R'\overset{-}{S}\overset{+}{Na} \longrightarrow R-S-R' + NaX$$

Na-Alkyl thiolate   Thio-ether

(b) Thio-ethers can also be prepared by heating alkyl halide with sodium or potassium sulphide.

$$2R-X + K_2S \longrightarrow R-S-R + 2KX$$

In place of sulphide corresponding mercaptides may be used when unsymmetrical thio-ethers may be obtained.

$$R-X + R'-SK \longrightarrow R-S-R + KX$$

9.6.2 Properties of Thio-ethers

9.6.2.1 Physical Properties

Thio-ethers are oily liquid with obnoxious smell. Their boiling points are to some extent higher than those of alkanes and ethers of comparable molecular weights. They are soluble in organic solvents.

9.6.2.2 Chemical Properties

(a) *Oxidation*: Unlike ethers which undergo oxidation at carbon forming hydro-peroxides, oxidation of thio-ethers occurs at sulphur forming *sulphoxides* and *sulphones* depending upon the nature as well as quantity of oxidising agent.

i. When mild oxidising agent like H_2O_2 is used the product is *sulphoxide.*

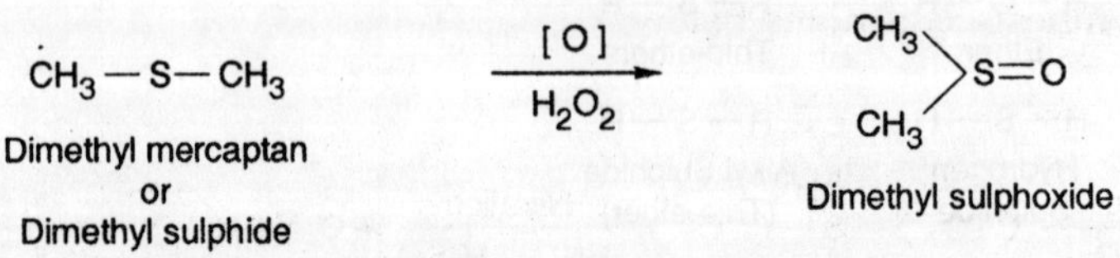

Dimethyl sulphoxide is used as a solvent in organic reactions.

ii. When strong oxidising agent such as $KMnO_4$ or HNO_3 is used in excess quantity, sulphoxide initially formed is further oxidised to *sulphone.*

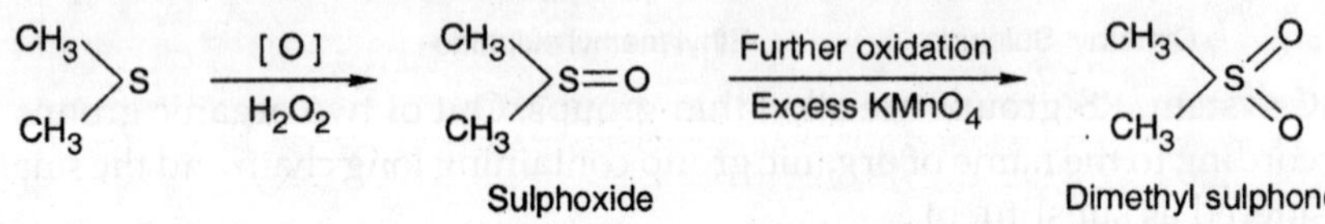

(b) *Alkylation of thio-ethers*: As sulphur is more nucleophilic in nature than oxygen, -thio ethers react with alkyl halides faster than ethers. The product obtained is *sulphonium salt.*

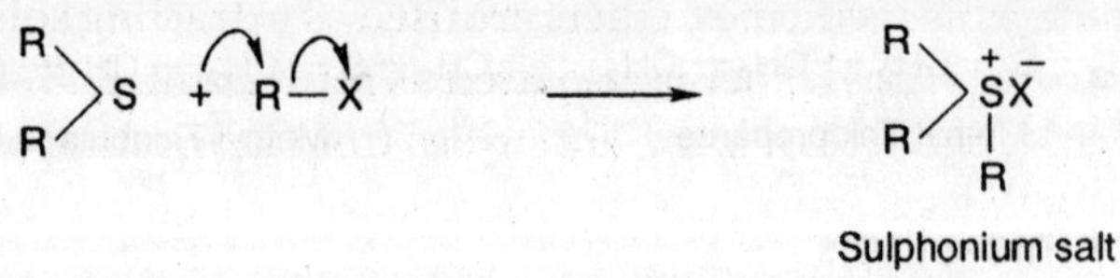

An important natural sulphonium salt is S-adenosyl methionine which acts as a key agent in certain biological processes.

9.7 Mustard Gas

It is a dichloro derivative of diethyl sulphide. It is poisonous and on exposure it can cause burns and blisters on skin. Its inhalation may affect lungs seriously. During World War I this gas was used as poisonous gas. It is prepared by the reaction between ethylene and sulphuryl chloride.

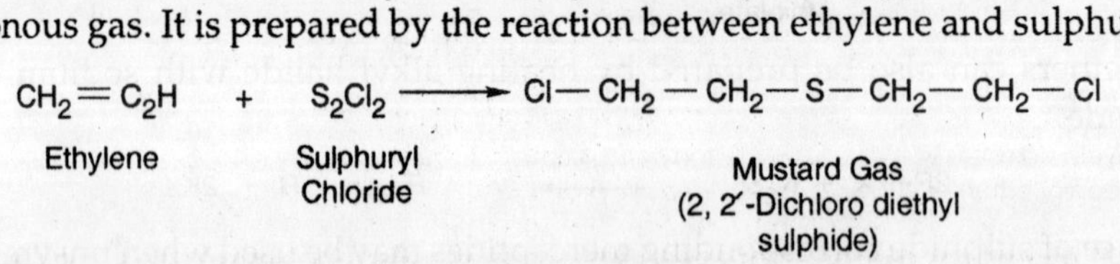

9.8 Uses of Ethers

The most significant use of ethers is in the field of medicine as general anaesthetics. Diethyl ether, commonly known as ether, is a safe and inexpensive general anaesthetic. But due to its low boling point, it is difficult to administer it in tropical temperature. However, divinyl ether (Vinethene) and methyl-propyl ether (**methopril**) were found to be more powerful and less irritating than diethyl ether as anaesthetics. They act faster and possess objectionable after-effects.

A large number of sulphone derivatives have been found to be effective for the treatment of leprosy. Incidentally, one such member chemically known as 4, 4'-diaminodiphenyl sulphone (dapsone) exhibited prophylactic activity against resistant **P. falciparum**. Dapose in conjuction with primethamine has been effectively used in the treatment of malaria caused by chloroquine resistant **P. falciparum**.

Dapsone is synthesised as noted below:

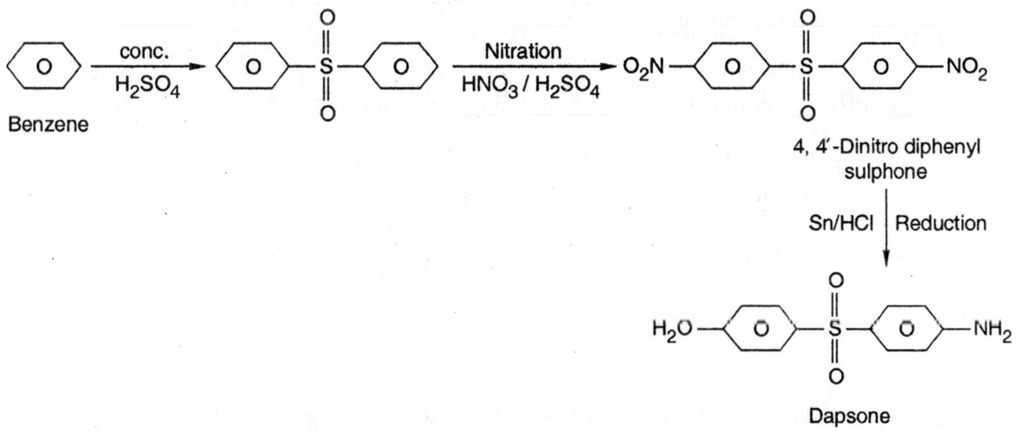

In addition to their uses as medicines, ethers are used as extracting solvents on large scale in industry and in laboratory. Deithyl ether is also used as refrigerant. B, B'-Dichloroethyl ether is used under the name **chlorex** for dissolving impurities from lubricating oils.

9.9 Epoxides

Epoxides are cyclic ethers in which oxygenatom is incorporated into a three-membered ring as indicated below:

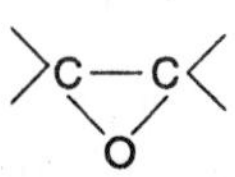

Epoxides are named as epoxy derivatives of alkanes. Thus,

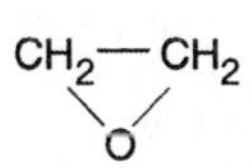

Ethylene oxide
(1, 2-epoxy ethane)

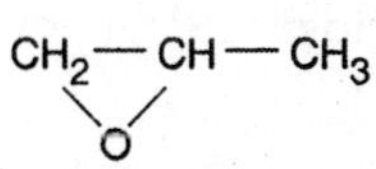

Propylene oxide
(1, 2-epoxy propane)

The most important member of epoxide family is ethylene oxide.

9.9.1 Preparation and Properties of Epoxides

Ethylene oxide is mainly prepared by two methods.

i. *Epoxidation of ethylene*: Epoxidation of ethylene is carried out with peroxy acids.

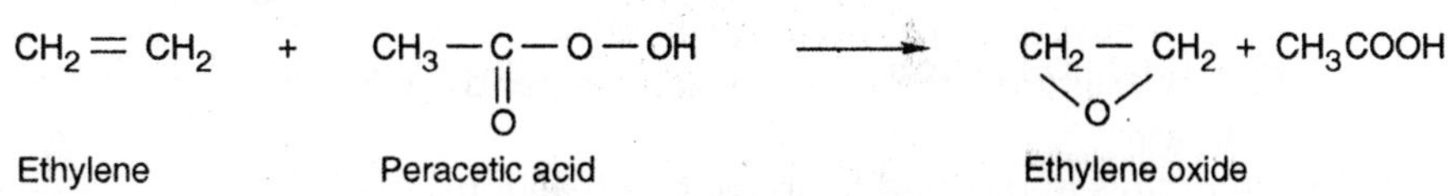

ii. *From halohydrin:*

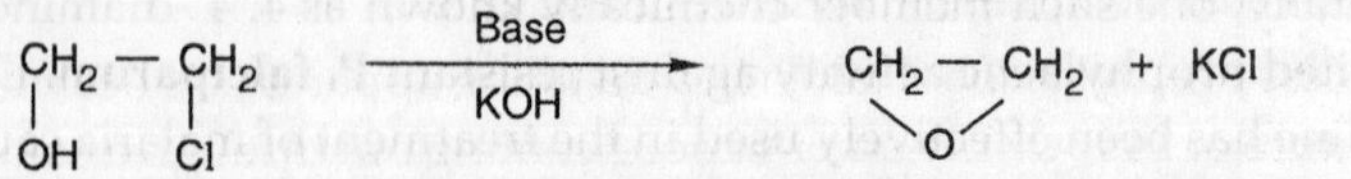

Properties of Ethylene oxide: Although ethers are less reactive but epoxides are relatively active. This is because the three-membered ring present in epoxides is highly strained and so readily undergoes ring opening reaction. Ring opening is generally carried out in presence of acidic catalyst, and the product is the glycol.

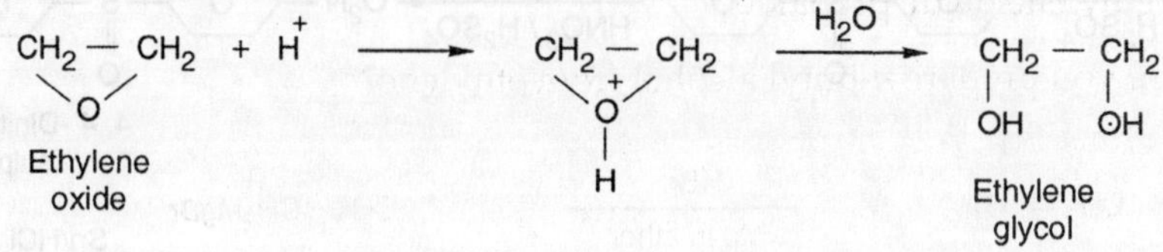

Ethylene oxide reacts with Grignard reagent to form primary alcohol. Thus,

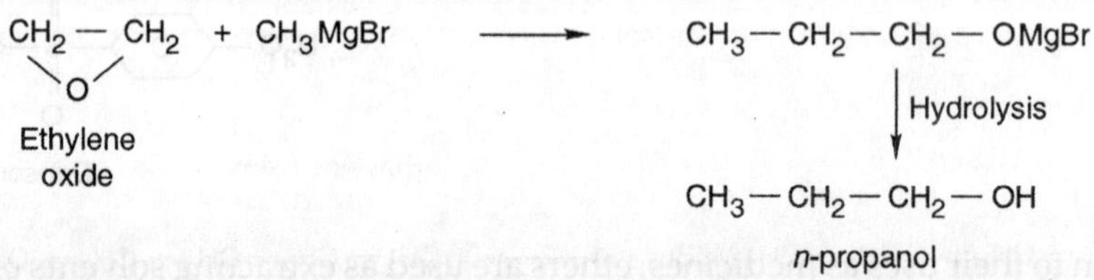

Uses of Ethylene oxide: Ethylene oxide is used in the preparation of (i) Synthetic fibre dacron, (ii) detergent and (iii) as drying agent in paints and varnishes.

Model Questions

1. Write the structural formulae of all the isomeric compounds that can be represented by the molecular formula, $C_4H_{10}O$. Write their IUPAC names.
2. Write notes on (a) Williamson's synthesis (b) uses of ethers.
3. Describe preparation of methyl ether using diazomethane.
4. Discuss the cleavage of ethers by acids.
5. Explain the basic character of ethers.
6. Explain why the boiling point of ethyl alcohol is higher than that of diethyl ether though they are of same molecular weight.
7. How will you distinguish between diethyl ether and ethyl alcohol?

Hints: (i) Ethyl alcohol responds to iodoform test.

$$\underset{\text{Ethanol}}{CH_3-CH_2OH} + I_2/NaOH \longrightarrow CH_3-CHO \longrightarrow \underset{\text{Iodoform}}{CHI_3}$$

(ii) Ethyl alcohol reacts with sodium metal to produce hydrogen gas.

$$\underset{\text{Ethanol}}{2CH_3-CH_2-OH} + 2Na \longrightarrow 2CH_3-CH_2ONa + H_2\uparrow$$

Diethyl ether fails to respond to above two reactions.

8. How will you synthesise diethyl ether from ethanol? How will you purify it? State its main noes. What do xin mean by anaesthetic ether.

Hints: Excess of ethyl alcohol taken in a distilling apparatus is heated with conc. H_2SO_4 at a temperature of 140 °C. The ether vapour coming out through a condenser is collected in a receiver immersed in ice.

Ether obtained above contains water, ethyl alcohol and sulphuric acid as impurities. It is shaken with dilute NaOH to remove sulphuric acid. The organic layer is collected and is repeatedly treated with $CaCl_2$ to remove ethyl alcohol and water.

12. How is ethylene oxide prepared?

13. How will you prepare *n*-butyl alcohol from ethylene?

Hints:

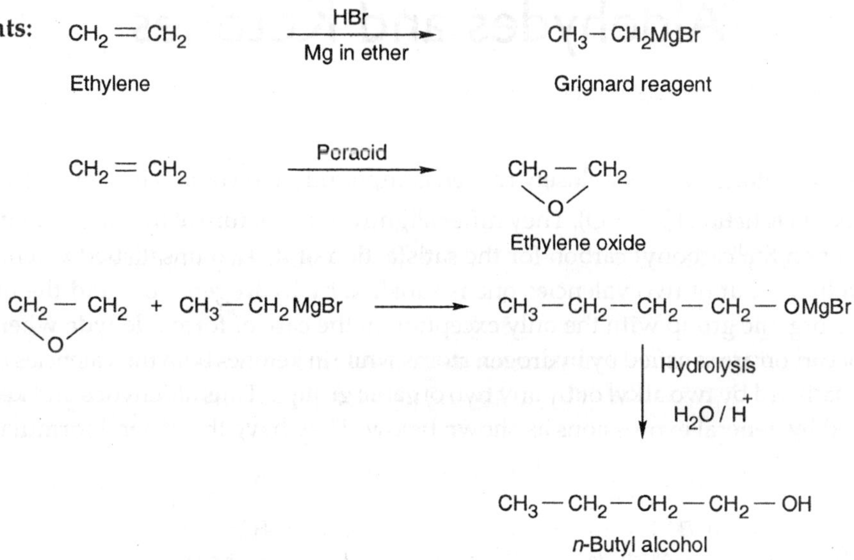

11. A compound, $C_4H_{10}O_3$, responds to the reactions of both an alcohol and an ether. When heated with excess of HI it forms di-iodoethylene (ICH$_2$—CH$_2$—I). Suggest the structure of the original compound.

12. (a) Give two methods for the preparation of ethers. (b) How will you prepare divinyl ether? Give its important uses.

13. What are thio-ethers? How are they prepared? Give some important uses of thio-ethers.

14. How would you prepare the following?
(a) Sulphone, (b) Mustard gas.
What are their uses?

CHAPTER TEN

Aldehydes and Ketones

Aldehydes and ketones are very closely related compounds and contain the common functional group, carbonyl function ($>C=O$). They differ slightly in the nature of the substituents required to be present on the carbonyl carbon for the satisfaction of its two unsatisfied valencies. In the case of aldehydes out of two valencies one is satisfied by hydrogen atom and the other by an alkyl or any organic group with the only exception in the case of formaldehyde where both the valencies of carbon are satisfied by hydrogen atoms while in ketones both the valencies of carbonyl carbon are satisfied by two alkyl or by any two organic groups. Thus aldehydes and ketones may be expressed by general expressions as shown below. They have the general formula, $C_nH_{2n}O$.

Aldehyde

Ketone

Some common members of aldehydes and ketones are:

Aldehydes:

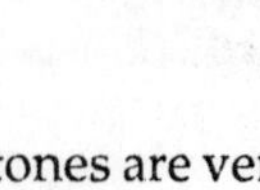

Formaldehyde

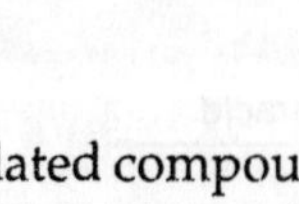

Acetaldehyde

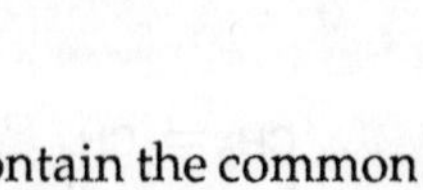

Propionaldehyde

Ketones:

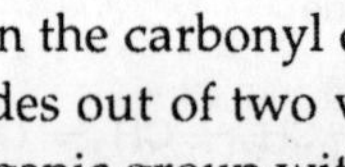

Acetone

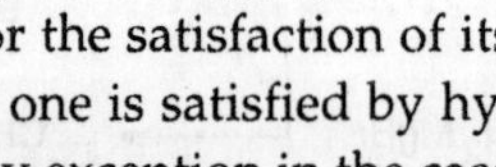

Butanone

10.1 Nomenclature of Aldehydes and Ketones

There are two systems by which both aldehydes and ketones are named.

i. *Common system*: In the common system aldehydes are named by adding the word *'aldehyde'* in place of *ic* of the name of carboxylic acid to be produced by the oxidation of the respective aldehydes. Thus.

Name of aldehyde	Name of acid produced on oxidation
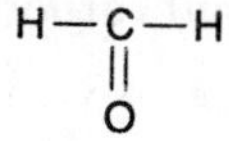 Formaldehyde	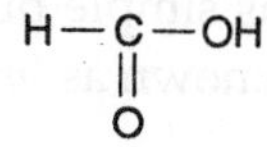 Formic acid
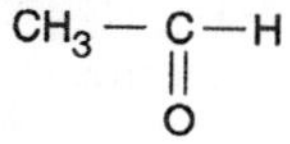 Acetaldehyde	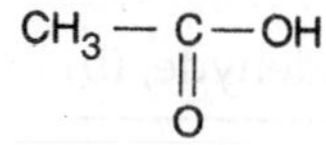 Acetic acid
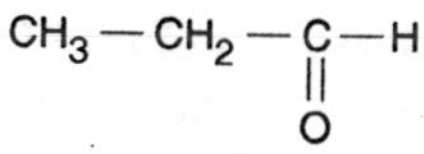 Proplonaldehyde	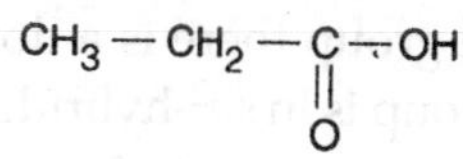 Propionic acid

But the names of ketones in this system are derived from the names of two groups attached to carbonyl carbon atom and adding the word *ketone*.

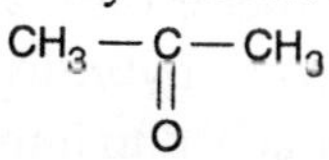

Acetone

(Dimethyl ketone)

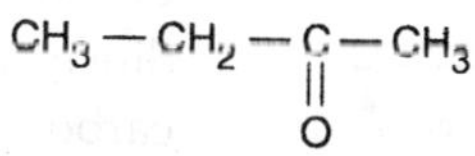

Butanone

(Ethyl methyl ketone)

ii. *IUPAC system*: According to IUPAC system, aldehydes are named by replacing the *'e'* of alkane with *'-al'*. Thus,

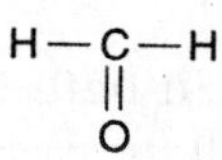

Formaldehyde

(Methanal)

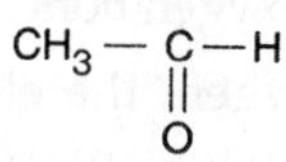

Acetaldehyde

(Ethanal)

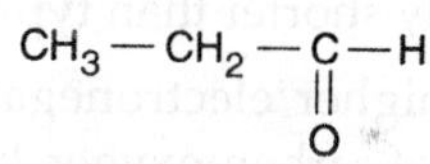

Propionaldehyde

(Propanal)

It may be pointed that aldehydic functional group 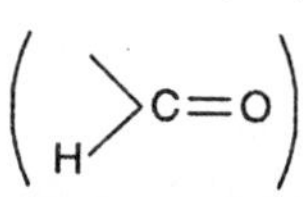 always resides at the terminal position of the chain and hence there is no need to indicate its position.

In IUPAC system names of ketones are obtained by replacing *'e'* from the names of longest alkane chain with *'-one'*. The position of keto-carbonyl carbon in the chain is indicated by number remembering that carbonyl carbon should be given lowest possible number.

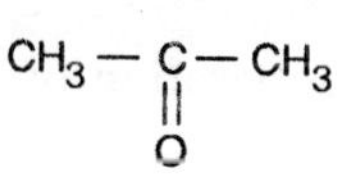

Acetone

(Propanone)

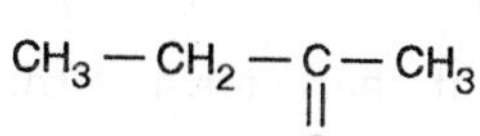

Butanone

(Butan-2-one)

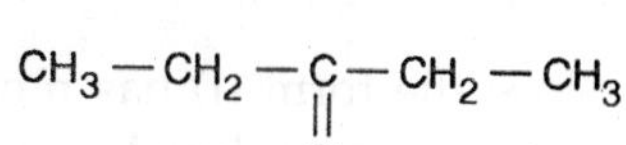

Diethyl ketone

(Pentan-3-one)

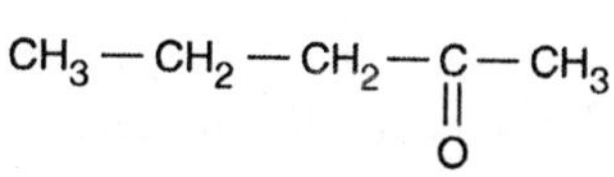

Methyl propyl ketone

(Pentan-2-one)

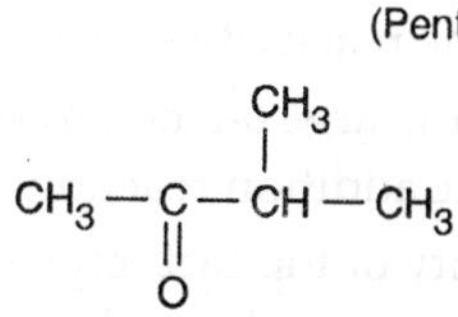

Isopropyl methyl ketone

(3-Methyl-butan-2-one)

It may be mentioned that when both the organic groups are identical, the ketone is designated as simple but if the two groups attached to carbonyl carbon are different, ketones are known as *'mixed'* or *'unsymmetrical'* ketones.

PROBLEM 10.1

Suggest the IUPAC names of the following:
(a) Isobutyraldehyde, (b) Ethyl isopropyl ketone, (c) Ethyl methyl ketone.

10.2 Structure and Bonding in Carbonyl Group

In carbonyl group there is a double bond between carbon and oxygen atoms. Carbon atom in carbonyl group is in sp^2-hybridised state. Out of two bonds between carbon and oxygen one is σ formed by the overlap of sp^2-orbital of carbon. Another bond between carbon and oxygen is a π-bond generated by the parallel overlap of unhybridised *p*-orbitals of carbon and oxygen. The remaining two sp^2-orbitals of carbon form two σ-bonds with other groups attached to it. Since carbon atom in carbonyl group is in sp^2-hybridised state, the carbonyl group and the atoms or groups attached to it must lie in the same plane. It has been observed that three sp^2-orbitals of carbon are inclined to each other at an angle of 120°. Thus, the structure of carbonyl group may be represented as shown in Fig. 10.1. Oxygen atom has two unpaired electrons. The average carbon-oxygen bond distance (1.22Å) is significantly shorter than typical carbon-oxygen bond distance (1.41Å).

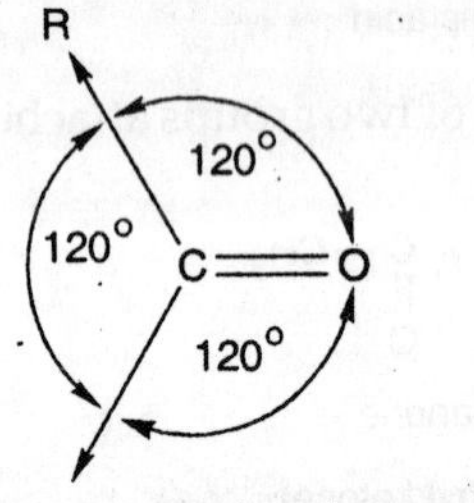

Structure of carbonyl group
Fig. 10.1

Due to higher electronegativity of oxygen, the electron density in both the σ -and π-components of carbon-oxygen bond is shifted toward oxygen. As a result the carbonyl group is polarised and carbon atom assumes slightly positive charge and oxygen atom gains partial negative charge. This polar character of carbonyl group is supported by dipole moment value (2.7D).

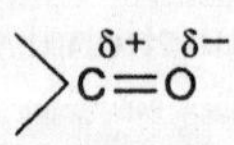

In terms of resonance the delocalisation of electrons in carbonyl group can be shown by two resonanting structures (I and II).

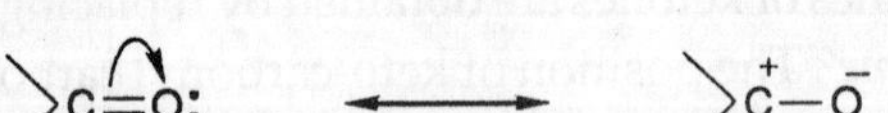

Since the form (I) has more covalent character and there is no separation of charges, it approximates more bonding nature in carbonyl group.

From the above structure and bonding in carbonyl group following conclusions may be drawn regarding the reactivity of carbonyl group:

i. The positive charge on the carbonyl carbon can readily attract the nucleophiles to undergo nucleophilic addition reaction and
ii. The planarity of the carbonyl group makes it easier for attacking nucleophiles to attach themselves from either side increasing thereby the reactivity of the carbonyl group. In fact, polarity and geometry are the two most significant aspects of carbonyl group regarding its reactivity.

10.3 Preparation of Aldehydes and Ketones

(a) Methods applicable for the preparation of both aldehydes and ketones:

1. *Oxidation Methods:* One of the most important and useful methods of preparation of carbonyl compounds both aldehydes and ketones is the oxidation method. In this method variety of chemical compounds can be utilised as the substrate as illustrated below:

   i. *Oxidation of Alcohols:* Oxidation of alcohols is one of the direct methods for the synthesis of carbonyl compounds. Aldehydes are obtained from the oxidation of primary alcohols while secondary alcohols yield ketone on similar reaction. Thus,

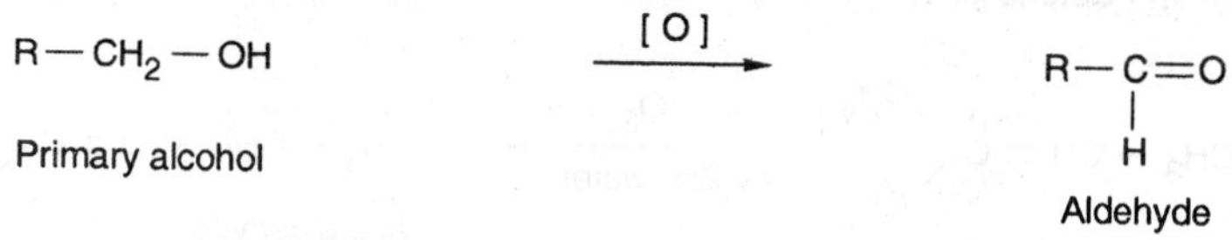

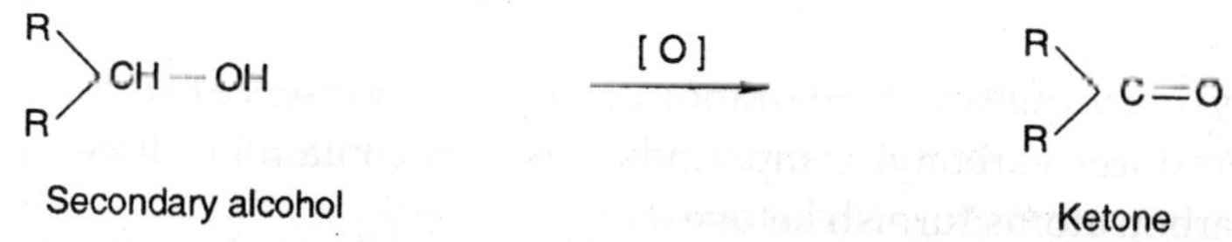

Oxidising agent commonly used is acid-dichromate. But sometimes alcohol vapours mixed with air may be passed over either heated silver or copper at 300 °C. It may be mentioned in this connection that as aldehydes are easily oxidisable to carboxylic acids, the use of excess of oxidising agent should be avoided.

   ii. *Oxidation of 1, 2- Diols and Alkenes:* Both aldehydes and ketones can successfully be prepared by the oxidation of alkenes to 1, 2-diols followed by the oxidative cleavage of diols so produced by lead-tetraacetate or periodic acid.

Cleavage of diol to carbonyl compounds is believed to take place as indicated below:

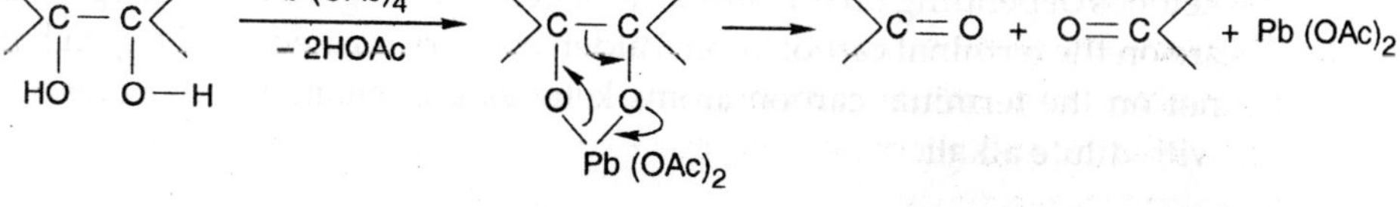

2. **Preparation of carbonyl compounds from unsaturated compounds**

i. *Ozonolysis of alkene*: Alkenes on treatment with ozone followed by decomposition with mild reducing agent like Zn-dust and water, or Zn and acetic acid yield aldehydes or ketones depending on the structure of alkenes.

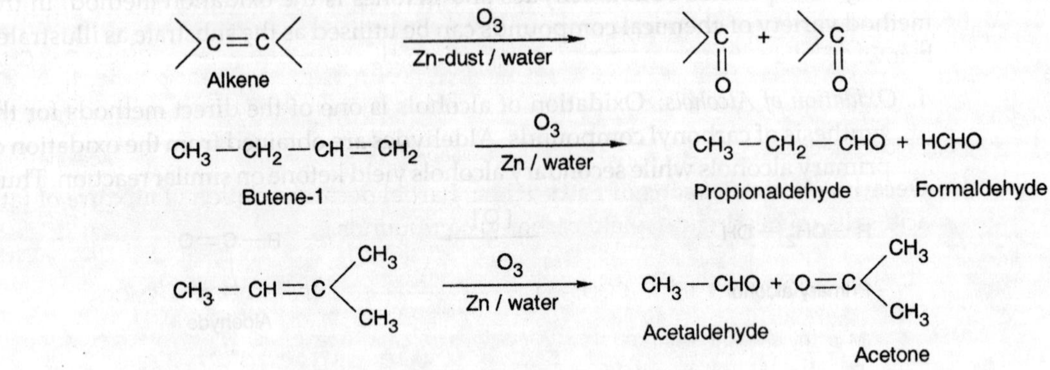

ii. *Hydration of alkynes*: Hydration of alkynes in presence of dilute H_2SO_4 and $HgSO_4$ produces carbonyl compounds. Alkynes containing three or more than three carbon atoms furnish ketones.

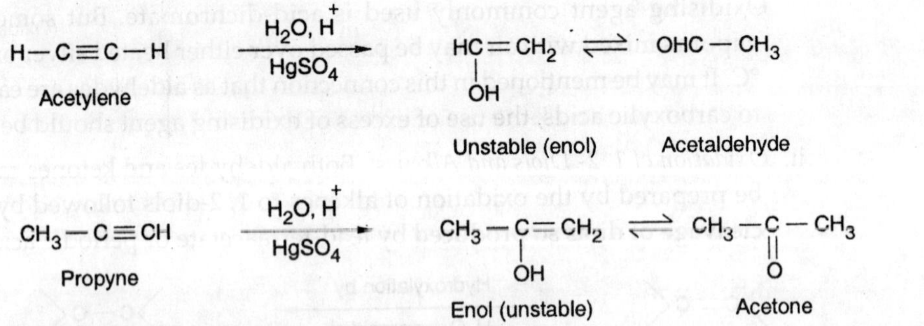

PROBLEM 10.2

Suggest the nature of alkene or alkyne from the following products:

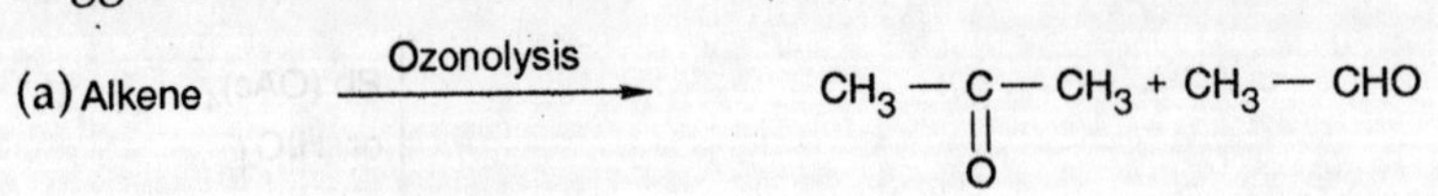

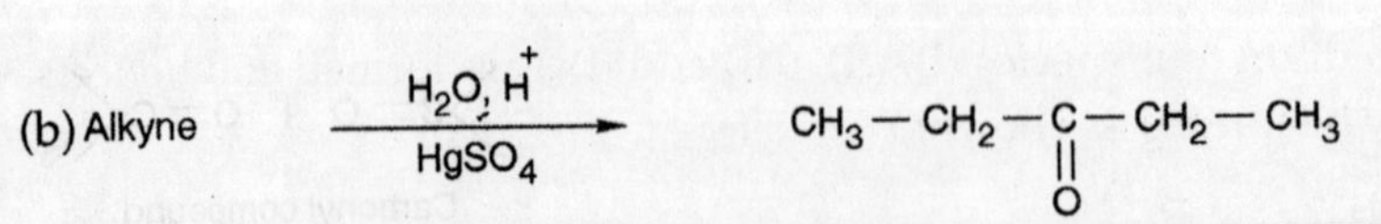

3. **Hydrolysis of gem dihalides:** Gem dihalides on hydrolysis yield aldehydes or ketones depending on the positions of gem dihalo groups. When gem dihalo groups are on the terminal carbon atoms aldehydes are formed. While gem halo groups are not on the terminal carbon atoms ketones are obtained. Hydrolysis is carried out with dilute alkali.

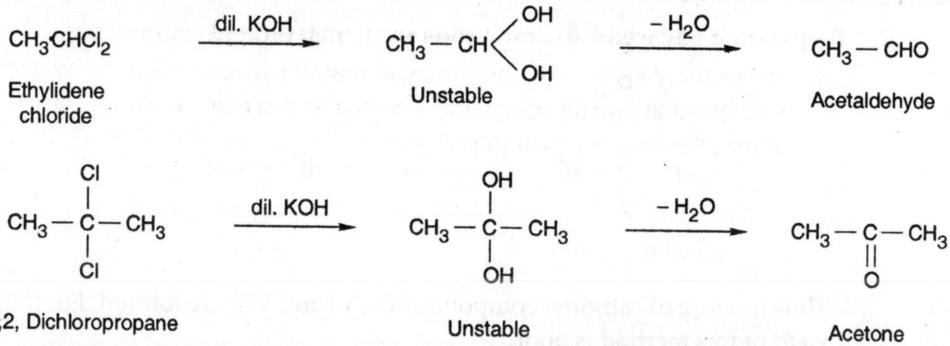

4. **Decarboxylation of salts of Fatty acids:** Partial decarboxylation of mixture of fatty acid salts on heating can yield carbonyl compounds.

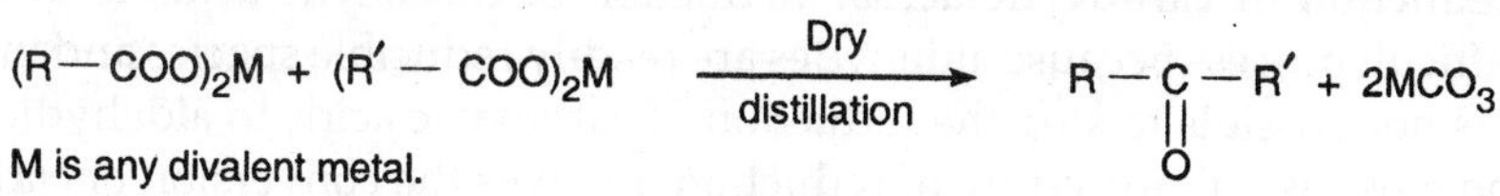

M is any divalent metal.

Mechanism of the reaction may be depicted as follows:

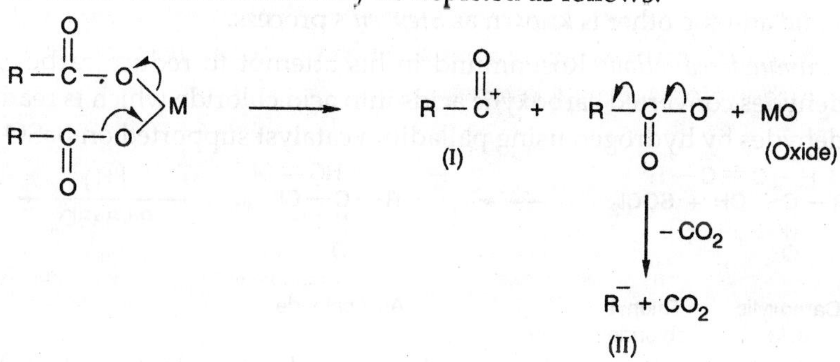

Similarly,

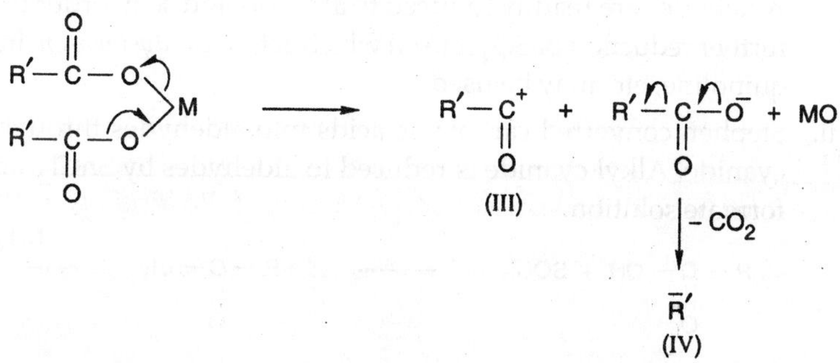

In reaction medium four species (I), (II), (III) and (IV) are formed and hence several products may be formed as shown:

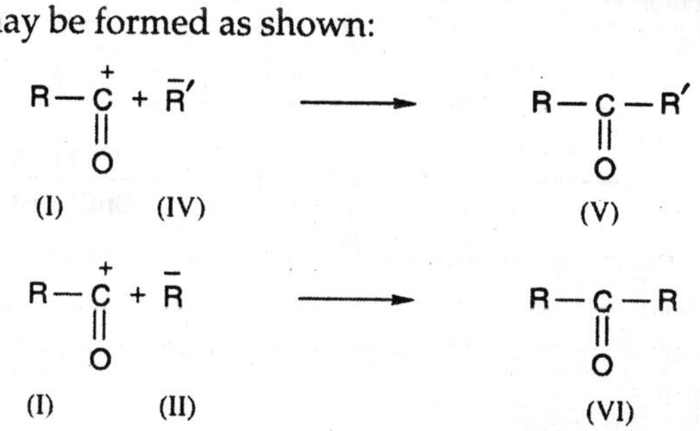

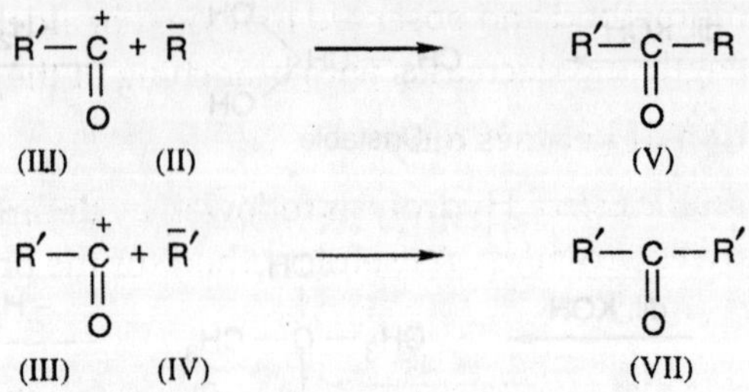

Thus mixture of carbonyl compounds (V, VI and VII) are formed. For this reason the yield of this method is poor.

(b) Methods applicable for the preparation of aldehydes only

Reduction of carboxylic acids: Reduction of carboxylic acids to aldehydes is a very difficult process because aldehydes are readily reducible species and in most of the cases it is not possible to stop the reduction of carboxylic acids to aldehydic stage. However, the most useful procedure of reduction involves the conversion of carboxylic acids to a derivative which is easily reduced to aldehydes. There are two methods—one is due to *Rosenmund* and the other is known as *Stephen's* process.

i. *Rosenmund reduction*: Rosenmund in his attempt to reduce carboxylic acids into aldehydes converted carboxylic acids into acid chloride which is readily reduced to aldehydes by hydrogen using palladium catalyst supported on $BaSO_4$.

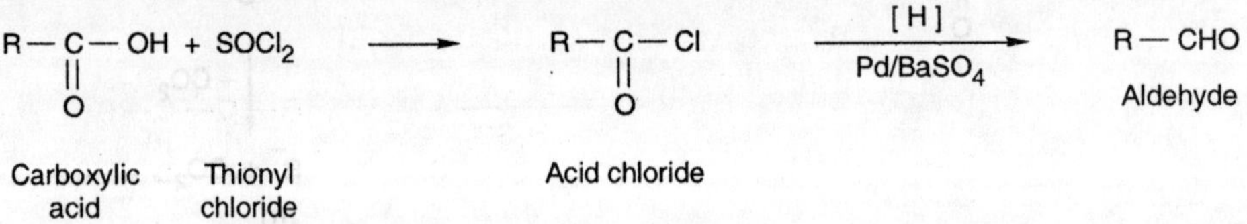

Aldehydes are readily reduced to alcohols and so in order to protect aldehydes from further reduction $BaSO_4$ is used which acts as *catalyst poison*. In place of $BaSO_4$, sulphur quinoline, etc. may be used.

ii. Stephen converted carboxylic acids into aldehydes through the formation of alkyl cyanide. Alkyl cyanide is reduced to aldehydes by $SnCl_2$ and HCl in ether or ethyl formate solution.

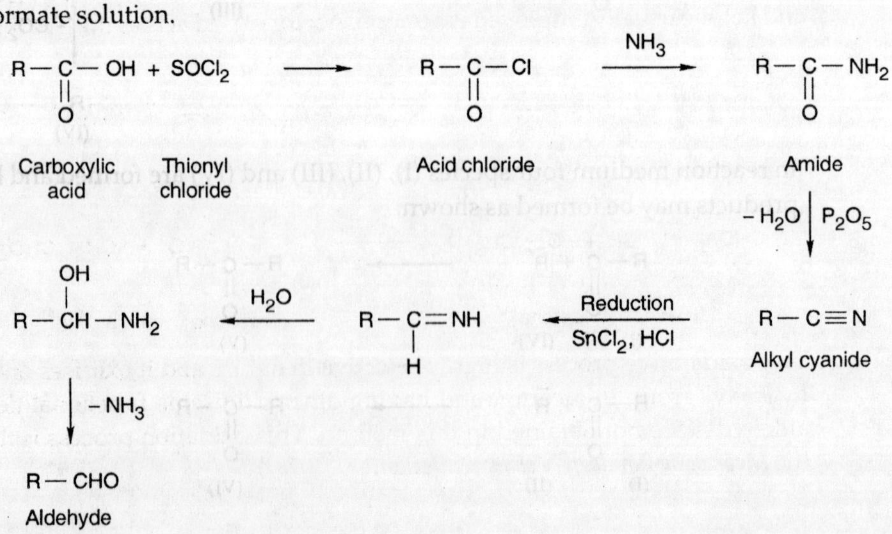

Turner modified this method and observed that yield of aldehydes increases with the increase in chain length and decreases with branching of the chain.

(c) Methods of preparation of ketones only

i. *Hydrolysis of Acetoacetic Ester*: Hydrolysis followed by decarboxylation of acetoacetic ester or its derivatives provides an useful method for the preparation of ketones.

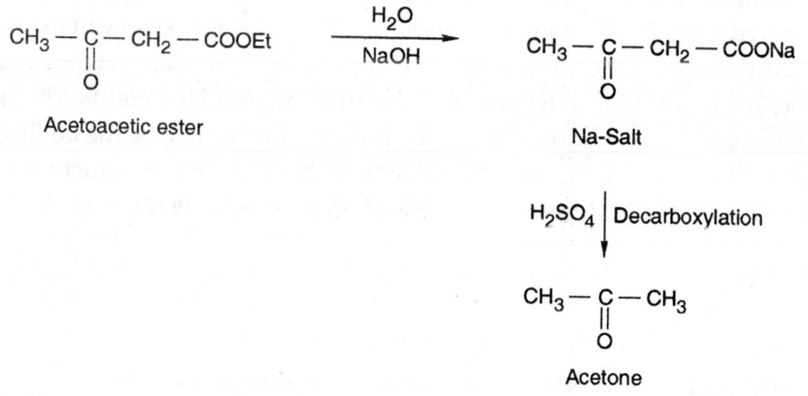

ii. *Pinacol-pinacolone transformation*: Pinacol-pinacolone rearrangement is a very common method of preparing ketones.

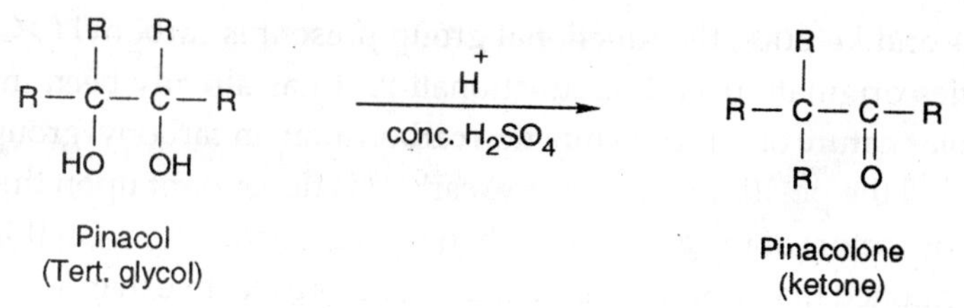

iii. *Oppenauer oxidation*: This process of oxidation of alcohols to carbonyl compounds is primarily suitable for ketones. In this oxidative process a ketone is used as oxidant in presence of a base. Base commonly used is aluminium tertiary butoxide $[(CH_3)_3CO]_3Al$ and ketone usually employed is acetone. Acetone used acts as the hydrogen acceptor.

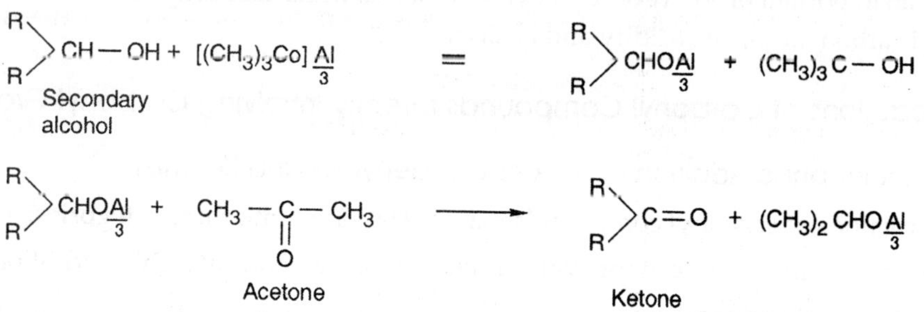

This oxidatative process is highly selective in nature and it oxidises only secondary hydroxyl group in a compound having other oxidisable functionalities. Normally aldehydes are not obtained in this method. This oxidation process is the reverse of the *Meerwein-Pondorff-Verley reduction*.

10.4 Physical Properties of Aldehydes and Ketones

The first and most active carbonyl compound, formaldehyde is a gas but other lower members are liquids. Lower members of aldehydes and ketones are soluble in water. An aqueous solution of formaldehyde is known as *formalin*. Because of the polar nature of carbonyl functionality intermolecular attractive force operates in carbonyl compounds. As a result their boiling points are higher as compared to hydrocarbons of comparable molecular weights. On the other hand, due to lack of hydrogen bond among themselves aldehydes and ketones have lower boiling points than alcohols and carboxylic acids of comparable molecular weights. Again, ketones have higher boiling points than aldehydes of comparable molecular weights. This is because the boiling point depends upon polarity—more the polarity, higher will be the boiling point. Since in general ketones are more polar than the aldehydes because of the inductive effects by two alkyl groups but in aldehydes inductive effect is offered by only alkyl group.

PROBLEM 10.3

Explain:

i. Boiling of acetone is 56 °C but propanol boils at 49 °C.

ii. n-butyl alcohol has higher boiling point than *n*-butyraldehyde.

10.5 Chemical Properties of Aldehydes and Ketones

Since in aldehydes and ketones, the functional group present is carbonyl (>C = O), their major chemical reactivities originate from this functionality. It has already been mentioned (Section 10.2) that due to polar nature of carbonyl function carbon atom in carbonyl group always develops a positive charge and the positivity of carbonyl carbon is dependant upon the electronic nature as well as size (steric factor) of the groups attached to this carbon atom. On this line of argument it has also been mentioned that in general aldehydes are more reactive than ketones. It is, therefore, reasonable to assume that since the positive charge can easily attract nucleophiles the most characteristic reactions of this family is the tendency to undergo *nucleophilic addition* reaction. However, carbonyl compounds can undergo other types of reactions as well. But before going into details of chemical activities of carbonyl compounds it is felt pertinent to mention in this connection an important property of carbonyl compounds which also originates from the positivity of carbonyl carbon atom, i.e., acidity and basicity.

10.5.1 Reactions of Carbonyl Compounds Directly Involving Carbonyl Group

10.5.1.1 Nucleophilic Addition Reactions of Aldehydes and Ketones

Addition reactions of carbonyl compounds may be classified into three categories:

(A) Simple addition (B) Addition with elimination of water and (C) Other addition reactions.

A. Simple addition reaction

1. *Addition reaction with sodium bisulphite* ($NaHSO_3$) and *hydrogen cyanide:* Both aldehydes and ketones react with these reagents to form bisulphite compounds and cyanohydrins as indicated:

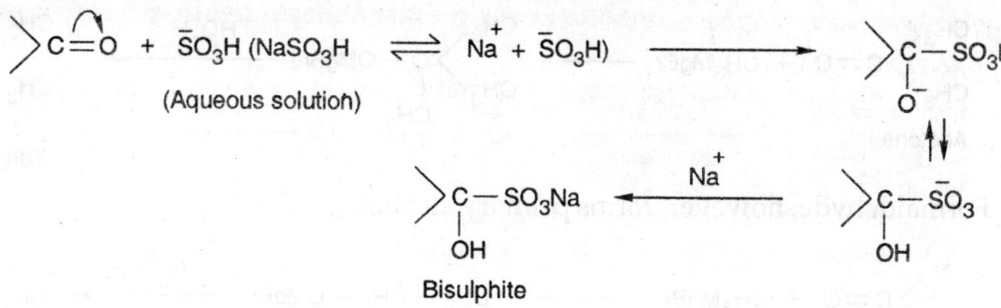

Similarly,

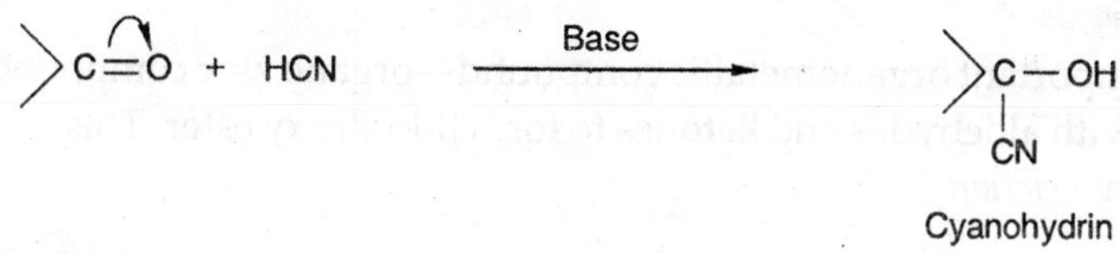

- *Comments:*

  i. It has been suggested that in aqueous solution $NaHSO_3$ forms corresponding anion $\bar{S}O_3H$ ($NaSO_3H \rightleftharpoons \overset{+}{Na} + \bar{S}O_3H$) which is stronger nucleophile.

  ii. Base used during the reaction with HCN facilitates the formation of $\bar{C}N$, i.e,

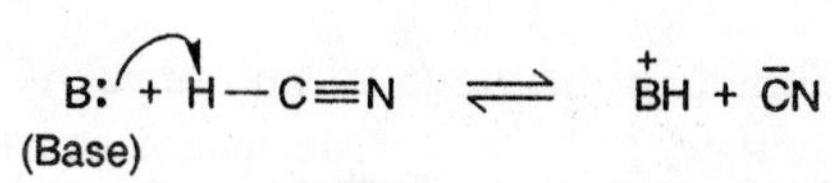

  iii. Almost all the aldehydes form additive compounds with $NaHSO_3$ but only a few lower members of ketones undergo such addition reactions. This is in accordance with the observed reactivity of carbonyl compound and in actual practice higher members (C_5 and onwards) do not react with this reagent and hence is utilised for distinguishing aldehydes and ketones.

2. *Addition reaction with Grignard reagent*: One of the most useful synthetic reaction utilising Grignard reagent is applicable to all the members of both aldehydes and ketones. The addition takes place in two steps. In the first step a Mg complex is formed which in the second stage is decomposed by acidiluted water to alcohols. Aldehydes form secondary alcohols while tertiary alcohols are formed from ketones.

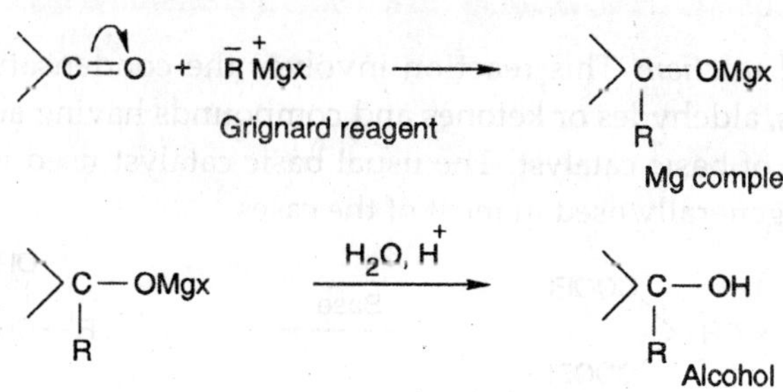

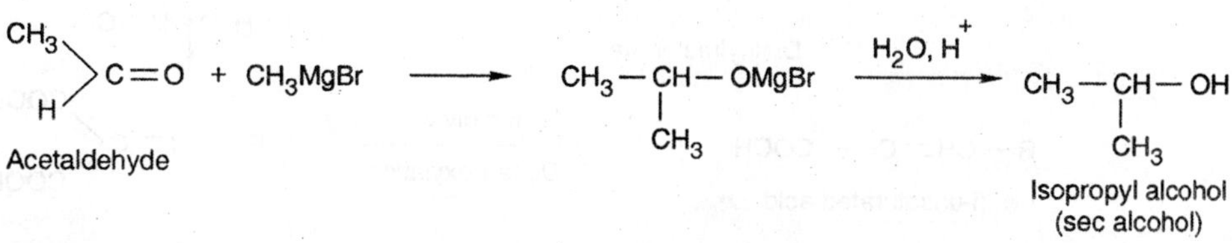

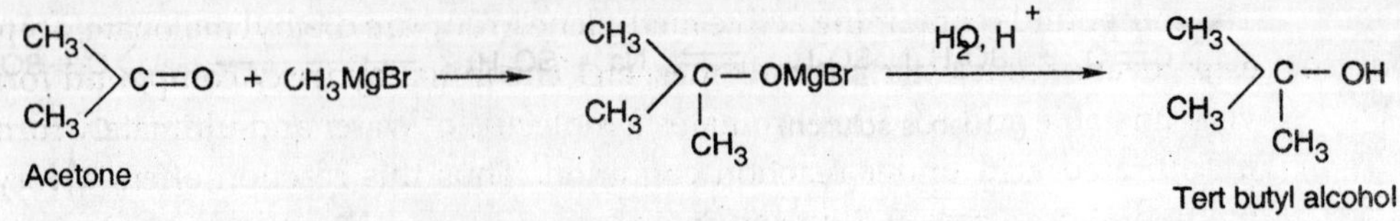

Formaldehyde, however, forms primary alcohol.

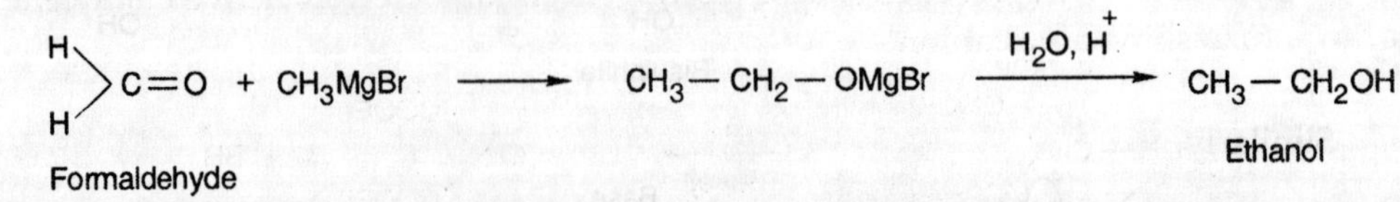

Another important organometallic compound—organo zinc compound of α-bromoester can react with aldehydes and ketones to form β-hydroxy ester. This reaction is known as *Reformatsky reaction*.

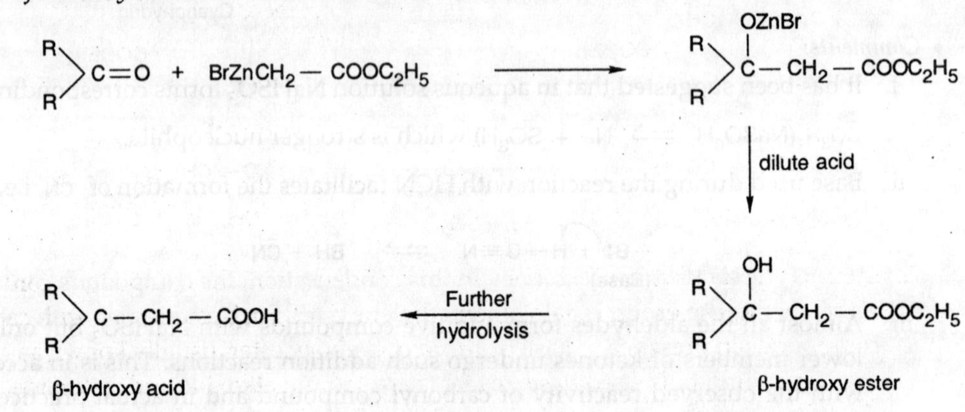

This reaction provides an useful method for the preparation of β-hydroxy acid.

3. *Reaction of carbonyl compounds with compounds having active methylene group:* Organic compounds having active methylene group can easily generate carbanion in presence of base and can serve as the source of nucleophiles. So it is expected that such organic compound may react with aldehydes and ketones to form carbon-carbon bond and as a result such reactions may suitably be employed for the preparation of variety of compounds having synthetic importance. Two such important reactions are discussed below:

   i. *Knoevenagel reaction*: This reaction involves the condensation between carbonyl compounds, aldehydes or ketones and compounds having active methylene group in presence of basic catalyst. The usual basic catalyst used is an amine. However, pyridine is generally used in most of the cases:

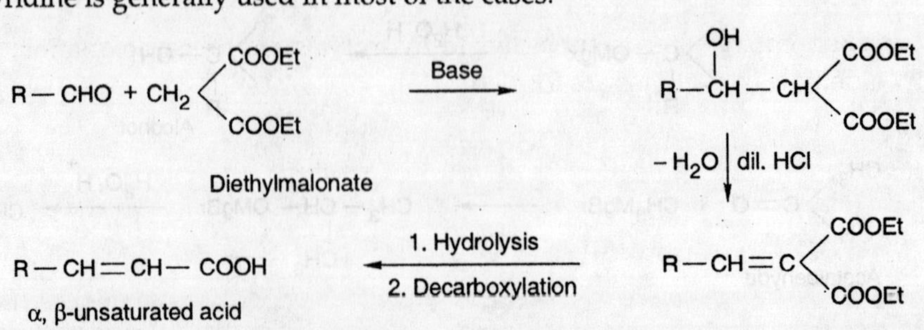

The compounds containing active methylene group are diethyl malonate, acetoacetic ester, cyanoacetic ester, nitroalkanes, etc. The initial hydroxy compound formed is very unstable and readily eliminates a molecule of water and ultimately forms α, β unsaturated acid under reaction condition. Thus this reaction offers a very good method of preparing α, β-unsaturated acid.

Mechanism: In presence of base a proton is eliminated from active methylene group furnishing a carbanion.

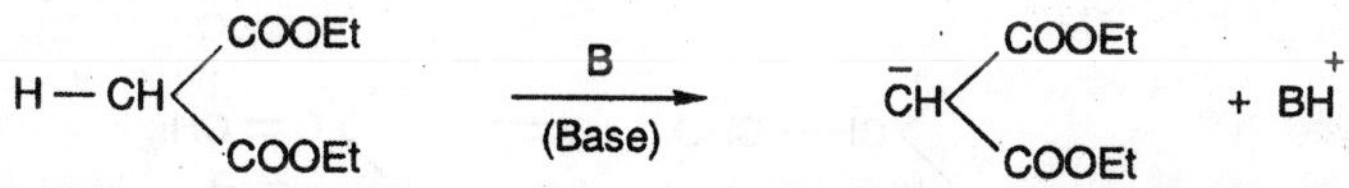

The carbanion thus produced combines with positively charged carbonyl carbon.

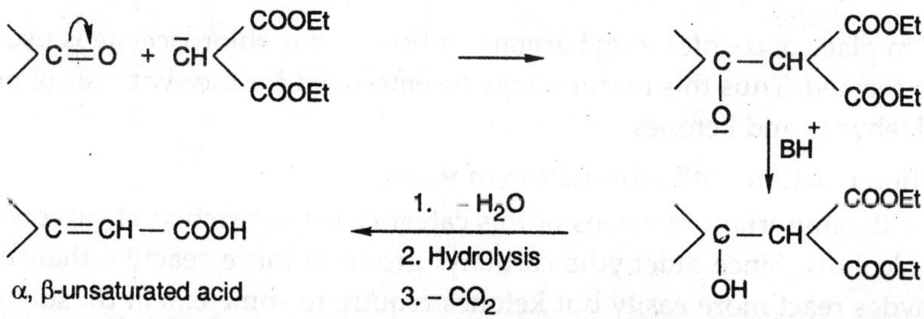

ii. *Darzens glycidic ester condensation*: In this condensation, the compounds containing active methylene group is halogenomethylene ester. Such esters react with carbonyl compounds in presence of base to afford α, β-epoxy ester, usually known as *glycidic ester*. The commonly used basic reagents are sodium alkoxide and sodamide. Thus,

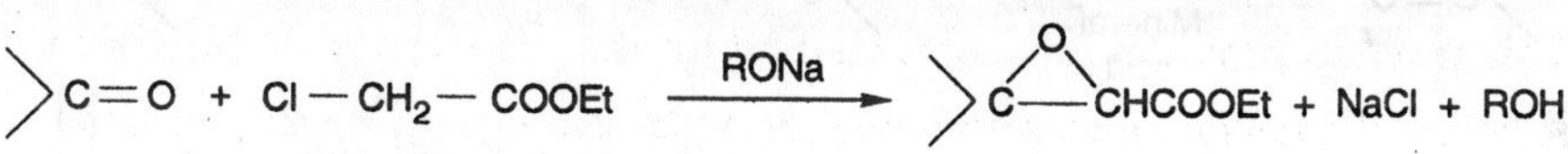

α-chloroethyl acetate

Mechanism: Halogenomethylene ester in presence of base forms carbanion which in the subsequent step combines with carbonyl carbon.

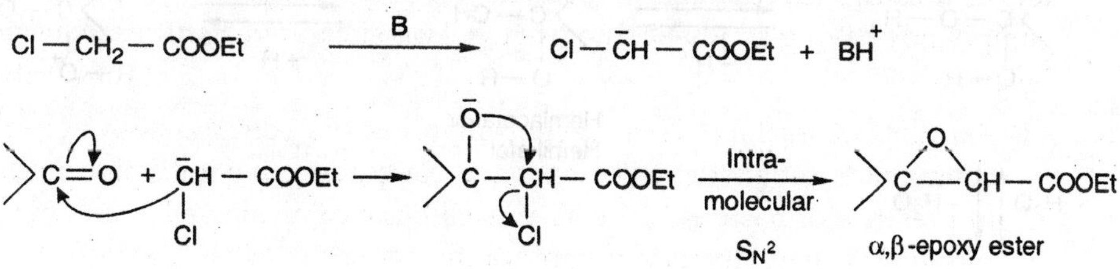

When epoxy ester is subjected to hydrolysis and decarboxylation, homologous aldehydes or ketones are formed.

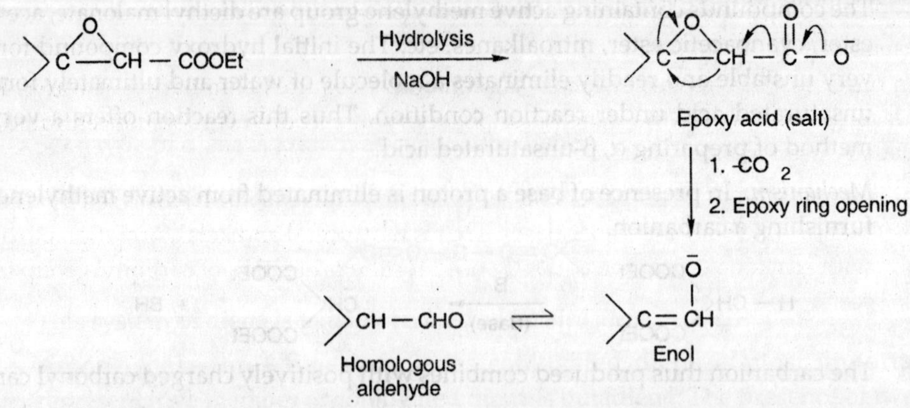

If in place of α-chloroethyl acetate, substituted α-chloroacetate is used, ketone will be formed. Thus this reaction may be employed for the synthesis of homologues of aldehydes and ketones.

B. Addition reaction with elimination of water

One of the important reactions of this category is the reaction of carbonyl compounds with alcohols. Since aldehydic carbonyl group is more reactive than keto carbonyl, aldehydes react more easily but ketones require to some extent drastic condition. The products are *acetals* in the case of aldehydes while products of ketones are termed as *ketals*. The reaction is usually catalysed by acids.

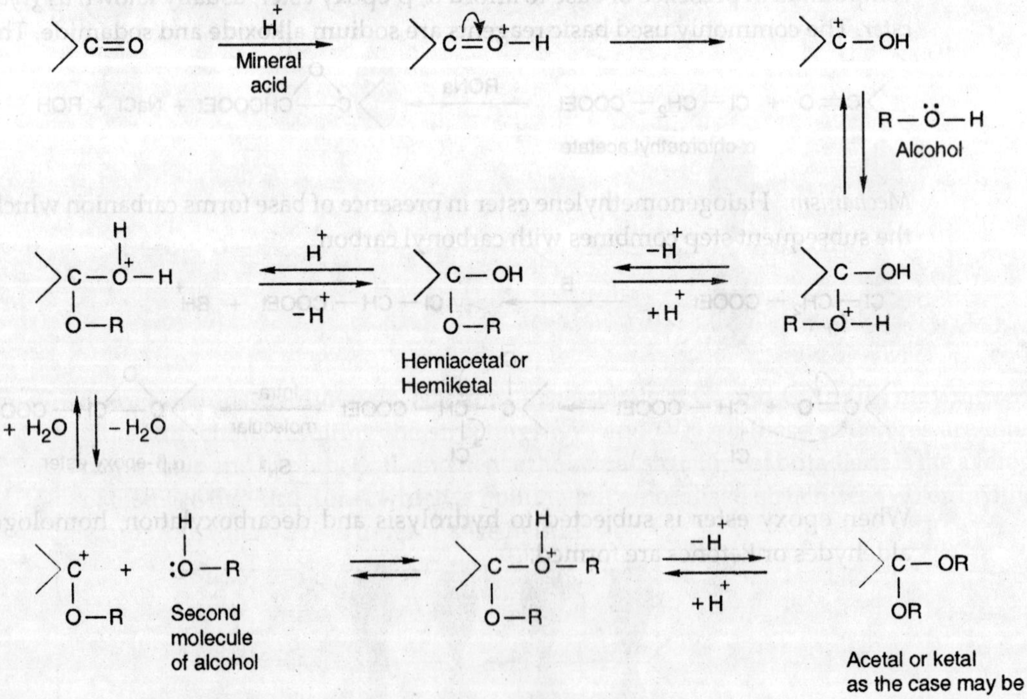

- *Comments*:

(a) In order to form acetals or ketals as seen above requires elimination of water. For this reason as well as for the increase of positivity of carbonyl carbon concentrated acid is usually used as catalyst.

(b) i. Since all the steps are reversible, acetals and ketals may be hydrolysed by dilute acid but they are stable towards bases. That is why acetal and ketal formation particularly with ethylene glycol is frequently used for the protection of carbonyl group in many reactions.

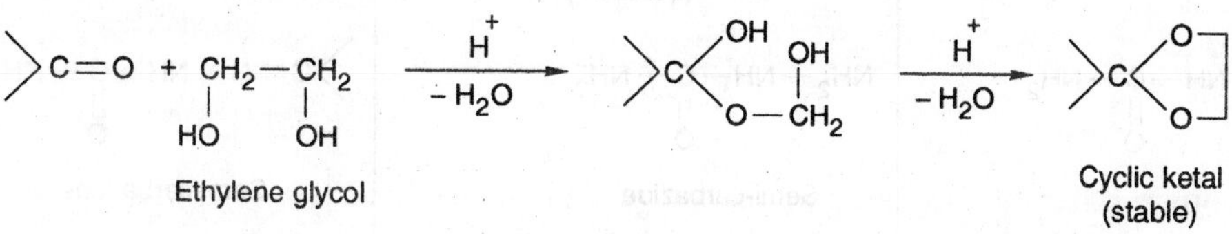

ii. *Reaction with* RNH_2 *derivatives*: Another important type of reaction of aldehydes and ketones with elimination of water is their reaction with a wide variety of chemical compounds of the type RNH_2. The products of the reaction are $>C=N—R$ and the reactions usually require the presence of acid catalyst. Thus,

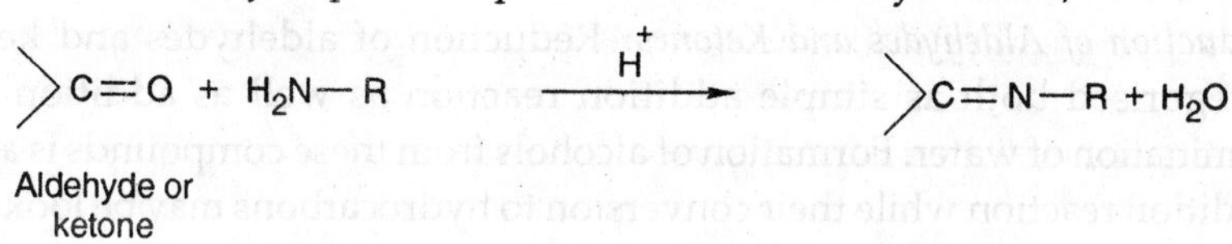

Mechanistically, reaction proceeds as under:

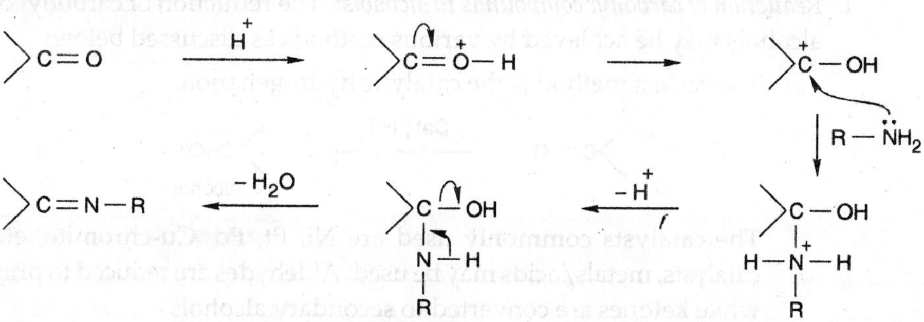

Different members of $R—NH_2$ series and the corresponding products formed are tabulated below:

Nature of R	Name of $R—NH_2$ member	Name of product
1. OH	NH_2OH Hydroxyl amine	$>C=N—OH$ oxime
2. NH_2	$NH_2—NH_2$ Hydrazine	$>C=N—NH_2$ Hydrazone
3. $NH—C_6H_5$	$NH_2—NH—C_6H_5$ Phenyl hydrazine	$>C=N—NH—C_6H_5$ Phenyl hydrazone

Nature of R	Name of R—NH_2 member	Name of product
4. 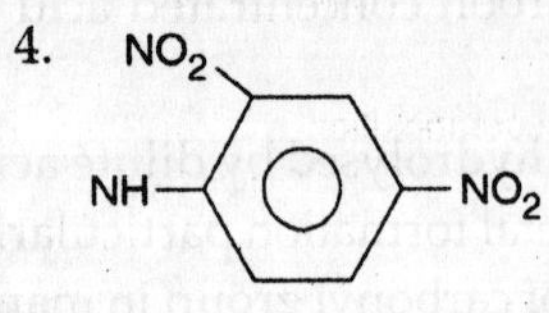	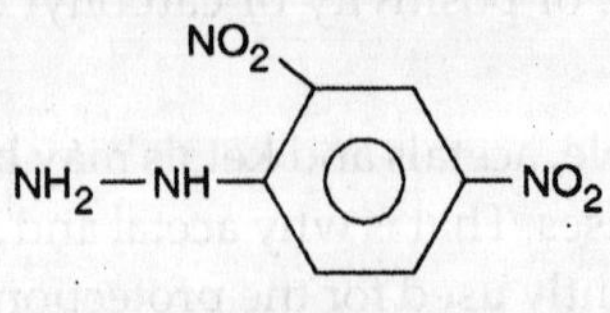 2, 4-Dinitrophenyl hydrazine (D.N.P.H.)	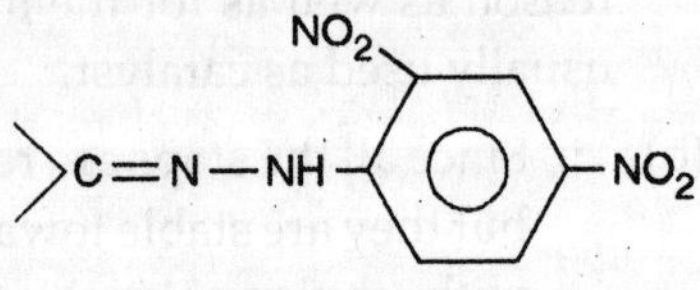 2, 4-Dinitrophenyl hydrazone
5. NH—C(=O)—NH_2	NH_2—NH—C(=O)—NH_2 Semi-carbazide	>C=N—NH—C(=O)—NH_2 Semi-carbazone
6. H	NH_3 Ammonia	>C=NH imine

C. Other type of addition reactions

(a) *Reduction of Aldehydes and Ketones*: Reduction of aldehydes and ketones may be categorised both as simple addition reaction as well as addition reaction with elimination of water. Formation of alcohols from these compounds is a case of simple addition reaction while their conversion to hydrocarbons may be looked upon as the addition reaction followed by elimination of water.

i. *Reduction of carbonyl compounds to alcohols*: The reduction of carbonyl compounds to alcohols may be achieved by various methods as discussed below:

(a) The easiest method is the catalytic hydrogenation.

$$>C=O \xrightarrow{\text{Cat [H]}} \underset{\text{Alcohol}}{>CHOH}$$

The catalysts commonly used are Ni, Pt, Pd, Cu-chromite, etc. In place of catalysts, metals/acids may be used. Aldehydes are reduced to primary alcohols, while ketones are converted to secondary alcohols.

(b) The reduction of carbonyl compounds to alcohols can also be achieved by the use of inorganic hydrides. The most widely used hydride is lithium aluminium hydride, $LiAlH_4$, commonly known as LAH. The reduction proceeds as under:

$$LiAlH_4 \rightleftharpoons \overset{+}{Li} + \overset{-}{Al}H_4$$

$$\overset{-}{Al}H_4 \rightleftharpoons AlH_3 + \overset{-}{H}$$

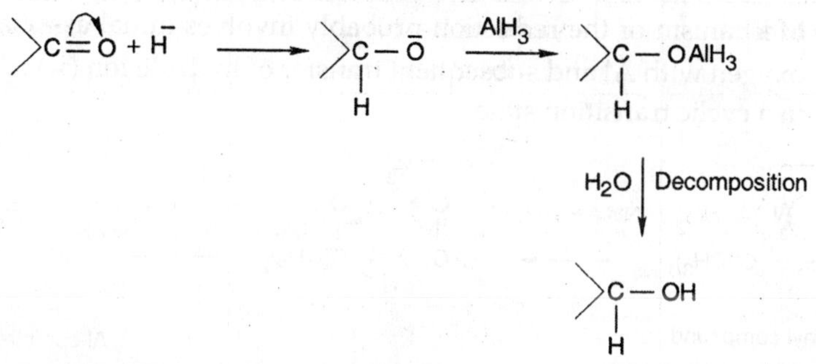

Reduction is carried out in ether solution and is specific for carbonyl group. So this reduction may be applied in presence of other reducible groups, such as NO_2, unsaturation, etc. Another important hydride is sodium borohydride, $NaBH_4$, which is also specific for carbonyl groups but is milder than $LiAlH_4$. The reaction path is similar to previous one.

(c) Bouveault and Blanc observed that metallic sodium in alcohol may successfully be used as a reducing agent for the conversion of carbonyl compounds into alchols.

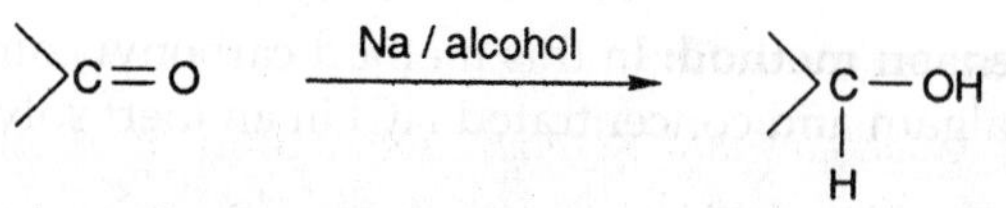

The mechanism of this reduction is a subject of much controversy. The most accepted mechanism of the reduction may be shown as:

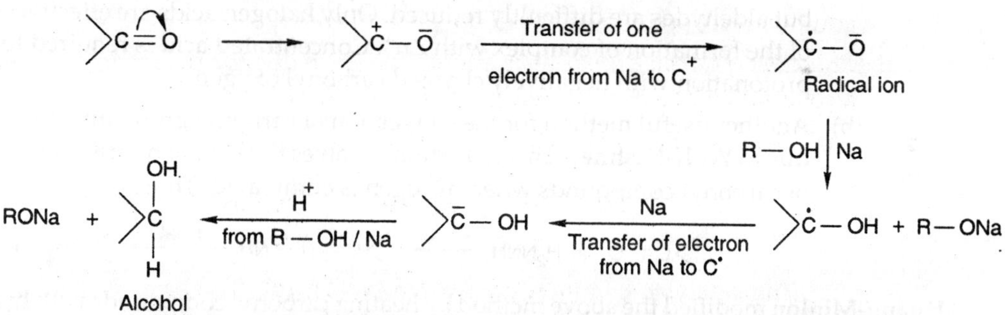

(d) Another most interesting method of reduction of carbonyl compounds to alcohols is due to Meerwein-Pondorff-Verley and is obviously known as Meerwein-Pondorff-Verley reduction. In this reduction carbonyl compounds are heated in isopropanol solution with aluminium isopropoxide. The isopropoxide is oxidised to acetone and the carbonyl group is reduced to alcoholic hydroxyl. It is a specific reducing agent only for the reduction of carbonyl compounds. This reduction is just a reverse process of *Oppenauer oxidation*. The first step of the reduction is the formation of Al-complex of alcohol which is decomposed by dilute H_2SO_4.

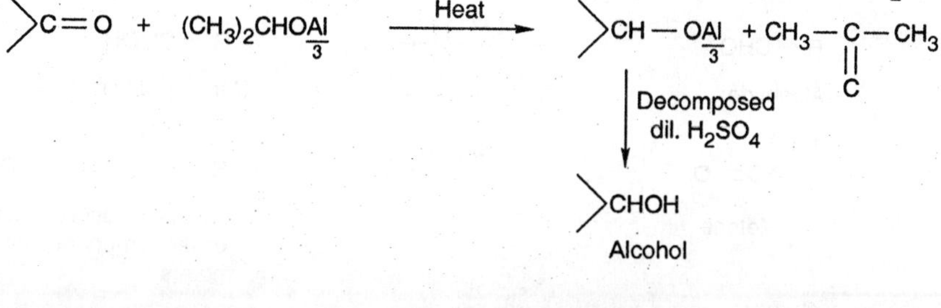

Mechanism of the reduction probably involves initial association of carbonyl oxygen with Al and subsequent transfer of hydride ion ($\bar{H}$) to carbonyl carbon in a cyclic transition state.

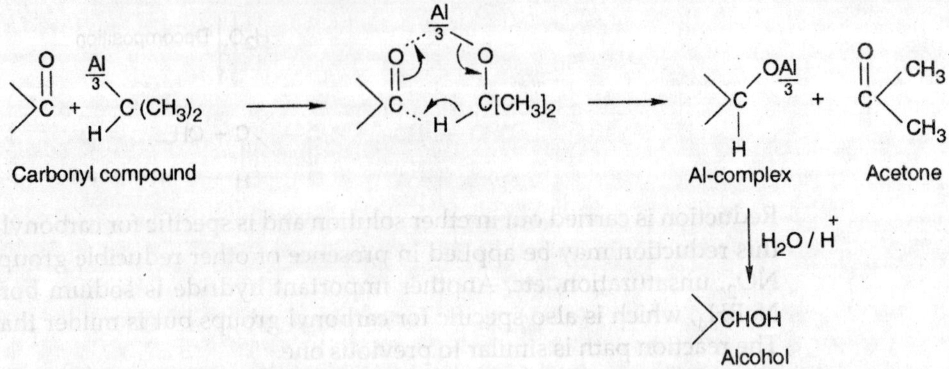

ii. *Reduction of carbonyl compounds to hydrocarbon*: Reduction of carbonyl compounds to hydrocarbons is carried out by following two important methods:

(a) **Clemmenson method:** In this method carbonyl compounds are reduced with zinc amalgam and concentrated HCl in an inert solvent.

$$>C=O \; + \; Zn / Hg / HCl \longrightarrow \; >CH_2$$

This reduction is a direct method and smoothly converts ketones to hydrocarbon but aldehydes are difficultly reduced. Only halogen acids are effective because of the formation of complex with Zn^+. Concentrated acid is required for initial protonation with negatively charged carbonyl oxygen.

(b) Another useful method for the conversion of carbonyl group into methylene is due to **Wolf-Kishner**. This reduction involves the heat of hydrazone derivative of carbonyl compounds when nitrogen is eliminated. Thus,

$$>C=O \; + \; H_2NNH_2 \longrightarrow \; >C=N-NH_2 \xrightarrow{\text{Heat}} \; >CH_2 \; + \; N_2$$

Huang-Minlon modified the above method by heating carbonyl compounds with hydrazine in ethylene glycol as solvent in presence of KOH at 150 °C.

10.5.1.2 Other Reactions of Carbonyl Compounds

10.5.1.2.1 Oxidation of Aldehydes and Ketones

i. Both aldehydes and ketones are oxidised to carboxylic acid. Aldehydes are oxidised without any loss of carbon atom but ketones form carboxylic acids containing lesser number of carbon atoms. For example,

$$\underset{\text{Aldehyde}}{R-CHO} \xrightarrow{[O]} \underset{\text{Carboxylic acid}}{R-COOH}$$

$$\underset{\text{Ketone}}{\overset{R}{\underset{R'}{>}}C=O} \xrightarrow{[O]} R-COOH + R'COOH$$

Carboxylic acid containing lesser number of carbon atom(s)

It may be mentioned in this connection that aldehydes require very mild oxidising agent, while in the case of ketones very strong oxidising agents like permanganate and dichromate are to be used. Due to this characteristic, by using a very mild oxidising agent both aldehydes and ketones may be easily distinguished. Two such very frequently used mild oxidising agents are ammoniacal $AgNO_3$ solution usually known as *Tollen's solution* (Tollen's test) and the other is *Fehling solution*.

In Tollen's test aldehydic compound is treated with ammoniacal $AgNO_3$ solution and is warmed in water bath, when aldehydes are oxidised to corresponding carboxylic acid and silver ion is reduced to metallic silver which appears as shining mirror on the wall of the reaction apparatus. For this reason this test is sometimes referred to as *silver mirror test*. Mechanism of the oxidation may be written as under:

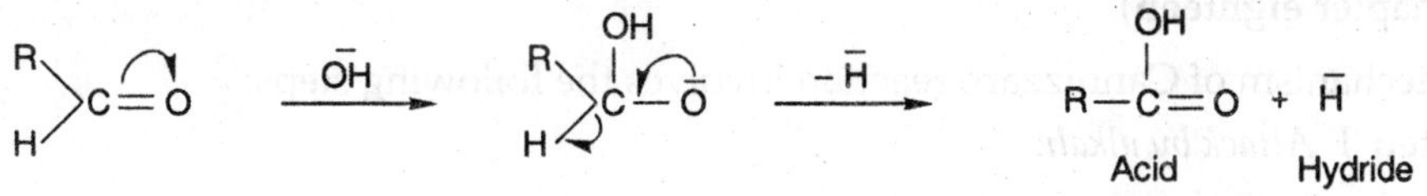

$$2\,Ag^{+} + \bar{H} \longrightarrow \underset{\text{Metallic silver}}{2\,Ag^{0}} + H^{+} \xrightarrow{\bar{O}H} H_2O$$

Oxidation of aldehydes with Fehling solution is carried out in the similar way. Aldehydes are warmed with Fehling solution in an water bath. Fehling solution is a mixture of equal volume of $CuSO_4$ solution in NaOH which is marked as Fehling solution A and solution of sodium-potassium tartarate (Rochelle salt) in NaOH marked as Fehling solution B.

Reaction proceeds in similar fashion. Hydride ion liberated from aldehyde in alkaline solution reduces Cu^{2+} to Cu^{+} which is precipitated as red cuprous oxide, i.e.,

$$2\,Cu^{++} + \bar{H} \longrightarrow 2\,Cu^{+} + H^{+}$$

$$2\,Cu^{+} + 2\,\bar{O}H \longrightarrow 2\,CuOH \xrightarrow{-H_2O} \underset{\text{Red}}{Cu_2O\downarrow}$$

Rochelle salt is used to stabilise Cu^{+} by complex formation. In place of Fehling solution sometimes Benedict solution is used. It is similar to Fehling solution but in place of Rochelle salt, sodium citrate in sodium carbonate solution is used, the function of which is identical to Rochelle salt. In this reaction same red precipitate of cuprous oxide is formed.

ii. *The Baeyer-Villiger Oxidation*: In this oxidation carbonyl compounds particularly ketones on oxidation with peracid form esters. Thus,

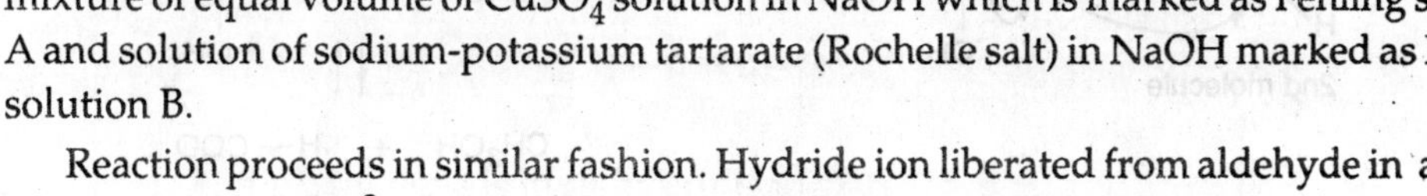

iii. *Cannizzaro Reaction*: It is a special type of reaction which is exhibited by a particular type of aldehydes. Cannizzaro observed that only those aldehydes which have no hydrogen atom at the carbon atom α to carbonyl carbon when treated with alkali undergo self oxidation-reduction reaction. Two molecules of such aldehydes are always involved, one of which is reduced to alcohol while the other is oxidised to corresponding carboxylic acid.

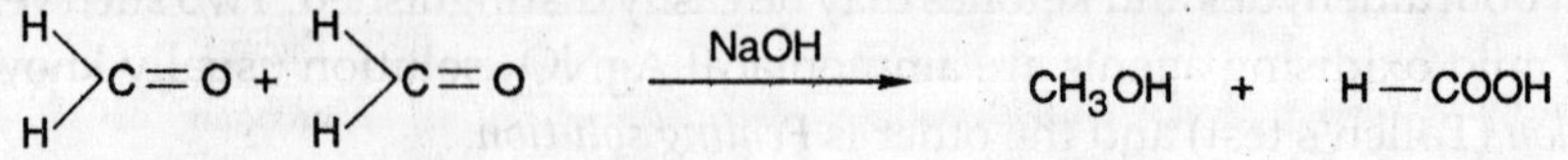

Formaldehyde Methanol Formic acid

A careful scrutiny reveals that formaldehyde and only a very few aliphatic aldehydes may have no α-H atom but invariably almost all the aromatic aldehydes do not have any α-H. For this reason *Cannizzaro reaction* is extremely common in aromatic aldehydes and that is why, this reaction has been discussed in detail with aromatic aldehydes (vide chapter **eighteen**).

Mechanism of Cannizzaro reaction involves the following steps:

Step I: *Attack by alkali*:

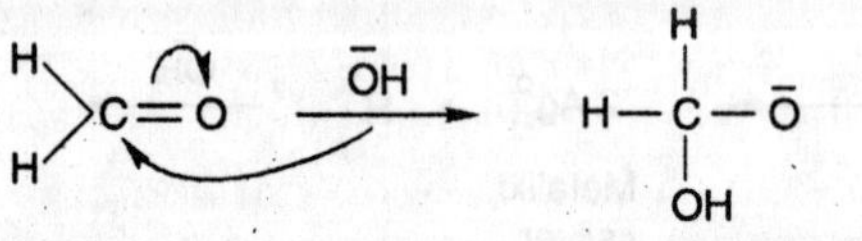

Step II: Transfer of hydride ion followed by oxidation reduction:

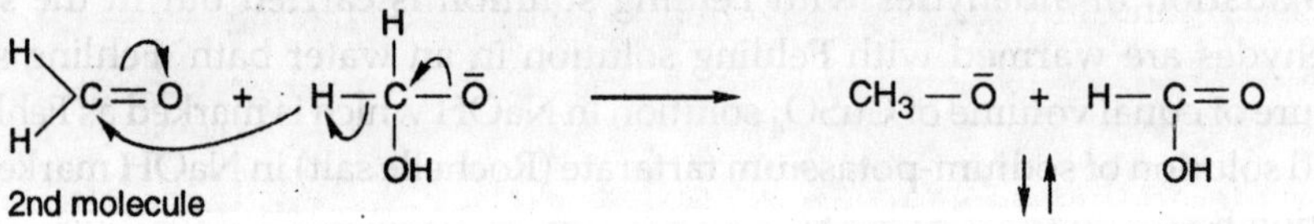

2nd molecule

Methanol Salt of formic acid

10.5.2 Reactions of Carbonyl Compounds due to the Influence of Carbonyl Group

It has been observed that due to electron withdrawing tendency of carbonyl group, hydrogen atom at α-carbon can be readily replaced by suitable reagent giving rise to some novel reactions. A few of such reactions are considered in sequel:

1. *Oxidation of α-carbon atom*: Aldehydes and ketones having methyl or methylene group at the α-position when subjected to oxidation by SeO_2 in acetic acid at room temperature are converted to α-dicarbonyl compounds.

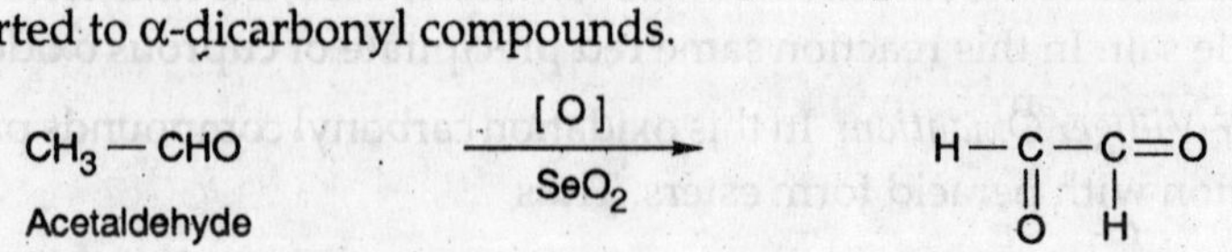

Acetaldehyde Glyoxal

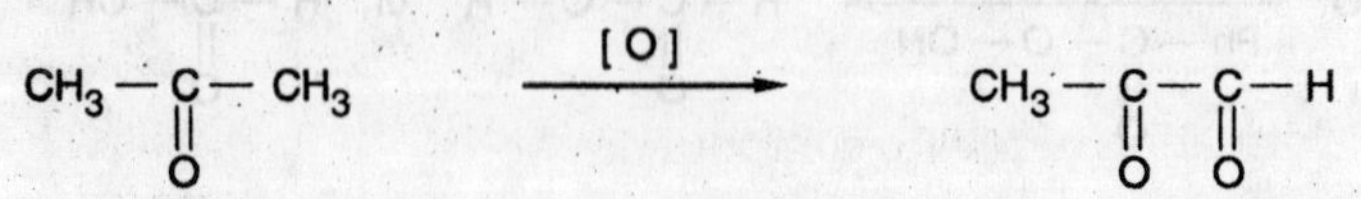

Acetone Methyl glyoxal

It is an useful method for the preparation of α-carbonyl compounds.

2. *Halogenation*: Reactions of carbonyl compounds having α-H atoms with free halogen is a very interesting phenomenon. This halogenation is usually carried out in presence of base as catalysts. Thus,

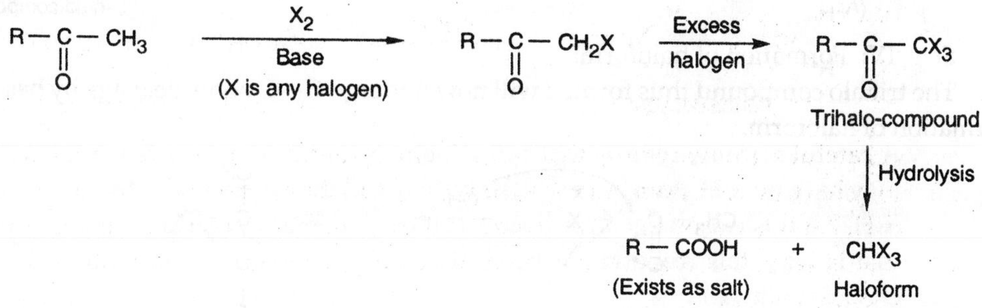

As evidenced from the above reaction path that *haloform* will be formed only when there are *three* hydrogen atoms at α-carbon atom, i.e., if the compound possesses keto-methyl $(-\underset{\underset{O}{\|}}{C}-CH_3)$ group. However, as alkaline halogen solution is a mild oxidising agent, organic compounds which originally do not contain $-\underset{\underset{O}{\|}}{C}-CH_3$, but under the mild oxidising condition may be converted to compounds having $-\underset{\underset{O}{\|}}{C}-CH_3$ functionality can undergo this reaction. Thus, ethanol, CH_3-CH_2-OH, isopropanol, $\begin{matrix}CH_3\\CH_3\end{matrix}\!\!>CHOH$ which are oxidised to acetaldehyde, $CH_3-\underset{\underset{O}{\|}}{C}-H$ and acetone, $CH_3-\underset{\underset{O}{\|}}{C}-CH_3$ respectively may undergo *haloform reaction*.

Mechanistically, haloform reaction proceeds via the following steps:

Step I: Formation of carbanion:

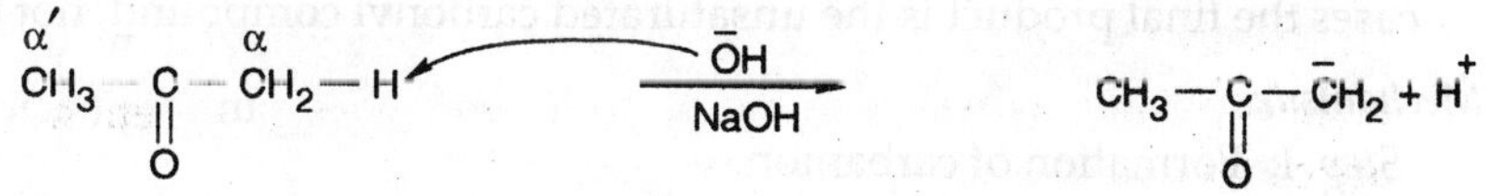

Step II: Formation of monohalo compound:

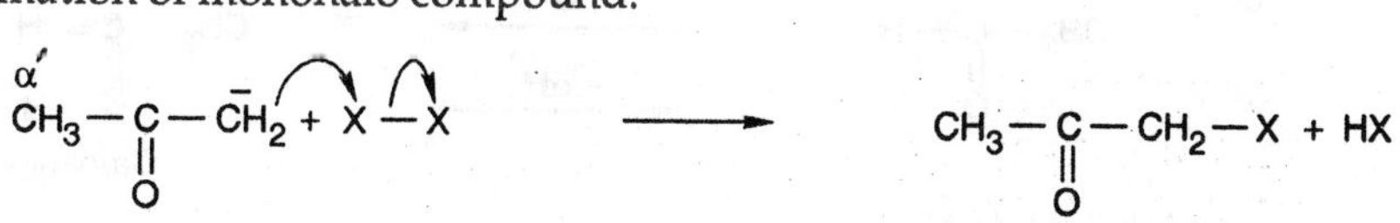

Monohalo compound (A)

Step III: Formation of trihalo compound:

As soon as the monohalogen derivative (A) is formed, in presence of excess of alkali, second molecule of halogen will preferentially attack α-carbon, not the α′-carbon. This is due to the fact that electron withdrawing effect of halogen increases the acidity of α-H. Hence, if there are two more α-H atoms, (A) will ultimately form trihalo compound.

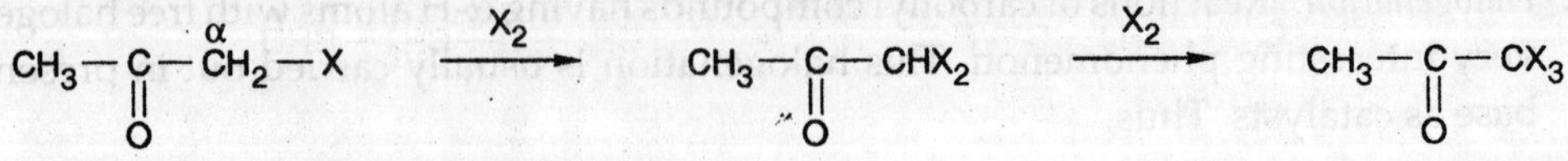

(A) Trihalo compound

Step IV: Formation of haloform:

The trihalo compound thus formed will now undergo C—C bond cleavage by base with the formation of haloform.

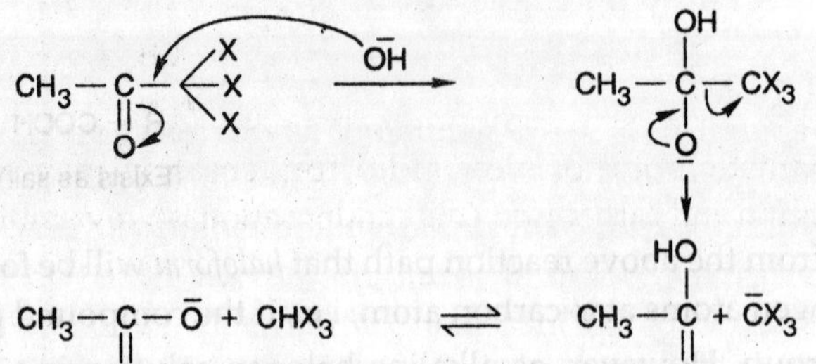

Haloform

Acid salt

3. *Aldol Condensation*: An important and interesting type of reaction undergone by carbonyl compounds having α-H is the *aldol condensation*. In this condensation reaction, two molecules of carbonyl compounds, (like or different) both having α-H atom are involved and the product is an aldol—β-hydroxy carbonyl compounds. This condensation process is induced by basic catalysts like NaOH, $Ba(OH)_2$, K_2CO_3 or dilute HCl. For example,

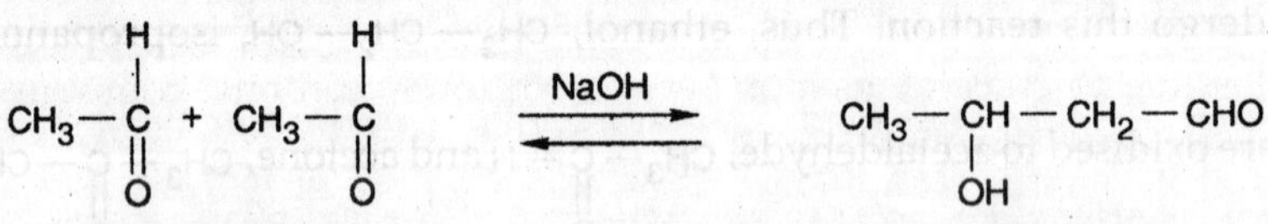

Acetaldehyde Aldol (β-hydroxy carbonyl)

The aldol obtained above is generally unstable and readily eliminates a molecule of water to form unsaturated compound and the elimination of water is so rapid that in some cases the final product is the unsaturated carbonyl compound, not the aldol.

Mechanism:

Step I: Formation of carbanion.

Carbanion

Step II: Formation of carbocation.

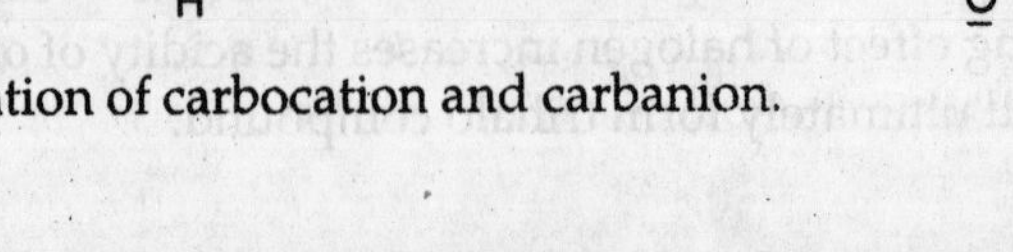

Step III: Combination of carbocation and carbanion.

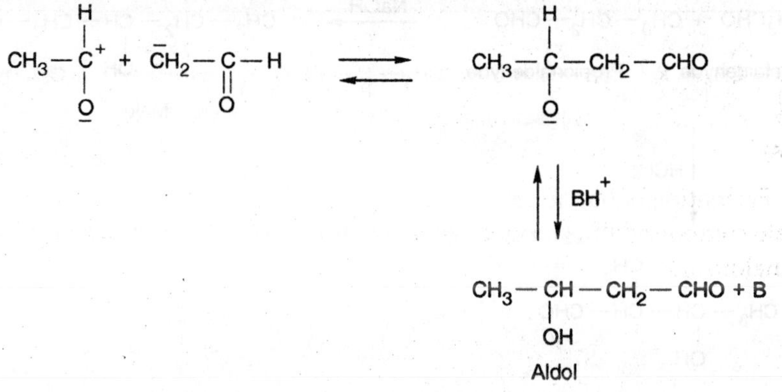

Thus, from mechanistic point of view aldol condensation may be looked upon as the combination of carbocation and carbanion. This condensation is a reversible reaction equilibriated between the products and reactants.

Scope and limitation:

(a) As defined above aldol condensation is only applicable for those carbonyl compounds which possess α-H atom.

(b) Since two molecules (like or different) are involved, the condensation may be divided into following categories:

Aldol condensation between (i) two identical aldehydes, (ii) two identical ketones, (iii) two different aldehydes, (iv) two different ketones and (v) an aldehyde and a ketone.

Nature of the product: Aldol condensation between two identical molecules (aldehydes or ketones) always affords a single product in predominant yield but when two different molecules (aldehydes or ketones) are involved the process becomes complicated and theoretically four products are possible. Such condensation between different carbonyl compounds is known as *crossed aldol condensation*. Thus,

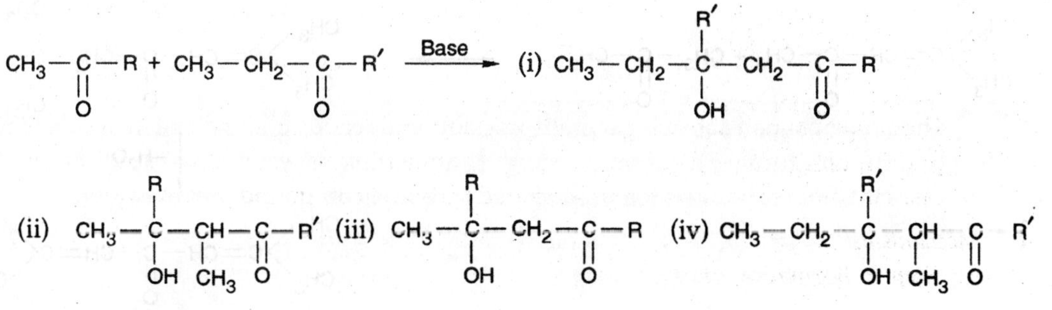

R and R′ may be any alkyl group or H atom.

Influence of reagent: By using suitable condensing agent, the predominancy of one of the products may be achieved. Thus,

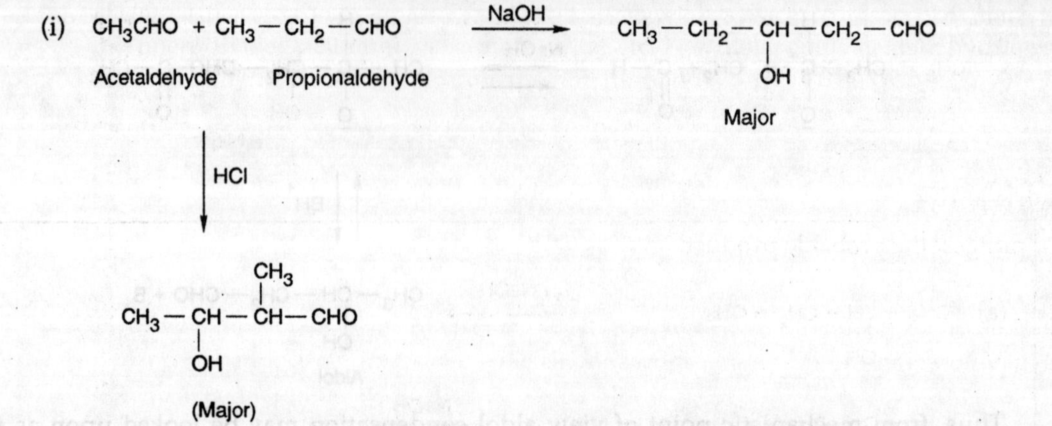

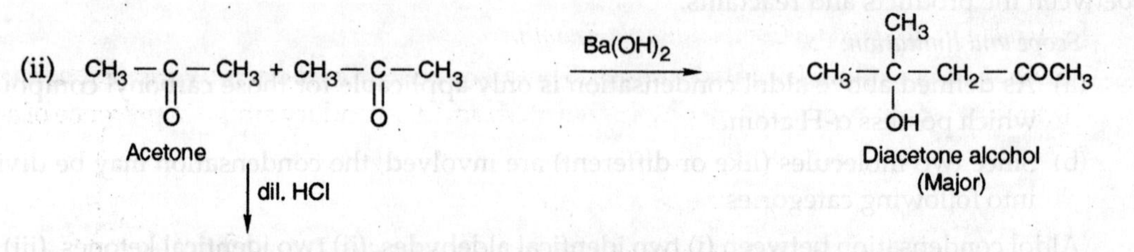

If excess acetone is used, mesityl oxide yields phorone, i.e.,

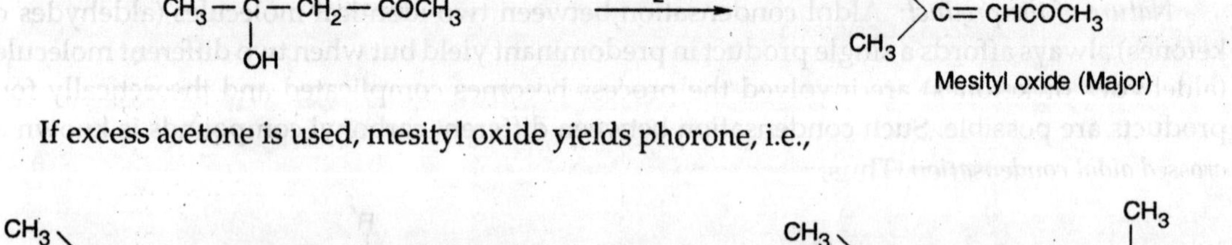

It has been observed that in most of the cases aldol may be made to predominate, if K_2CO_3 is used as condensing agent.

Further, when aldol condensation takes place between an aldehyde and a ketone, although theoretically four products are possible, yet since aldehydic carbonyl is more active, the carbocation will be generated from aldehyde while ketone will serve as the source of carbanion; consequently the major product will be

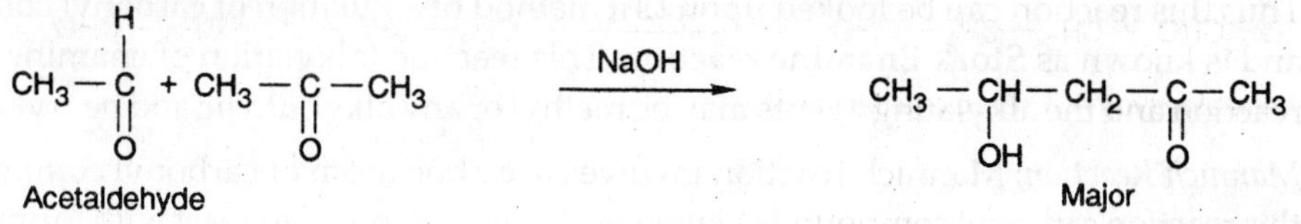

PROBLEM 10.4

Suggest the probable product:

(a) 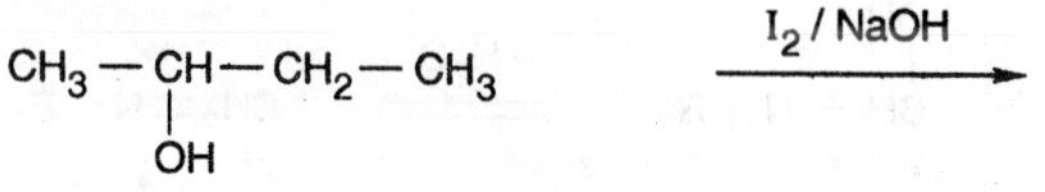

(b) 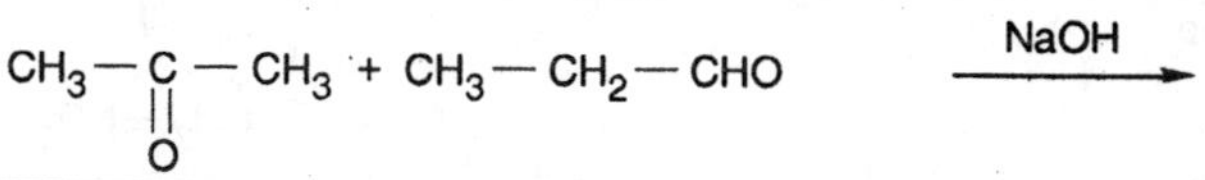

4. *Alkylation of Carbonyl Compounds via Enamine*

Enamine is α, β-unsaturated amines. These are generally formed by the reaction of a carbonyl compound having α-hydrogen atom and a secondary amine in presence of acid catalyst. Thus,

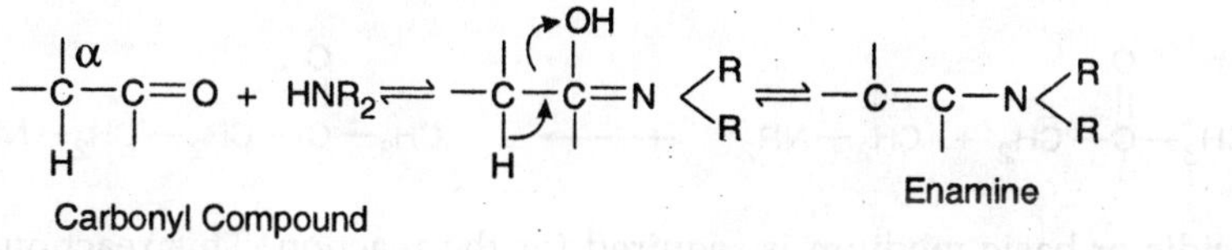

Enamines exist in resonance hybrid as shown below.

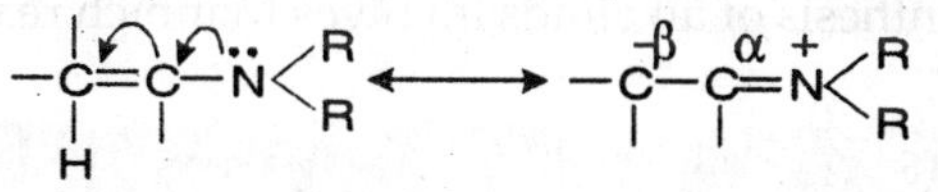

An examination of the resonance structures reveals that β-carbon atom behaves as a nucleophilic centre so that nucleophilic centre can be easily attacked by electrophiles, generally carbocations. The iminium ion that is formed is hydrolysed and the net result is the removal of the original amine and the formation of a carbonyl compound with an additional alkyl group at α-carbon atom.

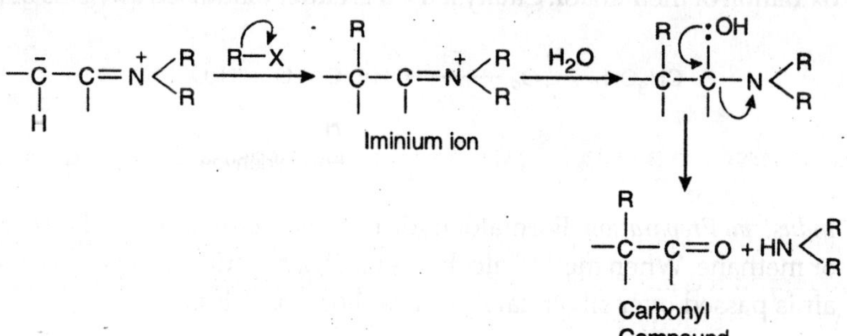

Thus this reaction can be looked upon as a method of alkylation of carbonyl compounds and is known as **Stork Enamine reaction**. This reaction (alkylation of enamine) is a SN^2 reaction and the alkylating agents may be methyl or any alkyl, allylic and benrylic halides.

5. *Mannich Reaction*: Mannich reaction involves α-carbon atom of carbonyl compounds. In this reaction carbonyl compounds having α-H atom is allowed to react with formaldehyde and an amine. The product formed is β-amino carbonyl compound usually known as *Mannich base*. Normally a secondary amine is preferred over primary amine.

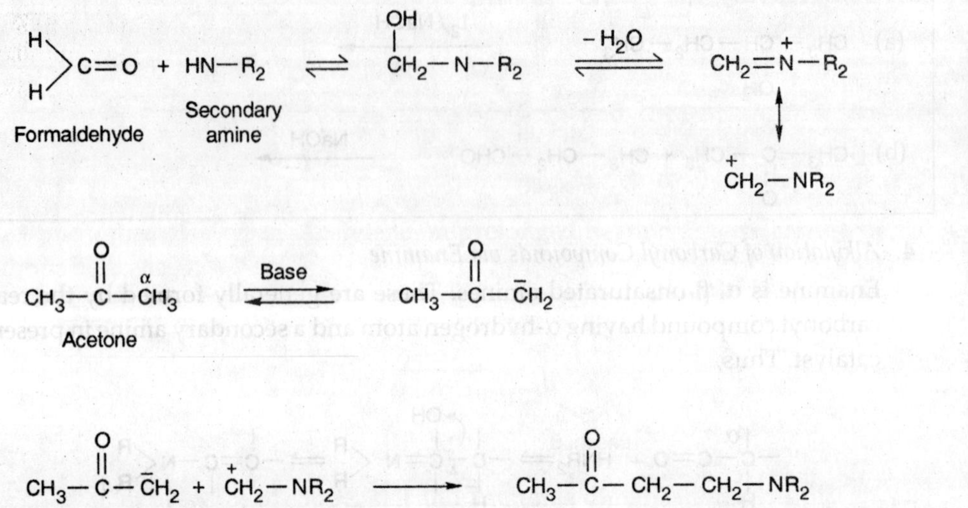

An acidic or basic medium is required for the reaction. This reaction is a satisfactory method for introducing a carbon atom in carbonyl compounds containing α-H atom. It has been observed that bio-synthesis of alkaloids involves Mannich reaction.

10.6 Some Individual Members

1. **Formaldehyde:** Formaldehyde is the first member of aliphatic aldehydic family. It is an important chemical utilised for variety of purposes. It is marketed in the form of 40 per cent aqueous solution known as *Formalin*. It is normally prepared by the following methods.

   i. *Laboratory Preparation*: In laboratory formaldehyde is prepared by the catalytic oxidation of methanaol. Catalyst used is either platinised asbestos or a platinum spiral.

$$CH_3OH + \frac{1}{2}O_2 \xrightarrow{Pt} \underset{\text{Formaldehyde}}{H-\underset{\displaystyle H}{\underset{|}{C}}=O} + H_2O$$

   ii. *Industrial Preparation:* Formaldehyde is manufactured by oxidation of either methanol or methane. When methyl alcohol is used, a mixture of vapour of methyl alcohol and air is passed over silver catalyst at 600-650 °C. Thus

$$CH_3OH + \frac{1}{2}O_2 \xrightarrow{Ag} H-\underset{\displaystyle H}{\underset{|}{C}}=O + H_2O$$

When methane is used as the starting matrial, air oxidation is carried out under pressure in the presence of molybdenum oxide as catalyst.

$$CH_4 + O_2 \longrightarrow H_2C{=}O + H_2O$$

• **Properties of Formaldehyde:** It is a colourless pungent smelling gas, readily soluble in water. It undergoes most of the reactions of aldehydic carbonyl compounds. However, it differs from other aldehydes in certain respects as discussed below.

(a) *Reaction with ammonia:* Formaldehyde when treated with ammonia *unlike other aldehydes forms a white crystalline substance* **hexamethylene tetramine**:

$$\underset{\text{Formaldehyde}}{6HCHO} + 4NH_3 \longrightarrow \underset{\text{Hexamethylene tetramine}}{(CH_2)_6N_4} + 6H_2O$$

Hexamethylene tetramine is a cyclic compound having the following structure

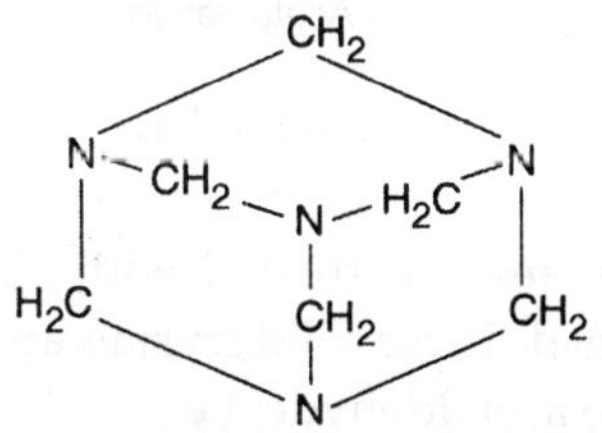

It is used in medicine under the name of *urotropine* or *aminoform* for the treatment of gout and rheumatism.

(b) Since formaldehyde has no α-hydrogen atom, on treatment with alkali it does not undergo aldol condensation but readily responds to *Cannizzaro reaction.*

$$2\ H_2C{=}O \xrightarrow{NaOH} \underset{\text{Methanol}}{CH_3OH} + \underset{\text{Sodium formate}}{HCOONa}$$

(c) *Polymerisation of Formaldehyde:* The most interesting characteristic of formaldehyde is its ready polymerisation to different useful compounds under different condition as depicted below:

i. When an aqueons solution of formaldehyde (formalin) is evaporated to dryness, it polymerises to a white crystalline solid, m.p. 122-123 °C. This polymer is known as *paraformaldehyde,* $(HCHO)_n$, H_2O, where n is about 6.50. Paraformaldehyde regenerates formaldehyde when heated. When a formaldehyde solution is treated with concentrated sulphuric acid, *polyoxymethylene* is obtained in solid form, $(HCHO)_n$, $H_2O(n > 100)$. It also reforms formaldehyde on heating.

When formaldehyde gas is allowed to stand at room temperature it slowly pohymerises to trioxymethyle (metaformaldehyde), $(HCHO)_3$ which is a white solid, m.p. 60-62 °C. It does not show any reducing proporties and is believed to have a cyclic structure as shown below:

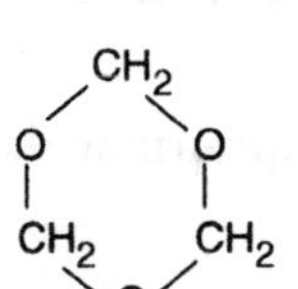

It is also known as trioxan. Trioxan is useful for generating formaldehyde since it is an anhydrous form of formaldehyde and is soluble in organic solvents.

It may be mentioned that as all the polymers can yield formaldehyde on heating, they are considered as an useful and convenient source of gaseous formaldehyde whenever required.

2. **Acetaldehyde (Ethanal):** Acetaldehyde, CH_3CHO, may be considered as a typical member of aldehyde family and exhibits practically all the reactions of aldehydes.

Preparation of Acetaldehyde: Following methods are generally utilised for its preparation:

i. In the laboratory, acetaldehyde is prepared by the oxidation of ethyl alcohol with dichromate and dlute sulphuric acid.

$$\underset{\text{Ethyl alcohol}}{CH_3CH_2OH} + [O] \xrightarrow[H_2SO_4]{K_2Cr_2O_7} \underset{\text{Acetaldehyde}}{CH_3CHO} + H_2O$$

Acetaldehyde, as soon as it is formed, is distilled away in order to avoid its further oxidation to acetic acid.

The crude aldehyde, thus, obtained is treated with ammonia when crystals of acetaldehyde-ammonia are obtained. These solid crystals are then distilled with dilute sulphuric acid to regenerate pure acetaldehyde, i.e.,

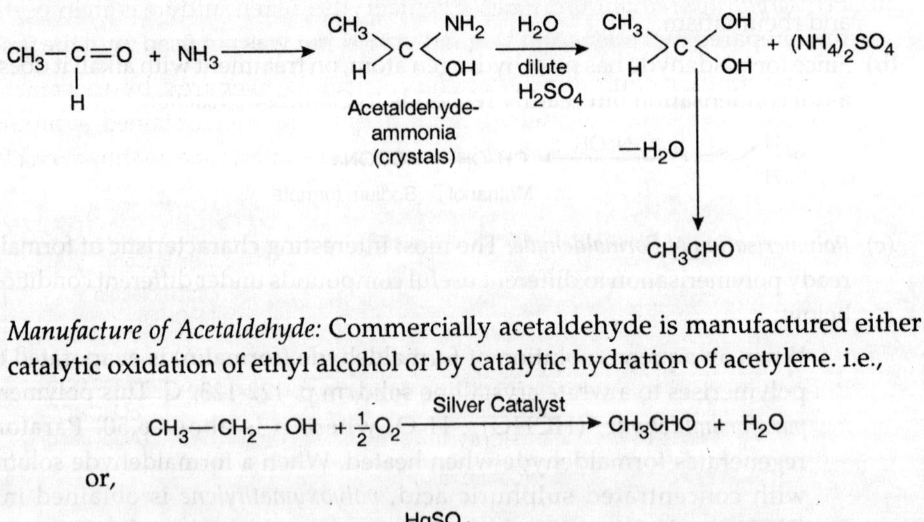

ii. *Manufacture of Acetaldehyde:* Commercially acetaldehyde is manufactured either by catalytic oxidation of ethyl alcohol or by catalytic hydration of acetylene. i.e.,

$$CH_3-CH_2-OH + \tfrac{1}{2}O_2 \xrightarrow{\text{Silver Catalyst}} CH_3CHO + H_2O$$

or,

$$CH \equiv CH + H_2O \xrightarrow[H_2SO_4\ \text{(dilute)}]{HgSO_4} CH_2=CH-OH \rightleftharpoons CH_3-CH=O$$

- **Properties of Acetaldehyde:** Acetaldehyde is a colourless pungent smelling volatite liquid, b.p. 20 °C. It is soluble in water, ethanol and ether. It responds to all the characteristic reactions of aldehydes. Like formaldehyde, it also undergoes *Polymerisation reactions* to form different products under different conditions.

i. On treatment with a few drops of concentrated sulphuric acid, it forms *paraldehyde* which exists in cyclic form.

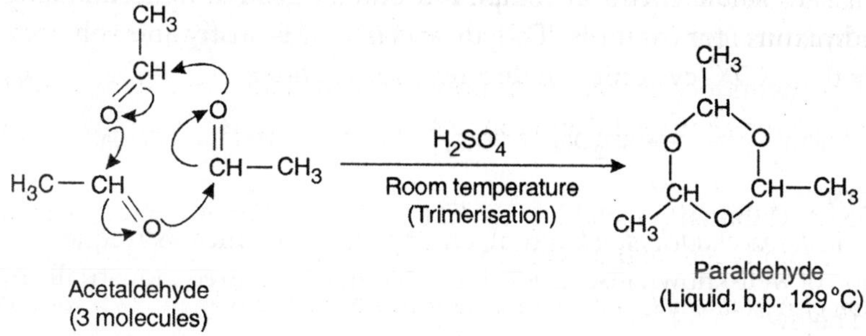

ii. When the above reaction is carried out at 0 °C in presence of the same reagent, concentrated sulphuric acid, four molecules of acetaldehyde are involved and a **tetramer** is obtained which is known as **metaldehyde**. It is a white solid, m.p. 245 °C.

$$4CH_3CHO \xrightarrow[0°C]{H_2SO_4} \underset{\text{Metaldehyde}}{(CH_3CHO)_4}$$

Metaldehyde exists in cyclic form as shown below:

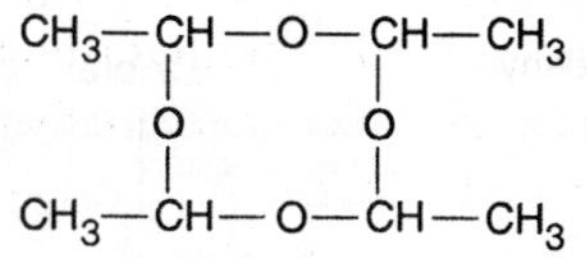

iii. *Pentaerythritol Tetranitrate (PETN)*: Pentaerythritol tetranitrate is an important explosive first prepared by Tollens and Wigand in 1891 but was not used until the first World War.

The mother compound, pentaerythritol, is prepared by the reaction between formaldehyde and acetaldehyde and the product thus obtained is nitrated with 99% HNO_3 at 15-20 °C followed by crystallisation from acetone as shown below:

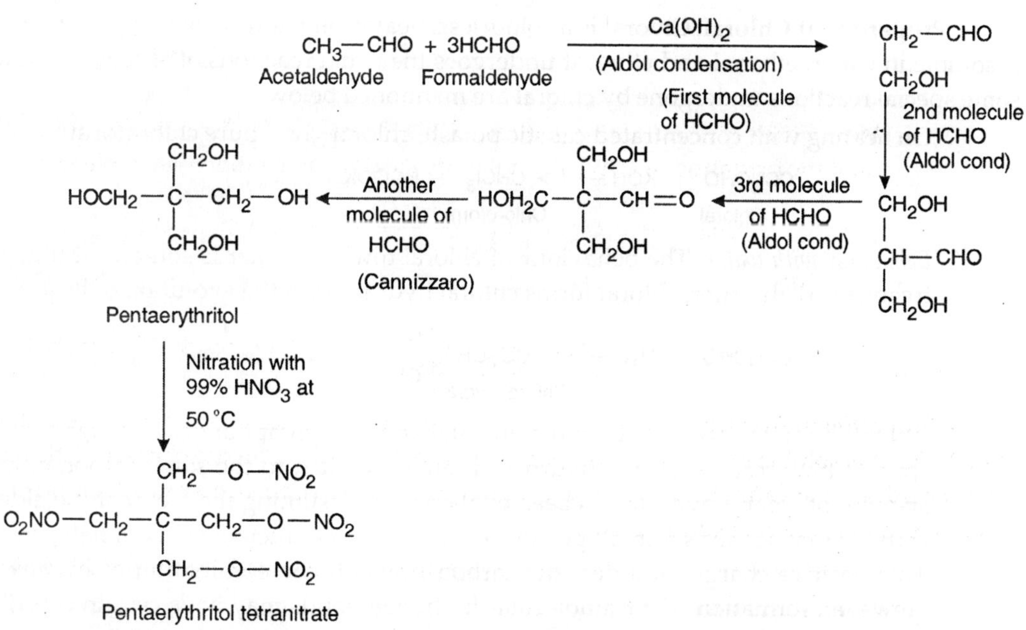

PETN is a very stable chemical compound but is sensitive to friction and is normally used in admixture, for example, TNT in *pentolites*. It is costly and is more sensitive but less stable than RDX (cyclonite). It decomposes as under:

$$\underset{\text{PETN}}{C(CH_2ONO_2)_4} \longrightarrow 4H_2O(g) + 3CO_2\uparrow + 2CO\uparrow + 2N_2\uparrow + 180\text{ kcal}$$

3. *Chloral (Trichloroacetaldehyde):* Chloral, an important chemical is frequently used for the preparation of well-known insecticide, DDT. It is manufactured industrially by the method discussed below:

• **Manufacture of Chloral:** It is manufactured by the reaction between chlorine and ethanol. Chlorine is allowed to pass first into cold ethanol and next into hot ethanol, heating at a temperature of 60 °C till the solution is saturated. Chloral alcoholate formed is separated as a crystalline solid. This is distilled with 85% sulphuric acid to get chloral. The reactions involved are as under:

$$\underset{\text{Ethanol}}{CH_3{-}CH_2{-}OH} \xrightarrow[-2HCl]{Cl_2} \underset{\text{Acetaldehyde}}{CH_3{-}CHO} \xrightarrow[-3HCl]{3Cl_2} \underset{\text{Chloral}}{CCl_3CHO}$$

$$\underset{\text{Chloral}}{CCl_3CHO} \xrightarrow{CH_3{-}CH_2OH} \underset{\substack{\text{Chloral alcoholate}\\ \text{(crystalline solid)}}}{CCl_3CH(OH).OC_2H_5}$$

$$\underset{\substack{\text{Chloral alcoholate}\\ \text{(crystalline solid)}}}{CCl_3CH(OH).OC_2H_5} \xrightarrow{85\%\ H_2SO_4} H_2O + C_2H_5HSO_4 + \underset{\substack{\text{Chloral}\\ \text{(oily liquid)}}}{CCl_3CHO}$$

The distillate is neutralised with calcium carbonate and redistilled.

• **Properties of Chloral:** Chloral is a colourless, heavy, oily liquid with a pungent odour. It is soluble in water, ethanol and ether. It undergoes the usual reactions of aldehyde. However, some special reactions undergone by chloral are mentioned below:

i. On heating with concentrated caustic potash, chloral gives pure chloroform.

$$\underset{\text{Chloral}}{CCl_3CHO} + KOH \longrightarrow \underset{\text{Chloroform}}{CHCl_3} + HCOOK$$

ii. *Behaviour with water:* The behaviour of chloral towards water is somewhat unusual on treatment with water, chloral forms chloral hydrate with the evolution of heat.

$$CCl_3CHO + H_2O \longrightarrow \underset{\text{Chloral hydrate}}{CCl_3CH\langle^{OH}_{OH}}$$

Chloral hydrate is one of the most unusual and rare compounds. It is highly stable in spite of the presence of two hydroxyl groups attached to the same carbon atom. The stability of chloral hydrate has been explained by assuming the fact that the aldehydic carbon atom acquires a small positive charge due to inductive effect of halogen atoms. This positive charge on aldehydic carbon prevents the elimination of hydroxyl ion. However, formation of intramolecular hydrogen bonds may have certain contribution towards its stability.

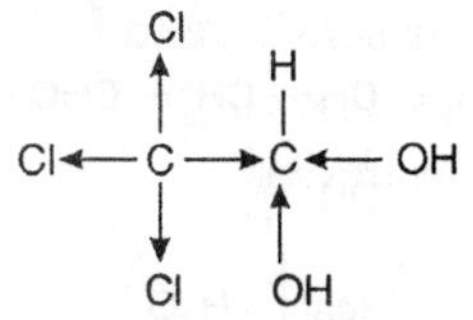

(Role of inductive effect)

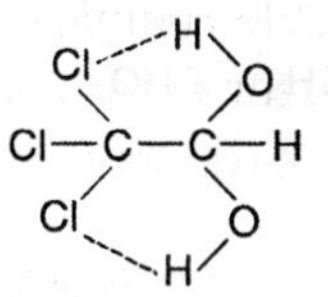

Intramolecular H-bonding

With alcohol chloral forms similar compound, chloral alcoholate.

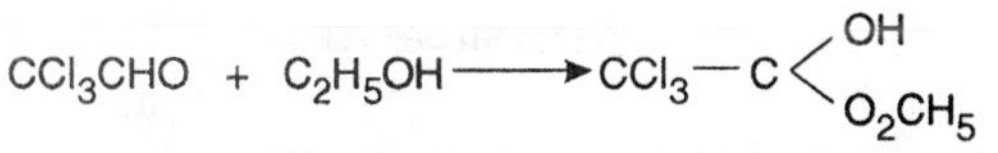

Chloral alcoholate

Chloral hydrate is used as a hypnotic and as a power stimulant.

10.7 Unsaturated Carbonyl Compounds

Unsaturated carbonyl compounds are those organic compounds in which in addition to a carbon-carbon double bond, there is a carbonyl function.

Among this type of carbonyl compounds, conjugated type, i.e., α, β-unsaturated carbonyl compounds are well known and well investigated. The important members of α, β-unsaturated carbonyl compounds are, mentioned below:

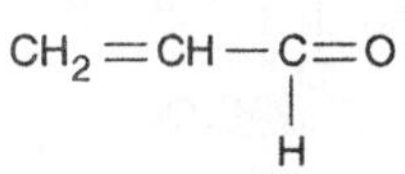

Acrolein (Acral dehyde)
(Propenal)

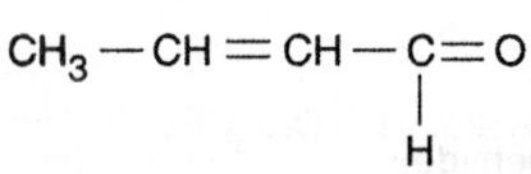

Crotonal dehyde
(2-Butenal)

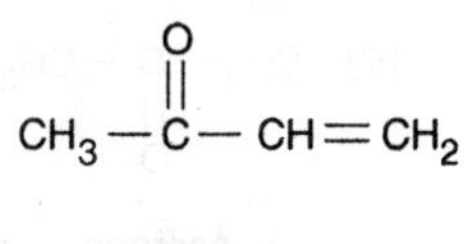

Methyl vinyl
ketone

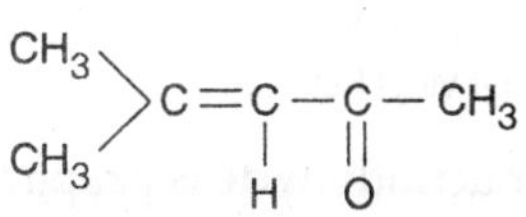

Mesityl oxide

Another important type of unsaturated carbonyl is the ketene in which carbonyl and unsaturation functions are cumulated, i.e., $H_2C=C=O$. Ketene may be aldoketene when one of the hydrogen atoms is replaced by any organic group: R—CH = C = O, and when both the hydrogen atoms are substituted by organic groups the ketene formed is known as keto ketene: $R_2C=C=O$.

10.7.1 α, β-Unsaturated Carbonyl Compounds

10.7.1.1 Methods of Preparation of α, β-Unsaturated Carbonyl Compounds

These carbonyl compounds are prepared by the following methods:

1. *Aldol condensation*

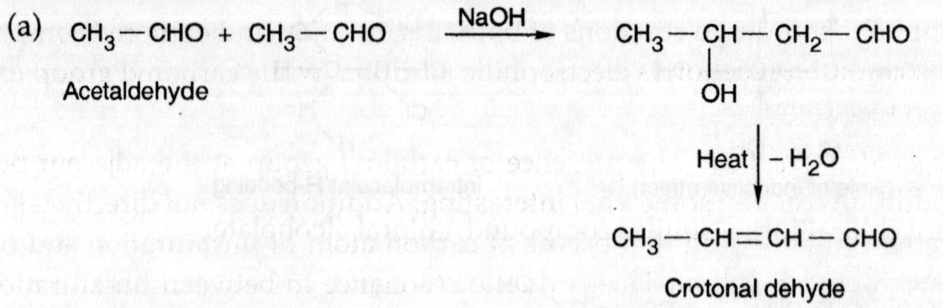

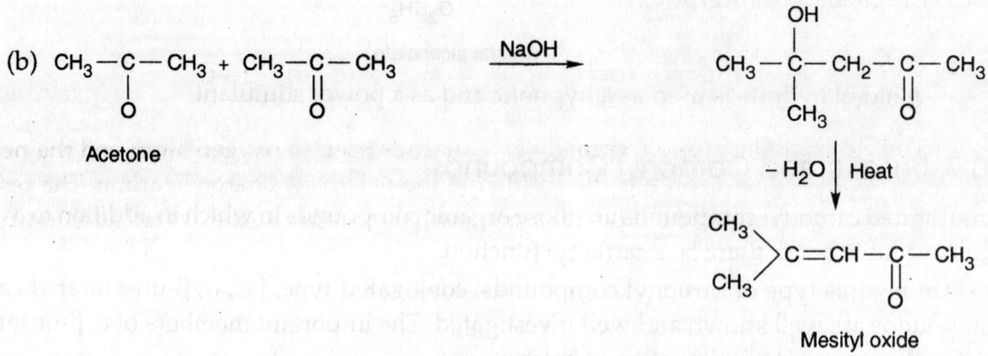

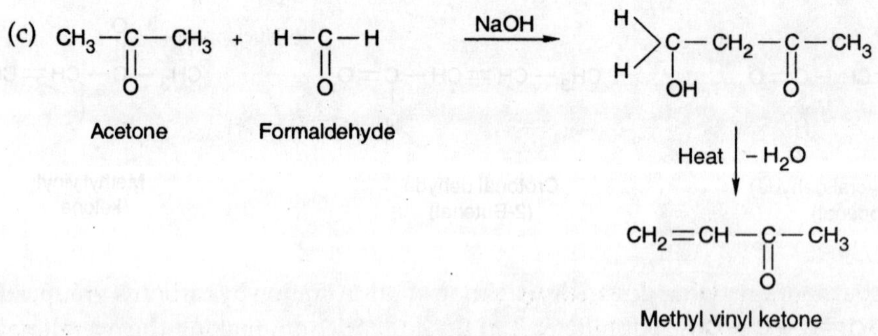

(d) *Specific method for the preparation of acrolein*: Acrolein or acraldehyde is prepared by a specific method. This method consists of dehydration of glycerol by heating with $KHSO_4$.

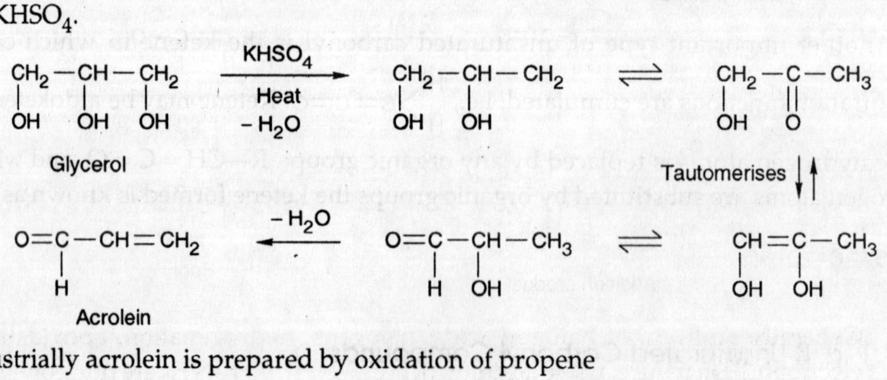

Industrially acrolein is prepared by oxidation of propene

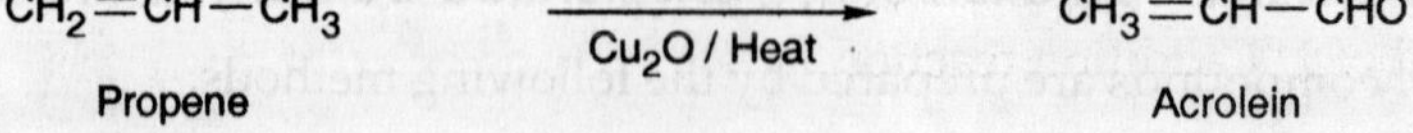

10.7.1.2 Properties of α, β-Unsaturated Carbonyl Compounds

These carbonyl compounds undergo reactions of both unsaturation and carbonyl compounds. For unsaturation the common reaction is electrophilic addition, while carbonyl group exhibits nucleophilic addition reactions.

(a) *Electrophilic addition reaction*: The presence of carbonyl group at the adjacent position makes the addition reaction somewhat interesting. Addition does not directly take place on unsaturation. Initially addition occurs at carbon atom of unsaturation and oxygen atom of the carbonyl function. This is due to resonance in between unsaturation and carbonyl function. Thus,

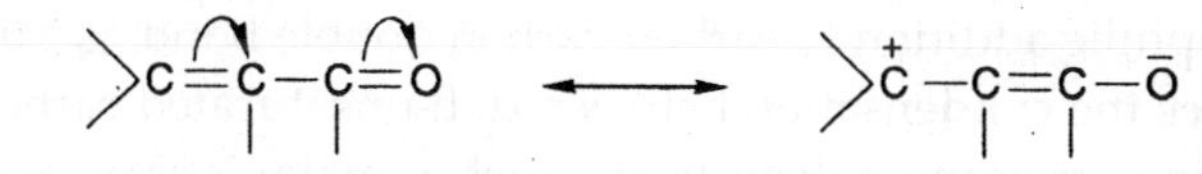

The electrophilic group (normally H^+) attaches itself to oxygen atom and the negative part of the addendenum is then added to the positively charged carbon. The resulting product is an enol and readily tautomerises to keto form. So the overall addition appears to be at carbon-carbon double bond.

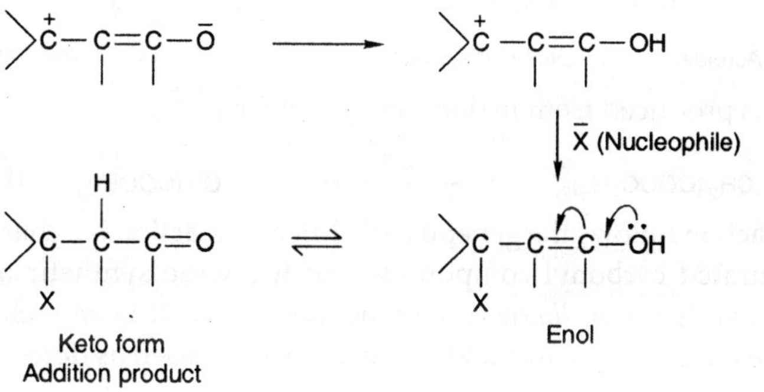

It may be mentioned that due to deactivation of unsaturation by carbonyl group, addition may be initiated by nucleophilic part of the addendenum making the overall nature of addition as nucleophilic. Thus,

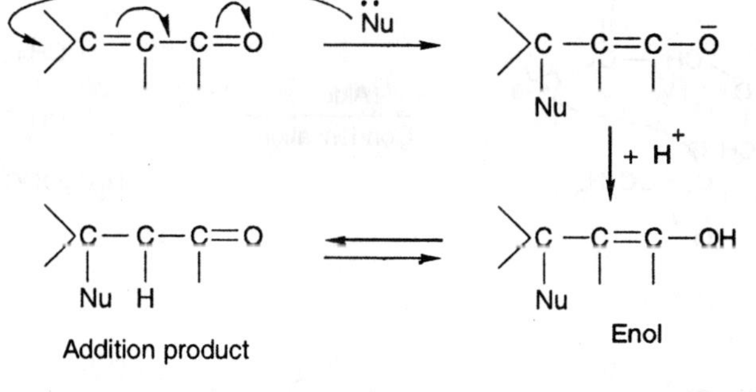

Generally addition of halogen acids, halogens, hydrogenation, epoxidation, etc. are electrophilic in nature, while addition of HCN, NH_3, NH_2-NH_2 are nucleophilic in nature. The addition at carbon-carbon double bonds whether electrophilic or nucleophilic addition is a kind of 1, 4 addition reaction.

PROBLEM 10.5

1. Explain why
   (a) vinyl alcohol is unstable.
   (b) vinyl chloride is inert.
2. Suggest the probable mechanism of
   (a) $(CH_3)_2-C=CH-COCH_3 + HBr$
   (b) $CH_3-CH=CH-CHO + HCN$

i. *Michael Reaction*: One of the most important reactions of α, β-unsaturated carbonyl of the type nucleophilic addition to carbon-carbon double bond, is Michael reaction. This reaction involves the condensation between α, β-unsaturated carbonyl compound and compound having active methylene group, such as malonic ester, aceto acetic ester, nitro alkane having α-H atom. In this reaction compound having active methylene serves as the source of carbanion (nucleophile) and the reaction is carried out in presence of base, alkoxide. Thus,

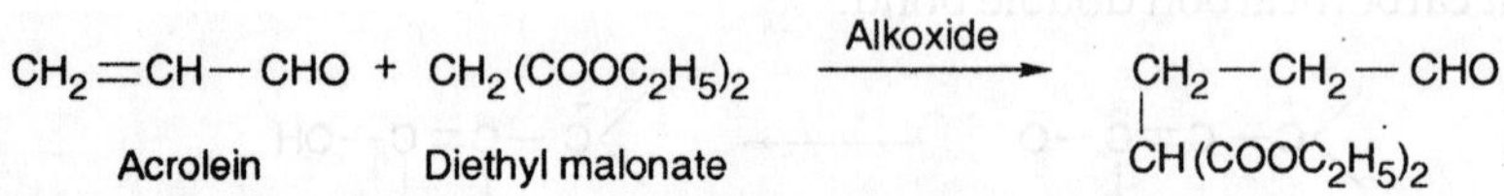

Carbanion is produced from malonic ester as below:

$$CH_2(COOC_2H_5)_2 \xrightarrow{\bar{O}R} \bar{C}H(COOEt)_2 + H^+$$

Next the reaction follows the general path. Michael reaction is a characteristic reaction of α, β-unsaturated carbonyl compounds and has wide synthetic applications. In this connection synthesis of *dimedone* may be mentioned. It is an well known reagent for quantitative estimation of formaldehyde. It is synthesised as described below:

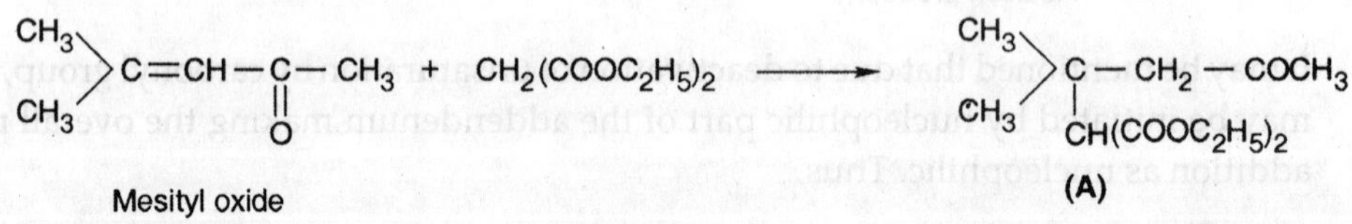

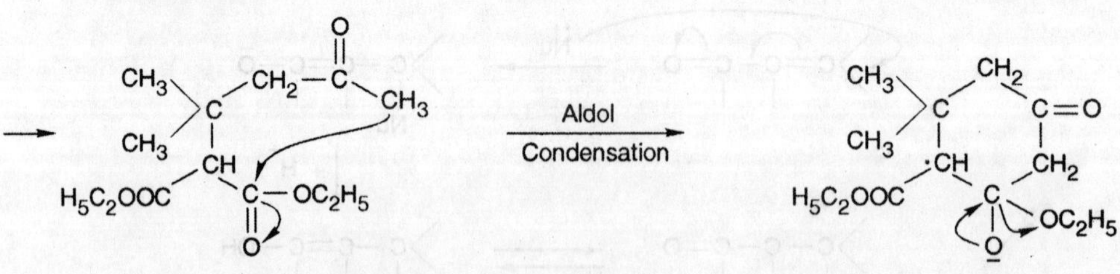

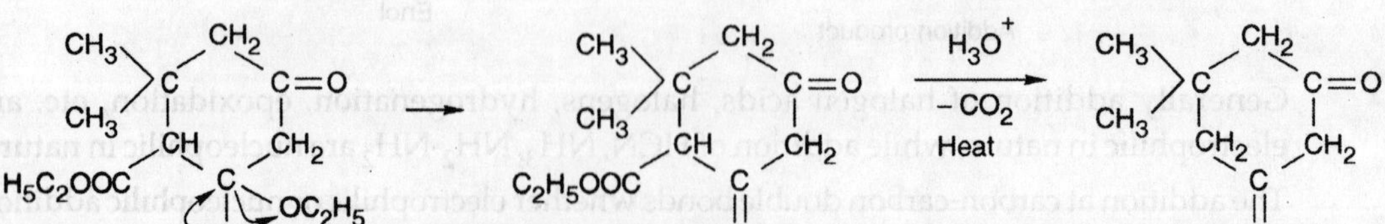

Dimedone

ii. *Diels-Alder Reaction*: It is another important reaction undergone by α, β-unsaturated carbonyl compounds. It can also be looked upon as proceeding through 1:4 addition. α, β-unsaturated carbonyl compounds in this reaction acts as *dienophile* and it adds to a *diene* to generate a cyclic compound. The reaction does not require any reagent, acidic or basic. It occurs only on heating. Recently this type of reaction has been classified as *pericyclic reaction* and is explained on the basis of conservation of orbital symmetry.

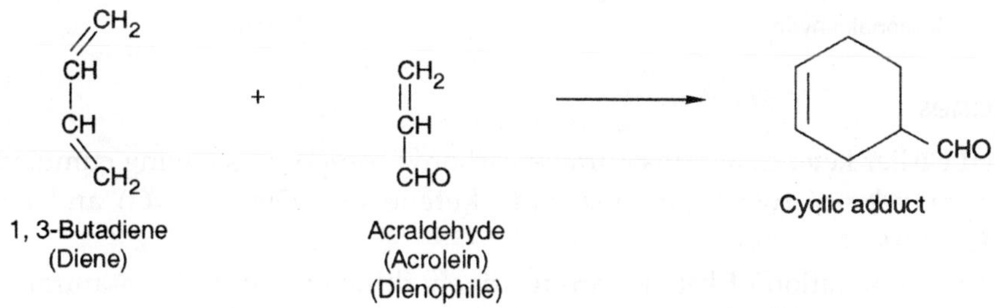

(b) *Nucleophilic addition to carbonyl compounds*: α, β-unsaturated carbonyl compounds can undergo nucleophilic addition at carbonyl group under certain conditions. Thus,

$$\underset{\text{Crotonaldehyde}}{CH_3-CH=CH-CHO} + HCN \longrightarrow \underset{\text{Cyanohydrin}}{CH_3-CH=CH-CH(OH)-CN}$$

$$\underset{\text{Acrolein}}{CH_2=CH-CHO} + HCN \longrightarrow \underset{\text{Cyanohydrin}}{CH_2=CH-CH(OH)-CN}$$

(c) *Some specific reactions*:

i. *Cannizzaro reaction*

$$\underset{\text{Acraldehyde}}{CH_2=CH-CHO + CH_2=CH-CHO} \xrightarrow[\text{Tischenko}]{Al(OC_2H_5)_3} \underset{\text{Allylacrylate}}{CH_2=CH-\overset{\overset{O}{\|}}{C}-OCH_2-CH=CH_2}$$

ii. *Retro aldol condensation*

$$\underset{\text{Acraldehyde}}{CH_2=CH-CHO} \xrightarrow{NaOH} \underset{\text{Formaldehyde}}{HCHO} + \underset{\text{Acetaldehyde}}{CH_3-CHO}$$

This retro aldol may be explained as under:

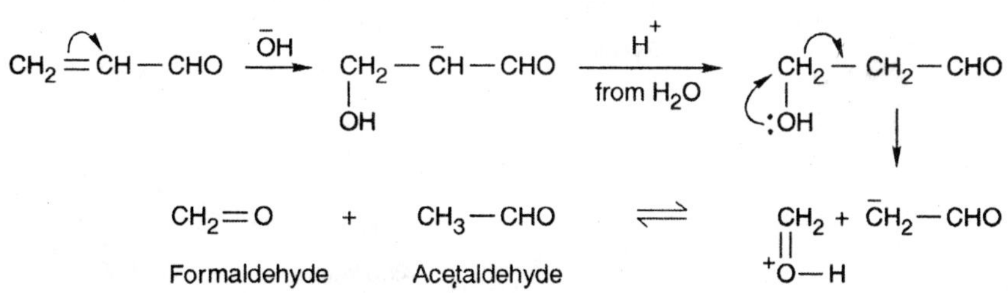

iii. *Selective reduction*

$$\underset{\text{Acraldehyde}}{CH_2{=}CH{-}CHO} \xrightarrow{LiAlH_4} \underset{\text{Allyl alcohol}}{CH_2{=}CH{-}CH_2OH}$$

iv. *Tollen's reaction*

$$\underset{\text{Crotonaldehyde}}{CH_3{-}CH{=}CH{-}CHO} \xrightarrow{Ag_2O} \underset{\text{Crotonic acid}}{CH_3{-}CH{=}CH{-}COOH} + Ag^{o}$$

10.7.2 Ketenes

As mentioned earlier ketenes are unsaturated carbonyl compounds having cumulated double bonds. They may be of two types, viz, aldo ketene ($R{-}CH{=}C{=}O$) and keto ketene [$(R)_2{-}C{=}C{=}O$)].

Preparation: Preparation of ketenes are relatively difficult than α, β-unsaturated carbonyl compounds. Following methods are usually adopted for their preparation:

i. *From carbonyl compounds*: When the vapour of carbonyl compound is passed over a coil of resistance wire heated to red hot, ketenes are formed.

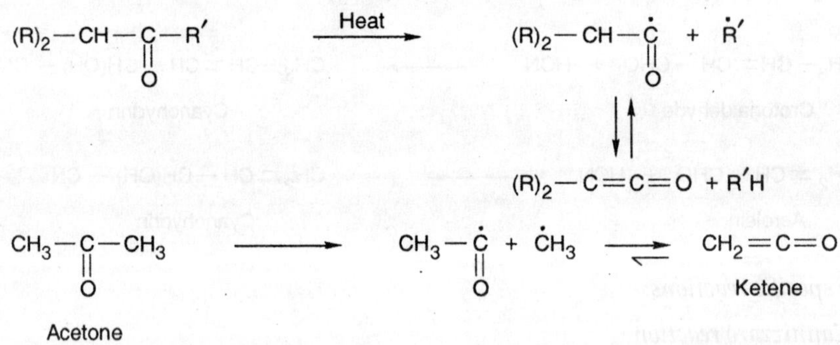

ii. *From acid chloride*: Acid chloride having α-H on refluxing in pyridine solution affords aldoketene.

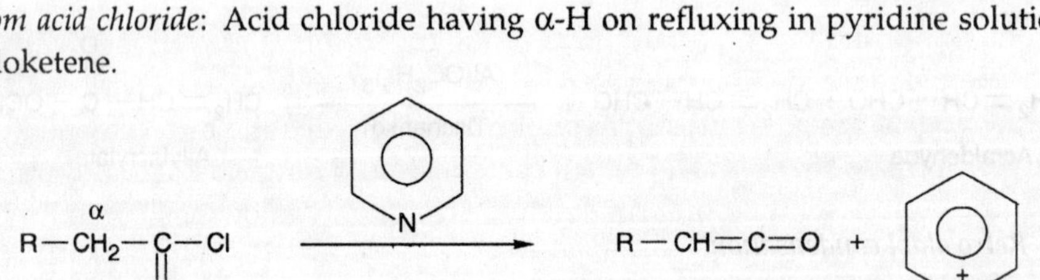

α-H is acidic and is abstracted in presence of base and so the reaction proceeds as below:

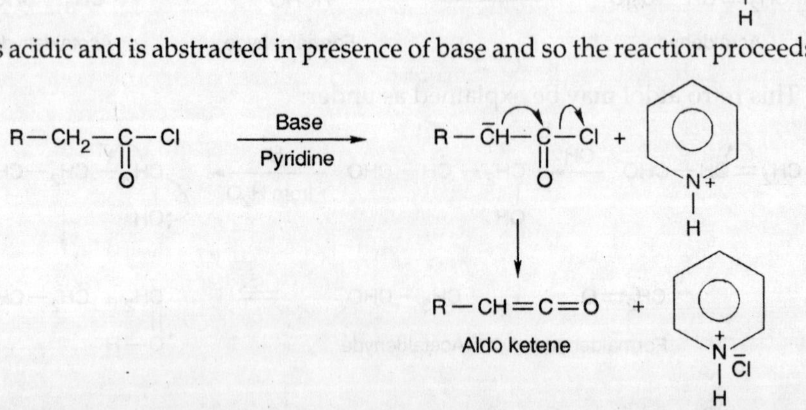

iii. *From α-halo acyl halide*: Treatment of α-halo acyl halide with metallic Zn readily affords ketene.

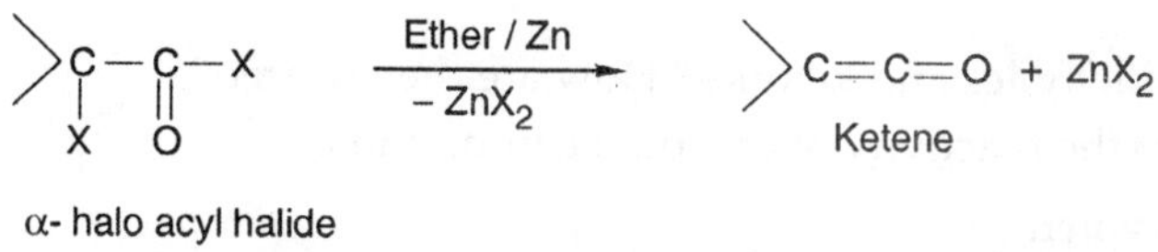

This method is considered as a general method.

Properties of Ketenes: Ketenes undergo some unusual reaction which may be summarised as below:

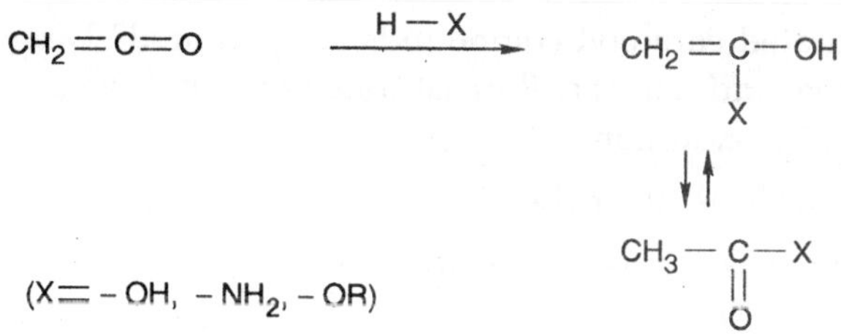

Depending upon the nature of X, variety of products may be obtained. Ketene is used as an useful acetylating agent.

Ketene is unsatable and readily dimerises.

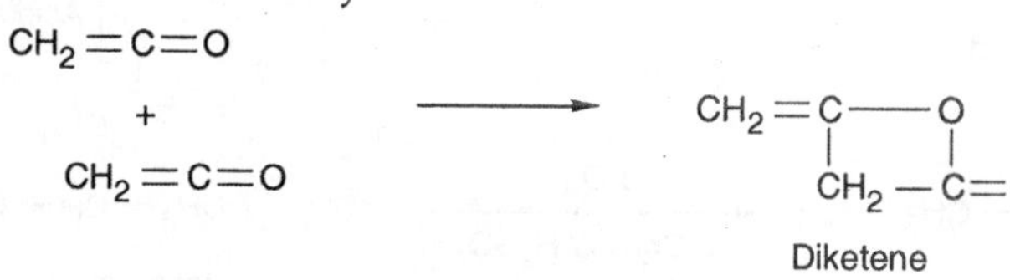

10.8 Uses of Carbonyl Compounds

Carbonyl compounds are an important class of organic compounds having pharmaceutical importance. Aldehydes are the first member of organic chemical used as hypnotics. Chloral (Tri chloro acetaldehyde) is a reiable and safe hypnotic. Paraldehydes and butyl chloral hydrate are strong sedatives. Formaldehyde is an excellent bactericide and fungicide. It is also employed for disinfection pupose. 40% solution of formal dehyde commonly known as **Formalin** is applied for hardening of skin and anatomical specimen and to prevent excessive perspiration. Paraldehyde is used as an active ingredient of contraceptive creams and glutaraldehyde known as **Cidex** is used as a sterilizing solution for equipments and surgical instruments. Most of the ketones were found to have hypnotic properties. α, β-Unsaturated ketones possess high diuretic activity and acrolin (α, β-unsaturated) is used as an insecticide. This class of organic compounds are also used for other purposes. Thus, formaldehyde is used for the preparation of phenol-formaldehyde and urea-formaldehyde resins. Acetone is employed for the preparation of medicinal compounds and as a solvent.

Model Questions

1. (a) What are aldehydes and ketones? How are they related?
   (b) Account for the reactivity of carbonyl compounds.
2. What happens when
   (a) acetaldehyde is treated with NaOH?
   (b) formaldehyde is treated with NaOH?
   (c) acetone is heated with barium hydroxide?
   (d) calcium acetate is heated?
3. How α, β-unsaturated carbonyl compounds are prepared? Discuss their characteristic reactions. Show that addition of α, β-unsaturated carbonyl compound at olefinic position proceeds through 1 : 4-addition.
4. What are ketenes? Discuss their chemisty.
5. How will you synthesise acetone from acetaldehyde?

Hints:

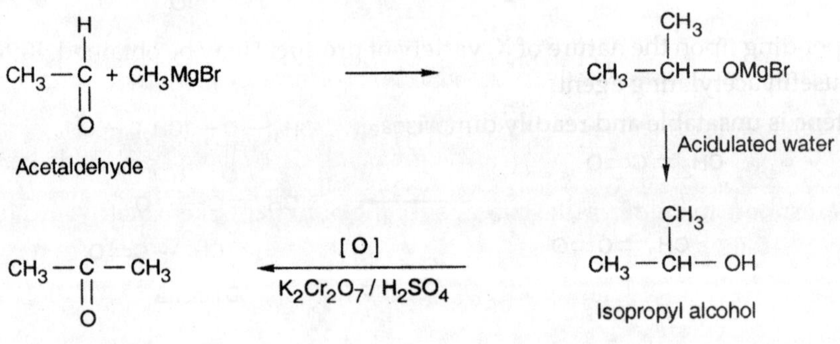

6. Describe the addition of sodium bisulphite to carbonyl compound. What is the utility of this reaction?
7. Write notes on:
   (a) Reformatsky reaction.
   (b) Aldol condensation.
   (c) Cannizzaro reaction.
   (d) Michael reaction.
   (e) Halogenation of carbonyl compounds.
   (f) Clemmenson reduction.
   (g) Wolf-Kishner reduction.
   (h) Oxidation of aldehydes with Tollen's reagent and Fehling solution.
   (i) Knoevenagel reaction.
   (j) Haloform reaction.
   (k) Meerwein-Pondorff-Verley reduction.
   (l) Diels-Alder reaction.
8. How would you distinguish a ketone and an aldehyde by chemical tests?

Hints: Tollen's reagent and Fehling solution.

9. Explain:
   (a) Alkenes undergo electrophilic addition reactions while carbonyl compounds undergo nucleophilic addition reaction.
   (b) Formaldehyde does not undergo aldol condensation.
   Hints: For aldol condensation presence of α-H is essential. Formaldehyde does not have any α-H atom.
   (c) Acetaldehyde undergoes aldol condensation but trimethyl acetaldehyde does not.
   Hints: Trimethyl acetaldehyde does not have α-H atom but acetaldehyde possesses α-H atom.

10. How would you distinguish the following pairs by simple chemical test?
   (a) CH_3CHO and $CH_3-\underset{\underset{O}{\|}}{C}-CH_3$
   (b) CH_3CHO and CH_3-CH_2-CHO
   (c) $CH_3-\underset{\underset{O}{\|}}{C}-CH_2-CH_2-CH_3$ and $CH_3-CH_2-\underset{\underset{O}{\|}}{C}-CH_2-CH_3$

   Hints: (a) Tollen's reagent and Fehling solution.
   (b) (c) Iodoform test — CH_3-CHO and $CH_3-\underset{\underset{O}{\|}}{C}-(CH_2)_2-CH_3$

   will respond to iodoform test because of the presence of keto methyl group but others do not have keto methyl group and so they will not respond to iodoform test.

11. Write all the possible isomers of the compound with molecular formula, C_4H_8O and give their IUPAC names.

12. Identify (A), (B) and (C).

$$CH_3-\underset{\underset{O}{\|}}{C}-CH_3 \xrightarrow{LiAlH_4} (A) \xrightarrow{SOCl_2} (B) \xrightarrow{Alc.\ KOH} (C)$$

Hints:

(A) $CH_3-\underset{\underset{OH}{|}}{CH}-CH_3$ Isopropyl alcohol (B) $CH_3-\underset{\underset{Cl}{|}}{CH}-CH_3$ Isopropyl chloride (C) $CH_3-CH=CH_2$ Propene

13. How will you synthesise acetaldehyde from formaldehyde?

Hints:

$$\underset{\text{Formaldehyde}}{\begin{matrix}H \\ H\end{matrix}\!\!>C=O} + CH_3MgBr \longrightarrow CH_3-CH_2-OMgBr$$

$$CH_3-CH_2-OMgBr \xrightarrow{\text{Decomposition with acidulated water}} \underset{\text{Ethanol}}{CH_3-CH_2OH}$$

$$\underset{\text{Ethanol}}{CH_3-CH_2OH} \xrightarrow[K_2Cr_2O_7\,/\,H_2SO_4]{[O]} \underset{\text{Acetaldehyde}}{CH_3CHO}$$

14. Write important pharmaceutical uses of carbonyl compounds.
15. How is formalin prepared? Give its properties and uses.
16. Give methods preparation, properties and uses of acetaldehyde.
17. How is chloral prepared? What are its properties and uses?
18. How is pentaerythritol tetranitrate prepared? Mention its main uses.

CHAPTER ELEVEN

Carboxylic Acids

Organic compounds containing carboxylic functionality ($-C(=O)-OH$) are known as carboxylic acids.

These acids are represented by the general structure

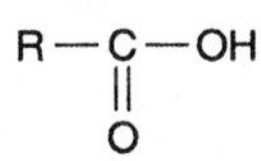

R may be either any alkyl or any aryl group. When R is any aliphatic organic group, the acid is aliphatic carboxylic, but if R is any aryl substituent, the corresponding acid is termed as aromatic carboxylic acid.

Classification: Depending upon the number of carboxylic groups present, carboxylic acids are classified as:

(a) *Monocarboxylic acids*: These compounds contain only one carboxyl function ($-C(=O)-OH$).

Some of the common members of aliphatic monocarboxylic acids are:

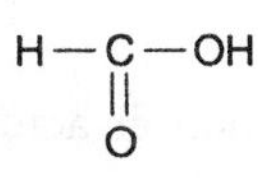

Formic acid

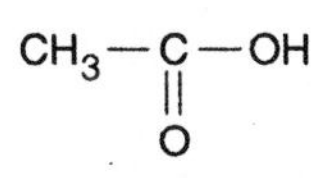

Acetic acid

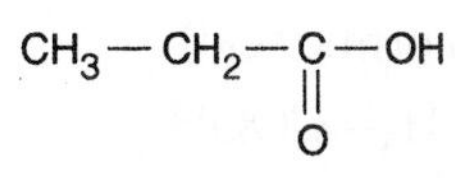

Propionic acid

(b) *Dicarboxylic acids*: In these acids two carboxylic groups are present. Some well known members are:

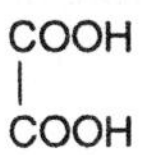

Oxalic acid

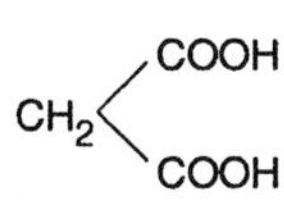

Malonic acid

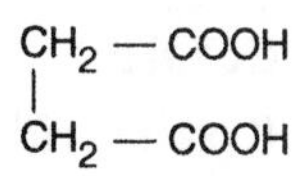

Succinic acid

(c) *Tricarboxylic acids*: As the name suggests they contain three carboxylic functions in their molecules. The most well studied member of this class is citric acid:

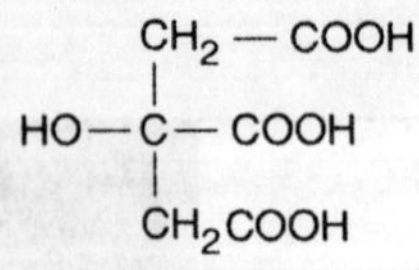

Citric acid

11.1 Monocarboxylic Acids

Among the carboxylic acids, monocarboxylic acids are the most common.

11.2 Nomenclature of Monocarboxylic Acids

There are two systems for naming carboxylic acids, viz, (i) *common system* and (ii) *IUPAC system*.

According to *common system*, names of carboxylic acids are derived from the source from which they are obtained. For examples.

Name	Source
$H—COOH$ Formic acid	*Formica* (ant)
$CH_3—COOH$ Acetic acid	Acetum (vinegar)
$CH_3—CH_2—CH_2—COOH$ Butyric acid	Butyrum (butter)
$CH_3—CH_2—CH_2—CH_2—COOH$ Valeric acid	Valerian (name of plant)
$CH_3(CH_2)_4—COOH$ Caproic acid (bad odour of goat)	Caper (goat)

In *IUPAC* system carboxylic acids are named by adding '—oic' to the name of alkane containing longest chain of carbon to which —COOH group is attached. For examples, (common names are: mentioned in parenthesis.)

Acid	Name
$H—COOH$ (Formic acid)	Methanoic acid
$CH_3—COOH$ (Acetic acid)	Ethanoic acid
$CH_3—CH_2—COOH$ (Propionic acid)	Propanoic acid
$COOH$ | $COOH$ (Oxalic acid)	Ethanedioic acid
$CH_2—COOH$ | $CH_2—COOH$ (Succinic acid)	Butanedioic acid

In the case of substituted acids, the position of the subsituent is indicated by number, the carboxylic carbon is always given number I. Thus,

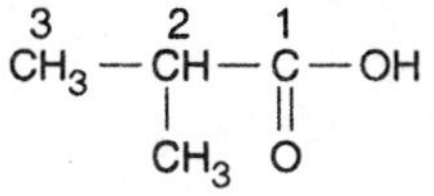

2-Methyl propane-I carboxylic acid

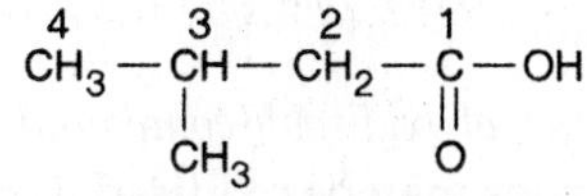

3-Methyl butane-I carboxylic acid

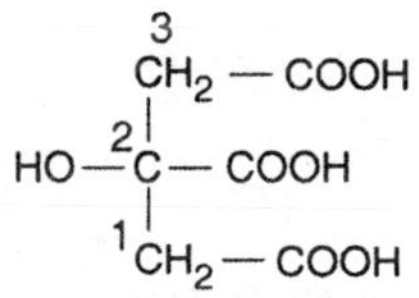

2-hydroxy propane-1, 2, 3 tricarboxylic acid (Citric acid)

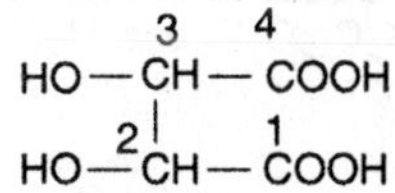

2, 3-dihydroxy butane dioic acid (Tartaric acid)

11.3 Structure of Carboxylic Group

Carboxylic group may be represented by the general structure(I) which resonates with the structure (II)

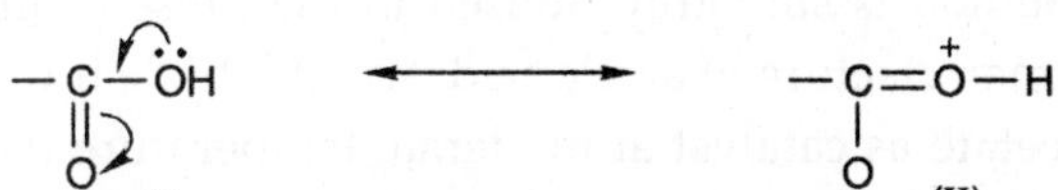

(I) (II)

Out of these two structures, structure (I) is stable because there is no separation of charges. Thus, carboxylic group is a resonance hybrid of structures (I) and (II) in which structure (I) has major contribution while the structure (II) makes minor contribution. The actual structure should be average of (I) and (II) and may be represented by the structure (III).

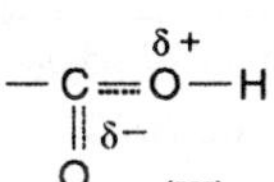

(III)

From molecular orbital point of view, structure (III) may be represented as (IV).

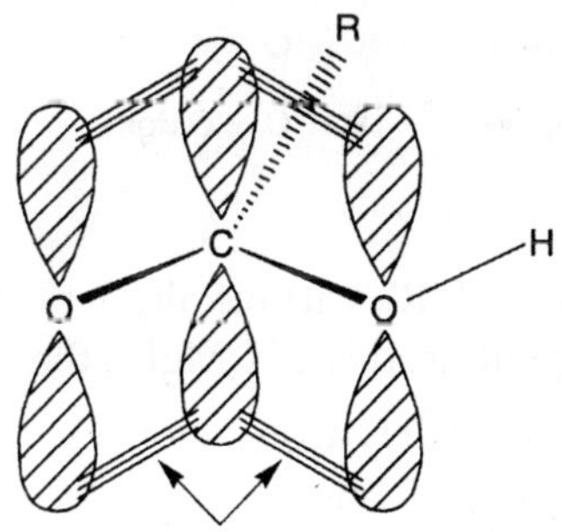

(IV)

The support in favour of resonance-hydrbid structure has been secured from bond length measurements. Carbon-oxygen bond length in carboxyl group has been found to be 1.22Å which is much shorter than normal carbon-oxygen σ-bond (1.30Å).

11.4 Methods of Preparation of Monocarboxylic Acids

Some of the most common and useful methods for the preparation of monocarboxylic acid are depicted below:

(a) *Oxidation of oxidisable compounds*: Easily oxidisable compounds like primary alcohols and aldehydes may be oxidised to carboxylic acids.

$$R-CH_2OH \xrightarrow[K_2Cr_2O_7\,/\,\text{conc. } H_2SO_4]{[O]} \underset{\text{Aldehyde}}{R-CHO} \xrightarrow[K_2Cr_2O_7\,/\,\overset{+}{H}]{[O]} \underset{\text{Acid}}{R-COOH}$$

Examples :

$$\underset{\text{Methanol}}{CH_3OH} \xrightarrow[K_2Cr_2O_7\,/\,\overset{+}{H}]{[O]} \underset{\text{Formaldehyde}}{H_2C{=}O} \xrightarrow[K_2Cr_2O_7\,/\,\overset{+}{H}]{[O]} \underset{\text{Formic acid}}{H-COOH}$$

$$\underset{\text{Ethanol}}{CH_3-CH_2OH} \xrightarrow[\text{conc. } H_2SO_4]{K_2Cr_2O_7} \underset{\text{Acetaldehyde}}{CH_3-CHO} \xrightarrow[K_2Cr_2O_7\,/\,\overset{+}{H}]{[O]} \underset{\text{Acetic acid}}{CH_3-COOH}$$

This oxidative method is smoothly utilised in the present time for the *manufacture of acetic acid*. In the manufacture of acetic acid, acetaldehyde is oxidised by air in presence of manganous acetate as catalyst at moderate temperature (60-70 °C). A concentrated solution of acetaldehyde is taken in a reaction flask to which small amount of manganous acetate is added. A current of air is allowed to pass through the reaction mixture, and the temperature is kept at 60-70 °C when crude acetic acid having 95 per cent concentration is obtained. This is purified by distillation. Reactions taking place are

$$\underset{\text{Acetaldehyde}}{CH_3-\overset{\displaystyle O}{\overset{\|}{C}}-H} \xrightarrow[Mn(OOCCH_3)_2,\ 60\text{-}70^{\circ}C]{O_2} \underset{\text{Acetic acid}}{CH_3-\overset{\displaystyle O}{\overset{\|}{C}}-OH}$$

(b) *By the action of Grignard reagent on carbon-dioxide*:

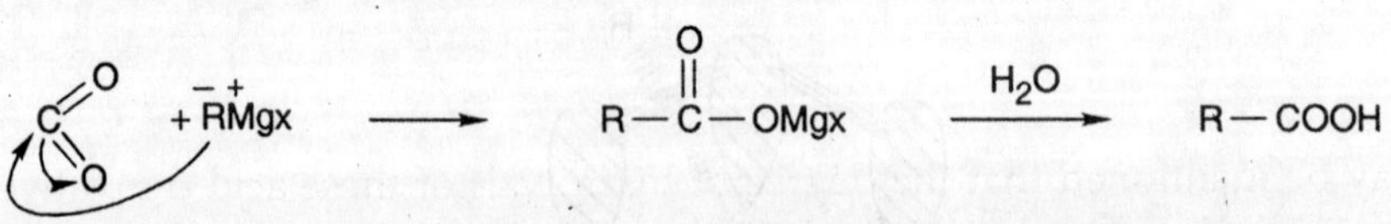

Depending upon the nature of 'R', various aliphatic carboxylic acids may be obtained. Thus, when Grignard reagent used is CH_3MgBr, the acid obtained is acetic acid.

(c) *Hydrolysis of nitriles* (cyanides): Hydrolysis of alkyl nitriles either by acids or alkalis, results in the formation of acids. Thus,

$$\underset{\text{Nitrite}}{R-C{\equiv}N} \xrightarrow[\text{Acid or alkali}]{H_2O} \underset{\text{Acid}}{R-COOH} + NH_3$$

(d) *Hydrolysis of acid derivatives*: Some carboxylic acid derivatives like acid chloride, acid amides, anhydrides and esters on hydrolysis in presence of acid or alkali furnish carboxylic acids.

i. 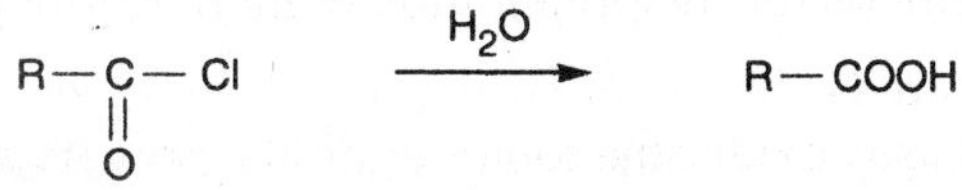

Acid chloride

ii. 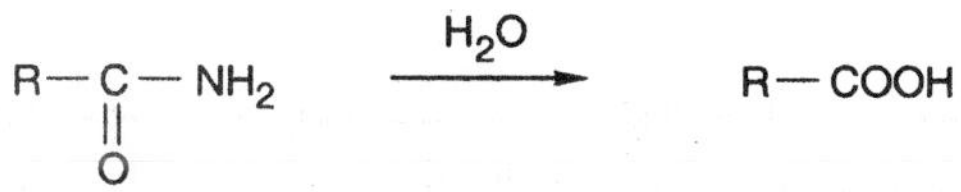

iii. 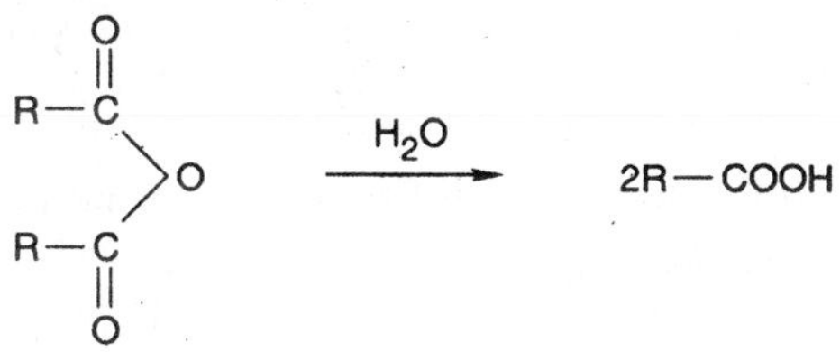

Acid anhydride

iv. 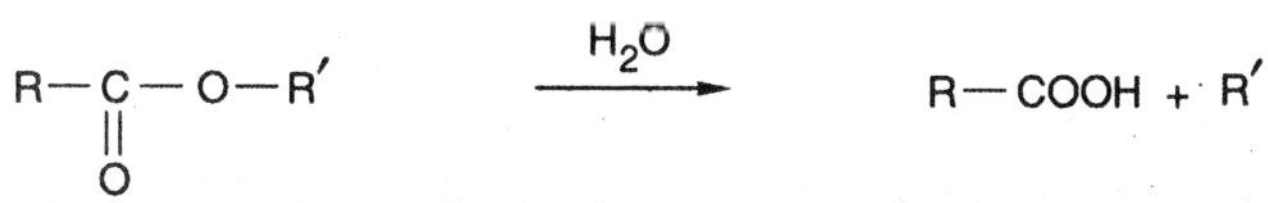

Depending upon the nature of R, variety of carboxylic acids may be formed in the hydrolysis of these acid derivatives. Mechanistic paths of hydrolysis of all these derivatives are similar involving the initial attack by water to carbonylic carbon followed by cleavage of carbon-hetero atom, i.e.,

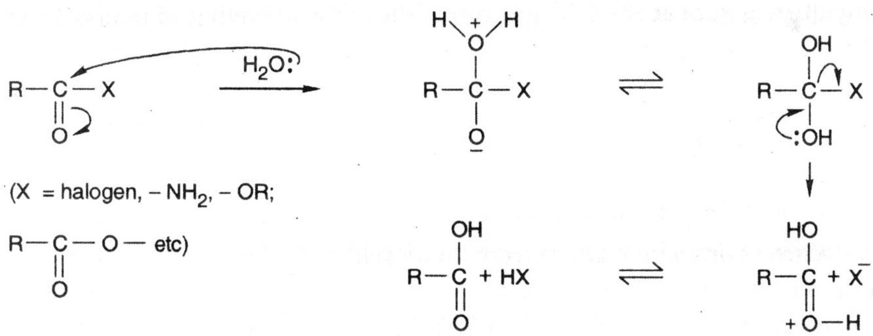

Acid

It may be mentioned that the degree of hydrolysis of these acid derivatives is not the same. The order of hydrolysis of these derivatives may be written as below:

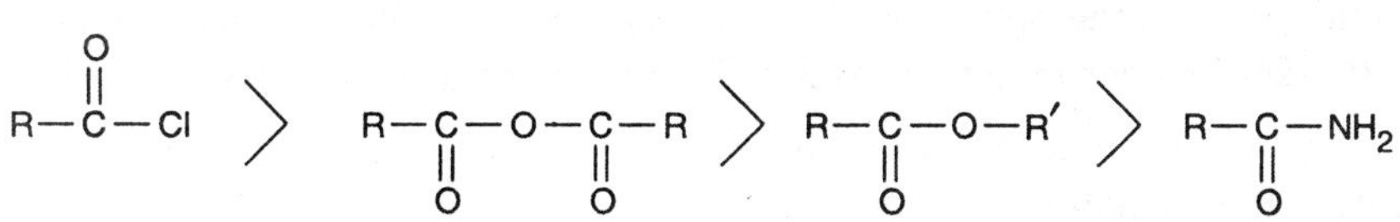

(e) *Decarboxylation of dicarboxylic acids*: Dicarboxylic acids particularly those in which both the carboxylic groups are connected to the same carbon atom are not so stable and hence if they are heated in presence of suitable catalyst can yield carboxylic acid by losing a molecule of carbon dioxide. Thus,

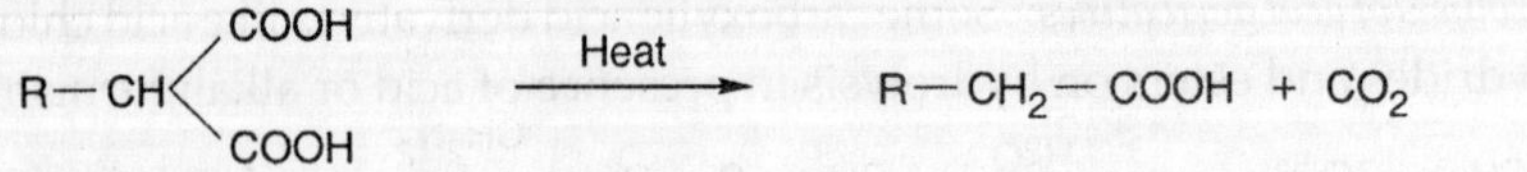

By this method, formic acid is prepared in laboratory using anhydrous glycerol as catalyst. In laboratory a mixture of anhydrous glycerol and oxalic acid taken in a flask is heated at a temperature of 110 °C when aqueous solution of formic acid is distilled over to a collector. Reaction taking place is given below:

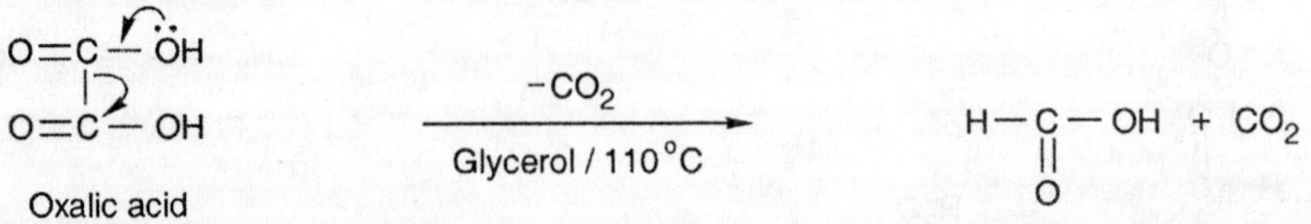

Oxalic acid

The aqueous formic acid is treated with lead carbonate when lead formate is obtained to which H_2S is allowed to pass when *anhydrous formic acid* is obtained. Anhydrous formic acid can also be prepared by heating sodium formate with sodium bislulphate, i.e.,

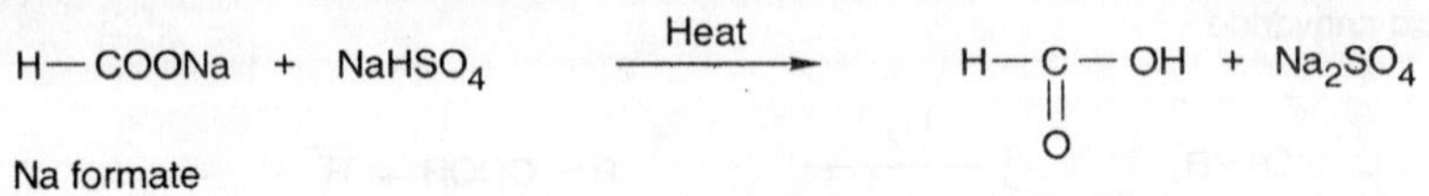

Na formate

Formic acid

(f) *By the reaction of carbon monoxide and alkoxide*: Salts of carboxylic acids may be obtained by the reaction between carbon monoxide and an alkoxide. Thus,

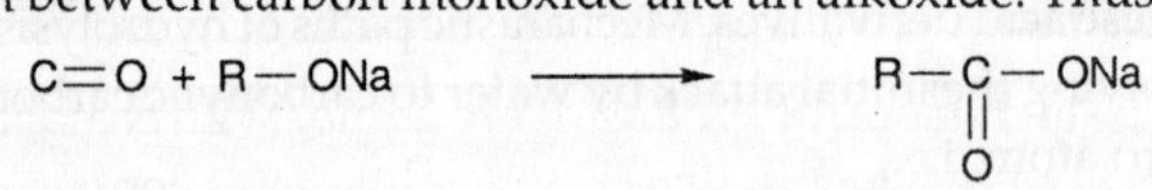

But if alkali is used in place of alkoxide, salts of formic acid is obtained. Thus,

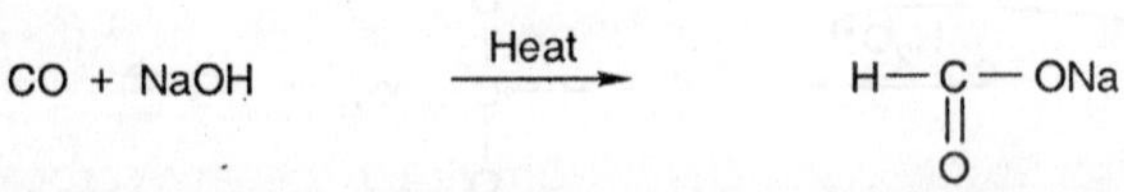

Na-formate

Formic acid is industrially prepared by this method.

(g) *Arndt-Eistert synthesis*: Starting from lower acid its higher homologue may be smoothly prepared by the application of this synthesis. This synthetic process involves the conversion of starting carboxylic acid into its acid chloride which on treatment with diazomethane furnishes diazomethyl ketone. Diazomethyl ketone formed is treated with Ag_2O followed by hydrolysis when higher acid is formed. Thus,

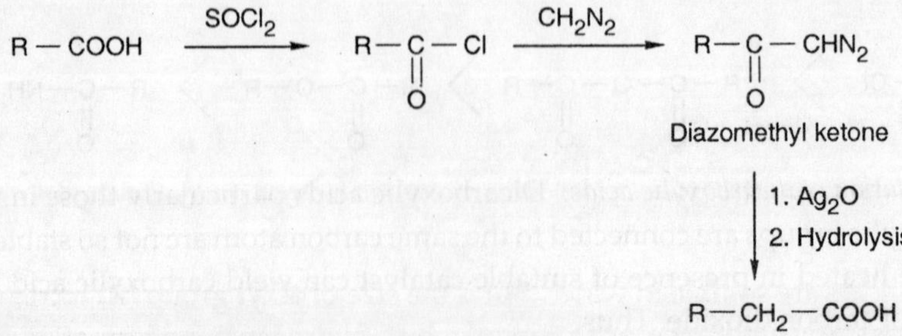

Diazomethyl ketone

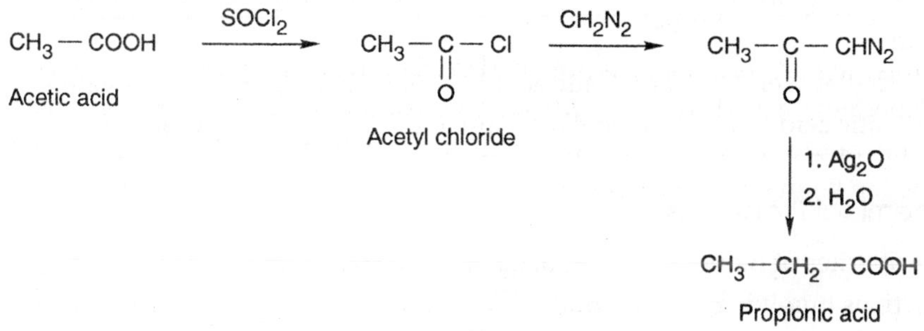

PROBLEM 11.1

(a) How will you prepare anhydrous formic acid?

(b) Complete the following reactions:

i. $CO + RONa \longrightarrow$

ii. $CH_3COOH + SOCl_2 \longrightarrow (A) \xrightarrow[\text{2. } Ag_2O]{\text{1. } CH_2N_2} (B)$

11.5 Properties of Monocarboxylic Acids

11.5.1 Physical Properties

Lower members (C_1—C_8) of monocarboxylic acids are liquids with characteristic odours. Formic, acetic and propionic acids have vinegar- like odours while acids containing C_4 to C_8 have goat-like odours. These acids are formed by bacteria and in trace amounts are present in the secretions of skin of mammals. Due to the difference in metabolic paths in different persons the odours coming out of different persons may be different. This difference enables the dog, specially trained for this purpose, to differentiate one person from other. Higher carboxylic acids are wax-like semisolids.

Carboxylic acids as a class has higher boiling points than alcohols of comparable molecular weights. This is due to their ability to form intermolecular hydrogen bonds as indicated below:

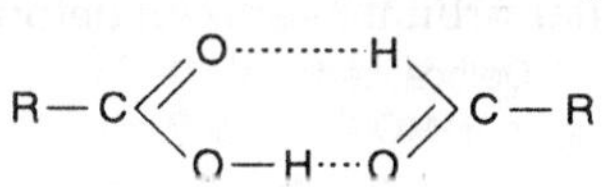

From the above it is evident that carboxylic acids exist as *dimers.* As a result the size and the molecular weights are doubled. Consequently they will have higher boiling points. But similar dimerisation is not possible in alcohols. Further, they can also form hydrogen bond with water as shown below:

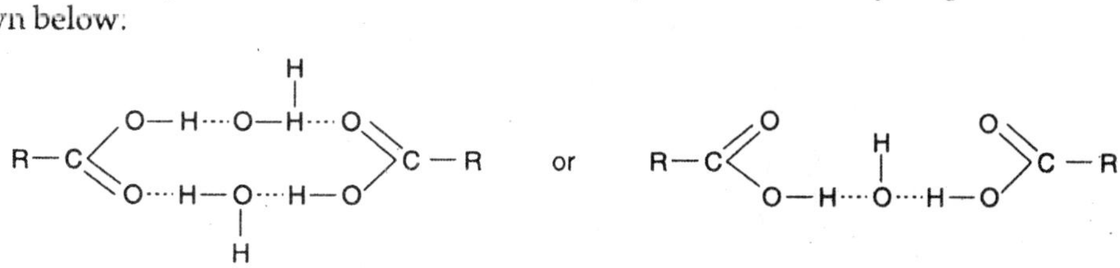

So carboxylic acids are soluble in water. But if the size of alkyl group (R) increases the long alkane chain creates steric hindrance, as a result of which hydrogen bond formation is disturbed. That is why higher members of monocarboxylic acids are insoluble in water.

Problem 11.2

Explain:
i. Molecular weight of propionic acid is double than the calculated value.
ii. Palmitic acid having molecular formula, $C_{18}H_{32}O_2$ is insoluble in water.

11.5.2 Chemical Properties

Chemical properties of monocarboxylic acids may be considered under following heads:

(a) Reactions involving, O—H bond.

(b) Reactions due to >C=O group.

(c) Reactions involving α-carbon atom.

(a) *Reactions due to* O—H *bond*: The most important property of carboxylic acids originating from O—H bond is their *acidity*. The acidity of carboxylic group primarily stems from the electron withdrawing tendency of > C = O bonding present in this functionality. As a result of such electron withdrawing tendency hydrogen atom attached to oxygen in O—H bond develops tendency to be released as proton, i.e.,

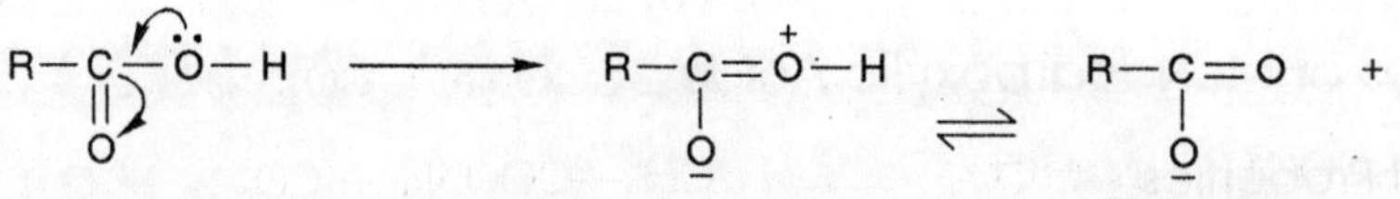

Again, the congugate base, the carboxylate anion that is formed can exist in resonance hybrid and hence is stabilised.

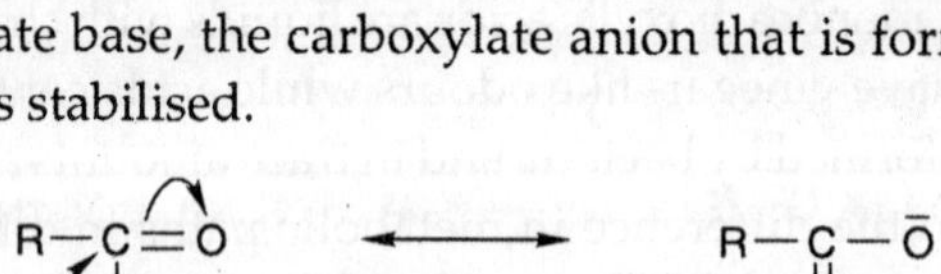

The molecular orbital picture also suggests that carboxylate anion is a stable species. *The carbon atom in this ion is in sp² state and forms σ-bonds with both the oxygen atoms and the unused p*-orbital of carbon overlaps with the *p*-orbitals of both the oxygen atoms forming an ideal delocalised molecular orbital as shown below:

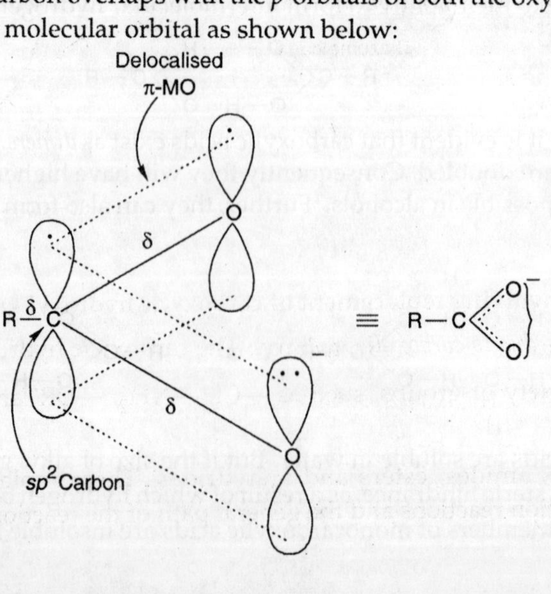

Thus, due to tendency of proton release as well as stability of conjugate base, carboxylic group and hence carboxylic acids possess perceptible acidity.

1. **Effect of substituents on Acidity:** The acidity of carboxylic group highly depends upon the nature of substituents on α-carbon atom. It has been observed that electron withdrawing substituent increases the acidity while presence of electron releasing group decreases the acidity. Thus, in the series.

$H-COOH$	CH_3-COOH	$Cl \leftarrow CH_2-COOH$
(I)	(II)	(III)
Formic acid	Acetic acid	Chloroacetic acid

The order of acidity is III > I > II.

The acidic character of carboxylic group is evidenced from the following reactions:

i. *Formation of salts:* Carboxylic acids react with alkalies and bicarbonates to form salts.

$$\underset{\text{Formic acid}}{H-COOH} + KOH \longrightarrow \underset{\text{Pot-formate}}{H-COOK} + H_2O$$

$$CH_3-COOH + KOH \longrightarrow \underset{\text{Pot-acetate}}{CH_3-COOK} + H_2O$$

$$H-COOH + NaHCO_3 \longrightarrow H-COONa + CO_2 + H_2O$$

$$CH_3-COOH + NaHCO_3 \longrightarrow CH_3-COONa + CO_2 + H_2O$$

ii. *Reaction with diazomethane:* Carboxylic acid when treated with diazomethane forms methyl ester replacing acidic hydrogen.

$$R-COOH + CH_2N_2 \longrightarrow \underset{\text{Methyl ester}}{R-COOCH_3} + N_2$$

Reaction occurs through the following path:

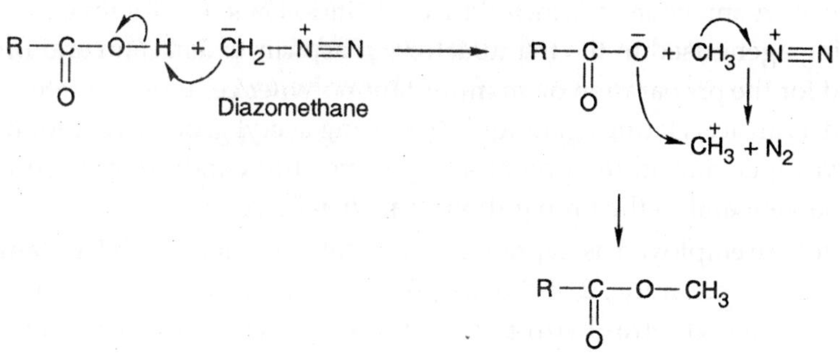

2. **Reactions involving replacement of carboxylic hydroxyl group:**

(a) *Reactions due to carboxylic hydroxyl:* The carboxylic hydroxyl group can be replaced by a variety of groups, such as —Cl, —NH_2, —OR′ and $O-\underset{\underset{O}{||}}{C}-R'$ forming acid chloride, amides, esters and anhydrides. These replacements are nucleophilic substitution reactions and the general path of the reaction may be traced as under:

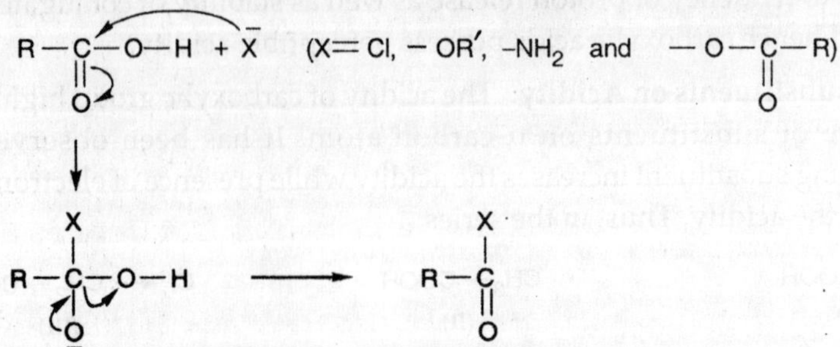

Thus,

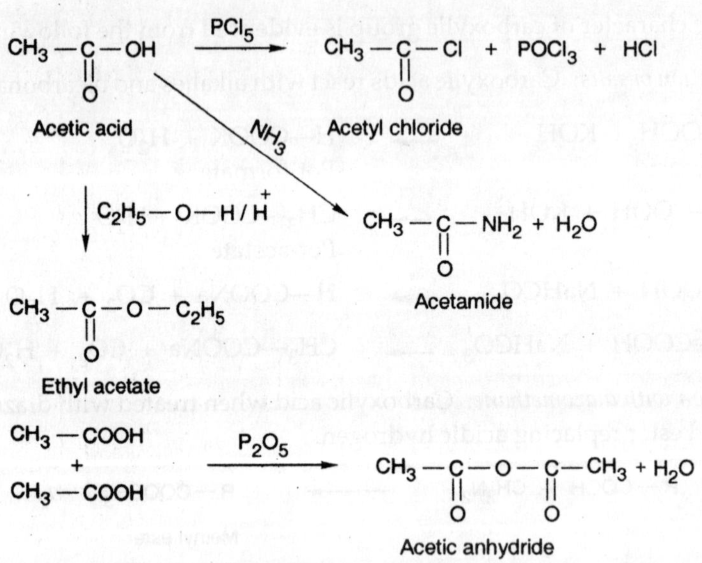

These acid derivatives are very useful reagents frequently employed in the preparation of variety of organic chemicals including medicines. Thus, acetic anhydride is an important acetylating agent used in the manufacture of aspirin, phenacetin and other drugs. It is also used for the preparation of an important polymer cellulose acetate. Acid chloride is also used as an acetylating agent for introducing acetyl group in compounds containing active hydrogen and in the preparation of dye-stuffs and pharmaceuticals. Esters are used as solvent and in the preparation of artificial essence.

Amides are employed as hypnotics and sedatives. Diethyl allyl acetamide (Novonal), diethyl bromo acetamide, 2, 4-dioxo-3, 3-diethyl tetrahydroxy pyridine (Persedon), 2, 4-dioxo-3, 3-diethyl tetra- hydropyridine (Methyprylon) are very effective and useful sedatives and hypnotics.

(b) *Reactions involving carboxylic carbonyl group*

i. The major reaction of carboxylic acids involving its carbonylic group is their *decarboxylation*. Carboxylic acids undergo decarboxylation reaction on heating. However, the ease of loss of CO_2 from carboxylic group depends upon the overall nature of the acids. It has been observed that decarboxylation proceeds smoothly if the heating is carried out in presence of sodalime. Thus,

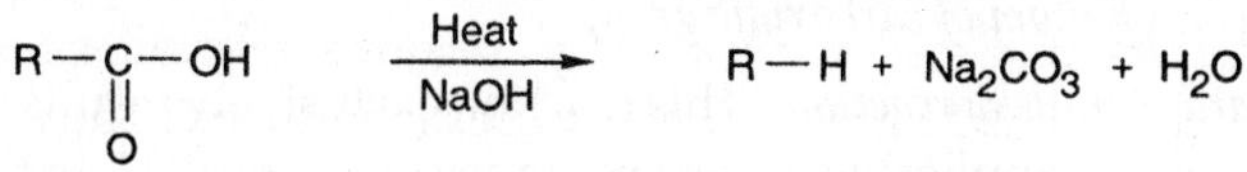

Mechanistically, decarboxylation takes place as under:

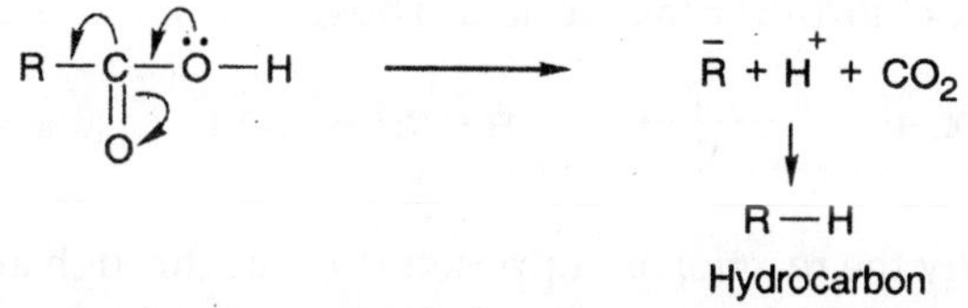

From the above path it is seen that decarboxylation is due to transmission of electrons from hydroxyl oxygen to alkyl group. So it is natural that higher the electron availability on hydroxyl oxygen, more rapid will be the decarboxylation. For this reason decarboxylation occurs smoothly in presence of sodalime. This is because carboxylic acids initially react with sodalime to form salt which readily ionises to yield carboxylate anion having higher electron density. Thus,

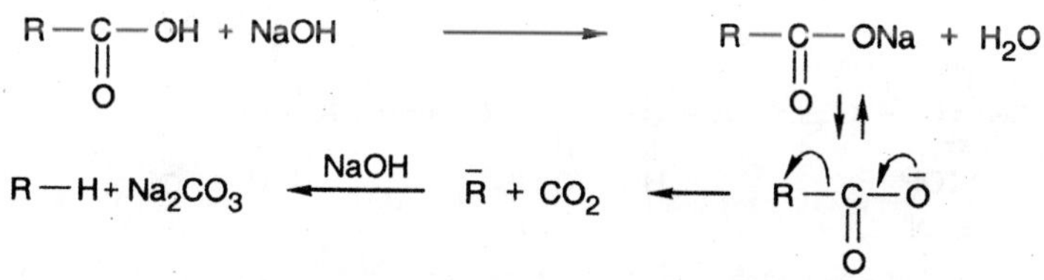

Decarboxylation of carboxylic acids has useful application in the synthesis of alkane (Kolbe synthesis), ketones (vide chapter **ten**) and in the preparation of alkyl halides.

ii. *Preparation of alkyl halides (Hunsdiecker Reaction)*: Silver salt of carboxylic acids on refluxing with bromine in carbon tetrachloride at 80 °C forms alkyl bromide. This is known as *Hunsdiecker reaction*.

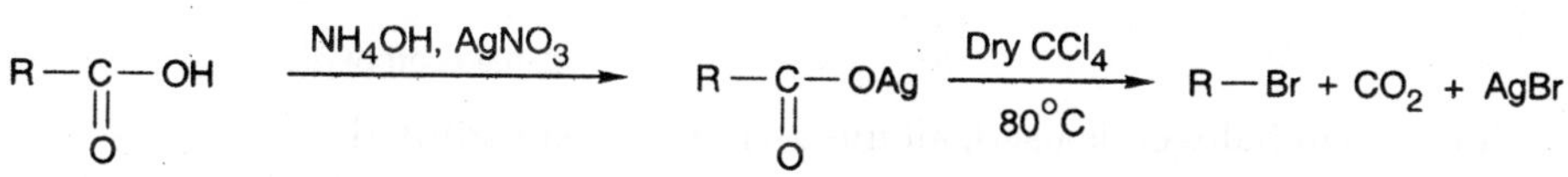

Mechanistically, this reaction may be explained as under:

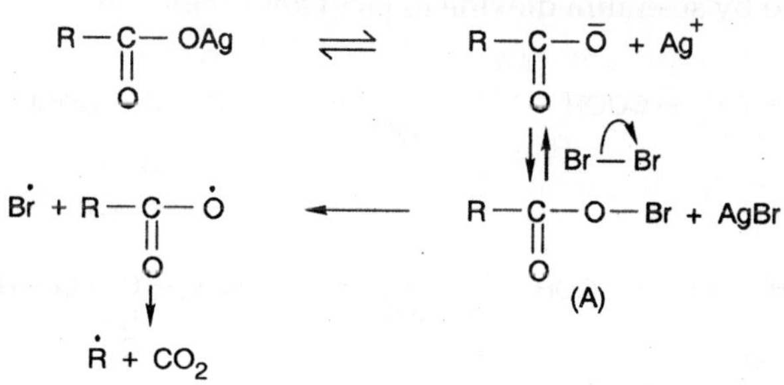

Now radical $\dot{R}$ combines with bromine salt (A):

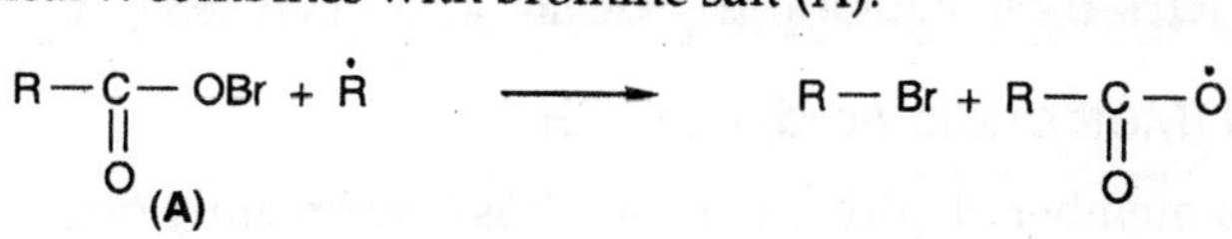

(c) *Reaction at α-carbon atom of carboxylic group:*

i. *Hell-Volhard-Zelinisky reaction*: This reaction exclusively results in the substitution at α-position and is applicable to carboxylic acids having α-H. In this reaction bromine or chlorine reacts smoothly in the presence of small quantity of phosphorous to form α-bromo- or α-chloro- carboxylic acid. Thus,

$$R-\overset{\alpha}{C}H_2-COOH \xrightarrow[P]{X_2} R-\underset{X}{\underset{|}{C}}H-COOH \quad \text{(where X = Cl or Br)}$$

Mechanistically the reaction is supposed to occur through an enol intermediate. The function of phosphorous is to act as halogen carrier by forming PX_3 with halogens, i.e,

$$2P + 3X_2 \longrightarrow 2PX_3$$

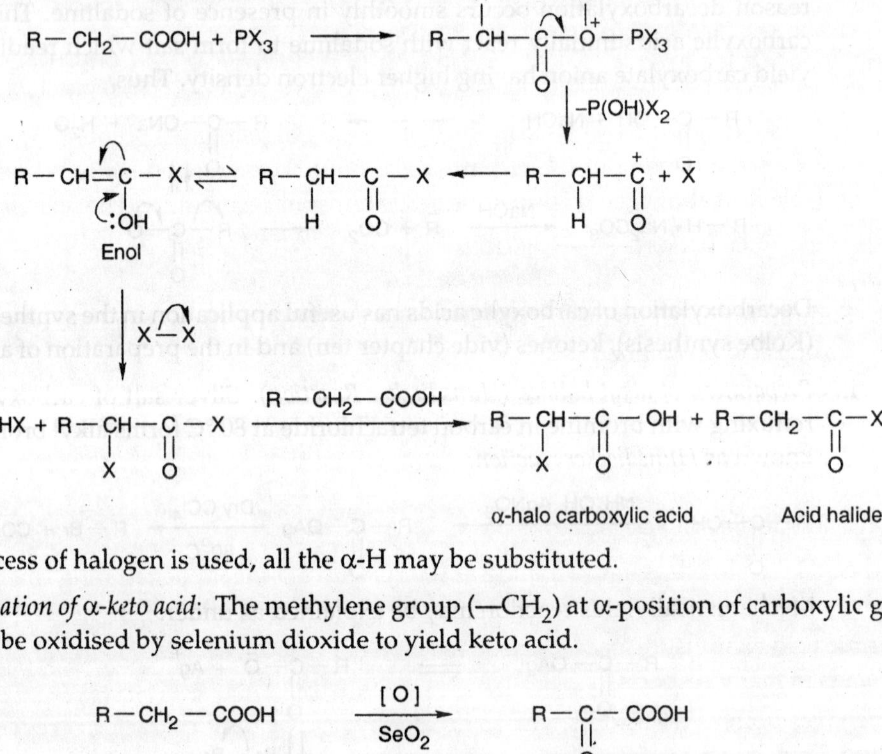

If excess of halogen is used, all the α-H may be substituted.

ii. *Formation of α-keto acid*: The methylene group ($—CH_2$) at α-position of carboxylic group may be oxidised by selenium dioxide to yield keto acid.

$$R-CH_2-COOH \xrightarrow[SeO_2]{[O]} R-\underset{O}{\underset{||}{C}}-COOH$$

α-keto acid

$$\underset{\text{Propionic acid}}{CH_3-CH_2-COOH} \xrightarrow[SeO_2]{[O]} \underset{\text{Pyruvic acid}}{CH_3-\underset{O}{\underset{||}{C}}-COOH}$$

11.6 Some Important Individual Members

11.6.1 Formic Acid (Methanoic Acid) HCOOH

Formic acid is the first member of fatty acid series. It is conveniently prepared by the following methods:

i. *Laboratory Preparation*: In laboratory formic acid is generally prepared by heating oxalic acid with glycerol at 100-110 °C. The reactions taking place are as under:

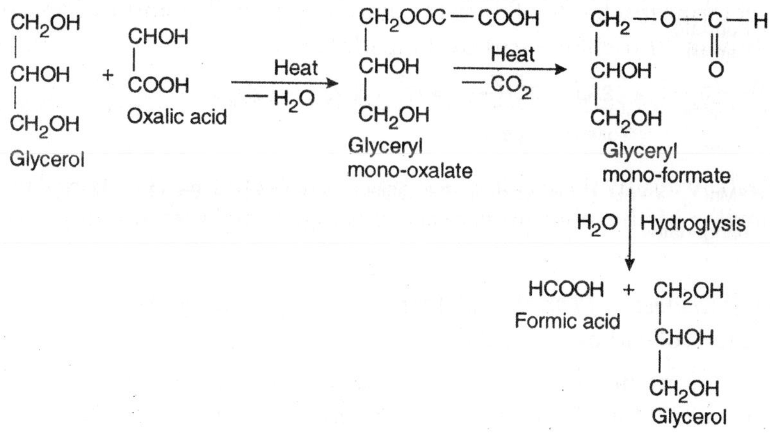

ii. *Industrial Preparation*: The most common industrial method of preparation of formic acid involves the heating of the mixture of carbon monoxide and sodium hydroxide in an autoclave at about 200 °C under the 6-10 atmospheric pressure. The yield is quantitative

$$\underset{}{CO + NaOH} \longrightarrow \underset{\text{Na-formate}}{HCOONa}$$

Sodium formate obtained is distilled with sodium hydrogen sulphate when anhydrous formic acid is obtained

$$HCOONa + NaHSO_4 \longrightarrow \underset{\substack{\text{Formic Acid} \\ \text{(Anhydrous)}}}{HCOOH} + Na_2SO_4$$

11.6.1.1 Properties of Formic Acid

Formic acid is a colourless liquid boiling at 100 °C with a pungent penetrating smell. It is highly corrosive producing blisters on the skin. It is soluble in water, ethanol and ether.

Formic acid exhibits the characteristic reactions of carboxylic acid. However, it differs from other acids in many respects.

It behaves both as an acid as well as an aldehyde. The dual character is revealed from its structure. Thus,

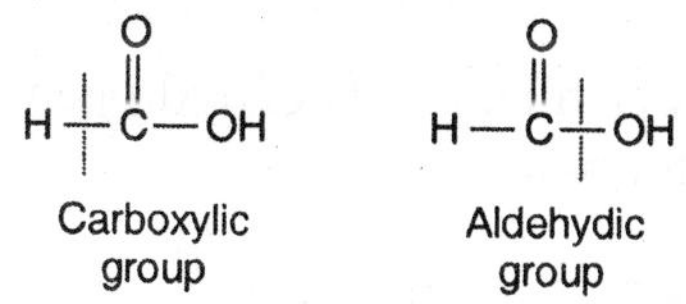

(a) i. *Aldehydic behaviour of formic acid*: Like other aldehydic compounds formic acid behaves as a strong reducing agent and reduces fehling's solution, Tollen's reagent, potassium permanganate, etc.

$$H-\underset{\underset{O}{\|}}{C}-\bar{O} + \underbrace{2Cu^{2+} + 5\bar{O}H}_{\text{Fehling's solution}} \longrightarrow C_3^{2-} + Cu_2O\downarrow + 3H_2O$$

Formate anion

$$H-\underset{\underset{O}{\|}}{C}-\bar{O} + \underbrace{2Ag^{+} + 3\bar{O}H}_{\text{Tollen's reagent}} \longrightarrow C_3^{2-} + 2Ag\downarrow + 2H_2O$$

$$H2MnO_4^- + 6H^+ \text{ (From acid)} + 5HCOOH \longrightarrow 2Mn^{2+} + 8H_2O + 5CO_2$$

Permanganate anion

ii. *Acidic Character of Formic acid:* Like other carboxylic acids it exhibits all the common reactions of carboxylic acids.

(b) Another important reaction of formic acid is that on dehydration with concentrated sulphuric acid it forms carbon monooxide in pure form.

$$HCOOH \xrightarrow{H_2SO_4} CO + H_2O$$

This reaction is utilised for the preparation of carbon monoxide in pure form in laboratory.

(c) Sodium or potassium salt of formic acid when heated at about 350 °C, it decomposes to form oxalate which on hydrolysis with dilute hydrochloric acid yields oxalic acid.

$$\underset{\text{Na-formate}}{2HCOONa} \xrightarrow[-H_2]{\text{Heat}} \underset{\text{Na-Oxalate}}{\begin{matrix}COONa\\|\\COONa\end{matrix}} \xrightarrow{HCl} \underset{\text{Oxalic acid}}{\begin{matrix}COOH\\|\\COOH\end{matrix}}$$

This reaction is used for the manufacture of oxalic acid.

11.6.1.2 Preparation of Anhydrous Formic Acid

Formic acid prepared in the laboratory or by the industrial process is not anhydrous in character. For preparation of anhydrous quality, aqueous solutions of formic acid is neutralised with lead carbonate (litharge) and the solution of lead formate obtained is filtered and evaporated to get the crystals of lead formate. These crystals are dried and heated at 100 °C in a current of hydrogen sulphide where anhydrous formic acid is distilled over.

$$\underset{\text{Pb-formate}}{(HCOO)_2Pb} + H_2S \longrightarrow 2HCOOH + PbS$$

Formic acid, thus, obtained may contain a very small quantity of hydrogen sulphide which is eliminated by redistilling it over some dry lead formate.

11.6.2 Acetic Acid (Ethanoic Acid), CH_3COOH

Acetic acid is one of the most common organic acid. It is the principal constituent of vinegar and hence its name (Latin *acetum*, vinegar).

Preparation of Acetic Acid: Following methods are generally utilised for its preparation.

11.6.2.1 Manufacture of Acetic Acid

The most economical method for the manufacture of pure acetic acid or **glacial acetic acid** is from acetylene. Acetylene is passed into an aqueous solution of sulphuric acid containing mercuric sulphate when acetaldehyde is formed.

$$\underset{\text{Acetylene}}{H-C\equiv C-H} + H_2O \xrightarrow[HgSO_4]{H_2SO_4} \underset{\text{Acetaldehyde}}{CH_3CHO}$$

The vapours of acetaldehyde are now mixed with air and the mixture is passed over manganese acetate at 65-70 °C when acetic acid is obtained.

$$CH_3CHO + \frac{1}{2}O_2 \xrightarrow[65\text{-}70°C]{\text{Mn-acetate}} \underset{\text{Acetic Acid}}{CH_3COOH}$$

Another method of manufacture of acetic acid is by **Wood distillation**. In this method, calcium acetate obtained during the manufacture of methanol by wood distillation, is distilled with dilute sulphuric acid when aqueous solution of acetic acid is obtained.

$$(CH_3COO)_2Ca + H_2SO_4 \longrightarrow 2CH_3COOH + CaSO_4$$

Dilute acetic acid so obtained is neutralised with sodium hydroxide and evaporated to get sodium acetate. This sodium acetate is fused and distilled with concentrated sulphuric acid when **glacial acid** (100%) is obtained. It may be mentioned that this method has now become obsolete.

More recently acetic acid is manufactured by **fermentation process**. This process is based upon the oxidation of fermented liquors (10-15% ethanol) by air under the influence of bacteria **mycoderma aceti**. A 3-7% solution of acid obtained is called **Vinegar**.

$$C_2H_5OH + O_2 \longrightarrow CH_3COOH + H_2O$$

Fermentation is carried out by the **quick vinegar process**. In this process, a large number of vats, filled with wooden shavings or twigs are arranged in series. Each vat has a perforated false bottom and a perforated cover. It is also provided with air inlet near the base. The wood shavings are impregnated with old vinegar containing bacteria. Dilute alcohol solution is then allowed to trickle down from the top. Air is drawn in through air inlets and moves upwards. The alcohol is oxidised to aceticacid. The heat generated in the process maintains the temperature at about 35 °C which is optimum for the proper development and activity of bacteria. The supply of air is carefully controlled—excess air admitted, if alcohol may be oxidised to carbon dioxide and water and if too little air is present oxidation may be stopped stop at acetaldehyde stage.

The liquor obtained from first vat is introduced at the top of second and so on.

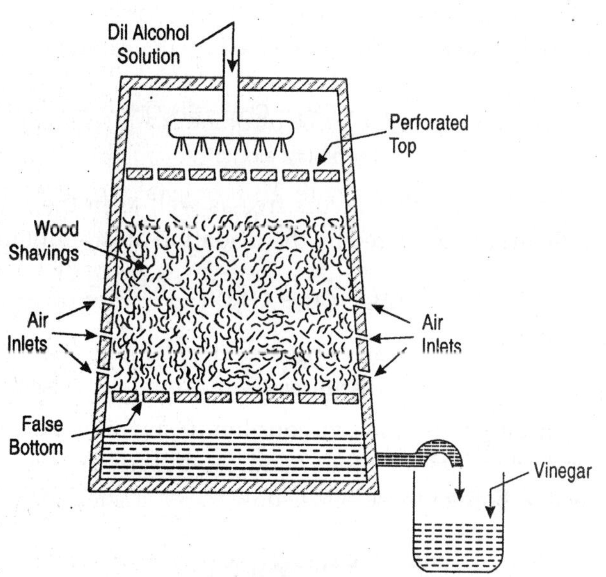

Fig. 11.1 : Manufacture of vinegar

This recirculation process gives at about 7-8 per cent acetic acid solution. This solution is neutralised by lime and the resulting solution is evaporated to dryness and pure acetic acid is obtained by the distillation of residue of calcium acetate with sulphuric acid. One of the vats used in quick vinegar process is shown Fig. 11.1.

11.6.2.2 Properties of Acetic Acid

At ordinary temperature acetic acid is a colurless liquid, b.p. 118 °C with a pungent smell. It is soluble in water, alcohol and ether. When sufficiently cooled, it forms ice-like crystals (m.p. 16 °C) and hence the name **glacial acetic acid**. It acts as a good solvent. Chemically it responds to all the characteristic reactions of carboxylic acids and is an important substance used for different purposes.

11.6.3 Propionic Acid (Propanoic Acid), $CH_3—CH_2COOH$

Propionic acid is industrially manufactured either by the catalytic air oxidation of *n*-propyl alcohol or by the reaction between ethylene, carbon monoxide and water at a high temperature and presure in the presence of a catalyst. Thus,

$$\underset{n\text{-Propanol}}{CH_3—CH_2—CH_2—OH} \xrightarrow{[\,O\,]} \underset{\text{Propionic Acid}}{CH_3—CH_2—COOH}$$

or

$$CH_2{=}CH_2 + H_2O + CO \longrightarrow CH_3CH_2—COOH$$

It is a colourless oily liquid, b.p. 140°C and is soluble in water, alcohol and ether. It undergres all the characteristic reactions of carboxylic acids.

11.6.4 Butyric Acid (Butanoic Acid), $CH_3CH_2CH_2COOH$

Two isomeric butyric acids are known—(i) *n*-Butyric acid and (ii) iso-Butyric acid (2-Methyl propanoic acid). *n*-Butyric acid, $CH_3—CH_2—CH_2—COOH$, occurs in butter as glyceryl ester. The typical smell of rancid butter is due to the liberation of butyric acid by the hydrolysis of glyceryl ester. It is manufactured by the catalylic oxidation of *n*-butyl alcohol.

$$\underset{n\text{-Butyl alcohol}}{CH_3—CH_2—CH_2—CH_2OH} \xrightarrow{[\,O\,]} \underset{n\text{-Butyric Acid}}{CH_3—CH_2—CH_2—CH_2OH}$$

iso-Butyric acid occurs free as well as in the combined state as esters in many plants. It is industrially prepared by the oxidation of iso-butanol

$$\underset{\text{Iso-Butanol}}{CH_3—\underset{\displaystyle CH_3}{\underset{|}{CH}}—CH_2OH} \xrightarrow{[\,O\,]} \underset{\text{Iso-Butyric Acid}}{CH_3—\underset{\displaystyle CH_3}{\underset{|}{CH}}—COOH}$$

n-Butyric acid is a viscous liquid smelling like rancid butter and is soluble in water, ethanol and ether. On the other hand, iso-butyric acid is a colourless oily liquid sparingly soluble in water. Both of these acids show the characteristic reactions of carboxylic acids.

11.6.5 Valeric Acids, $C_5H_{10}O_2$

Four structural isomers are possible and all of them are known.

i. normal (*n*-) Valeric acid, $CH_3-CH_2-CH_2-CH_2-COOH$, b.p. 187 °C.

ii. iso-Valeric acid, $(CH_3)_2CH-CH_2-COOH$, b.p. 195°C

iii. Ethyl methyl acetic acid or optically active valeric acid, $CH_3-CH_2-CH(CH_3)-COOH$, b.p. 175 °C

iv. Trimethyl acetic acid or Pivalic acid, b.p. 164 °C.

Among these isomeric acids, commonly known as valeric acid is isovaleric acid. It occurs in valerian root from which it is extracted by distillation in steam. The product which **contains also active valeric acid**, is used in pharamacy under the name **Acidum Valerianicum.**

Trimethyl acetic acid or Pivalic acid is prepared by the oxidation of pinacolone by means of sodium hypobromite.

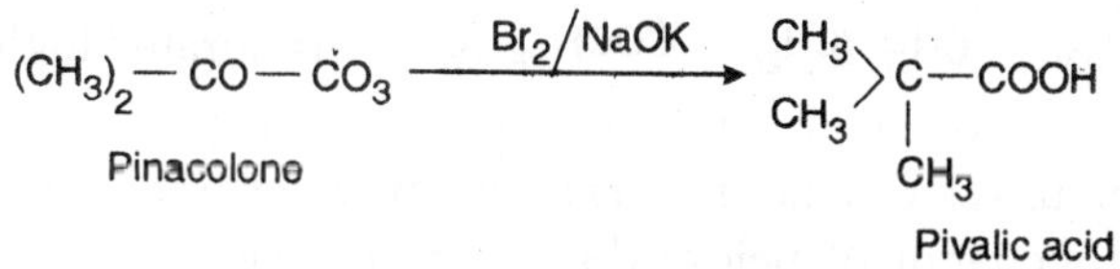

Normal valeric acid is generally prepared by the oxidation of normal amyl alcohol.

$$\underset{n\text{-Amyl alcohol}}{CH_3-CH_2-CH_2-CH_2-CH_2OH} \xrightarrow{[O]} \underset{n\text{-Valeric acid}}{CH_3-CH_2-CH_2-COOH}$$

Iso-Valeric acid is used for the large scale preparation of bromural which is used as a hypnotic.

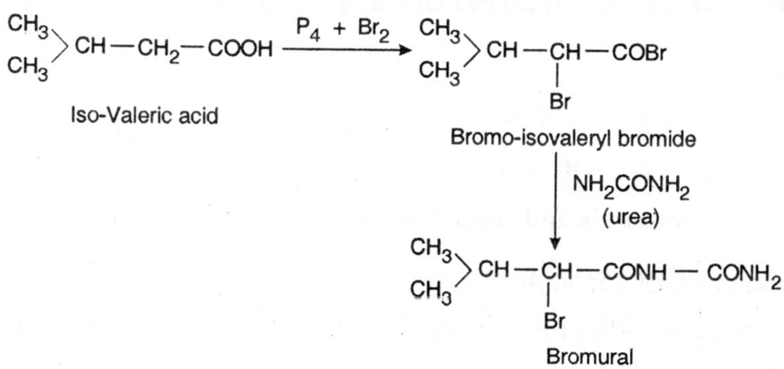

11.7 Higher Fatty Acids

The higher fatty acids occurring in nature usually contain even number of carbon atoms arranged in a chain. They generally occur in the form glyceryl esters in animal fats and vegetable oils. Some of the higher members occur in waxes as esters of monohydric alcohols. Among the large number of higher fatty acids important members are stearic, lauric, palmitic and oleic acids.

(a) **Palmitic Acid,** $C_{15}H_{31}COOH$ m.p. 64 °C occurs as its ester in palm oil. It is manufactured industrially by its hydrohysis of palm oil. The oil is hydrohysed by Twitchell process using Twitchell reagent (alkylaryl sulphuric acid) and dilute sulphuric acid. The crude palmitic acid, thus, obtained is purified by fractional crystallisation. Palmitic acid is a colourless waxy solid and has found many uses in industry. Thus (i) Myricyl palmitate, (ii) cetyl palmitate are the constituents of waxes and used in cosmetic and pharmaceutical preparations (iii) sodium and potassium salt of palmitic acid are used as soaps. (iv) It is also used in the manufacture of surface-active agents and plasticiser.

(b) **Stearic Acid:** It has the molecular formula, $C_{17}H_{35}COOH$. It is industrially prepared by the hydrolysis of tristearin a solid fat known as **tallow**. It is a colourless waxy solid, m.p. 65 °C. It is industrially very important. Thus its sodium and potassium salts are used as soaps. Zinc stearate is used as a mould lubricant in plastic industry, magnesium stearate used in paints and as component of cosmetics, dusting and talc powder. Aluminium stearate is used as an ingredient in polishes, to increase water-proofness and for waterproofing of fabrics, leather goods, etc. It is also used in the manufacture of plasticisers and surface-active agents.

(c) **Oleic Acid:** $CH_3-(CH_2)_7-CH{=}(CH_2)_7-COOH$. It is an unsaturated higher fatty acid and occurs in fats and oils as triolein (glyceryl ester) and is usually prepared by the hydrolysis of triolein. It is a colourless oily liquid, insoluble in water but soluble in alcohol and ether. Catalytic hydrogenation of aleic acid gives stearic acid.

$$\underset{\text{Oleic acid}}{CH_3-(CH_2)_7-CH{=}CH-(CH_2)_7-COOH} \xrightarrow{[2H]} \underset{\text{Stearic acid}}{CH_3-(CH_2)_{16}-COOH}$$

Oleic acid is the *cis* form, and the *trans* form is elaidic acid (m.p. 51 °C). Oleic acid responds to other reactions of carboxylic function and unsaturation.

11.8 Some Important Derivatives of Fatty Acids

11.8.1 Lactic Acid, $CH_3-\overset{\overset{\large H}{|}}{\underset{\underset{\large OH}{|}}{C}}-COOH$

Lactic acid occurs in sour milk and hence its name.

11.8.1.1 Preparation of Lactic Acid

Lactic acid may be prepared by the hydrolysis of either cyanohydrin of acetaldehyde or α-bromo propionic acid.

$$\underset{\text{Acetaldehyde}}{CH_3-CHO} + HCN \longrightarrow CH_3-CH\begin{matrix} CH \\ CN \end{matrix} \xrightarrow{H_2O} \underset{\text{Lactic acid}}{CH_3-CH(OH)COOH}$$

$$\text{Or } \underset{\alpha\text{-Bromo propionic acid}}{CH_3-\underset{\underset{Br}{|}}{CH}-COOH} \xrightarrow{H_2O} CH_3-CH(OH)-COOH$$

11.8.1.2 Manufacture of Lactic Acid

Lactic acid is manufactured by the fermentation of cane-sugar by microorganisms, **lactic acid bacillus** in the presence of powdered chalk. Chalk helps to keep the acidity below 1% and is necessary because even 1% free acid renders the bacilli inactive. Crystals of calcium lactate separate and are removed. Free lactic acid is regenerated from the calcium salt by the treatment of dilute sulphuric acid. Calcium sulphate is filtered off and the filtrate is distilled under reduced pressure to get free lactic acid.

The optimum conditions for fermentation are as under:

i. A neutral medium.

ii. Temperature must be kept in the range of 35 °C- 40 °C.

11.8.1.3 Properties of Lactic Acid

Lactic acid contains one asymmetric carbon atom and exists in three forms—D, L and dl. The racemic form (dl) is the ordinary lactic acid and it attributes sour taste to milk. It is a viscous syrupy liquid, soluble in water, alcohol and ether. Both dextro and laevo lactic acids melt at 26 °C. Chemically all the three varieties are identical excepting their behaviour towards light. All the three exhibit the properties of α-hydroxy acid and structurally they are α-hydroxy propionic acid ($CH_3-C^{*}H(OH)-COOH$). Some important reactions of lactic acid are **summarised** below.

$$\underset{\text{Lactic acid}}{CH_3-CH(OH)-COOH} \xrightarrow{ROH} \underset{\text{Lactate}}{CH_3-CH(OH)-COOR}$$

On heating it readily forms **lactide**. Two molecules are involved in the reaction.

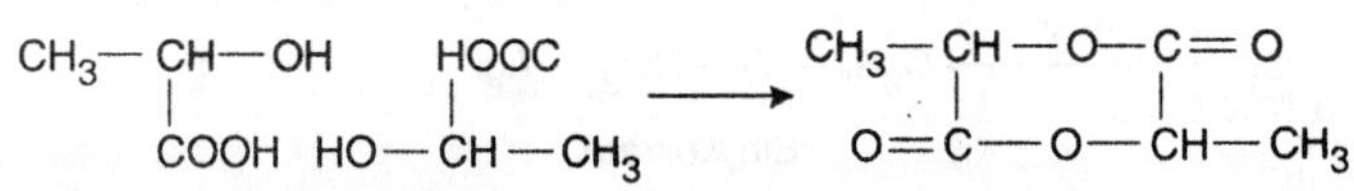

It is the general properties of α-hydroxy acids. On oxidation with milk oxidising agent like $FeSO_4$ and H_2O_2 (Fenton's reagent) it forms pyruvic acid.

$$CH_3-CH(OH)-COOH \xrightarrow{FeSOH_4\ +\ H_2O_2} \underset{\text{Pyruvic acid}}{CH_3-C(=O)-COOH}$$

But if strong oxidising agent is used, the product is acetic acid.

$$CH_3-CH(OH)-COOH \xrightarrow{KMnO_4} CH_3COOH + CO_2 + H_2O$$

It also undergoes other typical reactions of carboxylic group.

11.8.1.4 Uses of Lactic Acid

Lactic acid is extensively used as a mordant dye in **dyeing wool. It is also used for removing lime** from hides in tanning process. Lactic acid and its calcium salts find immense use in medicine. Its ethyl and butyl esters are used as solvents in plastic industry.

11.8.2 Ethyl Acetate ($CH_3COOC_2H_5$)

It is the ethyl ester of acetic acid. It is prepared in the laboratory as well as on a large scale by heating acetic acid and ethyl alcohol in the presence of concentrated sulphuric acid.

$$CH_3COOH + C_2H_5OH \xrightarrow{H_2SO_4} CH_3COOC_2H_5 + H_2O$$

It is a colourless liquid, b.p. 78 °C, with a characteristic smell. it is sparingly soluble in water but readily soluble in organic solvents. Chemically it gives all the reactions of esters. One important reaction of ethyl acetate is the Claisen condensation in which it forms ethyl acetoacetate. This β-ketoester is a very good source of carbanion and has been widely used for the synthesis of large number of organic compounds.

$$\underset{\text{Ethyl acetate}}{CH_3COOEt + CH_3COOEt} \xrightarrow{Na/EtOH} \underset{\text{ethyl acetoacetate}}{CH_3-\underset{\underset{O}{\|}}{C}-CH_2-COOEt} + EtOH$$

11.8.2.1 Uses of Ethyl Acetate

It is used as a solvent in the preparation of smokeless powder. It is largely used in the preparation of artificial fruit essences.

11.8.3 Ethyl Nitrate ($C_2H_5-O-\overset{\overset{O}{|}}{N}=O$)

Ethyl nitrate may be regarded as the ethyl ester of nitric acid. It is prepared by the following methods.

i. $\underset{\text{Ethyl iodide}}{C_2H_5I} + \underset{\text{Ag-nitrate}}{Ag-O-NO_2} \xrightarrow{\text{Heat}} \underset{\text{Ethyl nitrate}}{C_2H_5-O-NO_2} + AgI$

ii. $C_2H_5OH + HNO_3 \xrightarrow{\text{Urea}} C_2H_5-O-NO_2 + H_2O$

It is a colourless liquid, b.p. 88 °C with a pleasant smell. It is insoluble in water. On hydrolysis by boiling water it gives ethyl alcohol and nitric acid.

$$C_2H_5-O-NO_2 + H_2O \longrightarrow C_2H_2OH + HNO_3$$

When reduced with Sn and HCl it forms ethyl alcohol and hydroxyl amine.

$$C_2H_5ONO_2 \xrightarrow[+6H]{Sn/HCl} C_2H_5OH + \underset{\text{Hydroxyl amine}}{NH_2OH} + H_2O$$

11.8.4 Sodium Dioctyl Sulphosuccinate

It is an important synthetic detergent. It is manufactured by treating maleic anhydride with octyl alcohol followed by the treatment of the product with sodium bisulphite solution.

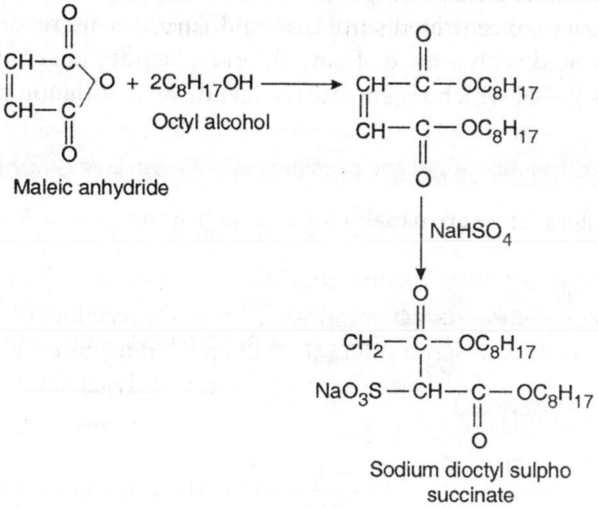

It is extensively used as a wetting agent in textile industry.

11.8.5 Sodium Lauryl Sulphate

Sodium lauryl sulphate is one of the most important synthetic detergent. It is manufactured from methyl laurate, lauryl alcohol and lauryl sulphate as shown below:

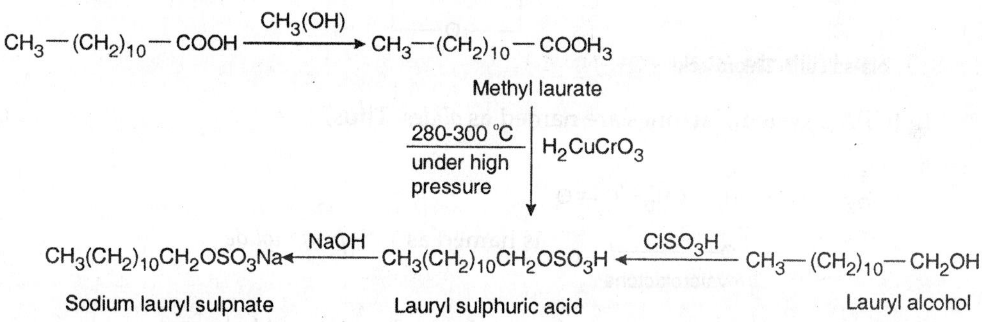

Lauric acid required in this synthesis is manufactured form by the hydrolysis of the esters present in coconut oil.

Sodium lauryl sulphate has excellent foaming characteristics and its effect on the skin is very mild. For this reason it is employed in the preparation of shampoos, cosmetics, toothpaste and light-duty household detergent.

11.8.6 Lactides and Lactones

Formation of lactides is a characteristic reaction of α-hydroxy acids. These are six-membered ring compounds formed by the reaction between two molecules of α-hydroxy acid and are named systematically as 3, 6-dialkyl-1, 4-dioxan-2, 5-dione

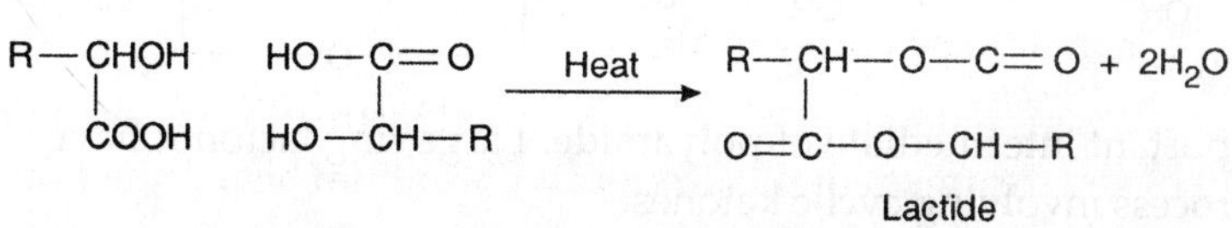

In some cases lactides are formed very easily, formed even by allowing the α-hydroxy acid to stand in desiccator over concentrated sulphuric acid. Lactides are readily hydrolysed to the acid by alkali. When heated with a trace of zinc chloride, lactides are converted to polyesters, HO—(—CHR—COO—)$_n$—H which regenerate the lactide on distillation under pressure.

11.9 Lactones

Lactones are internal esters. They are usually formed on heating γ- and δ-hydroxy acids. Thus,

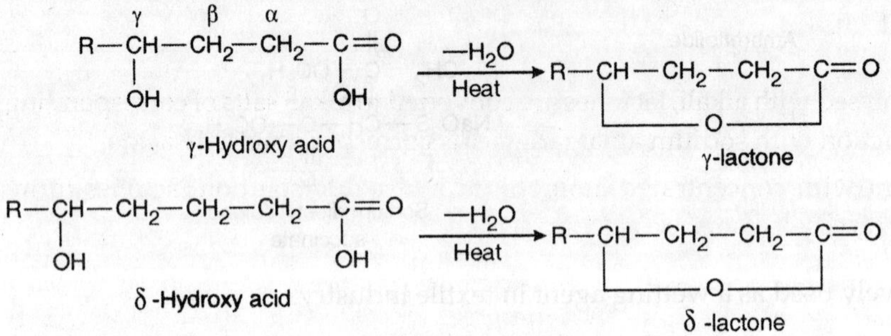

β-lactones from β-hydroxy acid can only be obtained under special circumstances. β-lactones are prepared by shaking the aqueous solution of the sodium salt of β-chloro acid with chloroform.

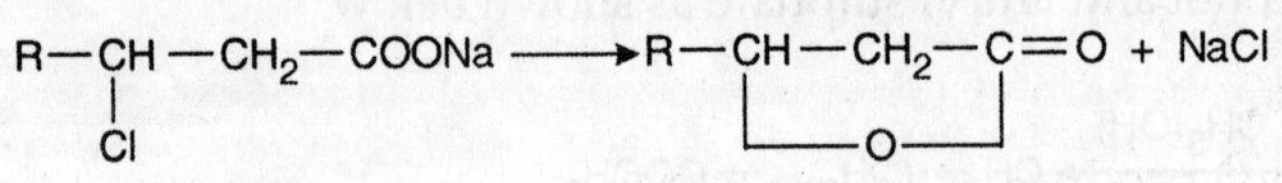

In IUPAC system, lactones are named as *olides*. Thus,

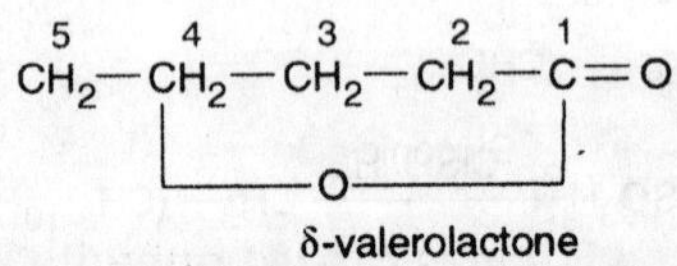

is named as 1, 5- *pentanolide*

Lactones may be prepared by other methods also as noted below:

i. *Rearrangements of unsaturated acid.*

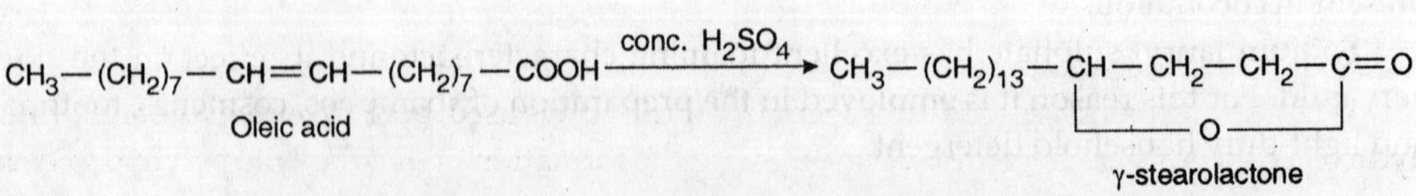

ii. *Oxidation of Glycols*: γ-butyrolactone is manufactured by oxidation of tetramethylene glycol over copper catalyst.

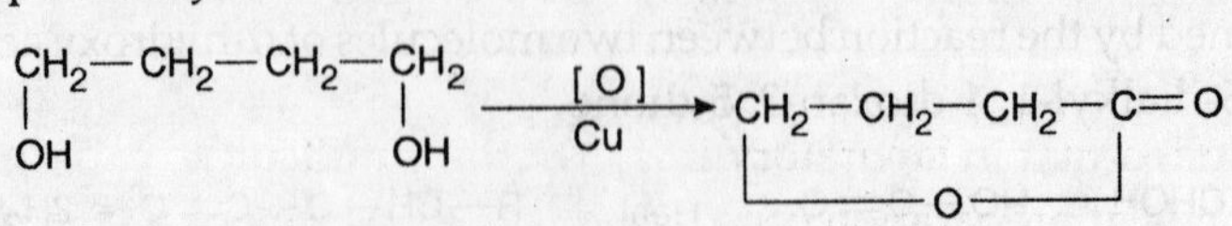

It is an important intermediate of polyamide. Large ring lactones have also been prepared by oxidation process involving cyclic ketones.

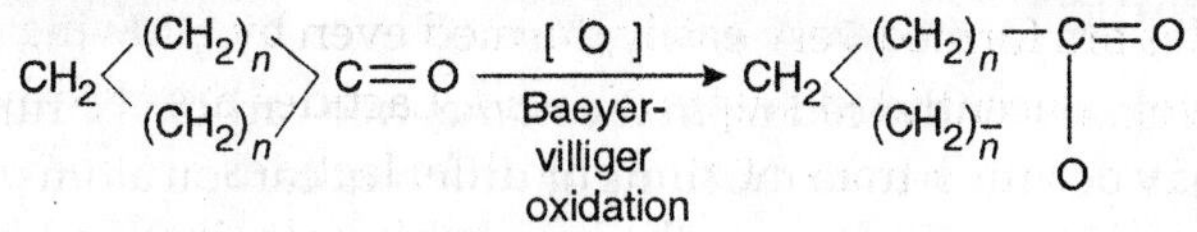

Some large ring lactones occur naturally.

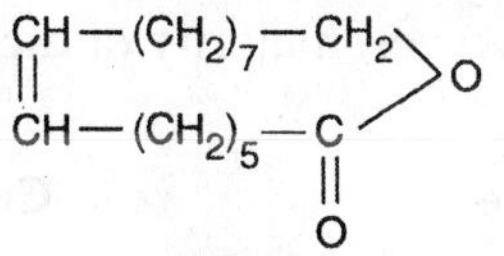

Ambrettolide

When hydrolysed with alkali, lactones are converted to alkali salts of corresponding hydroxy acid and on reduction with sodium amalgam yields corresponding fatty acids.

On treatment with concentrated **ammonium** hydroxide solution lactones form hydroxy amides, in some cases γ-lactams are also formed.

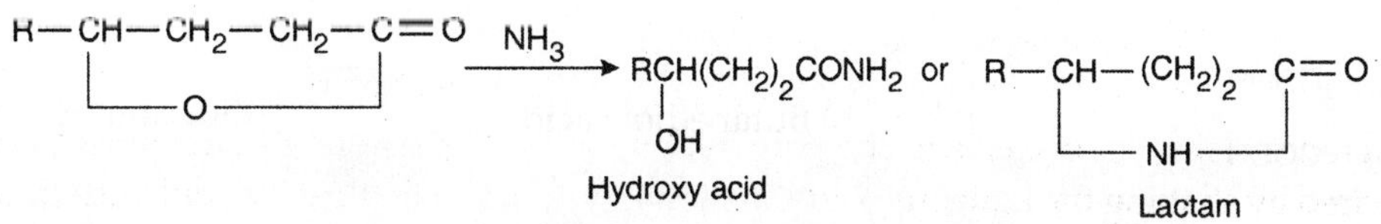

11.10 Gluconic and Glucuronic Acids

These two acids are the oxidation products of D(+)-glucose.

When treated with mild oxidising agent like bromine water aldehydic group of D(+)-glucose is oxidised with the formation of gluconic acid.

$$\underset{\text{D(+)-Glucose}}{CH_2OH-(CHOH)_4-CHO} \xrightarrow[Br_2-H_2O]{[O]} \underset{\text{Gluconic acid}}{\underset{\displaystyle OH}{\underset{|}{CH_2}}-(CHOH)_4-COOH}$$

For the preparation of gluconic acid in large scale, oxidation is carried out with mercuric oxide in the presence of calcium carbonate on glucose solution. Calcium gluconate is formed in 70-80% yield. Gluconic acid is also formed by the fermentation of glucose with **Aspergillus niger** or **Penicillium Chrysogenum**.

Gluconic acid is largely used medicinally in the form of γ-lactone.

When strong oxidising oxidising agent like nitric acid is used, both the aldehydic and primary hydroxyl functions are to carboxylic group with the formation of dicarboxylic polyhydroxy acid known as glucuronic acid.

$$\underset{\displaystyle OH}{\underset{|}{CH_2}}-(CHOH)_4-CHO \xrightarrow[HNO_3]{[O]} \underset{\text{Glucuronic acid}}{COOH\,(CHOH)_4-COOH}$$

It may be mentioned that in laboratory it is extremely difficult to carry out this oxidation. One of the best methods of preparation of this acid is to feed broneol, a tarpene alcohol to dogs and bornyl gluconate is excreted in the urine.

11.11 Dicarboxylic Acids

Dicarboxylic acids contain as is evidenced from the name, two carboxylic functionalities. These two carboxylic groups may be attached to the same or different carbon atoms. Dicarboxylic acids are obtained in pure crystalline solid form with sharp melting points and lower members are readily soluble in water. Because of this purity and ready solubility lower members such as oxalic and succinic acids are used as *standard substances for acid-base titrations*. In IUPAC system, dicarboxylic acids are named as *Alkanedioic acids*. However, majority of dicarboxylic acids are known by their common names. Thus,

Acid	IUPAC Name	Common Name
$COOH-COOH$	Ethanedioic acid	Oxalic acid
$COOH-CH_2-COOH$	Propanedioic acid	Malonic acid
CH_2-COOH / CH_2-COOH	Butanedioic acid	Succinic acid
CH_2-CH_2-COOH / CH_2-CH_2-COOH	Hexanedioic acid	Adipic acid

11.11.1 Properties of Dicarboxylic Acids

Due to the presence of two carboxylic groups they are stronger acids than monocarboxylic acids.

Dicarboxylic acids exhibit most of the properties of monocarboxylic acids. But since two carboxylic groups are present, both mono-and di-derivatives are formed. Thus,

$$\underset{\text{Oxalic acid}}{\begin{matrix} COOH \\ | \\ COOH \end{matrix}} \xrightarrow{NaOH} \underset{\text{Mono-sodium salt}}{\begin{matrix} COONa \\ | \\ COOH \end{matrix}} \xrightarrow{NaOH} \underset{\text{Disodium salt}}{\begin{matrix} COONa \\ | \\ COONa \end{matrix}}$$

Similar is the situation in the case of other derivatives—

$$\underset{\text{Mono-acid chloride}}{\begin{matrix} COCl \\ | \\ COOH \end{matrix}} \quad \underset{\text{Diacid chloride}}{\begin{matrix} COCl \\ | \\ COCl \end{matrix}} \quad \underset{\text{Mono-amide}}{\begin{matrix} CONH_2 \\ | \\ COOH \end{matrix}} \quad \underset{\text{Diamide}}{\begin{matrix} CONH_2 \\ | \\ CONH_2 \end{matrix}}$$

$$\underset{\text{Mono-ester}}{\begin{matrix} COOR \\ | \\ COOR \end{matrix}} \quad \underset{\text{Diester}}{\begin{matrix} COOR \\ | \\ COOR \end{matrix}}$$

However, an important type of reaction undergone by dicarboxylic acids—action of heat, requires to be discussed in detail.

11.11.1.1 Action of Heat on Dicarboxylic Acids

Action of heat on dicarboxylic acids solely depends upon the length of carbon chain in between two carboxylic groups. The products on heating may be mono-carboxylic acid, anhydride, cyclic ketone or polymers. It has been observed:

i. When there is either one or no carbon atom between the carboxylic groups, the product is monocarboxylic acid. Thus oxalic acids on heating furnishes formic acid.

$$\begin{array}{l} COOH \\ | \\ COOH \end{array} \xrightarrow[-\,CO_2]{\text{Heat}} \underset{\text{Formic acid}}{H-COOH}$$

ii. But when two or three carbon atoms are present in between two carboxylic groups anhydride is formed as the main product. Succinic acid on heating forms corresponding anhydride.

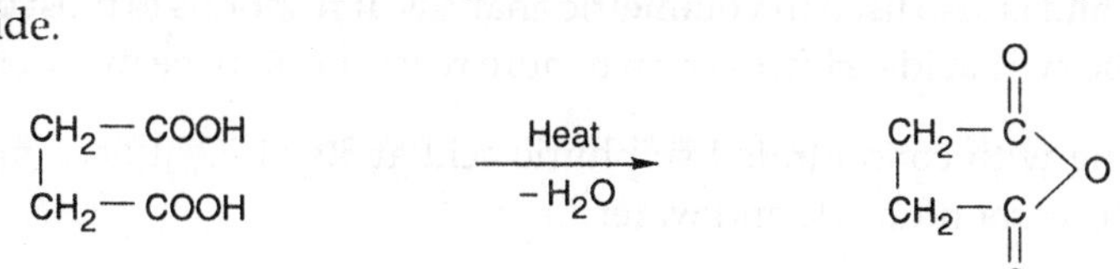

Succinic acid

Succinic anhydride

iii. Cyclic ketones are the predominant products in the case of presence of four to five carbon atoms in the chain.

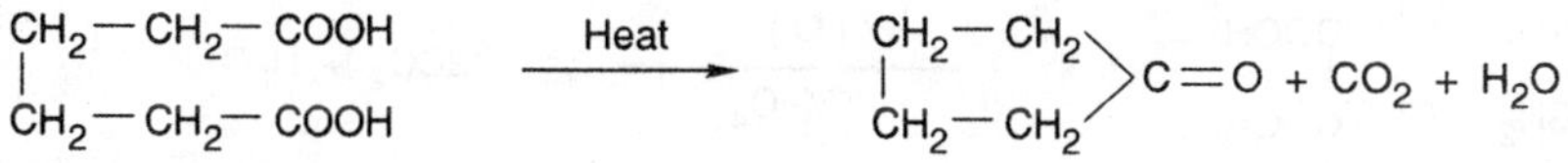

Adipic acid Cyclopentanone

When the chain contains more than five carbon atoms dimerisation is then preferred product. From the action of heat it is clear that the properties of dicarboxylic acids are primarily dependant on the length of carbon chain between the two carboxylic groups. It is, therefore, desirable that important members of this family should be described individually. Two most common members are oxalic and succinic acids.

11.11.2 Common Dibasic Acids

A. **Oxalic acid:** It is the simplest and most important member of dicarboxylic acid family. It occurs in *sorrel, rhubarb* and *tomatoe plants*. It has been observed that stones formed in kidney and bladder of human body are nothing but calcium salt of oxalic acid.

Preparation: It is prepared in the laboratory by the oxidation of cane sugar with concentrated nitric acid in presence of vanadium pentoxide as catalyst.

$$\underset{\text{Cane Sugar}}{C_{12}H_{22}O_{11}} + 18\,[O] \longrightarrow \underset{\text{Oxalic acid}}{6\,C_2H_2O_4} + 5H_2O$$

Oxalic acid thus produced is purified by crystallisation from hot water.

Manufacture of Oxalic acid: Oxalic acid is manufactured by heating sodium formate at a temperature of 350 °C. Sodium formate required in this manufacturing process is prepared by passing carbon monoxide under pressure into caustic soda.

$$\text{NaOH} + \text{CO} \longrightarrow \underset{\text{Sodium formate}}{\text{HCOONa}}$$

$$2\text{HCOONa} \xrightarrow[350\,^\circ\text{C}]{\text{Heat}} \underset{\text{Sodium oxalate}}{\begin{matrix}\text{COONa}\\ |\\ \text{COONa}\end{matrix}} + H_2$$

Sodium oxalate formed is mixed with calcium hydroxide when Ca-oxalate is precipated out. Calcium oxalate when decomposed with dilute sulphuric acid, free oxalic acid is formed. Oxalic acid crystallises as dihydrate, $\begin{matrix}\text{COOH}\\ |\\ \text{COOH}\end{matrix}.2H_2O$. It is used as mordant in dyeing and printing and is also used in volumetric analysis. It responds to most of the properties of mono-carboxylic acids. However, two more reactions may be mentioned.

i. On heating with concentrated sulphuric acid at 80-90 °C, it decomposes to carbon monoxide, carbondioxide and water.

$$\begin{matrix}\text{COOH}\\ |\\ \text{COOH}\end{matrix} \xrightarrow[\text{Heat}]{\text{conc. } H_2SO_4} CO + CO_2 + H_2O$$

ii. On oxidation with $KMnO_4$ it readily forms carbon dioxide and water.

$$\begin{matrix}\text{COOH}\\ |\\ \text{COOH}\end{matrix} \xrightarrow[KMnO_4]{[O]} 2CO_2 + H_2O$$

This oxidation is quantitative and for this reason it is employed for the standardisation of permanganate solution.

B. **Malonic acid:** Malonic acid is a colourless crystalline solid, mp 120 °C, soluble in water and alcohol but is sparingly soluble in ether. It responds to normal reactions of a dicarboxylic acid.

When heated at a temperature of 140-150 °C, it eliminates a molecule of carbon dioxide and forms acetic acid.

$$CH_2\begin{matrix}\diagup \text{COOH}\\ \diagdown \text{COOH}\end{matrix} \xrightarrow[140\text{-}150\,^\circ\text{C}]{\text{Heat}} \underset{\text{Acetic acid}}{CH_3COOH} + CO_2$$

But when heated with phosphorous pentoxide, a small amount of carbon suboxide is formed.

$$CH_2\begin{matrix}\diagup \text{COOH}\\ \diagdown \text{COOH}\end{matrix} \xrightarrow[-\,2H_2O]{P_2O_5} \underset{\text{Carbon suboxide}}{O{=}C{=}C{=}O}$$

However, malonic acid does not form a cyclic anhydride.

On treatment with nitrous acid followed by hydrolysis malonic acid forms *mesoxalic acid* (ketomalonic acid).

$$CH_2\begin{matrix}\diagup \text{COOH}\\ \diagdown \text{COOH}\end{matrix} \xrightarrow{HNO_2} (COOH)_2{-}C{=}NOH \xrightarrow{H_2O} \underset{\text{Mesoxalic acid}}{HOOC - C - CO - COOH}$$

Its diethyl or dimethyl ester (malonic ester) is a valuable synthetic reagent in organic chemistry.

Malonic acid is generally prepared by heating potassium chloroacetate with aqueous potassium cyanide, followed by hydrolysis with hydrochloric acid.

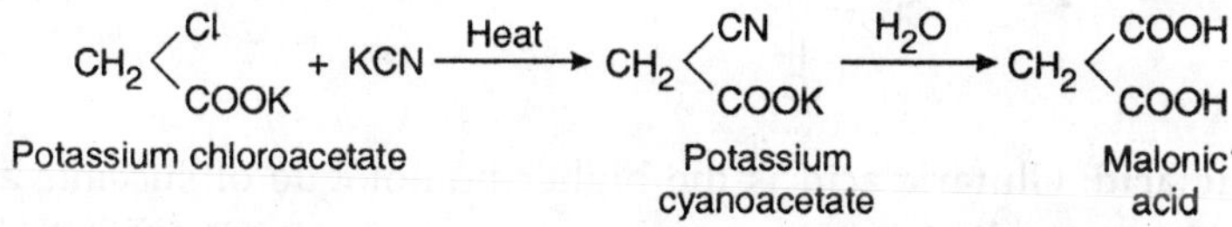

C. **Succinic acid:** Succinic acid is a solid crystalline compound soluble in water. It is usually prepared by the following methods.:

i. *From ethylene bromide:*

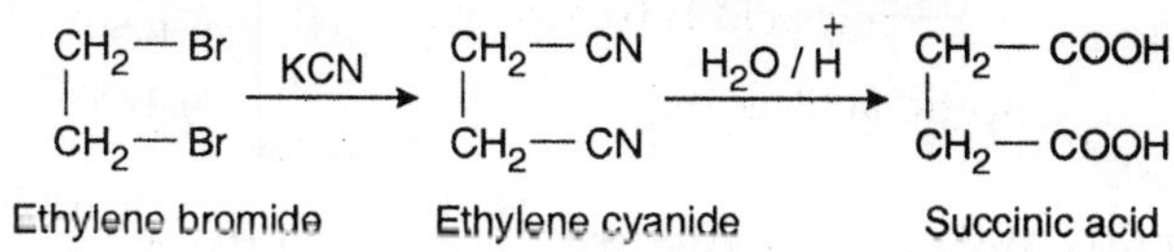

ii. *From malonic ester:*

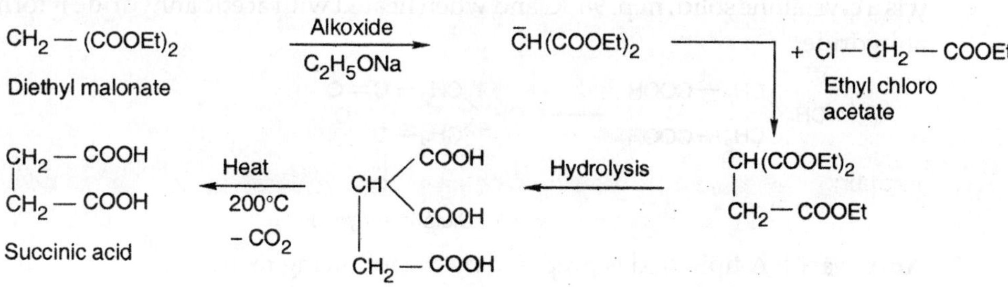

It responds all the reactions of monocarboxylic acids and its behaviour towards the application of heat has been mentioned earlier.

An important derivative of succinic acid is its N-Bromo derivative which is an useful reagent for brominating allylic carbon atom. It is prepared as:

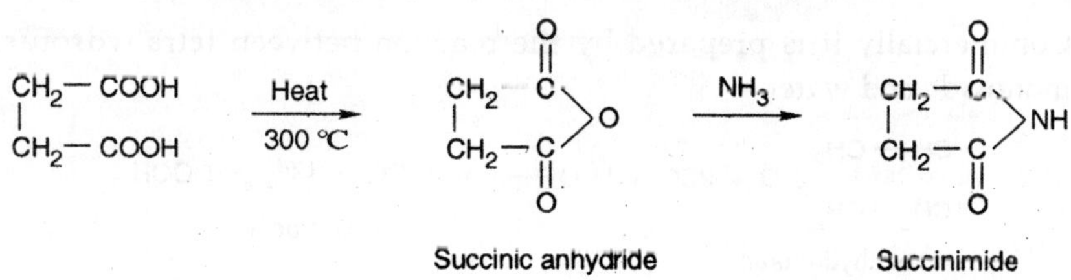

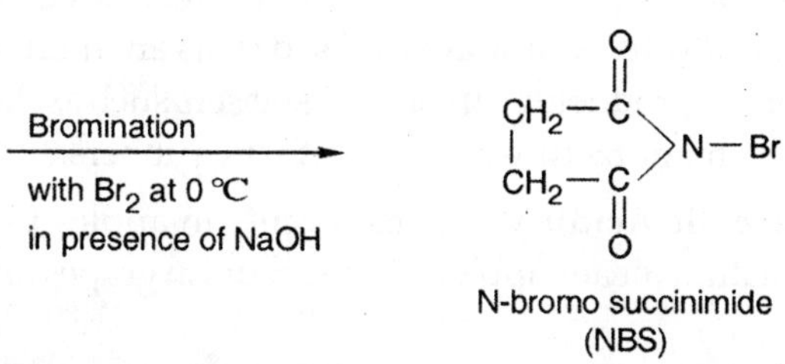

NBS readily brominates alkene at allylic position. Thus,

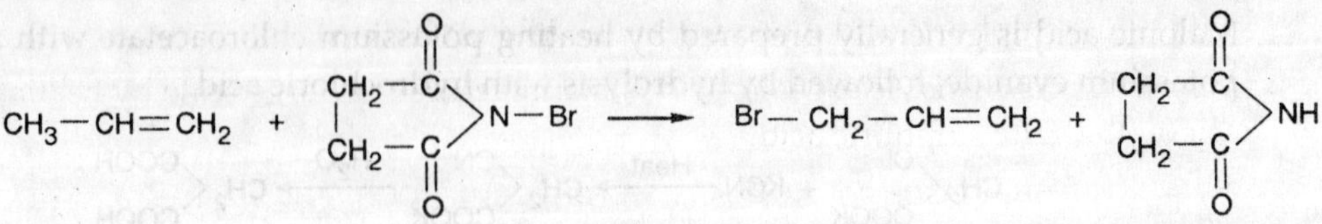

D. **Glutaric acid:** Glutaric acid is the higher homologue of succinic acid. It is normally prepared from malonic ester.

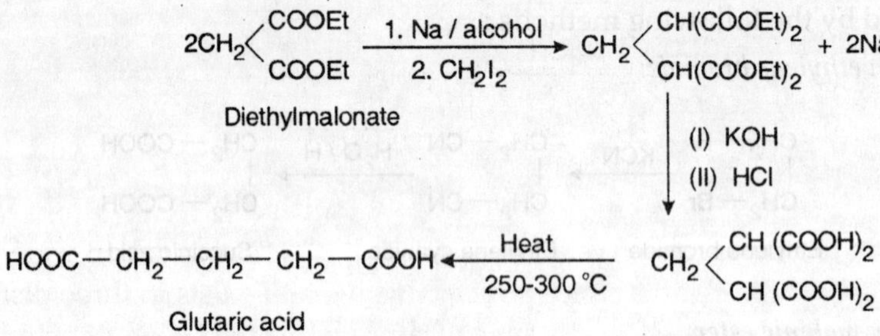

It is a crystalline solid, m.p. 98 °C and when heated with acetic anhydride it forms glutaric anhydride.

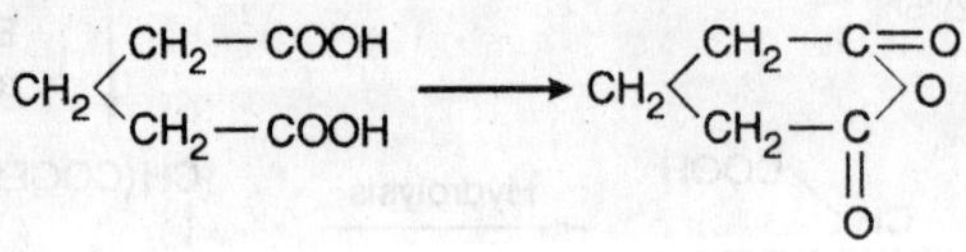

Glutaric anhydride

E. **Adipic acid:** Adipic acid is prepared by the following methods:

i. 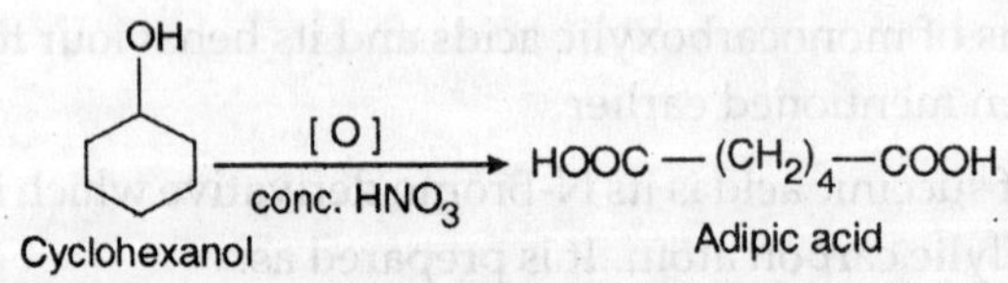

ii. Commercially it is prepared by the reaction between tetrahydrofuran, carbon monoxide and water.

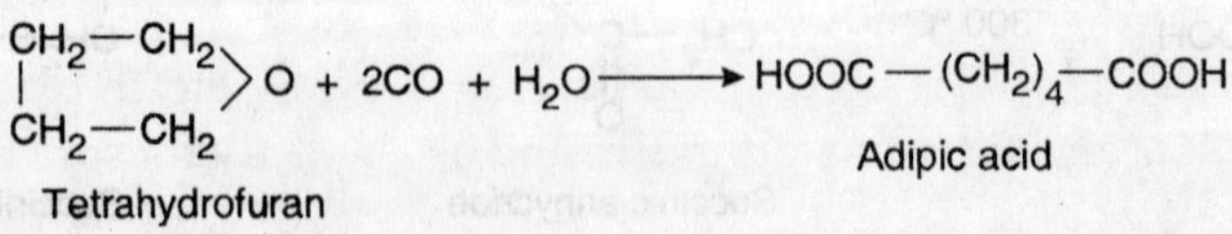

Adipic acid is a crystalline solid, m.p. 150 °C. On heating with acetic anhydride it forms a linear polymeric anhydride. Adipic acid is used (i) as an intermediate in the manufacture of nylon (ii) for the production of ester plasticisers such as dioctyl adipate (iii) as an intermediate in the manufacture of polyurethane rubbers.

F. **Malic Acid (Monohydroxy succinic Acid):** Malic acid occurs in apples from which its name has been derived (Latin, malum means apple). It also occurs in grapes and mountain-ash berries.

- *Isolation of Malic Acid:* Malic acid is isolated from mountain-ash berries by boiling their juice with lime. Malic acid is precipitated as calcium malate. It is filtered and is hydrolysed with dilute sulphuric acid when free malic acid is obtained.
- *Manufacture of Malic Acid:* Malic acid is manufactured on large scale by heating maleic acid with dilute sulphuric acid.

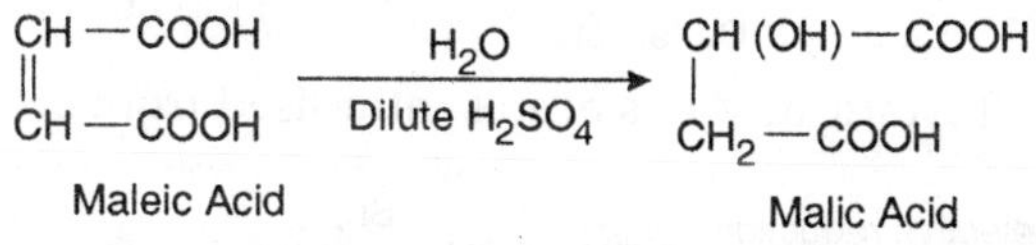

In *laboratory* it is prepared by heating bromo-succinic acid with silver hydroxide.

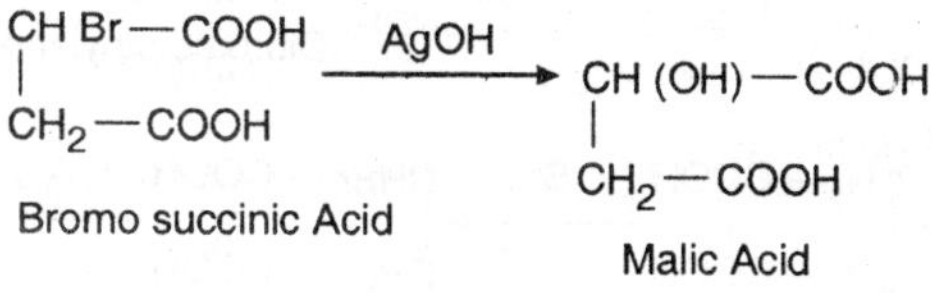

Malic acid is a colourless crystalline solid, m.p. 100 °C, soluble in water and alcohol. It has one choral centre and hence optically active and exists in three distinct forms. The naturally occurring malic acid is laevorotatory while the synthetic acid is as expected is racemic in character. Dextro form of malic acid may be obtained by the reduction of (+) tartaric acid with hydrogen iodide.

Chemically it behaves as an acid as well as a secondary alcohol. On heating it loses molecule of water and forms maleic anhydride and fumaric acid.

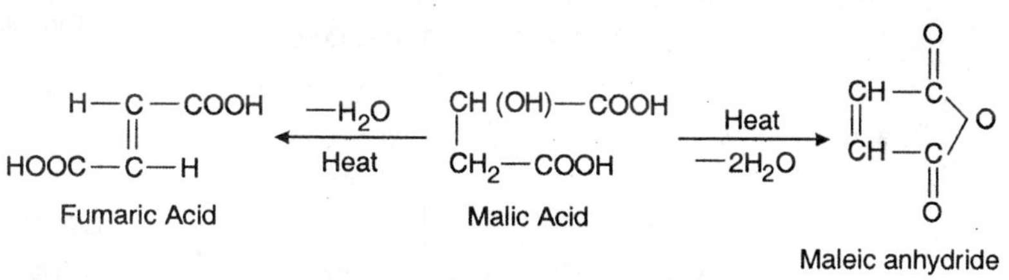

When reduced with hydroiodic acid it yields succinic acid.

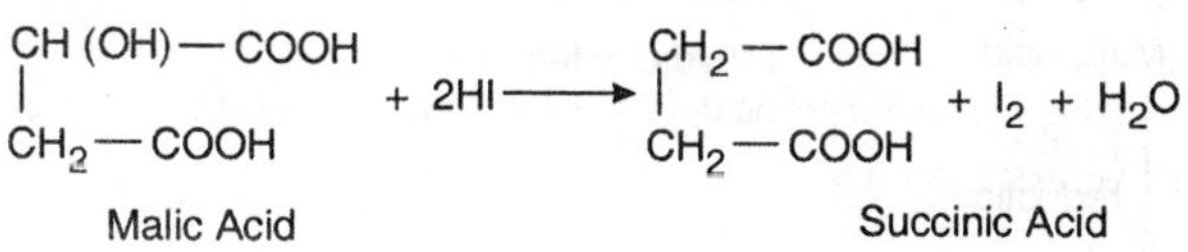

- *Uses of Malic Acid:* Malic is used in the beverages, jellies, etc. in place of citric acid and tartaric acid. It is also used as a purgative and as a remedy for sore throat.

G. **Tartaric Acid** (α, α′-Dihydroxy succinic acid or 2, 3-Dihydroxy butane dioic acid)

- *Preparation of Tartaric Acid:* Tartaric acid as such or as its potassium salt occurs in grapes, tamarind and berries. *Argol* which separates as crust during the fermentation of grape juice is impure acid, potassium tartrate. It is crystallised when pure white product, known as *Cream of tartar* is obtained. It is dissolved in water and is treated with lime till the solution is alkaline followed by the addition of calcium chlolide when calcium tartarate is precipitated. It is filtered and treated with measured amount of dilute sulphuric acid when free tartaric acid is liberated.

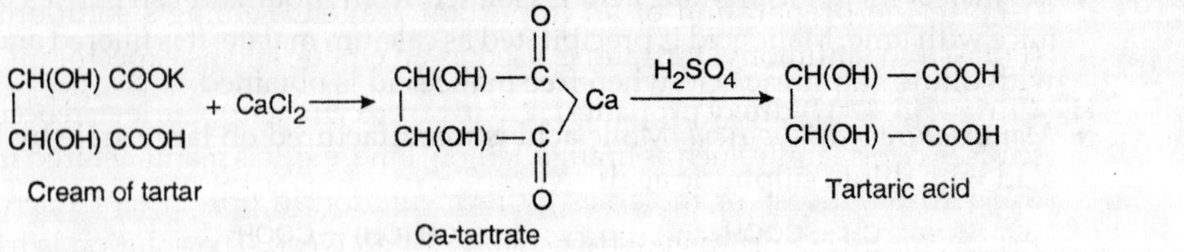

- *Synthesis of Tartaric Acid:* Tartaric acid has been synthesised from acetylene as under:

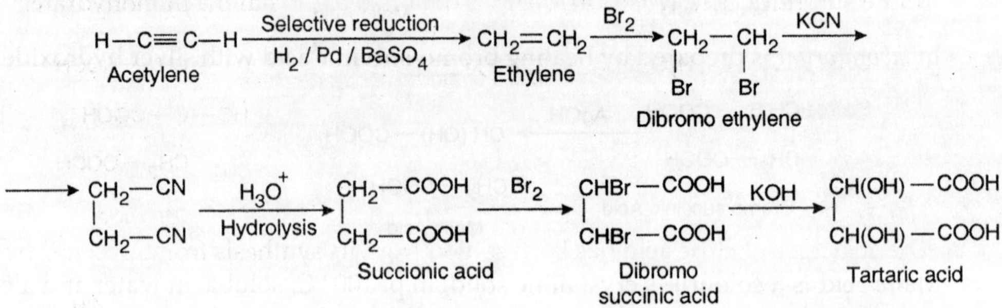

Tartaric acid is a white crystalline solid, m.p. 170 °C. It is soluble in water and alcohol but insoluble in ether. It has two chiral centres and exhibits optical activity. It exists in four isomeric forms (vide chapter **three**). Its major reactions are enlisted below:

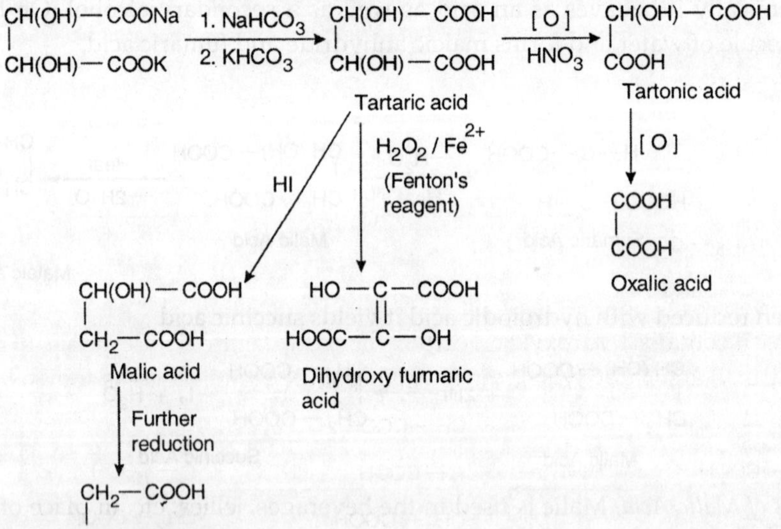

Tataric acid forms soluble complex salts with the hydroxides of heavy metals and thus prevents their precipitation. Thus copper sulphate is precipitated as copper hydroxide with sodium hydroxide but in presence of Rochelle salt solution remains clear due to the formation of complex Cu<(O—CH—COONa / O—CH—COOK) present in Fehling's solution.

- *Uses of Tartaric Acid:* Tartaric acid is used as mordant in dying and printing. Potassium hydrogen tartrate (cream of tartar) is used in drinks and baking powder. Rochelle salt is used in the preparation of an important reagent Fehling's solution. **Tartar emetic** (Potassium, antimonyl tartrate) is used as an emetic and as expectorant in medicine.

H. **Citric acid (2-Hydroxy propane-1, 2, 3 tricarboxylic acid):** Citric acid occurs in the unripe fruits of *citrus* family such as orange, lemon, lime, etc. It is manufactured from the solution of sucrose, glucose or molasses by fermentation in presence of micro-organism like *Aspergillus niger* or *citromyces plefferianus* for an week. The solution is treated with lime water when citric acid is precipitated as calcium salt. It is filtered and decomposed with dilute sulphuric acid when citric acid is obtained as crystalline monohydrate.

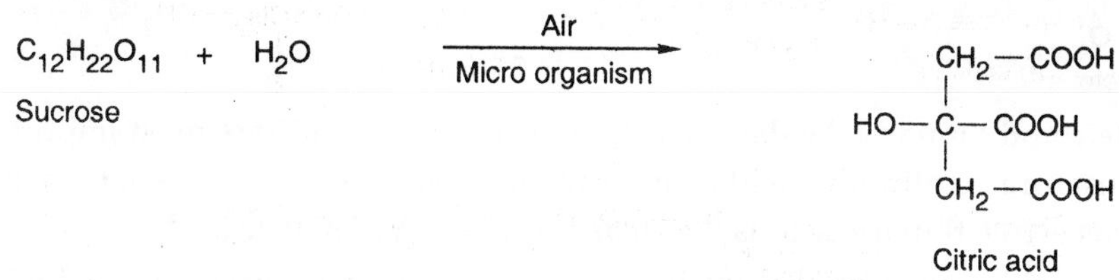

The structure of citric acid has been settled from its synthesis from glycerol.

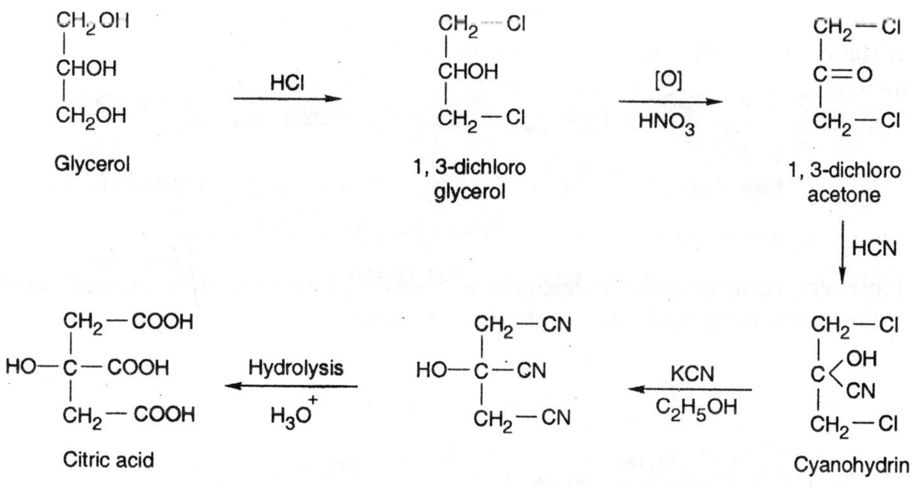

Since it contains hydroxyl and carboxylic groups citric acid responds to reactions of both hydroxyl and carboxylic groups which may be summarised as shown below:

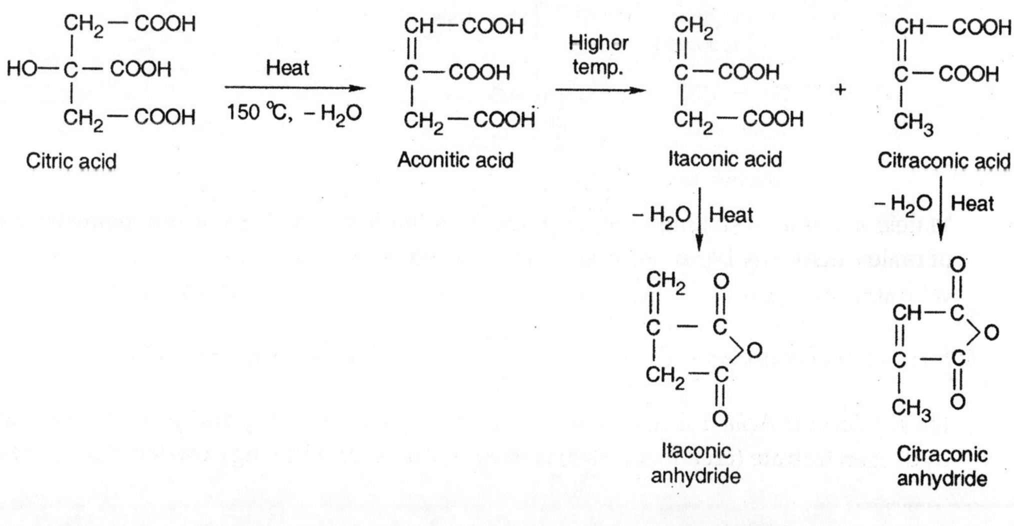

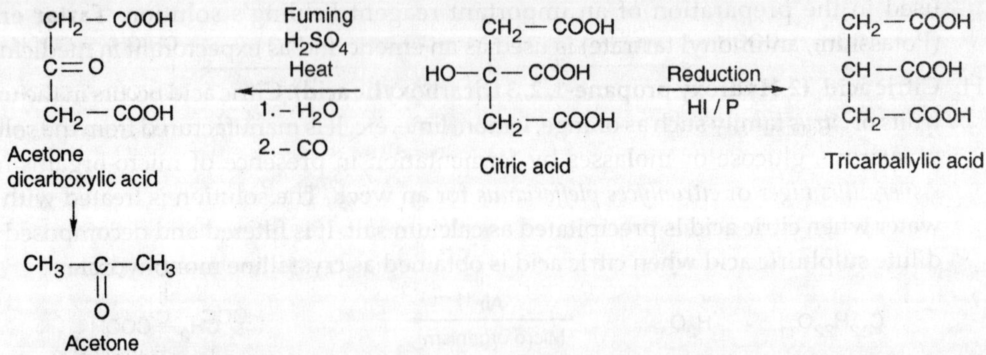

I. **Maleic and Fumaric Acids:** These two dicarboxylic acids are most important members of unsaturated aliphatic acids. These acids are isomeric to each other – maleic acid is *cis* isomer while fumaric acid is the *trans* counterpart of maleic acid.

Maleic acid is prepared by heating malic acid at 250°C fourwed by the hydrolysis of the anhydride formed.

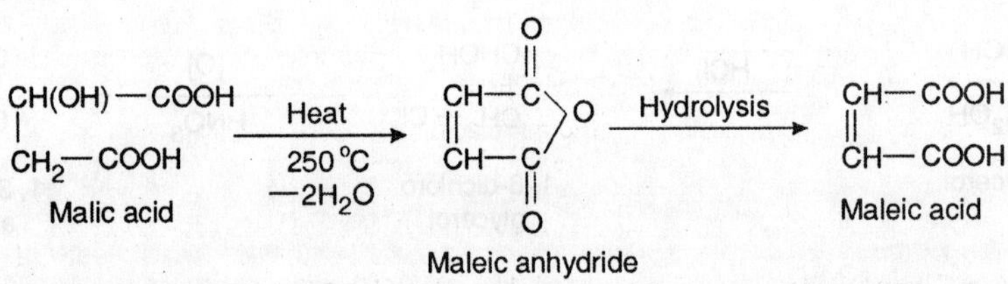

However, commercially maleic acid is prepared by the catalytic oxidation of benzene followed by hydrolysis of the anhydride formed.

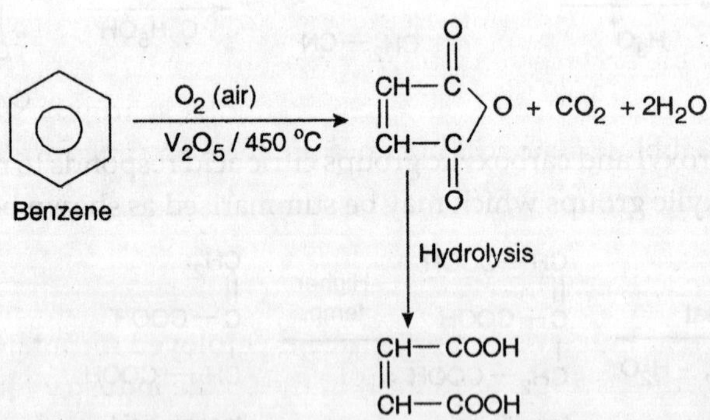

Maleic acid is a crystalline solid, m.p. 130 °C, soluble in water. Some important reactions of maleic acid may be summarised as discussed:

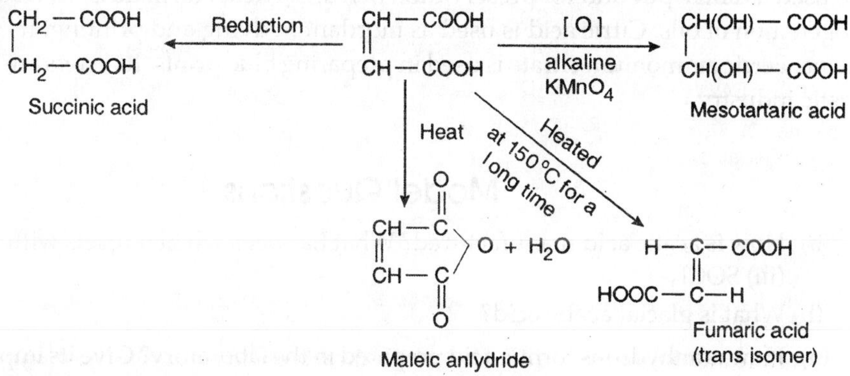

- *Uses of Maleic Acid:* Maleic anhydride is used for making varnishes and lacquers. It is also used to inhibit rancidity in milk powders, oils and fats.

  Fumaric acid is prepared by heating either maleic acid at 150 °C for a long time or bromo succinic acid with alcoholic caustic potash.

i. 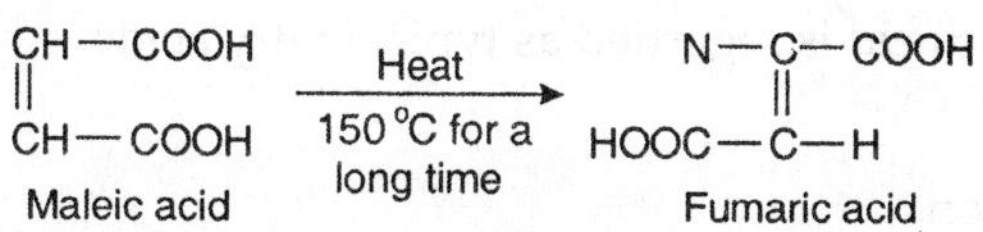

ii. 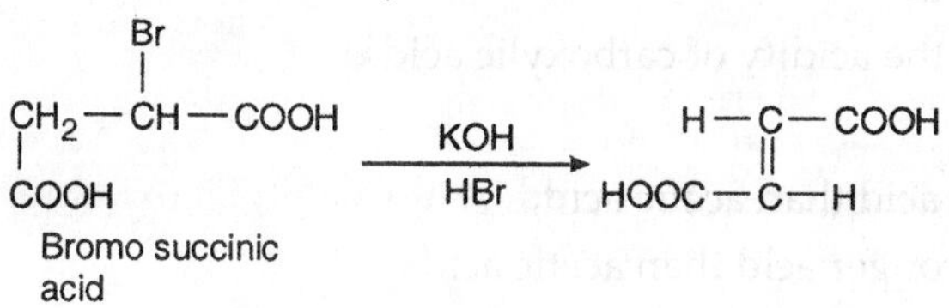

However, commercially it is prepared by the fermentation of glucose or other carbohydrates by the bacteria *Rhizopus nigricans*.

Fumaric acid is crystalline solid, m.p. 290 °C and is sparingly soluble in water. Chemically it resembles aaleic acid but does not form any anhydride of its own and this reaction differentiates this two isomers.

11.12 Uses of Aliphatic Carboxylic Acids

Aliphatic carboxylic acids are of immense importance and employed for many purposes. The first member of the family, formic acid, is used in (i) in the textile industry for certain dyeing processes (ii) rubber industry as a coagulant for latex (iii) the manufacture of plastics, water-proofing compounds, drugs etc. Acetic acid is employed for the preparation of cellulose acetate required for photographic films, for making vinegar and for coagulating rubber latex. Propionic acid is used in the manufacture of pharmaceuticals, herbicide,s etc. Sodium salt of citric acid when taken orally, forms a soluble complex with calcium ion which converts prothrombin into thrombin and so prevents blood clotting. Sodium, ammonium and calcium salts of propionic acid are active fungicides. Many other fatty acids such as caprylic [$CH_3(CH_2)_5$—CH_2—COOH] and undecylenic acid [CH_2=CH—CH_2—$(CH_2)_7$—COOH] possess strong antifungal properties. Of these undecylenic acid is best fatty acid which is used as topical fungicidal agent. Formic acid is also used as antiseptic and for preservation of fruits. Nickel formate is used as a catalyst in the hydrogenation of oils. Citric acid is used as mordant in dying and printing. Its salts are used in medicine. Ferric ammonium citrate is used in preparing blue prints. Its esters are used as solvents in plastic industry.

Model Questions

1. (a) How is acetic acid manufactured? What happens when it reacts with (i) PCl_5 (ii) P_2O_5 (iii) $SOCl_2$
   (b) What is glacial acetic acid?
2. (a) How is anhydrons formic acid prepared in the laboratory? Give its important reactions.
   (b) What happens when formic acid is treated with ammoniacal silver nitrate solution?
3. What happens when acetic acid is treated with ethyl alcohol in presence of sulphuric acid?
4. (a) How would you distinguish between formic acid and acetic acid?
   (b) Why acetic acid but not formic acid is regarded as typical fatty acid?
5. Write notes on
   (a) Hell-Volhard-Zelinisky reaction.
   (b) Acidity of carboxylic acid.
   (c) Effect of substitution on the acidity of carboxylic acids.
6. Explain:
   (a) Formic acid is a stronger acid than acetic acid.
   (b) Chloroacetic acid is a stronger acid than acetic acid.
   (c) Acetic acid is a stronger acid than propionic acid.
   (d) Boiling points of carboxylic acids are higher than corresponding alcohols?
7. How will you synthesise acetic acid from
   i. Acetylene?

Hints:

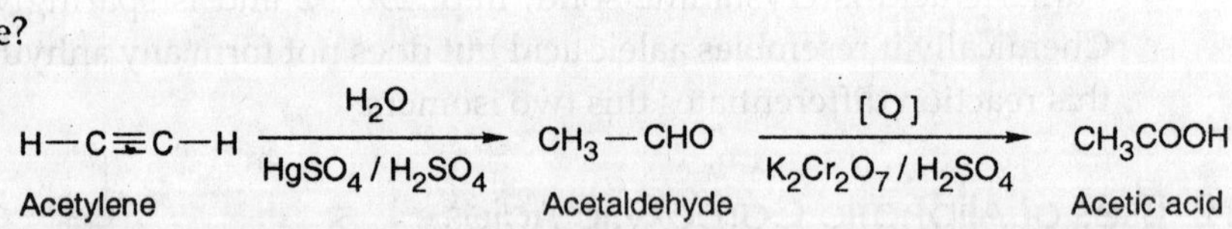

   ii. Propionic acid?

Hints:

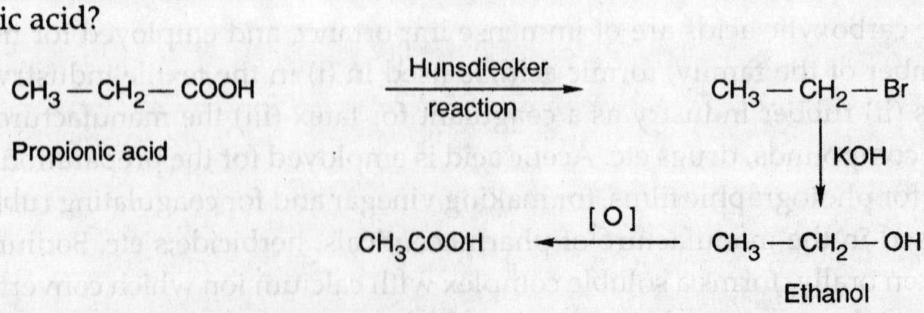

8. How will synthesise propionic acid from
   i. acetic acid?
   Hints: Arndt-Eistert synthesis

ii. Ethylene?

Hints: $CH_2{=}CH_2 + HBr \longrightarrow CH_3{-}CH_2{-}Br$

$$CH_3{-}CH_2{-}Br \xrightarrow[2.\ [O]]{1.\ KOH} CH_3{-}COOH \xrightarrow[\text{Eistert synthesis}]{\text{Arndt}} \text{Propionic acid}$$

9. How will you synthesise

(a) Glycine from acetic acid?

Hints: $CH_3{-}COOH \xrightarrow[\text{Zelinisky}]{\text{Helt-Volhard-}} Br{-}CH_2{-}COOH \xrightarrow{NH_3} \underset{\text{Glycine}}{H_2N{-}CH_2{-}COOH}$

(b) Acetone from acetic acid?

Hints: $\underset{\text{Acetic acid}}{CH_3{-}COOH} \xrightarrow{Ca(OH)_2} \text{Ca-salt} \xrightarrow{\text{Heat}} \underset{\text{Acetone}}{CH_3COCH_3}$

10. (a) Discuss the structure of carboxylic acid. Why carboxylic acids are stronger acid than alcohols?

(b) Explain why lower members of carboxylic acids are soluble in water but higher members are not.

11. Formic acid acts both as an aldehyde and as an acid — explain.

Hints: Like aldehyde formic acid is readily oxidised by mild oxidising agent.Thus ammoniacal $AgNO_3$ is reduced to Ag°.

$$H{-}COOH \xrightarrow[AgNO_3]{[O]} CO_2 + H_2O + Ag^o$$

Similarly, formic acid can reduce Fehling's solution.

$$HCOOH + CuSO_4 \longrightarrow \underset{\text{Red ppt.}}{Cu_2O} + CO_2 + H_2O + H_2SO_4$$

Again, formic acid reacts with NaOH and $NaHCO_3$ showing its acidic character.

12. Outline the synthesis of the following:

(i) $Me_2CH{-}CH_2{-}COOH$ and (ii) $Me_2CH{-}CH_2{-}CH(NH_2){-}COOH$ from malonic ester.

13. What happens when:

(a) Oxalic acid is heated?

(b) Oxalic acid is oxidised with $KMnO_4$?

(c) Malonic acid is heated?

(d) Succinic acid is heated?

14. How would you synthesise

(a) Oxalic acid from formic acid?

(b) Oxalic acid from ethylene?

(c) Malonic acid from acetic acid?

(d) Succinic acid from ethylene?

(e) N-bromo succinimide from succinic acid?

15. How would you distinguish oxalic acid and succinic acid?

Hints: Oxalic on heating forms carbon dioxide which can be precipitated with lime water but succinic acid does not form carbon dioxide, it forms anhydride.

16. What are hydroxy acids? How are they prepared? Give some important reactions of hydroxy acids.

17. What happens when

(a) lactic acid is heated?

(b) tartaric acid is treated with HI?

(c) tartaric acid is oxidised with HNO_3?

18. Give methods of preparation and properties of (i) Lactic acid (ii) tartaric acid (iii) citric acid.

19. How would you synthesise

(a) lactic acid from (i) acetaldehyde (ii) acetylene (iii) ethyl alcohol

(b) citric acid from glycerol?

20. (a) Starting from malic acid how would you prepare maleic and fumaric acid?

(b) How would you distinguish between maleic acid and fumaric acid?

CHAPTER TWELVE

Aliphatic Amines

Amines may be regarded as the derivatives of ammonia in which one or more or all the three hydrogen atoms are replaced by organic groups, such as alkyl or aryl. They are classified into the following three categories:

(a) *Primary amines*: In these amines only one hydrogen atom in ammonia is replaced by organic group and thus they may be represented by general formula, R—NH_2.

CH_3-NH_2 Methylamine

$CH_3-CH_2-NH_2$ Ethylamine

(b) *Secondary amines*: Amines containing $>$NH group are known as secondary amines, i.e., in these amines two hydrogen atoms in ammonia have been replaced by two same or different groups. Their general formula is

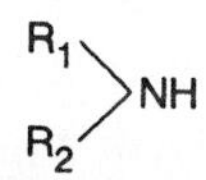

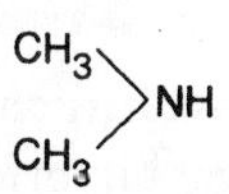

Dimethyl amine

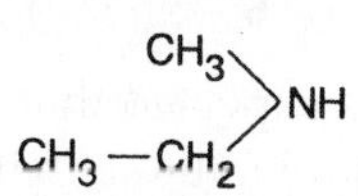

Ethyl methyl amine

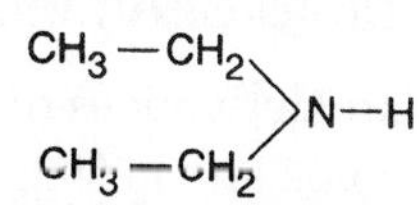

Diethyl amine

(c) *Tertiary amines*: In these amines all the three hydrogen atoms in ammonia have been replaced by three same or different alkyl or aryl groups. These amines have general expression,

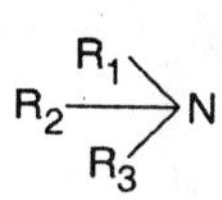

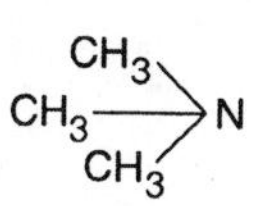

Trimethyl amine

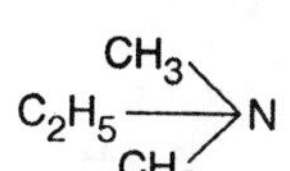

Dimethylethyl amine

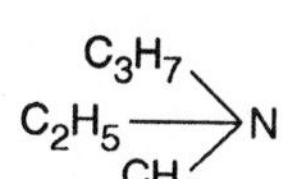

Ethyl methyl propyl amine

12.1 Nomenclature of Amines

Amines are generally named according to common system, i.e., by naming the group or groups attached to the nitrogen and adding at the end the word-'*amine*'. However, they may be named by IUPAC system of nomenclature. Names of some of the common amines in different systems may be summarised in the following table:

Compound	Common Name	IUPAC Name
CH_3NH_2	Methyl amine	Amino methane
$CH_3-CH_2-NH_2$	Ethyl amine	Amino ethane
$CH_3-\underset{\underset{\displaystyle CH_3}{\vert}}{CH}-NH_2$	Isopropyl amine	2-Methyl amino ethane
$\begin{matrix}CH_3\\CH_3\end{matrix}\!>\!NH$	Dimethyl amine	N-methyl amino methane
$\begin{matrix}CH_3\\CH_3-CH_2\end{matrix}\!>\!NH$	Ethyl methyl amine	N-methyl amino ethane
$\begin{matrix}CH_3\\CH_3\end{matrix}\!>\!\underset{\underset{\displaystyle CH_3}{\vert}}{N}$	Trimethyl amine	N, N-dimethyl amino methane
$\begin{matrix}CH_3\\CH_3\end{matrix}\!>\!\underset{\underset{\displaystyle CH_2-CH_3}{\vert}}{N}$	Ethyl dimethyl amine	N, N-dimethyl amino ethane

12.2 Structure of Amines

As amines are derivatives of ammonia, it is expected that they should have structure similar to that of ammonia and in fact, it has been found to be so. Nitrogen atom is sp^3-hybridised. One of the sp^3-hybridised orbitals is filled up with two electrons and so cannot participate in bond formation. Remaining sp^3-hybridised orbitals are directed towards the corners of a tetrahedron. Thus the shape of amines may be represented as

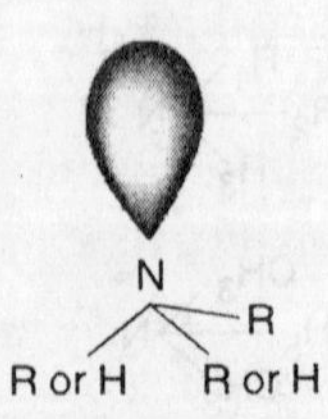

The bond angle C—N—C in trimethyl amine has been found to be 108°.

12.3 Stereochemistry of Amines

Since nitrogen atom in amine is tetrahedral in nature it is expected that amines may be dissymmetric in nature and hence may be resolvable into enantiomers. But in actual practice, amines have not yet been reported to exhibit any optical activity. This is because of the fact that the two enantiomers undergo rapid inversion in configuration due to very low energy barrier of only 6 kcal/mole between the two forms.

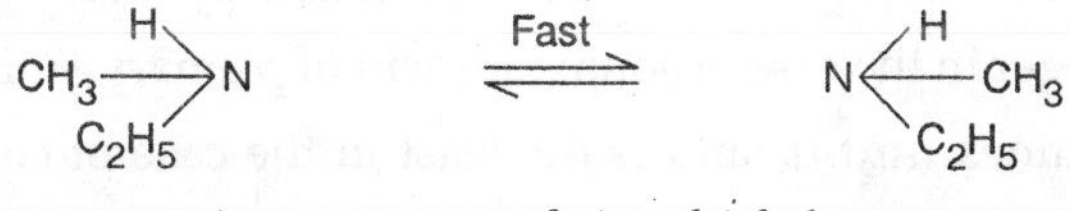

However, quaternary ammonium compounds in which four groups on nitrogen are arranged tetrahedrally can show optical activity. Because such inversion is not possible.

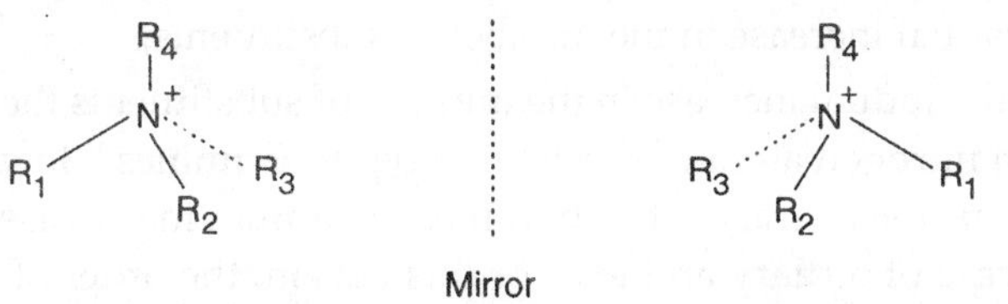

Similarly, nitrogen present in smaller rings cannot undergo inversion and so is resolvable into enantiomers.

PROBLEM 12.1

Which of the following compounds exhibit optical activity?

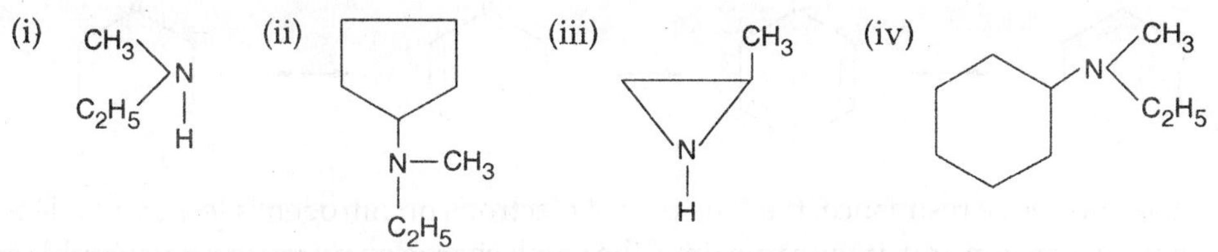

12.4 Basicity of Amines

Since amines are the organic derivatives of ammonia, it is highly reasonable to assume that amines may be basic in character. In fact, amines, like ammonia, give an alkaline reaction in aqueous solution and form salts with acids. In aqueous solution, amine exists in the following equilibrium:

$$RNH_2 + H_2O \rightleftharpoons R{-}\overset{+}{N}H_3 + \overset{-}{O}H$$

According to this modern concept the strength of any base depends upon the simultaneous fulfilment of two conditions: (i) avialability of electrons, (ii) stability of conjugate acid formed in solution. Any factor that can increase electron density of the species under consideration increases the basicity. Similarly, increase in the stability of conjugate acid increases the basic strength of the compound. But both these factors are to be considered simultaneously. Based on the above concept regarding the strength of the bases the observations noted in the table may be properly rationalised.

It has been observed that aliphatic secondary amine is most basic among ammonia, primary, secondary and tertiary amines, i.e., the order is

$$NH_3 < RNH_2 < (R)_2NH > (R)_3N > NH_3$$

The greater basicity of all the three types of amines than ammonia is attributable to the electron release by alkyl groups which increases the electron density on nitrogen and at the same time the conjugate acids formed are moderately stable, as a result of which the average effect of both the factors are greater in these amines than in ammonia, and amines are more basic than ammonia. But among the three types of amines, average effect of these two factors is not the same. In aqueous solution conjugate acids are stabilised by hydrogen bonding and such stabilisation is most stronger in the case of conjugate acid of primary amine $R—\overset{+}{N}H_3$, moderate in the case of secondary amines $(R)_2\overset{+}{N}H_2$ and is the least in the case of conjugate acid of tertiary amine $(R)_3\overset{+}{N}H$— the gradual decrease in stability of these conjugate acids is due to (i) availability of lesser number of hydrogen atom for hydrogen bond formation and (ii) gradual increase of steric strain due to gradual increase in the number of substituents.

On the other hand, gradual increase in the number of substituents there is gradual increase in electron density on nitrogen atom of these three types of amines. However, considering the effect of both the factors, the average effect becomes maximum in the case of secondary amines and it is least in the case of tertiary amines. For this reason, the order of basicity among three types of amines stands as

$$RNH_2 < (R)_2NH > (R)_3N$$

Weak basicity of aromatic amines is due to the resonance stabilisation as indicated below.

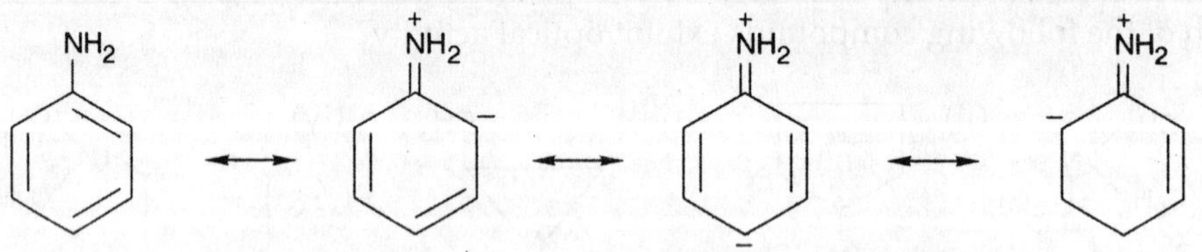

Owing to the above resonance, the lone pair of electrons on nitrogen is less available for co-ordinating with a proton and at the same time, the small charge on nitrogen atom would tend to repel a proton. Further, the conjugate acid, the anilinum ion is less stable than parent amine due to lesser number of resonating structures (only two).

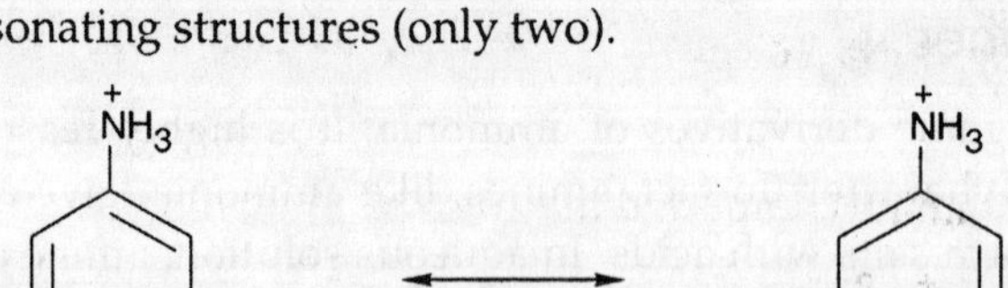

Anilinium ion

12.5 General Methods of Preparation of Aliphatic Amines

Some of the common methods for the preparation of amines are as described below:

1. *Alkylation of ammonia (Ammonolysis)*: This method is due to Hofmann. In this method, alkyl halides are treated with ammonia. By this method all the three types of amines can be prepared. Reactions taking place may be described as:

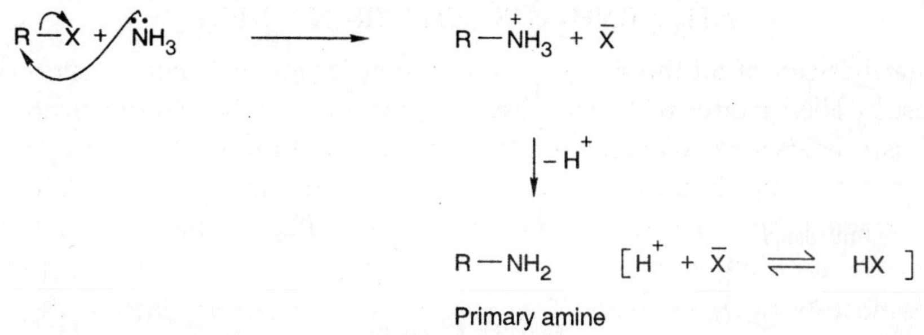

With excess alkyl halide reaction proceeds further forming secondary and tertiary amines.

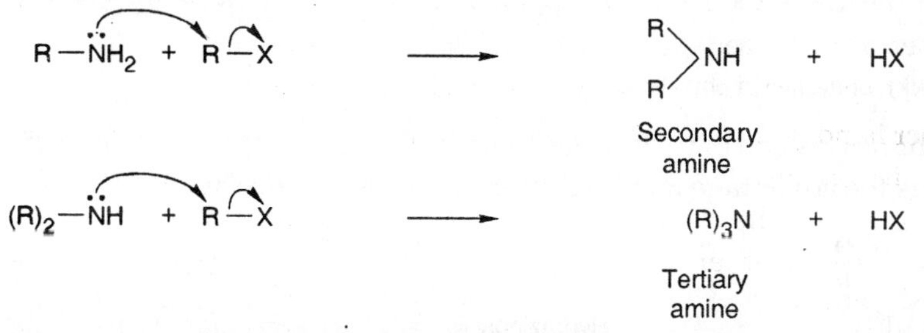

It may be mentioned that in presence of large excess of alkyl halide, reaction may proceed further yielding quaternary ammonium compound. So to get desired amine, controlled amount of alkyl-halide should be used.

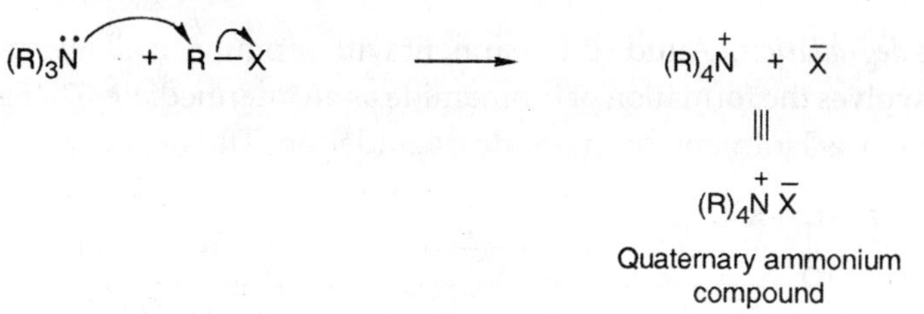

However, it has been observed that using large excess of ammonia, reaction may be stopped at primary amine stage, i.e.,

$$CH_3—Br + NH_3 \text{ (Excess)} \longrightarrow \underset{\text{Methyl amine}}{CH_3—NH_2} + HBr$$

By this method diamino compound may also be prepared.

$$\underset{\text{Dichloro ethane}}{Cl—CH_2—CH_2—Cl} + 2NH_3 \longrightarrow \underset{\text{Ethylene diamine}}{H_2N—CH_2—CH_2—NH_2} + 2HCl$$

2. *Gabriel Synthesis*: Pure primary amines can be prepared by this procedure. This process involves the alkylation of a derivative of ammonia in which two hydrogen atoms are temporarily replaced by blocking groups to prevent introduction of more than a single alkyl substituent. The cyclic substance, phthalimide is employed as ammonia derivative which possesses one hydrogen atom doubly activated by carbonyl groups and so this hydrogen atom is acidic in nature and is capable of forming metal salt. This salt when reacts with alkyl halides furnish alkylated phthalimide derivative. On hydrolysis with alkali, alkylated phthalimide liberates primary amine which is removed from the alkaline mixture by steam distillation. This method is also known as *Gabriel-phthalimide synthesis*.

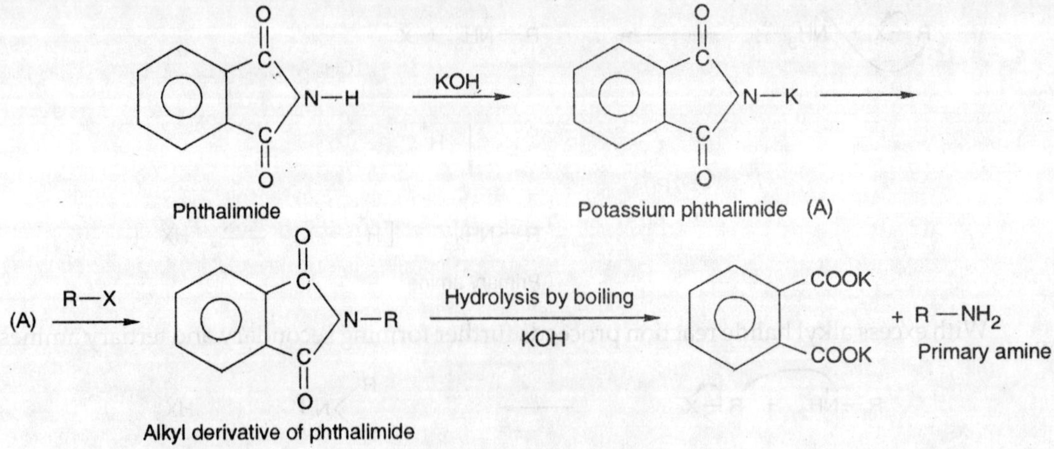

Somethimes instead of hydrolysis, hydrazinolysis is carried with hydrazine. Hydrazinolysis has the advantage that it requires mild condition. Thus,

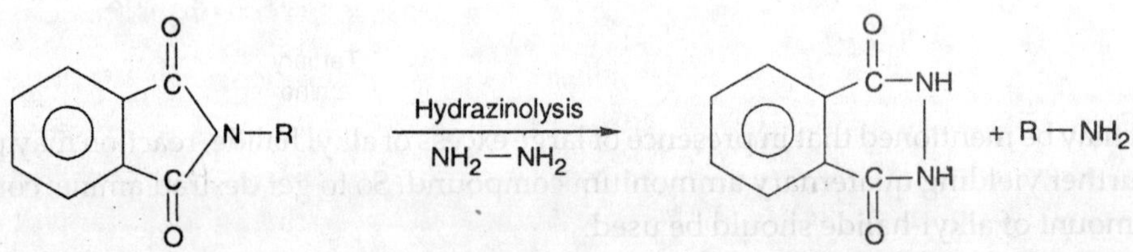

3. *Hofmann's degradation*: Amide on treatment with bromine in alkali furnishes amine. The reaction involves the formation of bromamide as an intermediate. That is why this method is also known as Hofmann bromamide degradation. Thus,

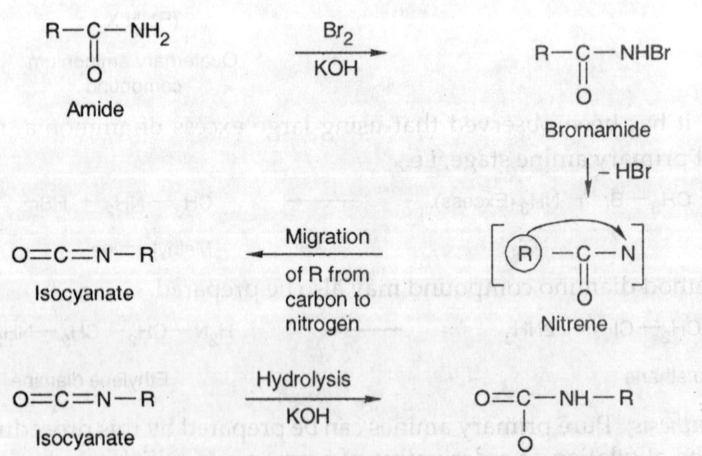

4. *Reduction of reducible compounds*: Easily reducible compounds like nitriles, oxime, amides and nitro compounds on reduction yield amines. Thus,

(a) *Reduction of nitrile*

$$\underset{\text{Nitrile}}{R-C\equiv N} \xrightarrow{\text{Reduction}} R-CH_2-NH_2$$

$$\underset{\text{Methyl nitrile}}{CH_3-C\equiv N} \xrightarrow{\text{Reduction}} \underset{\text{Ethyl amine}}{CH_3-CH_2-NH_2}$$

Reduction may be carried out either by catalytic reduction or by using reducing agent like sodium and alcohol. The latter reduction process is known as *Mendius reduction.*

(b) *Reduction of oxime*: Catalytic reduction of oxime forms amine.

$$\underset{\text{Acetaldoxime}}{CH_3-CH=N-OH} \xrightarrow{\text{Cat [H]}} \underset{\text{Ethyl amine}}{CH_3-CH_2-NH_2}$$

Sodium and alcohol can also be used as reducing agent in this reduction.

(c) *Reduction of amide*: Amide can be reduced to amine by catalytic reduction or by sodium and alcohol.

$$\underset{\text{Acetamide}}{CH_3-\underset{\underset{O}{\|}}{C}-NH_2} \xrightarrow[\text{or Na / alcohol}]{\text{Cat [H]}} \underset{\text{Ethyl amine}}{CH_3-CH_2-NH_2}$$

(d) *Reduction of nitro compound*: Reduction of nitro compound for the preparation of amines is a very common process particularly for the preparation of aromatic amines. In this reduction, variety of reducing agents may be used.

$$R-NO_2 \xrightarrow[\text{or Sn / HCl}]{\text{Cat [H]}} R-NH_2 + 2H_2O$$

(e) *Action of ammonia on alcohols*: When vapours of mixture of alcohol and ammonia is passed over heated alumina all the three types of amines are obtained.

$$\underset{\text{Ethanol}}{C_2H_5OH} + NH_3 \xrightarrow[350\text{-}400\ ^\circ C]{Al_2O_3} \underset{\text{Ethyl amine}}{CH_3-CH_2-NH_2} + H_2O$$

$$CH_3-CH_2-NH_2 \xrightarrow[Al_2O_3\,/\,350\text{-}400\ ^\circ C]{C_2H_5OH} (CH_3-CH_2)_2NH + H_2O$$

Similarly, tertiary amines may be obtained.

5. *Curtius reaction*: Curtius reaction may be utilised for the preparation of primary amines. When acyl azide is heated in a solvent, there is formation of amine through the formation of nitrene and isocyanate as in the case of Hofmann bromamide reaction. Thus,

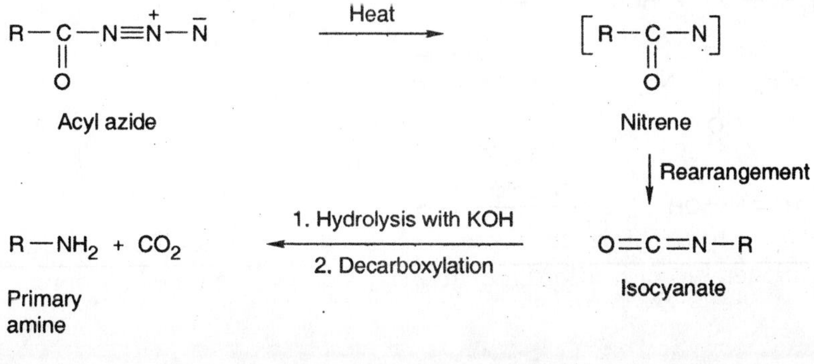

6. *Ritter method*: For the preparation of primary amines with tertiary alkyl group attached to nitrogen atom Ritter method is the best. This method involves the reaction of tertiary alcohol with alkyl cyanide in presence of strong sulphuric acid. Thus,

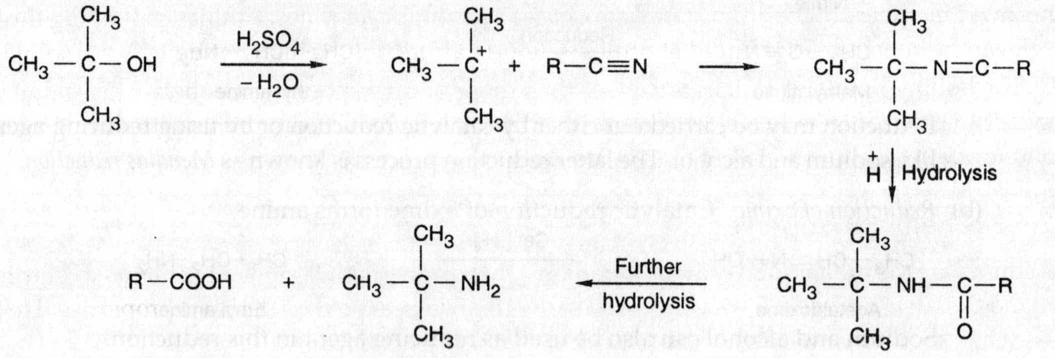

Butyl amine

7. *Some methods specific for secondary and tertiary amine*: A few methods are available for the preparation of secondary and tertiary amines.

   (a) *Preparation of secondary amines*

   i. $R-NH_2 + R-X \longrightarrow (R)_2NH + HX$

   ii. $R-N\equiv C \xrightarrow[4H]{Cat\,[H]} R-NH-CH_3$
   Isocyanide

   (b) *Preparation of tertiary amines*: Tertiary amines may be conveniently prepared by continuous alkylation of ammonia, primary or secondary amines by alkyl halides. However, trimethyl amine is most conveniently prepared heating paraformaldehyde with ammonium chloride.

$$\underset{\text{Paraformaldehyde}}{3(CH_2O)_3} \xrightarrow[\text{Heat}]{2NH_4Cl} 2(CH_3)_3\overset{+}{N}H\overset{-}{Cl} + 3CO_2 + 3H_2O$$

$$2(CH_3)_3\overset{+}{N}H\overset{-}{Cl} \xrightarrow{NaOH} \underset{\text{Trimethyl amine}}{2(CH_3)_3N}$$

PROBLEM 12.2

Suggest the probable product in the following reaction:

(a) $(CH_3)_3-C-OH + HCN \xrightarrow{H_2SO_4}$

(b) $CH_3-CH_2-\underset{\underset{O}{\|}}{C}-NH_2 \xrightarrow{Br_2\,/\,KOH}$

(c) $(CH_3)_2C=N-OH \xrightarrow{Na\,/\,alcohol}$

12.6 Properties of Amines

12.6.1 Physical Properties

The lower members of the amine family are gases and soluble in water. Amines containing three to eleven carbon atoms are liquid at ordinary temperature and the higher members are solids.

The boiling points of amines are lower than those of corresponding alcohols. This is due to the fact that nitrogen is less electro-negative than oxygen and so the probability of hydrogen bond formation in amines is less than in alcohols.

12.6.2 Chemical Properties

As amines are the organic derivatives of ammonia their properties are similar to ammonia centring around the basic nitrogen. It was discussed earlier that amines possess the basic properties. Their basic character is manifested by the following characteristic reactions:

(a) *Reactions with acids*: Amines react with acids to form salts. Salt formation with mineral acids is analogous to ammonium salt and is formed both in aqueous and anhydrous condition. Thus, when hydrogen chloride gas is passed into an ethereal solution of amine, salt of amine separates as white solid. Thus,

$$\underset{\text{Methyl amine}}{CH_3NH_2} + HCl \longrightarrow CH_3\overset{+}{N}H_3Cl$$

$$(CH_3)_2NH + HCl \longrightarrow (CH_3)_2\overset{+}{N}H_2Cl$$

$$(CH_3)_3N + HCl \longrightarrow (CH_3)_3\overset{+}{N}HCl$$

(b) *Reaction with nitrous acid*: One of the most important reactions of amines is with nitrous acid. The nature of the products depends very much upon whether the amine is primary, secondary or tertiary in character. Indeed, reaction of nitrous acid is used as a useful test for determining the primary, secondary or tertiary nature of amine. These three types of amines react differently with nitrous acid.

Primary amine reacts with nitrous acid to form initially an unstable diazonium compound which decomposes to evolve nitrogen. Nitrous acid is unstable and it is prepared *in situ* by reaction of sodium nitrite with hydrochloric acid, i.e.,

$$NaNO_2 + HCl \longrightarrow HNO_2 + NaCl$$

$$HNO_2 \equiv \dot{H}O{-}N{=}O + \overset{+}{H} \text{ (from HCl)}$$

$$\downarrow \text{Protonation}$$

$$H{-}\overset{+}{\underset{\underset{H}{|}}{O}}{-}N{=}O \xrightarrow{-H_2O} \underset{\text{Nitronium ion}}{\overset{+}{N}{=}O} + H_2O$$

This nitronium ion is active elctrophile and reacts with amine to form diazonium salt.

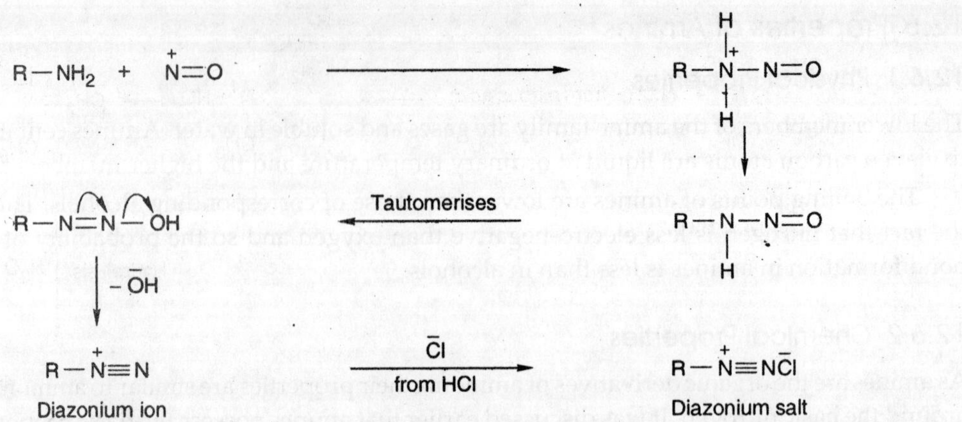

Diazonium ion or salt is very unstable. It readily undergoes decomposition with the evolution of nitrogen gas and generation of carbocation.

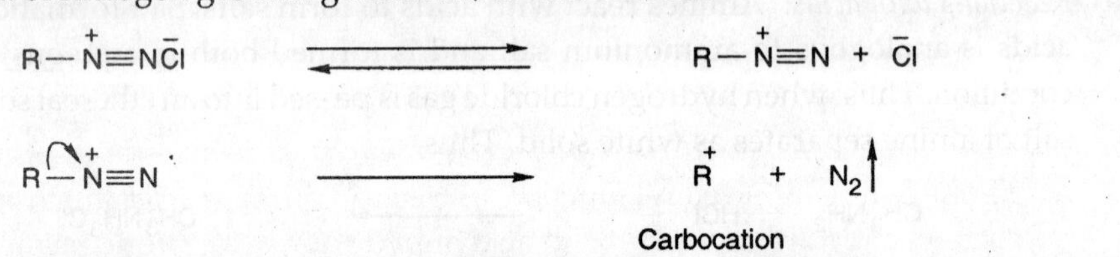

The carbocation formed combines with water in aqueous solution to form alcohol.

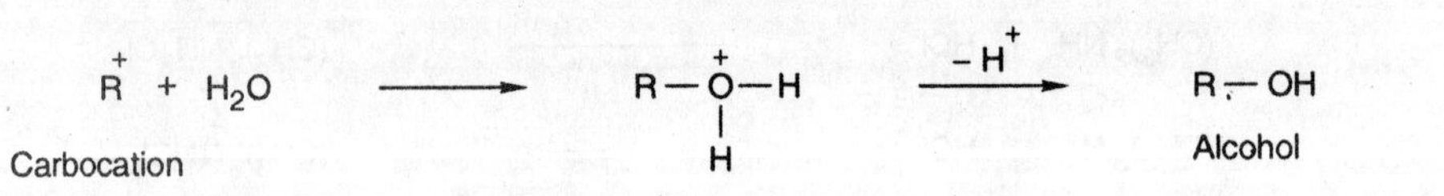

Thus, primary aliphatic amines normally yield primary alcohols on reaction with nitrous acid.

It may be mentioned that diazonium ions or salts of aromatic amines are to some extent stable due to participation of aromatic ring in resonance.

Secondary amines react with nitrous acid to form yellow oily compound insoluble in dilute mineral acid.

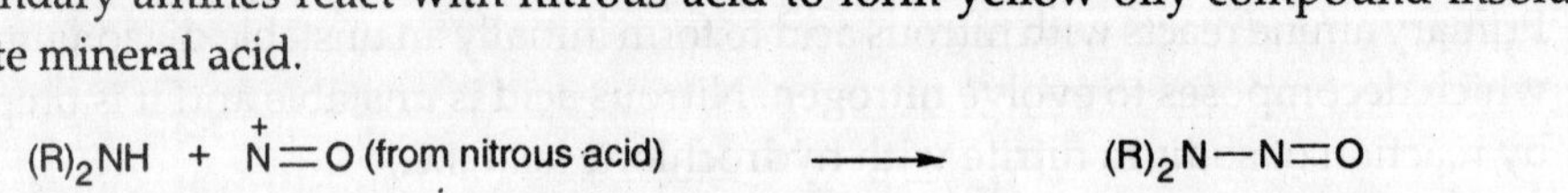

PROBLEM 12.3

Suggest the probable products in the following reactions:

(a) $CH_3-NH_2 + NaNO_2 + HCl \longrightarrow$

(b) $(CH_3)_2-NH + NaNO_2 + HCl \longrightarrow$

(c) $CH_3-CH_2-N(CH_3)(CH_3) + NaNO_2 + HCl \longrightarrow$

On the other hand, tertiary amine dissolves in nitrous acid without any evolution of nitrogen gas to give complex products.

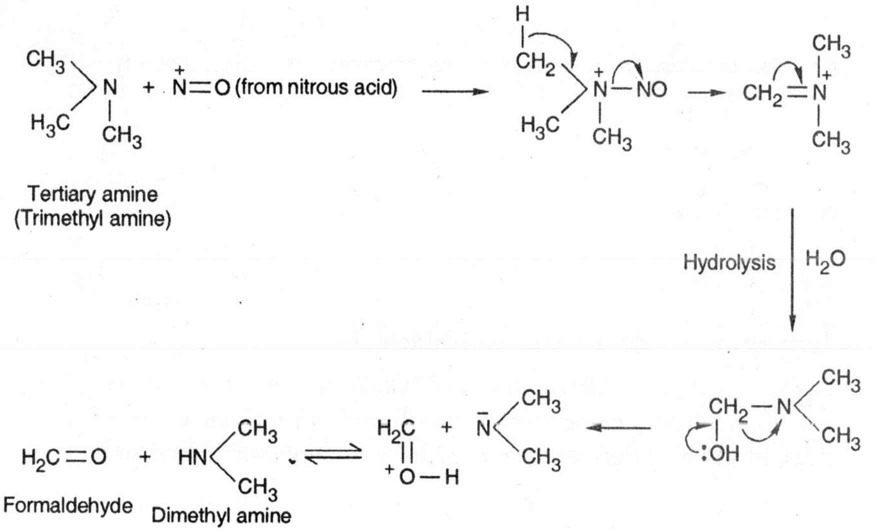

(c) *Reactions of Amines with compounds containing a carbonyl group*: Amines react with compounds having carbonyl function, as electron donor species (nucleophile). Examples of such reaction are available with acid anhydrides, acid chlorides and aldehydes. The general path of the reaction may be shown as below:

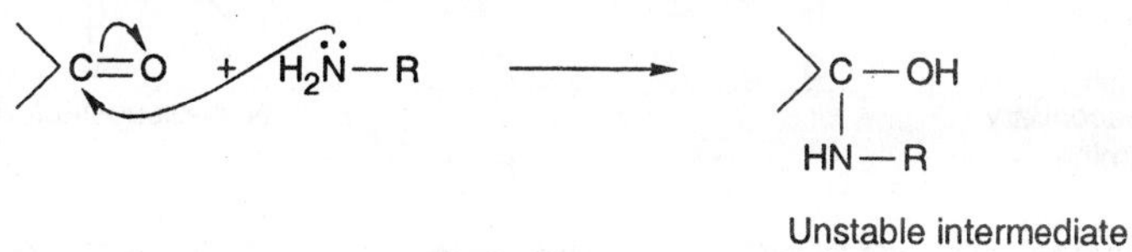

This unstable intermediate may eliminate water or hydrogen halide depending upon the nature of the amine and the carbonyl compounds.

i. When the carbonyl compound is an *aldehyde* and amine is *primary in nature*, normally elimination of water takes place forming a schiff-base, i.e.,

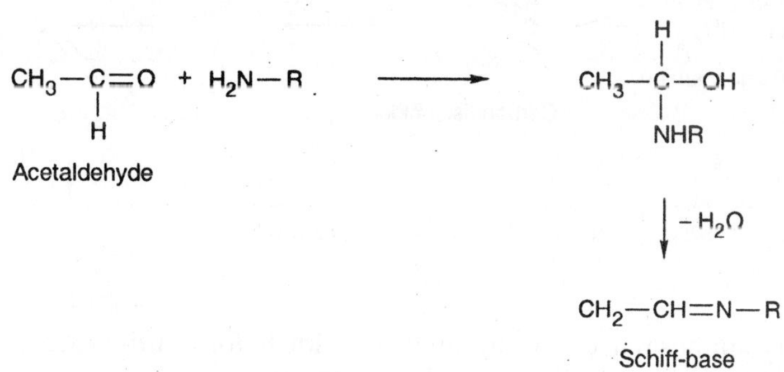

Secondary amines do not form any schiff-base with aldehydes. However, aldehydes having α-H atom can react with secondary amine yielding *enamines*.

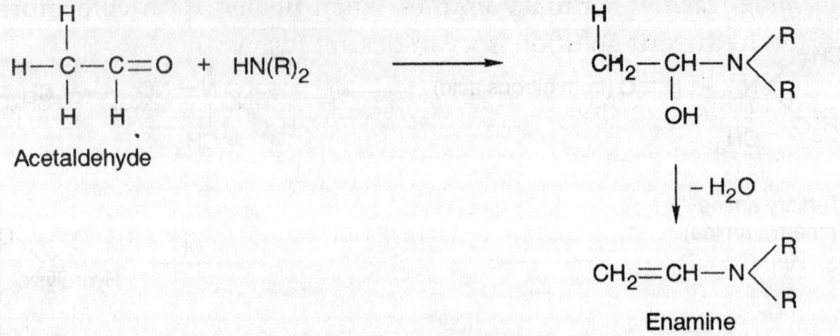

Tertiary amines do not react with aldehydes.

ii. *Reaction with acid-chloride and acid-anhydride*: Primary and secondary amines on reaction with acid-chloride and anhydride form acyl derivatives. But tertiary amines do not form acyl derivative as they have no replaceable hydrogen atom.

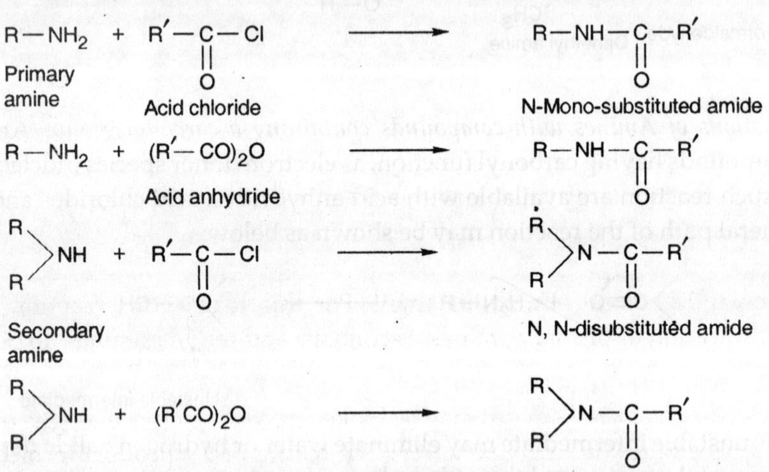

(d) *Reaction with carbon disulphide*: When *primary amine* is warmed with carbon disulphide in presence of mercuric chloride as catalyst, isothiocyanate is formed.

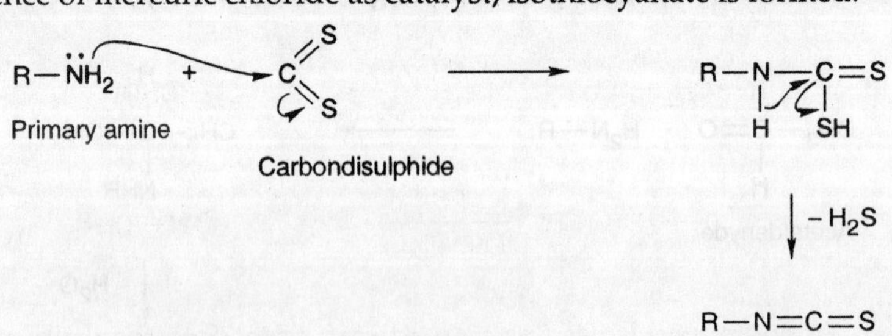

Secondary amines react with carbon disulphide to form dithiocarbamic acid.

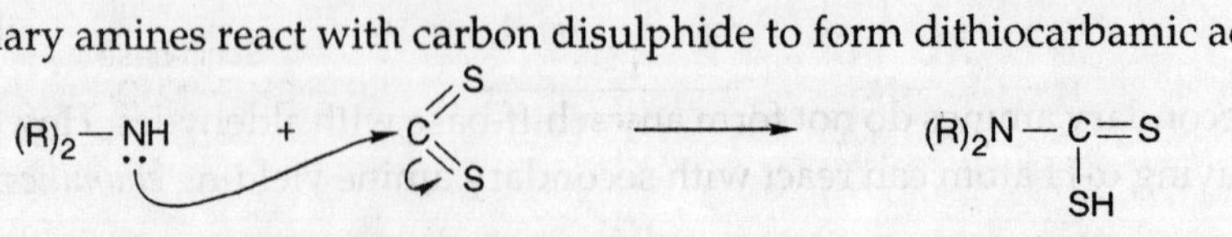

Tertiary amine do not react at all.

(e) *Carbylamine reaction*: Primary amines when heated with chloroform and alcoholic potassium hydroxide solution isocyanides are formed.

$$R-NH_2 + CHCl_3 + KOH \longrightarrow RNC + 2KCl + 3H_2O$$

Mechanistically the reaction may be explained as under:

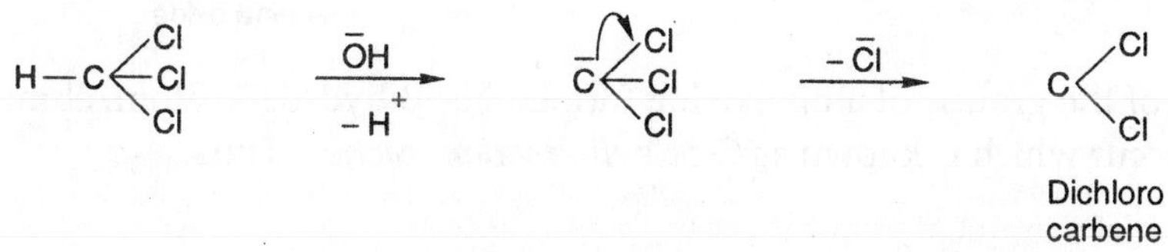

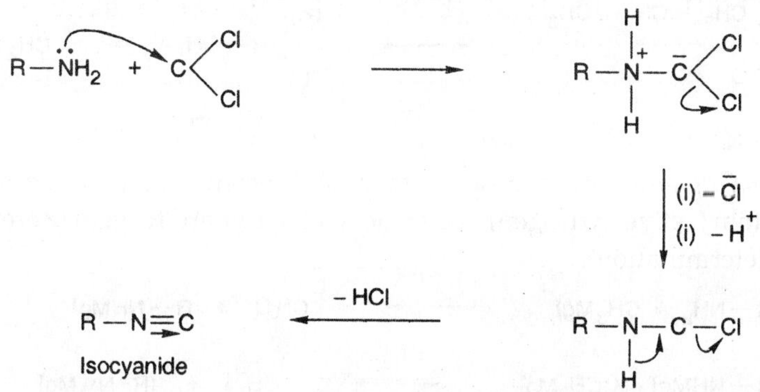

Isocyanide has an obnoxious smell. For this reason this reaction is employed for identification of primary amines. Secondary and tertiary amines do not respond to this reaction.

(f) *Oxidation of amines*: Amines may be looked upon as amino analogue of alcohols. So like alcohols amines undergo oxidation. The nature of the product formed depends on the nature of the oxidising agent.

Primary and secondary amines when oxidised with potassium permanganate solution aldehydes and hydroxyl amines are respectively formed. Thus,

$$R-CH_2-NH_2 \xrightarrow[KMnO_4]{[O]} R-CHO$$

$$R_2N-H \xrightarrow[KMnO_4]{[O]} R_2N-OH$$

However, when peracid is used as an oxidising agent both the primary and secondary amines yield hydroxyl amine, i.e.,

$$R-CH_2-NH_2 \xrightarrow[Peracid]{[O]} R-CH_2-NHOH$$

$$R_2NH \xrightarrow{[O]} R_2N-OH$$

Tertiary amines do not respond to $KMnO_4$ oxidation but when oxidised with peracid forms amine oxide.

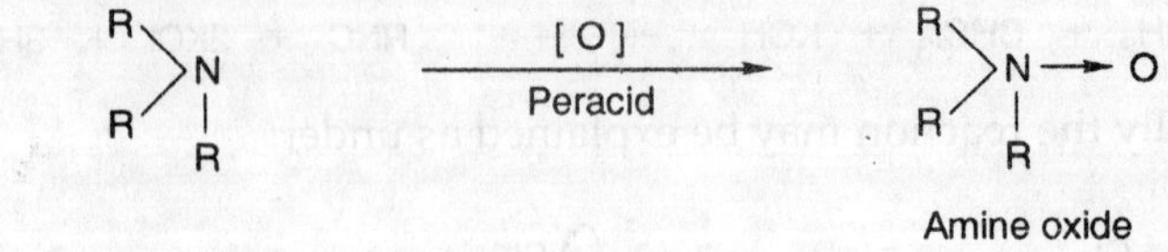

If one of the groups of amine oxide formed has β-hydrogen atom, elimination reaction may occur which is known as *Cope's elimination reaction*. Thus,

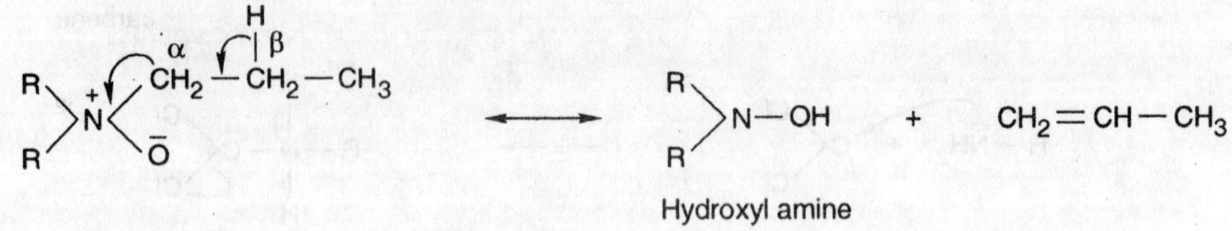

(g) *Reaction with Grignard reagent*: Since primary and secondary amines possess replaceable hydrogen atom (active hydrogen), they react with Grignard reagent (Zerewittinoff active hydrogen determination).

$$R{-}NH_2 + CH_3MgI \longrightarrow CH_4\uparrow + R{-}NHMgI$$

$$R{-}NHMgI + CH_3MgI \longrightarrow CH_4\uparrow + (R{-}N)_2MgI$$

$$R_2N{-}H + CH_3MgI \longrightarrow CH_4\uparrow + R_2NMgI$$

(h) *Mannich condensation reaction*: Only primary and secondary amines can participate in Mannich condensation reaction. Mannich condensation is a reaction of a compound containing at least one *active* hydrogen atom with formaldehyde and ammonia or ammonia derivatives. In this reaction active hydrogen atom is replaced by amino methyl group. Thus,

Step I:

Step II:

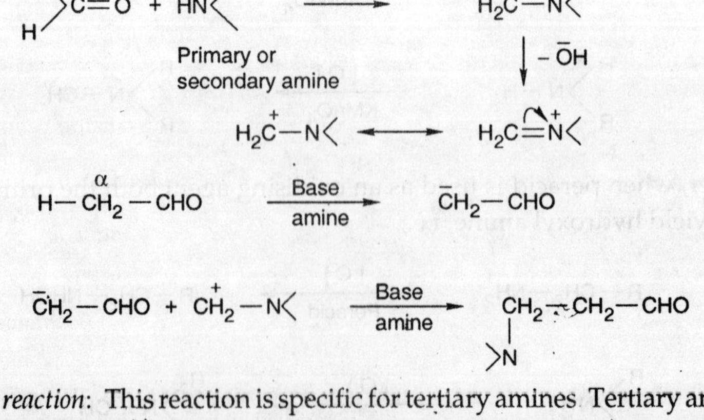

(i) *Von-Braun reaction*: This reaction is specific for tertiary amines Tertiary amines on reaction with cyanogen bromide afford a quaternary salt which on heating forms N, N-dialkyl cyanamide and an alkyl bromide. The dialkyl cyanamide when hydrolysed yields a **secondary amine**. Thus, this reaction may be considered as a method for the conversion of tertiary amine into a secondary amine and hence this reaction constitutes a method for the preparation of secondary amines.

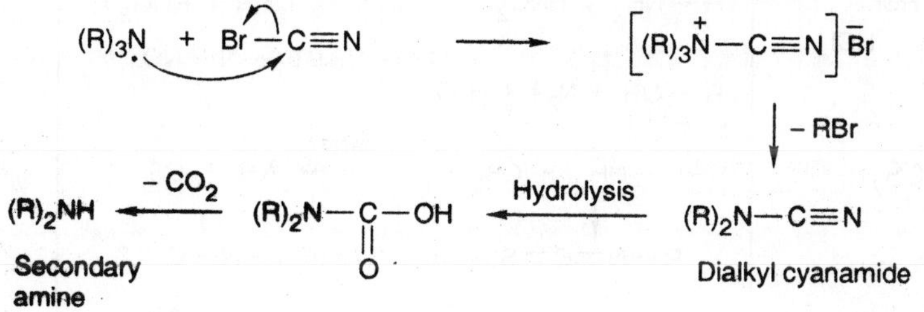

(j) *Exhaustive Methylation*: All the three types of amines when treated with alkyl halide form quaternary ammonium salt. Thus,

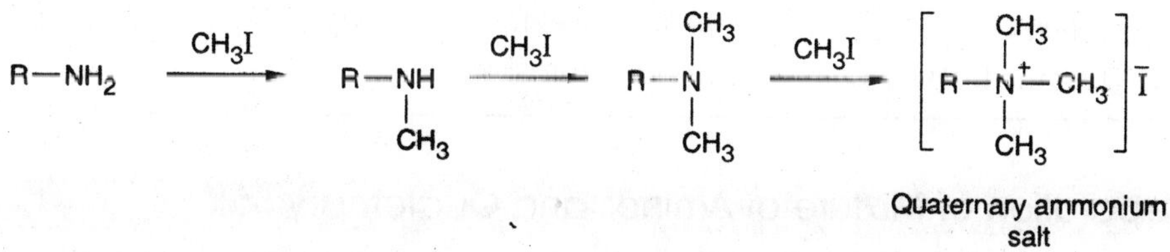

This is known as Hofmann's exhaustive methylation. When this quaternary salt is heated with moist silver oxide, tertiary amine and methyl alcohol are formed.

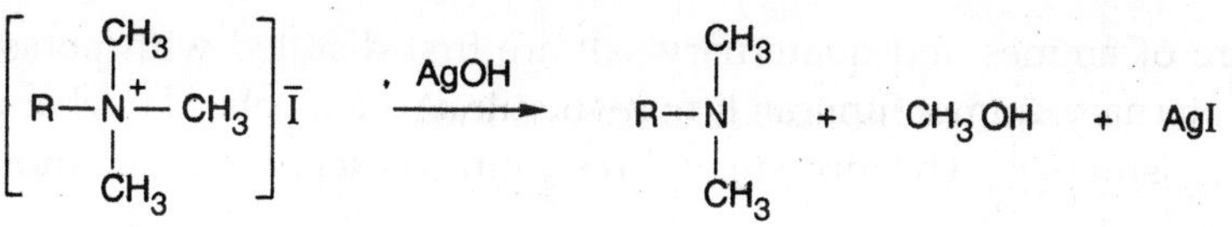

But if one of the four groups attached with nitrogen atom has a β-proton, olefin is the major product. It is known as Hofmann β-elimination reaction. Thus,

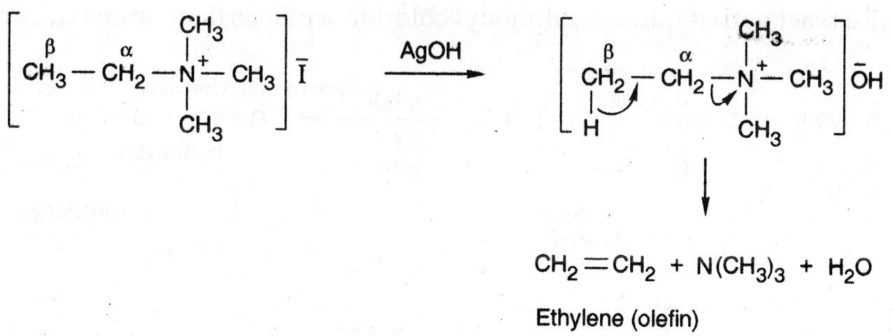

12.7 Differences between Primary, Secondary and Tertiary Amines

1. Action of HNO_2	Primary amine	Secondary amine	Tertiary amine
[$NaNO_2$ + HCl $\longrightarrow$ HNO_2 + HCl]	$R-NH_2 + HNO_2 \downarrow R-OH + N_2\uparrow + H_2O$	$(R)_2NH + HNO_2$ $(R)_2-N-NO$	$(R)_3N + HNO_2$ $(R)_3-N-NO$
2. Action of CS_2	$R-NH_2 + CS_2 \downarrow R-N{=}C{=}S$	$(R)_2NH + CS_2 \downarrow (R)_2-N-C(-SH){=}S$	No
3. Acylation	Yes Substituted amide	Yes Substituted amide	No
4. Isocyanide test (Carbyl amine test)	Yes	No	No

12.8 Separation of Mixture of Amines and Quaternary Salt

Most of the methods of preparation of amines are associated with the formation of mixture of amines and quaternary salts. Hence separation of these components is essential to get the pure amine.

The mixture of amines and quaternary salt are first distilled with potassium hydroxide solution. As quaternary ammonium salt is non-volatile, it is left behind unchanged but the three types of amines distill over. The mixture of three amines is separated into individual amine by the following methods:

1. *Hinsberg's method*: In this method of separation, mixture of amines is treated with aromatic sulphonyl chloride, preferably para-toluene sulphonyl chloride. Primary and secondary amines react with *p*-toluene sulphonyl chloride while tertiary amine does not react.

i. 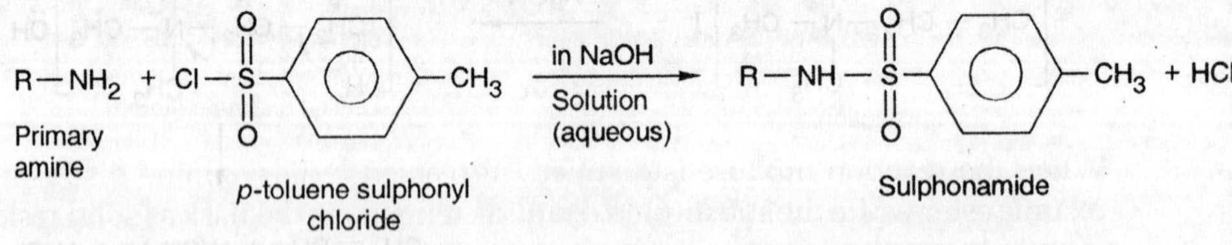

ii. 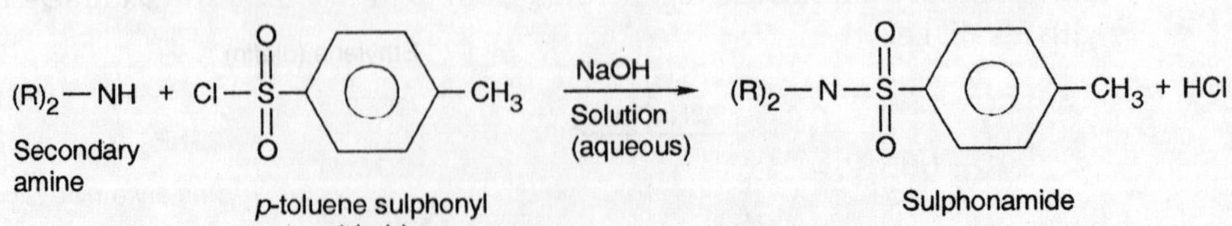

iii. $(R)_3N$ does not react

Tertiary amine

In alkaline solution, sulphonamide of primary amine gets dissolved but that of secondary amine does not. This is because sulphonamide of primary amine can tautomerise due to the presence of a hydrogen atom on nitrogen, i.e.,

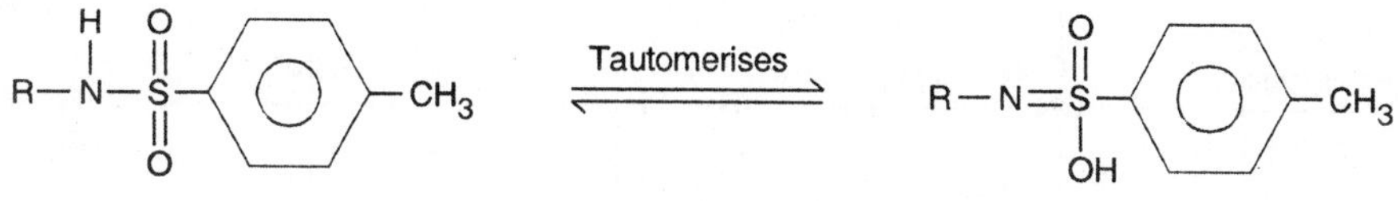

(in alkaline exists as salt)

Now this alkaline solution is extracted with ether when unreacted tertiary amine and sulphonamide of secondary amine being insoluble in aqueous medium pass into ether layer while sulphonamide of primary amine remains in aqueous layer. Aqueous layer is treated with 70% H_2SO_4 followed by the distillation with sodium hydroxide solution when primary amine free from other amines is separated out.

From the ether extract, ether is removed by evaporation and is distilled when tertiary amine being volatile distills over leaving behind the sulphonamide of secondary amine. The sulphonamide of secondary amine is hydrolysed with 70% H_2SO_4 when pure secondary amine is obtained after distillation over sodium hydroxide solution. General reactions taking place are as under:

$$\text{Sulphonamides of pr. and sec. amines} \xrightarrow[H_2SO_4]{70\%} \text{Salt of amines} \xrightarrow[NaOH]{\text{Distill}} \text{free amines}$$

2. *Hofmann's method*: This method involves the treatment of the mixture of amines with ethyl oxalate when primary amine forms crystalline solid substituted oxamide, secondary amine yields a liquid dialkyl oxamic ester while tertiary amine does not react with ethyl oxalate. Thus,

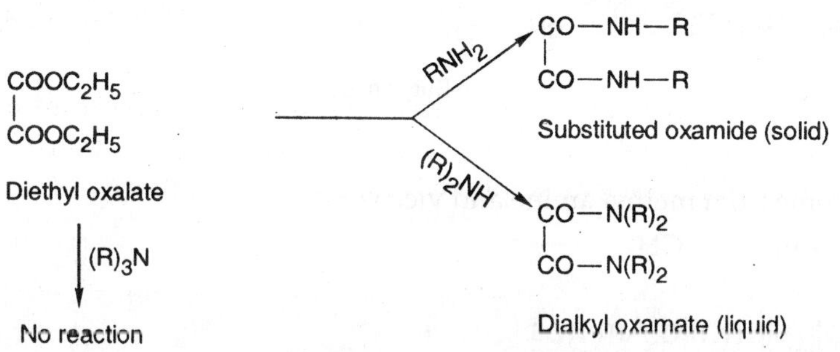

When the reaction mixture is distilled, unreacted tertiary amine distills first and then oxamic ester while the substituted oxamide remains in the flask as solid residue. Primary and secondary amines are regenerated from their oxamide and oxamic ester by boiling with alkali, i.e.,

$$\begin{matrix} CO-NHR \\ | \\ CO-NHR \end{matrix} \xrightarrow{2NaOH} \underset{\text{Disodium oxalate}}{\begin{matrix} COONa \\ | \\ COONa \end{matrix}} + \underset{\text{Primary amine}}{2RNH_2}$$

$$\begin{matrix} CO-N(R)_2 \\ | \\ CO-N(R)_2 \end{matrix} \xrightarrow{2NaOH} \begin{matrix} COONa \\ | \\ COONa \end{matrix} + \underset{\text{Secondary amine}}{2(R)_2NH}$$

12.9 Some Conversions

1. Stepping up and down in amine series is possible as shown below:

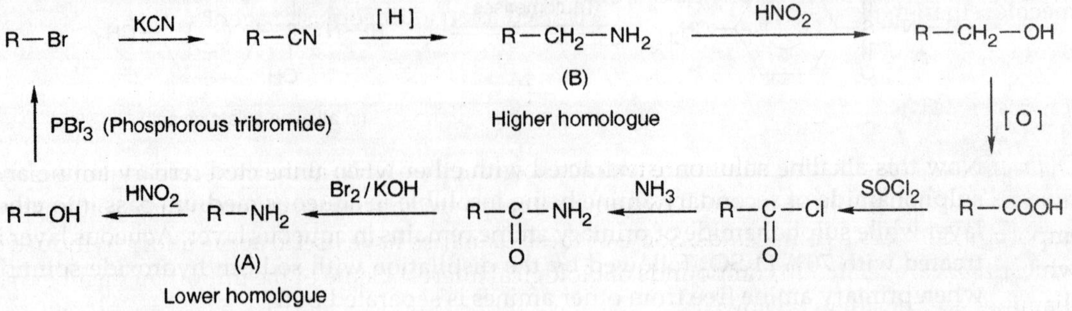

Thus, A → B shows stepping up, while B → A reveals stepping down.

2. Synthesis of *n*-propyl amine from *n*-propyl chloride.

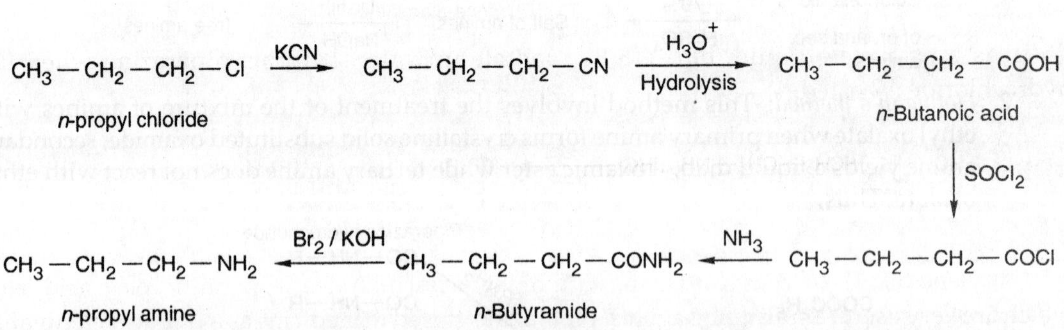

3. Ethyl amine from methyl amine and vice versa.
   Hint: As in 1, R = CH_3

12.10 Uses of Aliphatic Amines

Aliphatic amines are employed for variety of purposes as noted below. Methyl amine is usually used as refrigerant while ethyl amine is employed for dehairing of hides. It is also used as an accelerator in the vulcanization of rubber and as rocket fuels. Hexamethylene diamine is employed in the manufacture of nylon.

Aliphatic amines are also important in the field of medicine. Long chain amines are used as antioxidant, sterilizing and floating agents. Choline, an amino alcohol is a constituent of vitamin B complex and acts as a growth factor in chicks. Some of the members such as tauminoheptane ($CH_3-CH(NH_2)-CH_2-CH_2-CH_2-CH_2-CH_3$), methylhexamine ($CH_3-CH_2-CH(CH_3)-CH-CH(NH_2)-CH_3$) and cyclopentaminehydrochloride (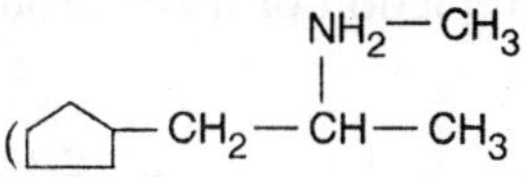) HCl are useful andregenic stimulants and mechlorethamine ($CH_3-N\langle^{CH_2-CH_2-Cl}_{CH_2-CH_2-Cl}$) is used as an antineoplastic agent.

12.11 Diamines

Diamines are those in which there are two amino groups (—NH_2) in the molecule. Out of a large number of diamines those in which two amino groups are attached to different carbon atoms are important and stable compounds. Some of these diamines have useful applications in industry while others are related to compounds of biological interest. Some of the important members of diamines are considered below:

12.11.1 Ethylene Diamine (1, 2-ethane diamine)

It is generally prepared by heating ethylene dichloride with ammonia under pressure.

$$Cl-CH_2-CH_2-Cl + 4NH_4 \longrightarrow \underset{\text{Ethylene diamine}}{NH_2-CH_2-CH_2-NH_2} + 2NH_4Cl$$

It is a colourless liquid, b.p. 118 °C, soluble in water. It forms piperazine when its hydrochloride is heated.

$$2\,HCl\,.\,NH_2-CH_2-CH_2-NH_2\,.\,HCl \xrightarrow{\text{Heat}} \underset{\text{Piperazine hydrochoride}}{HCl\,.\,HN\langle^{CH_2-CH_2}_{CH_2-CH_2}\rangle NH\,.\,HCl}$$

Ethylene diamine forms salt (soap) with higher acids like stearic, palmitic, oleic acid, etc. which are very useful emulsifying agents. Piperazine is used in medicine as a uric acid eliminant. It is also used as corrosion inhibitor, solvent for vat dye and as latex stabilisers.

12.11.2 Putrescine, Cadaverine and Hexamethylene Diamine

These are higher homologues of ethylene diamine. Putrescine is formed by the putrefaction of proteins in meat. However, it is conveniently synthesised as depicted below:

$$\underset{\text{Diethyl adipate}}{(CH_2)_4\langle^{COOEt}_{COOEt}} \xrightarrow[\text{Reflux}]{NH_2-NH_2} (CH_2)_4\left[(CONH-NH_2)\right]_2 \xrightarrow[NaNO_2\,/\,HCl]{HNO_2}$$

$$\longrightarrow (CH_2)_4\,(CON_3)_2 \xrightarrow[\text{Benzene Curtius rearrangement}]{\text{Heat}} (CH_2)_4\,(NCO)_2 \xrightarrow{\text{Aq. HCl}} \underset{\text{Putrescine}}{(CH_2)_4\,(NH_2HCl)_2}$$

It is a poisonous solid, m.p. 27 °C with obnoxius smell. It is soluble in water. It is closely related to amino acid, arginine and ornithine.

Cadaverine is also formed by the putrefaction of meat proteins. It is usually prepared as follows:

$$Br.(CH_2)_5-Br \xrightarrow{KCN} NO-(CH_2)_5-CN \xrightarrow{NO/C_2HO_5H} NH-(CH_2)_5-NH_2$$

Cadaverine is a poisonous, syrupy fuming liquid, b.p. 180 °C, with a bad smell and is soluble in water. It is the decarboxylation product of the amino acid, lysine.

Hexamethylene diamine is a colourless crystalline solid and is extensively used in the manufacture of nylon.

12.11.3 Ethylene Diamine Tetraacetate Hydrate

It is an important analytical reagent extensively used in the complexometric estimation of inorganic ions. It is normally prepared by the reaction between ethylene diamine and chloroacetic acid.

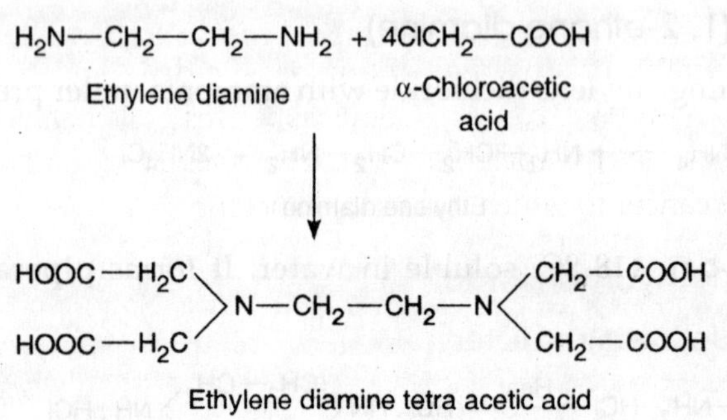

It is marketed as its disodium salt dihydrate

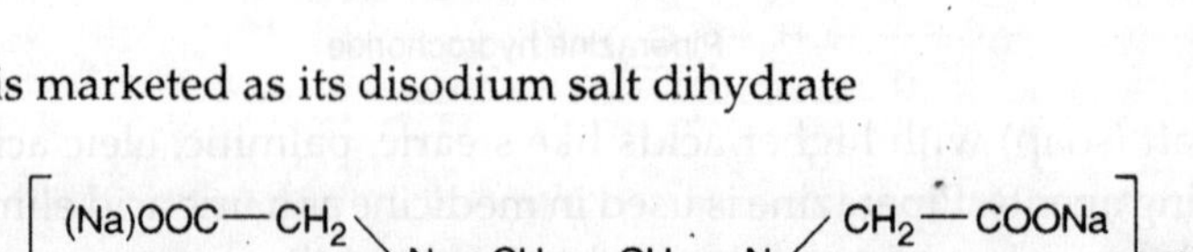

It is abbreviated as EDTA and its disodium salt is expressed as Na_2H_2Y. This disodium salt in aqueous solution readily ionises as:

$$Na_2H_2Y \rightleftharpoons H_2Y^{2-} + 2\overset{+}{Na}$$

The ion, H_2Y^{2-} formed is the active entity in forming the complex as

$$M^{n+} + H_2Y^{2-} \rightleftharpoons M^{(n-4)^+} + 2H^+$$

Using this reagent Zinc, Magnesium and Calcium ions are precisely estimated. This reagent is also used in the determination of hardness (permanent and temporary) in water.

12.12 Some Individual Members

12.12.1 Musteric Hydrochloride (Mechlorethamine Hydrochloride)

It is a hydrochloride of 2, 2′-dichloro-N-methyl diethyl amine and is known as *Nitrogen mustard*. It is a white hygroscopic powder stable up to 44 °C. It is readily converted to its active form when brought in contact with water and its solution is, therefore, prepared immediately before use. In aqueous solution it undergoes rapid intramolecular rearrangement with the loss of chloride anion (Cl^-) to form cyclic onium ion which then releases alkyl groups.

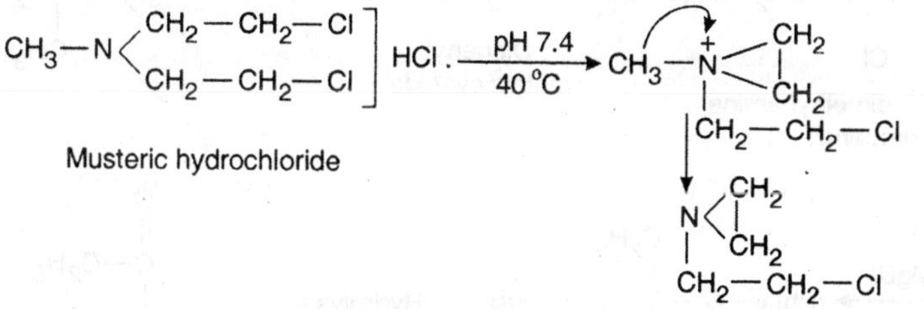

It is medicinally very important. It is used as antineoplastic drug and is applied in the treatment of lymphs sarcoma (a lymphatic cancer). Good responses have been obtained in the case of carcinomas of bronchi, breasts and ovaries. However, it has side effects and so it is restricted in the treatment of those type of cancer to which it is highly specific.

12.12.2 Dextropropoxyphene Hydrochloride

It is a tertiary amine having the following structure:

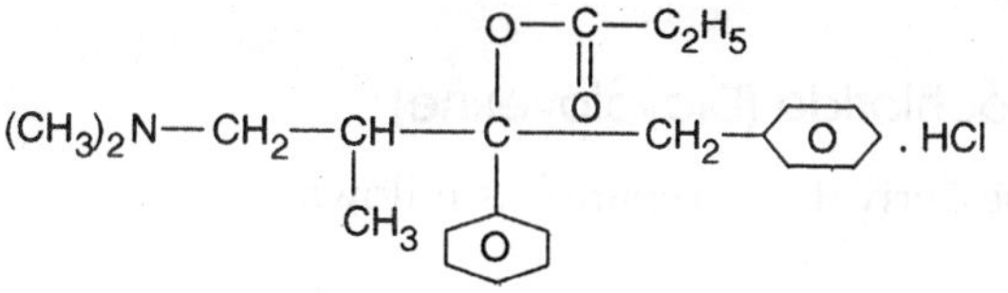

It is prepared by the interaction of propiophenone and dimethylamine in the presence of formaldehyde involving following steps.

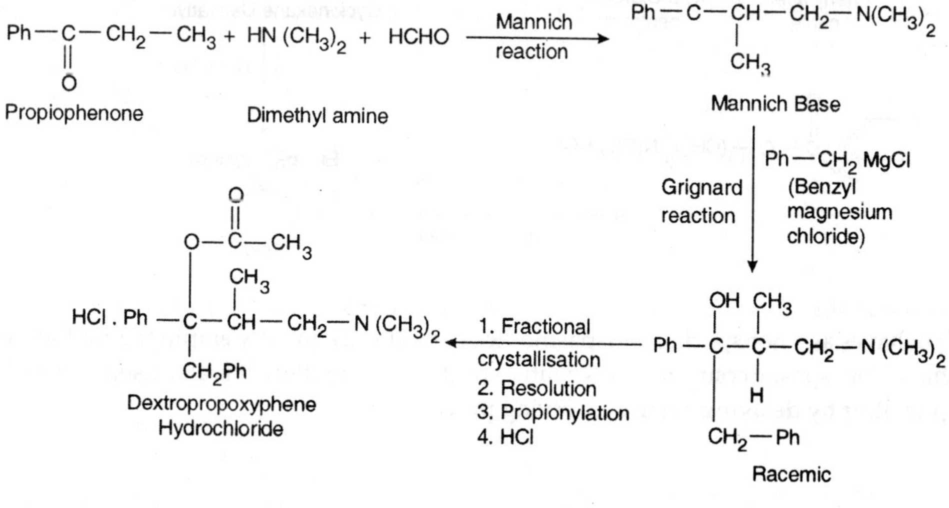

It is a narcotic analgesic possessing relatively milder actions. It is usually used to control mild to moderate pain and is primarily used with other analgesics having anti-inflammatory and antipyretic properties like aspirin and paracetamol.

12.12.3 Amidine (Methadone)

It is another tertiary amine derivative and is an useful analgesic. It is prepared as follows:

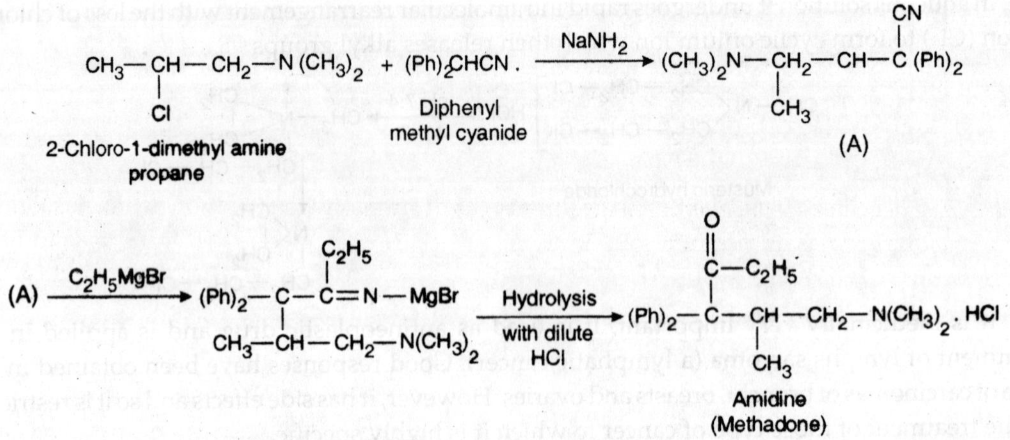

It is a potent narcotic analgesic having actions comparable to morphine. In addition, it exerts sedation and antitussive properties. It also helps temporary maintenance and treatment of dependance on narcotic drugs.

12.12.4 Dicyclomine Hydrochloride (Dicycloverine)

Dicyclomine is a tertiary amine derivative prepared as follows:

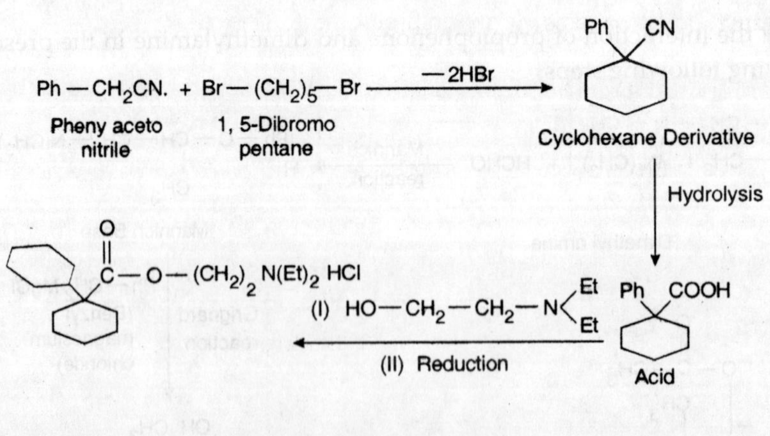

It behaves as a nonspecific antispasmodic agent. It is frequently employed for the treatment irritable colon, spastic colitis mucous colitis, spastic constitpation. It is also used in the diagnosis of peptic ulcer by delaying gastric emptying process.

12.13 Some Other Aliphatic Amines having Pharmaceutical Importance

(a) *Tauminoheptane:* Chemically it is 2-aminoheptane,

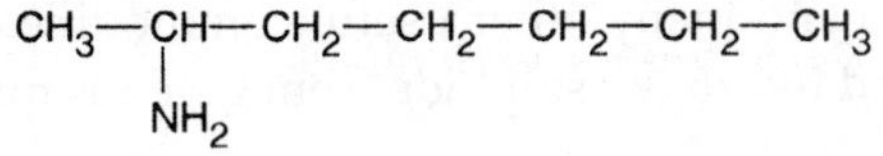

It is a vasoconstrictor and a sympathomimetic amine. It should be used with caution by those who have cardiovascular disease.

(b) *Methyl hexane amine:* Structurally it is 2-amino-4-methyl-hexane,

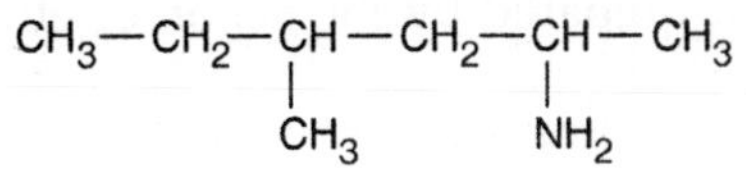

It is generally used as an inhalant for its local vasoconstrictor action on the nasal mucosa. It is used as an adjunct in the treatment of allergic or infectious rhinitis and sinusitis.

(c) *Isometheptene hydrochloride:* It exhibits antispasmodic and vasoconstrictors properties. Its other effects are bronchodilation, mydriasis, respiratory stimulation and shrinkage of nasal and pharyngeal mucosa. Structurally it is expressed as under:

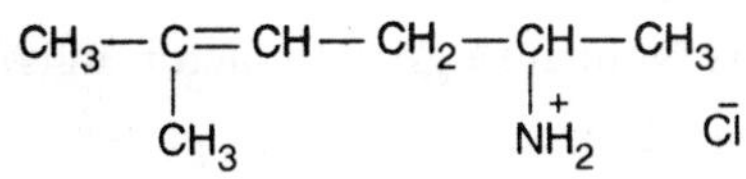

12.14 Alkanolamines

The most common alkonol amines are β-hydroxy amines. Some of the members of this clans of amines have been found to be useful industrial chemicals and some others are closely related to important biological compounds. Following are some of the important members of this group of amines.

12.14.1 Ethanolamines

Reaction of ethylene oxide with ammonia yields a mixture of ethanol amine (Cholamine or β-hydroxy ethanol amine), diethanol amine and triethanol amine which are separated by fractional distillation.

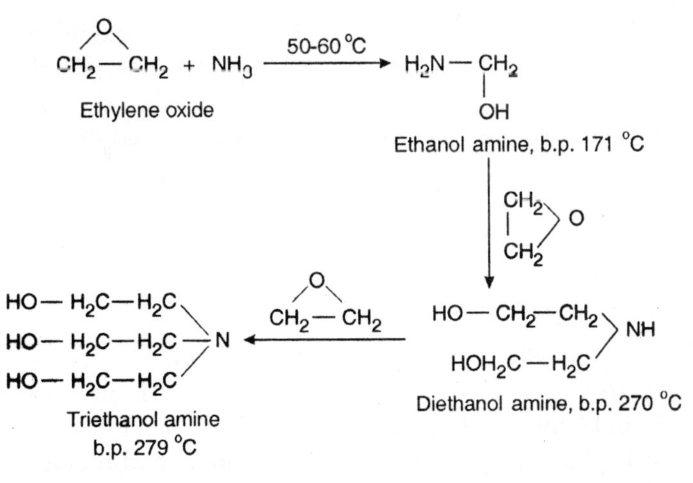

These ethanolamines are soluble in water and basic in nature. These compounds are usually sold as a mixture and can form soap with the higher fatty acids which are very good emulsifying agents and find application in the manufacture of shaving creams, hand lotions, dry-cleaning soaps, insective sprays, furniture polishes and many other useful commodities. They are also used for the removal of carbon dioxide and hydrogen sulphide from gaseous mixture.

12.14.2 Choline

Choline is a quaternary ammonium base related to ethanol amine. Chemically it is β-hydroxy ethyl trimethyl ammonium hydroxide. It is the part of molecular structure of **lecithine,** from which may be liberated by hydrolysis. It is best prepared by the action of ethylene oxide on trimethyl amine in aqueous solution.

$$\underset{\diagdown O \diagup}{CH_2-CH_2} + (CH_3)_3N + H_2O \longrightarrow \left[(CH_3)_3\overset{+}{N}-CH_2-CH_2-OH\right]\overset{-}{O}H$$

It is a colourless viscous liquid soluble in water and is strongly basic. On dehydration by boiling with barium hydroxide it forms *neurine* which is present in *brain.*

$$\left[(CH_3)_3N-CH_2-CH_2-OH\right]\overset{-}{O}H \xrightarrow{H_2O} \left[(CH_3)_3\overset{+}{N}-CH_2=CH_2\right]\overset{-}{O}H$$

Choline is present in vitamin B complex. It is Neurine a growth factor in chicks.

12.14.3 Acetyl Choline

Choline and acetyl choline are substances of great physiological importance. Administration of either compound produces a lowering of blood pressure, although acetyl choline is by far superior to choline in this action. The chlorides, bromides and other salts of both these quaternary ammonium bases are being extensively investigated in research on nerve physiology. Structurally it is represented as $\left[CH_3-\underset{\underset{O}{\|}}{C}H_2-O-CH_2-CH_2-\overset{+}{N}(CH_3)_3\right]\overset{-}{O}H$, and is usually prepared by acetylation of choline.

12.15 Urea and Ureides

Urea is physiologically very important and is the major metabolites of protein metabolism. An adult excretes daily 30 gm of urine. Historically urea is the first organic compound prepared from inorganic ingredients by Wöhler. It is highly useful as a fertiliser and raw materials for synthetic drugs.

Ureides are the N-acyl derivatives of urea is $R-\underset{\underset{O}{\|}}{C}-NH-\underset{\underset{O}{\|}}{C}-NH_2$

Ureides may be of two types, viz.,

i. Simple ureids
ii. Cyclic ureides.

Simple ureides are generally formed by the action of acid anhydrides or acid chlorides on vhile acid chlorides of dicarboxylic acids form cyclic ureides on reaction with urea. cyclic ontaining 5- and 6-membered rings may be looked upon as imidazole and pyrimidine respectively. Further, cyclic ureides may be mono- or diureides.

12.15.1 Preparation of Urea

Urea is generally prepared by the methods depicted below:

1. *Commercially* urea is prepared by the reaction involving carbon dioxide and liquid ammonia at a temperature of 200 °C and at about 100 atmospheric pressure.

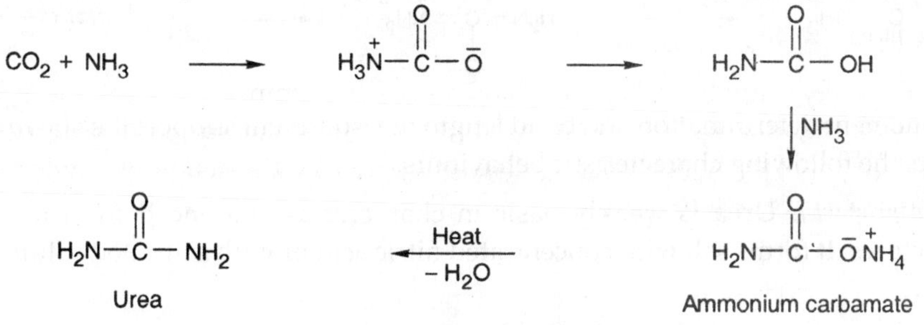

2. In the laboratory, urea is prepared by the action of ammonia on carbonyl chloride, alkyl carbonates or chloroformate.

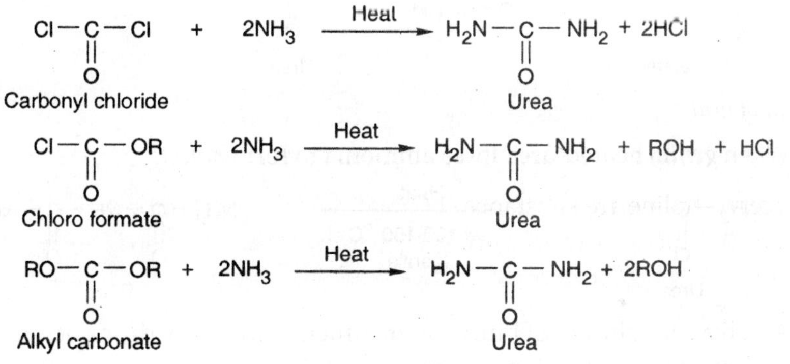

3. Wöhler prepared urea by evaporating a solution of potassium isocyanate and ammonium sulphate.

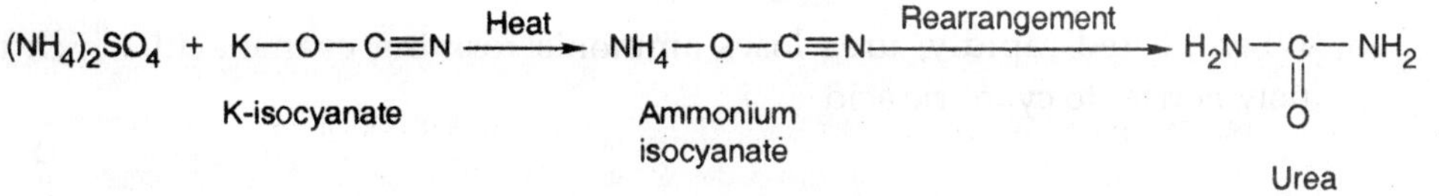

Rearrangement of ammonium isocyanate to urea may be interpreted as under:

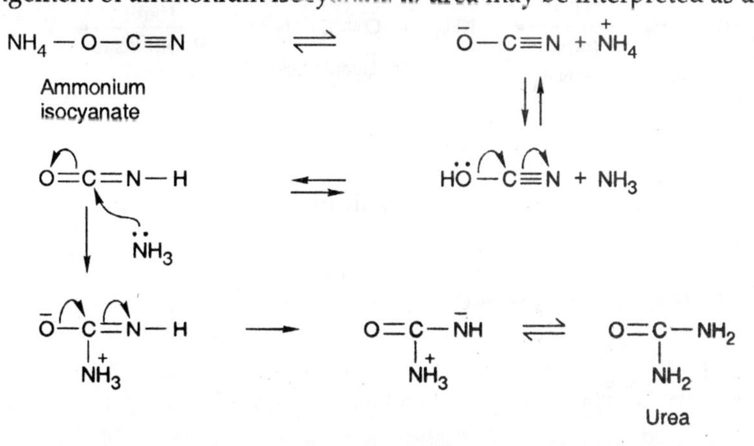

12.15.1.1 Properties of Urea

Urea is a white crystalline solid and melts at 135 °C. It is soluble in water.

Chemical Properties of Urea: Urea is a resonating molecule with the following contributing structures.

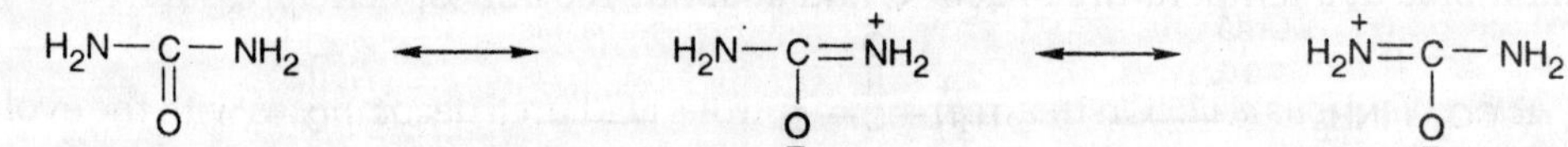

Dipole moment determination and bond length measurement support the above resonance. Urea exhibits the following characteristic behaviours.

i. *Basic property*: Urea is weakly basic in character as evidenced from its resonating structures. It forms salt with concentrated nitric acid or with saturated solution of oxalic acid.

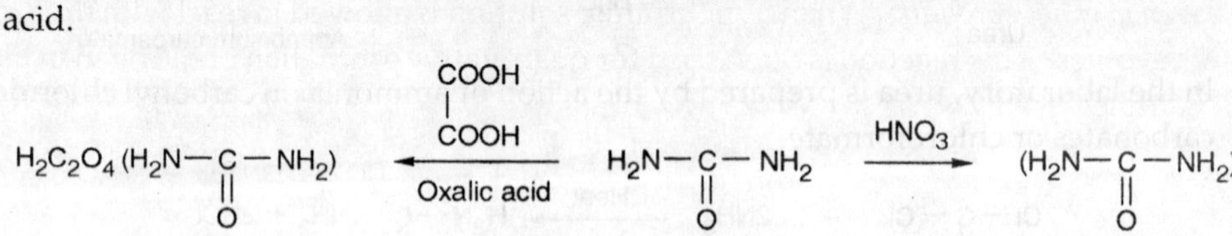

Urea oxalate　　Urea　　Ureanitrate

ii. *Action of heat*

(a) When *gently* heated urea loses ammonia to form *biuret*.

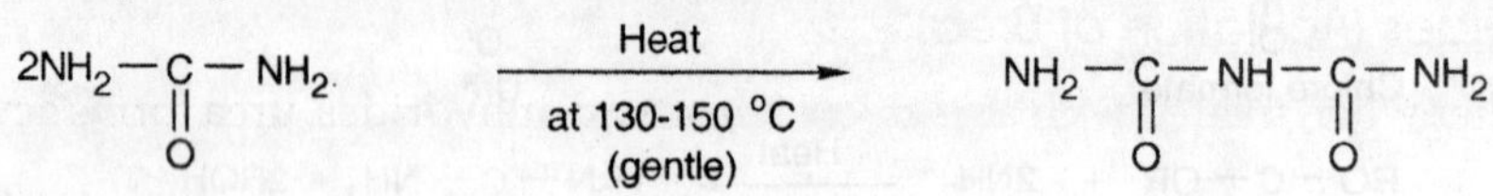

Urea　　Biuret

An alkaline solution of biuret on treatment with a few drops of aqueous solution of copper sulphate develops a violet colour. This is known as biuret test for compounds containing peptide linkage (—C(=O)—NH—), such as in proteins, urea and peptides.

(b) When heated rapidly, urea loses ammonia forming cyanic acid which readily polymerises to cyanuric acid.

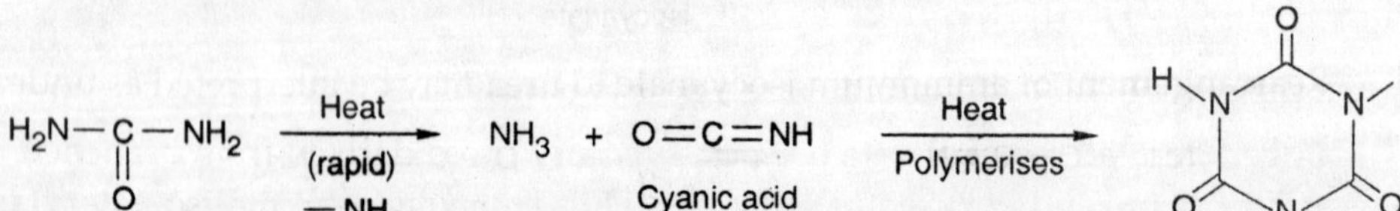

Urea　　Cyanuric acid

iii. *Hydrolysis*: On boiling with acid or alkali urea is hydrolysed to carbon dioxide and ammonia.

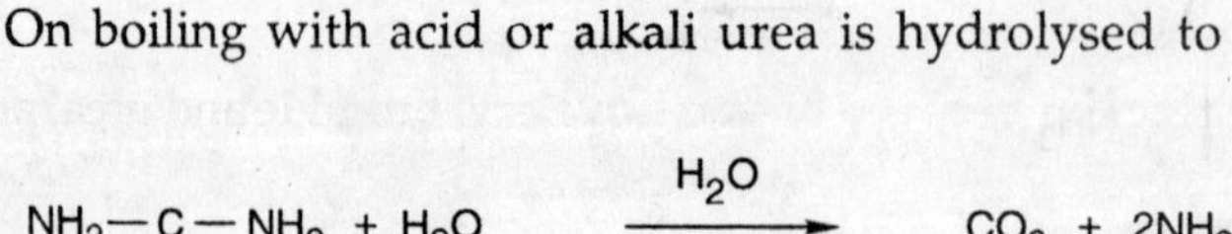

Urea

iv. *Reaction with hydrazine:* Urea reacts with hydrazine to form an useful reagent for detecting carbonyl compounds.

$$\underset{\text{Urea}}{H_2N-\overset{O}{\overset{\|}{C}}-NH_2} + \underset{\text{Hydrazine}}{H_2N-NH_2} \longrightarrow \underset{\text{Semicarbazide}}{H_2N-\overset{O}{\overset{\|}{C}}-NH-NH_2} + NH_3$$

v. *Action of nitrous acid*: On treatment with nitrous acid urea decomposes with the evolution of nitrogen.

$$\underset{\text{Urea}}{NH_2-\overset{O}{\overset{\|}{C}}-NH_2} + 2HNO_2 \longrightarrow CO_2 + 3H_2O + 2N_2\uparrow$$

vi. *Action of hypobromite*: When hypobromite solution is allowed to react with urea, nitrogen is evolved. This reaction is often used for quantitative estimation of nitrogen in biological samples.

$$\underset{\text{Urea}}{H_2N-\overset{O}{\overset{\|}{C}}-NH_2} \xrightarrow[NaOH]{NaOBr} N_2\uparrow + Na_2CO_3 + 3NaBr + 3H_2O$$

The mechanism of this reaction is analogous to Hofmann bromamide reaction.

12.15.2 Ureides (Acylation of Urea)

As stated earlier when treated with acid chlorides or acid anhydrides, urea forms acyl derivatives which are known as *ureides*.

$$NH_2-\overset{O}{\overset{\|}{C}}-NH_2 + R-\overset{O}{\overset{\|}{C}}-Cl \longrightarrow NH_2-\overset{O}{\overset{\|}{C}}-NH-\overset{O}{\overset{\|}{C}}-R$$

Dibasic acids or their acid chlorides under similar condition form cyclic ureides. Simple ureides are *neutral* in character and on hydrolysis by alkali generates urea and acid, i.e.,

$$NH_2-\overset{O}{\overset{\|}{C}}-NH-\overset{O}{\overset{\|}{C}}-R \xrightarrow{H_2O} NH_2-\overset{O}{\overset{\|}{C}}-NH_2 + R-COOH$$

On the other hand cyclic ureides are acidic in nature.

Halogen derivatives of simple ureides, specially those derived from branched chain acids are useful medicine and are used as sedatives. Thus *bromural* (α-bromo-iso-valeryl urea).

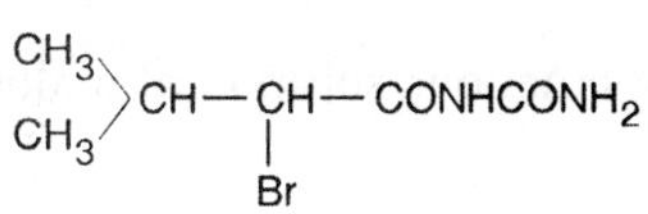

(prepared by the reaction between bromo isovaleryl bromide and urea) and *carbromal* (diethyl

bromo acetyl urea) 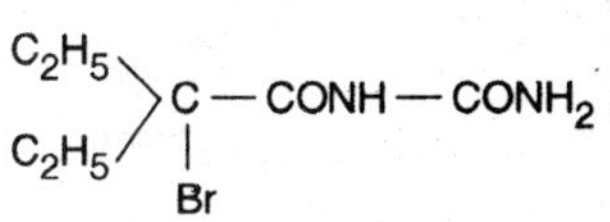 are important hypnotics.

12.15.2.1 Cyclic Ureides

Important cyclic ureides are parabanic acid, hydantoin, barbituric acid, alloxan, uracil.

i. Parabanic acid or oxal urea is formed by the action of oxalic acid or its chloride with urea.

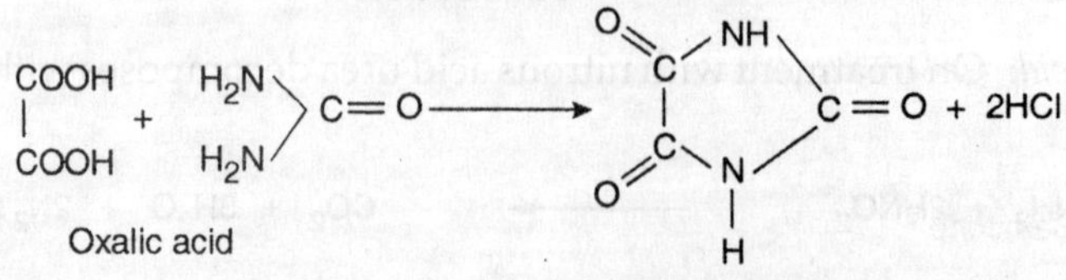

Oxalic acid

Parabanic acid (Oxal urea)

Parabanic on electrolytic reduction yields another cyclic ureide, *hydantoin*.

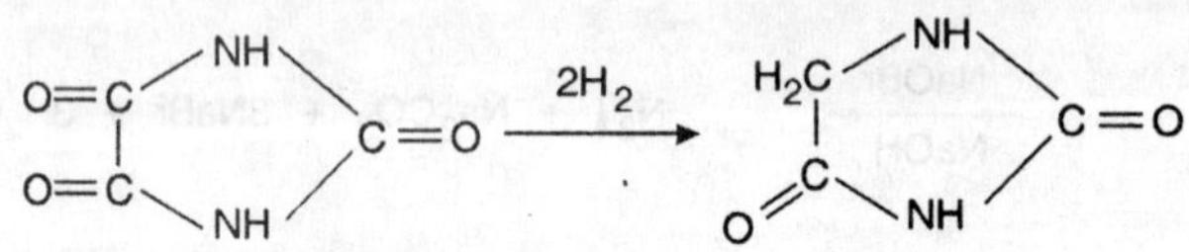

Parabanic acid → Hydantoin

ii. *Allantoin* which is an important decomposition production of uric acid is prepared from hydantoin.

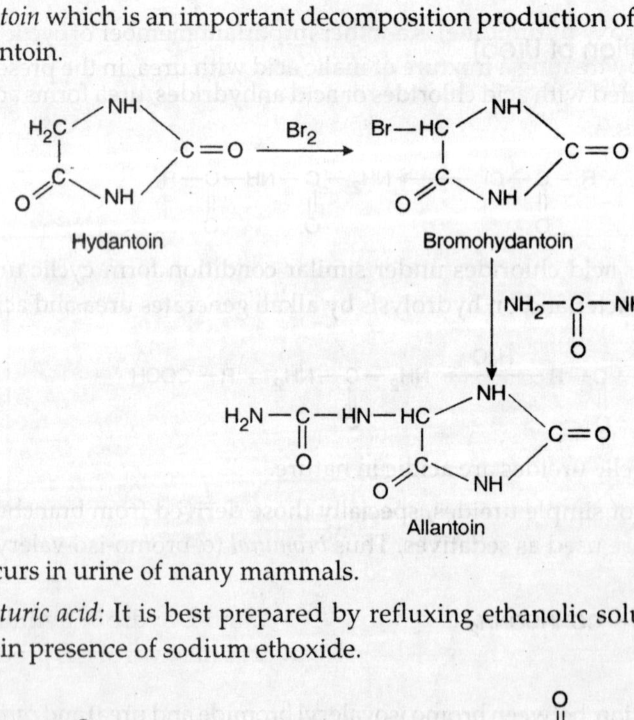

Hydantoin → Bromohydantoin → Allantoin

It occurs in urine of many mammals.

iii. *Barbituric acid:* It is best prepared by refluxing ethanolic solution of malonic ester and urea in presence of sodium ethoxide.

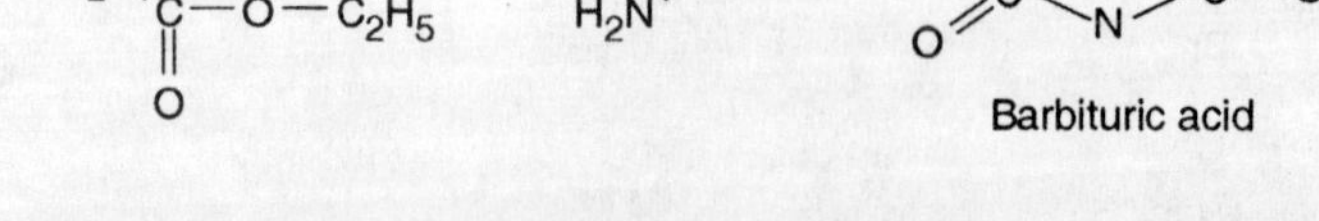

Barbituric acid

It is a colourless crystalline solid. Barbituric acid and its 5-substituted derivatives are used in medicine as hypnotics.

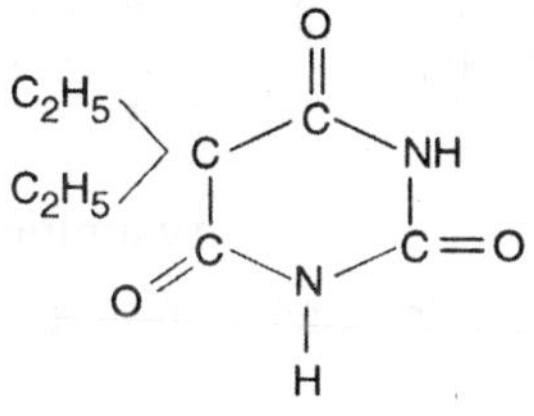

Barbitone

iv. *Alloxan* (mesoxal urea) has been discovered as an oxidation product of uric acid. On hydrolysis it forms mesoxalic acid and urea which settle its structure.

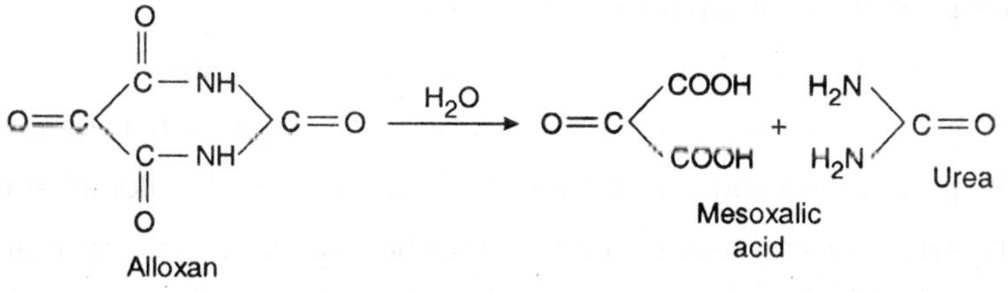

v. *Uracil* (2, 6-Dihydroxy pyrimidine) is another important member of cyclic ureide family. It is prepared by treating a mixture of malic acid with urea, in the presence of fuming sulphuric acid.

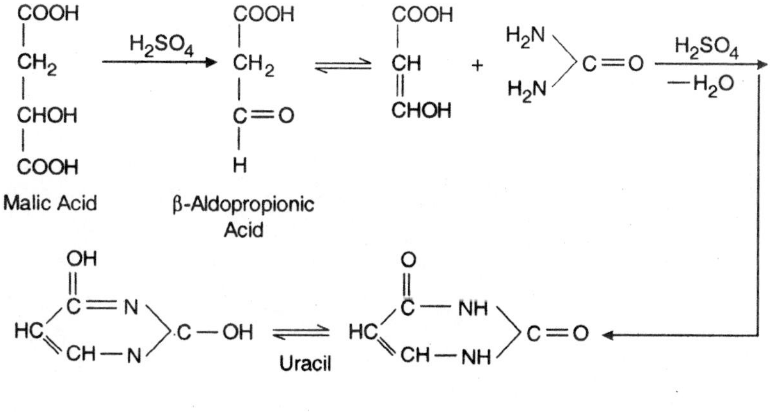

Uracil, thymine (5-methyluracil) and cytosine (4-amino-2-hydroxy pyrimidine are great physiological interest as they have all been isolated as the hydrolysis products of *nucleic acids*.

Model Questions

1. What are amines? How are they prepared? Describe some important reactions of amines.
2. Write the products of reaction of the following with HNO_2.
   (i) Diethyl amine (ii) Ethyl-dimethyl amine.
3. How will you distinguish between primary, secondary and tertiary amines?
4. Discuss the basicity of amines and show that the order of basicity of three types of amines is $RNH_2 < R_2NH > R_3N$.
5. Write notes on
   (a) Exhaustive methylation of amines and Hofmann's elimination.
   (b) Cope elimination
   (c) Hinsberg's method of separation of amines.
6. How will you separate primary, secondary and tertiary amines?
7. Describe Gabriels phthalimide synthesis. How will you prepare ethyl amine by this method?
8. Discuss the preparation and uses of some (a) diamines and (b) alkanol amines.
9. Discuss the synthesis and uses of some amines having medicinal importance.
10. What are ureides? Write what you know about parabanic acid, allantoin, barbituric acid? What are their medicinal importances.
11. How is urea prepared? State its uses. How will you detect its presence?

CHAPTER THIRTEEN

Esters of Synthetic Importance—Aceto-acetic Ester and Malonic Ester

13.1 Introduction

All the two esters, viz., malonic ester, and aceto-acetic ester possess hydrogen atom α- to carbonyl group. It is known that such hydrogen atom is acidic in nature and can be abstracted by a base with the formation of conjugate base, enolate ion which is stabilised by resonance.

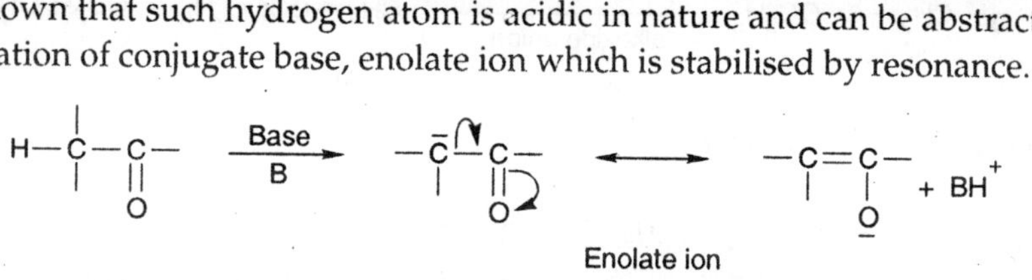

It is also known that greater the stability of conjugate base, more acidic will be the parent compound. Experimental results suggest that in the case of simple esters and ketones α-H atom are less acidic because of lesser capability of single carbonyl group to delocalise the anionic charge of the enolate ion. However, significant increase in acidity of α-H atom may occur if an electron withdrawing group like carbonyl, cyano, etc. is present at α-position to this acidic hydrogen (α-H). This is because in such situation, the anionic charge of the enolate ion can be delocalised by the carbonyl group already present as well as another electron withdrawing group as indicated below.

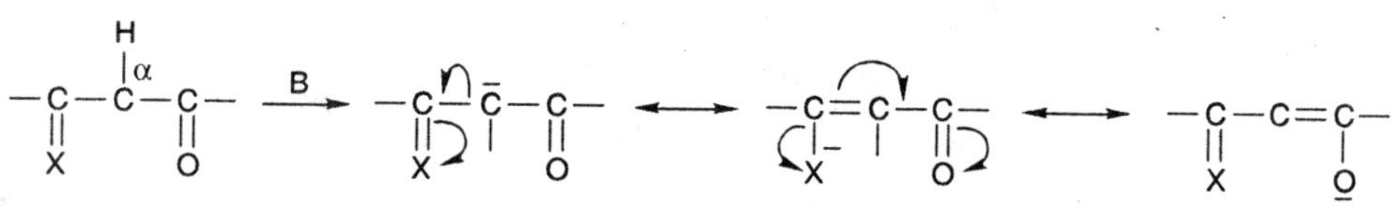

Thus, in such situation stable enolate ion will be formed which is highly susceptible to be attacked by electrophiles forming substitution product. By using different electrophiles a large number of organic compounds of synthetic importance can be synthesised. Therefore, such enolates will have significant utility in synthetic organic chemistry. A careful scrutiny of the esters under consideration have an additional electron withdrawing group (one ester group in the case of malonic ester and keto group in aceto acetic ester) at α-position in addition to ester functionality. Consequently, both these esters will have immense applications in synthetic organic chemistry and in actual practice it has been found to be so. It may be mentioned that $> CH_2$ group α to any electron withdrawing functionality is normally termed as *active methylene* group.

13.2 Aceto-acetic Ester

13.2.1 Preparation of Aceto-acetic Ester

The most important method for the preparation of aceto acetic ester and other β-keto ester is a reaction known as *Claisen condensation*. This condensation involves two molecules of esters which undergo self-condensation in presence of alkoxide bases. Thus ethyl acetate on treatment with sodium ethoxide affords aceto acetic ester—a β-keto ester.

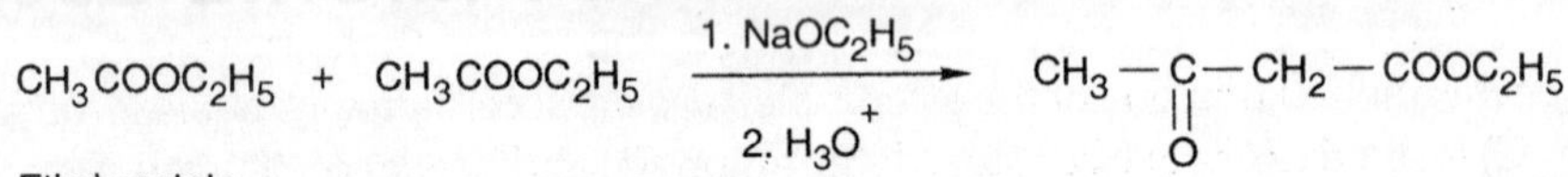

Ethyl acetate

Mechanism: Mechanistically Claisen condensation is similar to aldol condensation involving combination of carbocation ion and carbanion. Complete path may be traced as:

Step I: Generation of carbanion

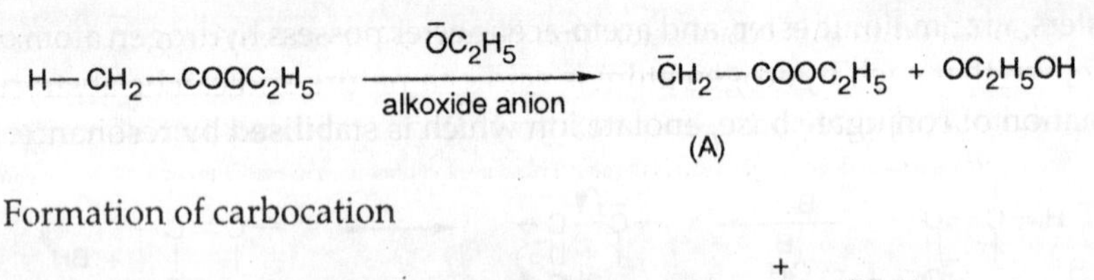

Step II: Formation of carbocation

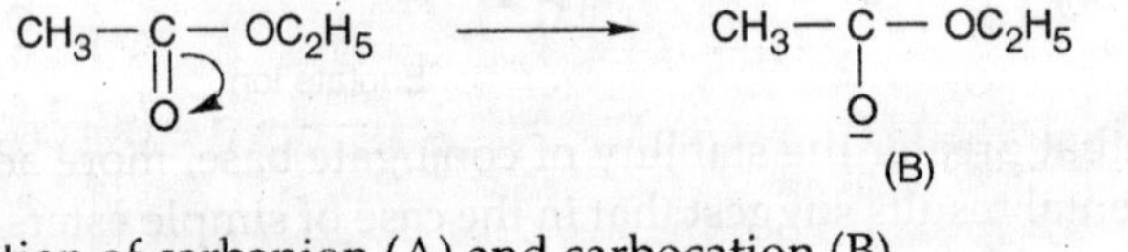

Step III: Combination of carbanion (A) and carbocation (B)

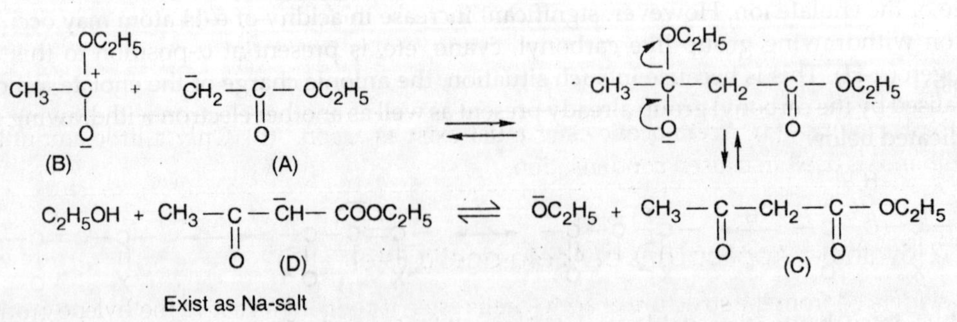

This condensation is a reversible reaction and the product (C) has the tendency to be reconverted to original components. For this reason, keto-ester (C) must be converted to its anion (D). In the above example aceto acetic ester is the exclusive product.

- **Quantity of Base Used**

Normally a gram equivalent of sodium is used but only a little ethanol is required to be added initially because more alcohol is liberated as soon as the reaction starts as evidenced from mechanism.

- **Scope and Limitation**

Claisen condensation may take place between two different ester molecules. Such condensation is termed as *crossed Claisen condensation*. If both the ester molecules possess α-H atom, like aldol condensation, mixed products are obtained and hence it is not encouraged. But if one of the esters does not contain α-H atom, exclusively one product is formed. Again, if an ester contains two ester functionalities, Claisen condensation may take place intramolecularly. In such situation the final product is a cyclic ketone. In fact, such intramolecular condensation is known as *Dickmann condensation*, normally employed for the preparation of cyclo alkanone.

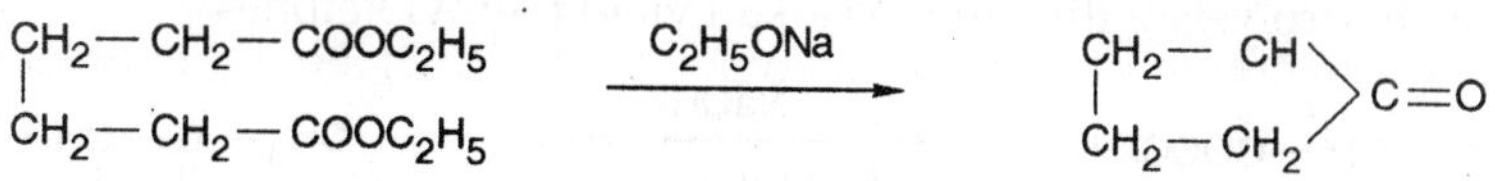

Diethyl adipate Cyclopentanone

It may be mentioned that one of the ester molecules must contain methylene group. Otherwise β-keto ester (C) formed cannot be converted into anion (D) and hence condensation is not favoured. That is why ethyl isobutyrate, $(CH_3)_2CH\text{-}COOC_2H_5$ fails to undergo Claisen condensation under normal condition. However, in such cases strong base is to be used so that the reaction becomes irreversible.

- **Comment**

It may be mentioned in this connection that β-keto ester cannot be directly prepared by the reaction between β-keto acid and alcohol. This is because β-keto acids are very unstable. The instability of β-keto acid due to the fact that free β-keto acid can form six-membered cyclic transition, state as a result of which ready decarboxylation occurs. Thus,

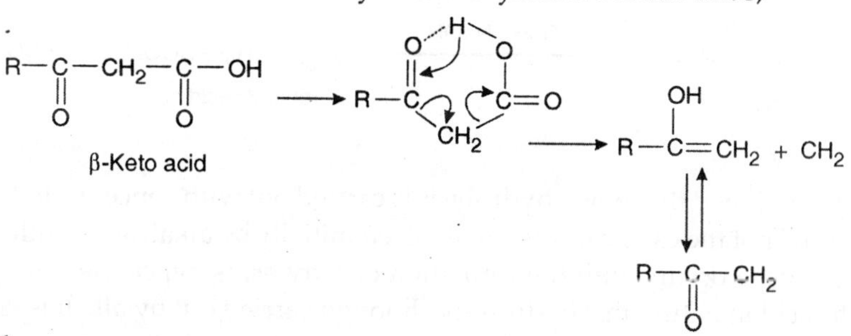

β-Keto acid

Problem 13.1

Explain why—(a) Aceto-acetic ester must exist as anion. (b) Only a little amount of ethanol is used in claisen condensation.

13.2.2 Synthetic Applications of Aceto-acetic Ester

As is evidenced from the structure of aceto-acetic ester, it contains an active methylene group, and two hydrogens of this methylene group are sufficiently acidic and as such readily replaceable by variety of electrophiles. Consequently, a large variety of organic compounds may be synthesised taking this ester as starting material. Synthesis of some of the important compounds are mentioned:

i. *Synthesis of mono and dialkyl derivatives*

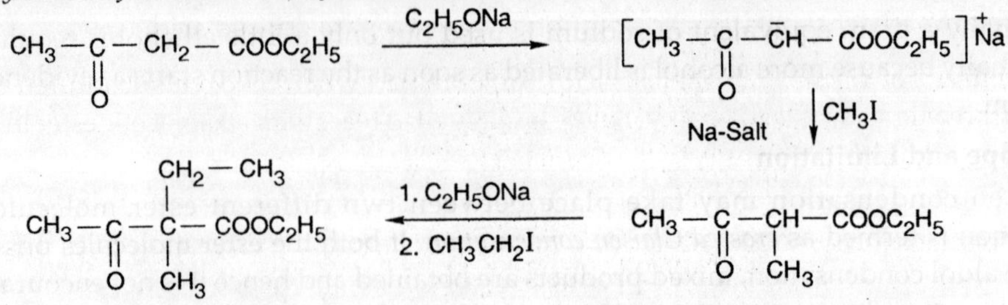

Na-Salt

Ethyl methyl aceto acetic ester (B)

Methyl aceto acetic ester (A)

ii. *Synthesis of methyl ketone:* The mono alkyl (A) and dialkyl derivatives (B) obtained above on ketonic hydrolysis with aqueous alkali yield methyl ketones.

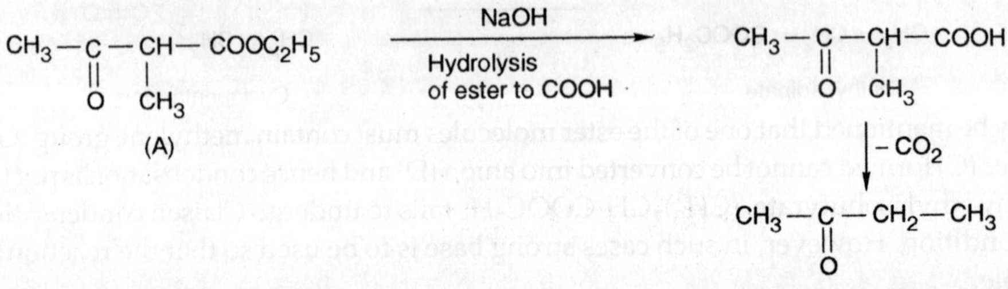

Ethyl methyl ketone

Depending upon the requirement for the preparation of mono or dialkyl derivatives, alkyl halides may be chosen.

iii. *Synthesis of mono carboxylic acids:* Acid producing hydrolysis of mono and dialkyl derivatives afford alkyl substituted acetic acid.

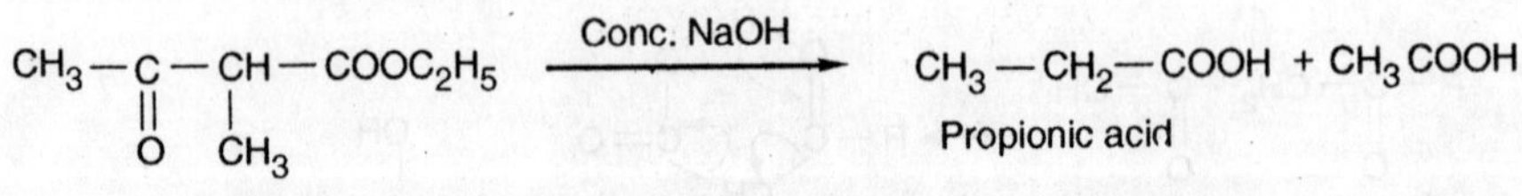

Propionic acid

It may be mentioned that when hydrolysis is carried out with concentrated alkali it is the keto carbonyl not the ester carbonyl is attacked initially by alkali as a result of which C—C bond cleavage occurs with the formation of fatty acids. Since the final products are carboxylic acid in nature this hydrolysis although carried out by alkali is known as acid hydrolysis meaning acid producing hydrolysis.

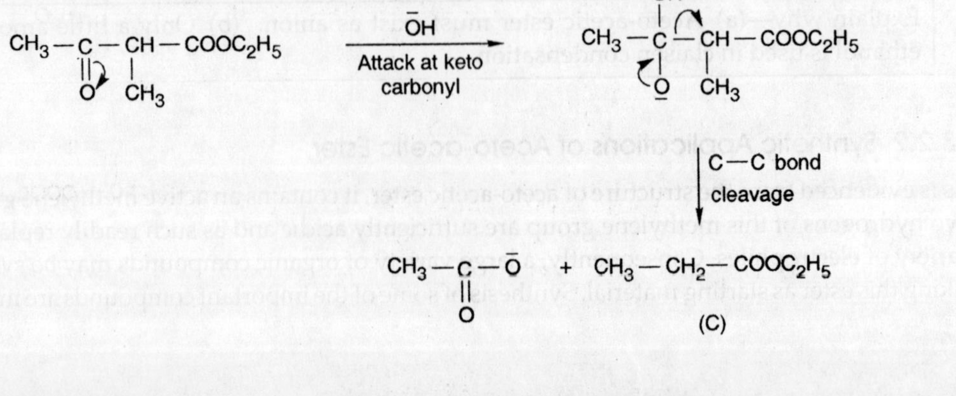

Ester (C) on normal hydrolysis by alkali furnishes corresponding acid. So if alkyl halides are properly chosen during alkylation we can prepare desired acid.

iv. *Synthesis of dibasic acid:* Dibasic acids are obtained when halogen substituted ester of a carboxylic acid instead of alkyl halide is allowed to react with aceto-acetic ester in presence of an alkoxide.

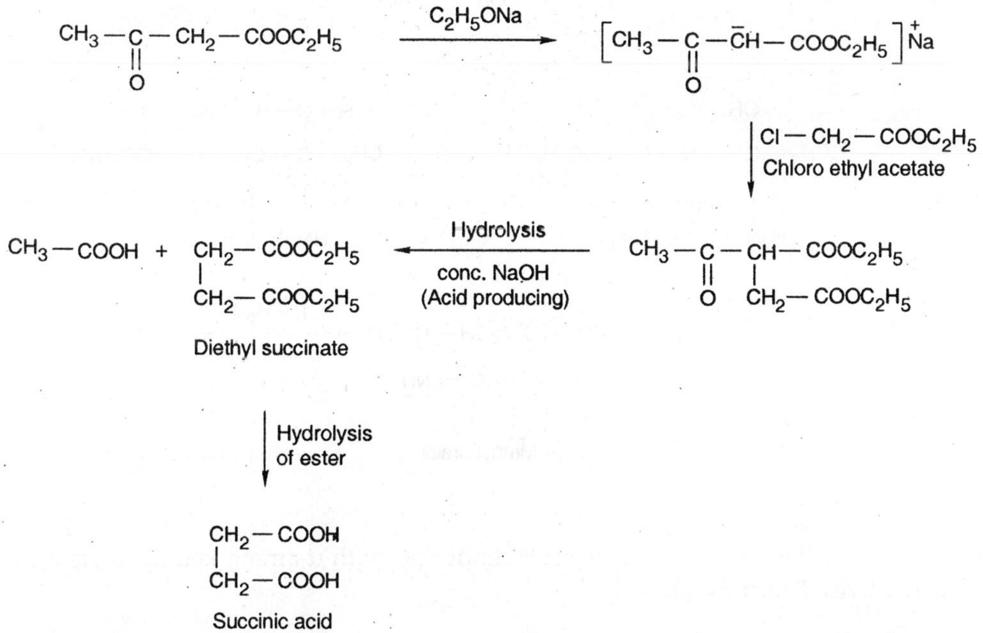

v. *Synthesis of α, β-unsaturated acids:* Knoevenagel reaction between an aldehyde or ketone in presence of base (pyridine) with aceto-acetic ester furnishes α, β-unsaturated acid.

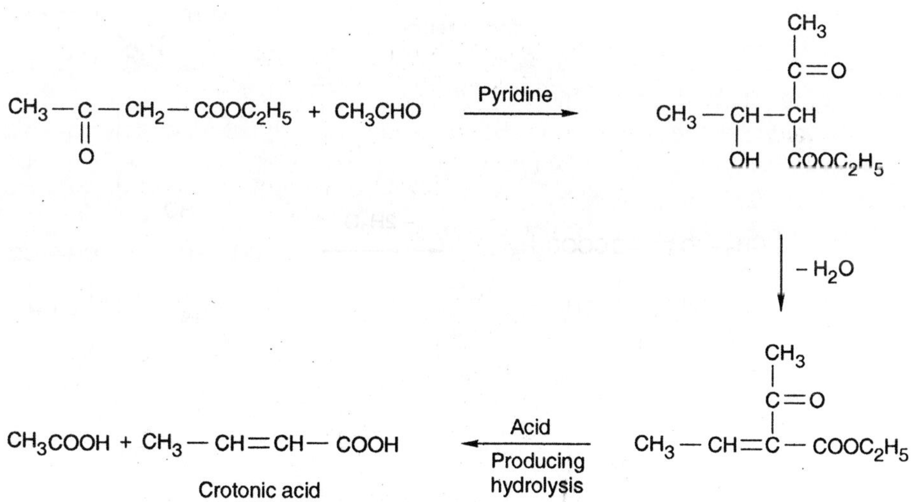

vi. *Synthesis of Cyclic Compounds:* Aceto acetic ester on reaction with urea forms uracil derivative

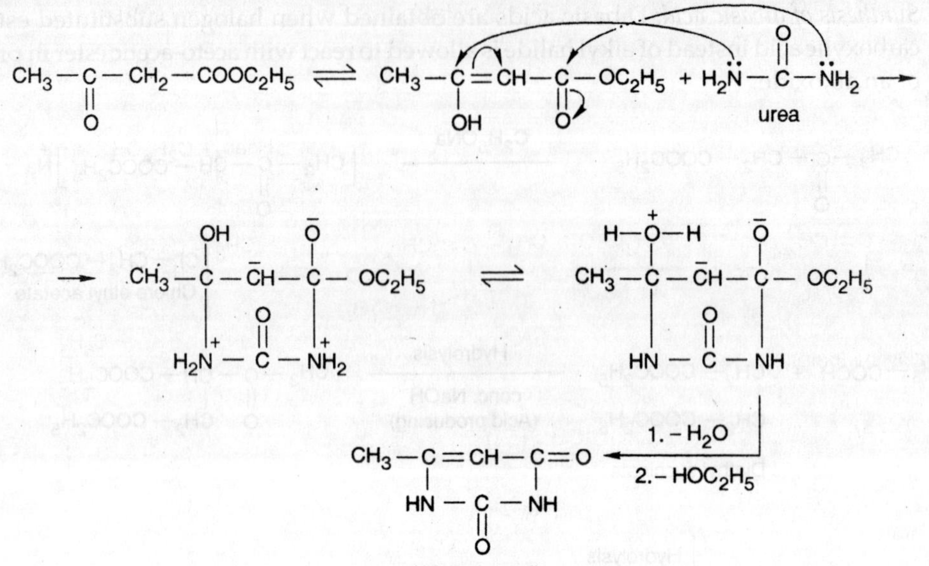

4-Methyl uracil

vii. *Synthesis of Pyrrole:* Aceto acetic ester condenses with α-amino ketone to yield Pyrrole derivatives (Knorr-Synthesis)

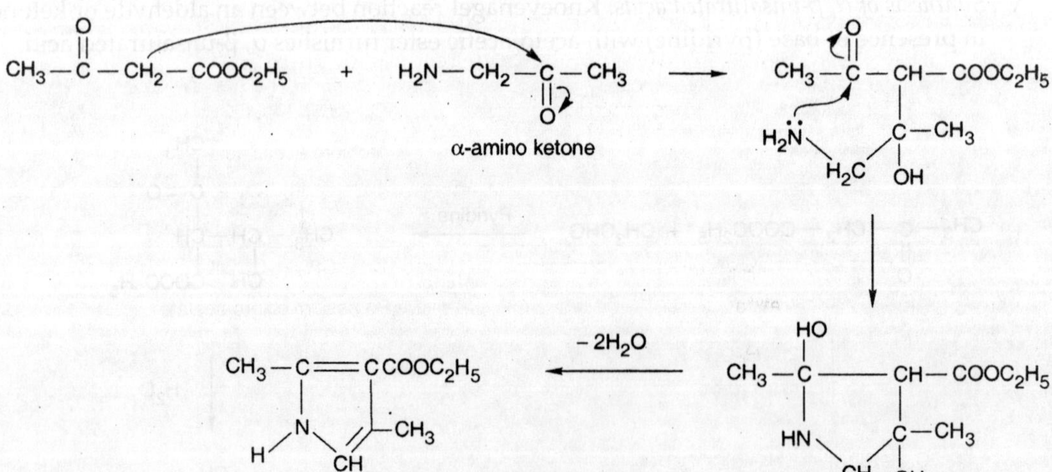

Pyrrole derivative

viii. Synthesis of Antipyrine

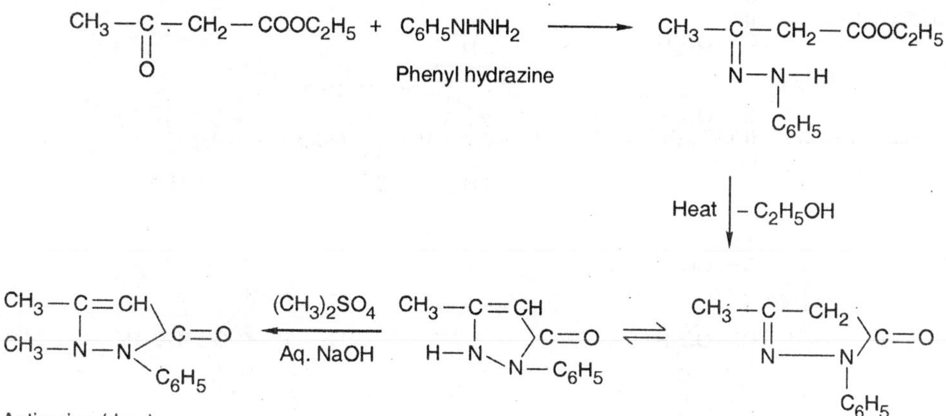

Antipyrine (drug)

13.3 Diethyl Malonate (Malonic Ester)

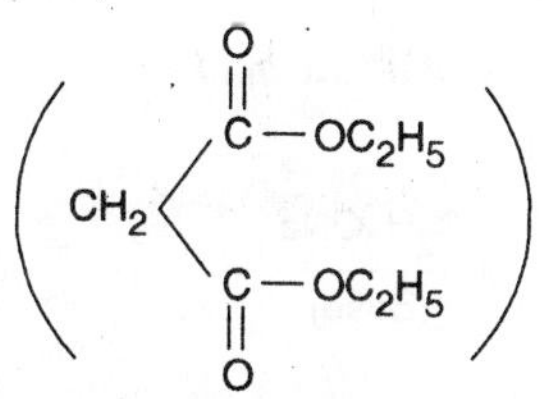

Like ethyl aceto-acetate it has immense synthetic importance.

13.3.1 Synthesis of Diethyl Malonate

It is synthesised by passing dry HCl gas through a solution of potassium salt of cyano acetic acid in ethanol. Cyano-acetic acid is usually obtained from acetic acid. Thus,

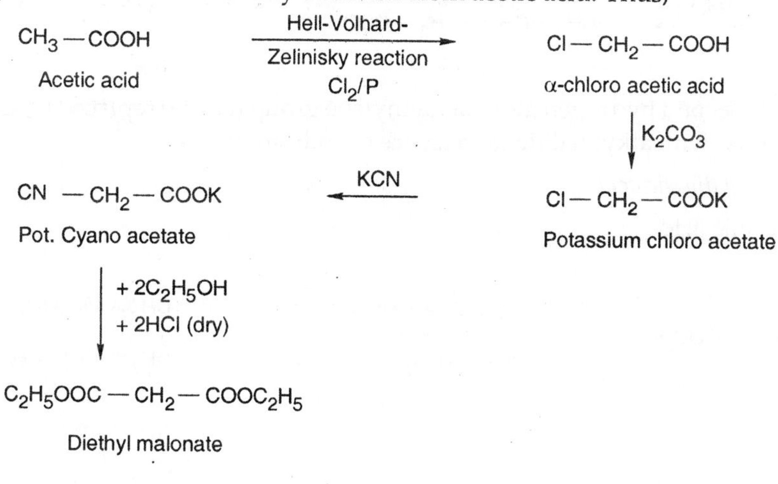

13.3.2 Applications of Diethyl Malonate

Like ethyl aceto-acetate it has acidic methylene hydrogen atoms. The acidic nature of methylene group arises from the fact that this group is flanked between two electron withdrawing ester carbonyl, as a result the anion formed by the removal of proton is stabilised by resonance.

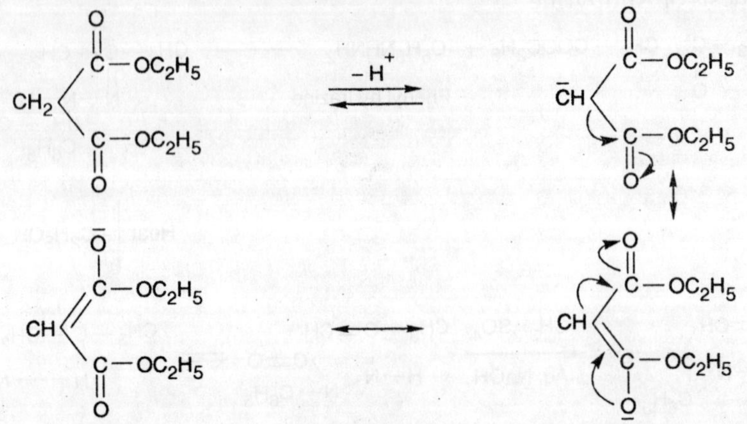

Formation of this stable anion can be employed as a very good source of carbanion and hence it can attack variety of electrophiles resulting in the formation of different compounds. Consequently, diethyl malonate has been utilised for the preparation of large number of organic compounds. Synthesis of a few of such compounds are described below.

i. *Synthesis of mono alkyl derivative of acetic acid*

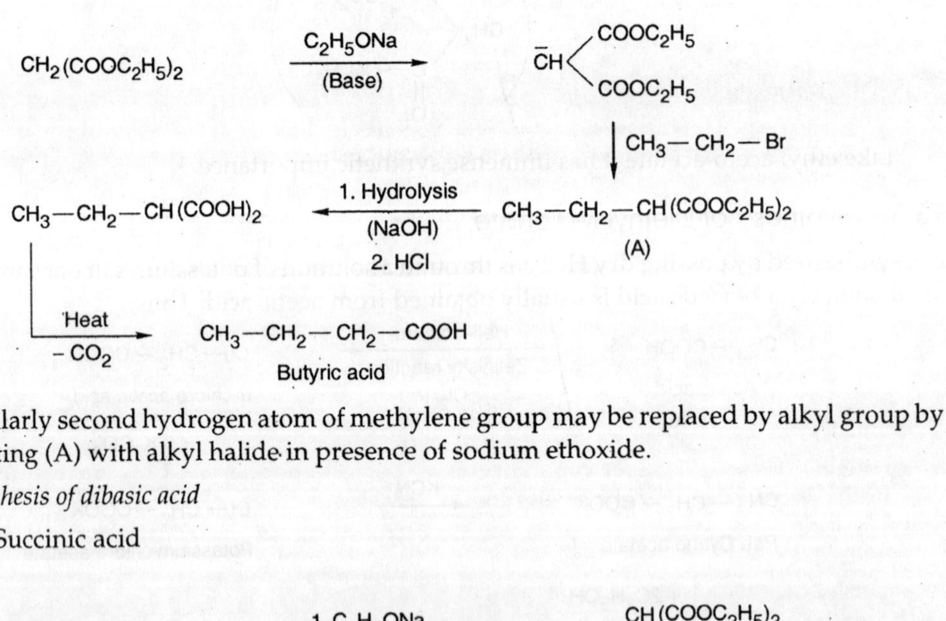

Similarly second hydrogen atom of methylene group may be replaced by alkyl group by treating (A) with alkyl halide in presence of sodium ethoxide.

ii. *Synthesis of dibasic acid*

(a) Succinic acid

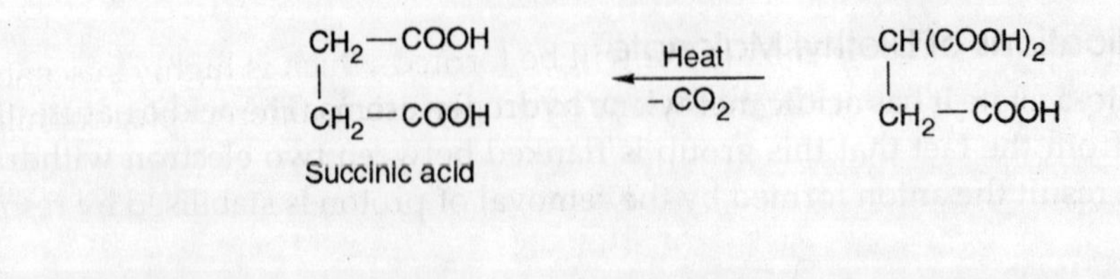

(b) Adipic acid

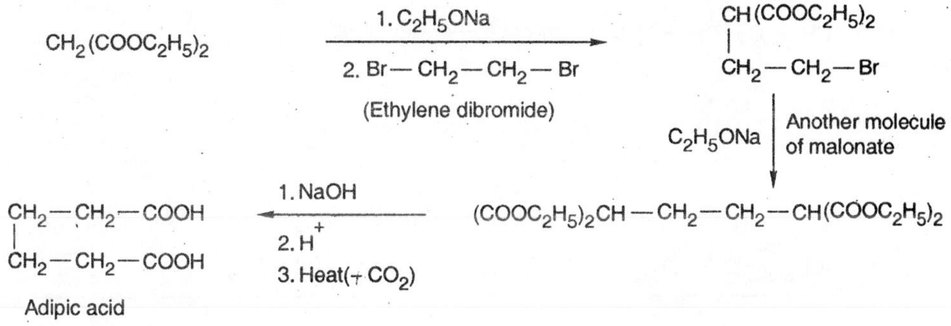

(c) Glutaric acid

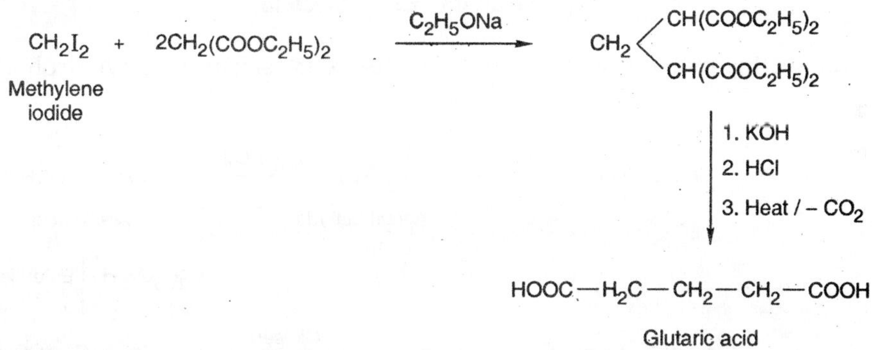

iii. *Synthesis of cyclo alkane carboxylic acid*

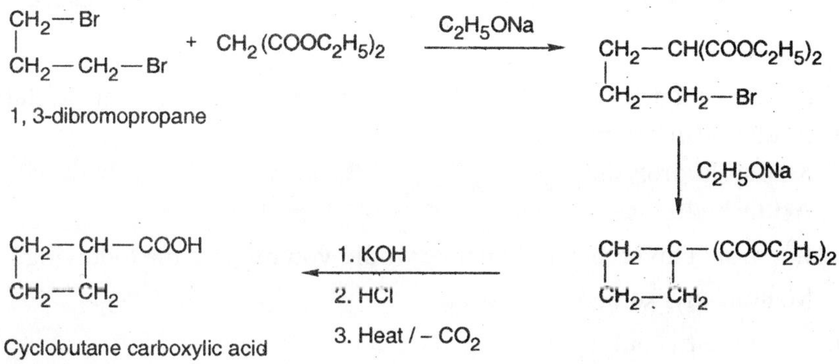

iv. *Malonyl urea*

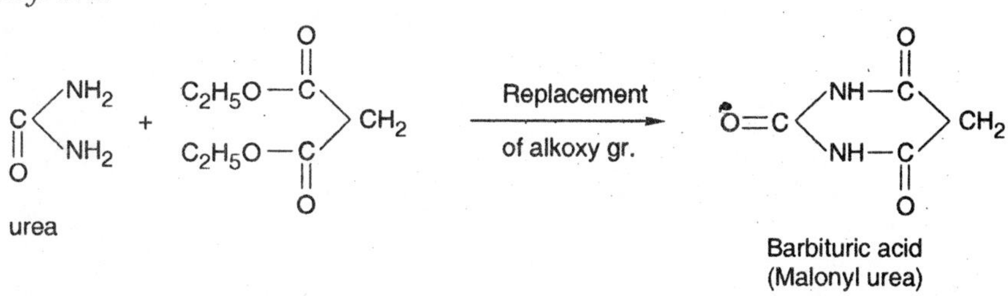

PROBLEM 13.2

Outline the synthesis of the following:

i. $CH_3-\overset{\overset{O}{||}}{C}-CH_2-CH_3$ from aceto-acetic ester.

ii. $CH_3-\overset{\overset{O}{||}}{C}-CH_2-\overset{\overset{O}{||}}{C}-CH_3$ from aceto-acetic ester.

iii. $CH_3-CH{=}CH-COOH$ from diethyl malonate.

iv. $(CH_3)_2-CH-CH_2-COOH$ from diethyl malonate.

Model Questions

1. Describe the method of formation of aceto-acetic ester from ethyl alcohol and sodium ethoxide.

Hints:

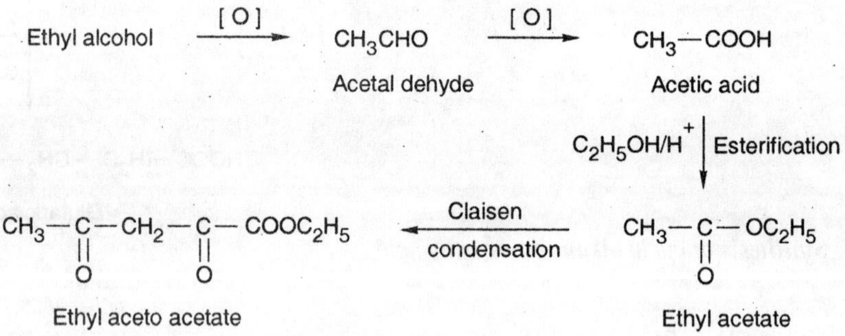

2. Describe giving mechanism the following properties of ethyl aceto acetate:
   i. Acidic nature of methylene
   ii. Ketonic hydrolysis
   iii. Acidic hydrolysis
3. Starting from ethyl aceto acetate how would you prepare the following?
   i. Methyl ethyl ketone
   ii. 2, 3-dimethyl butyric acid

Hints: 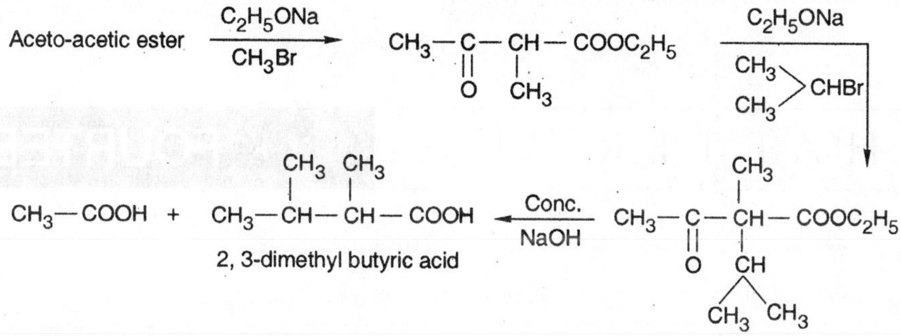

iii. Succinic acid
iv. Acetyl acetone

Hints: 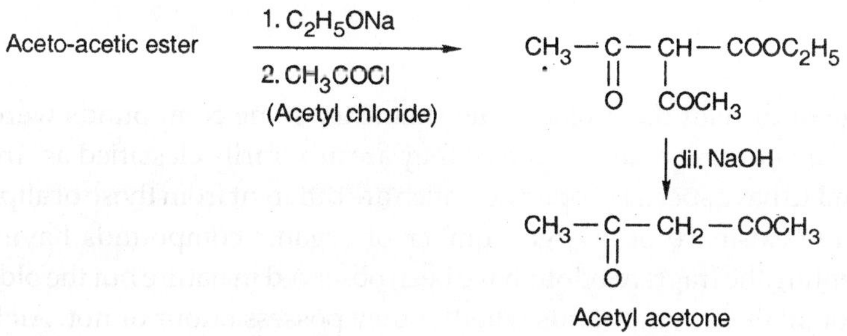

v. Crotonic acid
vi. 4-Methyl uracil
vii. Butanoic acid

Hints: 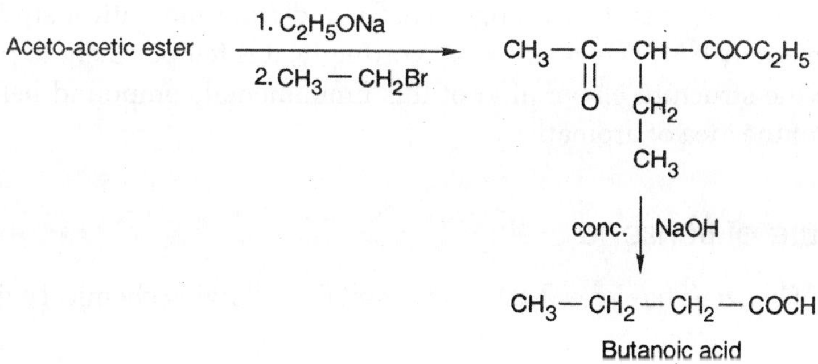

4. (a) Describe the reaction sequence depicting the synthesis of diethyl malonate.
   (b) Describe the properties of malonic ester.
   Hints: Acidic nature of methylene hydrogen and synthetic application.
   (c) How will you convert diethyl malonate into the following?
   (i) Succinic acid, (ii) Adipic acid, (iii) Barbituric acid (Malonyl urea), (iv) Glutaric acid.
5. Offer explanation: The ester ethyl aceto acetate is available in the market but not the corresponding carboxylic acid.

CHAPTER FOURTEEN

Aromatic Compounds

In the early age of development of organic chemistry some compounds were available which possessed fragrant odour, i.e., *aroma* and so they are arbitrarily classified as *Aromatic compounds*. They were found to have special properties which are different from those of aliphatic compounds. Subsequently the existence of a large number of organic compounds having similar special properties excepting the fragrant odour have been observed in nature but the older name *'aromatic'* was retained for all these compounds whether they possess odour or not. All these compounds were found to contain percentage of carbon and extremely low content of hydrogen indicating thereby their higher unsaturated character. They show some unusual behaviours such as extreme inertness towards addition, polymerisation and rapid oxidation reactions. They exhibit an interesting characteristic that they often afford benzene and its derivatives under the treatment of various procedures. For this reason benzene is considered as the most fundamental aromatic compound and in fact, it is that aromatic compound from the critical study of which a new concept—aromaticity has been emerged. Accordingly, it is felt pertinent to present here a short discussion on the structure elaboration of this fimdamental compound before going into the development of the idea of aromaticity.

14.1 Structure of Benzene

The structure of benzene has been established from the following chemical evidences and logical arguments.

1. Elemental analysis and molecular weight determination reveal the molecular formula of benzene as C_6H_6.
2. The extremely low content of hydrogen with respect to carbon suggests that the benzene molecule is highly unsaturated in nature.
3. Supportive evidence in favour of the presence of unsaturation has been secured from catalytic hydrogenation experiment.

$$\underset{\text{Benzene}}{C_6H_6} \xrightarrow[\text{Ni}]{\text{Cat [H]}} \underset{\text{Hexahydro benzene}}{C_6H_{12}}$$

Absorption of three mole equivalents of hydrogen not only confirms the presence of unsaturation but also indicates that there are three double bonds in benzene molecule.

4. *Nature of unsaturation*: Benzene molecule although is highly unsaturated yet it fails to undergo addition reactions which are very common to alkenes as indicated below.

(a) $C_6H_6 \xrightarrow{Br_2} \times$ (Bromine colour is not discharged)

(b) $C_6H_6 \xrightarrow{KMnO_4} \times$ (No decolourisation of $KMnO_4$ solution)

On the other hand, benzene readily undergoes substitution reactions characteristic of stable saturated aliphatic hydrocarbons. The above unusual behaviours of benzene clearly establish that the unsaturation present in benzene molecule is different from ethylenic one and it is unexpectedly a stable compound.

5. The hexahydro benzene (C_6H_{12}) formed during the catalytic hydrogenation can be expressed by the general formula, C_nH_{2n} which indicates the cyclic nature of the compound.

On the basis of above evidences, Kekule proposed the following structure (I) for benzene.

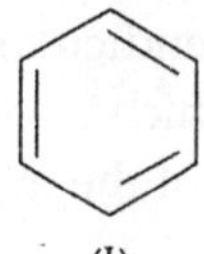

(I)

Drawbacks of Kekule structure: Kekule structure suffers from the following drawbacks:

i. It fails to explain the unusual stability.

ii. The structure (I) would produce five disubstituted benzene derivatives but in actual practice only three such disubstituted benzene derivatives are formed.

Kekule reconsidered his proposed structure and explained those anomalies by assuming that the double bonds are not static but dynamic in nature and accordingly benzene may be represented either by (I) or (II).

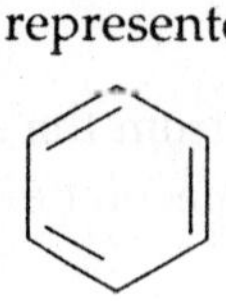

(I)

or

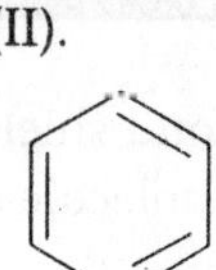

(II)

He further extended his views by suggesting that neither (I) nor (II) actually represent the benzene molecule but it is a mixture of (I) and (II) and always exists in equilibrium, i.e.,

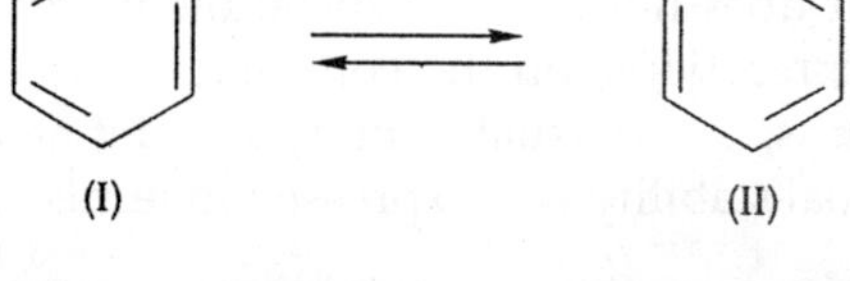

(I) (II)

Resonance Structure: With the advancement of the concept of resonance, Kekule, once again, proposed that benzene molecule is not an equilibrium mixture of (I) and (II), but it is a resonance hybrid of these two contributing forms. Thus, the structure of benzene stands as given below:

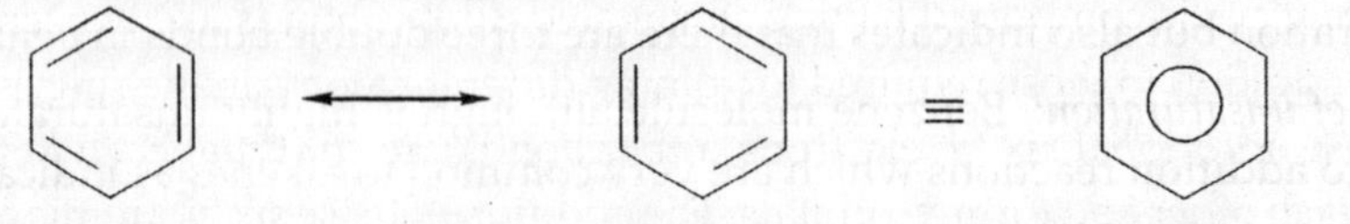

(I) (II) (III)

Hybrid structure

The above resonance structure has been supported by bond length measurement and other physical data.

14.1.1 Molecular Orbital Structure of Benzene

The Kekule resonance hybrid structure has further been substantiated by the modern *Molecular Orbital Theory*. All the six carbon atoms in benzene are in sp^2 hybridised state. Each of the six C—H σ-bonds is formed by the overlap of *s*-orbital of hydrogen atom with sp^2-orbital of carbon atom and each of the six C—C σ-bonds originates due to overlap of sp^2-orbitals of adjacent carbon atoms. Since all these σ-bonds are formed from the overlap of planar sp^2 orbitals, benzene molecule is planar. Again, in such planar benzene molecule six *p*-orbitals, one in each carbon atom are left. These six *p*-orbitals are perpendicular to the plane of σ-bonds and overlap each other laterally forming π-molecular orbital which is continuous throughout the ring of the molecule spreading both above and below the plane of the molecule as shown below:

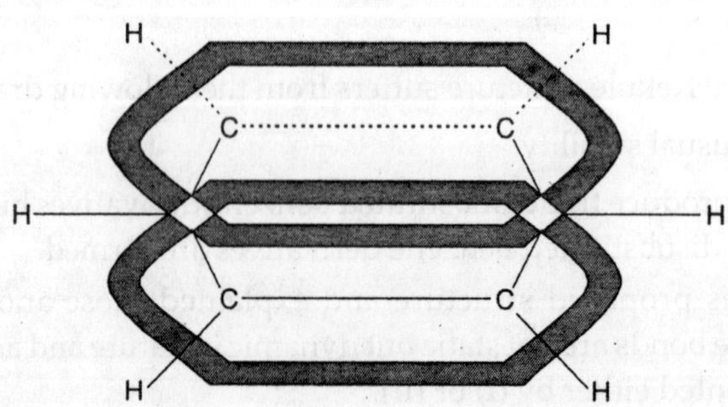

or

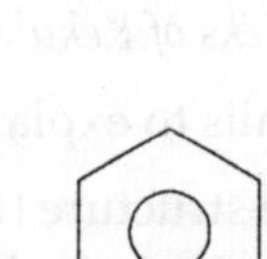

Short representation

This ring of π-electron cloud shields the ring atoms from the attack by the reagent and so unusual stability of benzene molecule originates. This molecular orbital structure is also known as delocalised structure.

14.2 Aromaticity or Aromatic Character

Since aromatic compounds furnish benzene in variety of reactions in the development of our present day ideas concerning aromaticity this hydrocarbon, benzene play the most significant role. A careful scrutiny of the structure of benzene reveals that aromatic character of benzene arises from the fact that (i) It does not exhibit typical olefinic reactions like rapid oxidation, addition and polymerization reactions, on the contrary, it smoothly undergoes substitution ractions. This chemical inertness, i.e., unusual stability was defined as the aromatic character. In the earlier concept, this unusual stability was expressed in terms of resonance energy and it has been opined that greater the resonance energy more is the aromatic character. But recently a vast number of organic compounds were found to be aromatic having very low resonance energy. Consequently many theories were advanced from time to time to account for the aromatic character.

One of the most popular and well accepted theories is the aromatic *Sextet* theory. According to this approach any cyclic compound having conjugated double bonds like benzene, if there are six '*p*' electrons in addition to those required for joining different atoms in the ring, is aromatic. Thus, in benzene these additional six '*p*' electrons (other bonds are sp^2 type) each left on each carbon atom, overlap each other and form π- orbitals. The addition of these six '*p*' atomic orbitals generates a new molecular orbital which is continuous throughout the whole ring as a result of which there is a formation of negative charges above and below the plane of the ring as shown below:

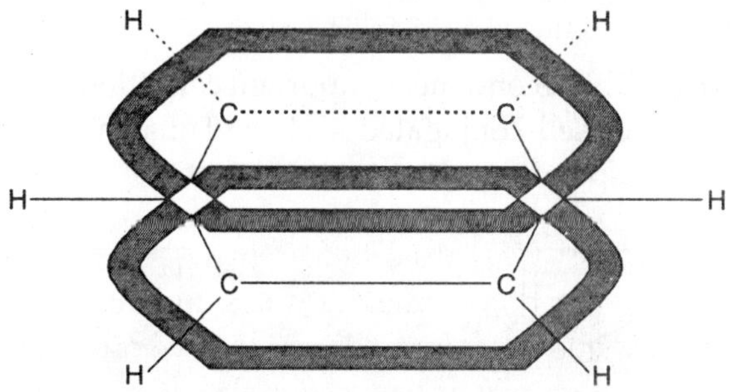

This ring of negative charges protects the ring atoms from the attack by the reagent and hence *unusual stability* originates. Formation of this type of molecular orbital is possible with homo- and heterocyclic compounds and so heterocyclic compounds such as pyridine, pyrrole and thiophene are aromatic in character. Even such sextet ring may be formed with the compounds having no carbon atom at all. Thus,

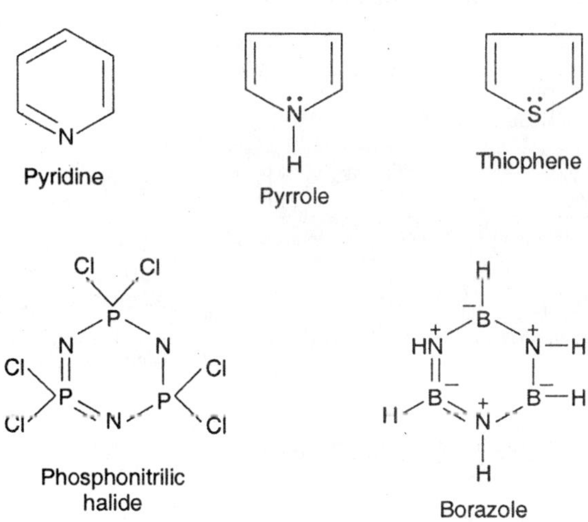

[In the case of pyrrole N atom donates two π - electrons and in thiophene S atom contributes two π– electrons towards the formation of sextet.]

From the above discussion it may appear that the aromatic character is only due to the existence of 6π– electrons in a closed circuit. However, there are certain compounds which contain either more or less than six π– electrons but are aromatic in nature. So a generalised approach has been put forward for aromatic character. According to this generalised view any cyclic compound containing conjugated double bonds is aromatic if it satisfies simultaneously the following two conditions.

i. *Planarity*: One of the most important conditions for aromaticity is the planarity. Thus cyclo-octatetraene has paired number of π-electrons in a closed system (ring) but is not aromatic, because it is not planar.

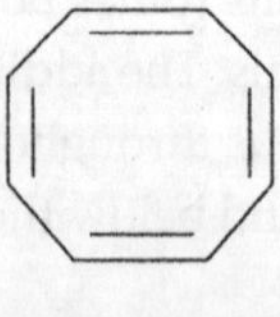

Cyclo-octatetraene

ii. *Pairing of π-electrons*: The second most important condition for aromaticity is the pairing of π-electrons in the closed conjugated system. Thus, cyclopentadienyl radical is not aromatic but the corresponding anion is aromatic.

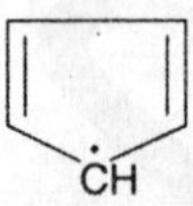

Cyclopentadienyl radical

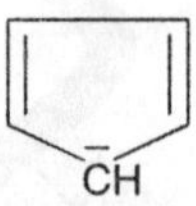

Cyclopentadienyl anion

From the consideration of all the prevailing facts Hückel proposed a rule for aromaticity. According to this rule any cyclic planar compound which contains $(4n + 2)$ π-electrons is aromatic where 'n' is any integer such as 0, 1 , 2, 3,... n. Thus, when $n = 0$, i.e, 2π-electron system may be aromatic and in fact, such aromatic compound is known. Some illustrated aromatic compounds are as below:

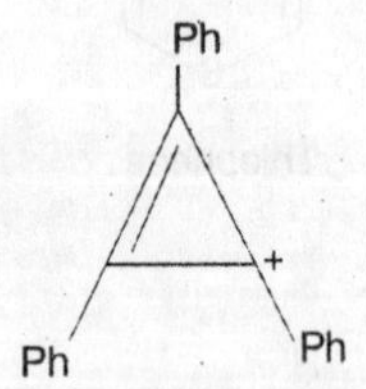

Triphenyl cyclopropylium ion ($n = 0$)

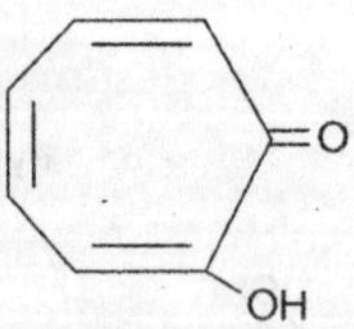

Tropolone

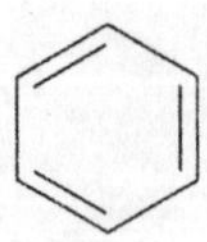

Benzene

6 π–electron system ($n = 1$)

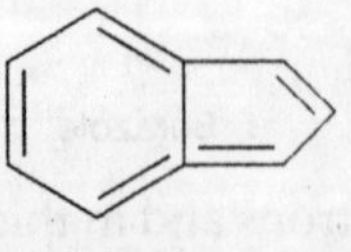

Azulene

6 π-electron system ($n = 1$)

(Azulene is considered as the combination of cyclopentadienyl anion and cycloheptatrienyl cation)

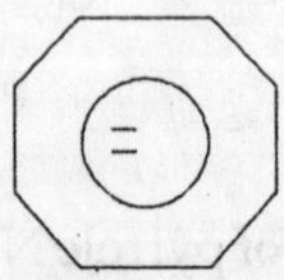

Cyclooctatrienyl dianion

10 π-electron system

($n = 2$)

It may be mentioned that in some cases Hückel's rule is not applicable as in the case of cyclobutadiene which according to Hückel's rule should be anti-aromatic but it may be aromatic under certain condition. That is why Hückel's rule is regarded as empirical.

14.3 Sources of Aromatic Compounds

Aromatic compounds are widespread in nature and have been found to occur both in animal world and in plant kingdom. Coal tar, a by-product of coal gas industry, is a very important source of aromatic compounds. Recently petroleum has been the main source of aromatic hydrocarbons. They may be prepared in the laboratory from aliphatic compounds but these methods are seldom applied for manufacturing purposes.

A. Aromatic Compounds from Coal Tar

- *Carbonisation of Coal*: Coal is the thermal decomposition product of trees burried under the earth's crust for a long time. When coal is heated in a steel retort in absence of air different compounds volatilise and are condensed. This process is known as *carbonisation or coking*. Generally following components are obtained.

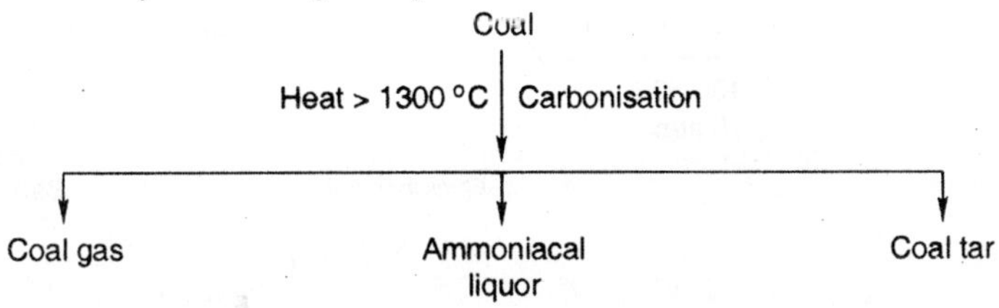

- *Distillation of Coal Tar:* The coal tar that is obtained is subjected to fractional distillation when following fractions are obtained.

Temperature range	Name of the fraction	Main constituents
up to 180 °C	Light oil	Benzene and its derivative, i.e., toluene, xylene, etc.
180-250 °C	Middle oil or Carbolic oil	Carbolic acid (phenol), and Naphthalene
250-300 °C	Heavy oil or Creosote oil	Cresols, Naphthalene, Quinoline
300-350 °C	Green oil or Anthracene oil	Anthracene, Carbazole
Residue	Residue or pitch	Carbon

- *Light oil Fraction*: This fraction is washed with caustic soda to remove acidic impurities and with concentrated sulphuric acid to eliminate basic impurities. It is finally thoroughly washed with water to remove the excess of acid and base and is then subjected to fractional distillation. The fraction up to 110 °C is known as benzol which contains benzene (70%), toluene and a little xylene.
- *Middle oil Fraction*: On cooling this fraction naphthalene crystallises out which is separated and purified. After the separation of naphthalene, phenol and cresol are isolated from the residue.

- *Heavy oil Fraction:* This fraction is primarily used for preserving timber and is sold in the market in the name of *cresote oil.*
- *Green oil Fraction:* This fraction has a green fluorescence and is known as green oil. Anthracene, phenanthrene and other polynuclear aromatic compounds are obtained from this fraction.
- *Pitch:* The residue left over in the retort is known as *pitch.* It is extensively used in the construction of road.

B. Petroleum as a Source of Aromatic Compounds

Nowadays aromatic compounds are manufactured from petroleum. The manufacturing process involves the cracking of petroleum in presence of oxides of chromium, vanadium and molybdenum supported alumina as catalysts.

The fraction containing up to eight carbon atoms is heated at a temperature of 400-500 °C at 15 atmospheric pressure when alkanes undergo cyclisation to form cycloalkanes. Cycloalkanes formed undergo dehydrogenation to yield aromatic compounds. Thus,

i. 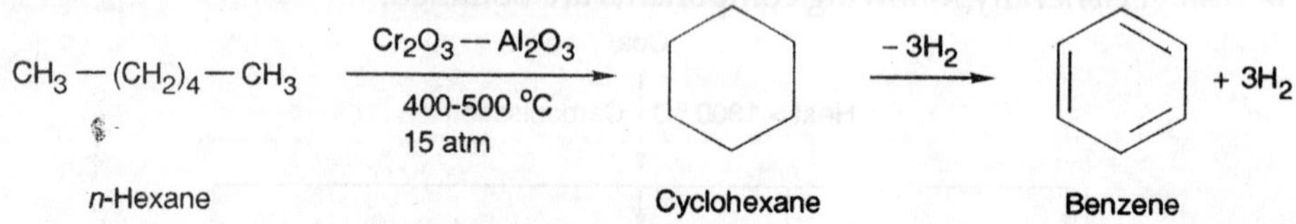

ii. 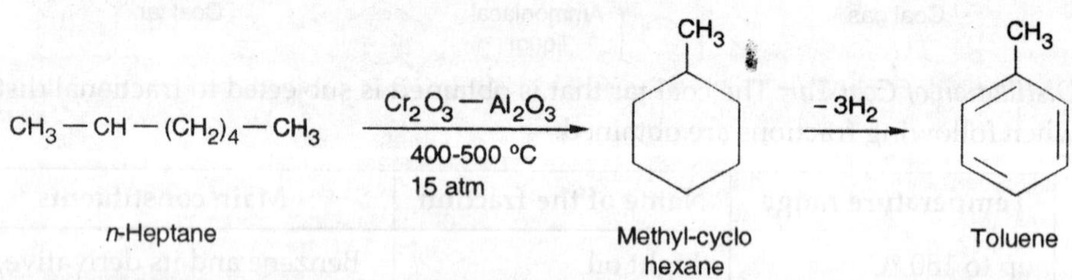

Similarly, other aromatic compounds may be prepared.

14.4 Classification of Aromatic Compounds

Like aliphatic compounds aromatic compounds may be classified on the basis of functional groups. Some examples of these classes along with their names and structures are mentioned below to make the readers familiar with the similarity of functional groups present in both aliphatic and aromatic compounds.

Hydrocarbons:

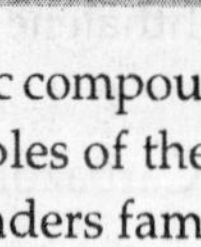

Benzene

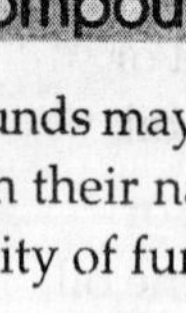

Toluene

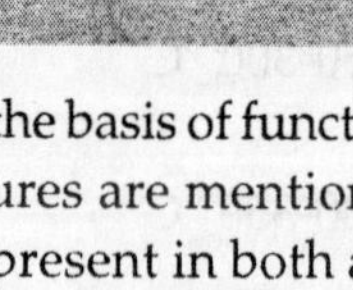

Ortho-xylene

Arylhalides:

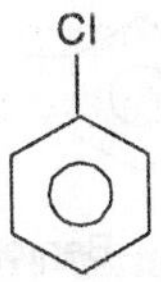

Chlorobenzene

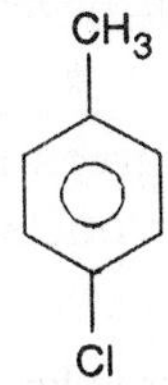

para-Chlorotoluene

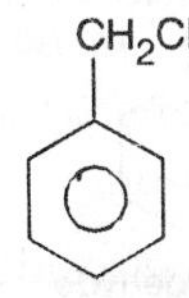

Benzyl Chloride

Sulphonic Acids:

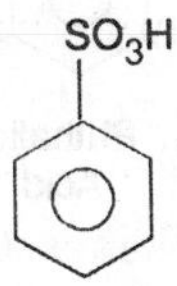

Benzene Sulphonic Acid

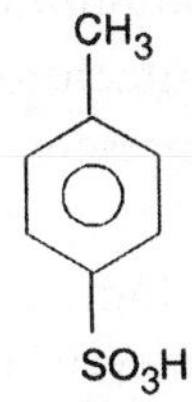

para-Toluene Sulphonic Acid

Nitro Compounds:

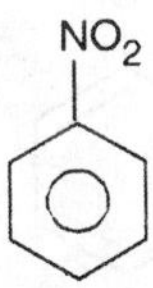

Nitro benzene

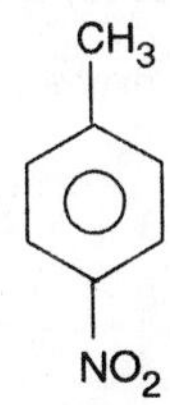

para-Nitrotoluene

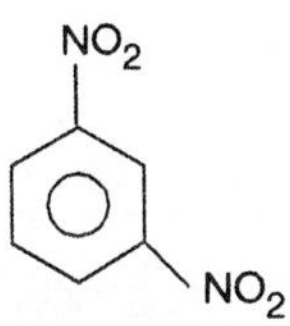

meta-Dinitro benezene

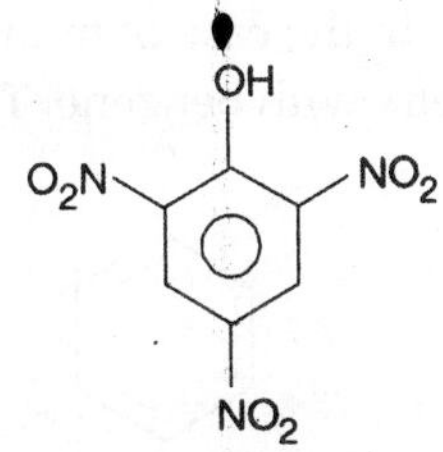

Picric Acid

Amino Compounds:

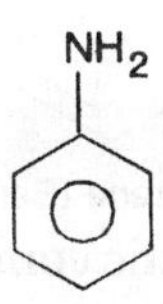

Aniline

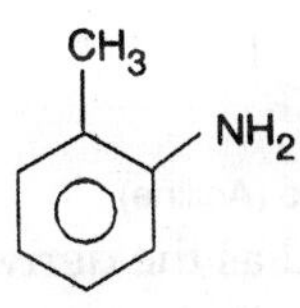

ortho-Toluidine

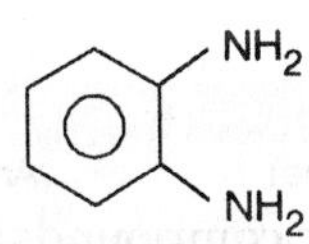

ortho-Phenylene diamine

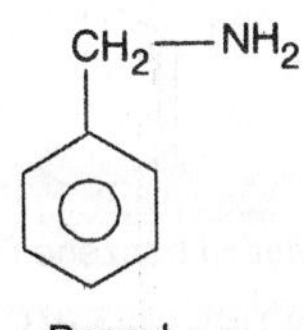

Benzyl amine

Hydroxy Compounds:

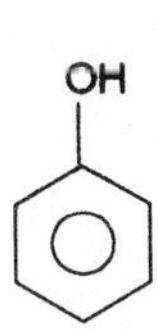

Phenol

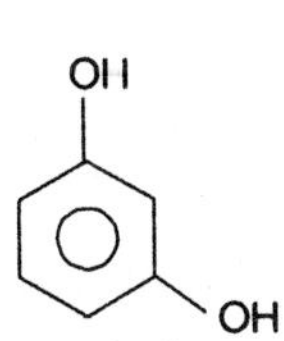

Resorcinol

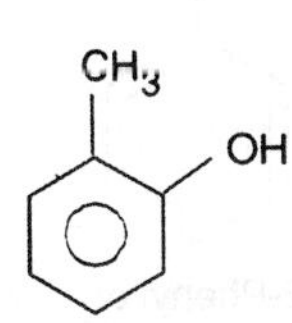

ortho-Cresol

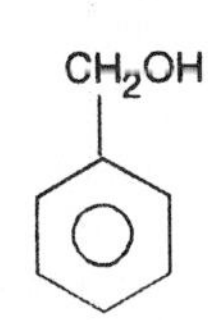

Benzyl alcohol

Carbonyl Compounds:

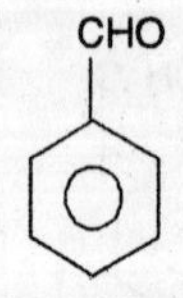

Benzaldehyde

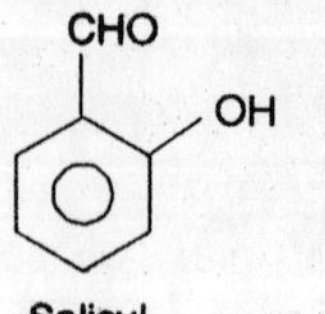

Salicyl aldehyde

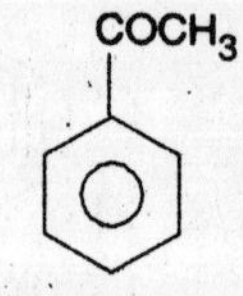

Acetophenone

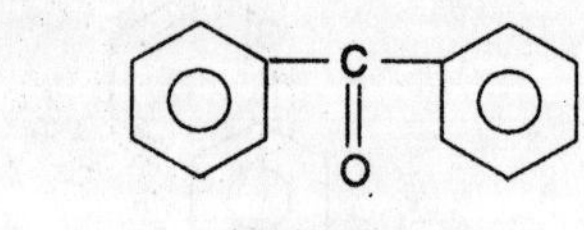

Benrophenone

Carboxylic Acids:

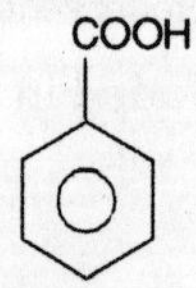

Benzoic Acid

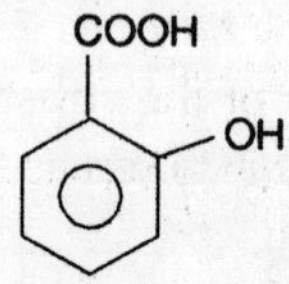

Salicylic Acid

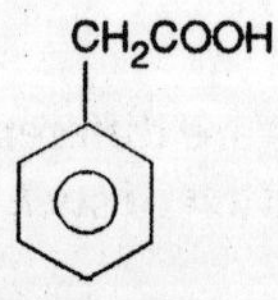

Phenyl acetic Acid

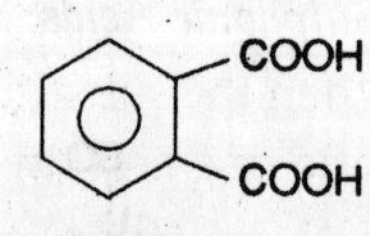

Phthalic Acid

14.5 Nomenclature of Aromatic Compounds

Aromatic compounds may be named by common or IUPAC system. However, common system of nomenclature is generally popular.

In the case of mono-substituted benzene derivatives, the name of the substituent is used as prefix with benzene. Thus,

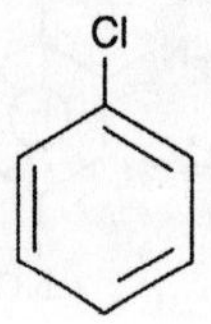

Chlorobenzene

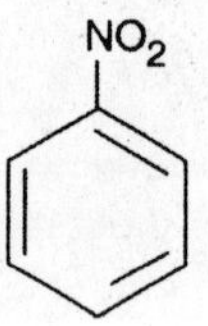

Nitrobenzene

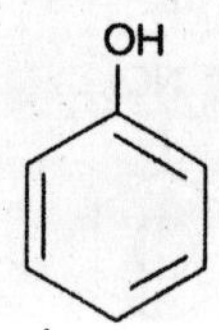

Hydroxy benzene or phenol

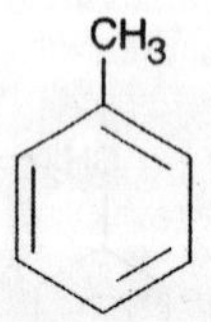

Methyl benzene (Toluene)

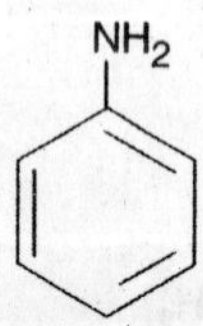

Amino benzene (Aniline)

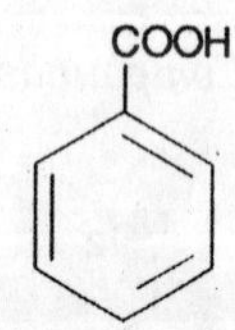

Carboxy benzene (Benzoic acid)

Sometimes aromatic compounds are named as the derivative of aliphatic compounds. The benzene ring is mentioned as a substituent. Like alkyl group, the corresponding aromatic group, C_6H_5 is named as phenyl, or aryl group and is indicated by Ph or Ar. Thus,

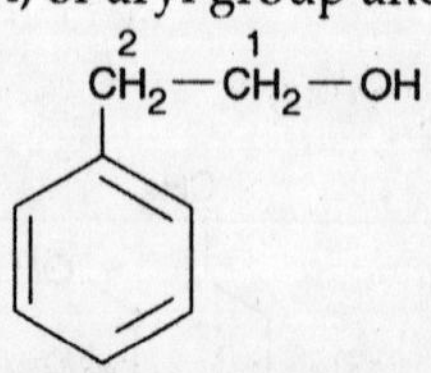

2-Phenyl or β-Phenyl ethanol

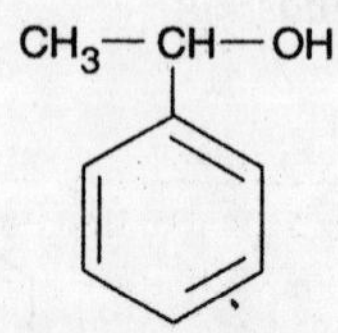

1-Phenyl or α-Phenyl ethanol

In naming the disubstituted benzenes, the positions of the substituents are indicated by number. However, in most of the cases, common system is used. The two substituents in benzene ring may be arranged in three different ways, the words ortho (*o*-), para (*p*-) and meta (+-) are used as prefixes. For example,

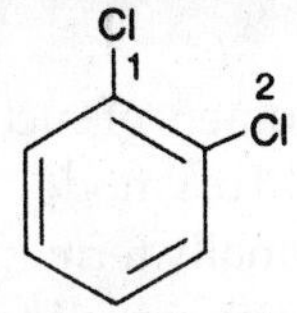

1, 2-Dichlorobenzene
(ortho dichlorobenzene
or *o*-dichlorobenzene)

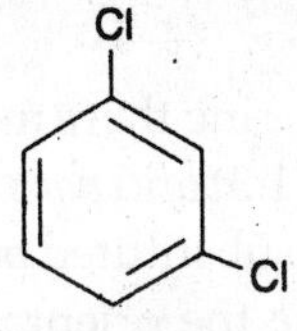

1, 3-Dichlorobenzene
(meta-dichlorobenzene
or *m*-dichlorobenzene)

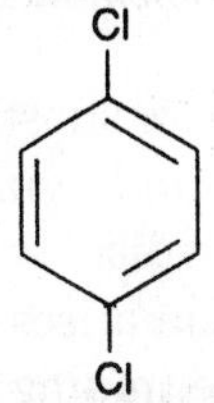

1, 4-Dichlorobenzene
(para-dichlorobenzene
or *p*-dichlorobenzene)

When the substituents are different, then one of the substituents is included in naming the aromatic ring and the position of such substituent is taken as I. Thus,

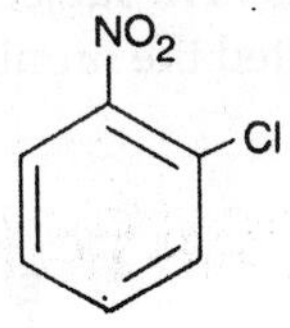

o-Chloronitrobenzene
or 2-Chloronitrobenzene

But in the case of substituted benzene if common name is available, then the name of other substituent is used as prefixes.

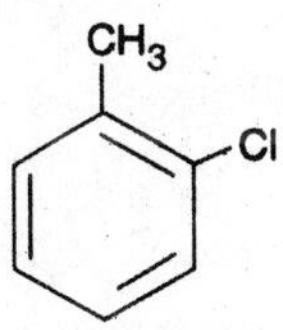

o-Chlorotoluene
or 2-Chlorotoluene

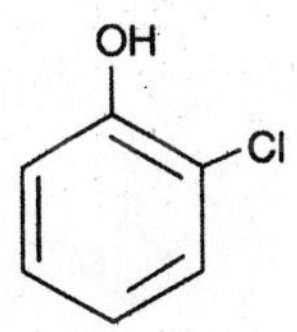

o-Chlorophenol
or 2-Chlorophenol

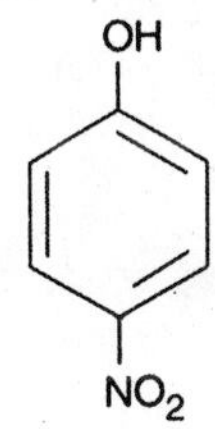

p-Nitrophenol
or 4-Nitrophenol

Similarly, higher substituted benzenes are named.

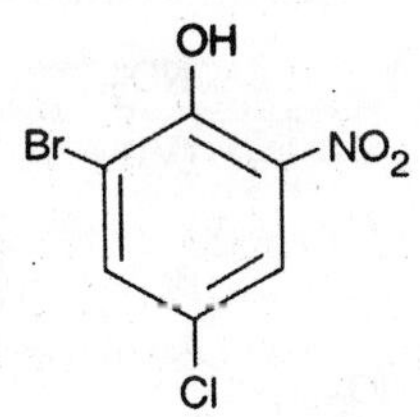

2-Nitro-4-chloro-6-bromophenol

PROBLEM 14.1

Suggest the names of the following:

(a)

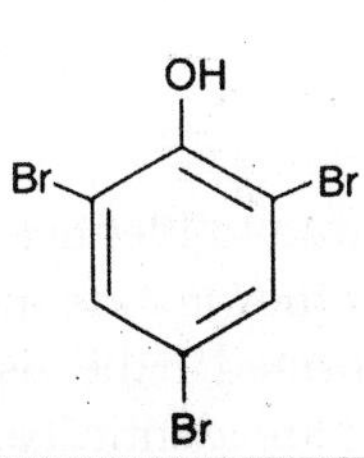

(b)

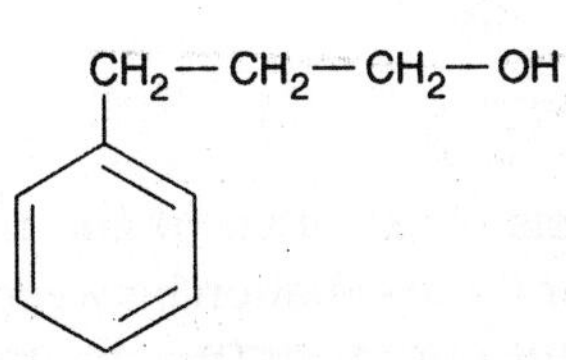

(c)

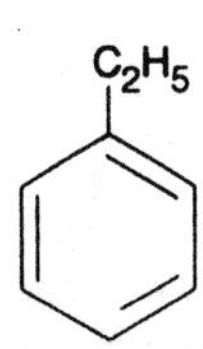

14.6 Orientation

When there are two substituents in benzene ring there may be three isomers of such disubstituted aromatic compounds, viz, *ortho* (1:2), *meta* (1:3) and *para* (1:4) isomers. This mode of arrangement of substituents in disubstituted and higher substituted benzene is normally termed as *orientation*. Now the question arises how to determine the orientation in aromatic ring. There are several methods for determining the orientation in benzene ring of which followings are most important.

(a) *Körner's absolute method*: This is the oldest and most reliable method for determining the orientation. The basic principle of this method is to convert a disubstituted aromatic compounds into trisubstituted products and counting the number of trisubstituted products so formed. In his experiment, Körner applied this principle in the determination of orientation of dibromobenzene. He subjected each isomer (ortho, meta and para) to the process of nitration and counted the number of isomeric nitro compounds formed as depicted below.

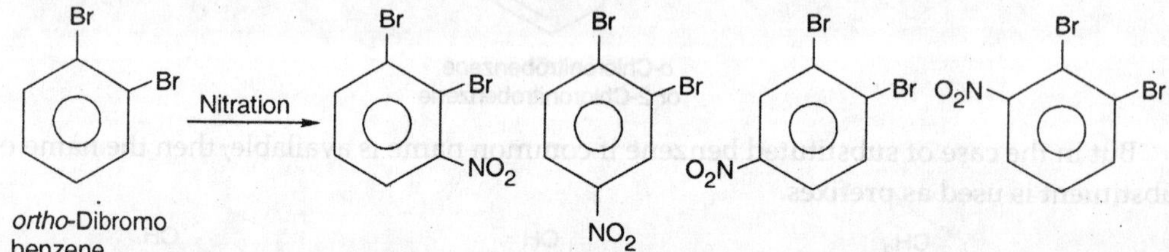

ortho-Dibromo benzene (I) (II) (III) (IV)

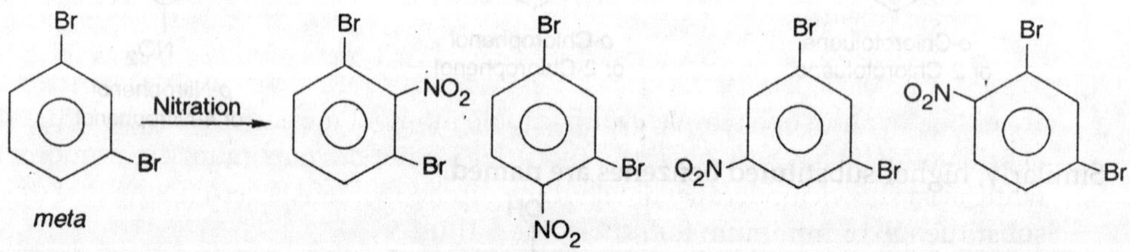

meta (V) (VI) (VII) (VIII)

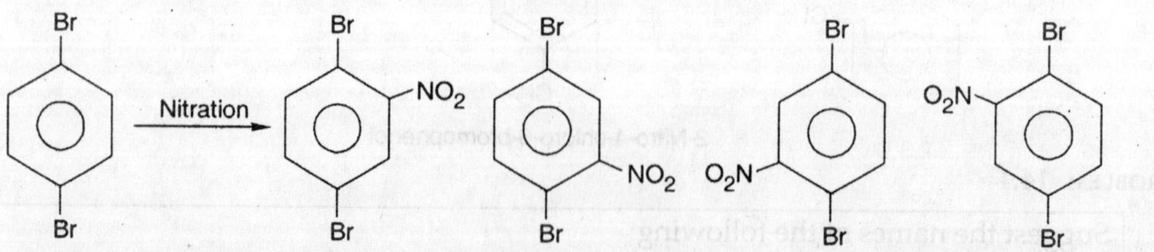

para (IX) (X) (XI) (XII)

Now a careful analysis reveals that (i) and (iv) are identical due to identical mode of arrangements. Similar is the situation between (II) and (III) and they are identical. Thus, the actual number of nitroproducts (trisubstituted derivative) formed in the case of ortho isomer is *only two* (I and II). Again, the products (VI) and (VIII) are identical and hence, meta isomer yields three nitroproducts (V, VI and VII). But all the products, (IX), (X), (XI) and (XII) are identical. Consequently. only one (IX) trisubstituted product is obtained in the case of para isomer.

On the basis of these observations Körner concluded that *ortho* disubstituted benzene forms two trisubstituted derivatives, *meta* gives three while only one trisubstituted benzene is obtained in the case of *p*-disubstituted benzene.

- *Drawbacks of Körner's method*: Körner's method suffers from the following defects:
  i. It is not applicable when the two substituents in disubstituted benzene are different.
  ii. It is a laborious process.

(b) *Relative method*: This method involves the conversion of disubstituted isomer of unknown orientation into a compound of known orientation or vice versa.

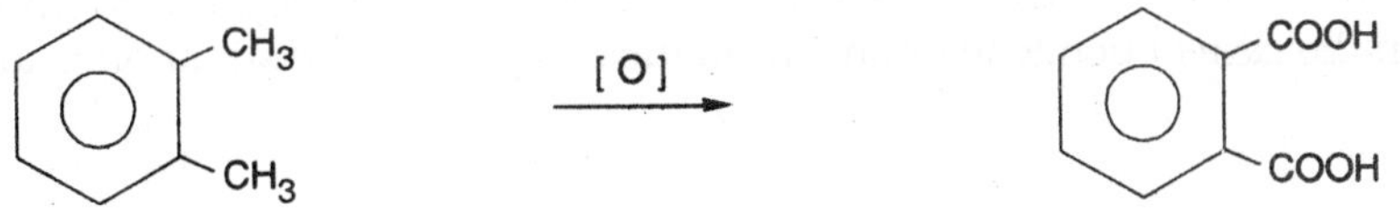

(Unknown) (*ortho*-isomer) — *ortho*-isomer (known)

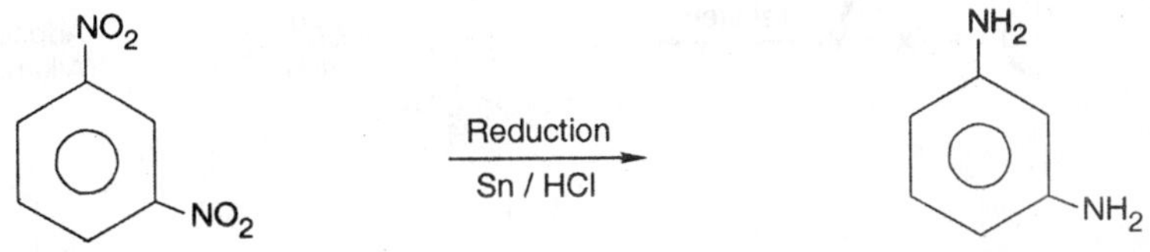

(Known) *m*-Dinitrobenzene — (Unknown) (*m*-Phenylene diamine)

(c) *Method of dipole moment measurement*: When two substituents in disubstituted benzene are either an atom or a simple group, dipole moment measurement may settle the issue of orientation. It has been observed that *ortho* isomer has maximum dipole moment value while *meta* shows moderate value but the dipole moment is zero (in the case of identical substituents) or minimum for *para* isomer. Thus,

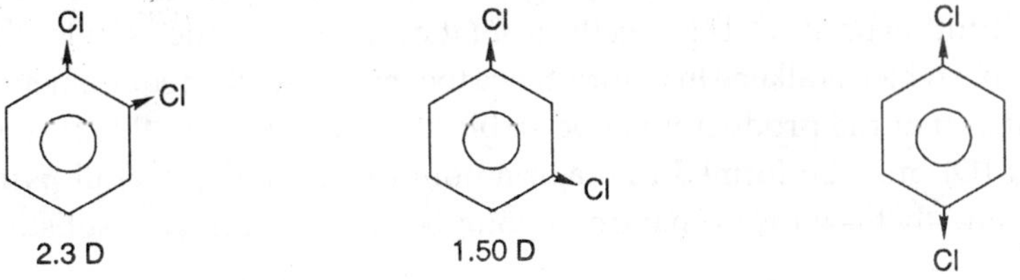

2.3 D   1.50 D   0

14.7 Reactions of Aromatic Compounds

Substitution Reactions of Aromatic Compounds: The most significant feature of aromatic compounds is their tendency to undergo substitution reactions with a number of reagents rather than addition reactions. This tendency of aromatic compounds is the reflection of their extra stability associated with their structures which may be envisaged as follows:

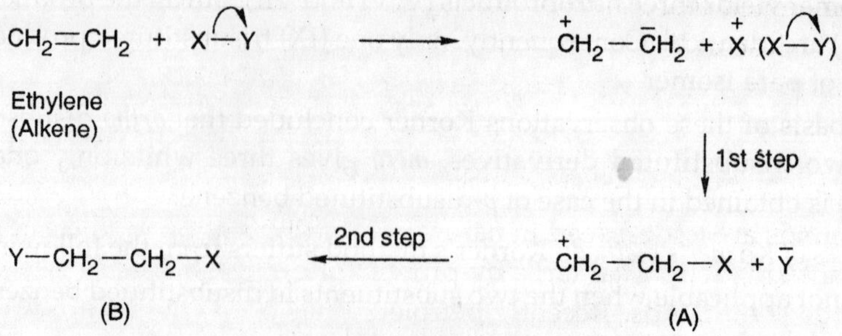

In the case of alkene, the carbocation (A) that is obtained in the first step of the reaction is stabilised by the combination with $\bar{Y}$ in the second step to form the product (B) making overall path an addition of XY to alkene.

But in the case of benzene or any aromatic compound, the situation is different.

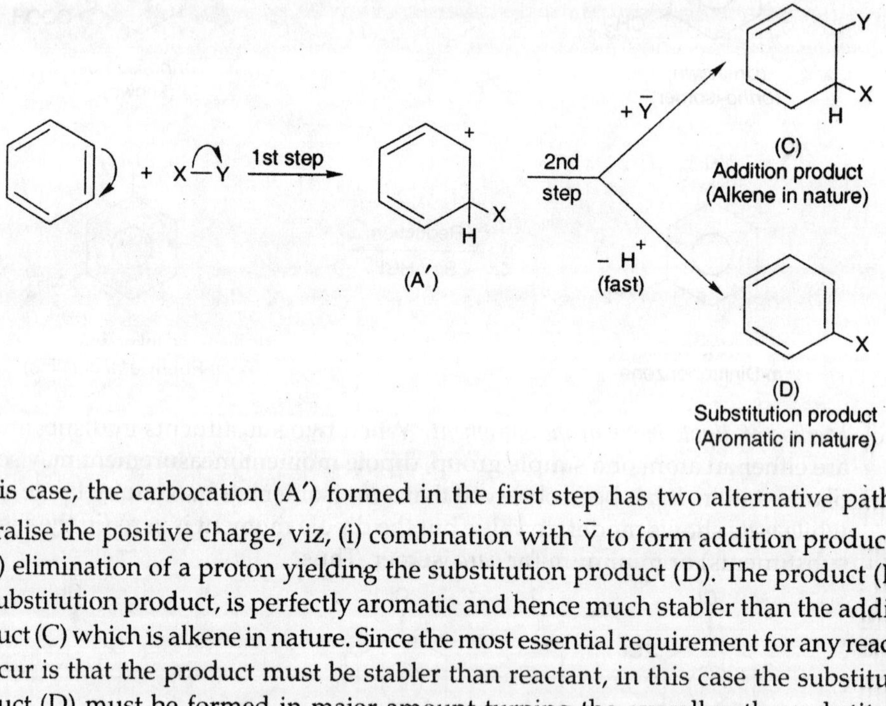

In this case, the carbocation (A′) formed in the first step has two alternative paths to neutralise the positive charge, viz, (i) combination with $\bar{Y}$ to form addition product (C) or (ii) elimination of a proton yielding the substitution product (D). The product (D)—the substitution product, is perfectly aromatic and hence much stabler than the addition product (C) which is alkene in nature. Since the most essential requirement for any reaction to occur is that the product must be stabler than reactant, in this case the substitution product (D) must be formed in major amount turning the overall path a substitution process and that is why aromatic compounds normally undergo substitution reaction.

(a) *Nature of Substitution Reactions*: It is an well established fact that in benzene and other aromatic compounds there exists a ring of electron clouds throughout the whole ring of the compounds which is spread over above and below the plane of the molecule (figure below) and this negatively charged electron cloud protects the ring carbon atoms from the attack by a nucleophile due to repulsion between similar charges but such electron cloud can accelerate the attack by an electrophile. Consequently aromatic compounds can readily undergo *electrophilic substitution reaction* and in fact, this has been found to be so in the overwhelming majority of aromatic compounds.

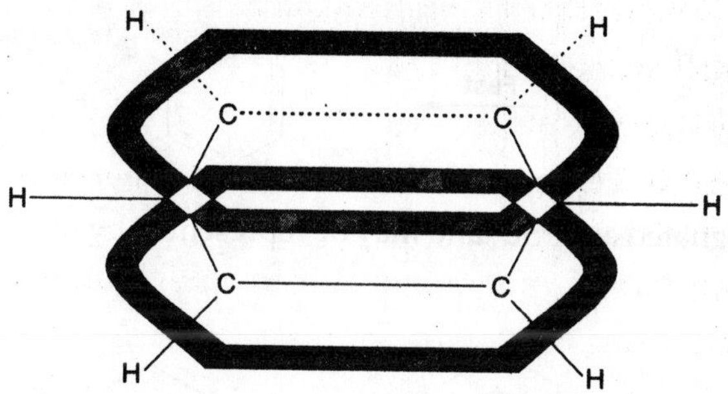

(b) *Mechanism of Aromatic Electrophilic Substitution Reactions*: Electrophilic substitution reactions in aromatic compounds may take place in two different paths as discussed below:

Stepwise Path: In this path attack by an electrophile to the aromatic compound and elimination of a proton from aromatic ring occur in two separate steps through the formation of an intermediate carbocation.

Step I: Attack by electrophile (E^+)

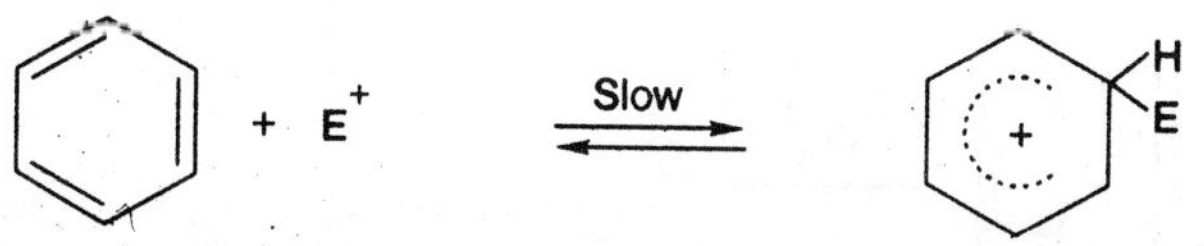

(A)
Carbocation (σ-complex)

Step II: Elimination of a proton

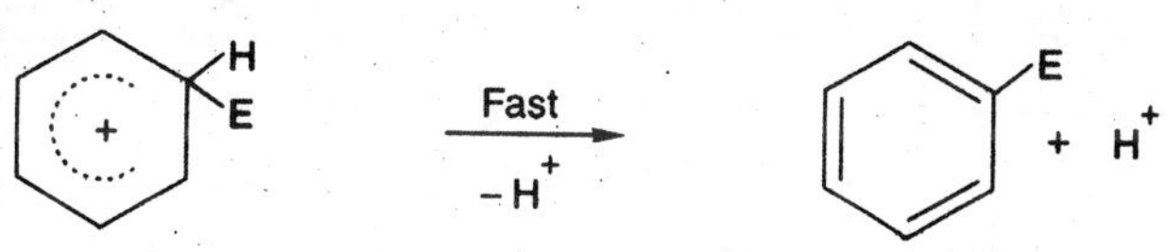

(A) Substitution product

Simultaneous Path: In simultaneous path attack by the electrophile and elimination of a proton take place simultaneously through a transition state.

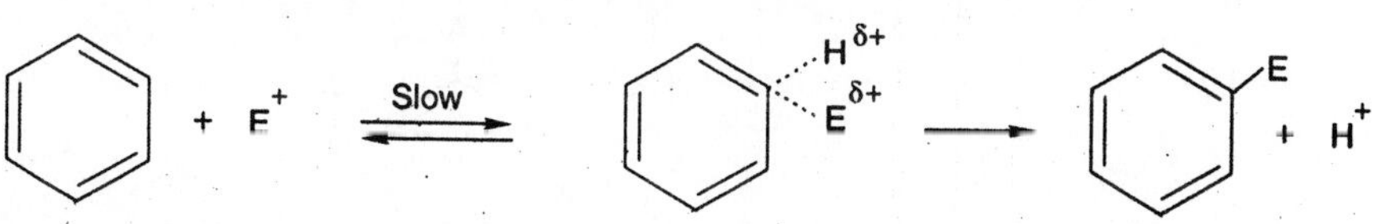

Transition state Product

Out of these two alternatives stepwise path has been found to be most rational and is the currently accepted mechanism for aromatic electrophilic substitutions and subsequently supported by experimental evidences. This stepwise path is very often written in localised bond-structure particularly in the case of substituted aromatic compounds for which localised bond-structure is most important. Thus,

Step I:

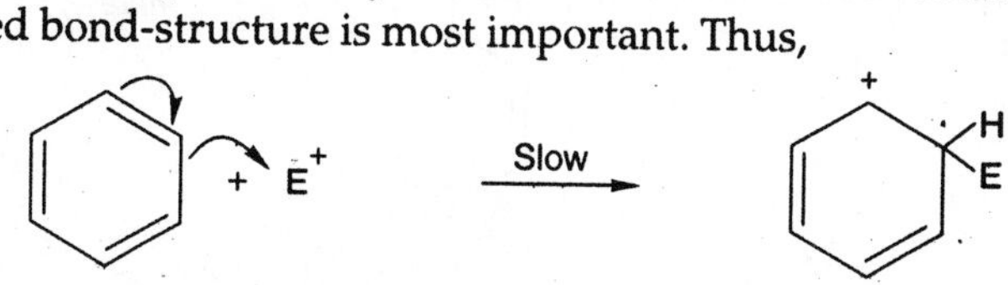

σ-complex

Step II: 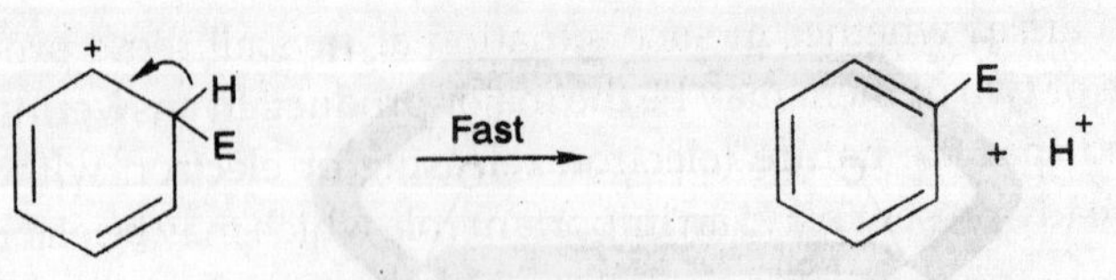

This path is designated as $ArSE^2$ and may be represented by the following energy profile diagram.

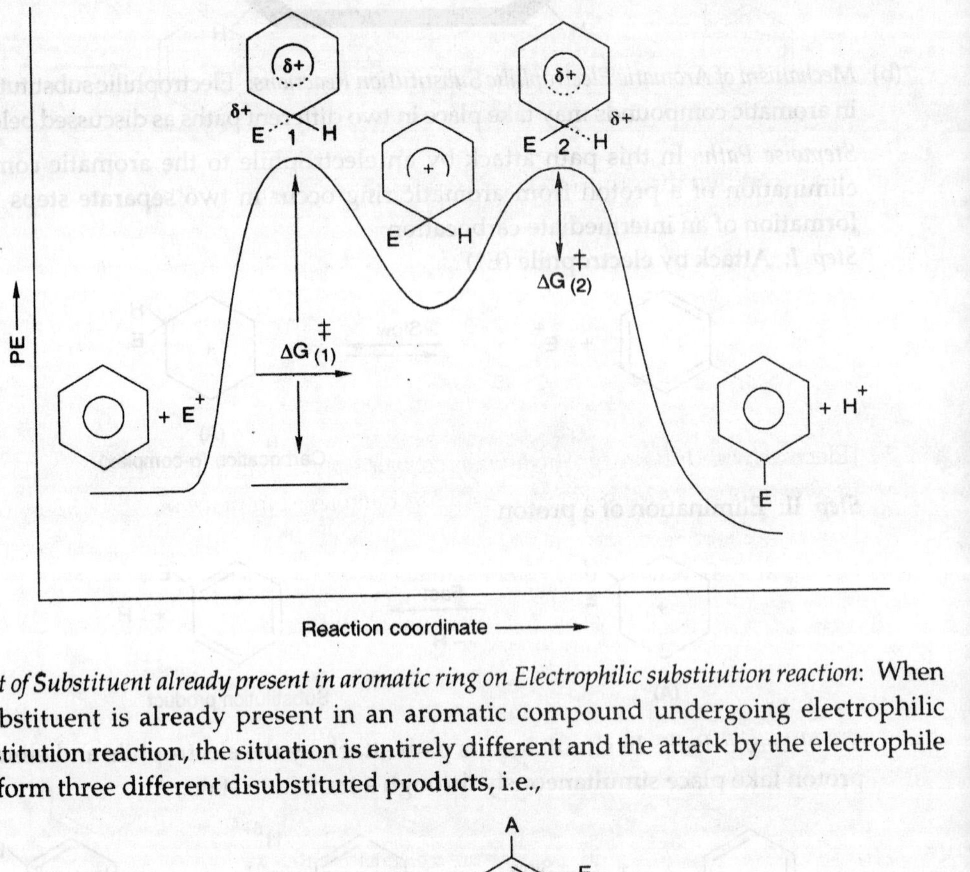

(c) *Effect of Substituent already present in aromatic ring on Electrophilic substitution reaction*: When a substituent is already present in an aromatic compound undergoing electrophilic substitution reaction, the situation is entirely different and the attack by the electrophile can form three different disubstituted products, i.e.,

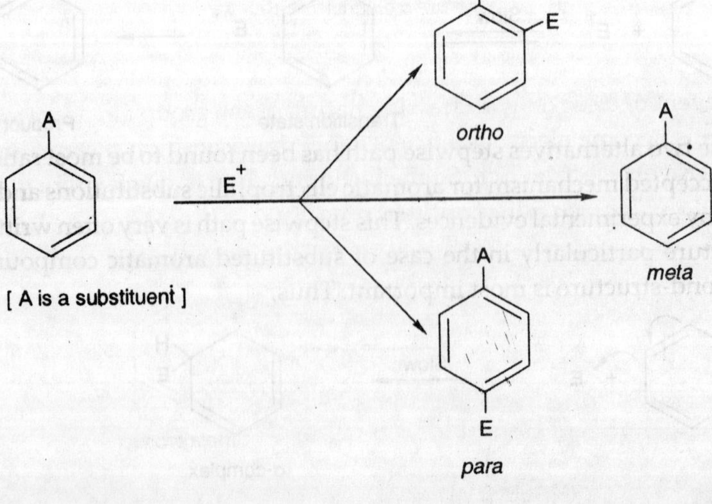

Now the question arises whether in such situation always all these products would be formed or any one or two of them may be the major product. In answering this question it may be mentioned that the nature (electron releasing or electron withdrawing) of the substituent (A) already present plays an important role which may be elaborated as below:

Case 1: When the group (A) is electron releasing in nature.

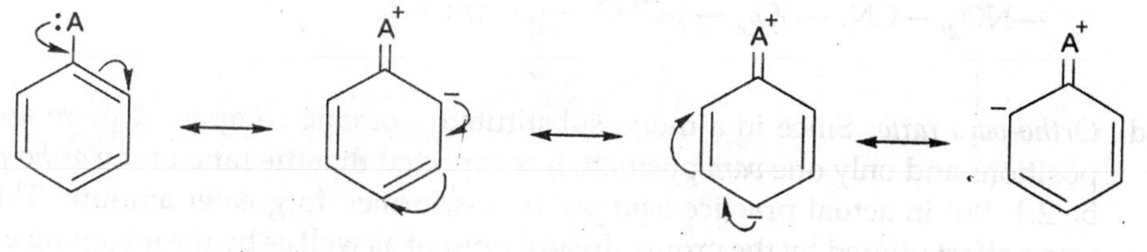

Case 2: When the group (A) is electron withdrawing in nature.

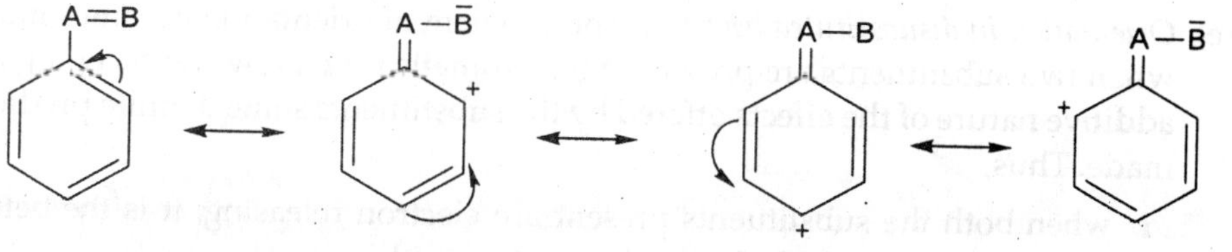

[Electron withdrawing group always contains more than one atoms having multiple bonds between them. For this reason, A=B has been used in place of A.]

From the above resonating structures it is, thus, evident that in the case of electron releasing nature of the group already present due to resonance, *ortho* and *para* positions become elctron rich, consequently incoming electrophile preferably enters at *ortho* and *para* positions forming *ortho* and *para* products, i.e.,

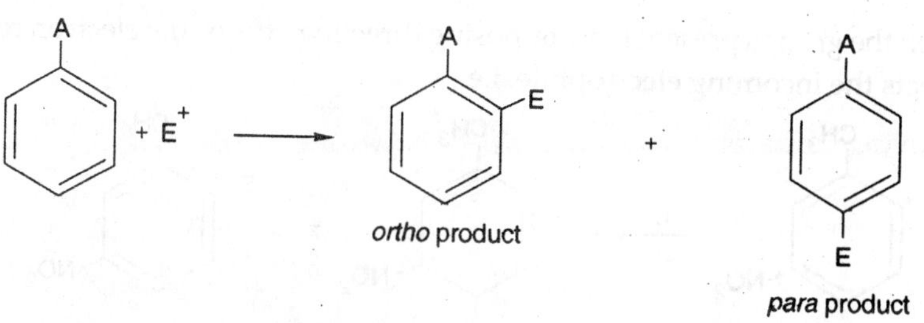

But in the event of electron withdrawing nature of the group already present, *ortho* and *para* positions become electron deficient while meta position remains unchanged and hence, is relatively electron rich. So the incoming electrophile favours the *meta* position for its attack yielding *meta* disubstituted product.

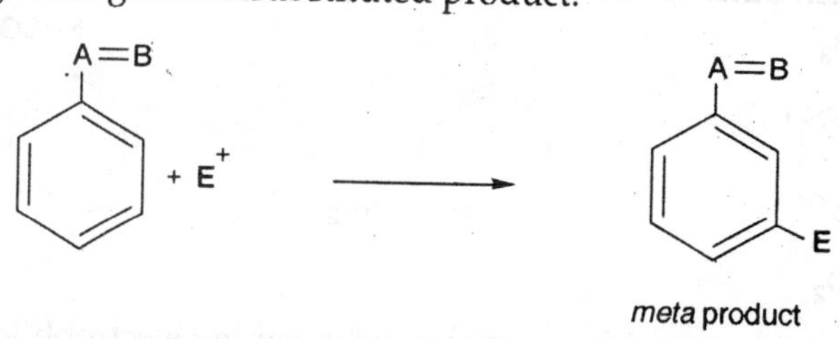

The first category of the group, i.e., electron releasing group is known as *ortho-para orienting or directing group* as it directs the incoming electrophile to enter at these positions. Some of the common *ortho-para* directing groups are—alkyl group, —OH,—NH_2, —NHR,—OR, —NHCOR, halogens, etc.

The other group, i.e., electron withdrawing group is termed as *meta orienting or directing group*: Commonly encountered *meta* orienting groups are:

$$-NO_2, -CN, -SO_3, ->C{=}O, -\underset{\underset{O}{\|}}{C}-OH, \text{etc.}$$

(d) *Ortho-para ratio*: Since in a mono-substituted aromatic compound there are two *ortho* positions and only one *para* position, it is expected that the ratio of the *ortho-para* should be 2:1. But in actual practice *para* product is formed in greater amount. This is due to steric effect offered by the group already present as well as by the incoming electrophile. It has been observed that larger the sizes of the substituent and the incoming electrophile, more is the decrease in the rate of formation of *ortho* product.

(e) *Orientation in disubstituted benzene*: The problem of orientation becomes much difficult when two substituents are present in the aromatic ring. However, keeping in mind the additive nature of the effects offered by the substituents some definite prediction can be made. Thus,

i. when both the substituents present are electron releasing, it is the better electron releasing group which directs the reaction path.

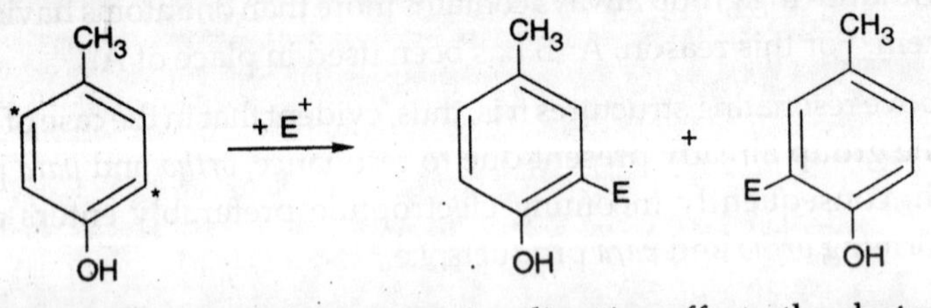

ii. when the groups present have opposing directing effects, the electron releasing group directs the incoming electrophile, i.e.,

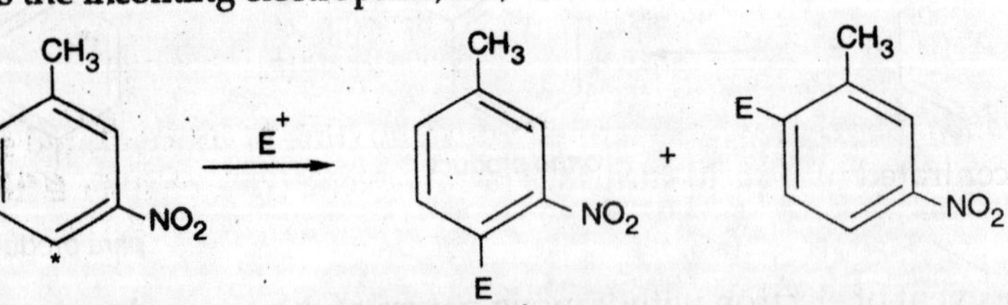

[Other ortho position is sterically hindered.]

iii. sometimes the locations of two groups may be such that their directing influence can reinforce each other towards a particular position.

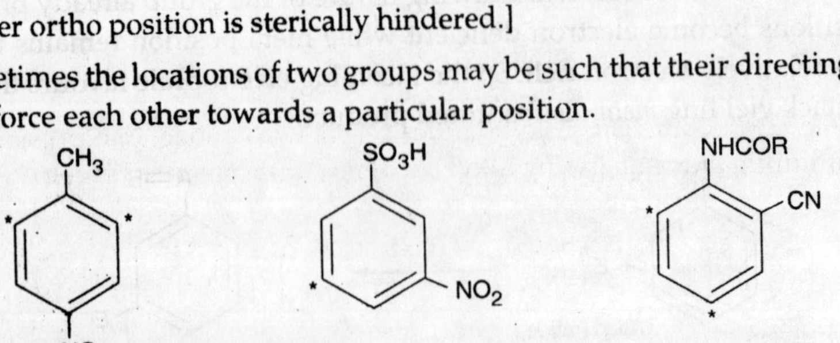

[*Positions are favoured for attack by the incoming electrophile.]

PROBLEM 14.2

1. Classify the following groups as *ortho/para* and *meta* director:
   $—CH_3$, $—NO_2$, $—OH$, $—NH_2$, $—CN$, >C=O, NHCOR
2. Predict the probable position of attack by an electrophile in the following compounds:

(a) 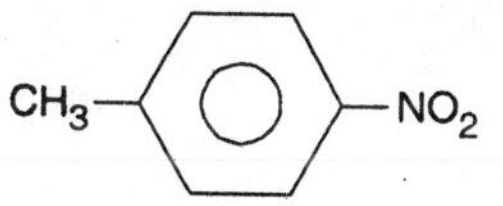

(b) 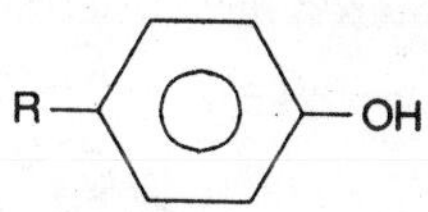

(f) *Some Representative Electrophilic Aromatic Substitution Reactions:* Electrophilic substitution reactions in aromatic compounds and electrophilic reagent are capable of wide variation. As a result electrophilic substitution reaction becomes highly significant. This type of substitution reaction is the principal method for the preparation of substituted derivatives of aromatic compounds both in the laboratory and industry. In this connection a few typical examples may be listed below, each of which has been discussed in more details in chapters **fifteen to nineteen.**

1. *Halogenation:* Halogen reacts with aromatic compound in presence ferric halide as a catalyst to afford halogen derivative (vide chapter **fifteen**).

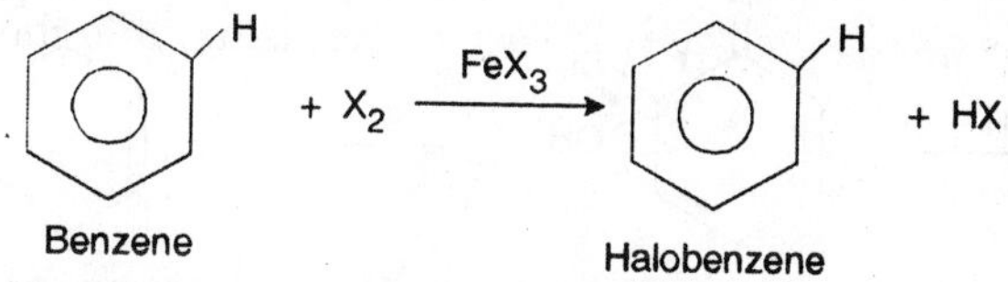

2. *Sulphonation:* Hot concentrated sulphuric acid reacts **with benrene to give benrene** sulphonic acid (vide chapter **fifteen**)

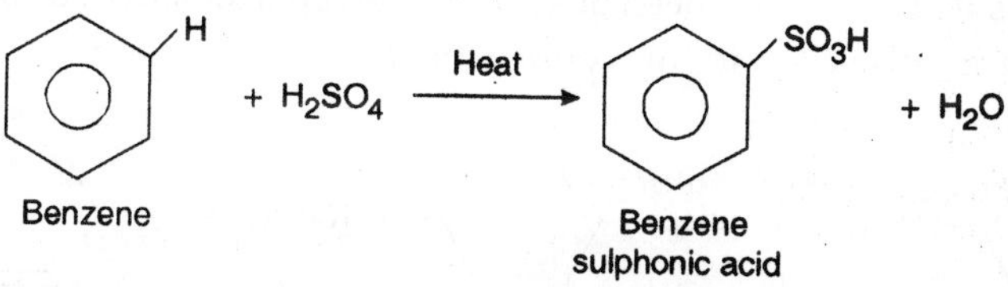

3. *Nitration:* Benzene when warmed with a mixture of concentrated sulphuric acid and concentrated nitric acid furnishes nitrobenzene (vide chapter **fifteen**)

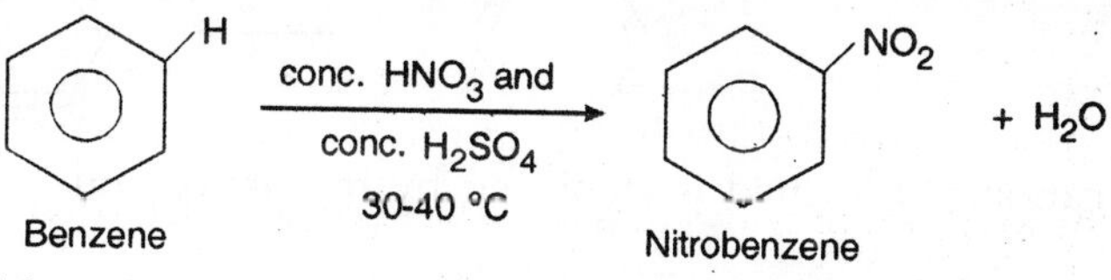

4. *Friedel-Crafts Reaction:* Alkyl halides reacts with benzene in presence of anhydrous aluminium chloride giving alkyl benzenes (vide chapter **fifteen**)

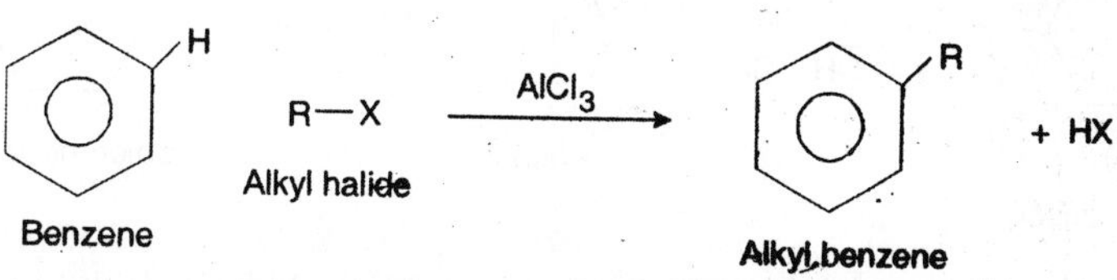

(g) *Aromatic Nucleophilic Substitution Reactions*: Although less common yet under certain conditions nucleophilic substitution reaction can take place in aromatic compounds. It has been observed that when electron withdrawing group is present in aromatic ring *ortho* and *para* positions become electron deficient. Hence at these positions nucleophile can enter. Thus,

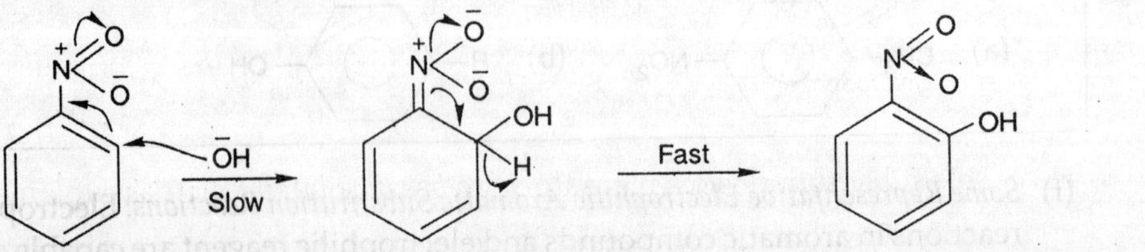

It is a bimolecular path and is extremely common in aromatic nucleophilic substitution reaction. Not only hydrogen at *ortho* and *para* positions is replaced but other substituents like halogens at these positions can be easily displaced. Thus, though normally chlorine in chlorobenzene cannot be replaced but chlorine in *ortho* and *para* nitrochlorobenzene is readily replaced.

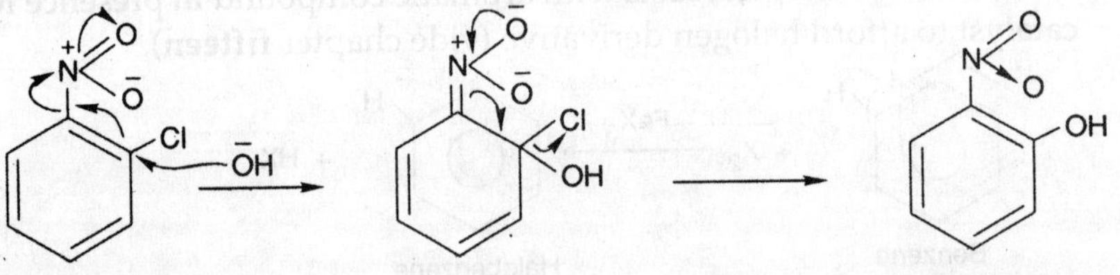

o-chloronitro benzene *o*-nitro phenol

This bimolecular path is represented as $ArS_{N}2$. In some cases unimolecular aromatic nucleophilic substitution has been observed. The replacement of diazonium group by a nucleophile may be cited in this connection, i.e.,

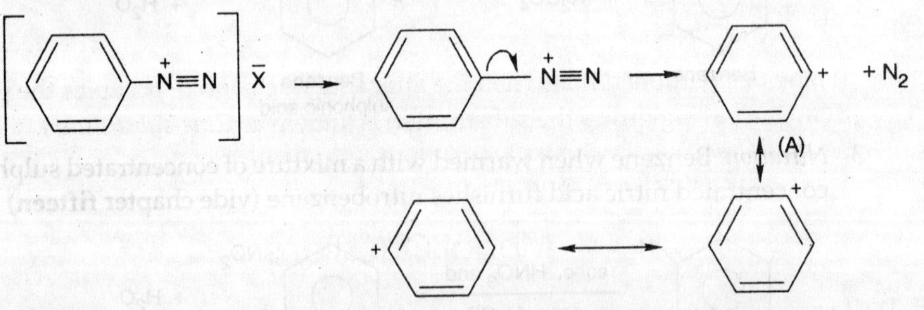

The phenyl cation (A) formed is stabilised by resonance and is attacked by any nucleophile.

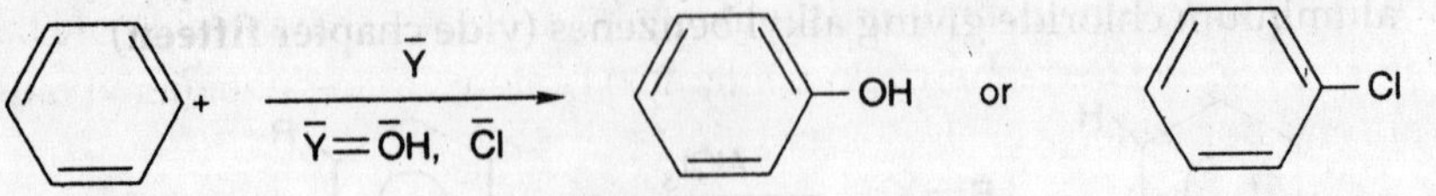

(A)

Phenyl cation

Phenol

Chlorobenzene

Sometimes by the use of strong base, replacement of group from aromatic ring may occur through nucleophilic path. For example,

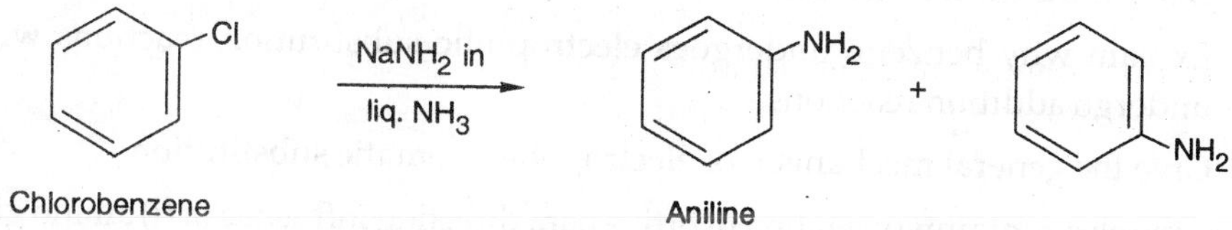

This substitution takes place through *benzyne intermediate* as explained below.

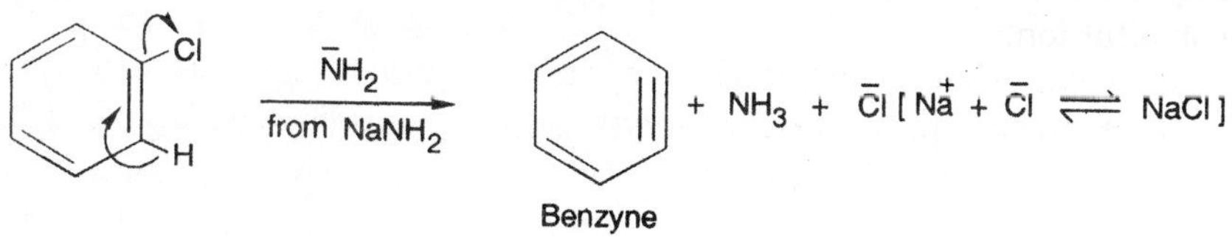

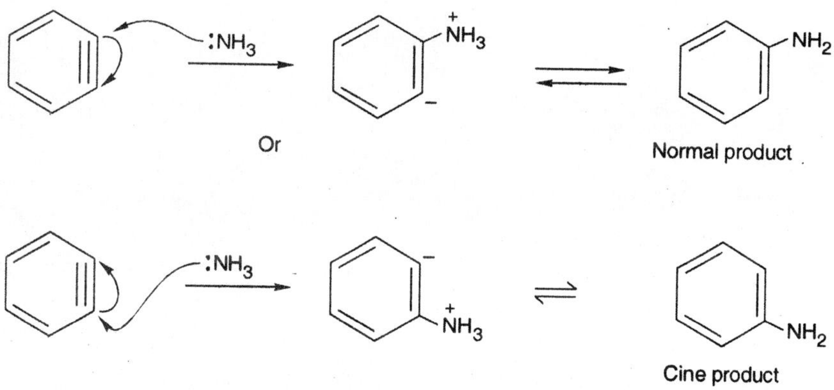

It may be mentioned that when the attacking nucleophile occupies the position other than the leaving group the substitution is known as *Cine-substitution.*

Model Questions

1. Write notes on the nomenclature of aromatic compounds.
2. What is aromaticity? State and explain the main points of Hückel's rule. How can this rule be employed to explain the aromaticity of organic compounds?
3. Which of the following compounds will exhibit aromatic character? Write their structural formulae. Cyclo-octatetraene, cyclo-pentadiexyl anion, Cyclo-pentadienyl radical, pyridine, pyrrole and borazole.
4. What are the main sources of aromatic compounds?
5. Write notes on:
   i. Coal tar distillation.

ii. Petroleum as a source of aromatic compounds.

iii. Körner's method of orientation.

6. Discuss the orbital structure of benzene.

7. Explain why benzene undergoes electrophilic substitution reactions whereas alkenes undergo addition reactions.

8. Give the general mechanism of electrophilic aromatic substitution.

9. Give electronic interpretation of ortho-para directing influence of (i) amino group (ii) alkoxy group.

10. Explain deactivating and meta directing nature of nitrogroup towards electrophilic substitut`ion.

CHAPTER FIFTEEN

Arenes and Their Halo, Sulphonic Acid and Nitro Derivatives

15.1 Arenes

Arenes are aromatic hydrocarbons based on benzene ring as a structural unit. Benzene is the first and most fundamental member of arenes. As mentioned earlier (vide chapter 14) the origin and development of the concept of *aromaticity* is centred around the discovery and the structure elucidation of benzene by Kekule. Later on, a large number of aromatic hydrocarbons (arenes) came into existence. Of these some commonly known members are toluene, xylene, ethyl benzene, styrene and trimethyl benzene.

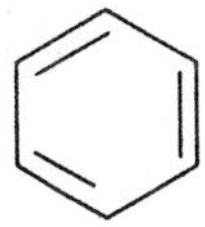
Benzene

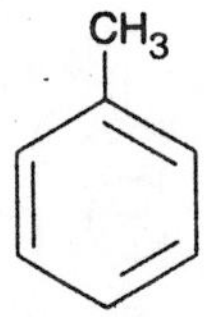
Toluene

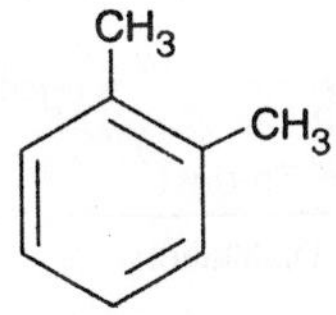
o-Xylene

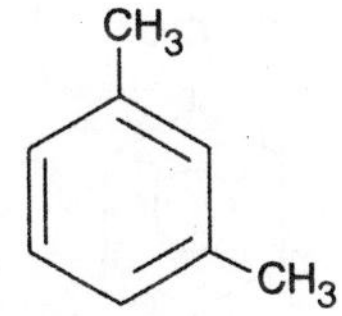
m-Xylene

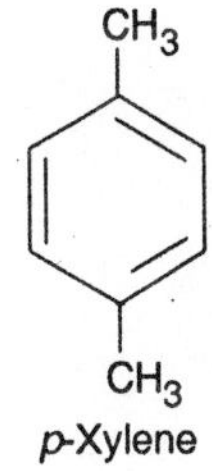
p-Xylene

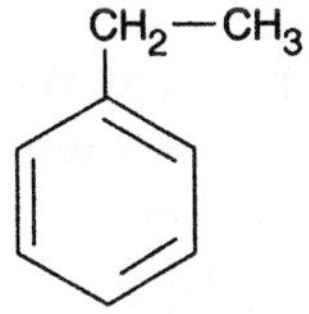
Ethyl benzene

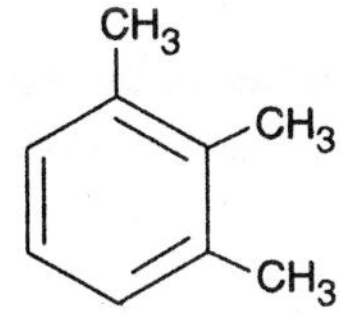
1, 2, 3-Trimethyl benzene

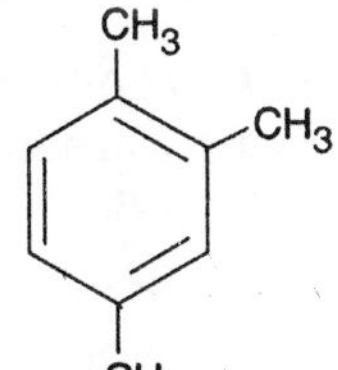
1, 2, 4-Trimethyl benzene

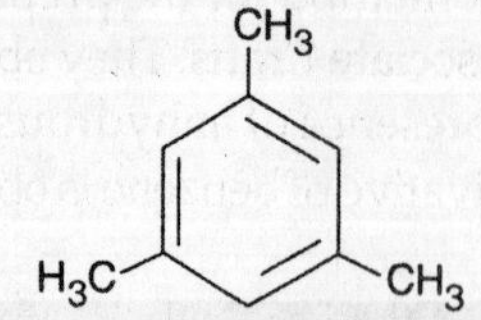

1, 2, 5-Trimethyl benzene

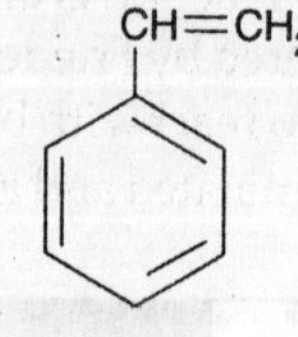

Styrene

15.2 Preparation of Arenes

Arenes are normally manufactured from coal tar or petroleum. However, some laboratory methods of preparation for arenes are available, a few of which are noted below.

1. *Decarboxylation of Aromatic Carboxylic Acids*: When aromatic carboxylic acids are heated with sodalime decarboxylation occurs with the formation of aromatic hydrocarbon.

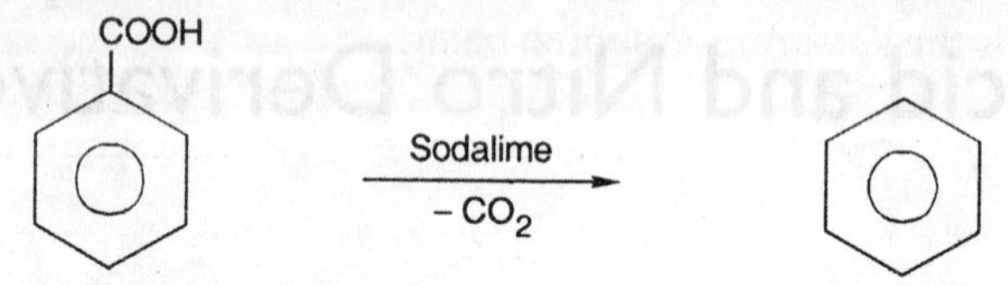

Benzoic acid → Benzene

2. *Distillation of Phenols*: Phenols on distillation with Zn-dust yield aromatic hydrocarbons.

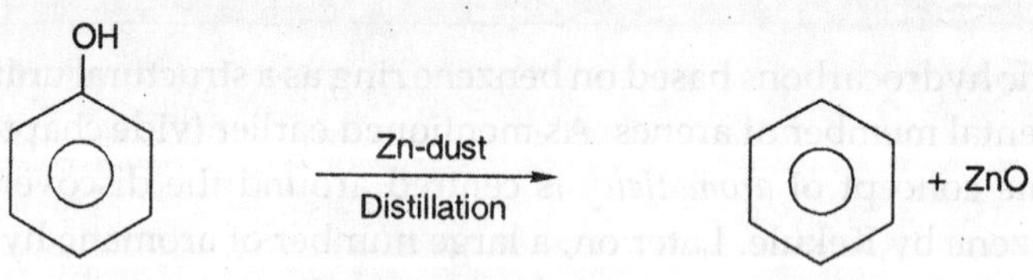

Benzene

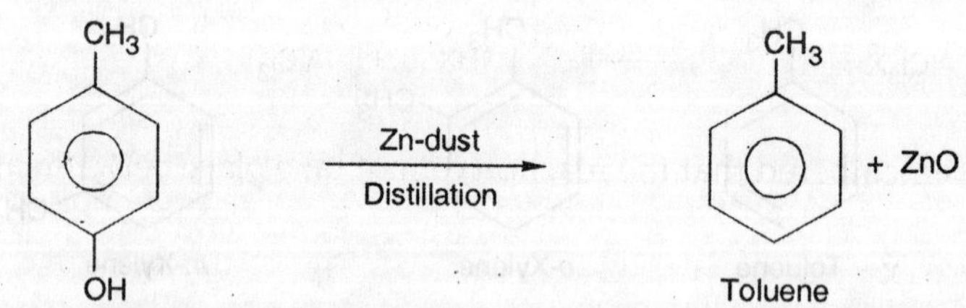

p-Methyl phenol → Toluene

3. *Wurtz-Fittig Reaction*: Homologues of benzene can be prepared by Wurtz-Fittig reaction involving warming of an ethereal solution of alkyl and aryl halide with metallic sodium.

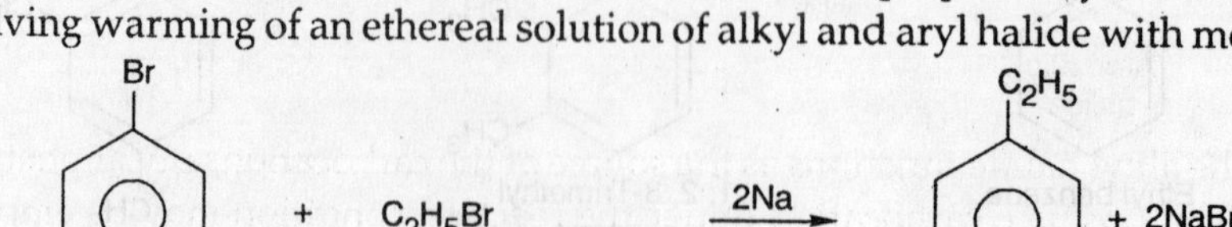

Bromo benzene + Ethyl bromide → Ethyl benzene

4. *Friedel-Crafts Reaction*: Friedel-Crafts reaction is an important method for the preparation of alkyl derivatives of benzene discovered by Friedel and his associate Crafts. They observed that when an alkyl halide is allowed to react with benzene in presence of anhydrous $AlCl_3$, a hydrogen atom of benzene ring is eliminated and an alkyl derivative of benzene is obtained.

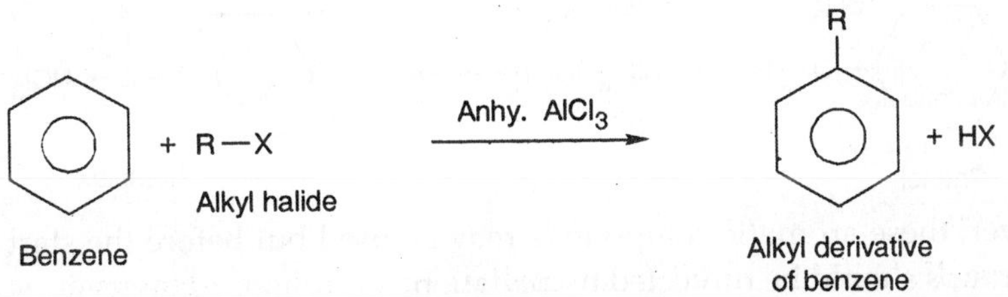

As there is formation of alkyl derivative of benzene, this reaction is also known as alkylation of aromatic hydrocarbon. Mechanistically, it is an electrophilic substitution reaction where alkyl halide acts as the source of electrophile (carbocation) and aromatic hydrocarbon is the substrate as shown below.

Step 1: $R—X + AlCl_3 \longrightarrow \overset{\delta+}{R}\cdots\cdots X \cdots\cdots \overset{\delta-}{AlCl_3} \longrightarrow \overset{+}{R} + \overset{-}{AlCl_3X}$

Step 2:

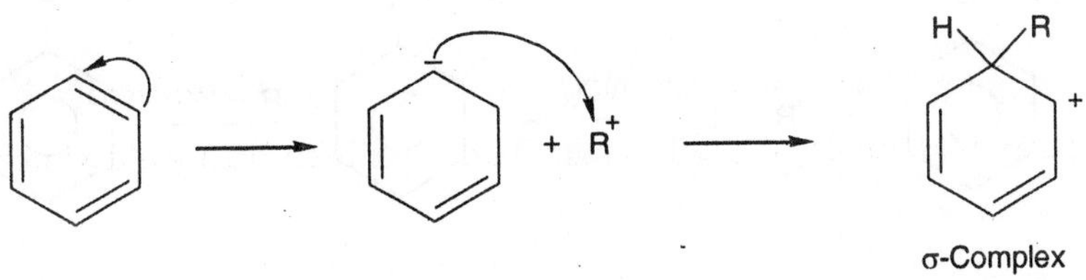

Step 3:

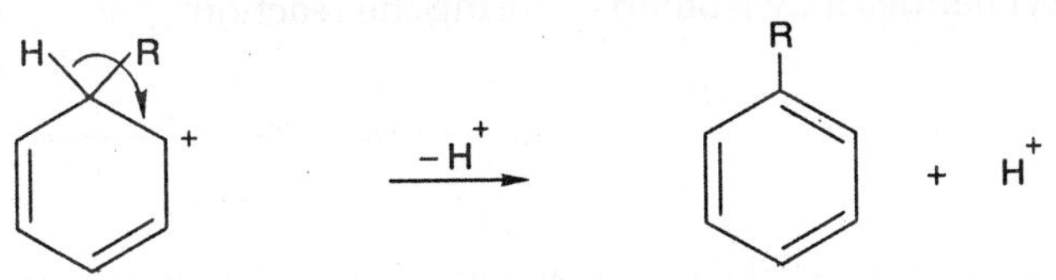

Step 4: $\overset{-}{AlCl_3X} + \overset{+}{H} \longrightarrow HX + AlCl_3$

- *Comments:*

i. It may be remembered that the reaction cannot take place between alkane and aromatic halide, i.e.,

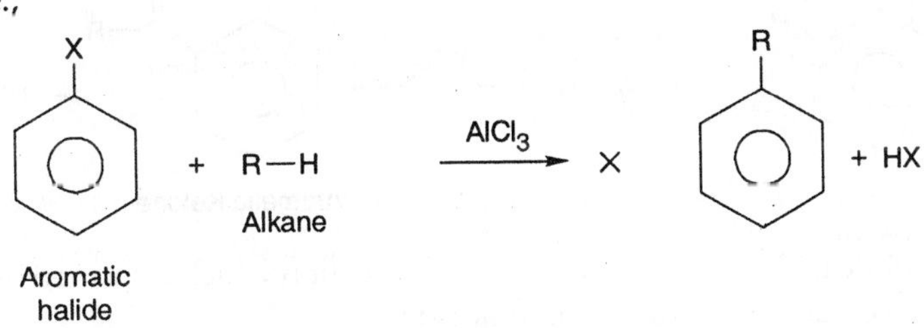

Since the alkyl halide functions as the source of the carbocation, any aliphatic compound which can produce carbocation under the reaction condition may be employed in this reaction. Thus, alkenes, alcohols, acid-chlorides, acid anhydrides in addition to alkyl halides have been employed in this reaction to obtain variety of substituted aromatic compounds other than alkylated compound.

ii. Any aromatic compound may be used as the substrate in this reaction. But those containing hydroxyl and amino groups may complicate the reaction. This is because the lone pair of electrons in these compounds may form inorganic complex with $AlCl_3$ which make them insoluble in common organic solvents.

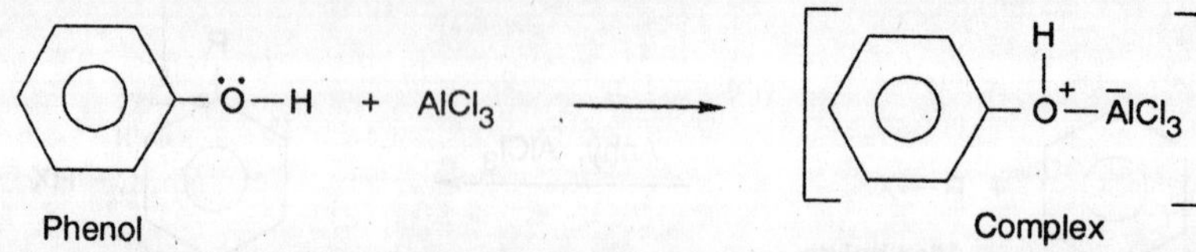

However, these aromatic compounds may be used but before the start of the reaction such groups should be protected by acylation.

iii. Different Lewis acidic catalysts such as $AlCl_3$, $ZnCl_2$, $FeCl_3$, $TiCl_4$, BF_3, concentrated H_2SO_4, $SnCl_4$ may be used for the reaction but most commonly used catalyst is anhydrous $AlCl_3$.

iv. Friedel-Crafts reaction has some drawbacks, viz,

(a) It cannot be stopped at desired stage, i.e.,

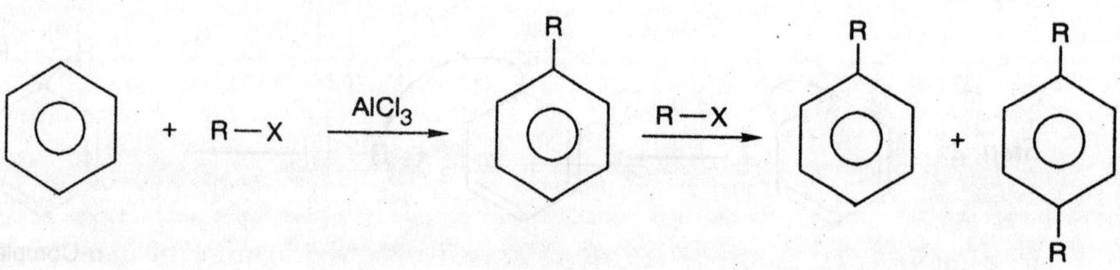

(b) Certain alkyl halides may isomerise during the reaction:

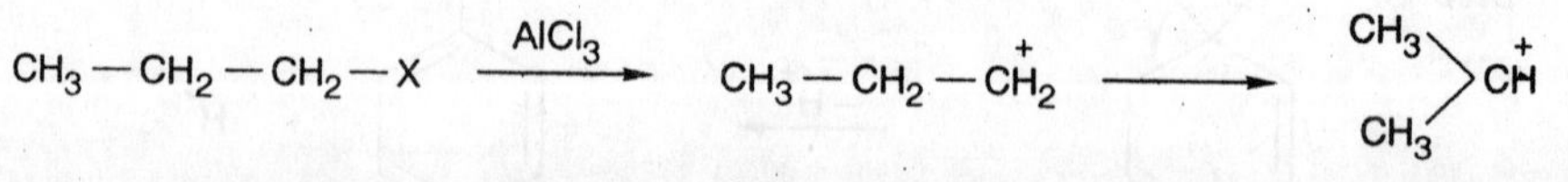

v. An important aspect of Friedel-Crafts reaction is the acylation of arenes. Sometimes this is referred to as Frieded-Craft acylation reaction. In this reaction primarily acyl halide is used as the source of carbocation. The reaction proceeds as under:

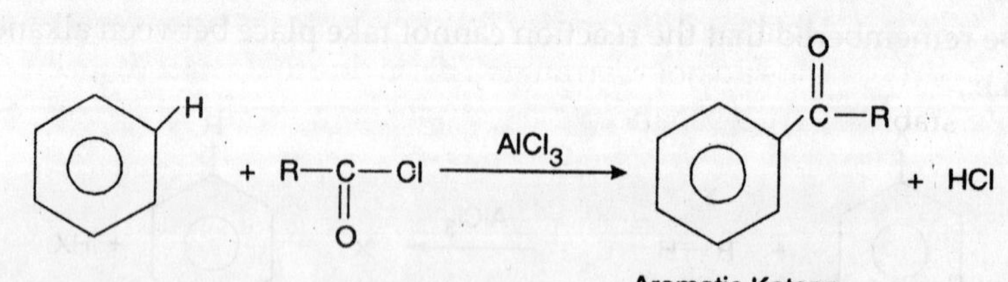

The electrophile in this reaction is the acyl carbocation which is formed by the coordination of an acyl chloride with aluminium chloride.

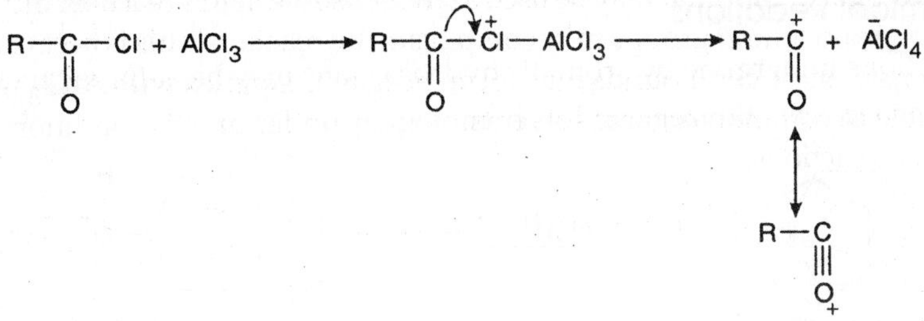

(A)

The acyl carbocation (A) in the next step reacts with arene as shown below:

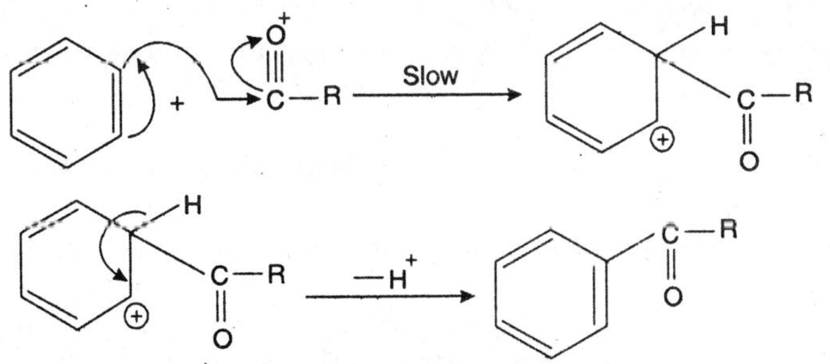

$$\overset{+}{H} + \overset{-}{Al}Cl_4 \longrightarrow AlCl_3 + HCl$$

In place of acylchloride carboxylic acid anhydride may be used to generate acyl carbocation. Thus,

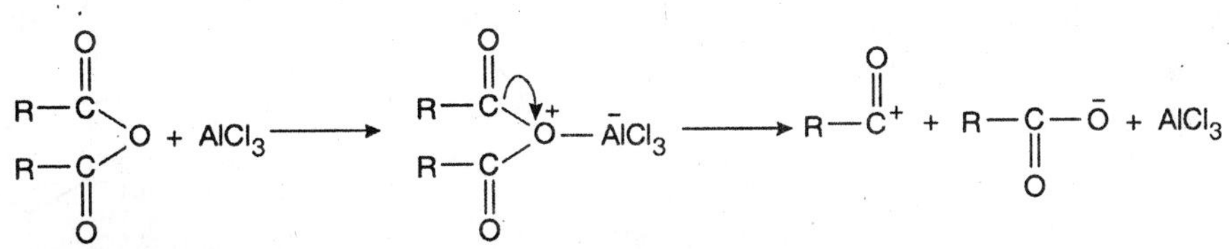

Acidanhy dride

It may be mentioned that the difference of Friedel-Crafts acylation reaction from alkylation is that acyl carbocations do not rearrange. This is due to the fact that acyl carbocation(A) is strongly stabilised by resonance.

15.3 Properties of Aromatic Hydrocarbons (Arenes)

15.3.1 Physical Properties

Lower members of aromatic hydrocarbons are liquid but higher members are crystalline solids. They burn with sooty flame due to the high content of carbon. They are insoluble in water but soluble in organic solvents. Some of the aromatic hydrocarbons have fragrant odour. The boiling point increases with the increase in the carbon content. They are used as solvents for fats, resins and for the preparation of insecticides and expolsives.

15.3.2 Chemical Reactions

Chemical reactions undergone by aromatic hydrocarbons may be of three types.

1. *Addition reaction:* Benzene and its homologues under drastic condition undergo certain addition reactions.

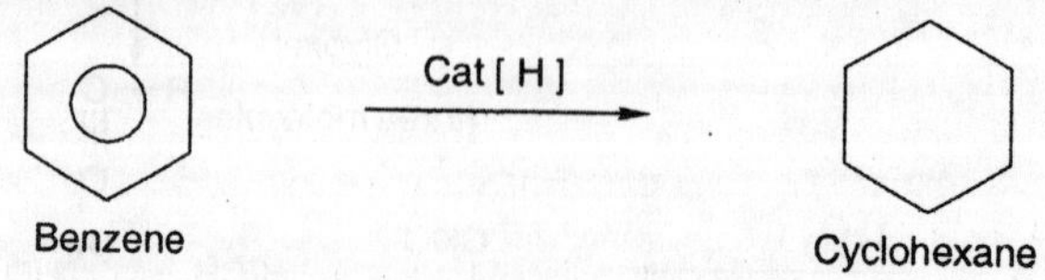

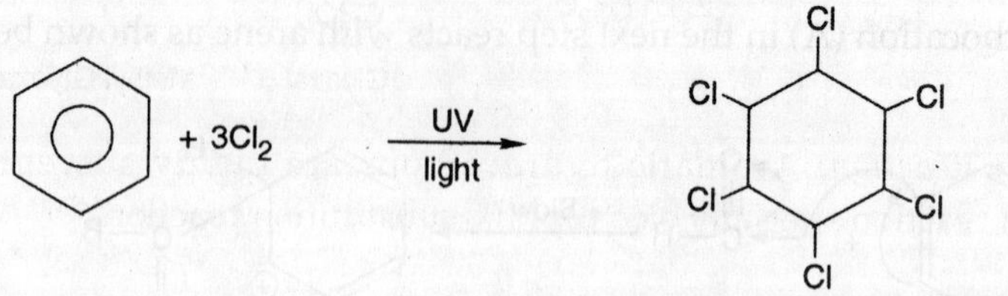

Benzene hexachloride is a powerful insecticide. The addition takes place through radical path, i.e.,

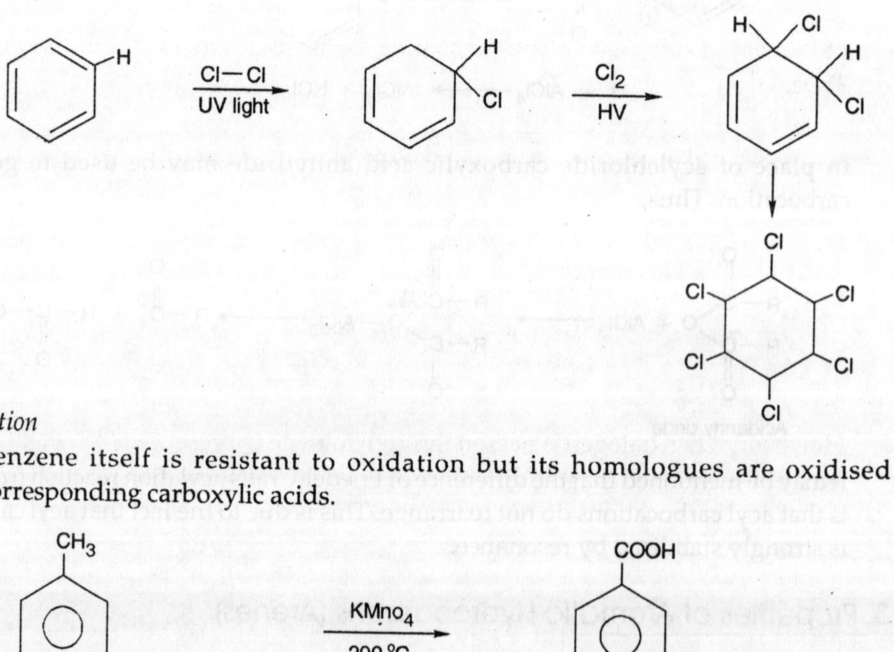

2. *Oxidation*
   i. Benzene itself is resistant to oxidation but its homologues are oxidised to corresponding carboxylic acids.

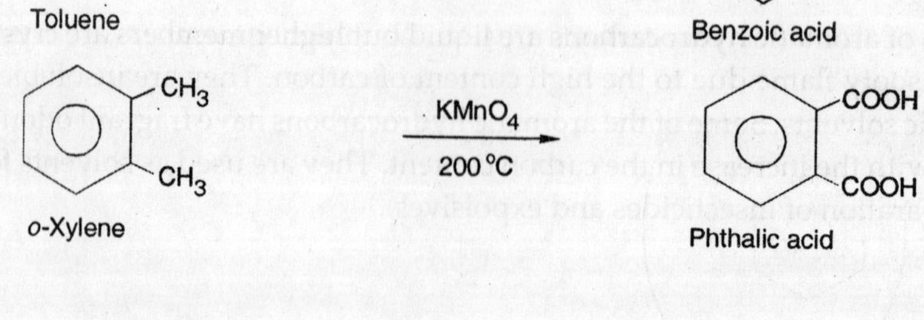

ii. Aromatic hydrocarbons undergo ozonolysis reaction. Thus,

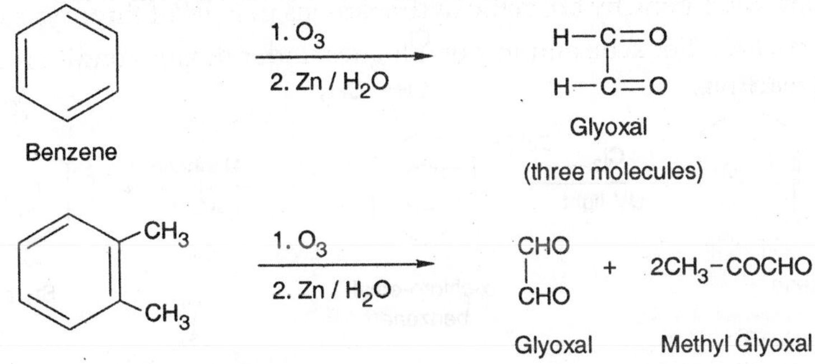

3. *Substitution Reaction:* Aromatic hydrocarbons are highly susceptible to undergo substitution reaction specially electrophilic substitution reaction.

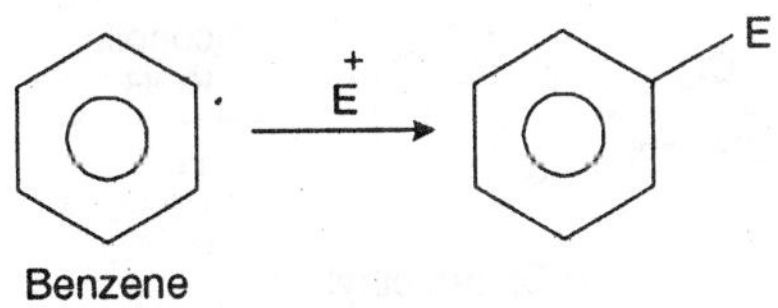

In the case of side chain arenes, incoming electrophile enters at ortho and para position. Thus,

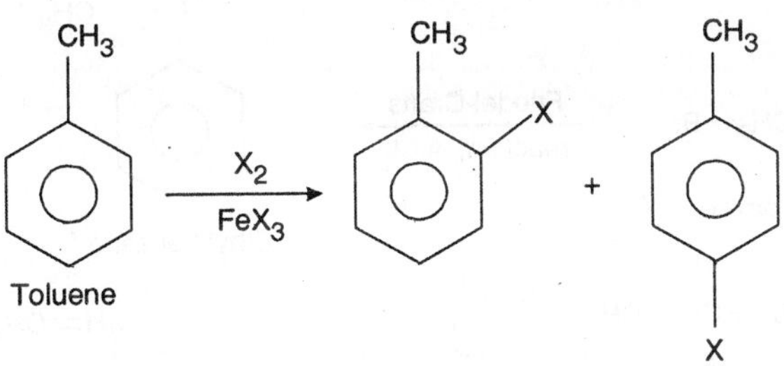

However, when halogen is passed through toluene in presence of UV-light halogenation occurs at side chain.

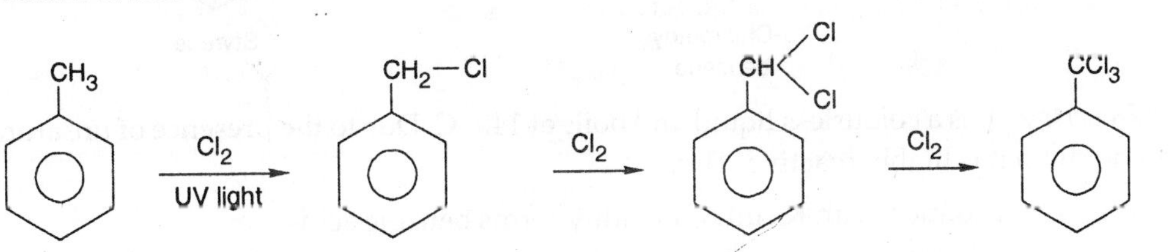

Benzyl chloride Benzal chloride Benzo trichloride

15.4 Styrene

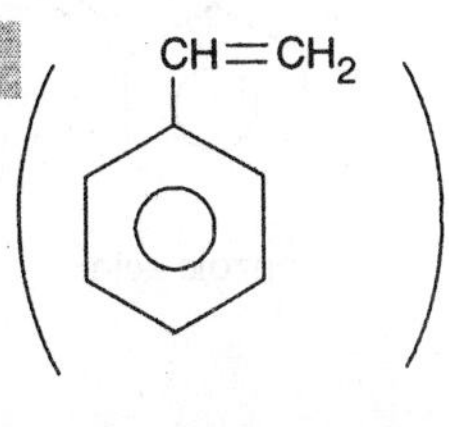

Styrene is industrially very important chemical compound and is extensively used in the synthesis of polystyrene polymer. It is commonly prepared by the following methods:

i.

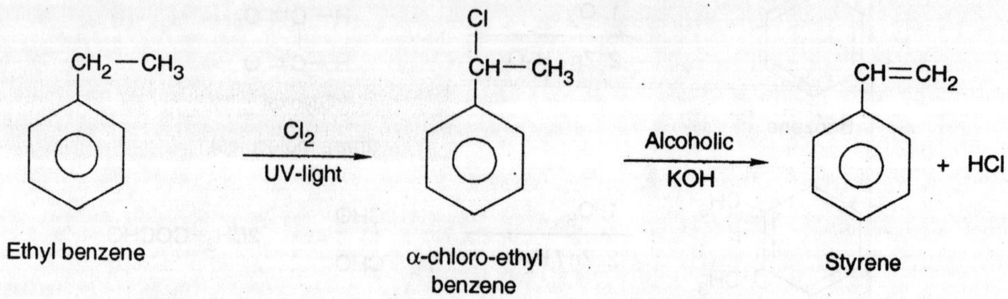

ii.

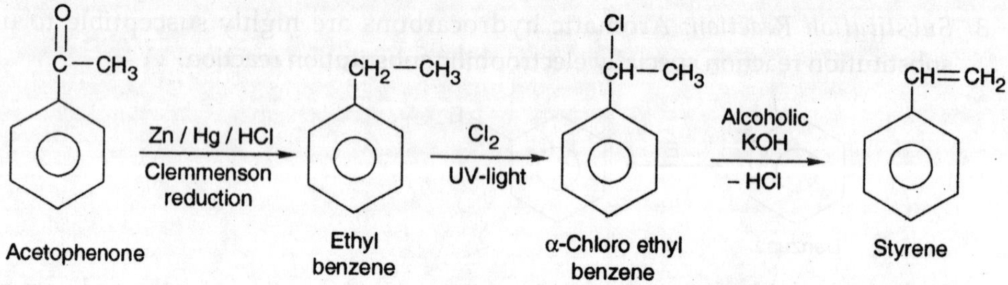

iii. It can also be prepared from benzene adopting the following sequence of reactions:

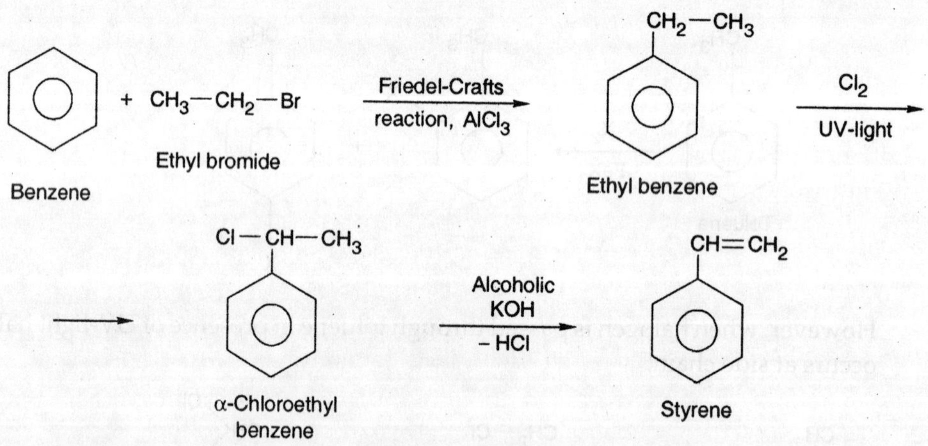

Properties: It is a colourless liquid and boils at 140 °C. Due to the presence of unsaturation in the side chain it is highly reactive. Thus,

i. On oxidation with $KMnO_4$ it readily forms benzoic acid.

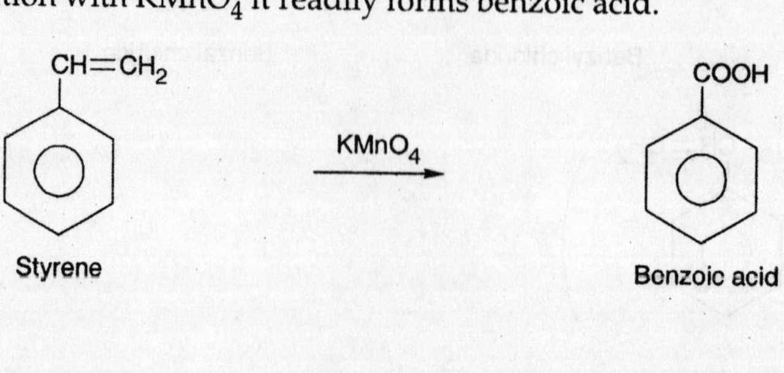

ii. Halogen acids in presence of H_2O_2 affords β-phenyl ethyl halide.

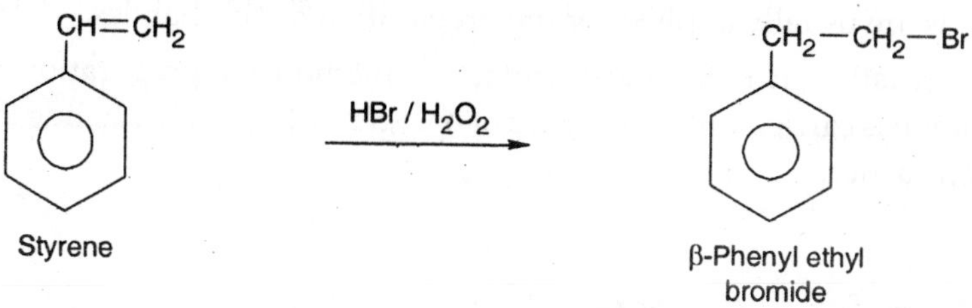

iii. When treated with halogen in carbon tetrachloride, dihalo compound is formed.

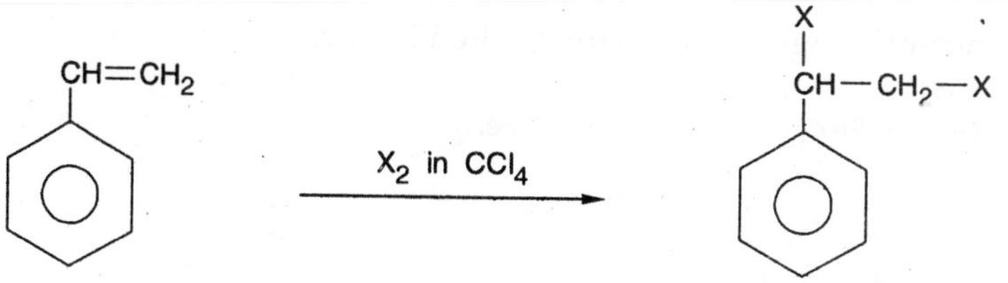

iv. The most important reaction of styrene is its polymerisation reaction. It readily polymerises in presence of peroxide.

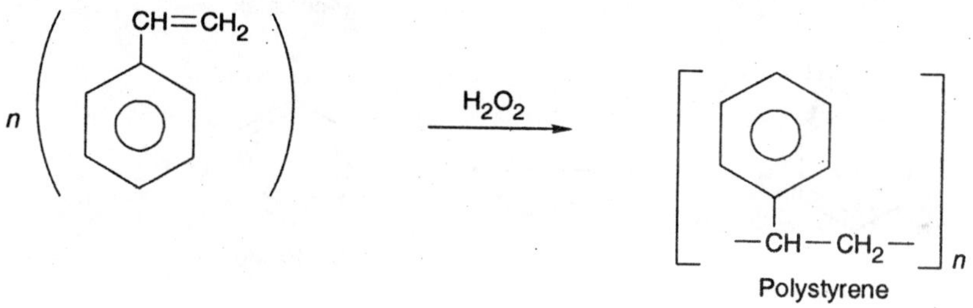

15.5 Uses of Arenes

Benzene and toluene are used as solvents for fats and resins. They are also used as starting materials for a variety of commercial products like trinitro benene (T.N.B.) and trinitro toluence (T.N.T.) which are important explosives. Toluene is used for the preparation of saccharin (an artificial sugar) and some drugs like tolbutamide (a hypoglycemic drug). Xylenes are used as solvents in lacquer industry while styrene is an important raw material in synthetic plastic and rubbcr industries.

15.6 Halo Derivatives (Aryl Halides)

15.6.1 Aryl Halides

Aryl halides are those in which halogens are present in the aromatic ring.

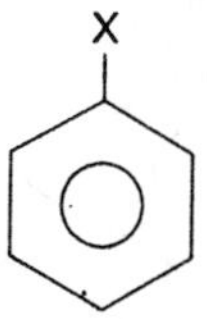

Aryl halide

15.6.1.1 Preparation of Aryl Halides

Following methods are usually applied for the preparation of aryl halides.

1. *Direct halogenation:* It is the most important method for preparation of aryl halides. Halogenation is carried out in presence of halogen carrier. Ferric halide is generally used as halogen carrier.

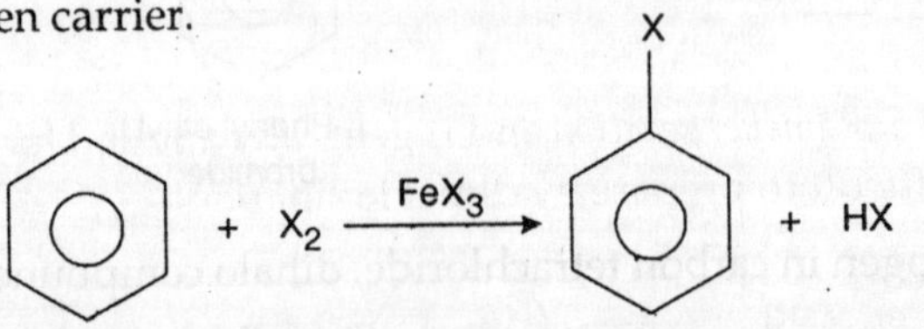

Mechanistically halogenation occurs as cited below:

Step 1: $X{-}X + FeX_3 \rightleftharpoons \overset{+}{X} + \overset{-}{Fe}X_4$

Step 2:

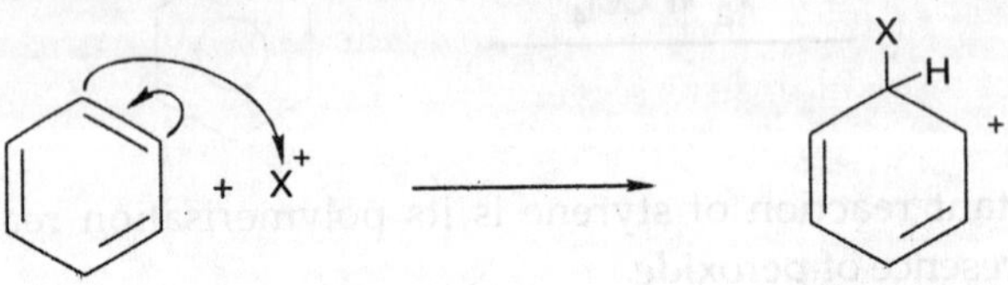

σ-complex

Step 3:

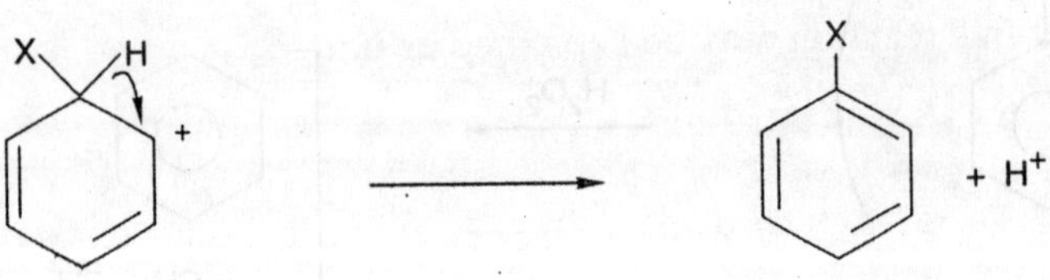

Aryl halide

Step 4: $\overset{-}{Fe}X_4 + \overset{+}{H} \rightleftharpoons HX + FeX_3$

In this method chloro and bromo compounds can be smoothly prepared. But iodo compound cannot be prepared. This is because of the reversibility of iodination reaction. However, in presence of HNO_3 or peracid iodo compound may be prepared. The function of such oxidising agent is to remove HI as soon as it is formed. Thus,

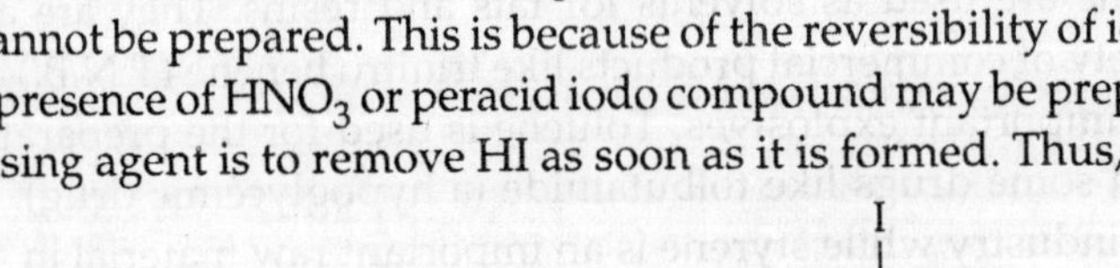

$$2HI + HNO_3 \rightleftharpoons H_2O + I_2 + HNO_2$$

2. *From Diazonium compound*: Aromatic diazonium salts on decomposition in presence of metal halides afford aryl halides.

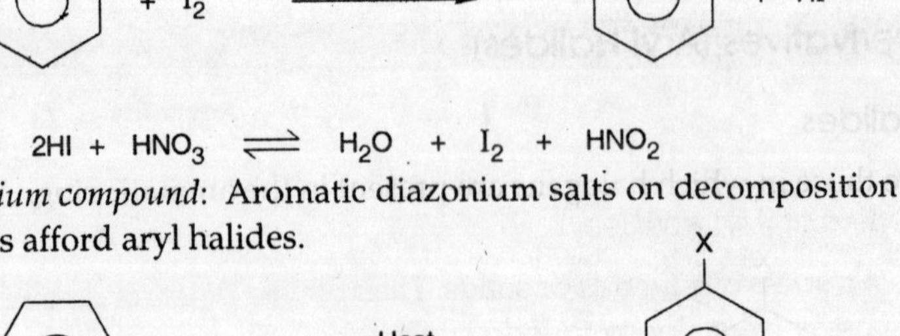

Aromatic diazonium salt

Aryl halide

Mechanism of the reaction may be depicted as below:

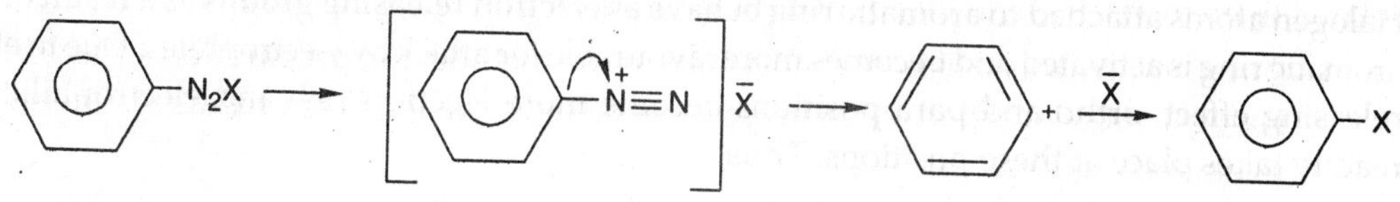

This reaction is known as *Sandmeyer reaction* and is generally applied for the preparation of aryl iodide which is difficult to prepare by direct iodination.

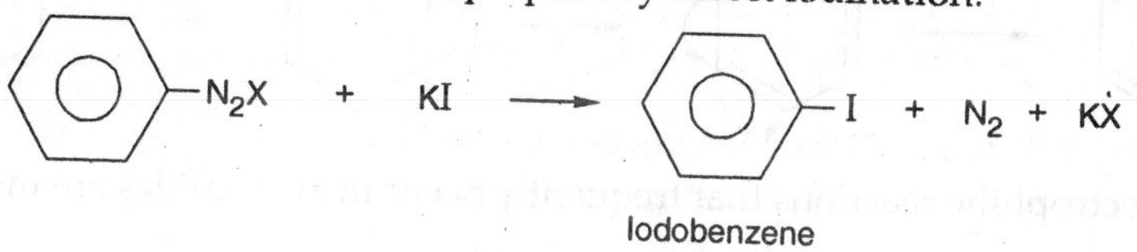

3. *Hunsdicker Method*: By heating silver salt of aromatic carboxylic acid with bromine in presence of carbon of tetrachloride as solvent.

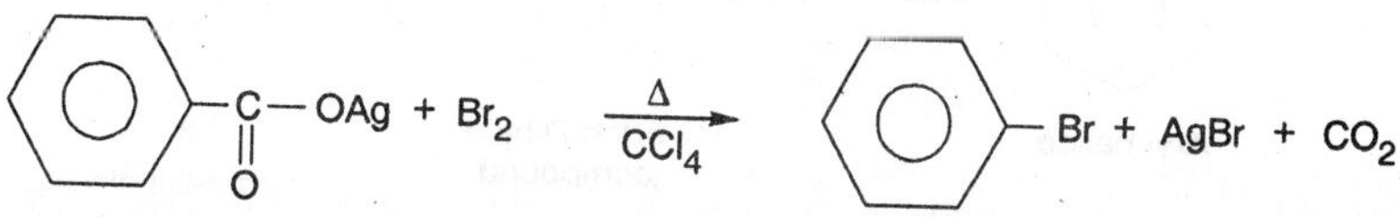

Mechanistically this reaction may be explained as under:

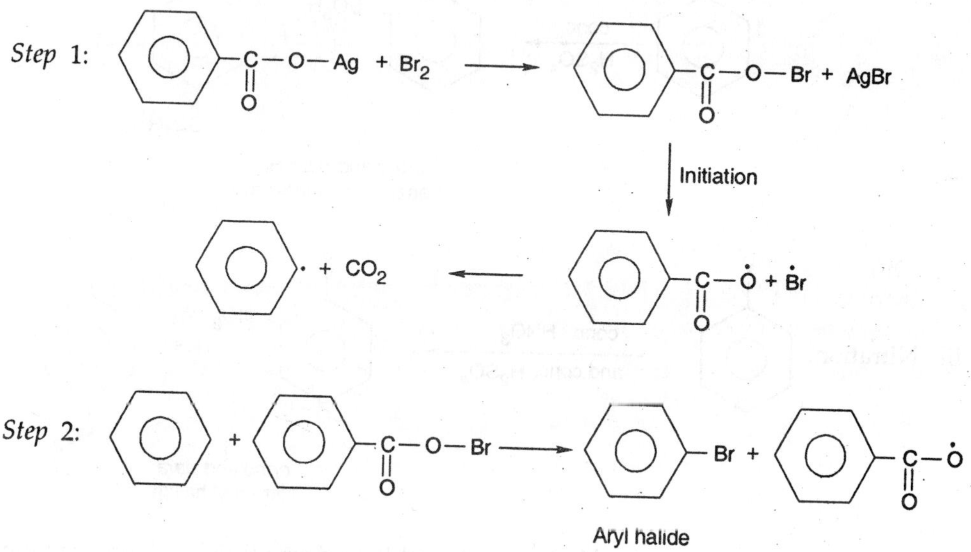

15.6.1.2 Properties of Aryl Halides

Aryl halides are colourless oily liquids or solids. Their boiling points and melting points gradually increase as one passes from fluoro to iodo compounds. They are soluble in common organic solvents but isoluble in water.

Chemical Properties: Chemical properties of aryl halides may be of two types—involving (i) aromatic ring and (ii) halogens.

15.6.1.2.1 Reactions Involving Aromatic Ring

Halogen atoms attached to aromatic ring behave as electron releasing groups as a result of which aromatic ring is activated and becomes more favourable for attack by electrophiles. Due to electron releasing effect, ortho and para positions become more electron rich and electrophilic attack readily takes place at these positions. Thus,

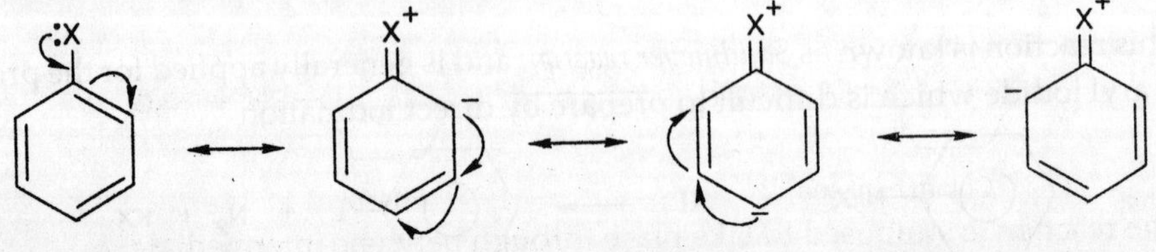

Common electrophilic reactions that frequently occur in aryl halides are mentioned below:

i. Halogenation:

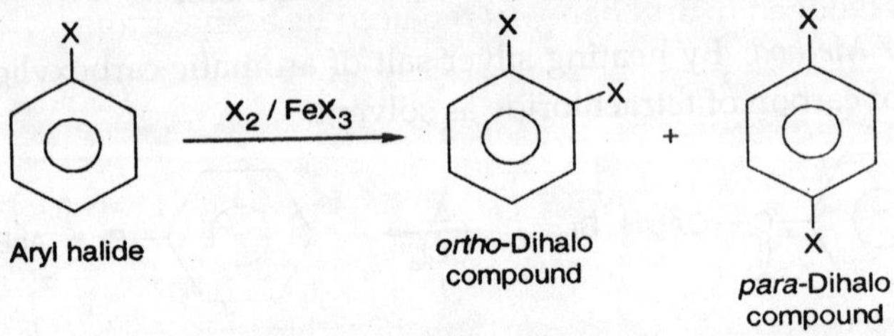

ii. Sulphonation:

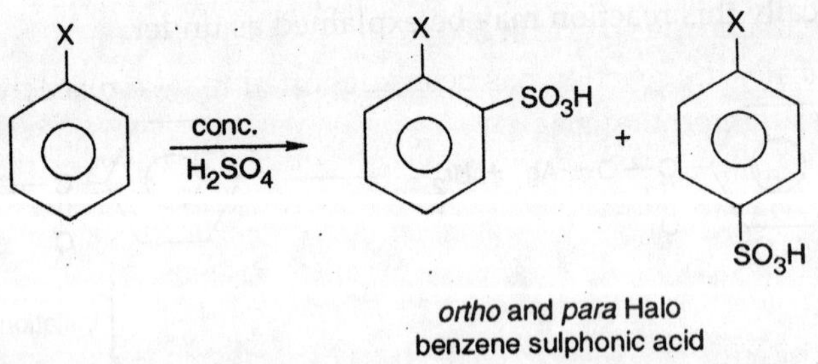

iii. Nitration:

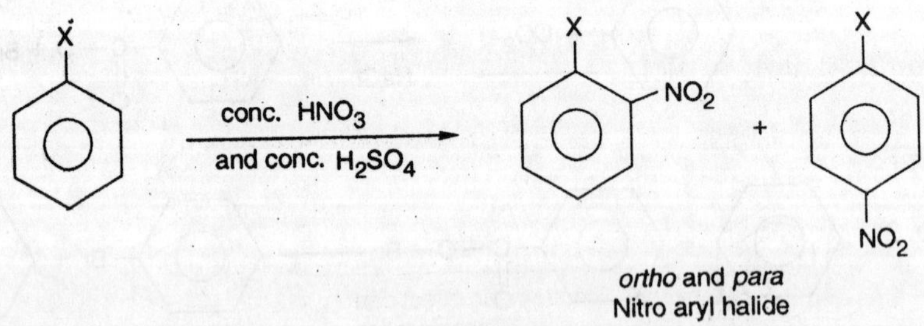

iv. Friedel-Crafts reaction: Aryl halides can readily undergo Friedel-Crafts reaction, i.e.,

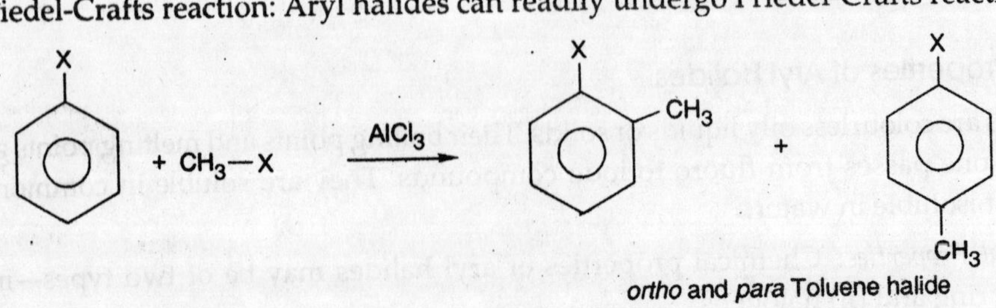

15.6.1.2.2 Reactions Involving Halogens

Halogen atoms in aromatic ring are tightly bound to aromatic ring because of the resonance as shown above. So they cannot be readily replaced. However, under certain conditions halogens may be replaced as described below:

i. *Drastic condition*: When heated with alkali at a high temperature, halogen may be replaced yielding phenol.

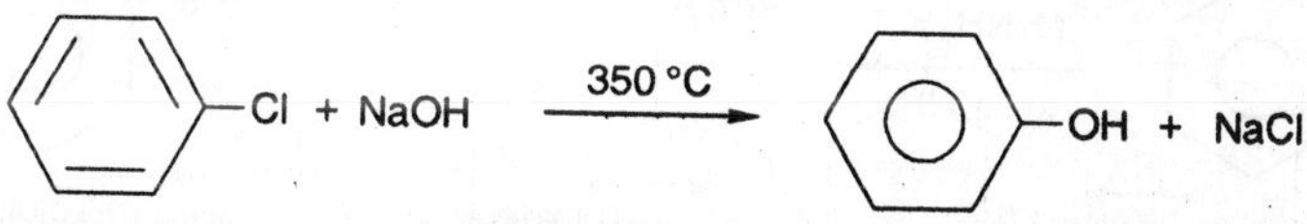

Chloro benzene Phenol

The reaction is supposed to take place through benzyne intermediate.

ii. *By the use of certain reagent*: When warmed with sodium or potassium amide in liquid ammonia halogen in aryl halide is replaced by amino group.

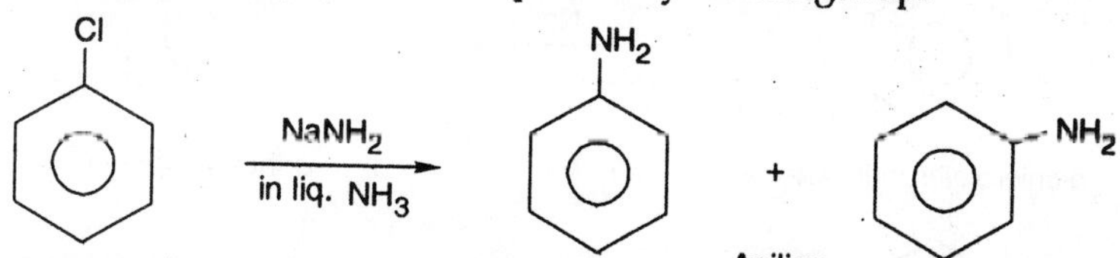

Aniline

The same reaction may also be carried out by heating aryl halide with aqueous ammonia in presence of cuprous oxide at 200 °C.

Mechanistically the reaction has been suggested to take place through the formation of benzyne as an intermediate.

Step 1:

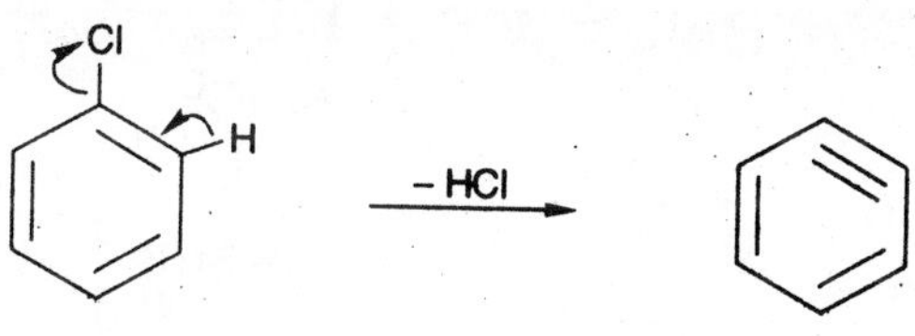

Aryl halide Benzyne

Step 2: $NaNH_2 + HCl \longrightarrow NaCl + NH_3$

Step 3:

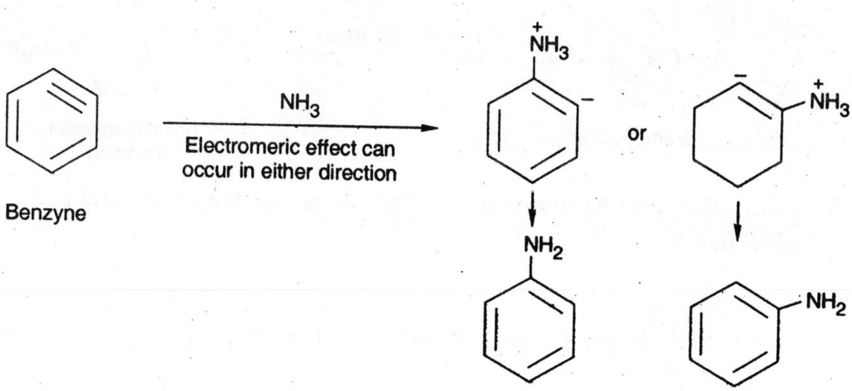

(A) Aniline (B)

Amino group may be at the position where halogen was connected (A) or it may be attached to the adjacent position forming (B). Formation of the product (B) during this substitution reaction is known as *Cine-substitution*. When a substituent is present in aryl halide, the products (A) and (B) become different.

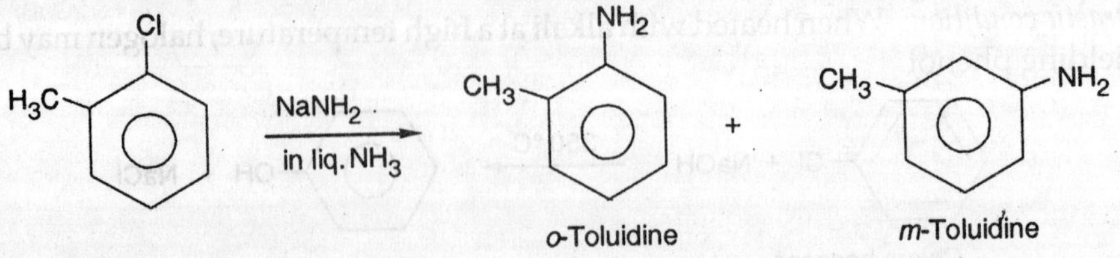

iii. *In the presence of strong electron-withdrawing group*: When strong electron withdrawing group is present at *ortho* and *para* positions, halogen may be replaced. i.e.,

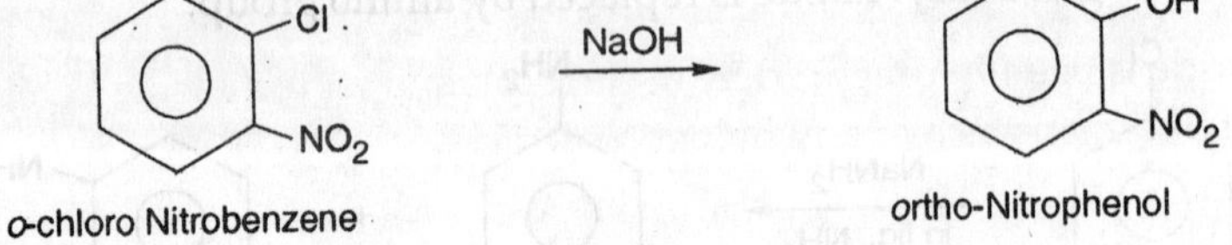

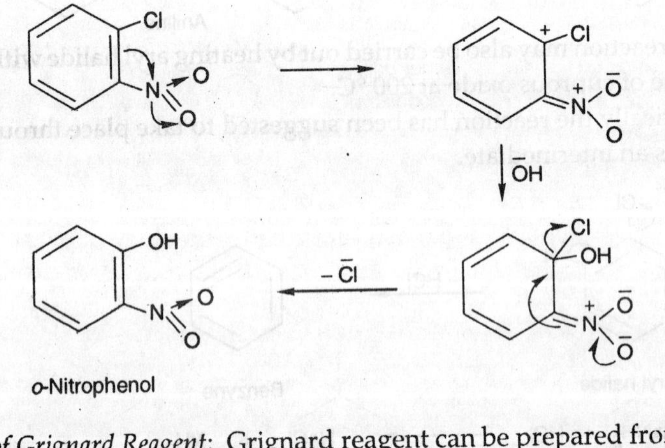

iv. *Formation of Grignard Reagent*: Grignard reagent can be prepared from aryl halide.

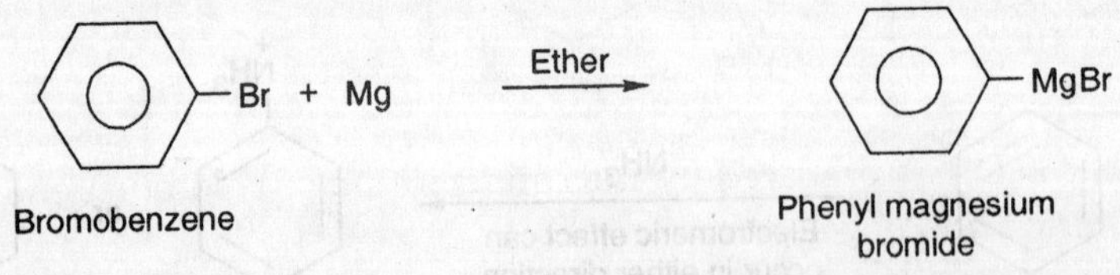

v. *Wurtz-Reaction*: Aromatic nuclear halide is capable of undergoing *Wurtz reaction* with alkyl halide.

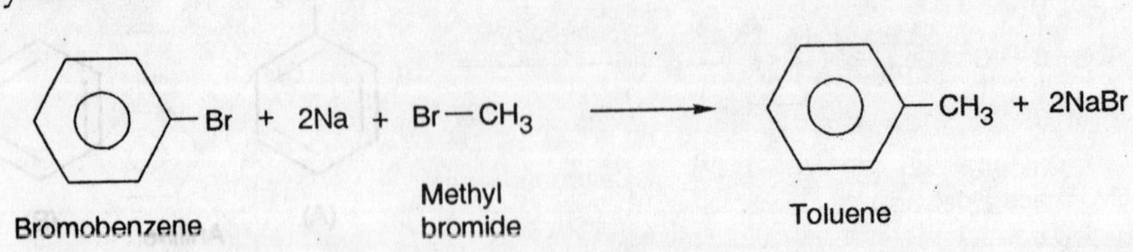

vi. *Ullmann Reaction*: Aryl halide when heated with metallic copper, biphenyl is formed. This reaction is known as *Ullmann reaction.*

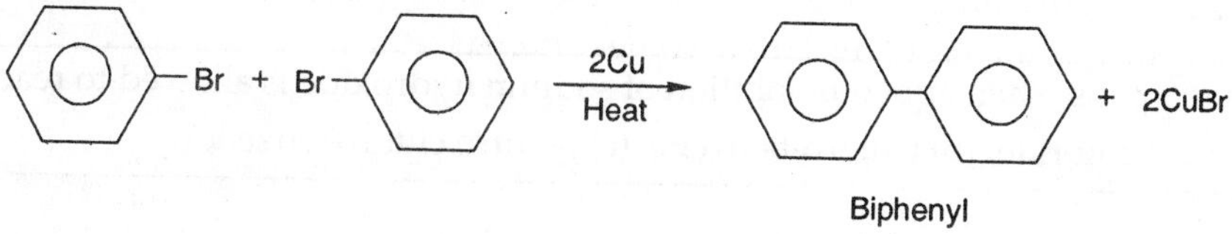

15.7 Side-Chain Aromatic Halide

There are some aromatic halides in which halogens are not attached to the phenyl ring but are connected to the side chain. These are known as side chain aromatic halides. Two most important members of this type of halides are benzyl chloride and 2, 2-di (*p*-chloro-phenyl)-1, 1, 1-trichloro ethane (D. D. T).

Benzyl chloride is usually prepared by boiling toluene with chlorine at high temperature in presence of light but in absence of any halogen carrier.

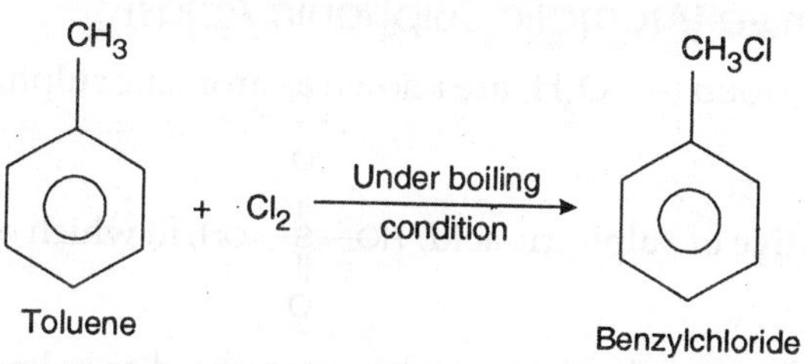

If excess of chlorine be present reaction proceeds further.

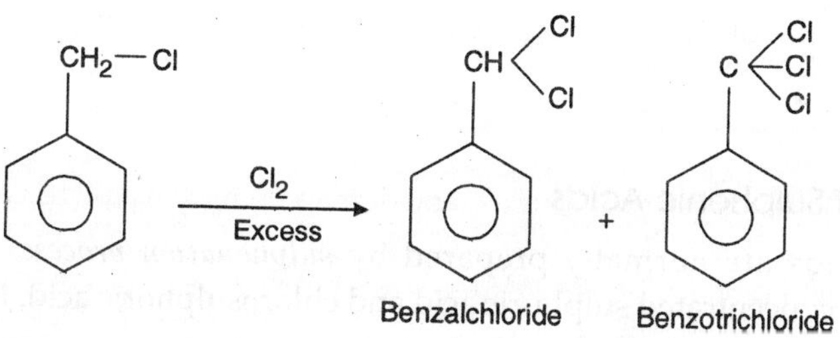

Other member D.D.T is prepared by the condensation of chlorobenrene with choloral in presence of sulphuric acid.

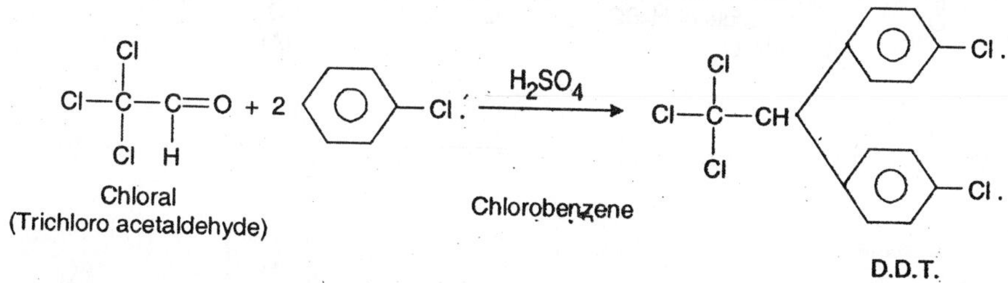

D.D.T. is an effective insecticide.

Side-chain aromatic halides are closely similar to alkyl halide and can be readily substituted by variety of groups resulting in the formation of different compounds as shown below:

PROBLEM: 15.1

> What happens when aqueous solution of sodium hydroxide is allowed to react with (a) Benzyl chloride, (b) Chloro-benzene, (c) *p*-Nitro chlorobenzene?

15.8 Uses of Aromatic Halides

Aryl-halides are used as starting materials for the synthesis of many organic compounds. Chlorobenzene is an important intermediate for the manufacture of D.D.T., D.D.D. [(1, 1-dichloro-2, 2-bis (*p*-chloro phenyl) ethane] which are used as insecticide. Besides, methoxy chlor [1, 1, 1-trichloro-2, 2-bis (*p*-methoxy phenyl)] ethane, perethane [1, 1-dichloro-2, 2-bis (*p*-ethyl phenyl) ethane and D.F.D.T (1, 1, 1-trichloro-2, 2-bis (*p*-fluoro phenyl)] ethane are also used as insectides. Benzene hexachloride (B.H.C.) is a strong insecticide.

15.9 Sulphonic Acid Derivative (Aromatic Sulphonic Acids)

Arenes containing sulphonic acid group (—SO_3H) are known as aromatic sulphonic acids. They may be looked upon as the derivative of sulphuric acid, 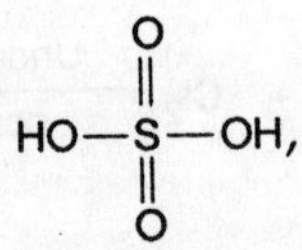 in which one —OH group has been replaced by aryl group. Structurally they may be represented as below:

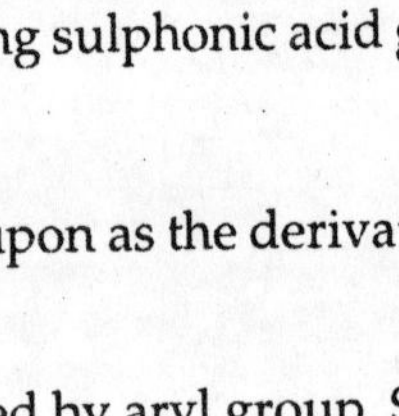

15.9.1 Preparation of Sulphonic Acids

Aromatic sulphonic acids are normally prepared by *sulphonation process*. Most common sulphonating agents are concentrated sulphuric acid and chlorosulphoric acid. Mechanistically, sulphonation proceeds as under:

Step I:

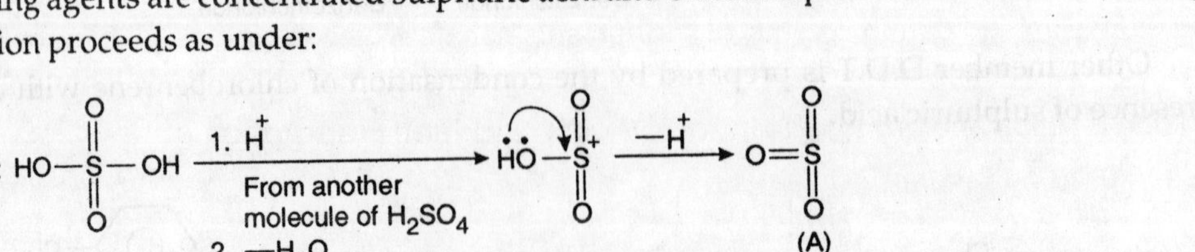

Step 2:

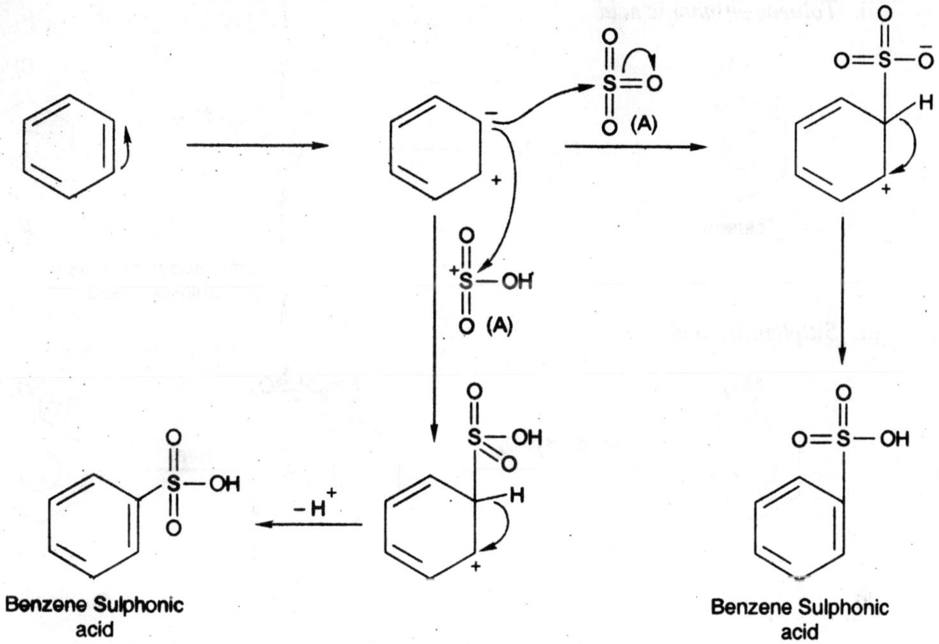

When chlorosulphonic acid is used, path becomes as shown below:

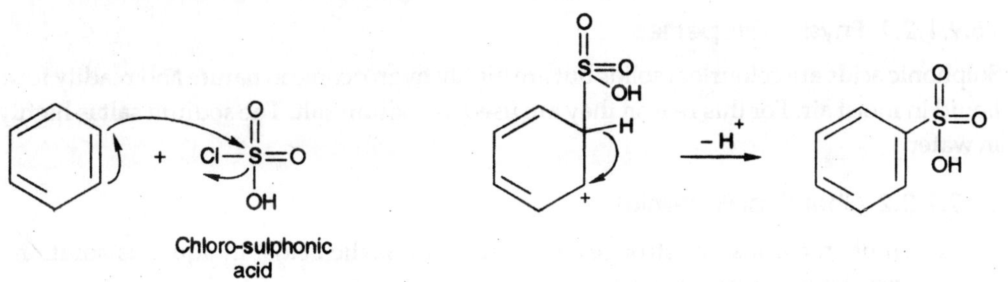

Sometimes fuming sulphuric acid (oleium) is used for sulphonation.

Sulphonic acid is usually isolated after the sulphonation reaction. The reaction product is diluted with cold water and is treated with calcium hydroxide when unused sulphuric acid is removed as calcium sulphate which is precipitated and filtered. The filtrate is then treated with sodium carbonate when excess of calcium hydroxide is precipitated out and filtered. The filtrate is evaporated to obtain crystals of sodium sulphonate which is used as such in the reaction.

15.9.1.1 Some Common Sulphonic Acids and Their Preparation

i. *Benzene Sulphonic acid*

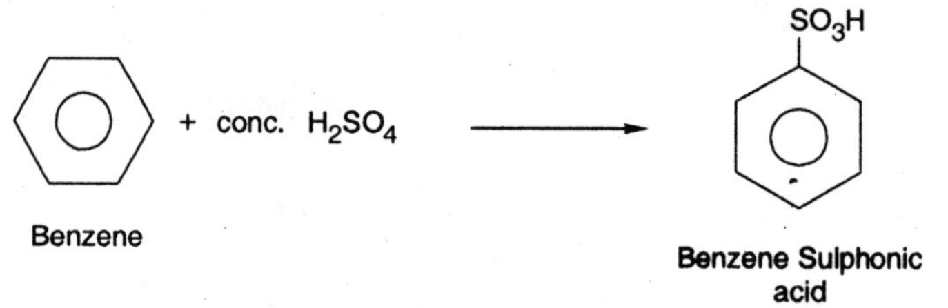

ii. *Toluene sulphonic acid*

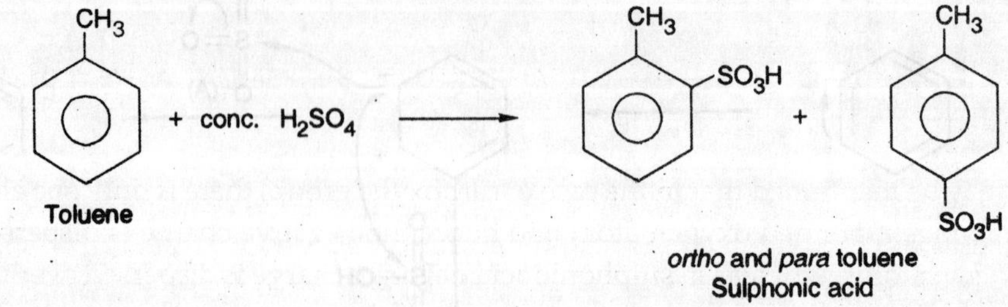

iii. *Sulphanilic acid*

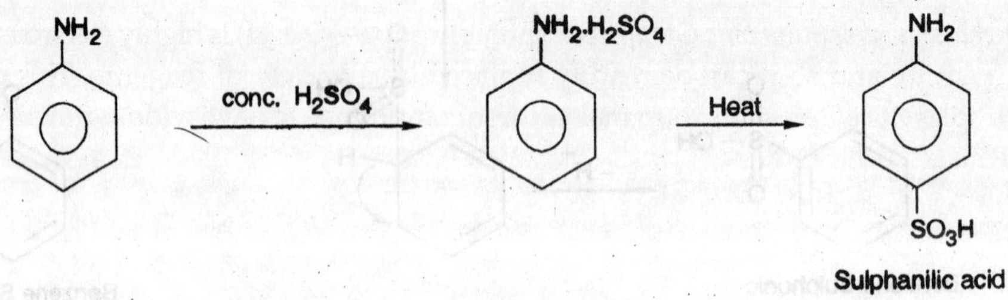

15.9.1.2 Properties of Aromatic Sulphonic Acids

15.9.1.2.1 Physical Properties

Sulphonic acids are colourless solids but are highly hygroscopic in nature and readily form syrupy liquid in moist air. For this reason they are used as sodium salt. The sodium salt is highly soluble in water.

15.9.1.2.2 Chemical Properties

1. Sulphonic acids are stronger acid than carboxylic acids. In aqueous solution they are completely ionised as under:

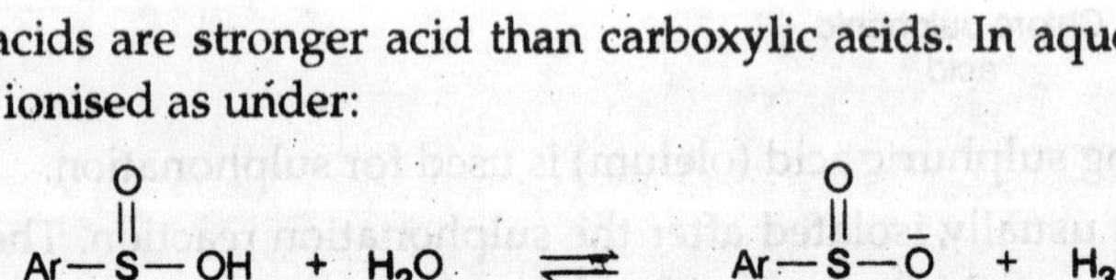

The acidity of sulphonic acid originates from the release of protons and due to the presence of two electron withdrawing π-bonded oxygen atoms at the same sulphur atom elimination of proton becomes very rapid.

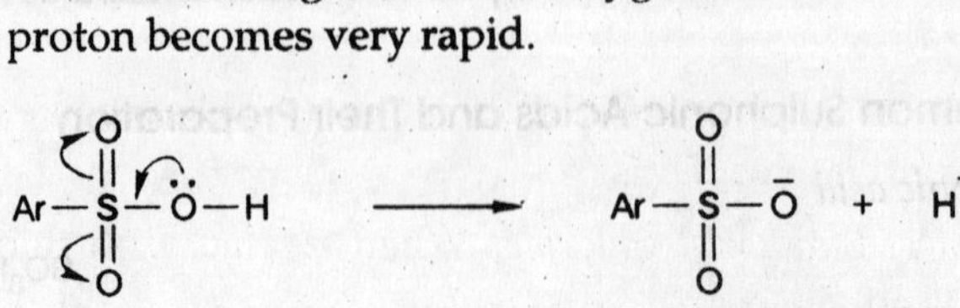

Conjugate base

Further, the conjugate base is stabilised by resonance.

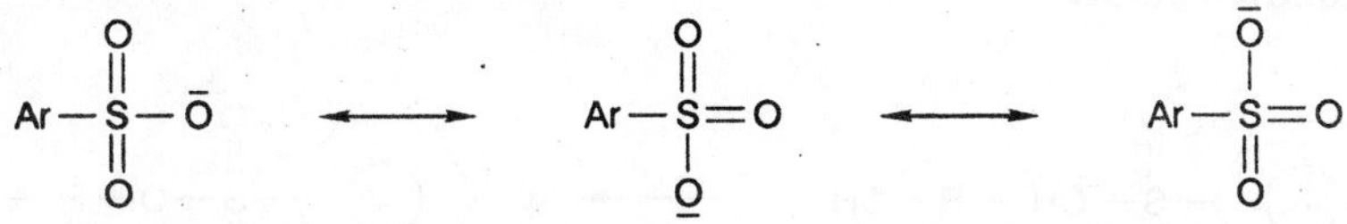

It may be mentioned that in the case of carboxylic group, there is only one electron withdrawings π-bonded oxygen atom and hence the negative charge is dispersed over two oxygen atoms, whereas in sulphonic acid negative charge is dispersed over three oxygen atoms. So the conjugate base of sulphonic acid is more stable than carboxylate ion. For this reason sulphonic acids are stronger acids than carboxylic acids.

2. *Replacement of Sulphonic Group*: Sulphonic group (—SO_3H) is highly electron withdrawing in nature and so it can be readily replaced by a variety of reagents. This characteristic property of sulphonic group makes these compounds to have wide synthetic applications. Thus,

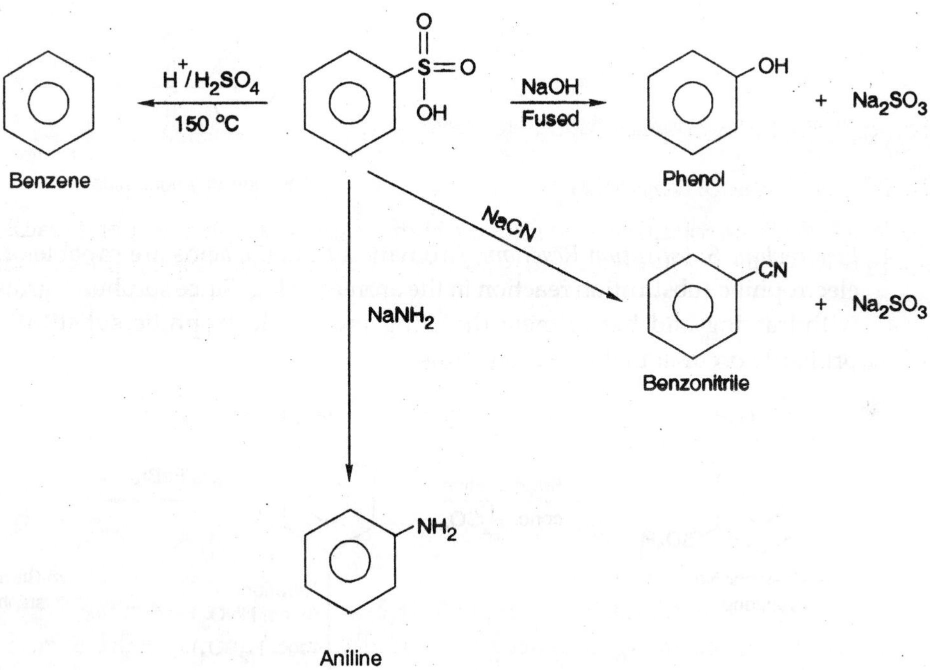

3. *Reaction due to Sulphonic group*: Sulphonic group behaves like carboxylic group and can form similar derivatives. Thus,

   (a) *Formation of Sulphonyl Chloride*: When treated with thionyl chloride, sulphonyl chloride is obtained.

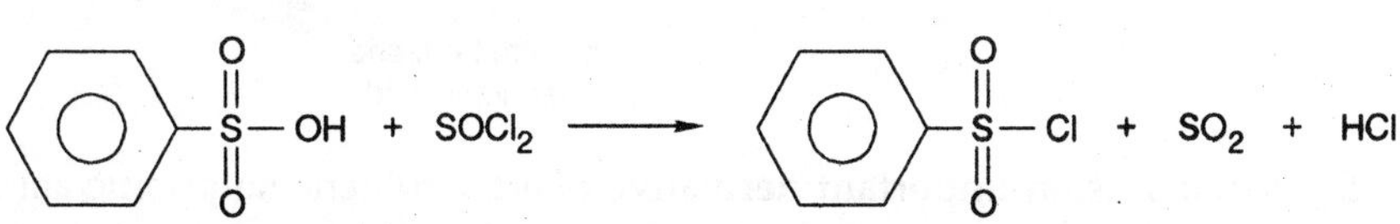

Phosphorous pentachloride can also be used in place of thionyl chloride.

(b) *Formation of Ester and Amide*: Like carboxylic group, they can form esters and amides as shown below:

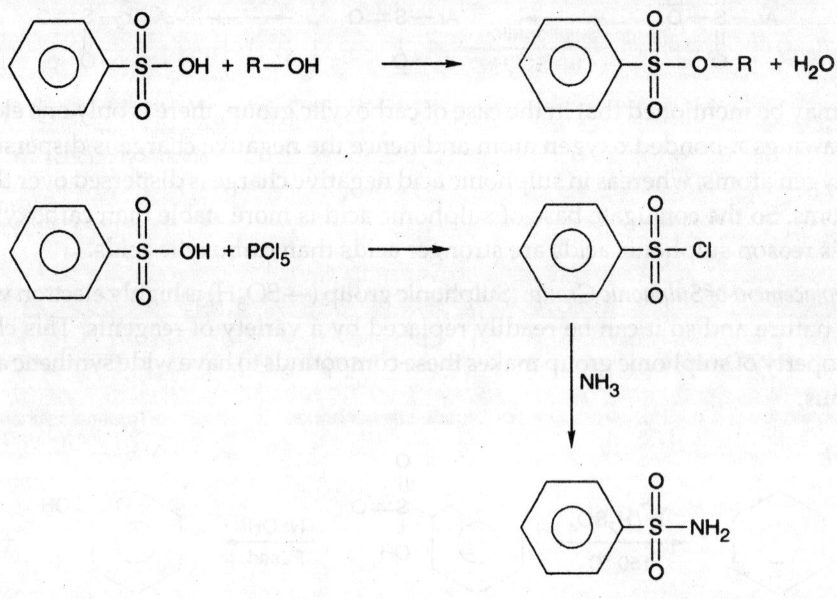

Benzene Sulphonamide

4. *Electrophilic Substitution Reaction*: Aromatic sulphonic acids are capable of undergoing electrophilic substitution reaction in the aromatic ring. Since sulphonic group is electron withdrawing and hence meta directing group, electrophilic substitution reactions primarily occur at meta position. Thus,

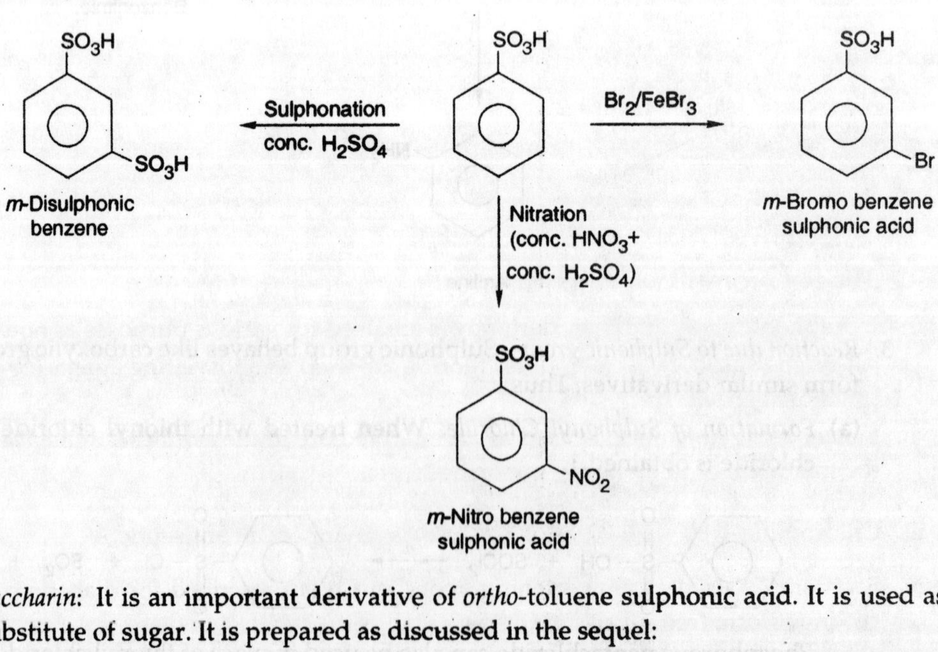

Saccharin: It is an important derivative of *ortho*-toluene sulphonic acid. It is used as a substitute of sugar. It is prepared as discussed in the sequel:

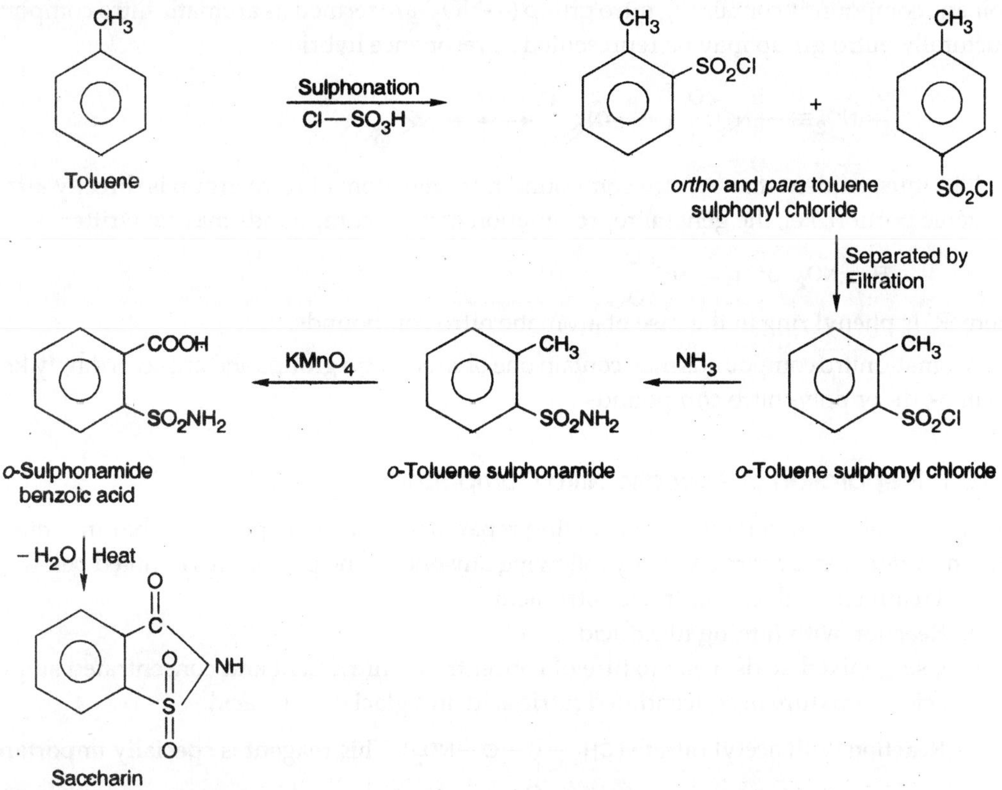

Saccharin reacts with NaOH to form sodium salt which is actually marketed.

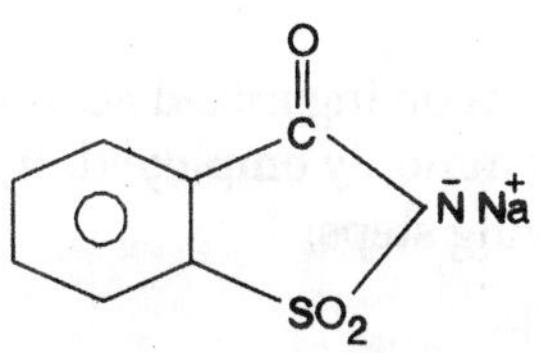

Na-Salt

15.9.2 Uses of Aromatic Sulphonic Acids

Aromatic sulphonic acids and their derivatives are used for various purposes as noted below:

i. *p*-Toluene sulphonic acid and its chloride are used as a tosylating agents for protecting functional groups.

ii. Benzene sulphonamide is used as an intermediate in the synthesis of *Sulpha Drugs* for the treatment of pneumonia, gonorrhoea, etc.

iii. Chloromine-T ($CH_3-C_6H_4-SO_2\bar{N}Cl\,\overset{+}{Na}$) is an important antiseptic.

iv. Saccharin is used as a sweetening agent and it is prescribed for diabetic patients for getting calorie-free sugar.

v. They are employed extensively in synthetic organic chmistry.

15.10 Nitro Derivative (Aromatic Nitro Compounds)

Aromatic compounds containing nitro group (—NO_2) are termed as aromatic nitro compounds. Structurally, nitro group may be represented as resonance hybrid.

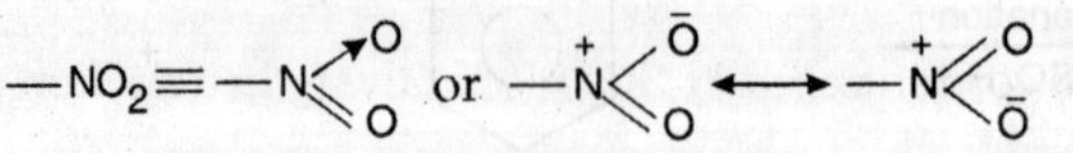

It is, thus, evident that in nitro compound nitrogen atom of nitro group is directly attached to organic portion, i.e., the general representation of nitro compounds may be written as

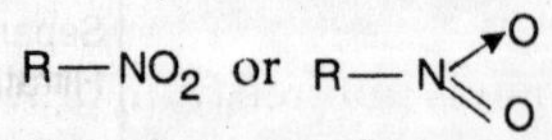

where 'R' is phenyl ring in the case of aromatic nitro compounds.

Aromatic nitro compounds may contain one or more nitro groups and are accordingly known as mono-, di- or poly- nitro compounds.

15.10.1 Preparation of Aromatic Nitro Compounds

The most useful and important method for the preparation of nitro compounds is the direct nitration. Direct nitration may be carried out by following any one of the procedures as noted below:

i. Treatment with concentrated nitric acid
ii. Reaction with fuming nitric acid
iii. Using mixed acids, i.e., mixture of concentrated nitric acid and concentrated sulphuric acid or mixture of concentrated nitric acid and glacial acetic acid.
iv. Reaction with acetyl nitrate ($CH_3-\underset{\underset{O}{\|}}{C}-O-NO_2$). This reagent is specially important for the introduction of nitro group at the *ortho*-position in the case of nitration of substituted benzene and for only mono nitro derivative. However, special care is to be taken during its use as it explodes on heating.

Among all the above processes of nitration, reaction involving mixed acids of concentrated nitric and sulphuric acids is the most successful and is commonly employed. It is believed that the nitration by mixed acids proceeds through the following steps:

Step 1: Generation of active electrophilic nitro group.

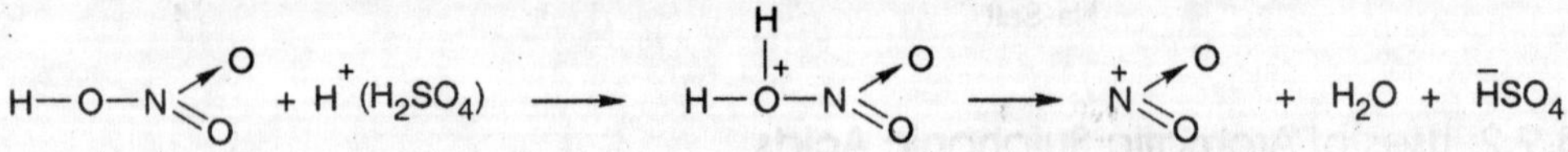

Nitronium ion

Step 2: Attack by nitronium ion to aromatic ring.

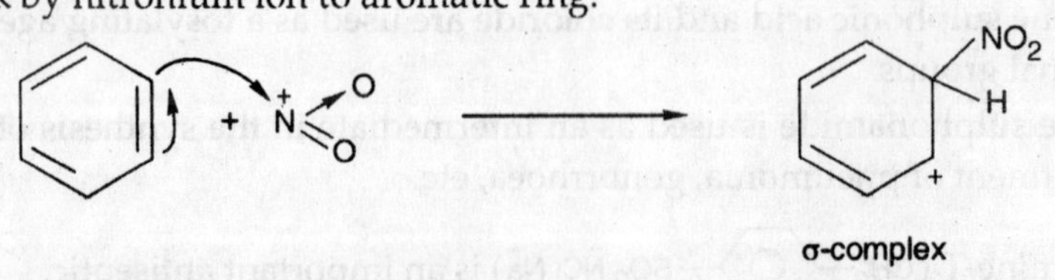

σ-complex

Step 3:

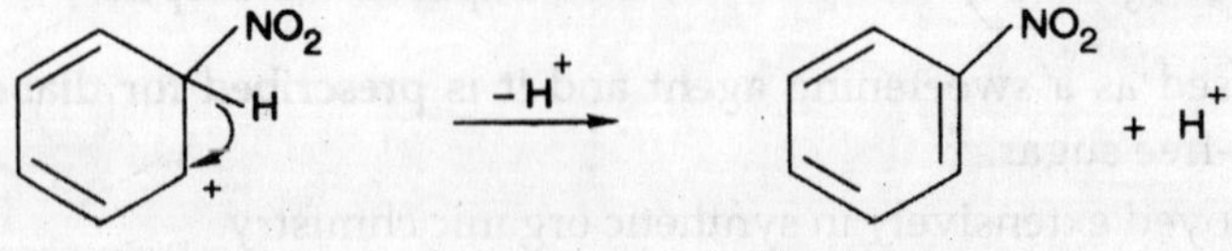

Nitro benzene

Step 4: $$\overset{+}{H} + \overline{H}SO_4 \rightleftharpoons H_2SO_4$$

It may be mentioned that the same nitronium ion is beleived to be formed during the nitration with fuming HNO_3.

Sometimes BF_3 is used, instead of concentrated H_2SO_4, as catalyst, the function of which is to form nitronium ion as indicated below:

$$H—O—N\begin{smallmatrix}\nearrow O\\ \searrow O\end{smallmatrix} + BF_3 \longrightarrow N\begin{smallmatrix}\nearrow O\\ \searrow O\end{smallmatrix} + HO—\overline{B}F_3$$

Drawbacks of Direct Nitration: The process of direct nitration is not free from drawback. It is not applicable in the case of substituted aromatic compounds. Ortho and para dinitro benzenes and para-nitro benzoic acid cannot be prepared by this method because direct nitration of nitrobenzene and benzoic acid would always yield *m*-isomer. However, such compounds may be prepared by adopting indirect routes. Thus,

i. 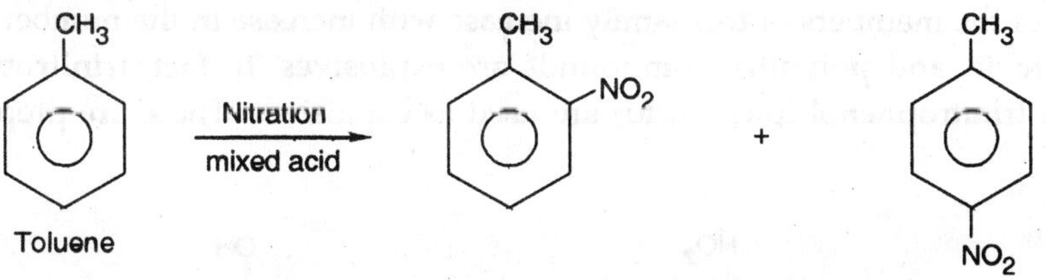

o and *p*-Nitro toluene

ii. 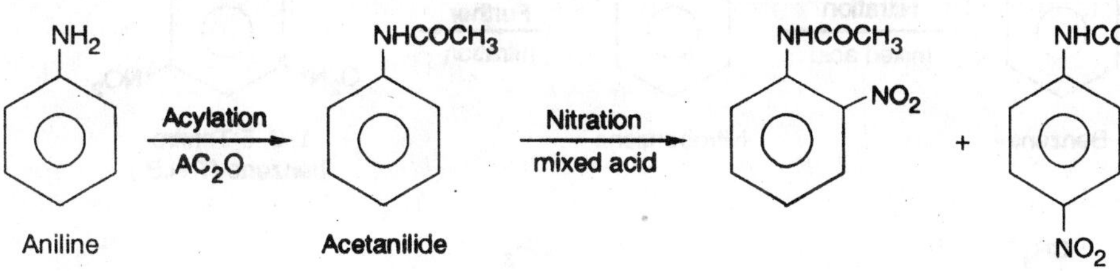

o and *p*-Nitro acetanilide

Two isomers are separated by distillation.

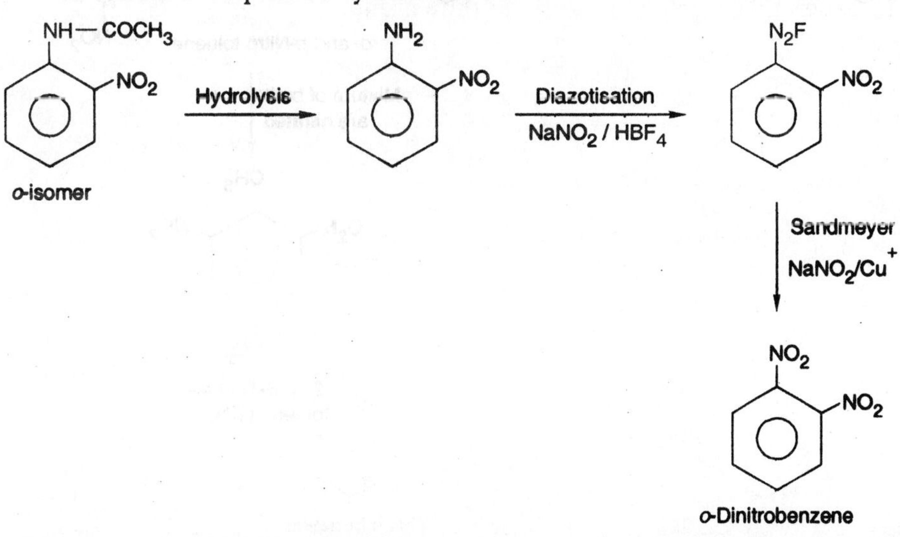

o-Dinitrobenzene

After separation each of the isomers is subjected to oxidation.

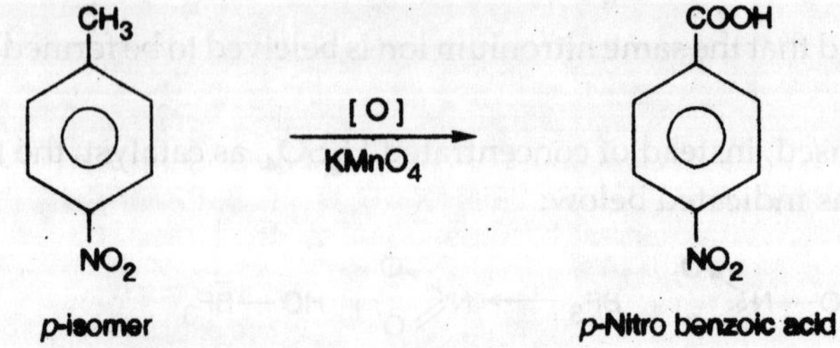

15.10.2 Properties of Aromatic Nitro Compounds

15.10.2.1 Physical Properties

A few lower members are pale yellow liquids but others are yellow crystalline solids. Melting and boiling points of the members of this family increase with increase in the number of nitro groups. They are toxic, and polynitro compounds are explosives. In fact, trinitrobenzene, trinitrotoluene and trinitrophenol (picric acid) are used as explosives. These are prepared by direct nitration.

i. 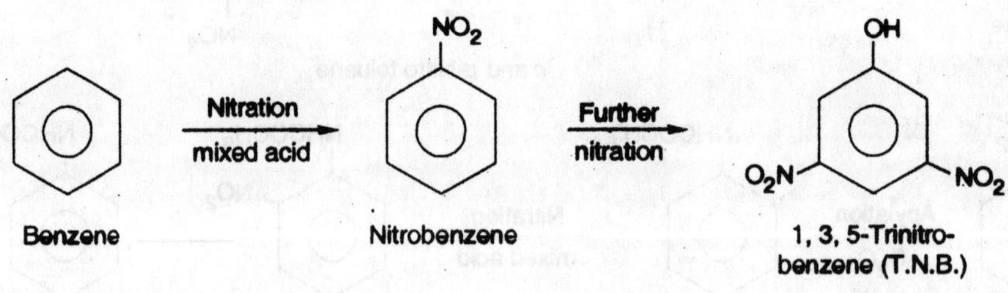

ii. 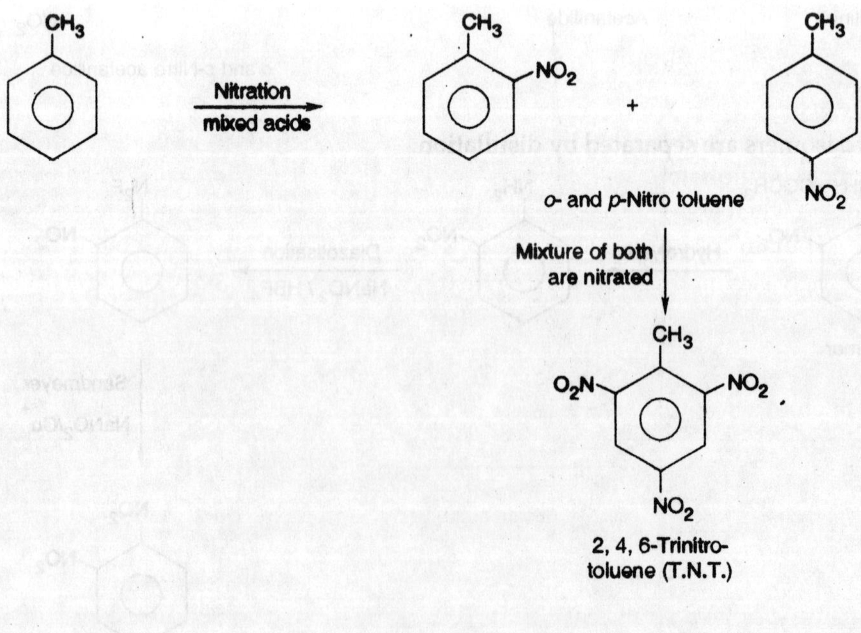

iii.

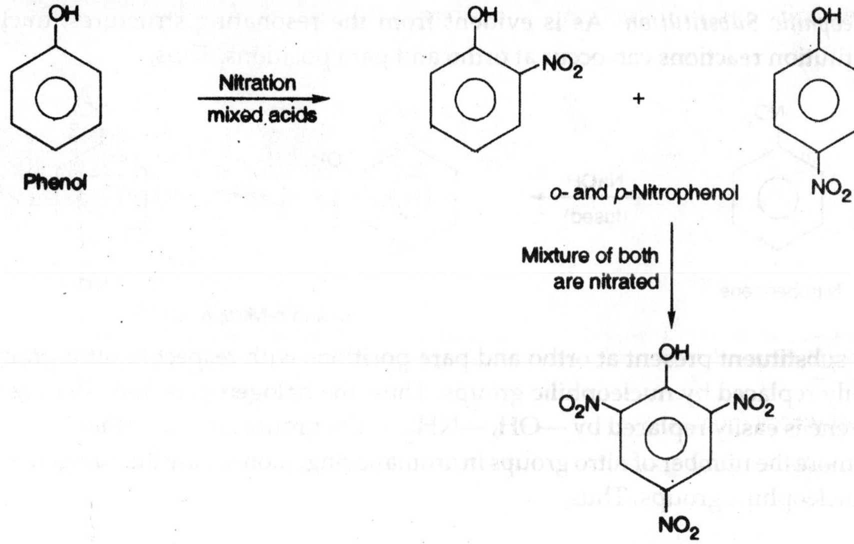

2, 4, 6-Trinitrophenol
(Picric acid)

15.10.2.2 Chemical Properties

Chemical properties of aromatic nitro compounds may be considered under two headings.

15.10.2.2.1 Reactions of Aromatic Ring Due to the Influence of Nitro Group

Since the nitro group is electron withdrawing in nature it deactivates the aromatic ring particularly its *ortho* and *para* positions, but *meta* position as it remains intact is relatively elctron rich as is envisaged from the following resonating structures.

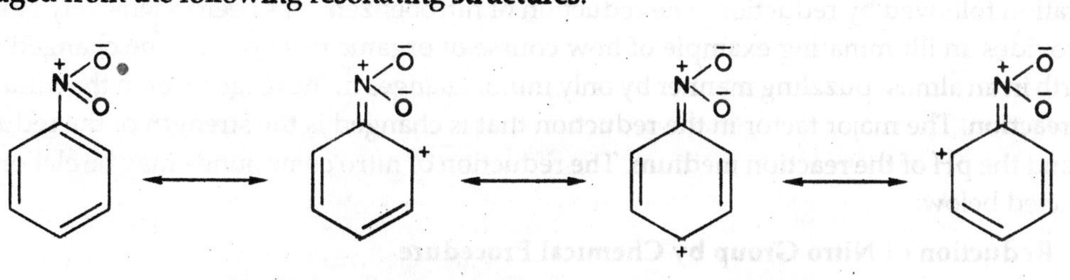

i. Accordingly *electrophilic substitution* may occur at *meta* positions, i.e.,

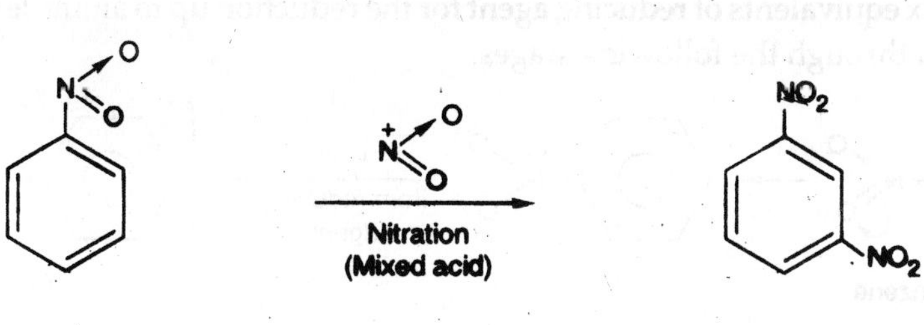

m-dinitrobenzene

ii. *Nucleophilic Substitution*: As is evident from the resonating structures, nucleophilic substitution reactions can occur at ortho and para positions. Thus,

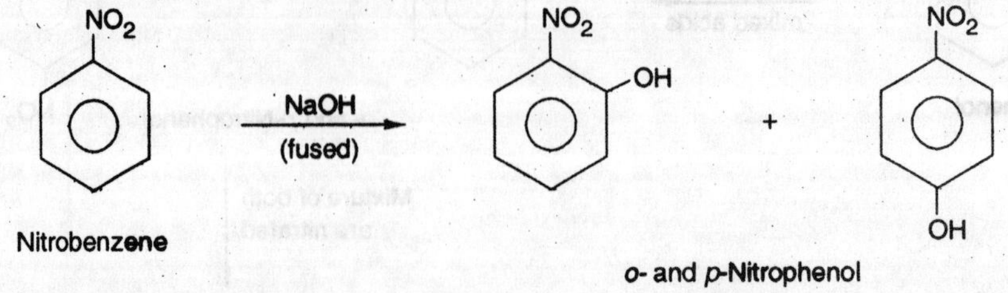

Any substituent present at ortho and para positions with respect to nitro group can be readily replaced by nucleophilic groups. Thus, the halogen in *o*- and *p*-halogeno nitrobenzene is easily replaced by —OH, —NH_2, —CN groups. It has further been observed that more the number of nitro groups in aromatic ring, more easily the halogen is replaced by nucleophilic groups. Thus,

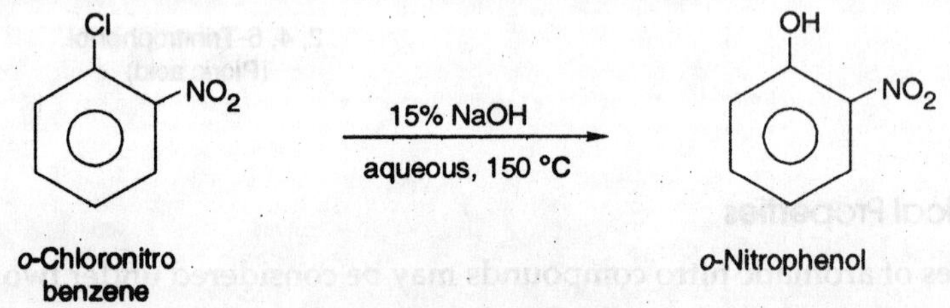

15.10.2.2.2 Reactions Due to Nitro Group: Reduction of Aromatic Nitro Compound

The most important reaction of nitro compounds having synthetic significance involves the reduction of nitro group, particularly to the amine level. In fact, amines are normally prepared by nitration followed by reduction. The reduction of nitrobenzene has been extensively studied and provides an illuminating example of how course of organic reactions can be changed back and forth in an almost puzzling manner by only minor changes in the reagents or in the condition of the reaction. The major factor in the reduction that is changed is the strength of the reducing agent and the pH of the reaction medium. The reduction of nitro compounds may be elaborated as depicted below:

A. Reduction of Nitro Group by Chemical Procedure

(a) *In acidic condition*: When reduction of nitro compound is conducted in acidic solution, it requires six equivalents of reducing agent for the reduction up to amine level and appears to proceed through the following stages:

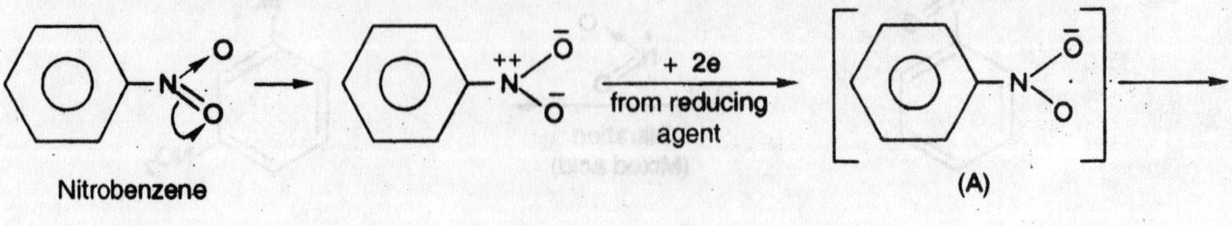

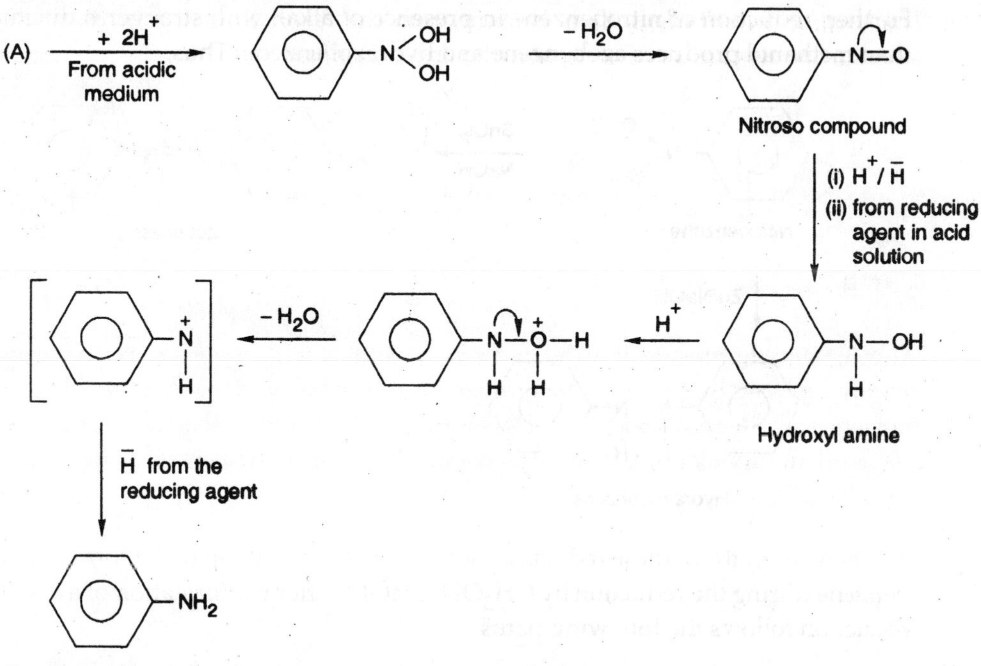

Amine (Aniline)

- *Comments*
  i. A large variety of reducing agents may be used. Commonly used such reducing agents are Sn/HCl, $SnCl_2$/HCl, Zn/HCl, etc.
  ii. In weak acid solution, the major product is amine but when strong acid solution is used the major product becomes *p*-aminophenol.

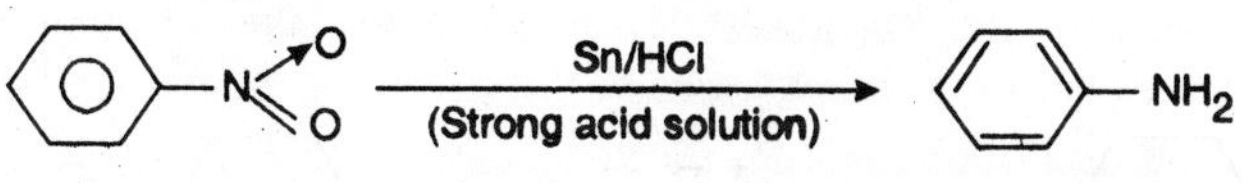

p-Amino phenol

(b) ***Reduction in neutral and alkaline conditions:*** In neutral or alkaline solution, the reducing power of the reagents towards nitro group is less than in acid solution. Typical examples are the reduction of nitrobenzene with Zn and NH_4Cl and NaOH in CH_3OH.

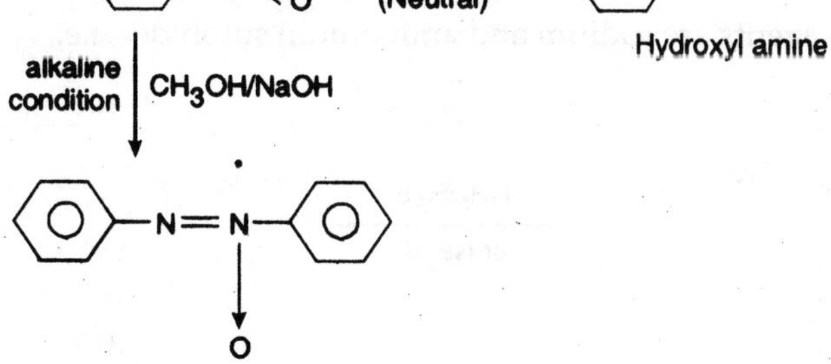

Azoxy benzene

Further, reduction of nitrobenzene in presence of alkali with stronger reducing agents than methanol produces azobenzene and hydrazobenzene. Thus,

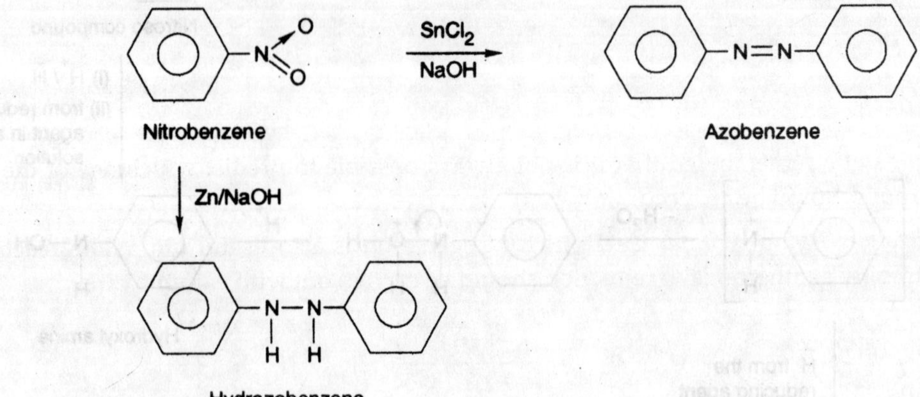

Nitrobenzene — Azobenzene — Hydrazobenzene

Mechanistic paths of these reductions follow the same path up to the formation of azoxy benzene during the reduction by $CH_3OH/NaOH$. After the formation of azoxy benzene reduction follows the following paths.

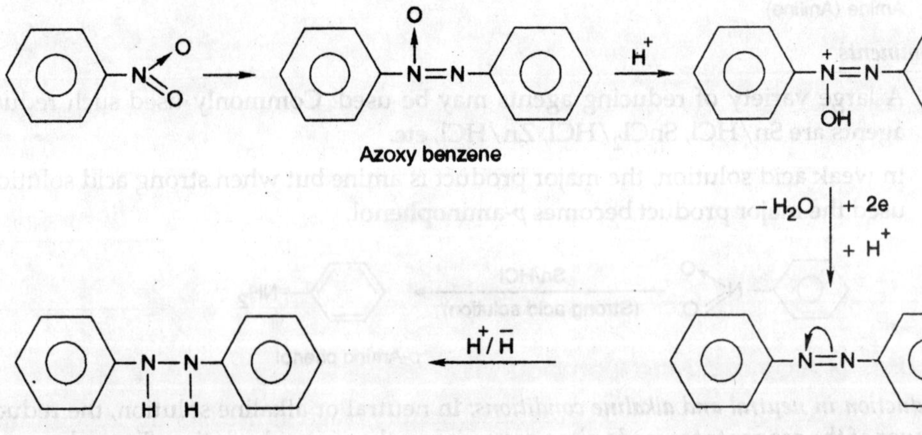

Azoxy benzene — Azobenzene — Hydrazo benzene

(c) *Selective Reduction*: One of the nitro groups in dinitro compound can be selectively reduced by the use of some specific reducing agents.

Such reducing agents are sodium and ammonium sulphides, i.e.,

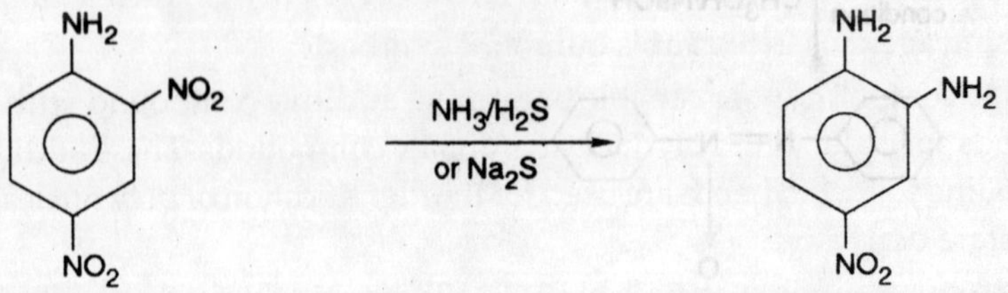

2, 4-Dinitro aniline — 4-Nitro-orthophenylene diamine

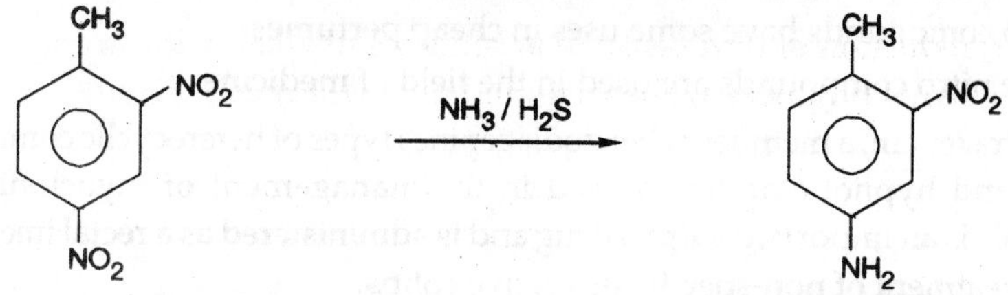

2, 4-Dinitro toluene 2-Nitro *p*-toluidine

It may be remembered that it is not always possible to predict which one of the nitro groups would be reduced.

(d) *Catalytic Hydrogenation*: Catalytic hydrogenation is also useful but as the reaction is strongly exothermic the reduction should be carried out with extreme care.

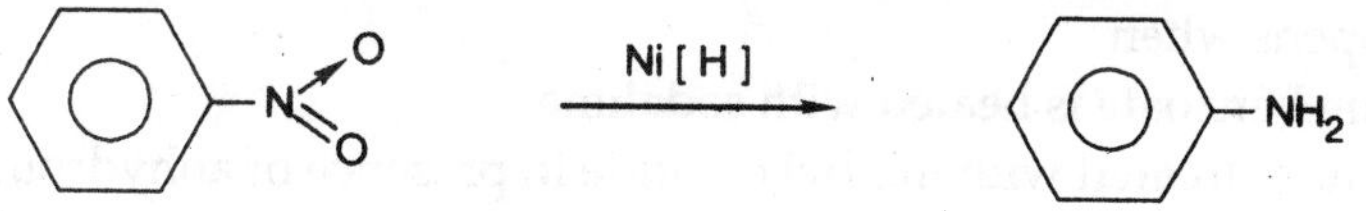

B. Electrolytic Reduction

It has been proposed that the course of reduction of nitro compound through electrolytic path has been supposed to follow the path of reduction in acid solution, i.e., the major product is the amine.

PROBLEM 15.2

Suggest the product:

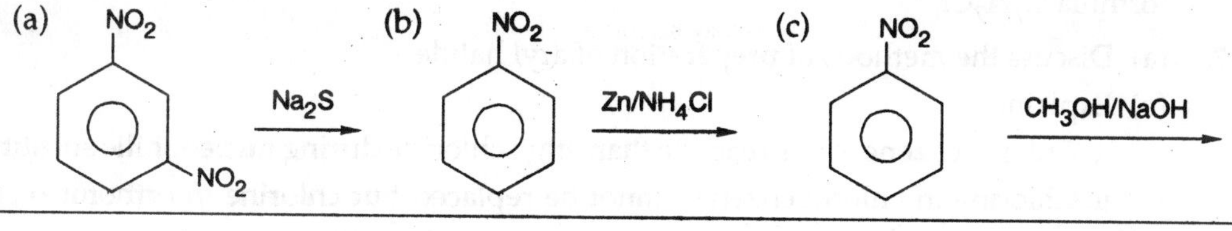

15.10.3 Uses of Aromatic Nitro Compounds

(a) Many nitro compounds are very useful laboratory reagents used for the identification of organic compounds. For example (i) 2, 4-dinitrophenyl hydrazine is the most important reagent for the identification of carbonyl compounds (ii) 3, 5-dinitrobenzoyl chloride is employed for the identification of hydroxy group (iii) 2, 4-dinitrofluoro benzene is widely used in protein chemistry for the analysis of N-terminal of amino acid. It is generally known as Sanger's reagent.

(b) Nitro compounds find some use as solvents as in Friedel-Crafts reaction.

(c) As oxidising agent as in Skraup's quinoline synthesis.

(d) Many nitro compounds are capable of forming additive compound with certain organic compounds specially with polynuclear aromatic compounds. These additive compounds are crystalline solid and hence are used for the identification of poly nuclear hydrocarbons as for picrate derivative.

(e) Some nitro compounds such as T.N.B., T.N.T. are widely used as explosives.

(f) Nitro compounds have some uses in cheap perfumes.

(g) Some nitro compounds are used in the field of medicine.

Thus, nitrazepam, a member of benzodiazepines types of heterocyclic compound is employed as sedative and hypnotic and also used in the management of myoclonic seizures. Nitrosulphathiazole is an important sulpha drug and is administered as a rectal injection as an adjunct in the local treatment of non-specific ulcerative colitis.

Model Questions

1. How is benzene prepared? Describe its important reactions.
2. What happens when
   (a) Sodium benzoate is heated with sodalime
   (b) Benzene is treated with methyl chloride in presence of anhydrous $AlCl_3$.
   (c) Chlorine is passed through bioling toluene.
   (d) Benzyl chloride is treated with NaOH.
3. How will you prepare styrene from benzene? Give some of its uses.
4. Write short note on Friedel-Crafts reaction.
5. How are aromatic halogen compounds classified?
   Hints: Nuclear and side chain halides.
6. Write the structures and names of all possible isomers of aromatic halides with molecular formula C_7H_7Cl.
7. (a) Discuss the methods of preparation of aryl halide.
   (b) Explain:
      i. Chlorobenzene is less reactive than ethyl chloride during nucleophilic substitution.
      ii. Chlorine in chlorobenzene cannot be replaced but chlorine in orthonitro chlorobenzene can be.
      iii. Chlorobenzene is less reactive than benzyl chloride.
8. What is benzyne? Describe mechanism for aromatic nucleophilic substitution.
9. How will you synthesise the following?
   (a) D.D.T. from chlorobenzene
   (b) Benzyl alcohol from bromobenzene
   (c) Benzoic acid from bromobenzene.
   Hints: (b) and (c):

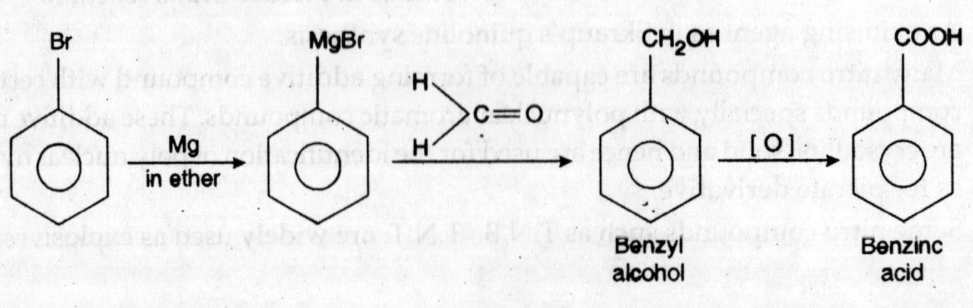

10. (a) What are sulphonic acids? How are they prepared?
(b) Give mechanisim of sulphonation.

11. How will you prepare the following?
(a) Benzene sulphonyl chloride
(b) Saccharin
(c) *p*-Toluene sulphonic acid from benzene
(d) Phenol from benzene sulphonic acid
(e) Sulphanilamide from aniline
(f) T.N.T. and T.N.B. from benzene.
(e) **Hints:**

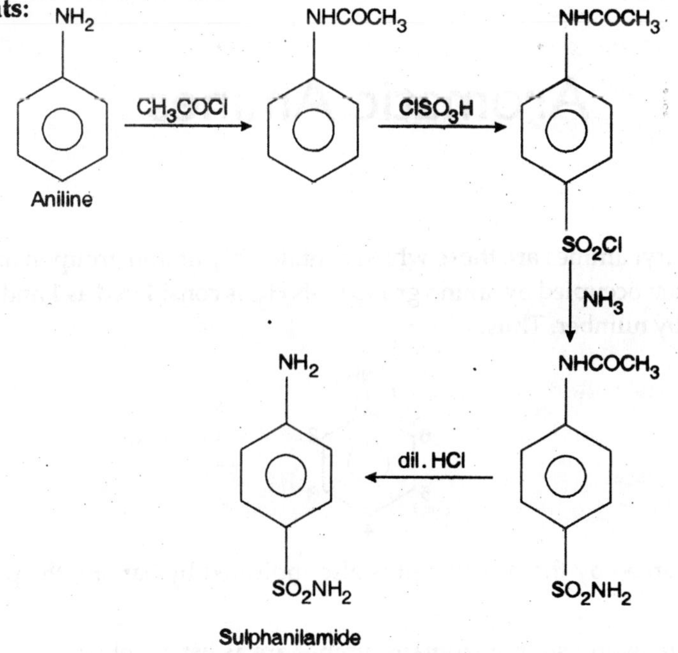

12. What are nitro compounds? How are they prepared? Suggest mechanism of nitration.

13. Describe the properties of nitro compounds.

14. Account for: Nitrobenzene undergoes both electrophilic and nucleophilic substitution reactions.

CHAPTER SIXTEEN

Aromatic Amines

Aromatic amines or aryl amines are those which contain only amino group in aromatic ring. In aryl amine, the position occupied by amino group (—NH_2) is considered as 1 and the substituent present is indicated by number. Thus,

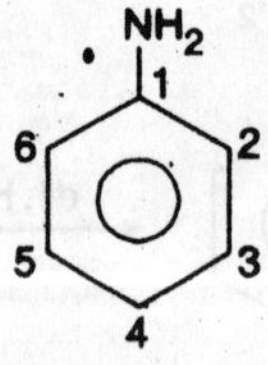

The position occupied by the substituent is also indicated by naming the position as *ortho*, *meta* and *para*.

Some of the common and simple aromatic amines are as listed below:

Compound	**Common name**	**IUPAC Name**
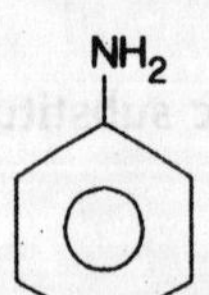	Aniline	Amino benzene
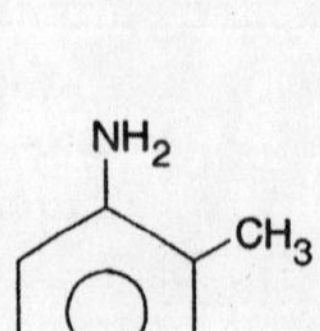	*o*-Toluidine	2-Methyl aniline

Compound	Common name	IUPAC Name
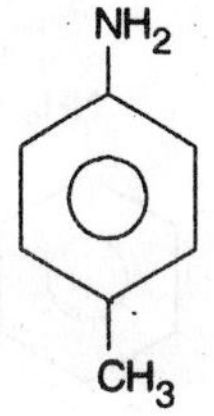	*p*-Toluidine	4-Methyl aniline or *p*-Methyl aniline
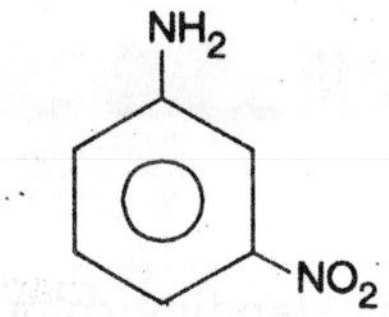	—	3-Methyl aniline or *m*-Nitro aniline

Like aliphatic amine, aryl amine may be primary, secondary and tertiary in nature. In the case of secondary and tertiary amines, they are simple if all the groups attached to nitrogen atom are aryl groups or they may be mixed when both alkyl and aryl groups are connected to nitrogen atom. Thus,

Simple aryl amine:

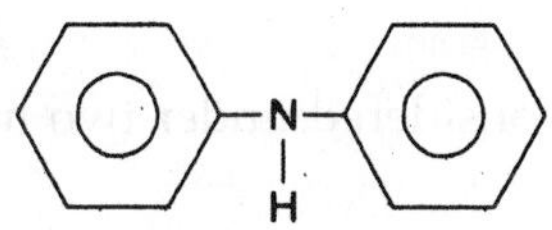

Diphenyl amine

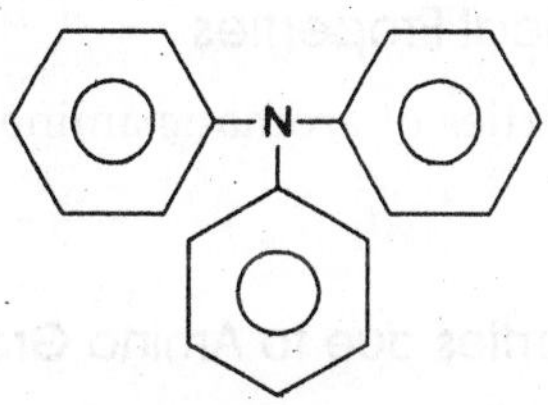

Triphenyl amine

Mixed aryl amine:

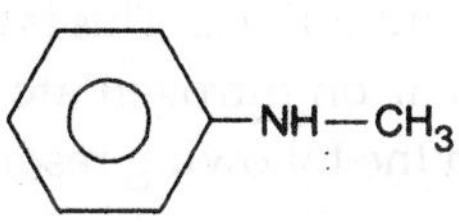

N-Methyl aniline

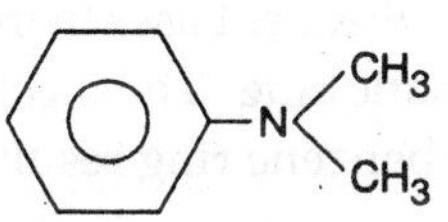

N, N-Dimethyl aniline

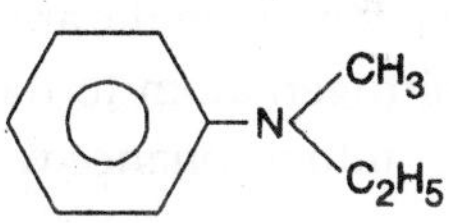

N-Ethyl, N-Methyl aniline

16.1 General Methods of Preparation of Aromatic Amines

Aniline and different substituted anilines are prepared by adopting the following methods:

1. *Reduction of Nitro Compounds*: This is the most common method of preparing aromatic amines. Variety of reducing agents may be used for the purpose of reducing nitro group. Commonly used such reducing agents are (i) metal/acid (ii) NH_4HS for specific reduction of only one nitro group (iii) Na/CH_3OH and (iv) $SnCl_2/HCl$, (v) catalytic reduction (vide reduction of nitro compound chapter **fifteen**). The general path of the reduction is

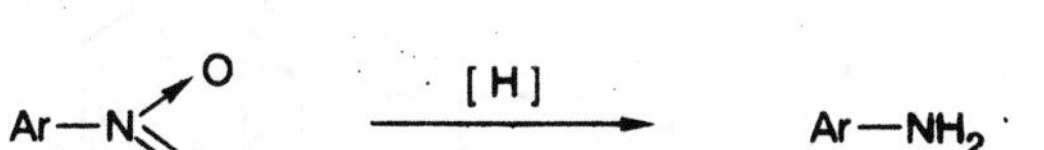

[Ar = aryl group]

2. *Hofmann degradation* (vide chapter twelve): Hofmann degradation is another important method for the preparation of aromatic amines.

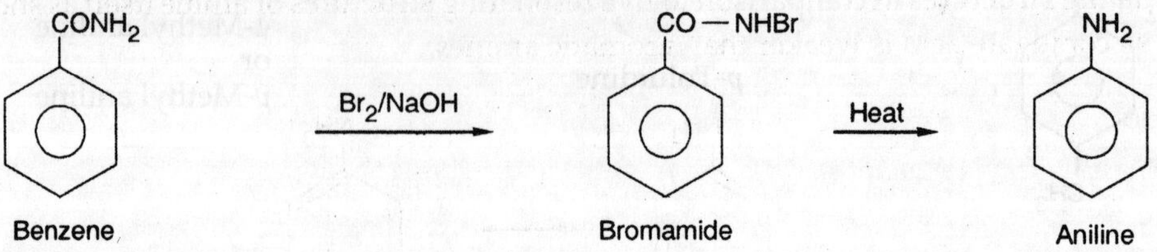

16.2 Properties of Aromatic Amines

16.2.1 Physical Properties

Aromatic amines are generally either colourless liquids or solids but on long standing colour gradually changes to pale yellow to deep yellow and ultimately to red. They are capable of forming intermolecular hydrogen bonding. Because of this intermolecular hydrogen bonding and high molecular weights their boiling points are relatively high. They are toxic and some of them are carcinogens. They are sparingly soluble in water but highly soluble in organic solvents.

16.2.2 Chemical Properties

Chemical properties of aromatic amines may be considered under two headings as described below:

16.2.2.1 Properties due to Amino Group

The most significant properties of aromatic amines that arises from amino group is their *basicity*. The basicity of these compounds originates from the lone pair of electrons on nitrogen atom. However, aromatic amines are weaker bases than aliphatic amines. This is due to the attachment of nitrogen atom to the aromatic ring. The electron pair on nitrogen atom in aromatic amine enter into resonance with the benzene ring resulting in the following resonating structures.

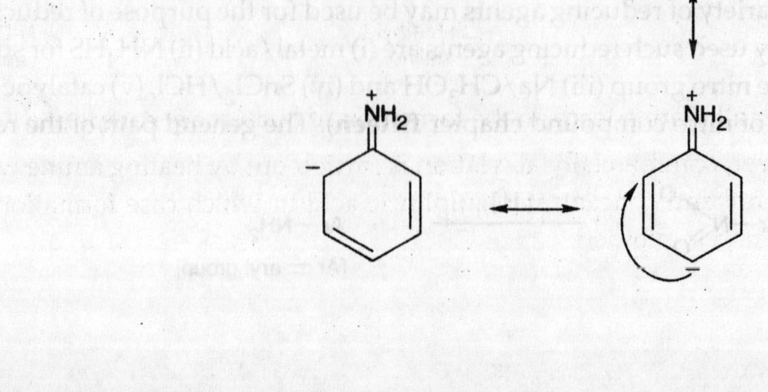

As a result of such resonance lone pair on nitrogen atom in arómatic ring is not easily available for coordinating with the proton. Further, the conjugate acid (protonated amine) has only two resonating structures in comparison to five resonating structures of amine itself as shown earlier and so conjugate acid is weaker than aromatic amines.

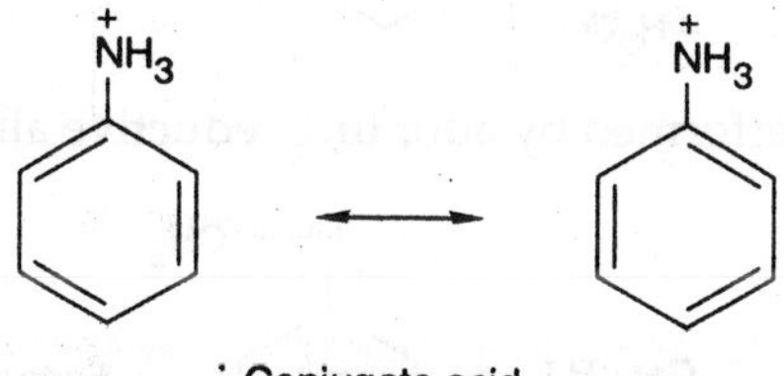

Conjugate acid

Due to above two facts aromatic amine becomes a weaker base than aliphatic amine where no such resonance occurs.

It may be mentioned that the substitutents either on the nitrogen atom or in the ring has significant influence on the basicity of aromatic amines. Increase in the number of alkyl groups on nitrogen atom increases the basicity. Again, presence of electron releasing group in the aromatic ring increases the basicity while electron withdrawing group decreases the basicity. It has been observed that the effect, either increasing or decreasing basic strength becomes maximum when the substituent is present at ortho position.

The basic character of aromatic amines is revealed from the following reactions:

(a) *Reaction with acid*: With mineral acids aromatic amines form salts. Thus,

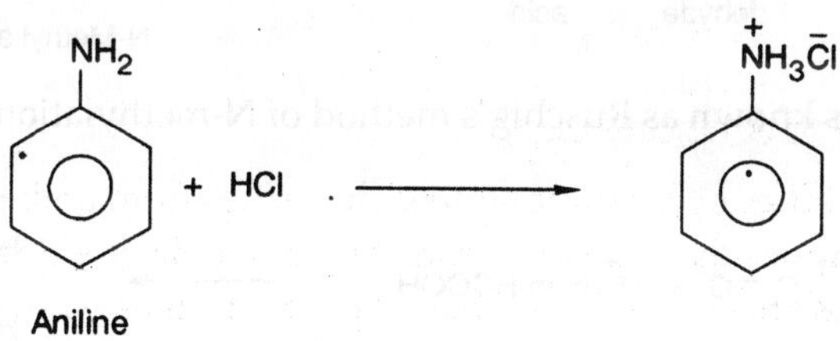

(b) *Alkylation*

i. Alkylation of aromatic amines is usually carried out by the treatment of amines with alkyl halide and in this reaction nitrogen atom of amine with its lone pair of electrons plays the key role. Thus,

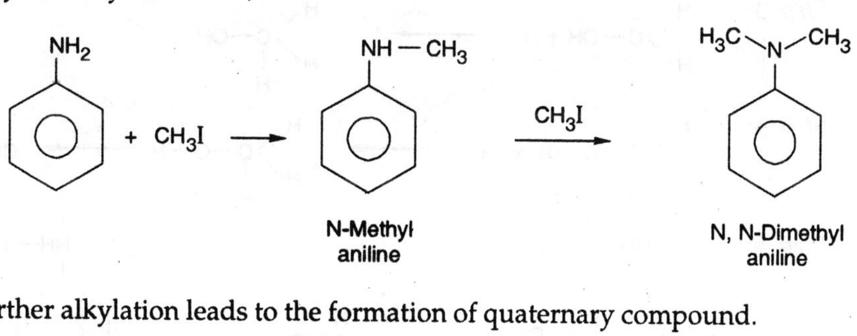

Further alkylation leads to the formation of quaternary compound.

ii. However, commercially alkylation is carried out by heating amine with the mixture of alcohol and concentrated sulphuric acid in which case formation of quaternary compound is avoided.

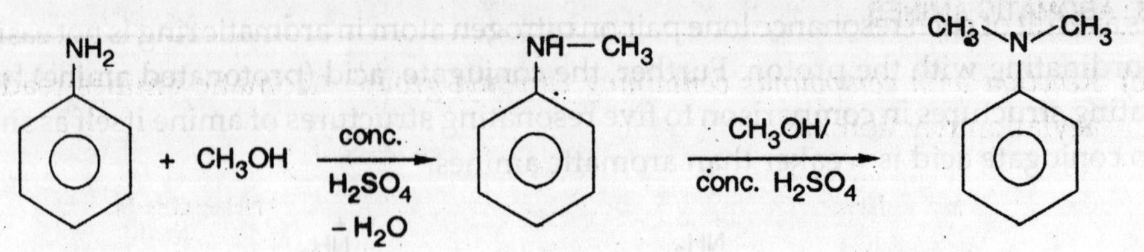

iii. Alkylation is also performed by adopting reductive alkylation procedure, i.e.,

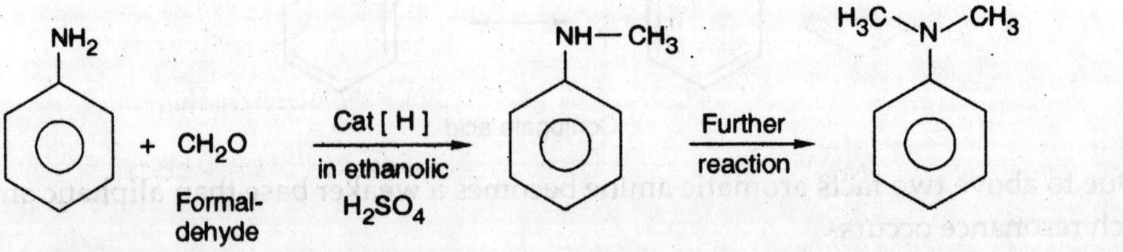

It may be mentioned that in the case of N-methylation commonly mixture of formaldehyde and formic acid is used which is a very useful and usually an adopted procedure, i.e.,

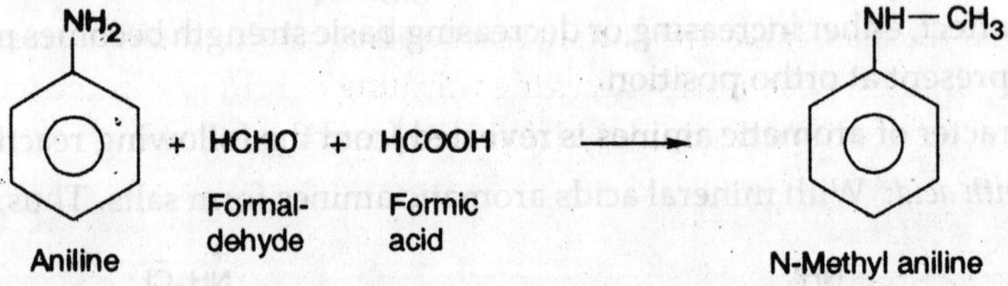

This process is known as Ruschig's method of N-methylation and may be explained as under:

Step 1:

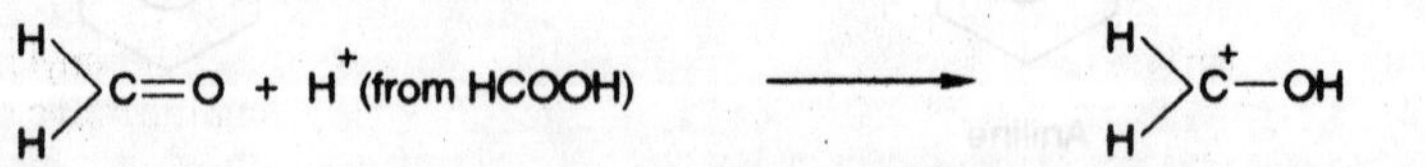

Step 2:

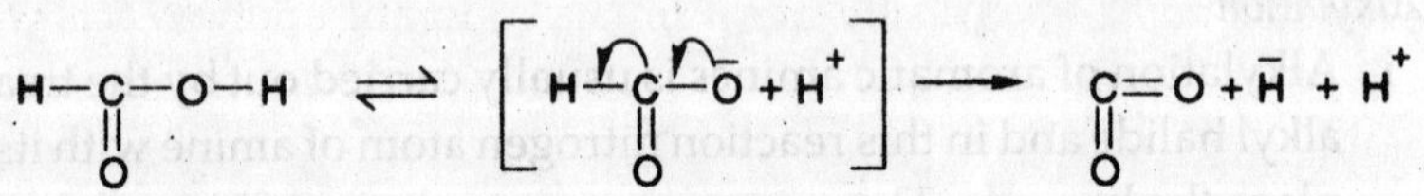

Step 3:

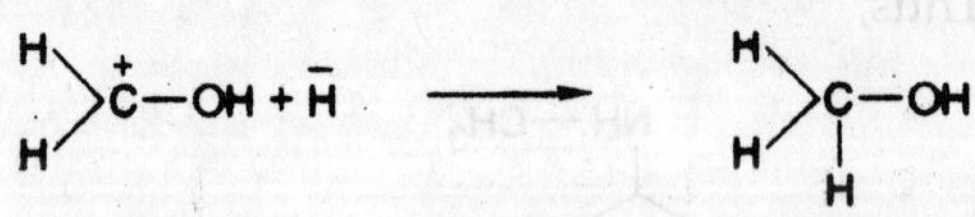

Step 4:

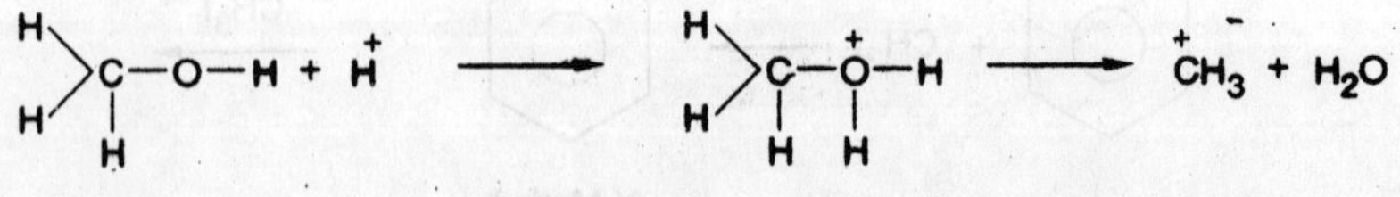

Step 5:

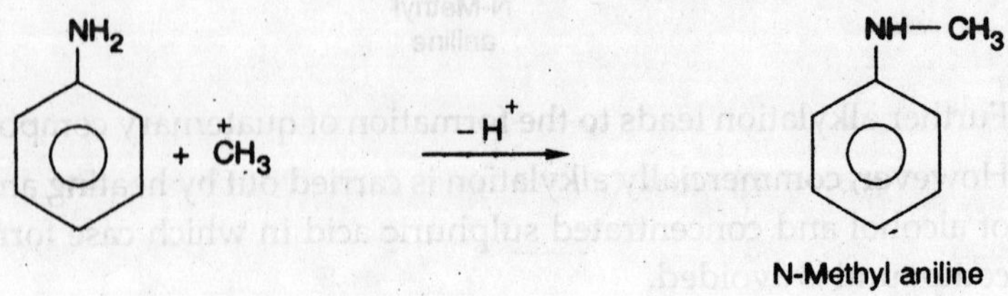

(c) *Reaction with compounds containing carbonyl group*: Aromatic amines readily undergo acylation reaction, i.e.,

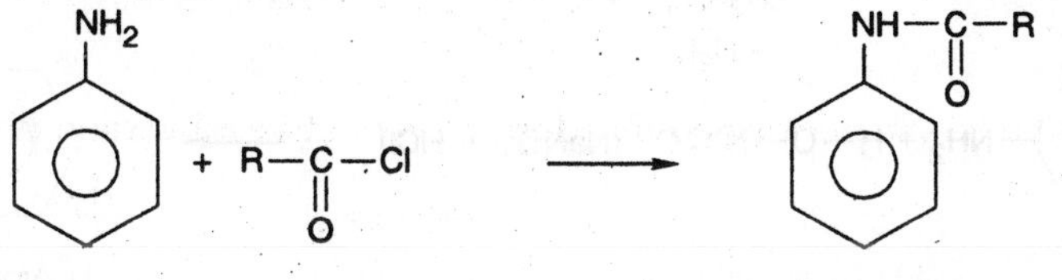

N-acyl aniline

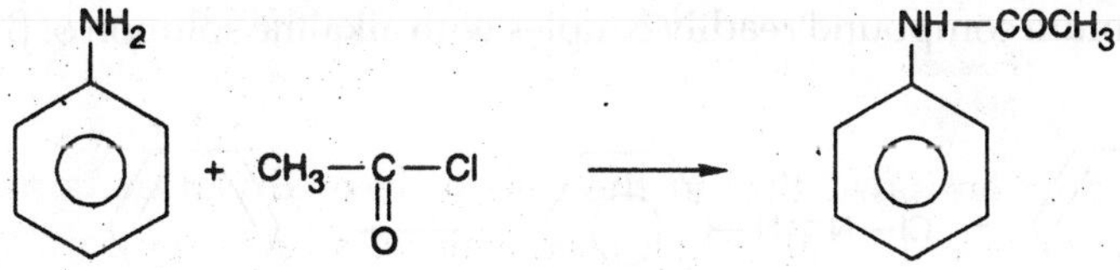

Acetanilide

(d) *Carbyl amine reaction*: It is an important reaction frequently employed for the identification of primary amines. Reaction involves the warming of primary amine with chloroform in presence of ethanolic potassium hydroxide (vide chapter **twelve**).

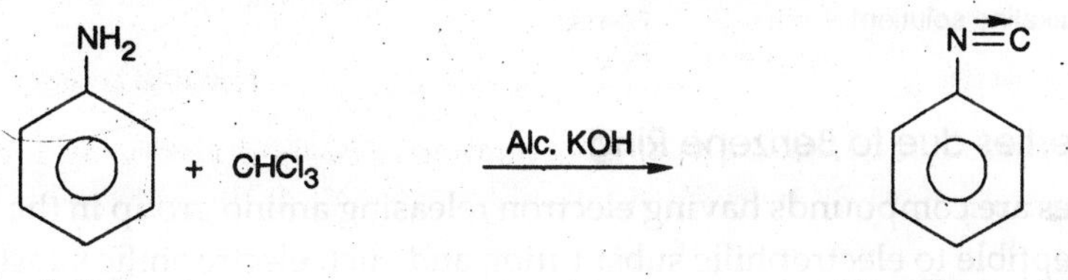

Aniline

Phenyl isocyanide (characteristic obnoxious odour)

(e) *Reaction with carbon disulphide*: Primary aromatic amine reacts with carbon disulphide.

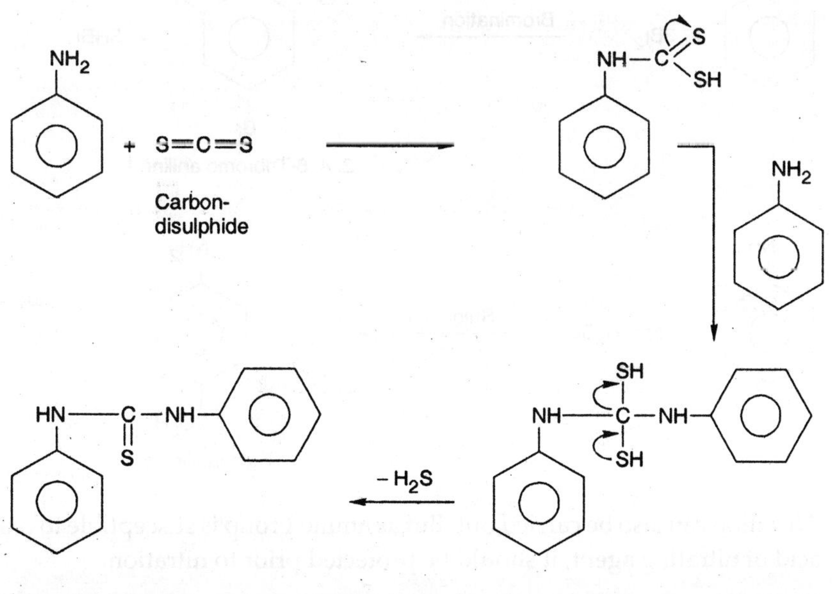

(f) *Diazotisation*: It is one of the most significant reaction of primary aromatic amine having wide synthetic and analytical application. It is frequently used for identification of primary amines and is known as *dye test*. Thus,

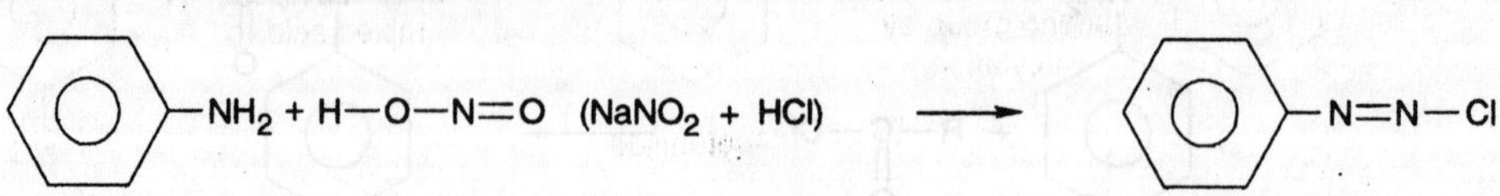

Aromatic diazonium chloride

This diazonium compound readily couples with alkaline solution of β-Naphthol forming a red dye.

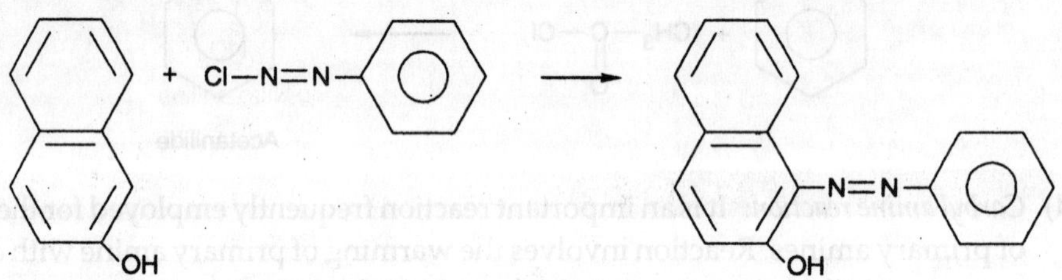

β-Naphthol (alkaline solution) Azo dye

16.2.2.2 Properties due to Benzene Ring

Aromatic amines are compounds having electron releasing amino group in the ring. Hence they are highly susceptible to electrophilic substitution and such electrophilic substitution reactions generally take place at ortho and para positions. Thus,

(a)

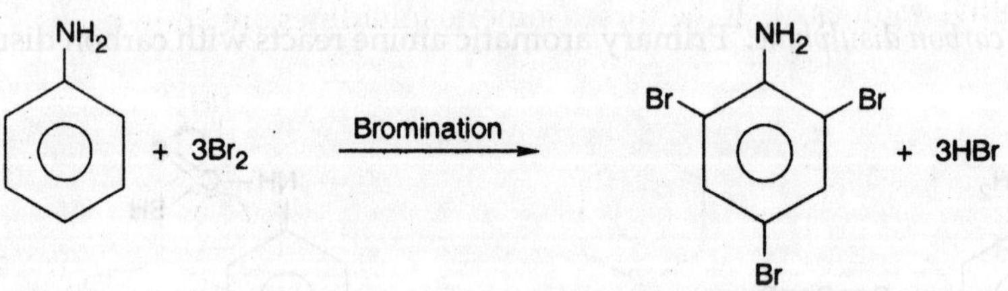

2, 4, 6-Tribromo aniline

(b)

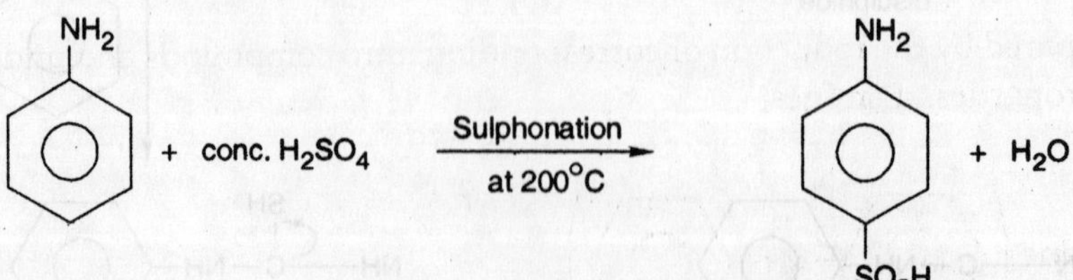

Sulphanilic acid

(c) Nitration can also be carried out. But as amino group is susceptible to oxidation by nitric acid of nitrating agent, it should be protected prior to nitration.

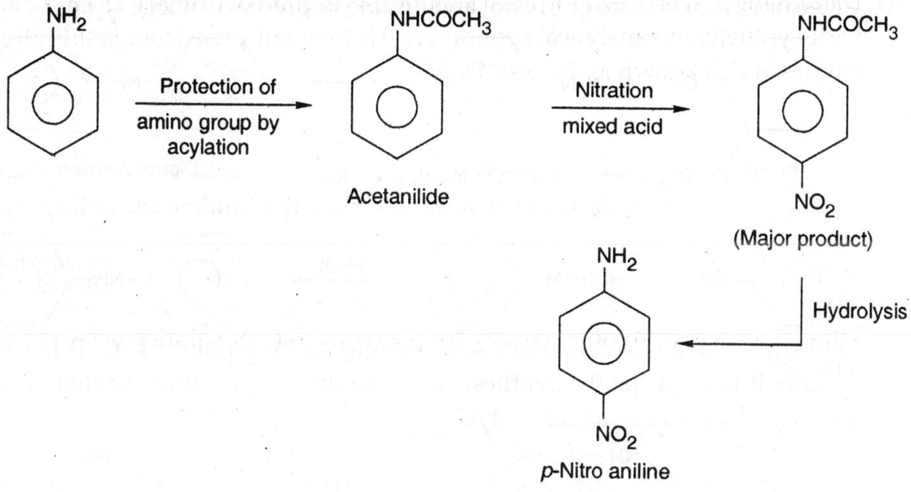

16.3 Some Important Aromatic Amines

1. Aniline

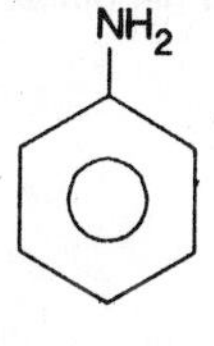

It is a colourless liquid but on long standing becomes reddish. It is used for the synthesis of azodyes and in the manufacture of antioxidants drugs, and plastic. It undergoes all the typical reactions of aromatic amines.

2. *Toluidines* (Methyl anilines): All the three isomeric toluidines are known, i.e.,

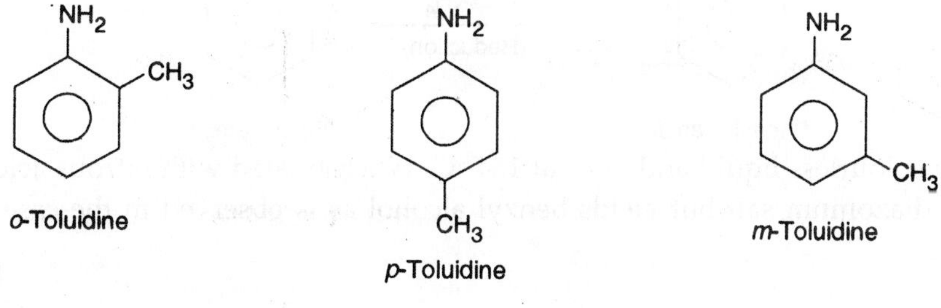

They are prepared by the reduction of corresponding nitro compounds and undergo all the typical properties of amines.

3. Diphenyl amine

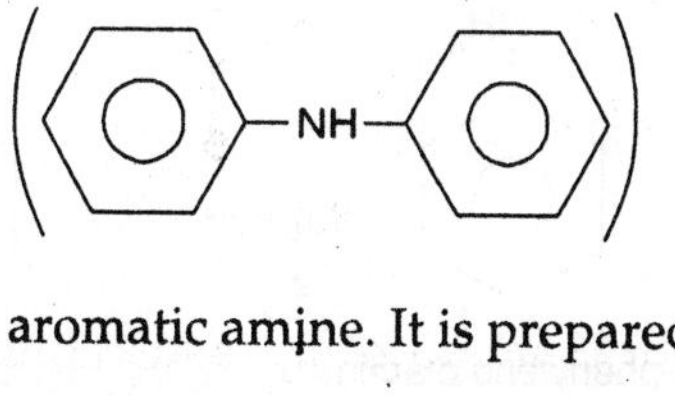

It is a secondary aromatic amine. It is prepared by the following methods:

By heating the mixture of phenol and aniline in presence of $ZnCl_2$, i.e.,

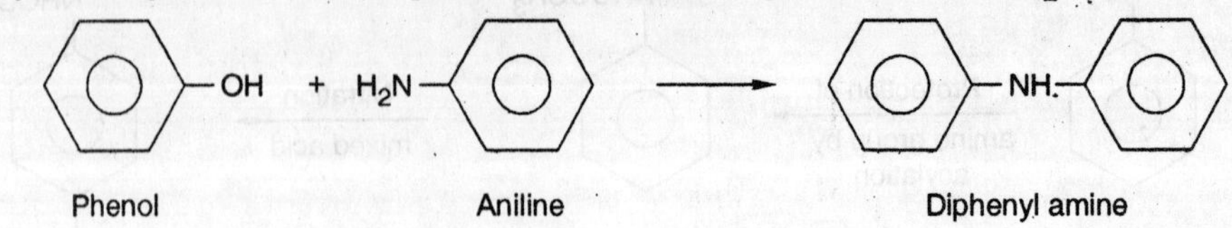

Industrially it is manufactured by heating a mixture of aniline and aniline hydrochloride.

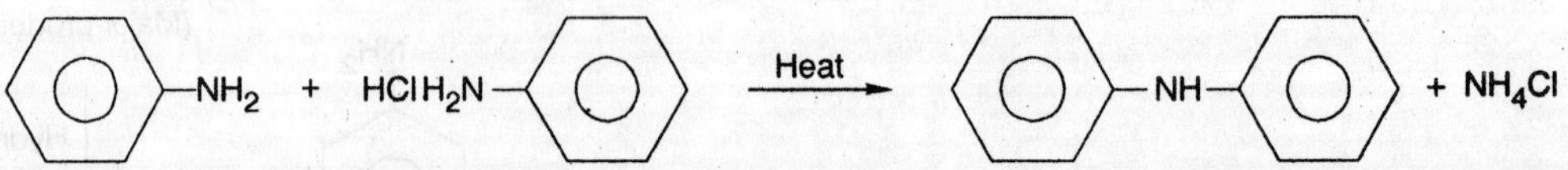

Diphenyl amine is a colourless solid having melting point 54 °C. It is less basic than aniline. It is used for the synthesis of some dyes. Thus when heated with sulphur, it forms phenothiazine, an azine dye.

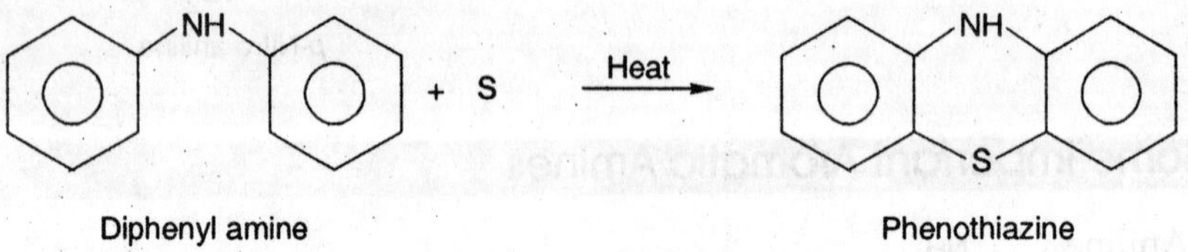

4. *Benzyl amine* 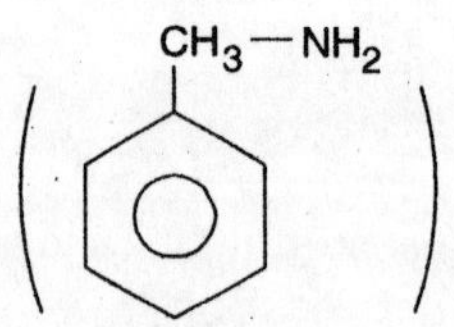

In this amine amino group is at the side-chain and so it behaves as an aliphatic amine. It is prepared by the reduction of pheny cyanide.

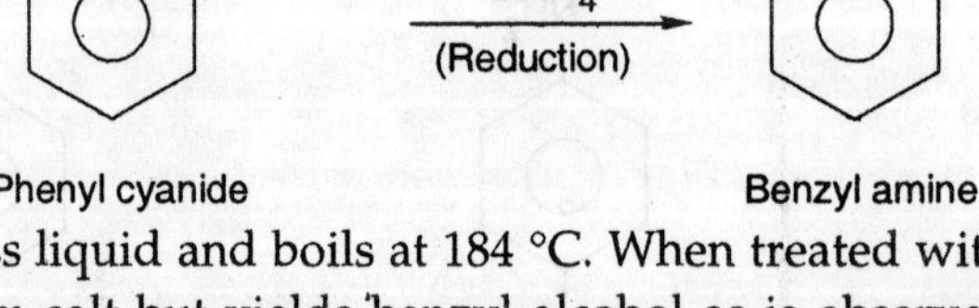

It is a colourless liquid and boils at 184 °C. When treated with nitrous acid it does not form diazonium salt but yields benzyl alcohol as is observed in the case of aliphatic amines.

16.4 DIAMINES

Aromatic diamines are known as phenylene diamines. Three isomeric phenylene diamines are known. They are

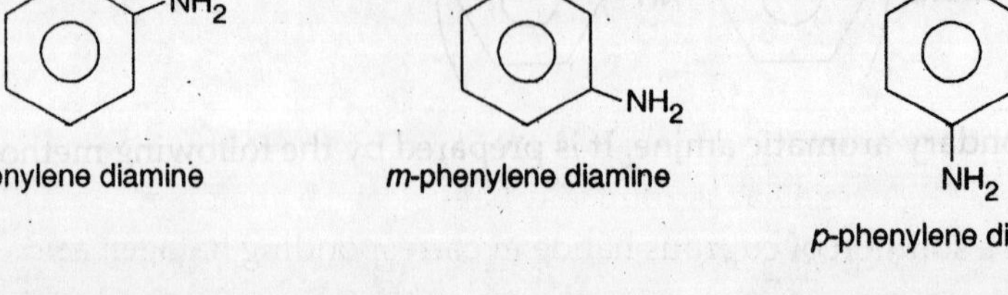

They are prepared by the reduction of corresponding nitroanilines and serve as the starting materials for the preparation of different types of dyes.

16.5 Aromatic Diazonium Compound

Aromatic diazonium compounds are synthetically a very important class of compounds. It is usually formed by the reaction of nitrous acid with primary aromatic amines.

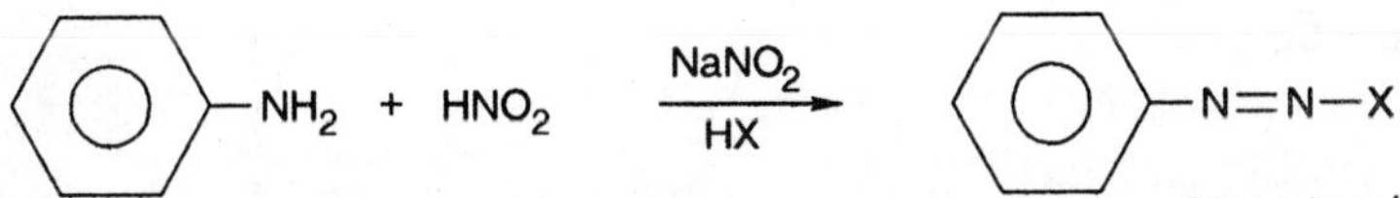

Diazonium salt

The structure of diazonium salt is a subject of much controversy. However, after much investigations it has been suggested that it exists as geometrical isomers having the structures.

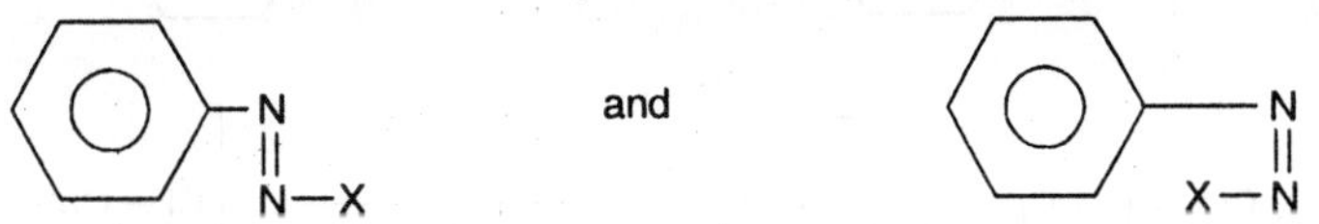

Anti Syn

The corresponding ion, diazonium ion, exhibits resonance as shown below:

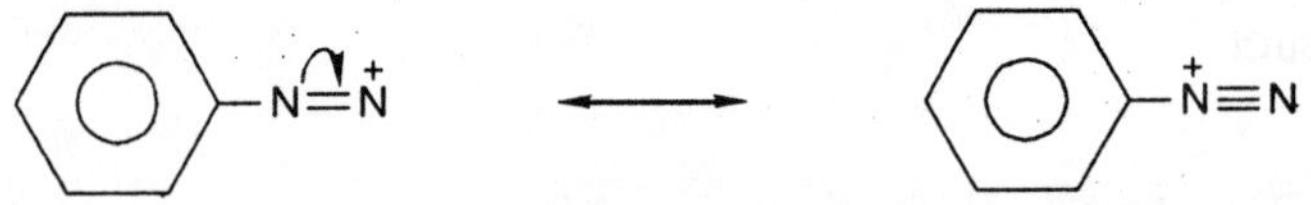

Such resonance may be extended to aromatic ring and for this, diazonium ion of aromatic amine is to some extent stabilised and is stabler than corresponding ion of aliphatic amines. Although stabilised to some extent due to extended resonance, yet it is sufficiently unstable and can be replaced by variety of groups. Owing to this characteristic aromatic diazonium compouds are extensively utilised in synthetic organic chemistry.

Reactions of Aromatic Diazonium Compounds: Properties of aromatic diazonium compounds may be considered under two headings as depicted below.

A. Reactions involving replacement of —N_2X group by other group with the evolution of nitrogen

i. *Formation of hydrocarbon*: Diazonium salt when warmed with alcohol, aromatic hydrocarbon is formed.

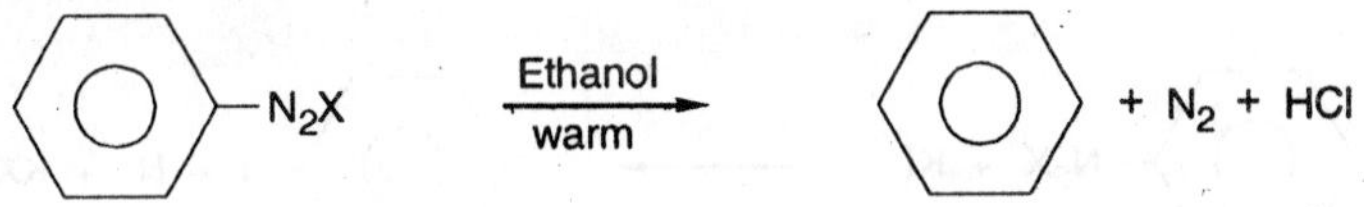

Diazonium salt Benzene

ii. *Formation of Phenols*: Diazonium salts offer an excellent method of preparing phenol. When diazonium salt is boiled with water, phenol is formed.

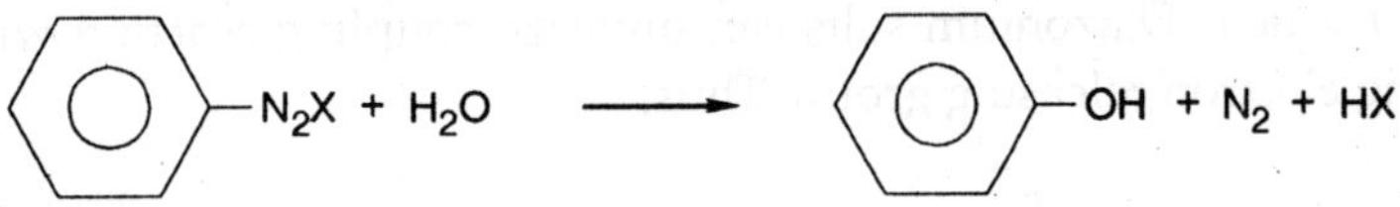

Phenol

iii. *Sandmeyer Reaction*: Diazo group may be replaced by halogen when its solution is passed through a solution of cuprous halide in corresponding halogen acid. Thus,

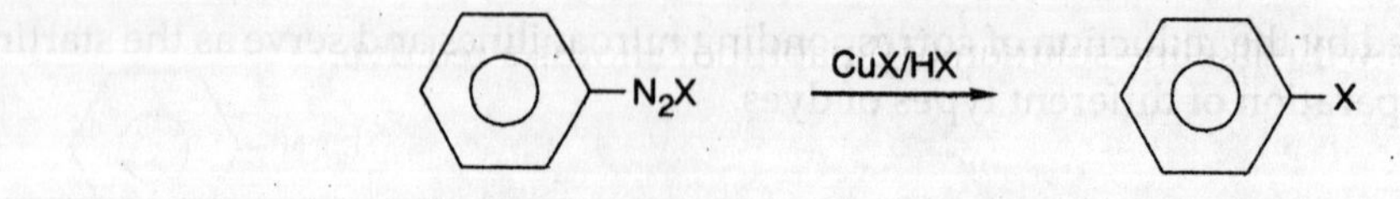

Halobenzene

This reaction is known as Sandmeyer reaction. The mechanistic path of this reaction has been suggested as elaborated below:

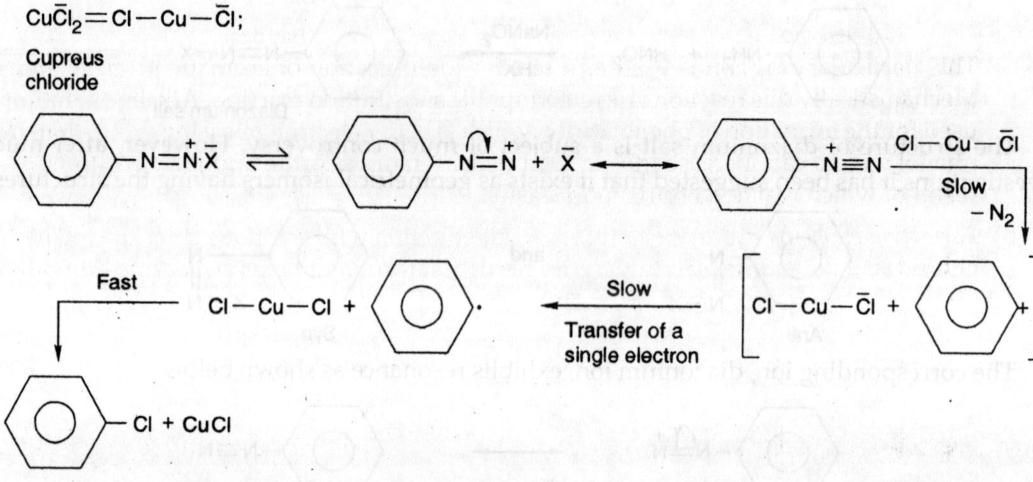

Sandmeyer reaction can also be carried out with KCN and cuprous cyanide (CuCN).

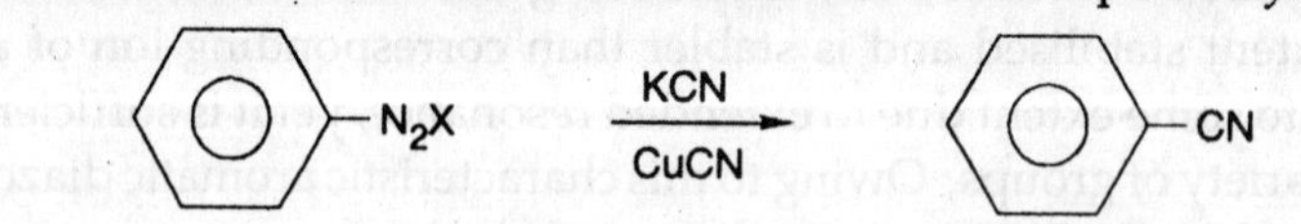

Phenyl cyanide

Sandmeyer reaction may also be carried out in presence of copper powder. Thus,

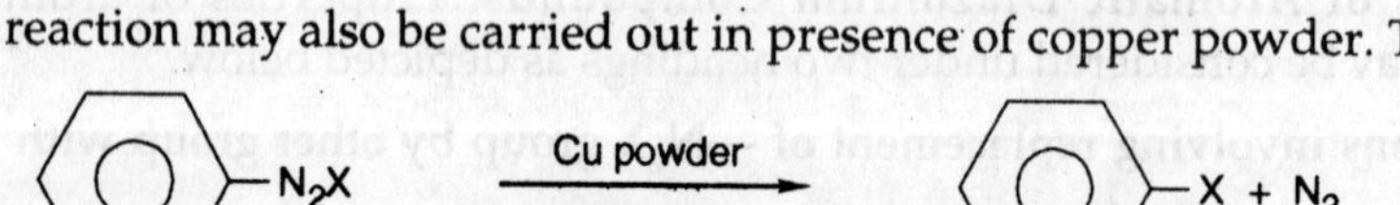

In some cases replacement of N_2X group takes place without using cuprous salt or copper powder. Thus,

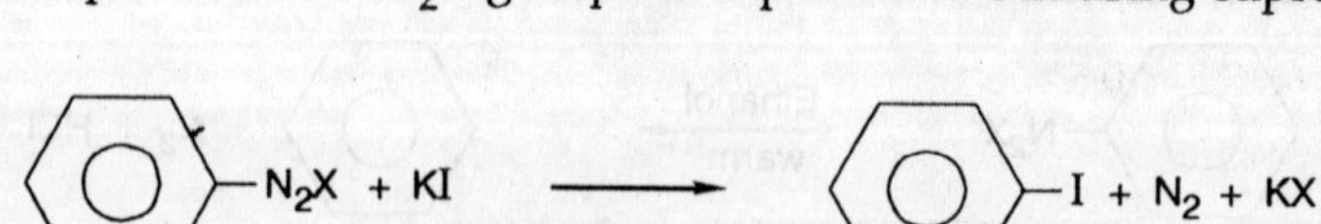

This is the best way of preparing aromatic nuclear iodo compound.

B. Reactions involving retention of nitrogen atom

(a) *Coupling reaction*: Diazonium salts can undergo coupling reaction with aromatic ring containing electron releasing group. Thus,

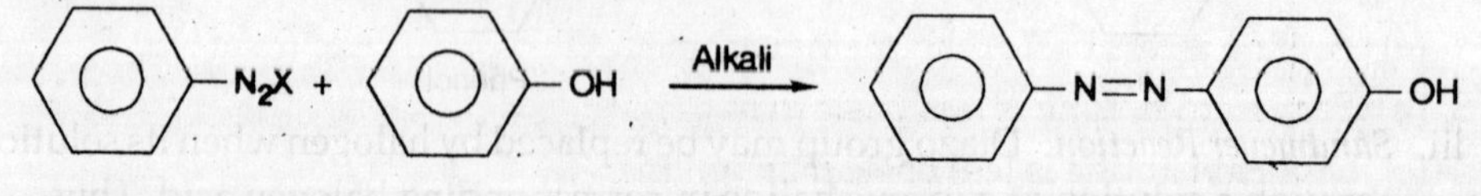

Such reaction with alkaline solution of β-naphthol affords a red dye.

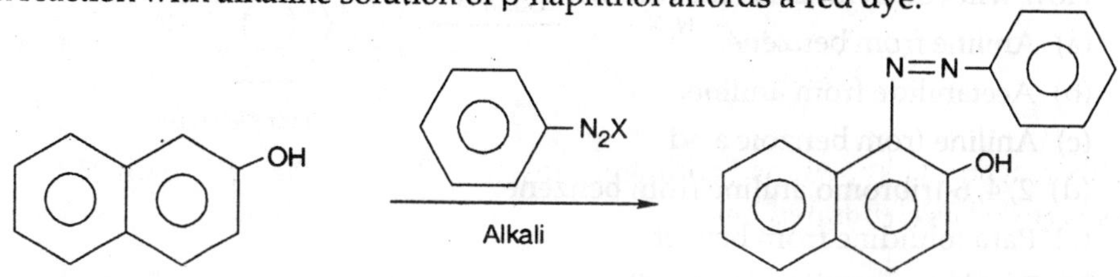

β-Naphthol   Red dye

This particular reaction is used as a test for identification of aromatic primary amine. Mechanistically this reaction is an electrophilic substitution reaction. Alkaline solution is used for the formation of phenolate ion which is better electron releasing group than free phenol and so can increase the electron density more at ortho and para positions as a result of which reaction occurs more easily.

(b) *Formation of phenyl hydrazine derivative*: On reduction with stannous chloride and hydro chloric acid diazonium salt undergoes reduction forming phenyl hydrazine derivative.

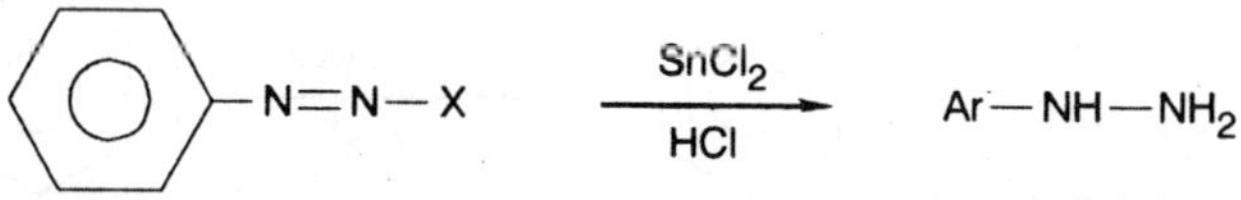

16.6 Uses of Aromatic Amines

Aromatic amines particularly aniline is widely used as a starting material for different types of compounds. Aromatic diamines are extensively used for the preparation of azo (bismark brown), azine (methylene blue), phenazine, etc dyes. However, the most mentionable uses of amines are in the field of medicine. Many aromatic amines or their derivatives such as acetanilide, exalgin (N-methyl acetanilide), *p*-aminophenol are important antipyretic. Again, phenacetin, para-acetamol, and enphorin which are the derivatives of aniline are used as analgesic.

Model Questions

1. Discuss some methods of preparation of aromatic amines. Explain why aromatic amines are less basic than aliphatic counter part.
2. What happens when aniline is treated with the following?
   (a) $NaNO_2/HCl$ at 0-5 °C.
   (b) Bromine water.
   (c) Chloroform and alcoholic potassium hydroxide.
3. How will you distinguish:
   (a) Aniline and ethyl amine.
   (b) Aniline and N-Methyl aniline.
   (c) Aniline and benzyl amine.
4. Explain why
   (a) Aniline is less basic than methyl amine.
   (b) Para nitro-aniline is less basic than aniline.
   (c) Diphenyl amine is less basic than aniline.

5. How will you synthesise the following:
   (a) Aniline from benzene.
   (b) Acetanilide from aniline.
   (c) Aniline from benzoic acid.
   (d) 2, 4, 6-tribromo aniline from benzene.
   (e) Para toluidine from benzene.
   (f) Para bromo aniline from aniline.

   Hints: (f)

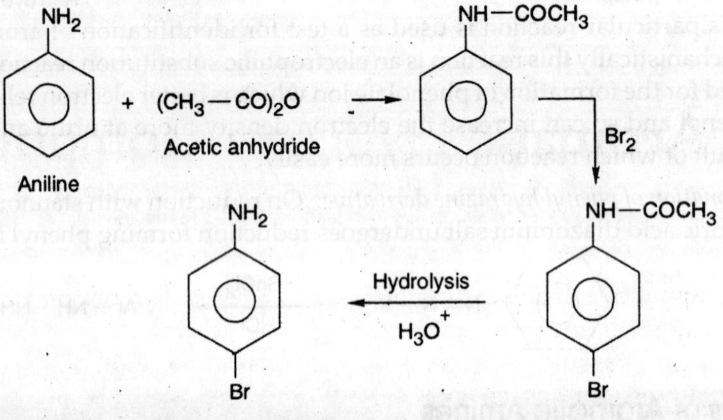

p-Bromo aniline

6. How benzene diazonium chloride is prepared in the laboratory?
   Hints: Aniline is dissolved in an aqueous solution of hydrochloric acid in a beaker and it is placed in an ice bath. To it aqueous solution of sodium nitrite is gradually added keeping the temperature of the reaction mixture at 0-5 °C. The solution of benzene diazonium chloride thus obtained is ready for next reaction.
7. Discuss the synthetic application of benzene diazonium compound.
8. Write notes on
   (a) Diazotisation.
   (b) Sandmeyer reaction.

CHAPTER SEVENTEEN

Aromatic Hydroxy Compounds

Aromatic compounds containing hydroxyl functions are known as aromatic hydroxy compounds and may be classified under two categories:

i. Aromatic alcohols are those which have hydroxyl functions only in the side-chain and

ii. *Phenols*: In phenols hydroxyl groups are directly lined to aromatic ring, i.e., they are nuclear hydroxy compound.

Of these two categories phenols are most important both from academic as well as synthetic point of view.

17.1 Phenols

Phenolic compounds may be classified under three groups, viz., (i) Monohydric phenol, (ii) Dihydric phenol and, (iii) Trihydric phenol. Among these monohydric phenols are of frequent occurrence and extensively studied compounds of this family.

17.1.1 Monohydric Phenols

As the name reveals, these phenols contain only one hydroxy group in the aromatic ring and may be represented by the structure shown below:

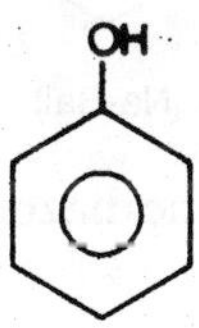

Monohydric phenol
or phenol

17.1.1.1 Methods of Preparation of Monohydric Phenols

Monohydric phenyls are generally prepared by the following methods:

(a) *From coal tar*: Middle oil fraction of coal tar contains phenolic substances which on fractional distillation affords phenols.

(b) *Fusion of sulphonic acids with alkali*: Aromatic sulphonic acids when fused with potassium or sodium hydroxide, phenols are formed.

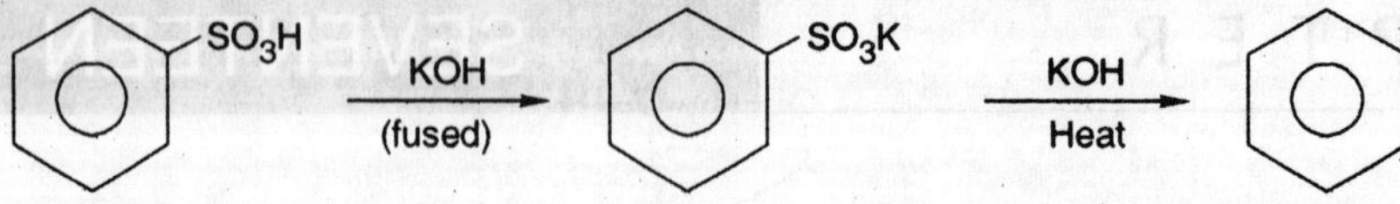

Benzene sulphonic acid — K-Salt — Phenol

(c) *Drastic treatment of aromatic nuclear halides*: Aromatic nuclear halides on hydrolysis with sodium or potassium hydroxide under drastic condition yield phenols.

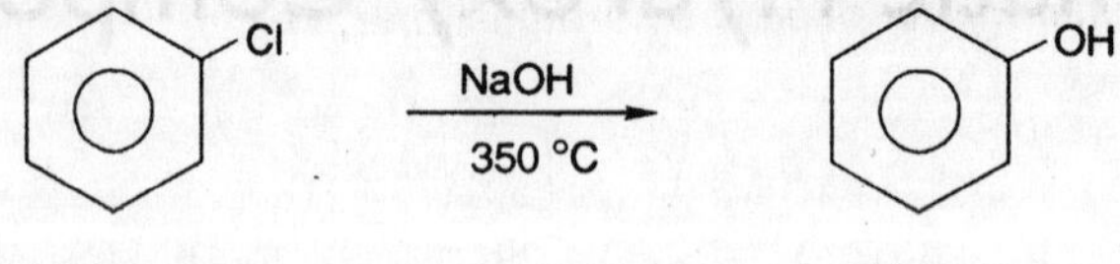

Chlorobenzene — Phenol

(d) *From aromatic nuclear halogen compounds containing electron withdrawing group*: Halogen in aromatic ring can be easily replaced by hydroxyl group under normal condition if there is deactivating (electron withdrawing) group in the ring. Thus,

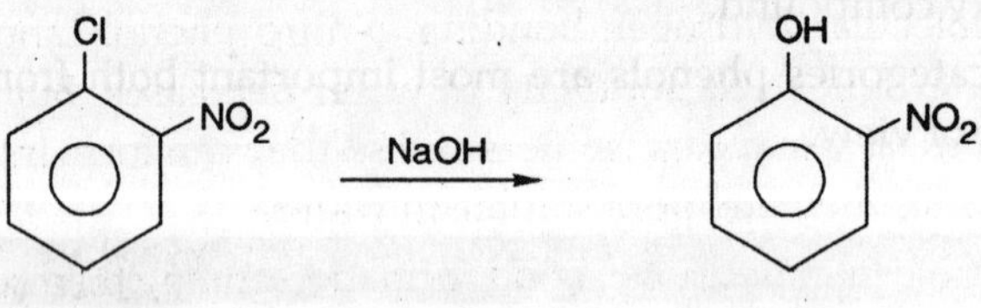

o-Nitro chloro-benzene — *o*-Nitro-phenol

(e) *Decarboxylation of phenolic acids*: Phenols can be prepared by the decarboxylation of phenolic acids by heating with sodalime.

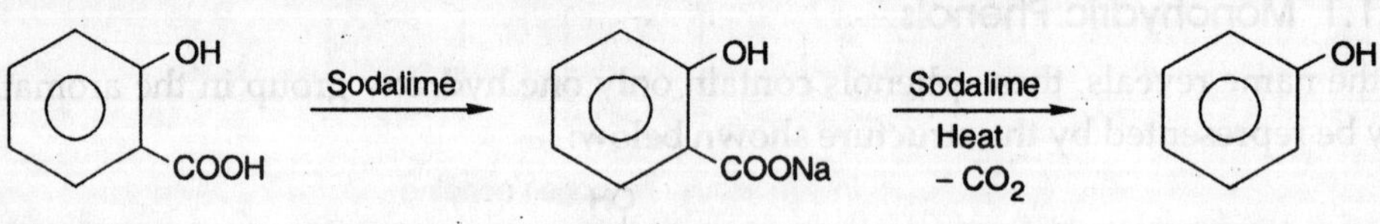

Salicylic Acid — Na-Salt — Phenol

(f) *From aromatic diazonium salts*: Aromatic diazonium salt in aqueous solution on distillation furnishes phenol.

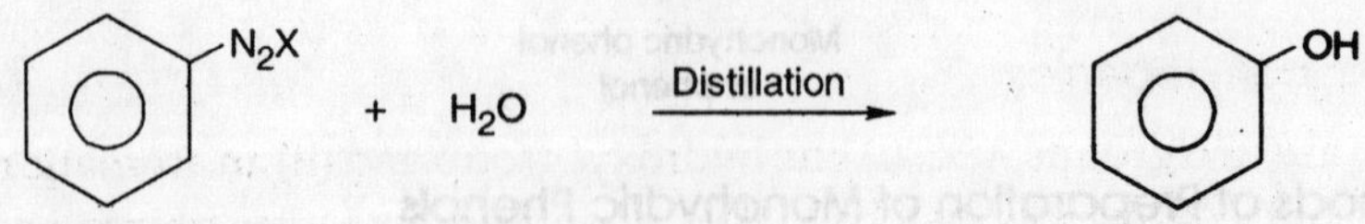

Diazonium Salt — Phenol

17.1.1.2 Properties of Monohydric Phenols

17.1.1.2.1 Physical Properties

Phenols may be solids or liquids with characteristic carbolic odour. That is why simple phenol is known as carbolic acid. They are soluble in water due to formation of intermolecular hydrogen bonding with water.

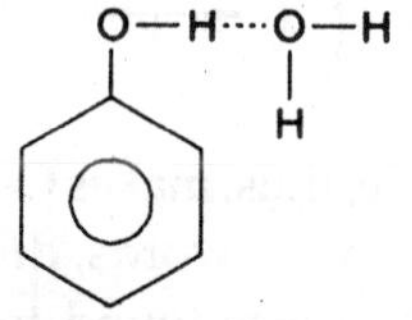

Hydrogen bonding

However, *ortho* nitrophenol is less soluble than its *meta* and *para* isomers. This is due to formation of *intramolecular hydrogen bond* by *ortho* isomer, i.e.,

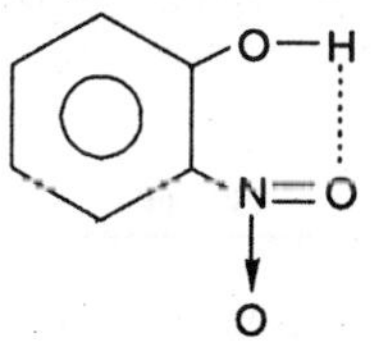

o-Nitrophenol

Intramolecular hydrogen bond formations

Due to this intramolecular hydrogen bonding, *o*-nitro phenol cannot form *intermolecular hydrogen* bond with water and so its solubility in water decreases. But no such *intramolecular hydrogen bond* is formed in *meta* and *para* isomers and so they can form intermolecular hydrogen bond with water and hence they are more soluble in water.

Again, due to intermolecular hydrogen bond formation among themselves by simple phenol, they can exist as associated molecules. So in general, simple phenols have higher boiling points than toluene or other aromatic liquid hydrocarbons.

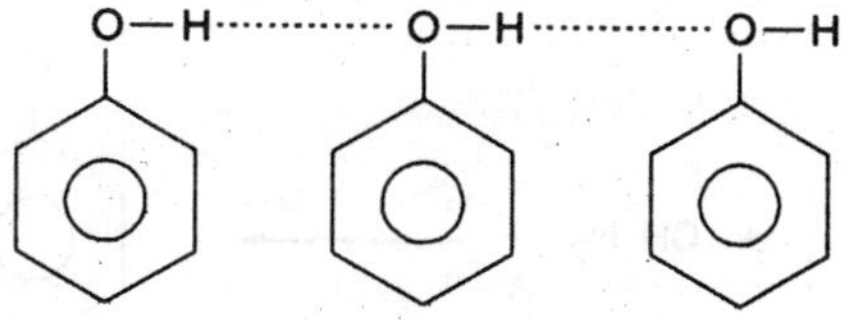

Intermolecular hydrogen bonding

However, *o*-nitrophenol, as it is incapable of forming intermolecular hydrogen bonding, cannot exist as associated molecules, consequently its boiling point is lowered as compared to simple phenols or its *meta* and *para* isomers which as mentioned can form associated molecules due to intermolecular hydrogen bonding.

17.1.1.2.2 Chemical Properties

In phenols, there are two groups, viz., (i) one hydroxyl group and (ii) an aromatic nucleus. Hence the chemical activities of phenols may be looked upon from two view points, i.e.,

i Effect of aromatic nucleus upon hydroxyl group.

ii. Influence of hydroxyl function on the aromatic nucleus.

A. Effect of aromatic ring upon hydroxyl group:

Since hydroxyl group is directly linked to the aromatic ring it participates in resonance with the aromatic ring and so phenol exists as resonance hybrid of the following contributing structures.

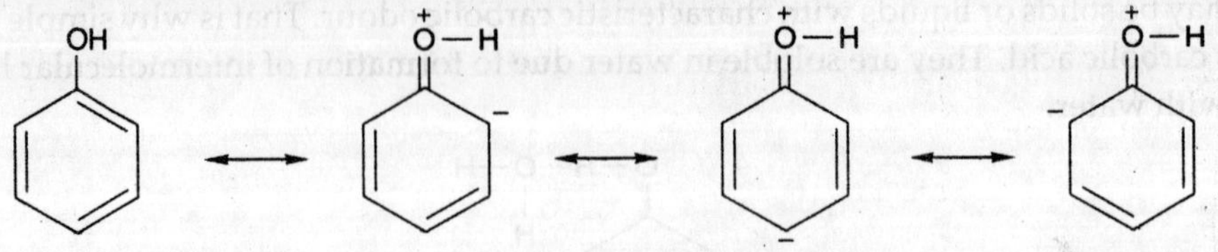

Acidic Nature: The above resonance, thus, makes O—H bond very weak and hence hydrogen atom can be readily replaceable. Or in other words, due to above resonance phenols behave as proton donar, i.e., acidic and in fact, it was found to be so. The acidic nature of phenols is manifested by its following behaviours.

(a) Phenols react with litmus solution when blue litmus turns red.

(b) In alkaline solution it readily dissolves forming salt.

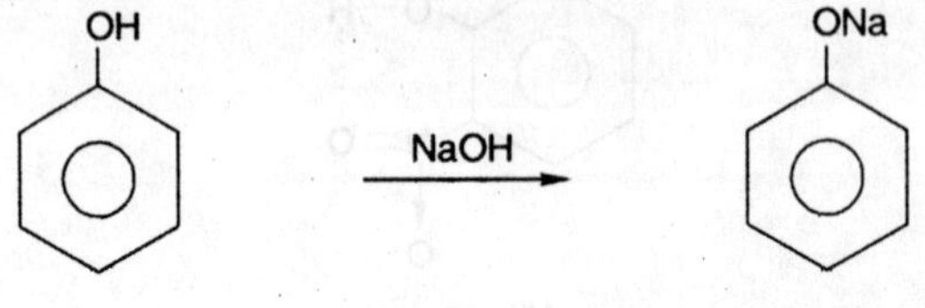

Na-Phenate

(c) They smoothly undergo acetylation and benzoylation reaction.

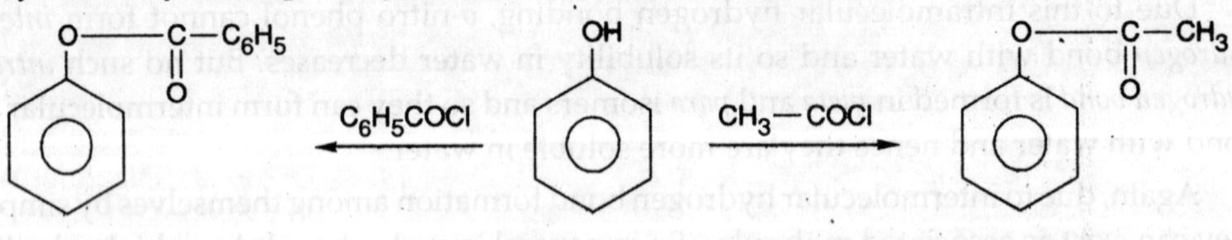

Phenylbenzonate Phenyl acetate

(d) Like carboxylic acid it can be methylated by diazomethane.

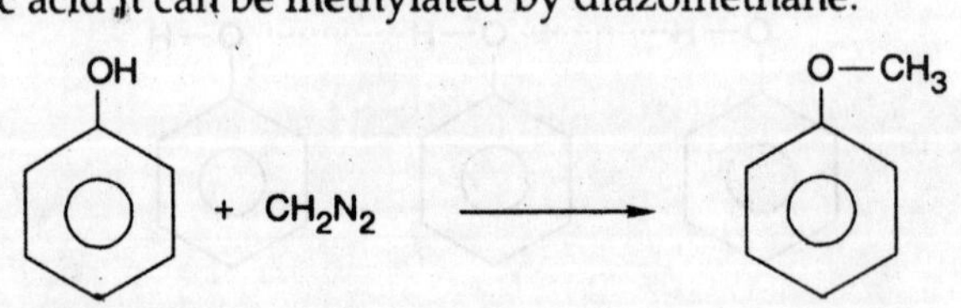

Mechanistically, this methylation may be explained as under:

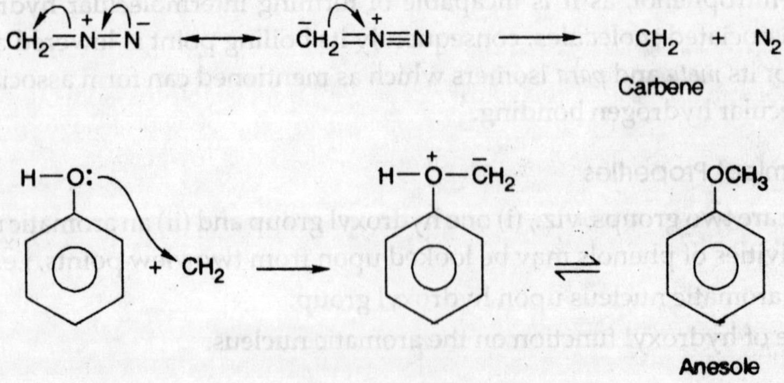

Effect of substituent on acidity of phenol: It may be mentioned that acidity of phenol depends upon the nature of the substituents present in the aromatic ring. Thus, when electron withdrawing group is present, due to its electron withdrawing effect acidity of phenolic hydroxyl is increased, i.e.,

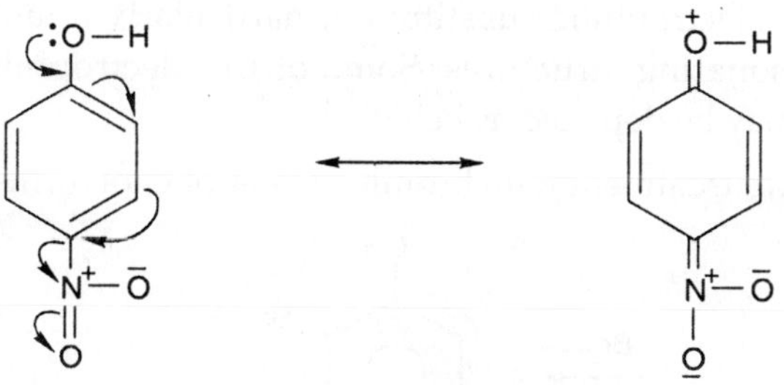

That is why nitrophenol is more acidic than simple phenol. It may be remembered that since OH group is *ortho* and *para* directing in nature, enhancement of acidity becomes maximum when such electron withdrawing group or groups are present at *ortho* and *para* positions with respect to phenolic hydroxyl function. Again, it has been observed that with the increase in the number of electron withdrawing groups in the ring, acidity increases. For this reason the order of acidity of the following series stands as under:

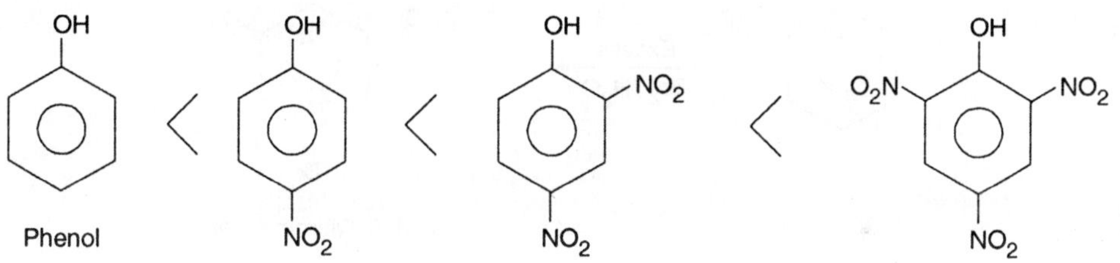

Phenol < *p*-Nitrophenol < 2, 4-dinitrophenol < Picric acid

Thus, picric acid is a very strong acid. Further, as expected acidity of phenol decreases when electron releasing group is present in the ring. Thus, amino phenol is less acidic than phenol. This is due to the fact that the electron releasing group present may also participate in resonance along with aromatic ring. As a result, lone pair of electron on oxygen atom of phenolic hydroxyl is not fully contributed towards resonance which reduces the acidity to some extent, i.e.,

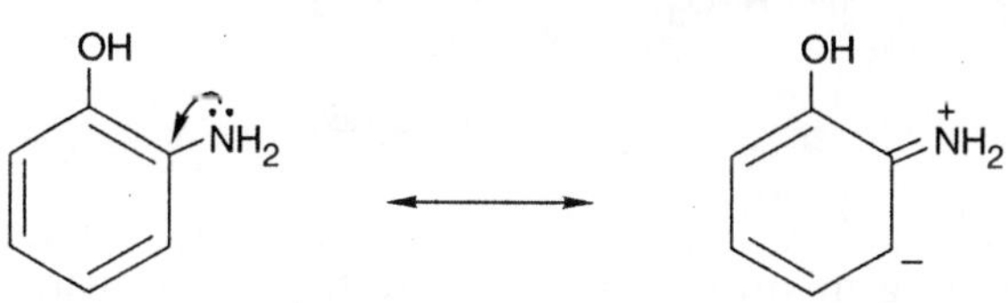

Thus, effect of substituent on the acidity of phenol may be expressed as under:

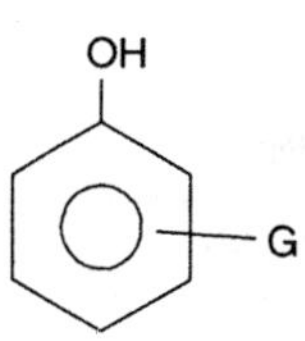

G is any group at *ortho* and *para* positions

When G is electron withdrawing, acidity increases but when it is electron releasing in nature, acidity of phenol is decreased.

B. Influence of hydroxyl function on aromatic ring:

As hydroxyl group is electron releasing, in general it activiates the aromatic ring. Accordingly, phenol highly favours electrophilic substitution, particularly at *ortho* and *para* positions as envisaged from its resonating structures. Some of the electrophilic substitution reactions undergone by phenol may be depicted as below:

(a) *Halogenation*: On treatment with bromine water phenol forms bromo compound.

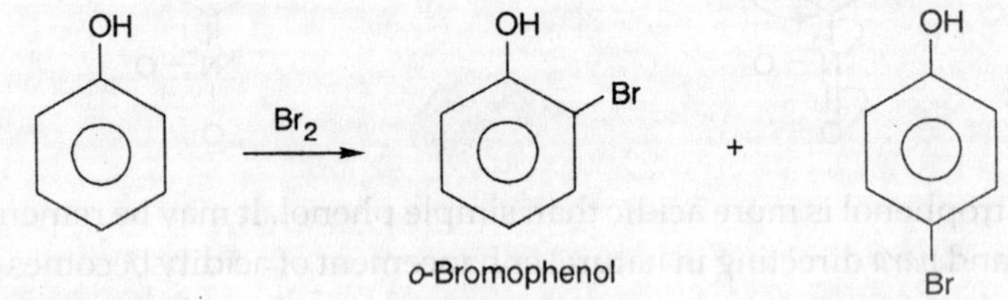

o-Bromophenol

p-Bromophenol

In presence of excess of bromine water, tribromophenol is formed.

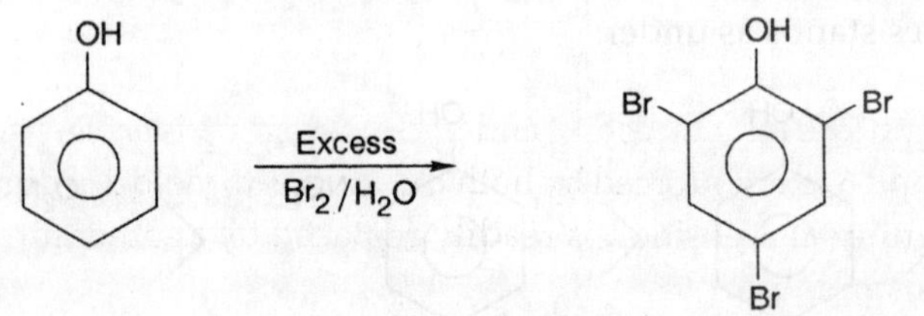

2, 4, 6-Tribromophenol

This reaction is employed for the quantitative estimation of phenol.

(b) *Nitration*: When nitration is carried out with concentrated nitric acid, mono-nitrophenols are formed.

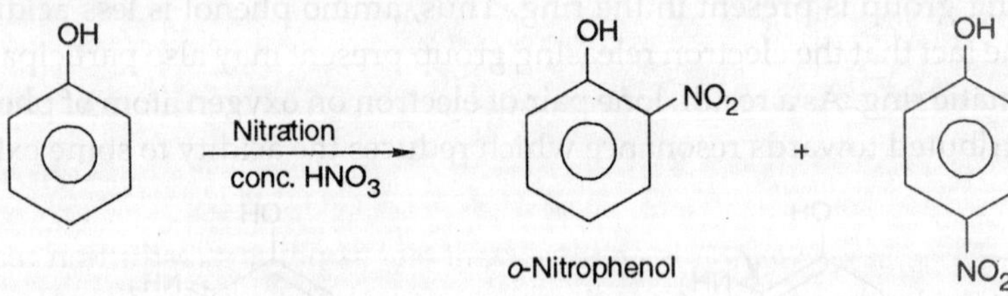

o-Nitrophenol

p-Nitrophenol

But when nitrating mixture is used as nitrating agent, trinitrophenol (picric acid) is obtained.

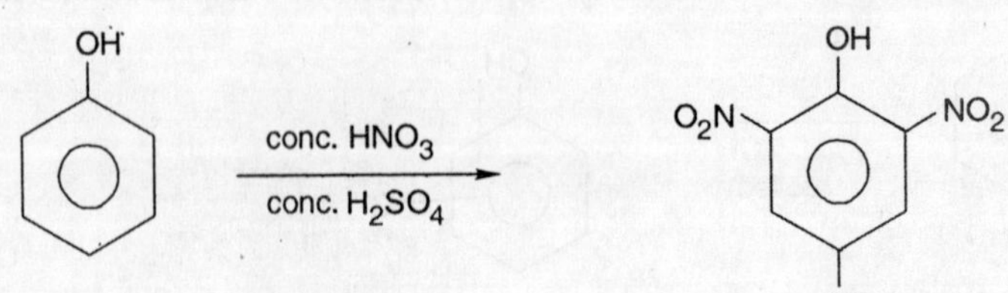

2, 4, 6-Trinitrophenol (Picric acid)

Formation of picric acid in presence of mixed acid is due to the fact that in this reaction initially concentrated sulphuric acid reacts with phenol to form parahydroxy sulphonic acid.

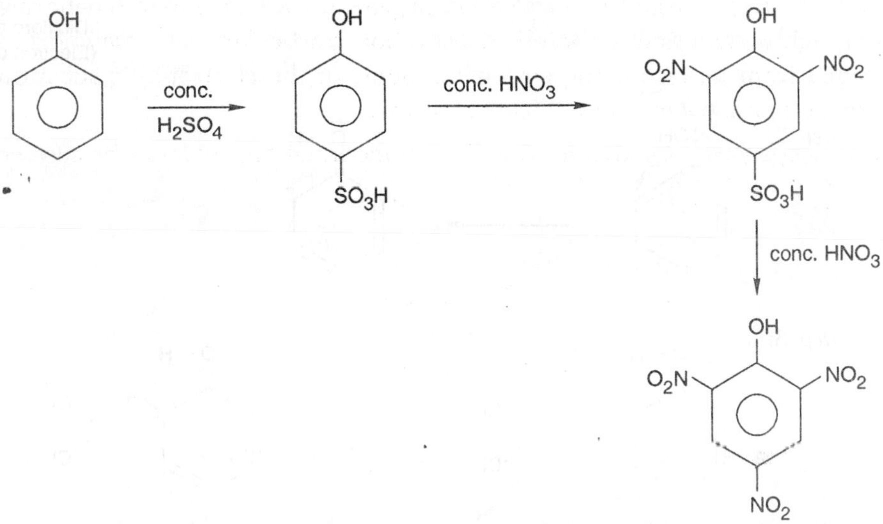

Sulphonic group is *meta* directing and hydroxyl group is *ortho*/*para* orienting. As a result positions 2 and 6 are reinforced by both the groups to yield 2, 6 dinitro compound. Finally sulphonic group at 4 position is readily replaced by another nitro group to form easily the trinitro compound.

(c) *Sulphonation*: Phenols readily undergo sulphonation reaction to afford *ortho* and *para* hydroxy sulphonic acids.

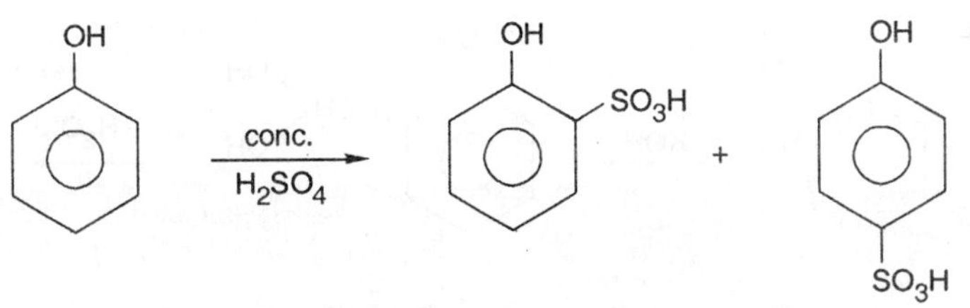

(d) *Reimer-Tiemann reaction*: It is an important electrophilic substitution reaction of phenol and is frequently employed for the preparation of phenolic aldehydes. The reaction is carried out by boiling phenol with chloroform in alcoholic potassium hydroxide solution.

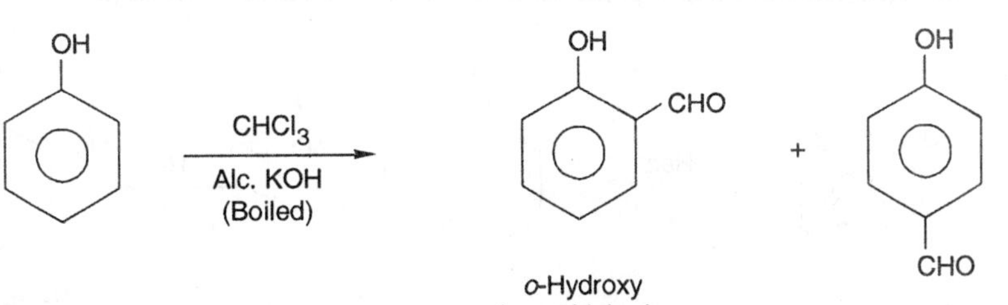

o-Hydroxy benzaldehyde (Salicyldehyde)

p-Hydroxy benzaldehyde

Mechanistically the reaction is believed to proceed as under:

Step 1:

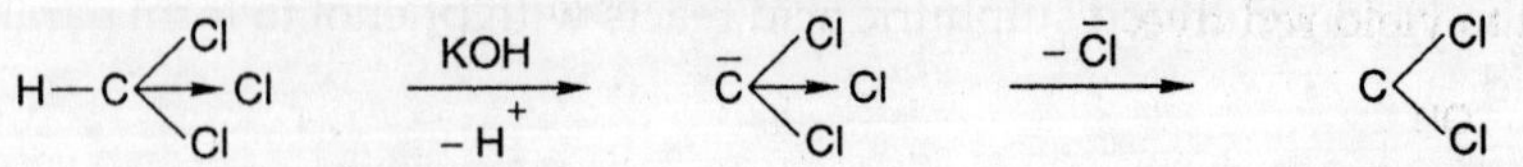

Dichloro-carbene
(Electron deficient)

Step 2:

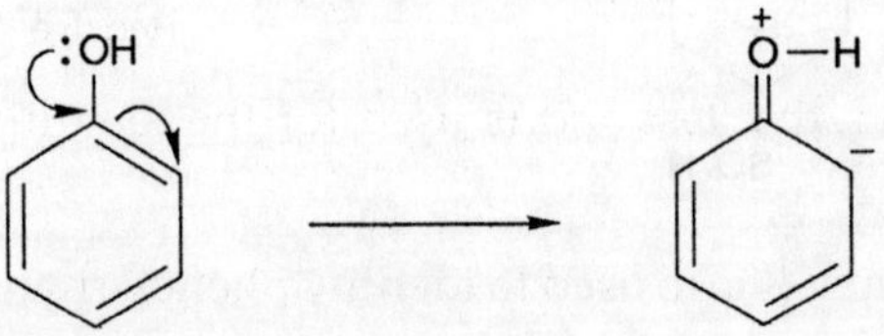

Step 3:

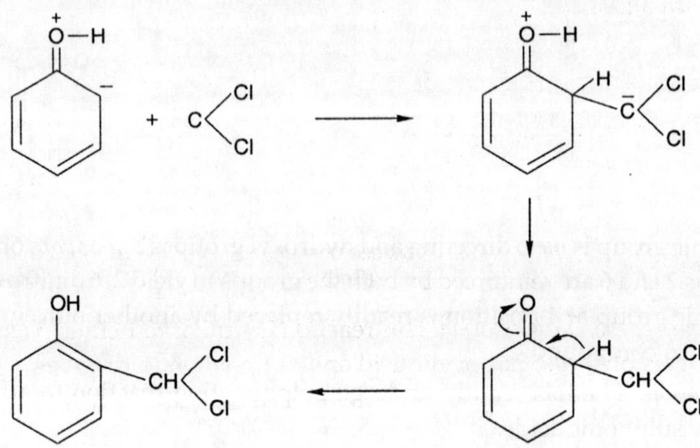

Step 4:

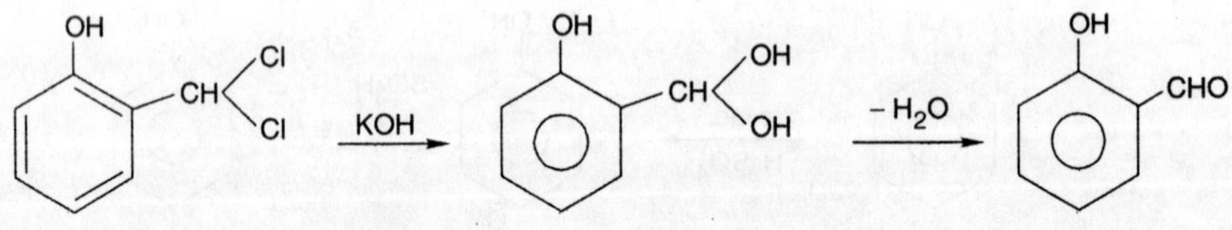

o-Hydroxy
benzaldehyde

Similarly, *p*-isomer is formed.

(e) *Kolbe-Schmidt reaction*: It is an electrophilic substitution reaction where carbon dioxide serves the function of electrophile to form hydroxy carboxylic acid.

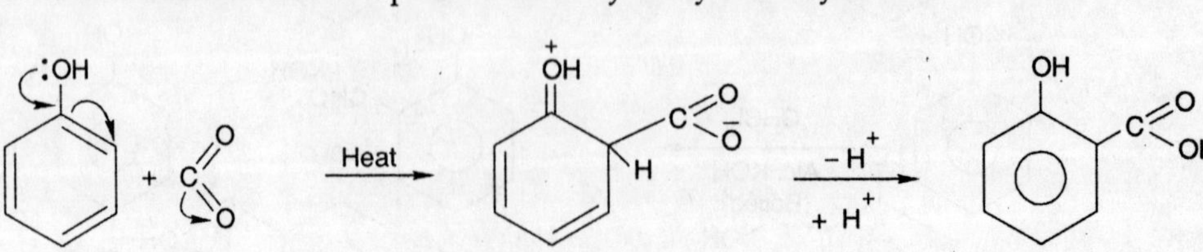

Salicylic acid

(f) *Coupling reaction*: Alkaline solution of phenol in cold condition can couple with diazonium salt to yield red dye.

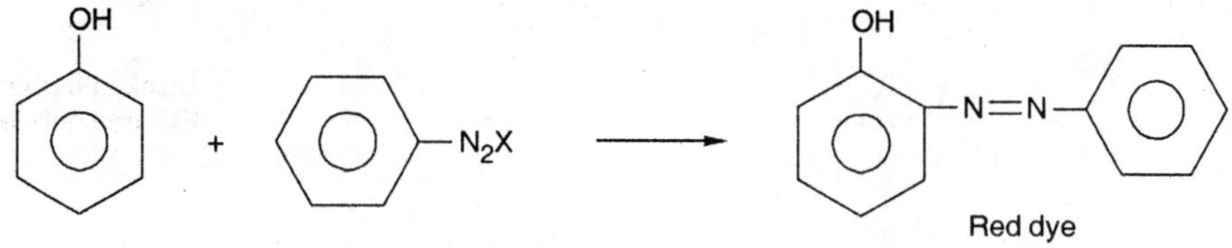

This reaction is known as back dye test and is used for the identification of phenolic hydroxyl group.

(g) *Leibermann-reaction*: This reaction is also used to identify phenolic hydroxyl group and is carried out initially treating phenol with nitrous acid and next the product formed is treated with alkali.

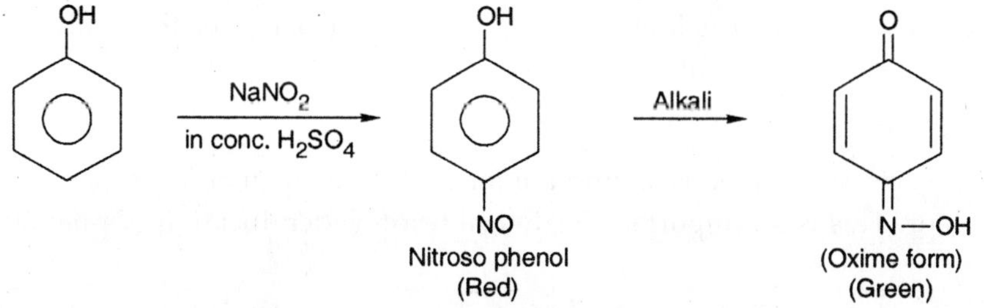

(h) *Reaction with carbon tetrachloride:* This reaction is similar to Reimer-Tiemann reaction but the product is phenolic carboxylic acid and not phenolic aldehydes.

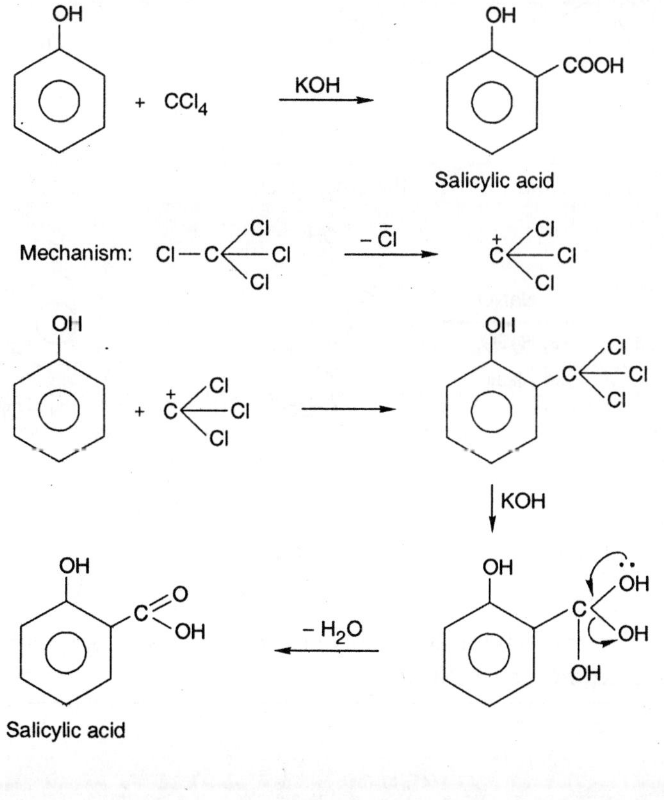

(i) *Reaction with formaldehyde*: Phenol on treatment with formaldehyde in presence of acid or alkali, phenol-formaldehyde polymer known as *bakelite* is formed.

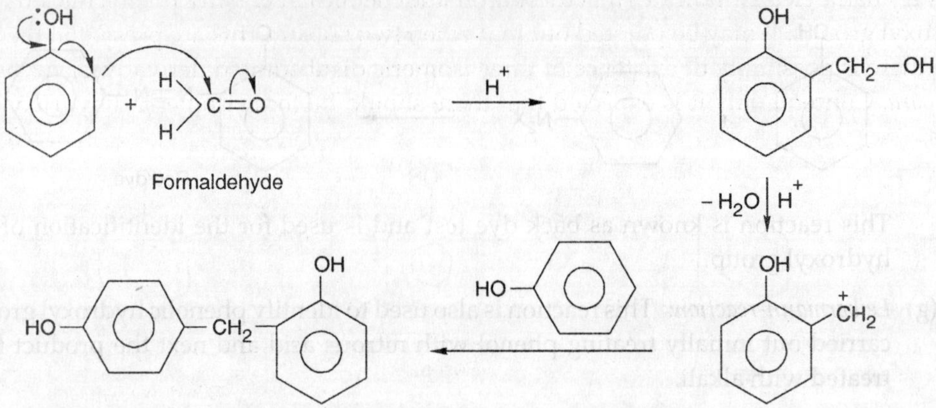

Further molecules of formaldehyde and phenol react to lengthen the chain and ultimately a resinous polymer, bakelite, is obtained.

- *Other type of reactions*

i. Phenol reacts with aqueous solution of ferric chloride to generate violet, green or wine red colour. This is an important analytical test for identification of phenolic hydroxyl group.

ii. When distilled with Zn-dust, phenol forms aromatic hydrocarbon.

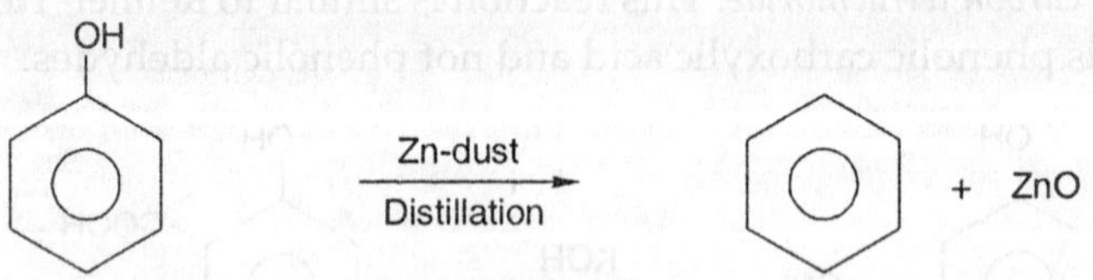

PROBLEM 17.1

(a) Suggest the mechanism of the following reactions:

i.

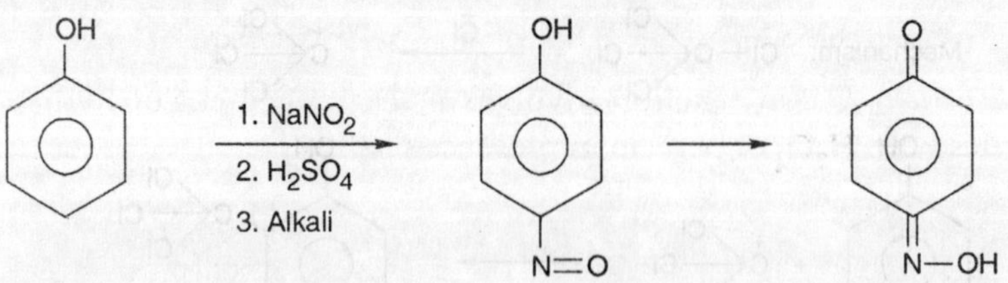

ii.

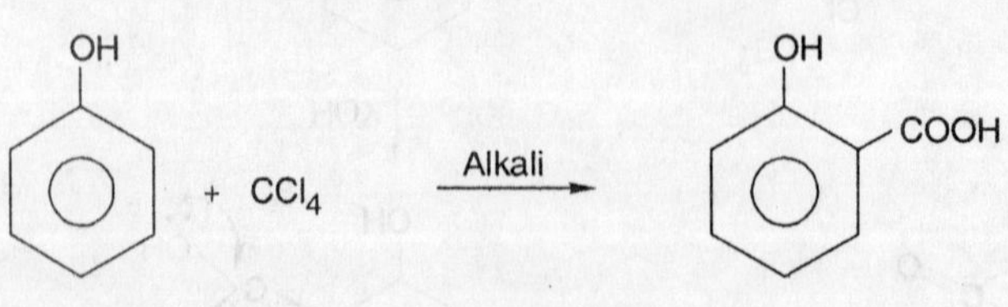

(b) Explain why picricacid is formed in mixed acid ($HNO_3 + H_2SO_4$) but only mononitrophenol is formed in conc. HNO_3.

17.2 Dihydroxy Benzenes

The very name clearly indicates that these aromatic chemicals contain a phenyl nucleus with two hydroxyl groups. It may be pointed out that when two substituents are present in the aromatic ring, there is possibility of existence of three isomeric disubstituted derivatives, viz, *ortho*, *meta* and *para*. Consequently it is expected that there should be three isomeric dihydroxy benzene. Thus,

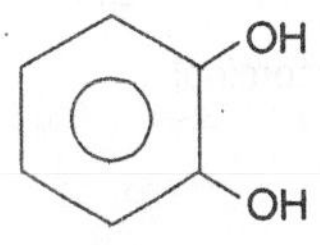

o-Dihydroxy benzene (Catechol)

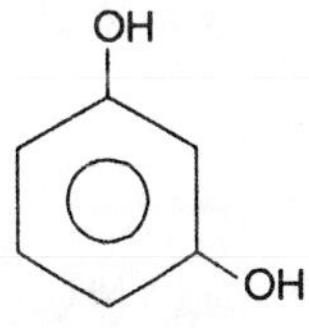

m-Dihydroxy benzene (Resorcinol)

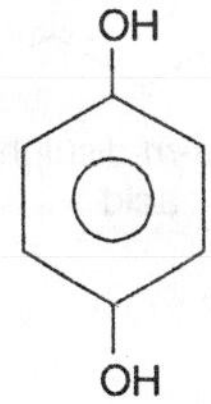

p-Dihydroxy benzene (Quinol)

17.2.1 Preparation of Dihydroxy Benzenes

1. *Catechol:* Catechol is prepared mainly by the following methods:

(a) *Fusion of phenol sulphonic acid with alkali*

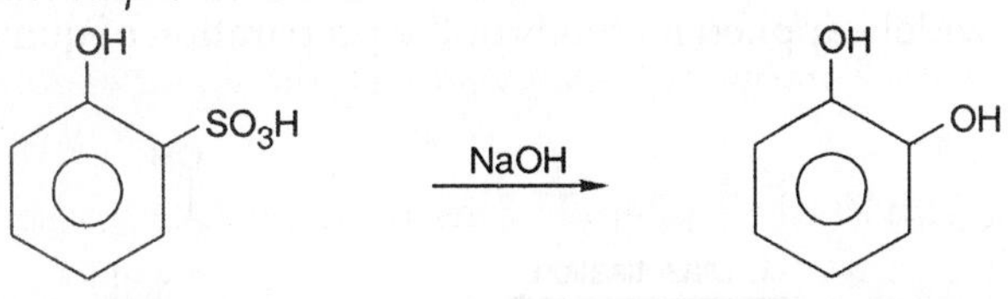

o-Hydroxy benzene sulphonic acid — Catechol

(b) *Hydrolysis of ortho chlorophenol*

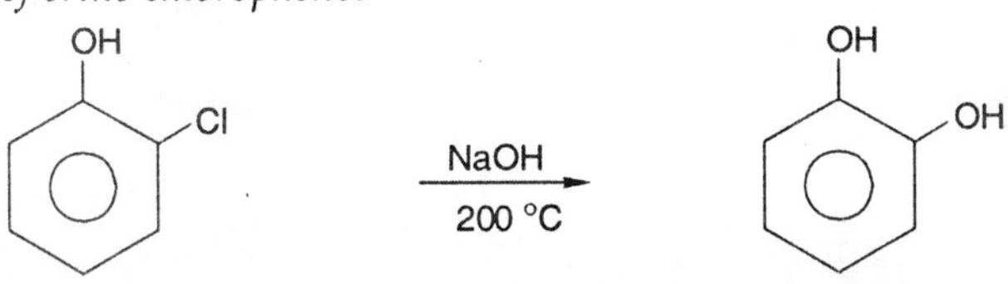

o-Chloro phenol — Catechol

(c) *Dakin reaction*: Dakin reaction involves a rearrangement of hydroxy aromatic aldehydes with H_2O_2 or peracid in presence of alkali.

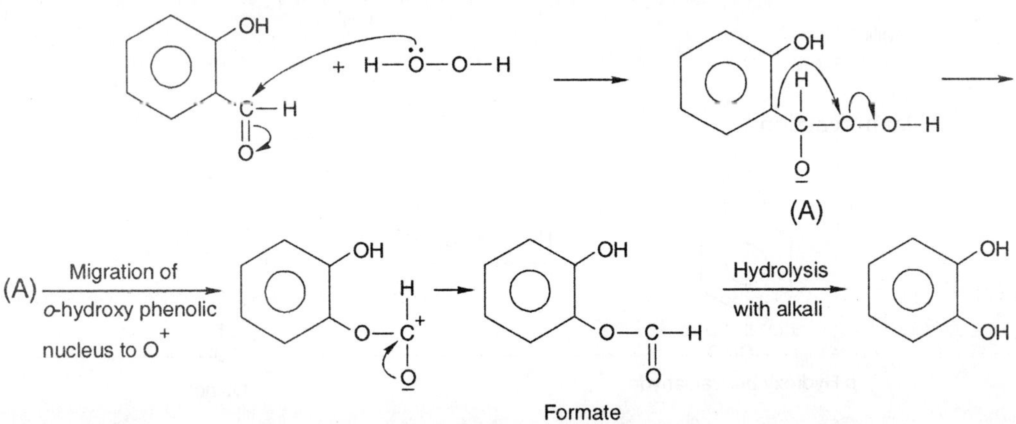

It is analogous to Baeyer-Villiger reaction. This reaction is also applicable to *p*-hydroxy benzal-dehyde.

2. *Resorcinol*: Resorcinol is most conveniently prepared by the following methods:

(a)

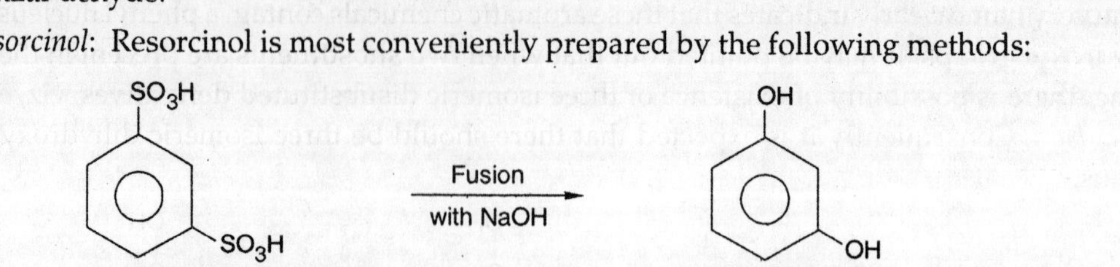

Benzene-*m*-disulphonic acid → Resorcinol

(b)

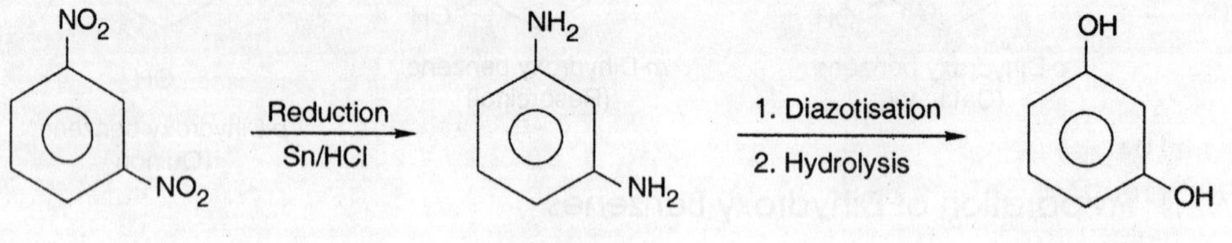

m-Phenylene diamine → Resorcinol

3. *Quinol*: Most widely applied methods of the preparation of quinol are as noted below:

(a)

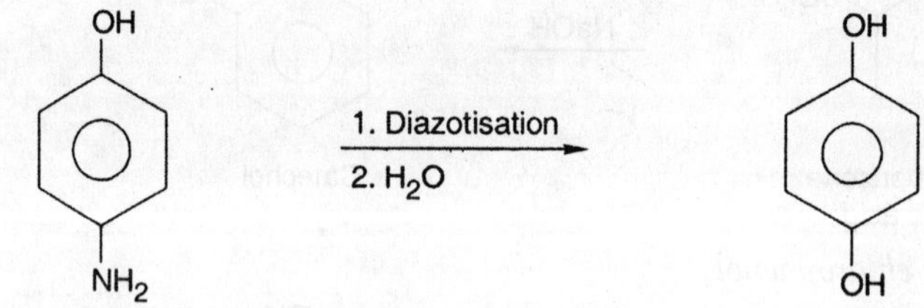

p-Aminophenol → Quinol

(b)

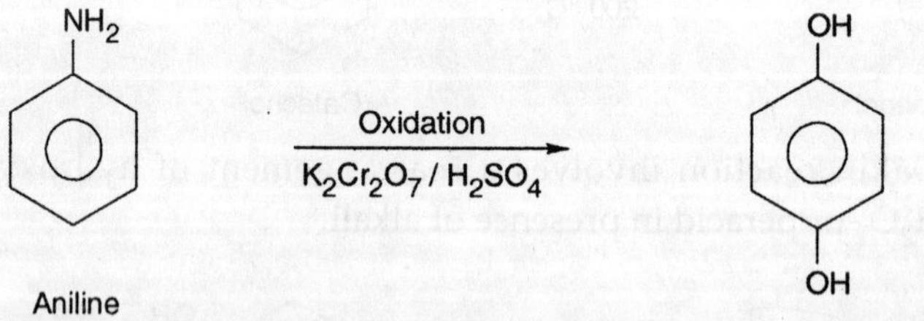

Aniline → Quinol

(c) Dakin reaction

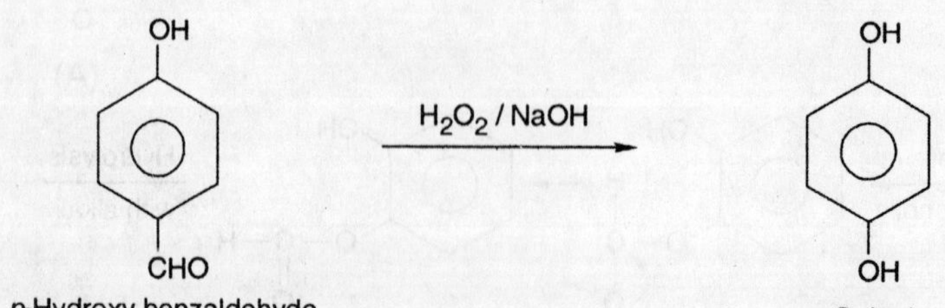

p-Hydroxy benzaldehyde → Quinol

17.2.2 Properties of Dihydroxy Benzenes

All these isomeric dihydroxy benzenes are colourless solids in the pure state and are soluble in water, ethanol and ether. They are highly oxidisable substances and are oxidsed by Fehling's solution, Tollen's reagent and even by ferric chloride solution. Catechol and quinol are oxidised to corresponding quinones while resorcinol furnishes a very complex-oxidation product of unknown structure.

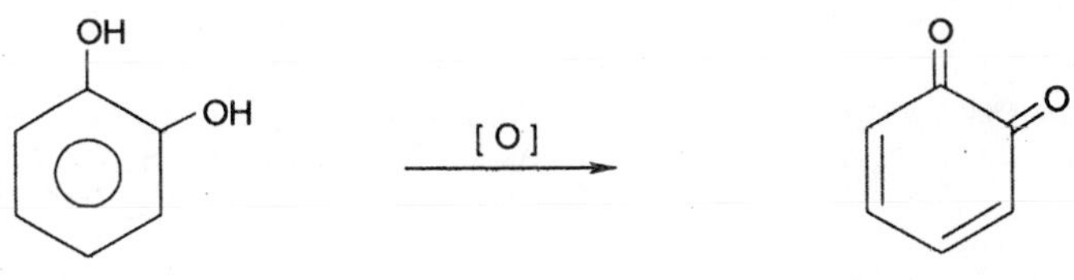

Catechol o-Benzoquinone

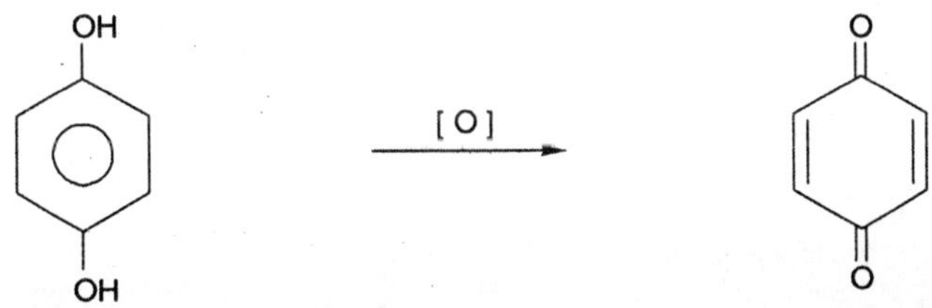

p-Benzoquinone

Electrophilic Substitution Reactions: It may be mentioned that the presence of two hydroxyl groups makes the aromatic ring highly active towards electrophilic substitution reaction. Some interesting electrophilic substitution reactions of these phenols are noted below:

i.

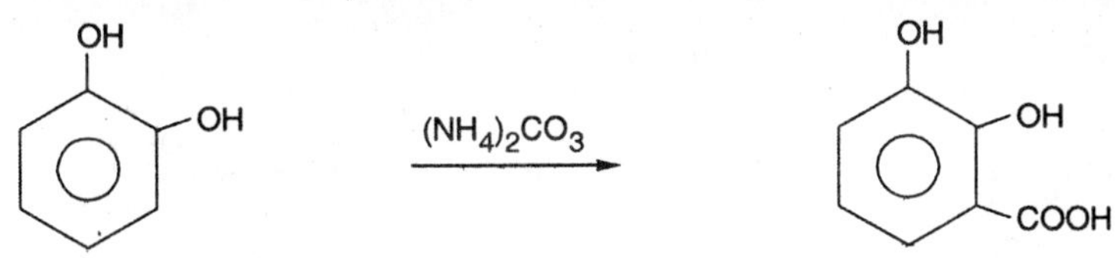

Catechol Protocatechuic acid

ii.

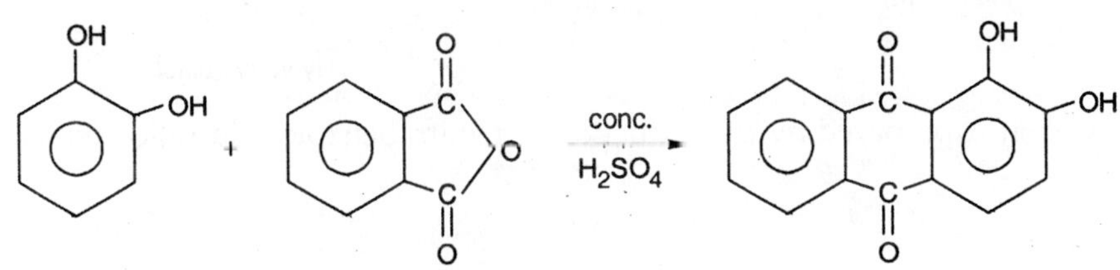

Phthalic anhydride

iii.

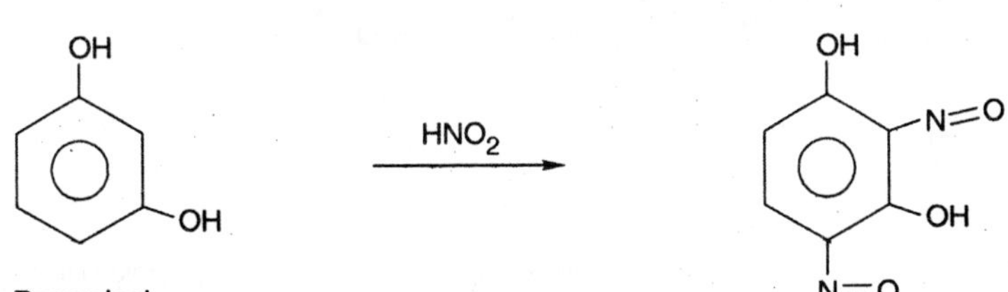

Resorcinol Dinitroso-resorcinol

iv.

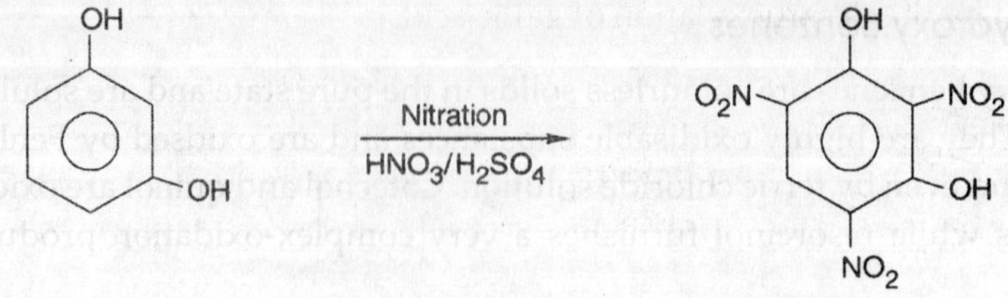

Styphnic acid

v.

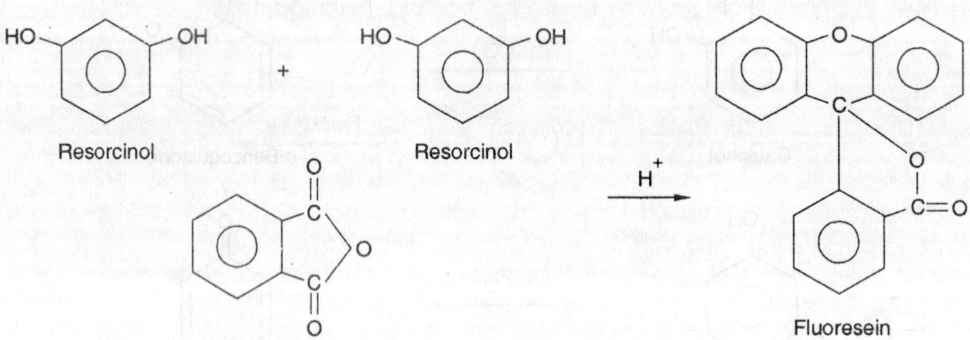

Phthalic anhydride

17.3 Trihydric Phenols (Trihydroxy Benzenes)

The most important members of trihydric phenols are phloroglucinol, pyrogallol and hydroxy quinol.

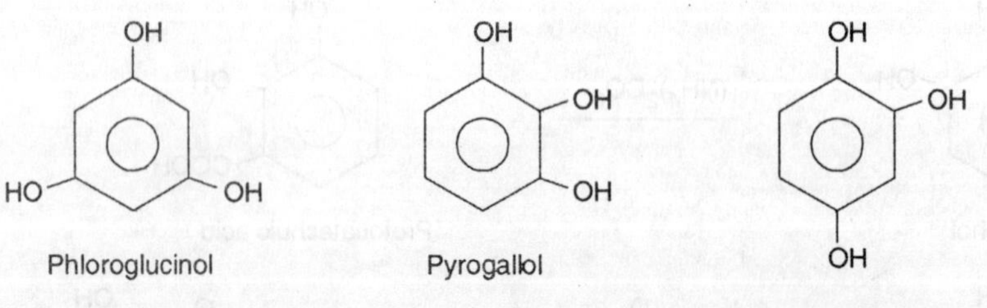

Phloroglucinol: It is prepared by the reduction of trinitrobenzoic acid followed by boiling with water.

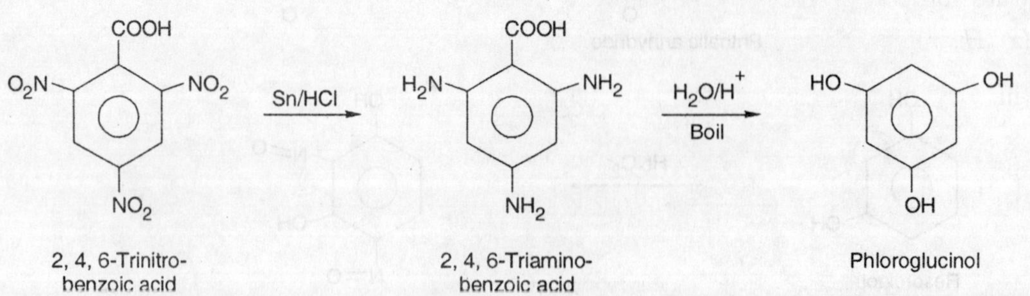

Pyrogallol: It is prepared by the decarboxylation of gallic acid.

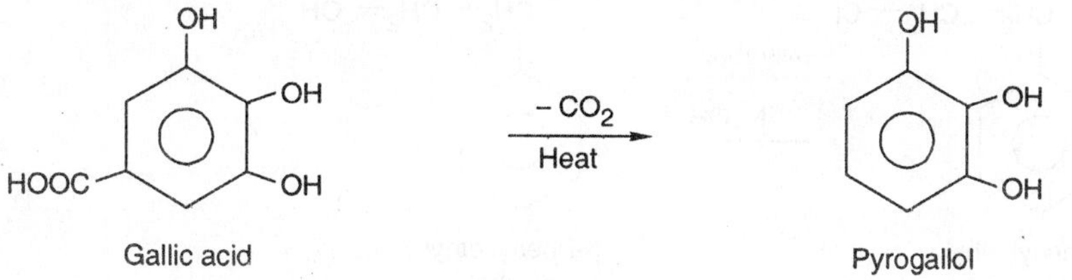

Hydroxy quinol: It is obtained by the acetylation of *p*-benzoquinone.

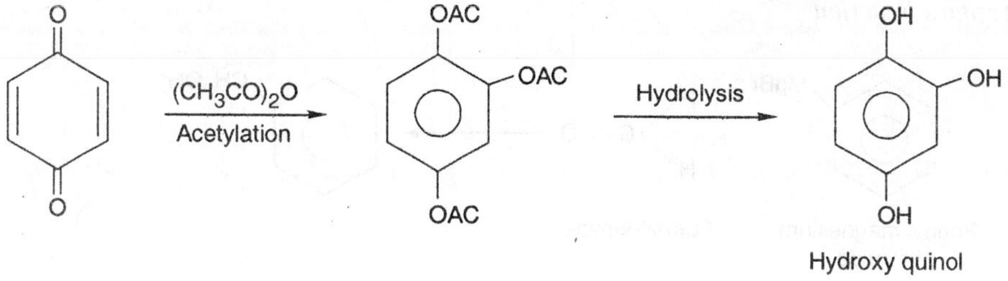

PROBLEM 17.2

> How will you prepare the following:
> (a) Protocatechnic acid, (b) Styphnic acid, (c) Fluorescein?

17.4 Aromatic Alcohols

In these compounds hydroxyl function is present in the side chain. Two most common members of this class of alcohol are as mentioned below:

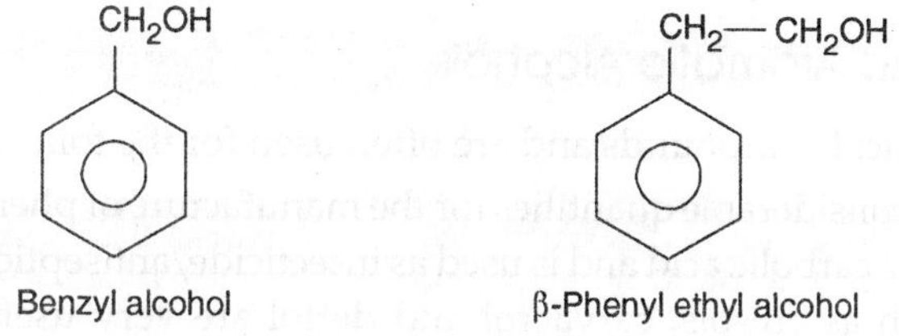

17.4.1 Preparation of Aromatic Alcohols

They are normally prepared by the following methods:

(a) *Hydrolysis of aromatic side chain halides:*

i.

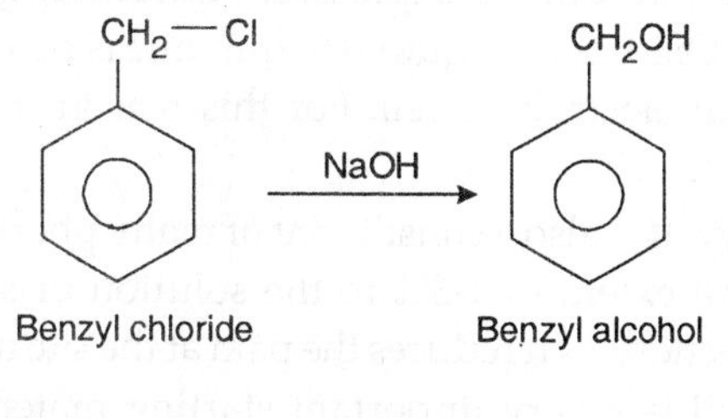

ii. 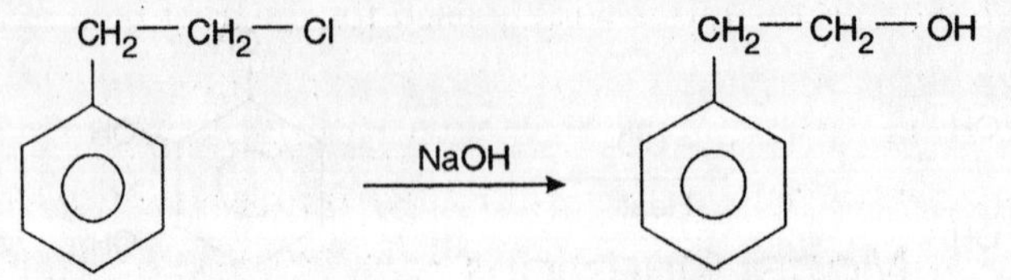

β-Phenyl ethyl chloride β-Phenyl ethyl alcohol

(b) *Grignard Reaction*

i. 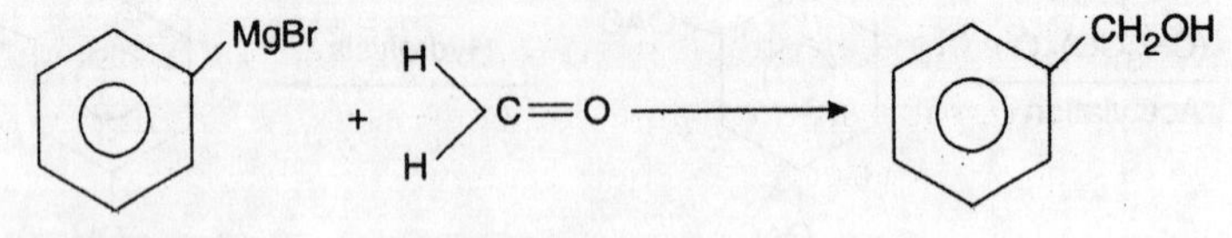

Phenyl magnesium bromide Formaldehyde

ii. 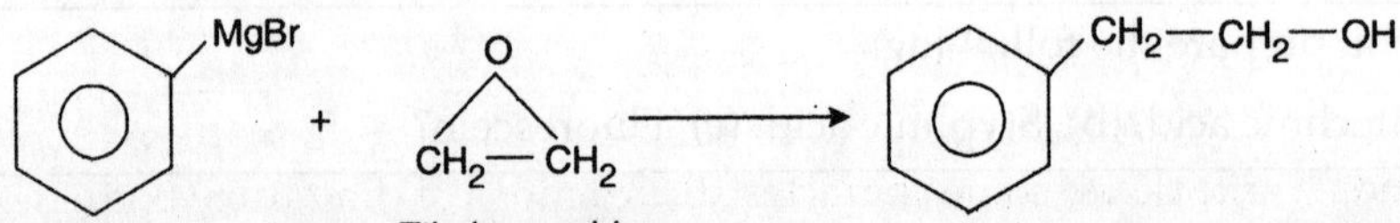

Ethylene oxide

17.4.2 Properties of Aromatic Alcohols

These alcohols are closely similar to aliphatic alcohols and undergo most of the characteristic reactions of aliphatic alcohols.

17.5 Uses of Phenols and Aromatic Alcohols

Phenols are very useful chemical compounds and are often used for the following purposes:

Simple phenol is used in considerable quantities for the manufacture of phenol formaldehyde resin. It is commonly known as carbolic acid and is used as insecticide, antiseptic and disinfectant. Some alkylated phenols such as cresols, carvacrol and dettol are very useful antiseptics. *p*-Aminophenol is an intermediate for the preparation of *phenacetin* which is an useful drug with antipyretic and analgesic actions. Caprokol, a phenolic compound, is a well known urinary antiseptic. It is commonly used for the treatment of ascariasis and tapeworm infections. A few phenolic compounds as for examples chloro-carvacrol and butyphen are strong anthelmintic drugs. Nitrophenols are used as insecticides in agriculture for controlling plant pests and weeds. Picric acid (Trinitrophenol) is used for the preparation of explosives. Catechol, quinol and pyrogallol are used as photographic developer. Oxidation of quinol to quinone is reversible and rapid and can produce a potential difference in electrolytic cell. For this reason it is used as electrode known as *Quinhydrone* electrode.

Benzyl alcohol is used in perfumery industry. It is also a constituent of many pharmaceutical preparations. i.e., benzyl alcohol is added to an extent of 1-3% to the solution or suspension intended for intramascular or subscutaneous injections as it reduces the pain at the site of injection. Benzhydrol [Diphenyl carbinol, $(C_2H_5)_2CHOH$] is a very important starting material for the synthesis of an important class of drugs known as *antihistaminics*. Benadryl, for example, is the β-dimethyl aminoethyl ether of benzhydrol and is widely used for the treatment of cough and cold.

Model Questions

1. What are phenols? Give their classification.
2. Describe some common methods of preparation of phenols.
3. Explain:
   i. Phenol is acidic while ethyl alcohol is not.
   ii. Introduction of nitrogroup in aromatic ring increases the acidity of phenols while introduction of CH_3 group decreases their acidity.
4. What happens when
   (a) Phenol is heated with Zn-dust?
   (b) Phenol is treated with bromine water?
   (c) Phenol is treated with carbon tetrachloride in NaOH?
5. What are dihydroxy benzenes? Give important methods of preparation of these compounds. Write down some characteristic reactions of dihydroxy benzene.
6. Write notes on:
   (a) Reimer-Tiemann reaction.
   (b) Uses of phenols.
7. In what respects phenol resembles and differs from ethyl alcohol? How is phenol converted into (i) picric acid (ii) salicylic acid and (iii) salicylaldehyde.
8. What are aromatic alcohols. How it differs from phenol? Discuss some methods of preparation of aromatic alcohols.
9. How will you synthesise the following?
   (a) Benzyl alcohol (b) β-phenyl ethanol (c) α-phenyl ethanol.

CHAPTER EIGHTEEN

Aromatic Carbonyl Compounds

In aromatic carbonyl compounds carbonyl group ($\rangle C{=}O$) is directly connected to aromatic rings. As expected, they may be of two types—(i) Aldehydes and (ii) Ketones. Thus,

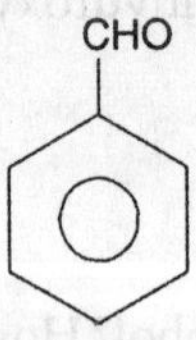

Benzaldehyde

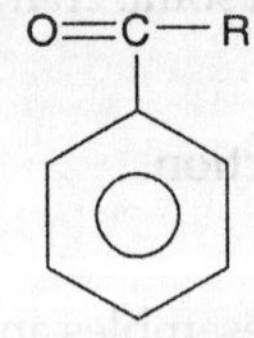

Aromatic Ketone
(R may be any alkyl or phenyl group)

In general, aromatic carbonyl compounds are less active than their aliphatic counterparts. This is due to the participation of carbonyl group in resonance with aromatic ring which appreciably reduces the positive charge on carbonyl carbon.

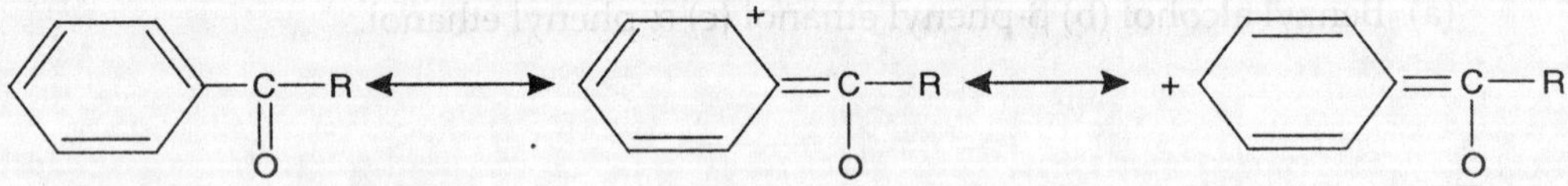

(R=H or any group)

It may be mentioned that the presence of electron releasing group reduces the activity while electron withdrawing group when present increases the activity.

Some of the most common members of aromatic carbonyl compounds are as listed below:

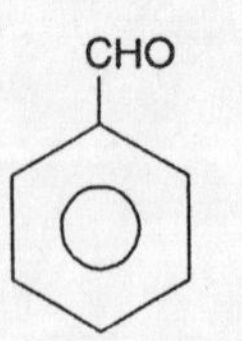

Benzaldehyde

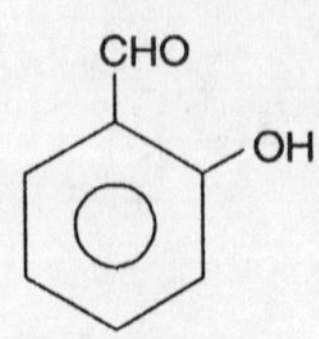

Salicylaldehyde

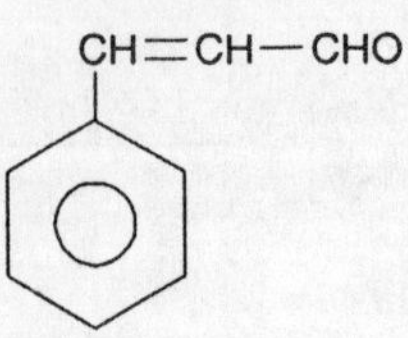

Cinnamaldehyde

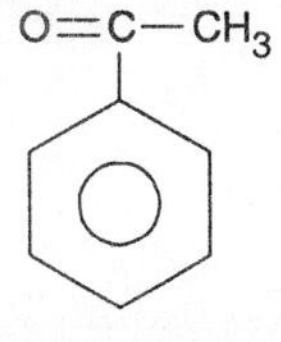

Acetophenone

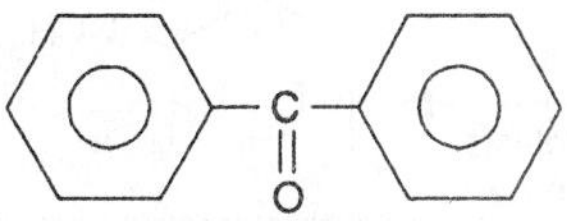

Benzophenone

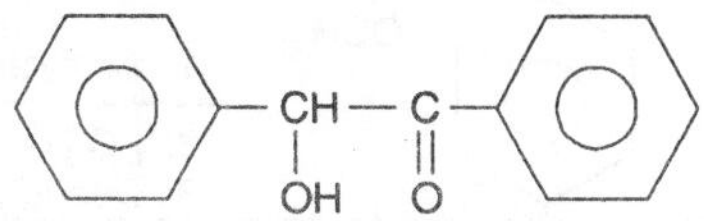

Benzoin

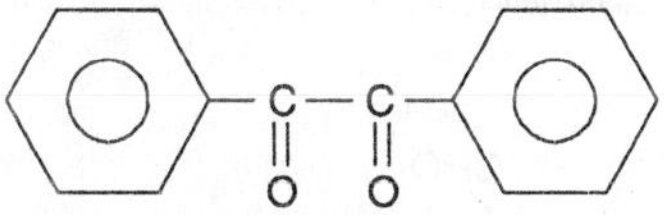

Benzil

18.1 Methods of Preparation of Aromatic Carbonyl Compounds

General methods as discussed in the case of preparation of aliphatic carbonyl compounds are equally applicable for the preparation of aromatic carbonyl compounds. However, there are some special methods for the preparation of aromatic carbonyl compounds which are described below:

18.1.1 Preparation of Aromatic Aldehydes

1. *Gattermann synthesis:* In this method aromatic compound is treated with a mixture of hydrocyanic and hydrochloric acids in presence of aluminium chloride, and the intermediate complex formed is decomposed by water.

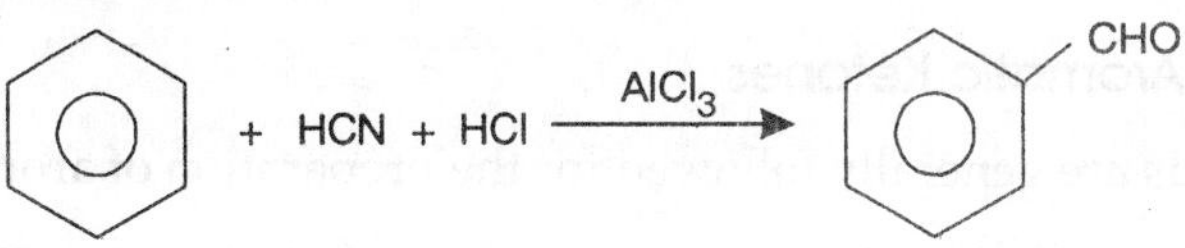

Benzaldehyde

2. *Gattermann-Koch synthesis:* This process involves reaction of aromatic hydrocarbon with a mixture of carbon monoxide and hydrochloric acid in presence of aluminium chloride. Thus,

$$CO + HCl \longrightarrow H-\underset{\underset{Cl}{|}}{C}=O$$

Formyl chloride

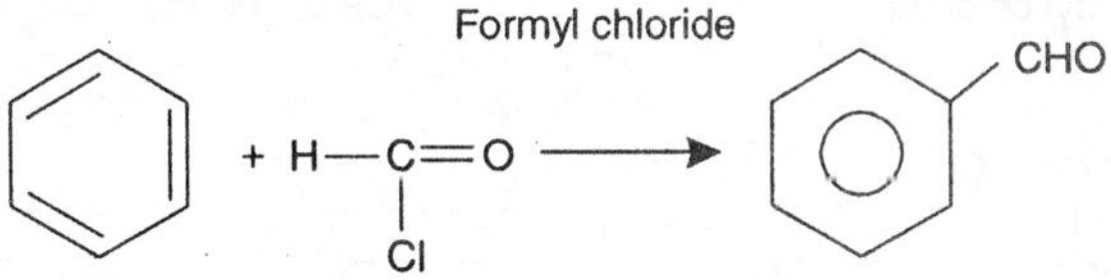

Benzaldehyde

3. Oxidation or ozonolysis of olefinic compound:

i. 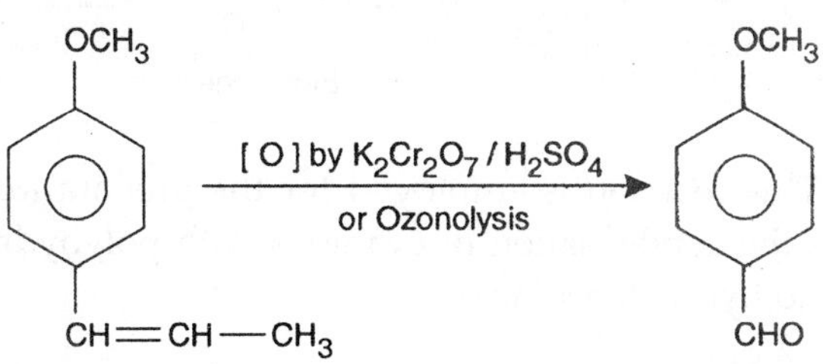

Anethole Anisaldehyde

ii.

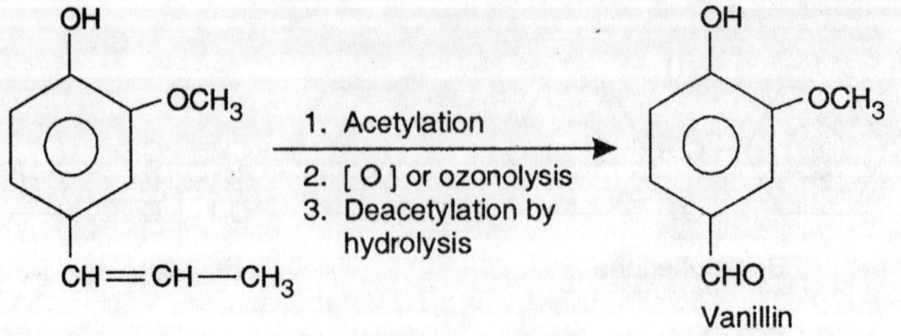

iii.

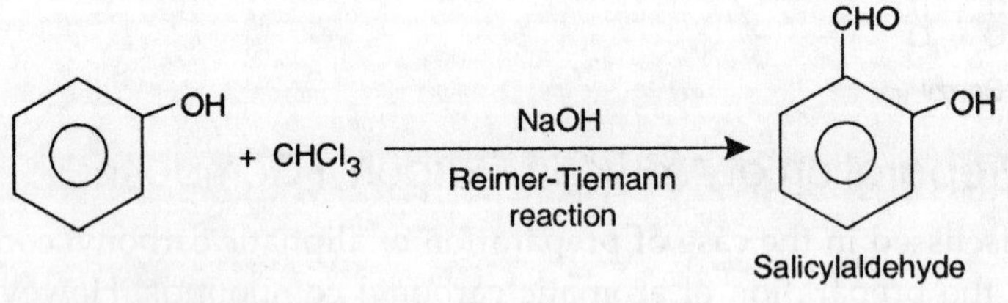

4. Claisen Condensation: This condensation is normally used for the preparation of αβ *unsaturated aromatic aldehyde*. Thus,

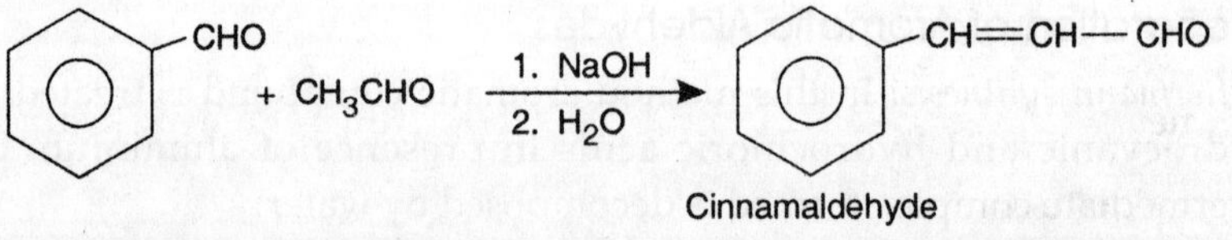

18.1.2 Preparation of Aromatic Ketones

Following special methods are generally followed for the preparation of aromatic Ketones.

1. *Friedel-Crafts Reaction:* It is the most common method for preparing aromatic Ketones.

i.

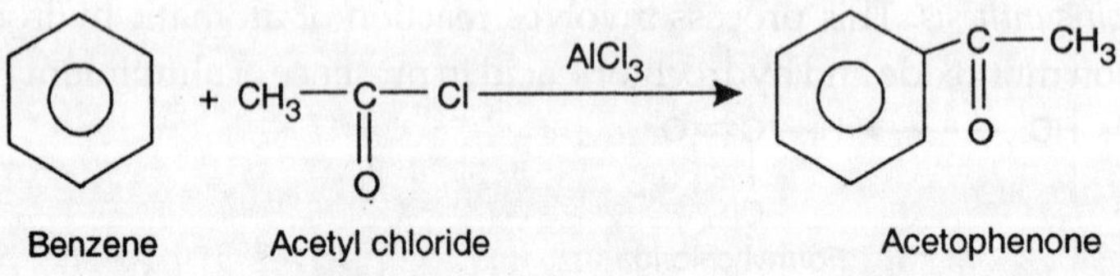

ii.

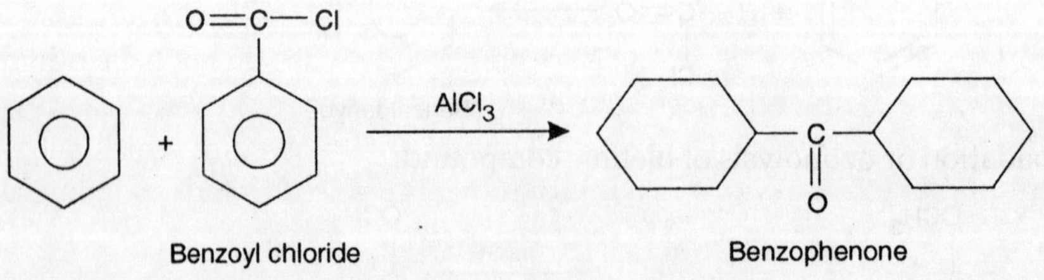

2. *Houben-Hoesch Synthesis*: This reaction is employed for the preparation of phenolic ketones. Reaction involves the condensation of cyanides with polyhydric phenols in presence of zinc chloride and hydrochloric acid.

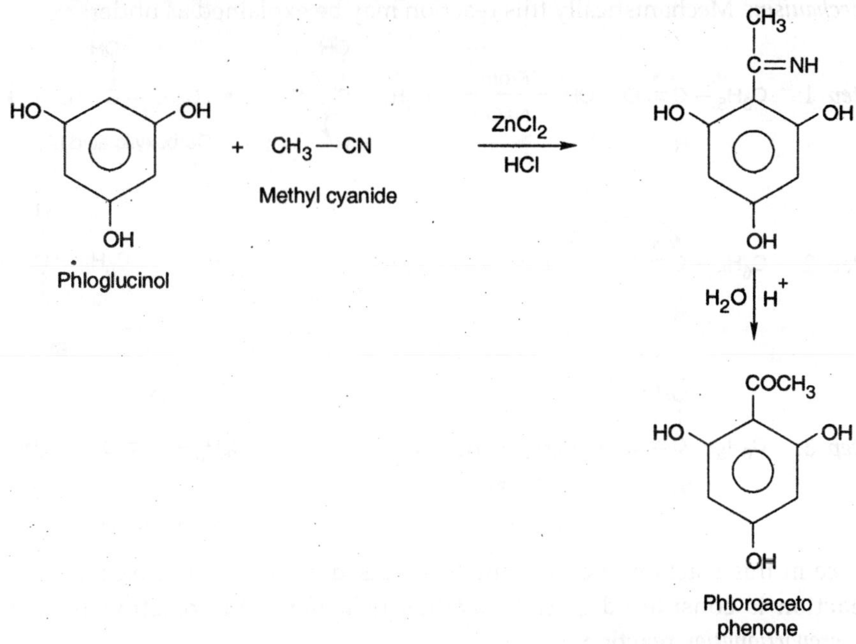

This method, in fact, is an extension of Gatter mann's aldehyde synthesis.

18.2 Properties of Aromatic Carbonyl Compounds

Aromatic carbonyl compounds have properties similar to those of aliphatic carbonyl compounds with some exceptions due to lesser activity originating from the attachement of aromatic ring.

18.2.1 Properties of Aromatic Aldehydes

Aromatic aldehydes although exhibit similar properties like aliphatic aldehydes but differ in the following respects:

1. They do not reduce Fehling's and Tollen's solutions.
2. They do not undergo aldol condensation among themselves in presence of alkali but undergo *cannizzaro reaction*. It is a characteristic reaction of all the aromatic aldehydes. This is because this reaction involves aldehyde having no hydrogen atom at α-position with respect to aldehydic group. As aromatic aldehydes do not have α-hydrogen atom, this reaction frequently occurs in aromatic aldehydes. In Cannizzaro reaction, two molecules of aldehydes having no α-H atom are involved of which one is oxidised to corresponding carboxylic acid while the other is reduced to corresponding alcohol. Thus,

$$\underset{\text{Benzaldehyde}}{C_6H_5CHO} + C_6H_5CHO \xrightarrow{NaOH} \underset{\text{Benzoic acid}}{C_6H_5COOH} + \underset{\text{Benzyl alcohol}}{C_6H_5CH_2OH}$$

Mechanism: Mechanistically this reaction may be explained as under:

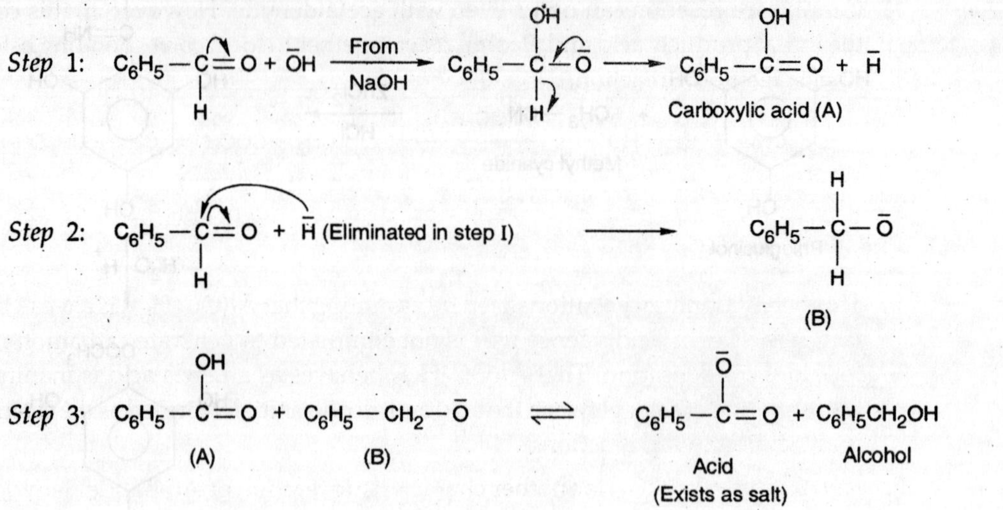

Since in this reaction one molecule is oxidised and another molecule is reduced, this reaction is considered as *self-oxidation reduction*. This reaction is also termed as *disproportionation* reaction.

It may be mentioned in this connection that Cannizaro reaction may occur between two different aldehydes having no α-H atoms. Such reaction is known as *crossed Cannizzaro reaction*. In this case more active aldehyde is oxidised while the other is reduced to alcohol. Thus,

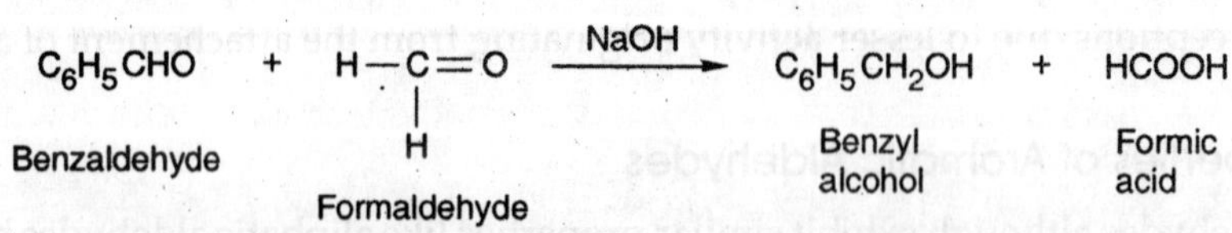

It has been observed that Cannizzaro can take place intramolecularly. For example,

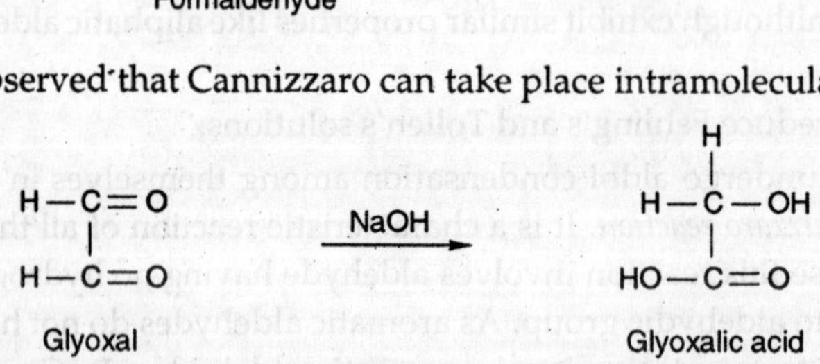

Further investigations have revealed that Cannizaro reaction may occur with aldehydes having α-H under certain conditions. Thus,

i. Hauserman observed that when isopropionaldehyde is heated with sodium hydroxide at a temperature of 200 °C, self-oxidation-reduction takes place.

$$(CH_3)_2\overset{\alpha}{C}HCHO \xrightarrow[200\ ^\circ C]{NaOH} (CH_3)_2CHCOONa + (CH_3)_2CHCH_2OH$$

This may be explained by assuming that α-H atom in the above molecule is highly crowded and due to this steric hindrance, α-H is not easily abstracted to form carbanion. So occurrence of aldol condensation is restricted.

ii. Tischenko reported that if aluminium ethoxide is used instead of sodium hydroxide. Cannizzaro reaction can occur even with acetaldehyde. However, in this condition the initial products acid and alcohol react together to form corresponding ester in the final stage of the reaction.

$$CH_3CHO + CH_3CHO \xrightarrow{Al(OC_2H_5)_3} [CH_3-COOH + CH_3-CH_2OH] \longrightarrow \underset{\text{Ester}}{CH_3COOC_2H_5}$$

This behaviour may be rationalised by assuming that $Al(OC_2H_5)_3$ is a weak base—in fact, it is a Lewis acid. Hence α-H is not eliminated to generate carbanion required for aldol condensation. That $Al(OC_2H_5)_3$ behaves as a Lewis acid is manifested by the formation of ester between the acid and alcohol initially formed as the esterification is an acid catalysed reaction.

3. *Benzoin condensation*: This is another characteristic reaction of aromatic aldehyde. In this reaction two molecules of aromatic aldehydes condense together in presence of potassium cyanide and the final product is aromatic α-hydroxy-ketone, usually known as benzoin.

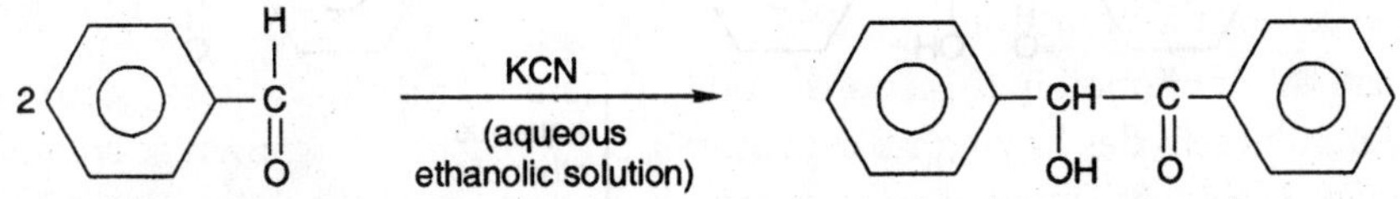

Benzaldehyde Benzoin

(a) Mechanistically this reaction may be interpreted as traced below:

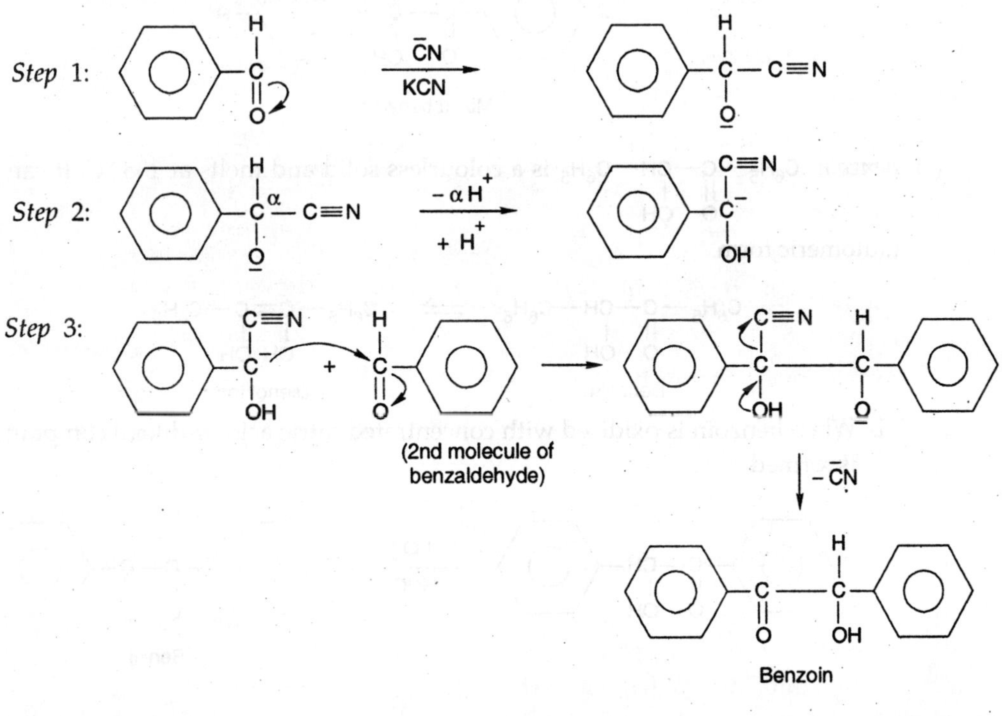

Benzoin

(b) *Comments*:

i. **Benzoin condensation may take place between two different aromatic aldehydes to form mixed benzoins.**

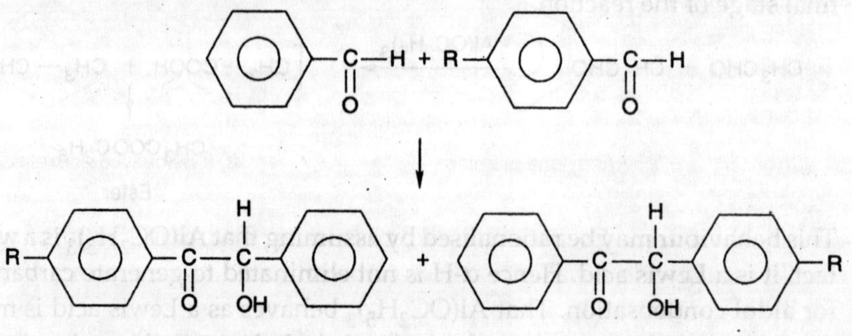

ii. **Benzoin condensation is reversible in nature. It is evidenced from the fact that when benzoin formed between two molecules of benzaldehyde, is treated with a different aromatic aldehyde, mixed benzoin is formed, i.e.,**

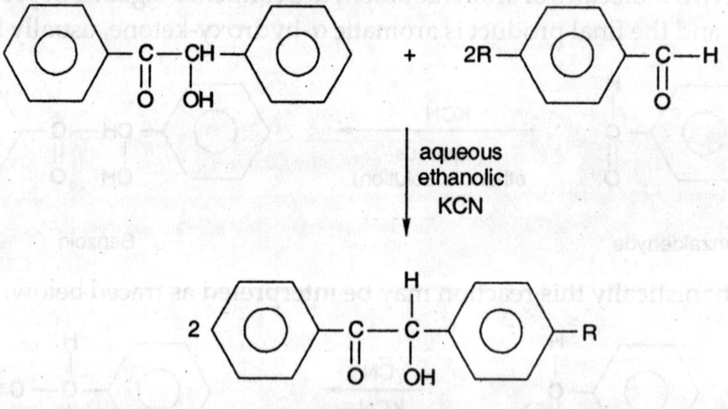

Mixed benzoin

(c) *Benzoin*, $C_6H_5-\underset{\underset{O}{\|}}{C}-\underset{\underset{OH}{|}}{CH}-C_6H_5$ **is a colourless solid and melts at 138 °C. It can exists in tautomeric form.**

$$\underset{\text{Benzoin}}{C_6H_5-\underset{\underset{O}{\|}}{C}-\underset{\underset{OH}{|}}{CH}-C_6H_5} \rightleftharpoons \underset{\text{Dienol form}}{C_6H_5-\underset{\underset{OH}{|}}{C}=\underset{\underset{OH}{|}}{C}-C_6H_5}$$

i. **When benzoin is oxidised with concentrated nitric acid, α-diketo compound benzil is formed.**

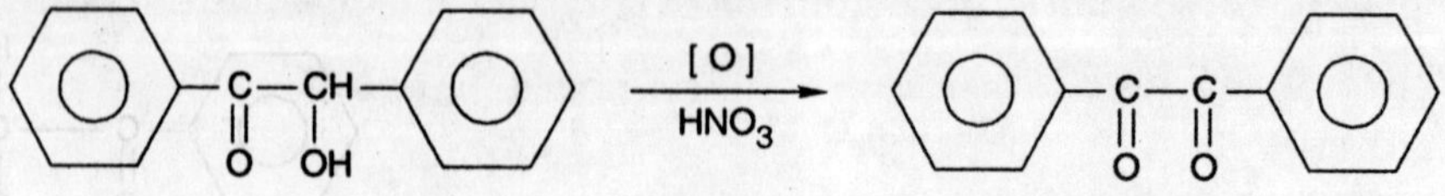

Benzil

ii. Benzil like aliphatic α-diketones condenses with *ortho* phenylene diamine to form quinoxaline derivative.

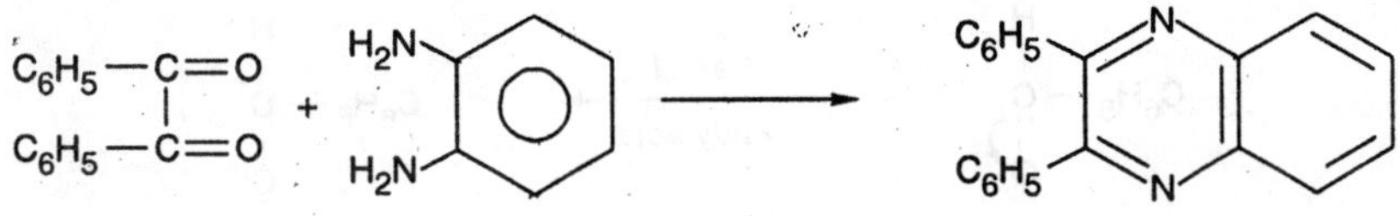

Benzil *o*-Phenylene diamine 2, 3-diphenyl quinoxaline

iii. Benzil when heated with ethanolic, potassium hydroxide solution undergoes a rearrangement and forms α-hydroxy carboxylic acid.

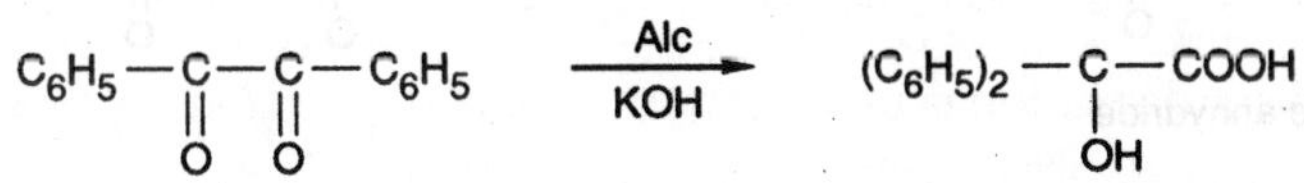

Benzilic acid

The accepted mechanism of this rearrangement may be written as under:

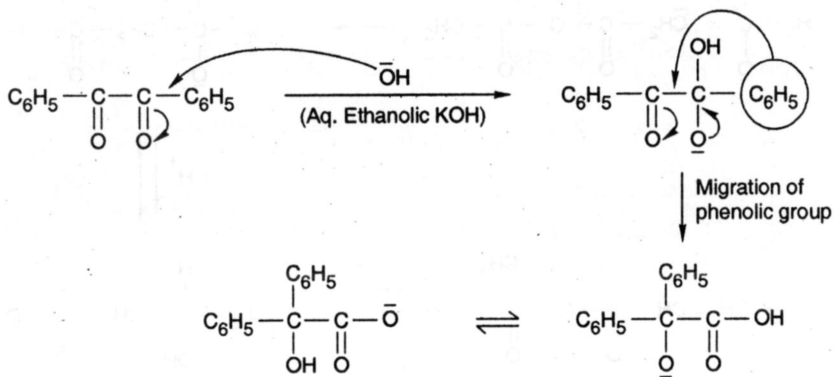

Benzilic acid
(Exists as salt)

This rearrangement may also be carried out in presence of alkoxide but in that condition the product is not an acid but an ester.

4. *Perkin Reaction*: It is also an important reaction frequently encountered in aromatic aldehydes. It is analogous to aldol condensation but the required carbocation is always generated from the aldehydic part of the condensation reaction. As aromatic adehydes do not possess any α-hydrogen atom they always serve as the source of carbocation and that is why this reaction is normally observed in aromatic aldehydes. The other component of this condensation reaction is the anhydride of fatty acid. The reaction is carried out in presence of sodium or potassium salt of fatty acid at temperature of nearly 200 °C. Thus,

$$\underset{\text{Benzaldehyde}}{C_6H_5CHO} + \underset{\text{Acetic anhydride}}{(CH_3CO)_2O} \xrightarrow{CH_3COONa} \underset{\text{Cinnamic acid}}{C_6H_5-CH{=}CH-COOH}$$

(a) The accepted mechanism of Perkin reaction may be described as below:

Step 1: Formation of carbocation:

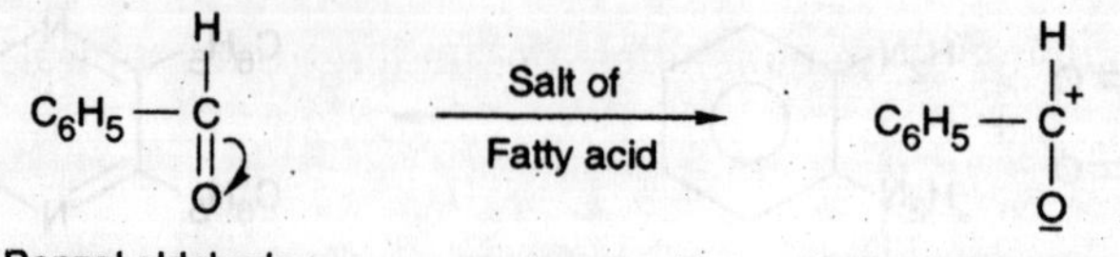

Benzal aldehyde

Step 2: Formation of carbanion:

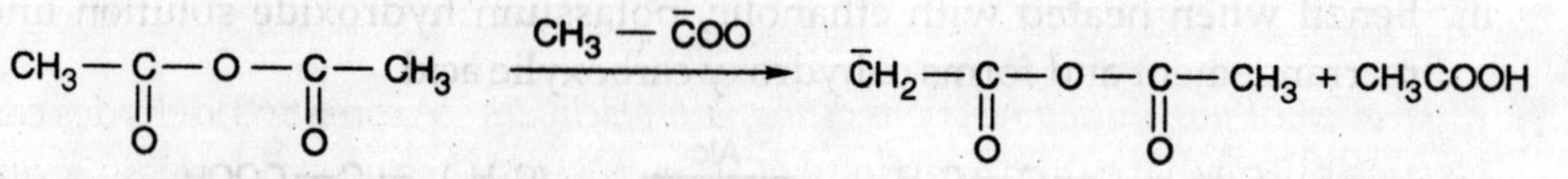

Acetic anhydride

Step 3: Combination of carbocation and carbanion:

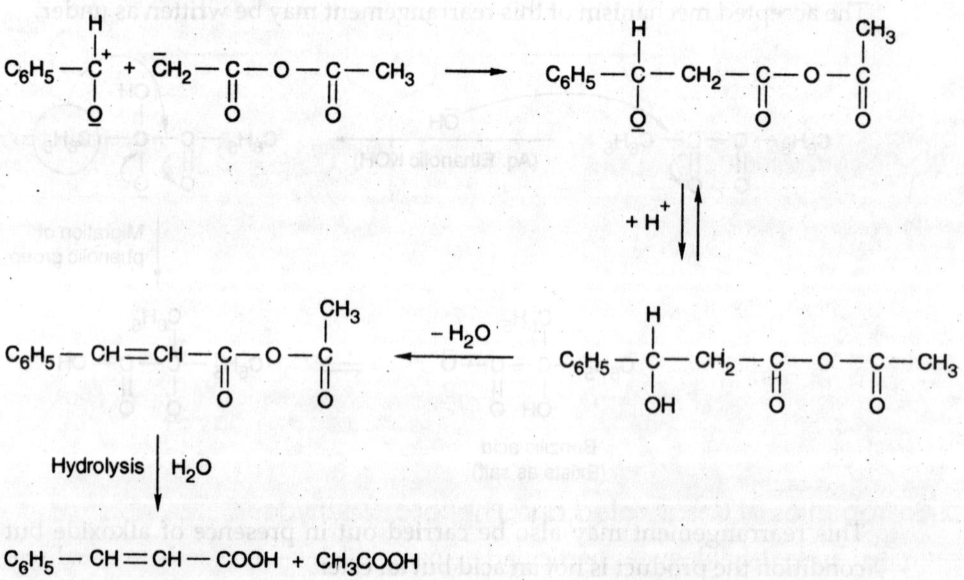

(b) *Comments*

i. Salt of fatty acid acts as base.

ii. However, salt can also act as a source of carbanion. So if anhydride and salt are of different fatty acids, mixed products may be obtained and so complications may arise regarding the separation of products. Hence in order to avoid such complications, salts and anhydride of the same fatty acid are normally used in this reaction.

iii. Perkin reaction is a significant method for the preparation of α, β-unsaturated acid.

iv. Acid anhydride should have two α-hydrogen atoms in order to get unsaturated acid.

5. *Claisen Reaction*: Aromatic aldehydes undergo aldol condensation with aliphatic aldehydes or ketones having α-hydrogen atom in presence of alkali with the formation of α, β-unsaturated aldehyde or ketone.

$$C_6H_5CHO + CH_3CHO \xrightleftharpoons{NaOH} C_6H_5-CH=CH-CHO$$

Cinnamaldehyde

6. Like aliphatic aldehydes aromatic aldehydes undergo other typical reactions of aldehydes. Thus,

(a) $C_6H_5CHO \xrightarrow{[O]} C_6H_5COOH$

Benzoic acid

(b) $C_6H_5CHO \xrightarrow{[H]} C_6H_5CH_2OH$

Benzyl alcohol

7. *Electrophilic Substitution reactions of aromatic aldehydes*: Aromatic aldehydes can undergo electrophilic substitution reactions at *meta* position because aldehydic group is *meta*-orienting. Some of the electrophilic substitution reactions may be summarised as under:

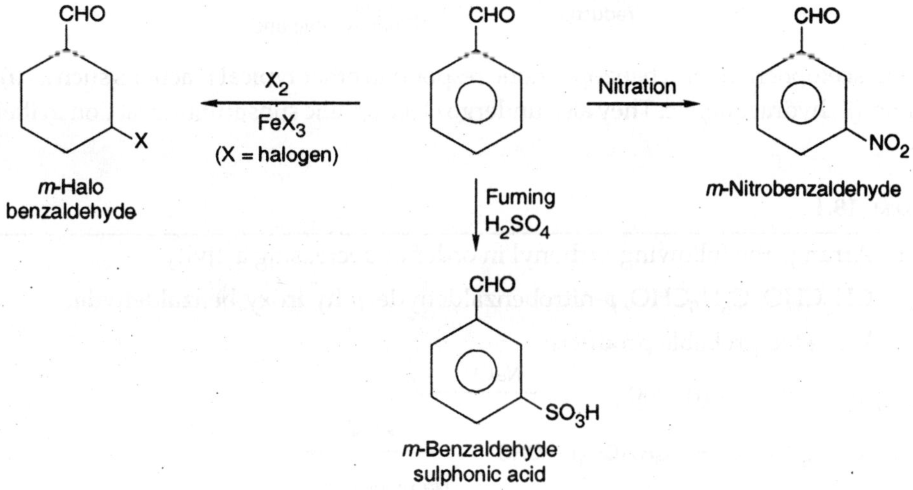

18.2.2 Properties of Unsaturated and Phenolic Aldehydes

Unsaturated aromatic aldehydes particularly cinnamaldehyde responds to usual reactions of unsaturation and an aldehydic group. Thus, it reacts with bromine water to form dibromo derivative and on oxidation with ammoniacal silver nitrate solution it yields cinnamic acid. However, on vigorous oxidation with potassium permanaganate benzoic acid is formed by the cleavage of carbon-carbon double bond.

Phenolic aldehyde, salicylaldehyde, is a liquid with boiling point 200 °C. It responds to ferric chloride colour reaction of phenol and typical reactions of aldehydic group. It can form intramolecular hydrogen bond as a result of which it has higher boiling point and less solubility than those of its *para* and *meta* isomers.

18.2.3 Properties of Aromatic Ketones

Representative member acetophenone is a liquid, (boiling point 203 °C) while benzophenone is a colourless solid (melting point 50 °C) Both of them exhibit usual properties of aliphatic ketones.

i. $$\underset{\text{Acetophenone}}{C_6H_5COCH_3} \xrightarrow[\text{alc. KOH}]{\text{Zn}} \underset{\text{Methyl benzyl alcohol}}{C_6H_5-CH(OH)-CH_3}$$

$$\underset{\text{Benzophenone}}{C_6H_5COC_6H_5} \xrightarrow[\text{KOH}]{\text{Zn/alc.}} \underset{\text{Benzhydrol}}{C_6H_5-CH(OH)-C_6H_5}$$

ii. $$C_6H_5COCH_3 \xrightarrow[\text{Clemmenson reduction}]{\text{Zn/Hg/HCl}} \underset{\text{Ethyl benzene}}{C_6H_5-CH_2-CH_3}$$

$$C_6H_5COC_6H_5 \xrightarrow[\text{Clemmenson reduction}]{\text{Zn/Hg/HCl}} \underset{\text{Diphenyl methane}}{C_6H_5-CH_2-C_6H_5}$$

Both acetophenone and benzophenone respond to other typical reactions such as (i) formation of oxime, (ii) hydrazone, etc. They also undergo electrophilic substitution reaction in their aromatic rings.

PROBLEM 18.1

1. Arrange the following carbonyl in order of decreasing activity.

   CH_3CHO, C_6H_5CHO, *p*-nitrobenzaldehyde, *p*-hydroxy-benzaldehyde.

2. Write the probable products:

   (a) $HCHO + C_6H_5CHO \xrightarrow{\text{NaOH}}$

   (b) $C_6H_5CHO + C_6H_4(CH_3)-CHO \xrightarrow{\text{KCN}}$

   (c) $C_6H_5CHO + (CH_3-CO)_2O \xrightarrow{\text{Na-propionate}}$

18.3 Uses of Aromatic Carbonyl Compounds

Benzaldehyde is used as a flavouring agent and as a perfume. It is also used for the synthesis of an well-known dye *malachite green*. Anisaldehyde and vanillin are used as flavouring agents. Acetophenone and benzophenone are used in perfumery industry. Acetophenone is an useful drug and is used as hypnotic under the trade name *'hypnone'* other aromatic ketones are used as mild sedative

Model Questions

1. What happens when benzaldehyde is heated with the following:

   (a) Concentrated NaOH solution.

   (b) Alcoholic KCN.

   (c) Acetic anhydride in presence of sodium acetate at 180 °C.

2. How will you synthesis
   (a) cinnamic acid from benzaldehyde?
   (b) diphenyl methane from benzophenone?
   (c) salicylaldehyde from phenol?
   (d) ethyl benzene from acetophenone?
3. Write notes on:
   (a) Perkin reaction
   (b) Cannizzaro reaction
   (c) Benzoin condensation
   (d) Claisen-Schmidt reaction
   (e) Uses of aromatic carbonyl compounds.
4. Discuss the methods of preparation of phenolic aldehydes. Discuss the properties of salicylaldehyde.

CHAPTER NINETEEN

Aromatic Carboxylic Acids

In aromatic carboxylic acid carboxylic function is directly linked to aromatic ring. The common names of aromatic carboxylic acids originate from the parent aromatic hydrocarbons. For example, benzene and benzoic acid, naphthalene and naphthoic acid etc. Substituted aromatic acids are named either using prefixes, *ortho, meta* or *para* or using number. The position of carboxylic group is always considered as I. Like aliphatic carboxylic acids, these acids may be dicarboxylic in nature. Some of the extremely common aromatic acids are listed below:

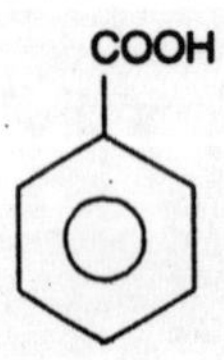

Benzoic acid

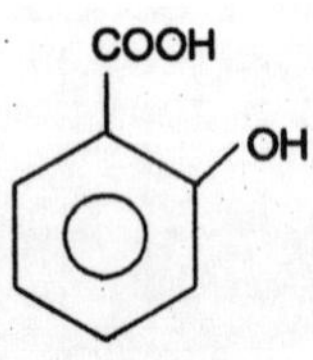

o-Hydroxy benzoic acid
(Salicylic acid)

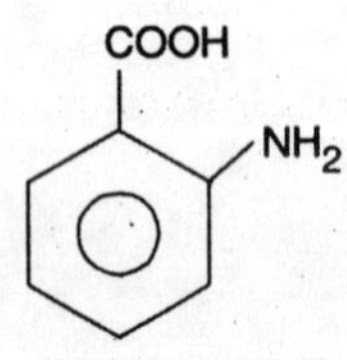

o-Amino bezoic acid
(Anthranilic acid)

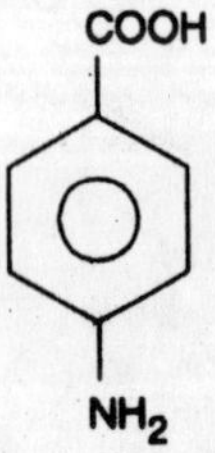

p-Aminobenzoic acid

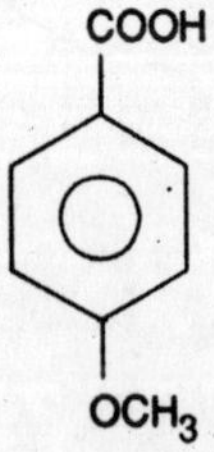

p-Methoxy benzoic acid
(anisic acid)

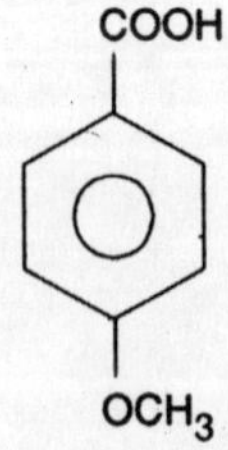

p-Toluic acid

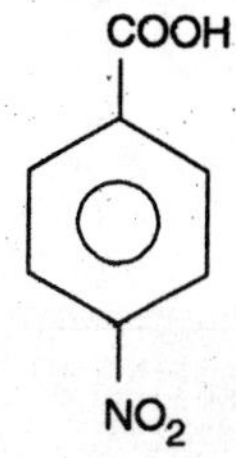

p-Aminobenzoic acid

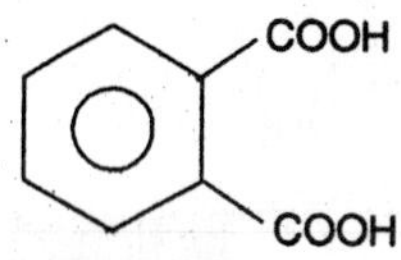

Phthalic acid

19.1 Methods of Preparation of Aromatic Carboxylic Acids

These acids are commonly prepared by the methods depicted below:

1.

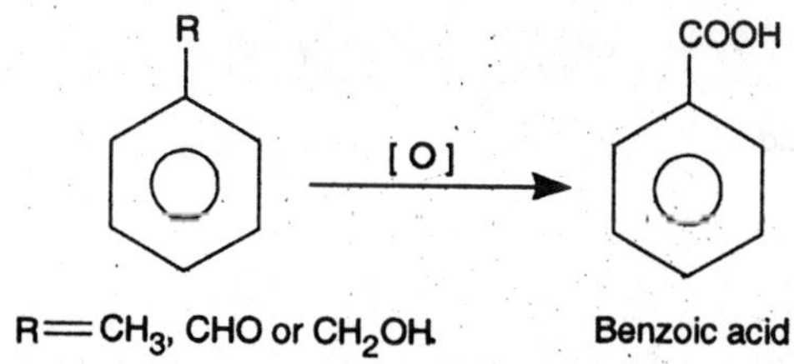

2.

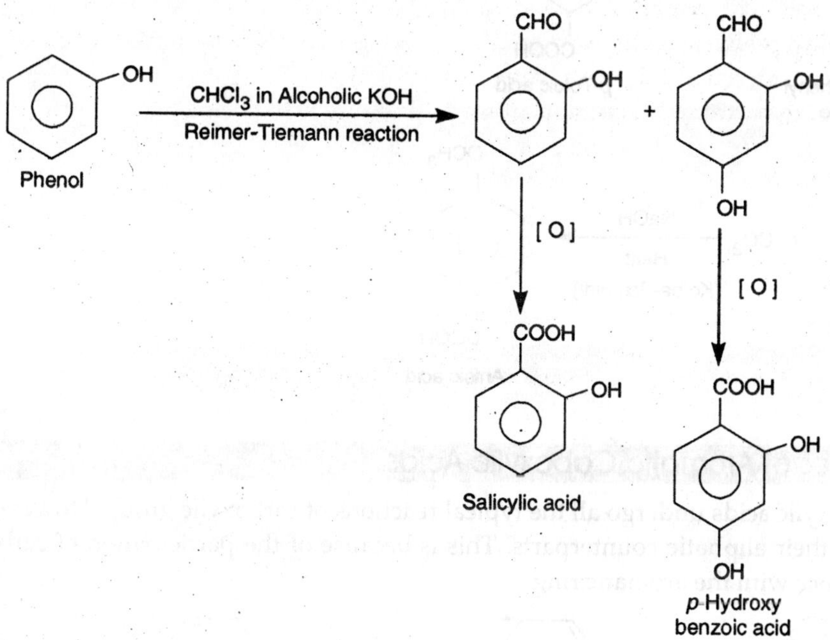

3.

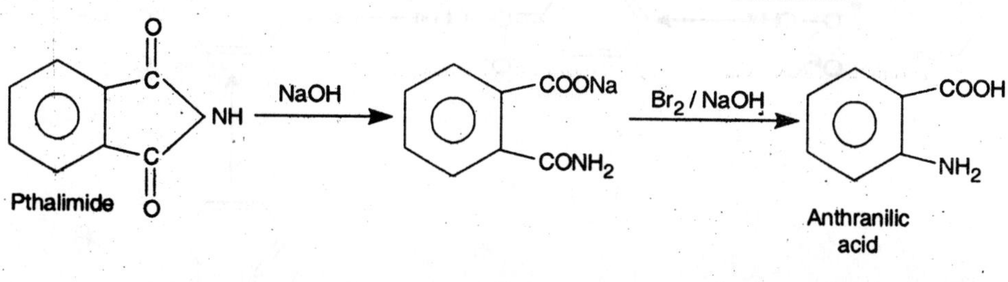

4. 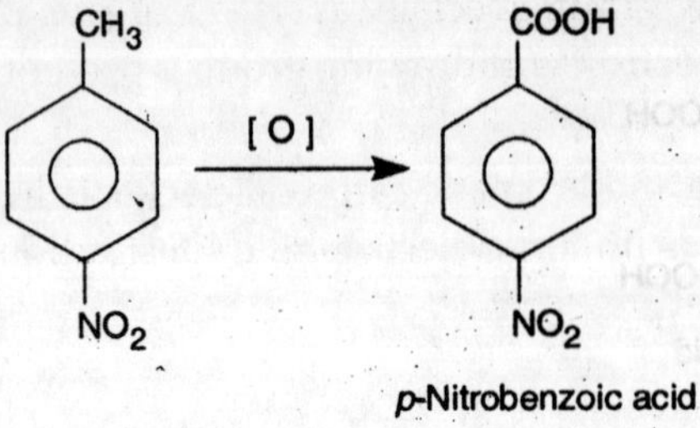

5. 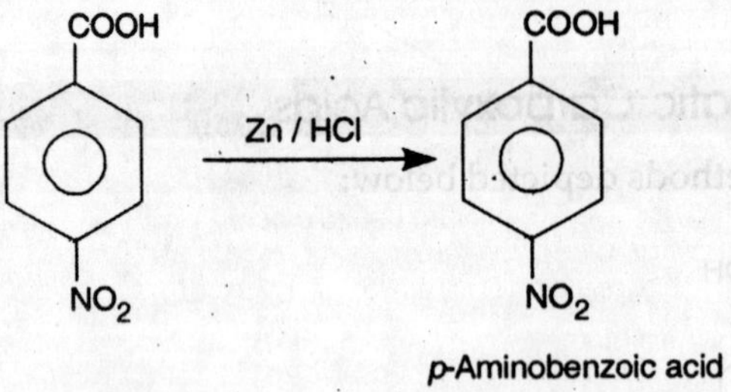

6. 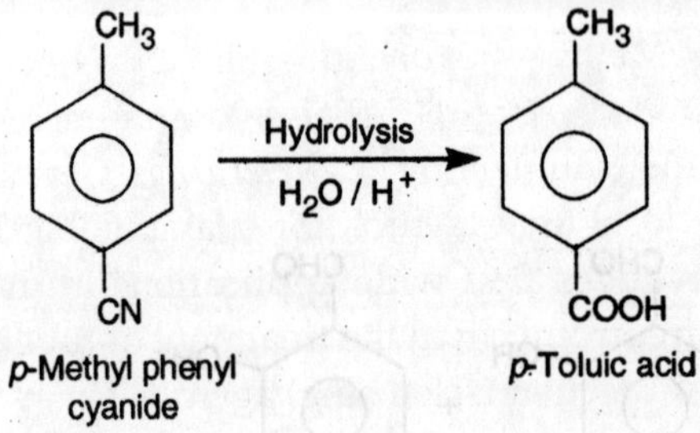

7. 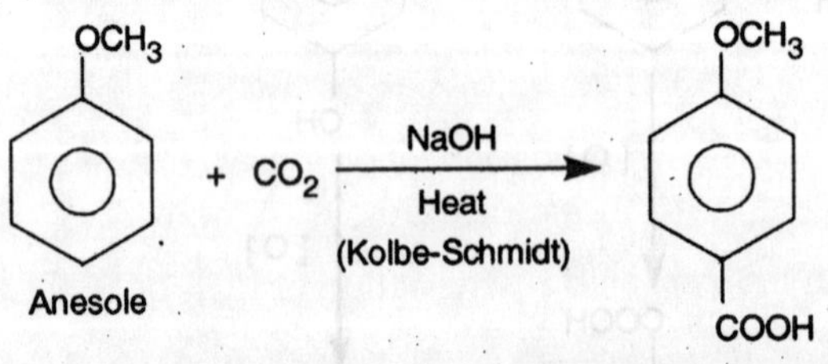

19.2 Properties of Aromatic Caboxylic Acids

Aromatic Carboxylic acids undergo all the typical reactions of carboxylic group. However, it is less acidic than their aliphatic counterparts. This is because of the participation of carboxylic group in resonance with the aromatic ring.

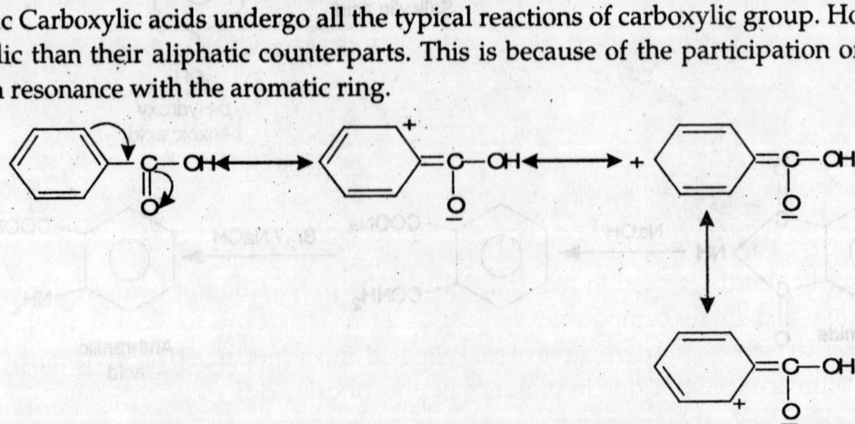

As expected, the presence of electron releasing group specially at *ortho* and *para* positions decreases acidity while acidity is enhanced when electron withdrawing group is present at these positions.

Another point of difference between aliphatic and aromatic carboxylic acids is in the fact that due to the presence of aromatic ring these acids undergo electrophilic substitution at *meta* position as carboxylic group is meta orienting in nature.

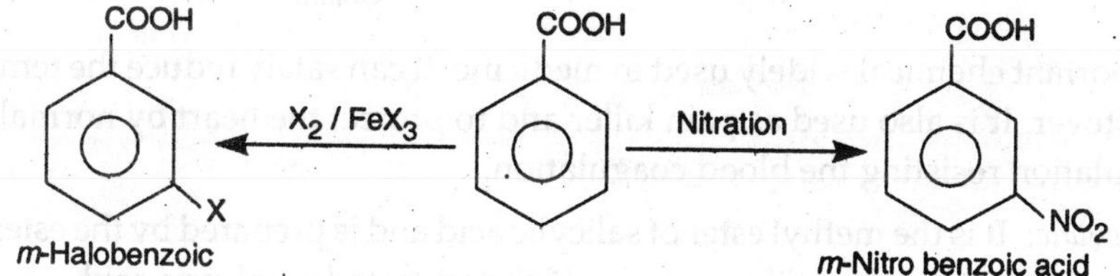

19.3 Uses of Aromatic Carboxylic Acids

Sodium benzoate is used as a preservative in foods. Methyl ester of anthranilic acid is extensively used in perfumery while its para isomer, i.e., *p*-aminobenzoic acid (PAB) is a constituent of vitamin B-complex and folic acid. This acid is also used in the manufacture of *sulpha drugs*. Certain esters of *p*-amino benzoic acid are used extensively as local anaesthetics, for example, benzocaine, novocaine (procaine). Salicylic acid and its derivatives find wide applications in medicine. *p*-Amino salicylic acid (PAS) is used along with streptromycin in the treatment of tuberculosis. Sodium salt of salicylic acid is also used as a cardiovascular (sclerosing) agent.

19.4 Some Important Derivatives of Aromatic Carboxylic Acids

A few derivatives of aromatic carboxylic acids are used for variety of purposes. Their preparations and uses are described below.

(a) *Benzoyl chloride*: It is prepared from benzoic acid by the action of PCl_5 or $SOCl_2$.

i. 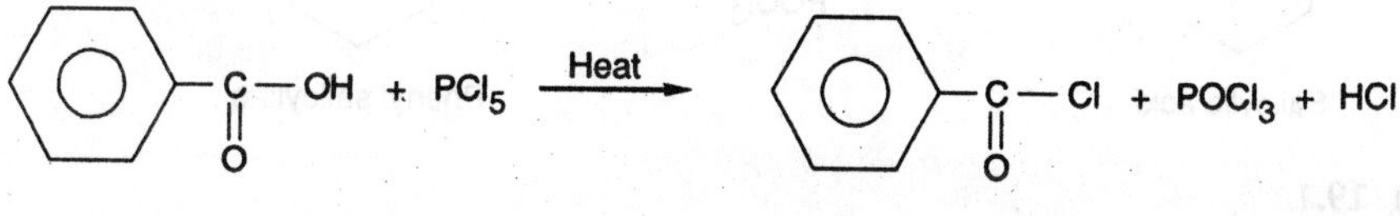

Benzoyl chloride

ii. 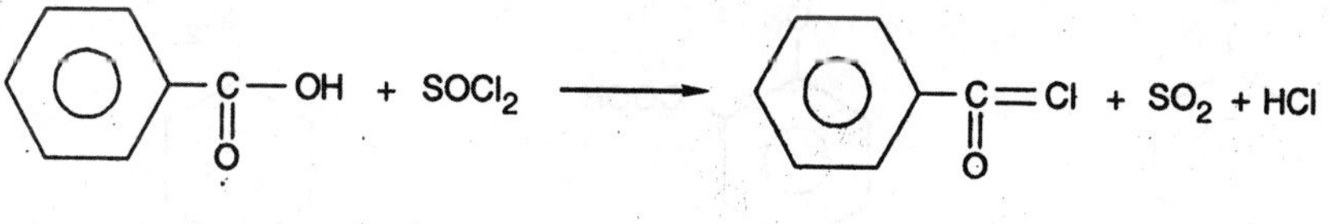

Benzoyl chloride

Benzoyl chloride is used in tear gas and for the preparation of benzoyl derivatives of hydroxy and amino compounds.

(b) *Aspirin*: It is the acetyl derivative of salicylic acid and is prepared by acetylation of salicylic acid with acetic anhydride in presence of phosphoric acid.

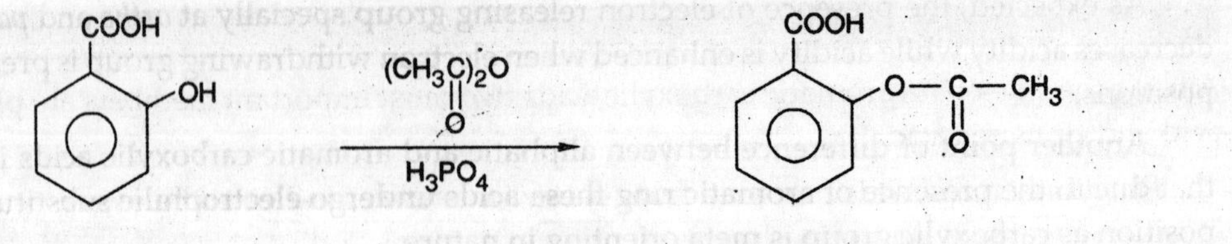

Salicylic acid — Acetyl salicylic acid (Aspirin)

It is an important chemical widely used in medicine. It can safely reduce the temperature caused by fever. It is also used as pain killer and to protect the heart by normalising the blood circulation resisting the blood coagulation.

(c) *Methyl salicylate*: It is the methyl ester of salicylic acid and is prepared by the esterification of salicylic acid with methanol in presence of concentrated sulphuric acid.

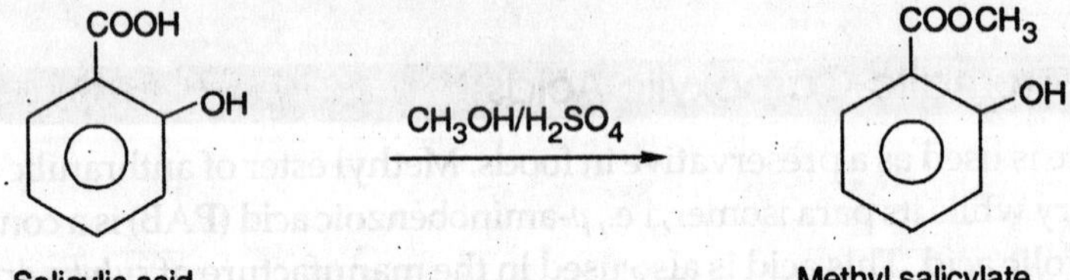

Salicylic acid — Methyl salicylate (Oil of Wintergreen)

It is also known as *oil of wintergreen*. It is used for the preparation of ointments for sprains, aches, etc.

(d) *Phenyl salicylate*: Phenyl salicylate is an important antiseptic and is prepared by the action of phenol on salicylic acid.

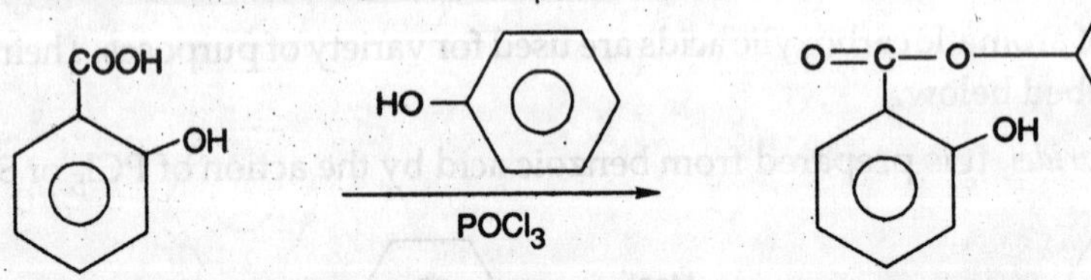

Salicylic acid — Phenyl salicylate

Problem 19.1

1. Arrange the following in order of their acid strength:

i.

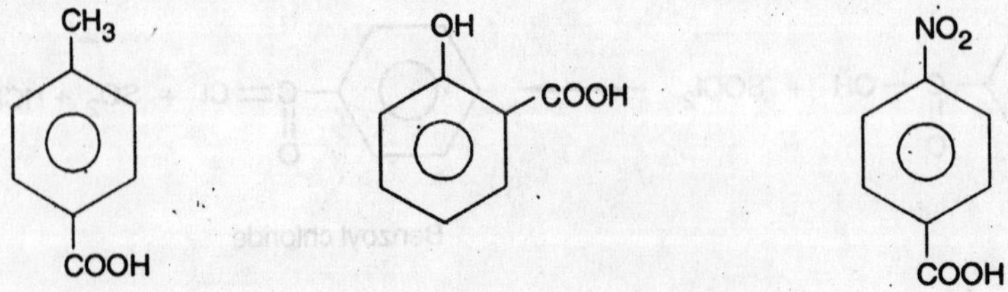

2. How will you prepare aspirin? What are its uses?

19.5 Side-Chain Aromatic Carboxylic Acids

Among the side-chain aromatic carboxylic acids two most important members are phenyl acetic acid and cinnamic acid.

Phenyl acetic acid: It is prepared from benzyl chloride as indicated below:

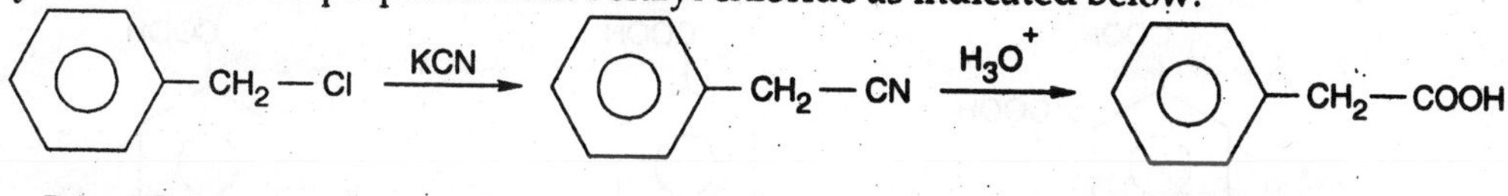

Benzyl Chloride Phenyl acetic acid

It is more acidic than benzoic acid as carboxylic group is not directly connected to aromatic ring. On oxidation it forms benzoic acid.

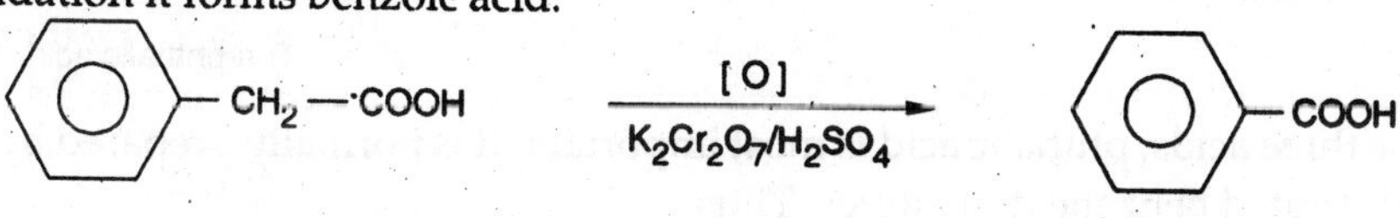

Phenyl acetic acid Benzoic acid

Cinnamic Acid: It is prepared by the following methods.

i. *Perkin reaction*

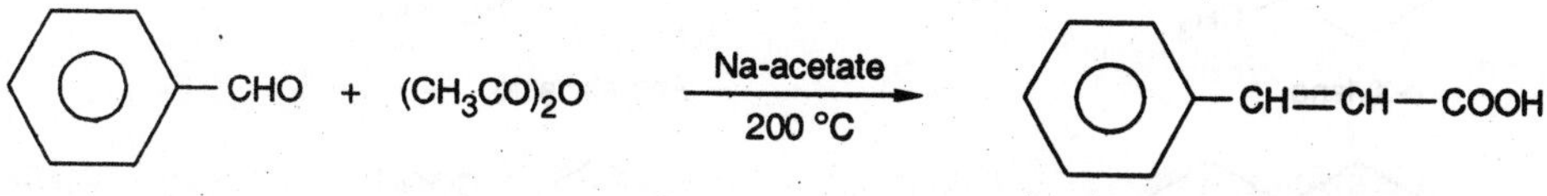

Benzaldehyde

ii. *Claisen reaction*

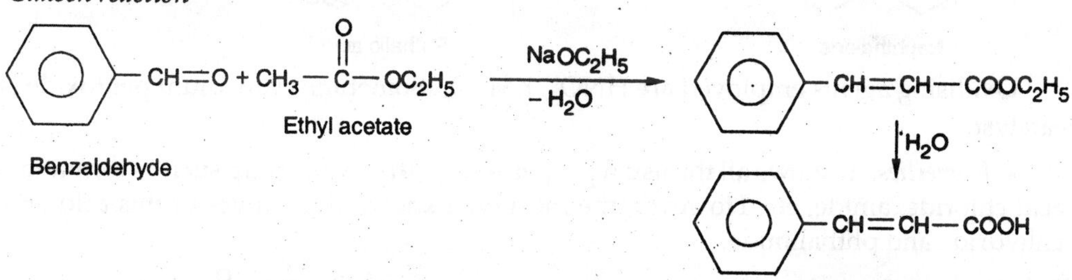

Ethyl acetate

Benzaldehyde

Cinnamic acid

It exsibits all the properties of carboxylic group as well as unsaturation. For example,

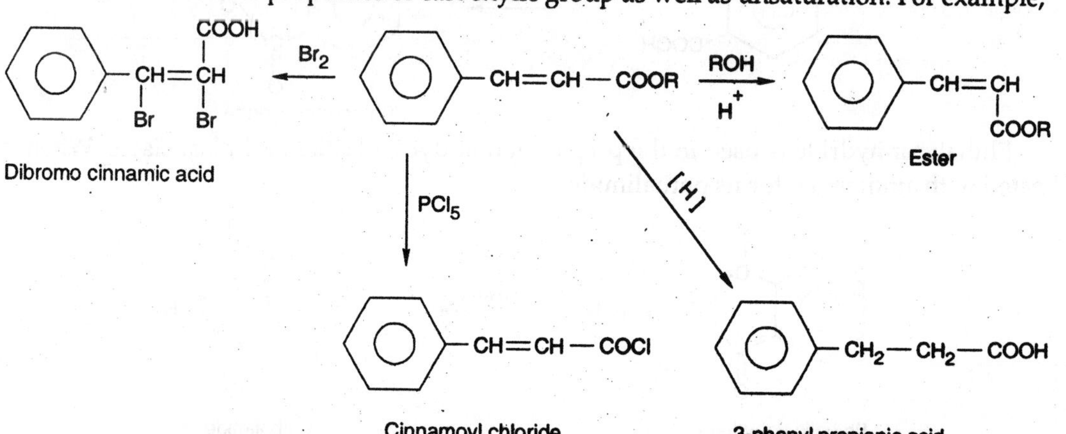

Dibromo cinnamic acid

Ester

Cinnamoyl chloride 3-phenyl propionic acid

It can also undergo electrophilic substitution reaction.

19.6 Aromatic Dicarboxylic Acids

All the three possible isomeric dibasic aromatic acids are known.

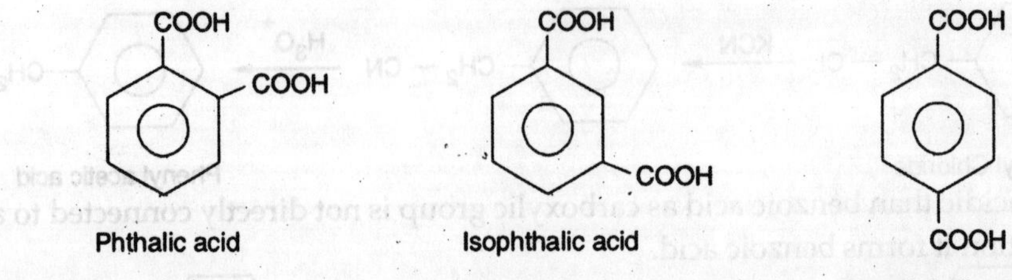

Phthalic acid Isophthalic acid Terephthalic acid

Of these three acids, phthalic acid is most important. It is normally prepared by oxidation of suitably substituted benzene derivatives. Thus,

i. 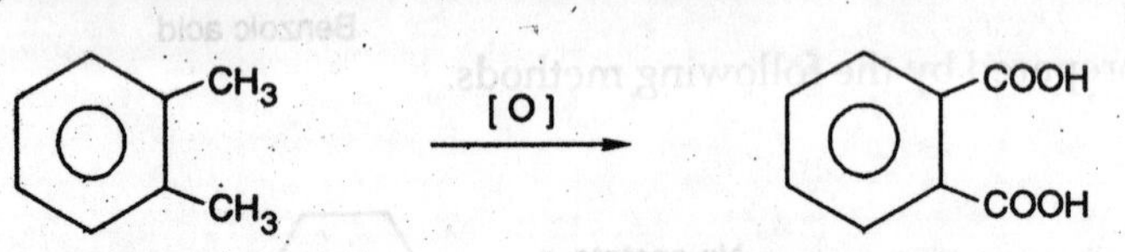

o-Xylene Phthalic acid

ii. 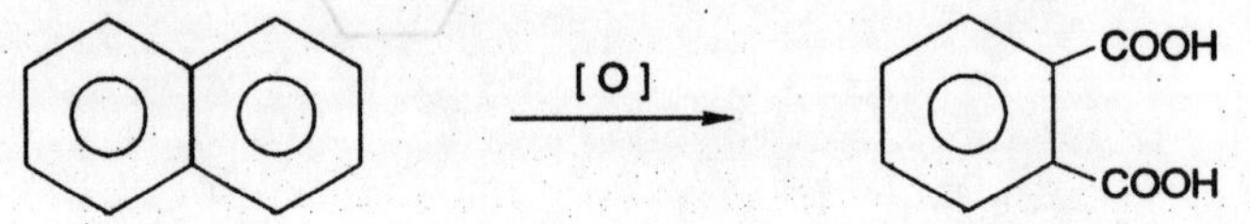

Naphthalene Phthalic acid

Oxidising agents employed are HNO_3, $KMnO_4$. Sometimes vanadium pentoxide is used as catalyst.

• *Properties*: It shows all the usual properties of carboxylic group such as formation of ester, acid chloride, amide, etc. However, the most well known derivatives of this acid are phthalic anhydride and phthalimide.

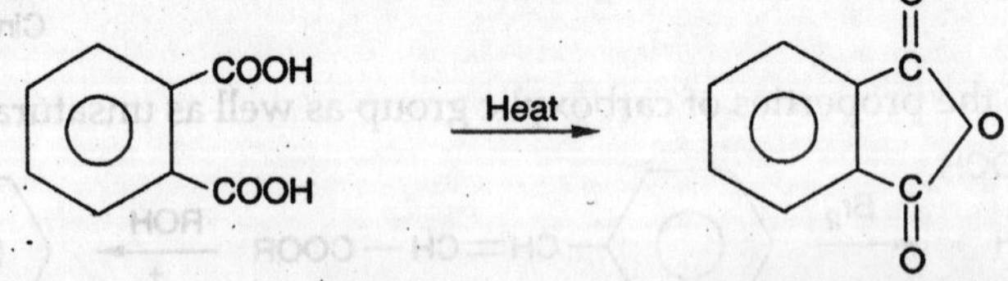

Phthalic anhydride

Phthalic anhydride is used in the preparation of dyes, plastics and plasticisers. When it is heated with ammonia it forms phthalimide.

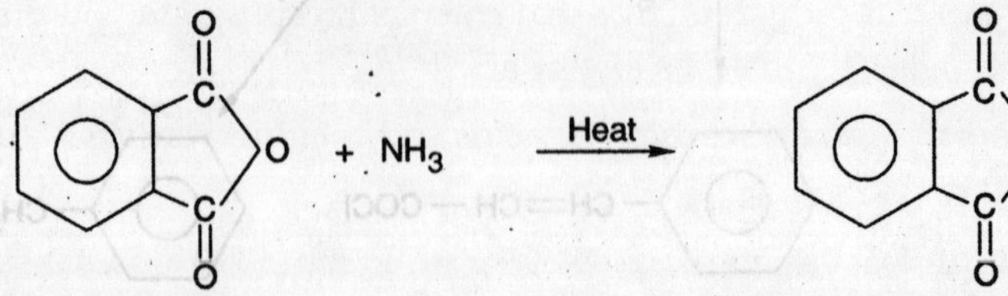

Phthalic anhydride Phthalimide

Phthalimide is used for the preparation of amino acids in the method known as *Garbriel's* ***phthalimide synthesis***.

Terephthalic acid and isophthalic acid are similarly prepared by the oxidation of *p*-xylene and *m*-xylene respectively.

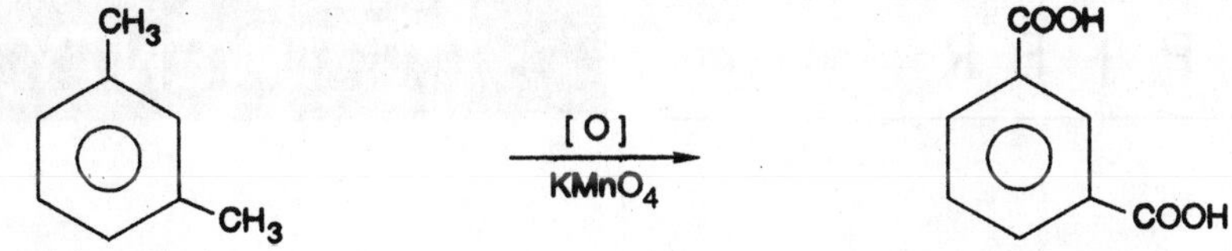

m-Xylene acid — Isophthalic acid

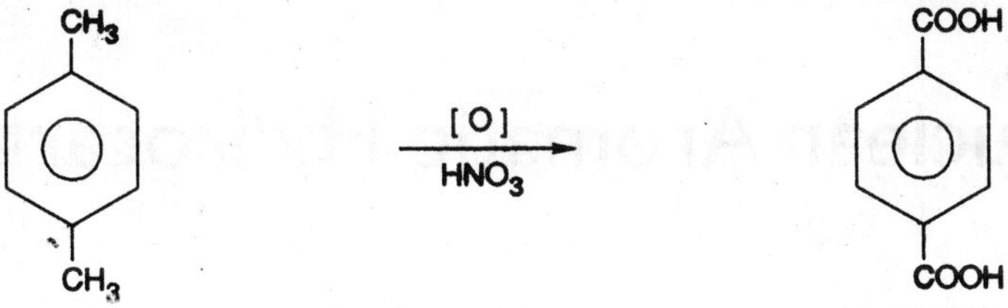

p-Xylene — Terephthalic acid

Terephthalic acid is used in the manufacture of polyester known as *Terylene*.

Model Questions

1. (a) How benzoic acid is prepared?
   (b) Explain:
      i. Nitration of benzoic acid gives *m*-nitrobenzene acid.
      ii. Benzoic acid weaker than acetic acid.
2. How will you synthesise the following?
   (a) Benzoic acid from benzene.
   (b) Phthalic acid from benzene.
   (c) *p*-Toluic acid form benzene.
   (d) Salicylic acid from phenol.
   (e) Aspirin from phenol.
   (f) Methyl salicylate from phenol.
   (g) Phenyl acetic acid from toluene.
3. How is phthalic acid prepared? Mention some of its properties.
4. How is cinnamic acid prepared? By what chemical tests would you distinguish between benzoic acid, cinnamic acid and salicylic acid?
5. Discuss the uses of aromatic carboxylic acids and their derivatives.

CHAPTER TWENTY

Polynuclear Aromatic Hydrocarbons

Polynuclear aromatic hydrocarbons are those in which there are more than one benzene rings in the molecules. They are generally of two types as described below:

1. *Fused polynuclear aromatic hydrocarbons*: In these hydrocarbons different benzene rings are fused together at *ortho* positions. The most common members of this group are napthalene, anthracene and phenanthrene.

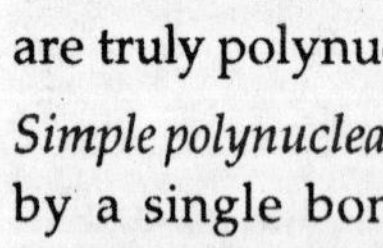

Naphthalene

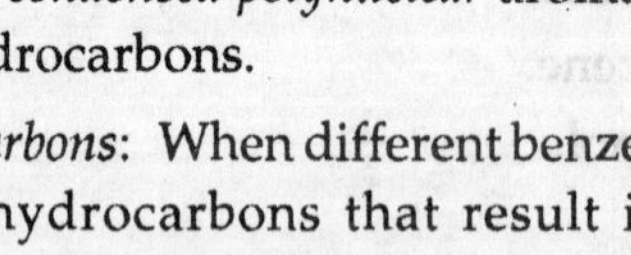

Anthracene

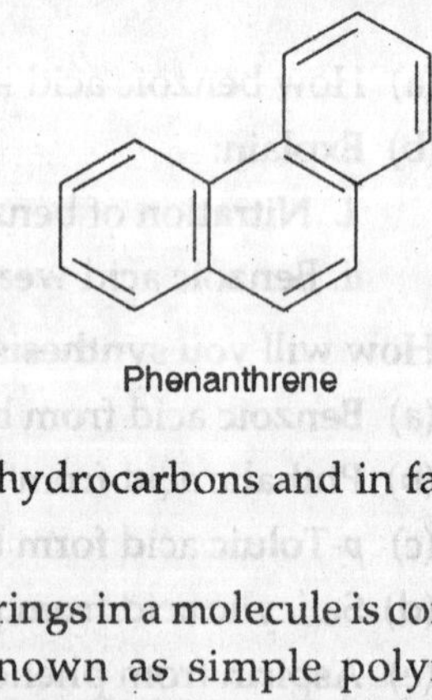

Phenanthrene

These are also known as *condensed polynuclear* aromatic hydrocarbons and in fact, they are truly polynuclear hydrocarbons.

2. *Simple polynuclear hydrocarbons*: When different benzene rings in a molecule is connected by a single bond, the hydrocarbons that result is known as simple polynuclear hydrocarbons. They are not true polynuclear compounds as they may be looked upon monophenyl or biphenyl derivatives of benzene. Some important members of this family are biphenyl, triphenyl, diphenyl methane.

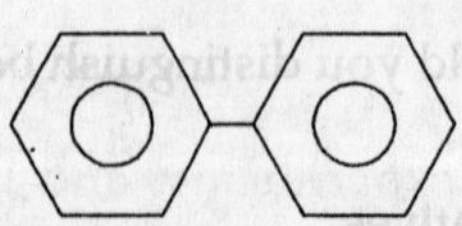

Biphenyl or phenyl benzene

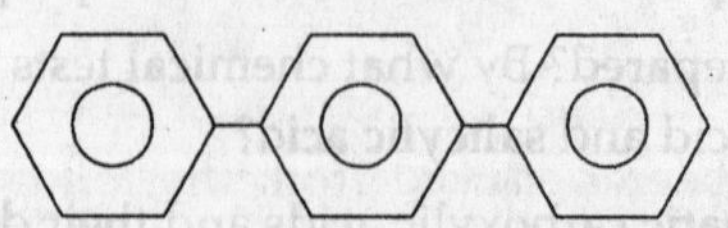

Triphenyl or 1, 4-diphenyl benzene

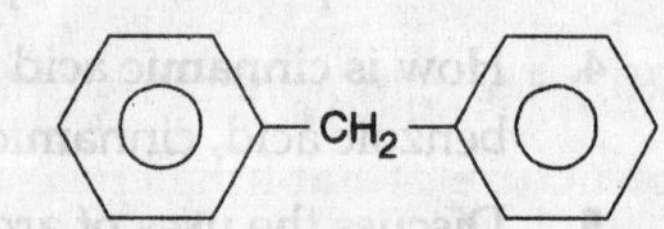

Diphenyl methane

20.1 Condensed Polynuclear Aromatic Hydrocarbons

20.1.1 Naphthalene ($C_{10}H_8$)

It is the most abundant constituent of coal tar and is important as a source of phthalic and anthranilic acids which are intermediates to various dyes such as azo, indigo, triphenyl methane, etc. Naphthalene is used as moth replellant and insecticides. Hydrated naphthalene is used in motor fuels, lubricant and as a solvent.

20.1.1.1 Isolation of Naphthalene

It is isolated from the middle oil fraction of the coal tar in pure form according to following flow sheet.

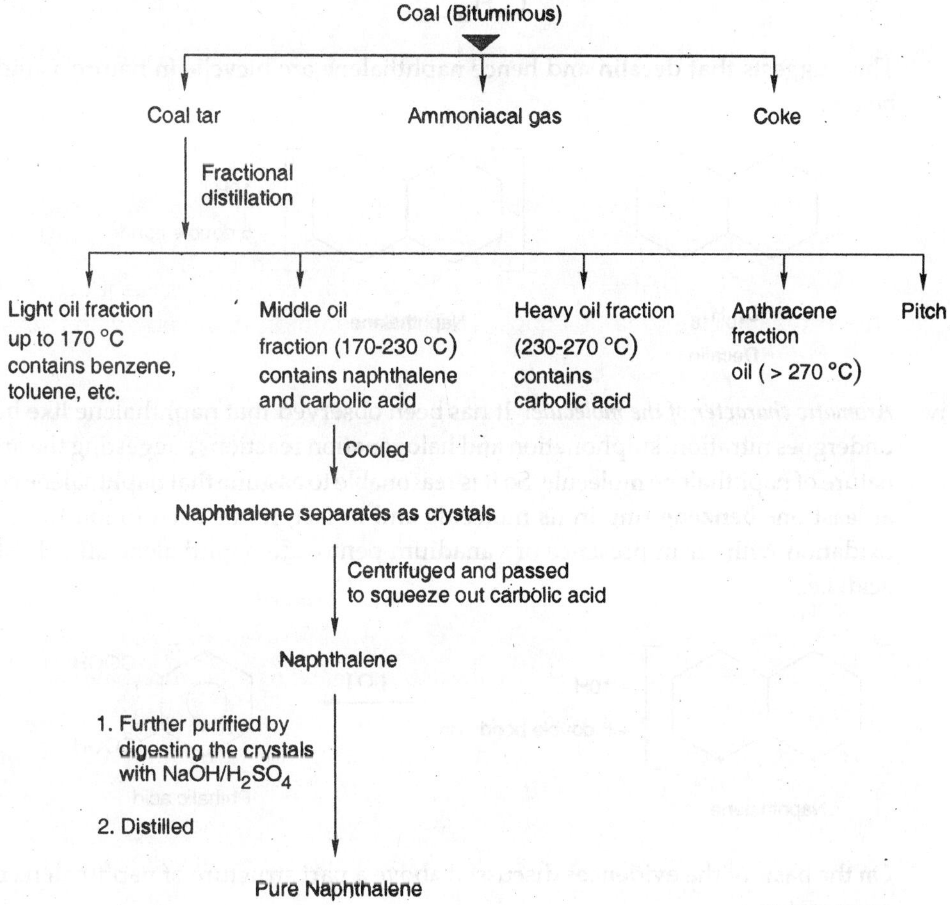

20.1.1.2 Structure of Naphthalene

Structure of naphthalene has been deduced from the following experimental and logical arguments.

i. Analytical data and molecular weight determination reveal that naphthalene has the molecular formula, $C_{10}H_8$.

ii. Extremely low content of hydrogen suggests that naphthalene molecule is highly unsaturated. Experimental evidence in favour of such assumption has been secured from catalytic hydrogenation. On catalytic hydrogenation naphthalene absorbs five mole equivalents of hydrogen and forms completely saturated hydrocarbon, decalin.

$$\underset{\text{Naphthalene}}{C_{10}H_{18}} \xrightarrow[\text{Cat [H]}]{5[H_2]} \underset{\text{Decalin}}{C_{10}H_{18}}$$

iii. Further, the completely saturated hydrocarbon, decalin has the molecular formula, $C_{10}H_{18}$ which can be expressed by the general formula,

$$C_nH_{2n-2.}$$

This suggests that decalin and hence naphthalene are bicyclic in nature as indicated below:

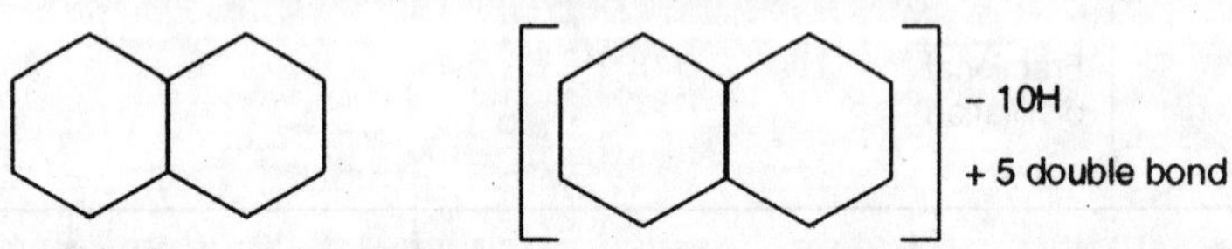

$C_{10}H_{18}$ Decalin   Naphthalene

iv. *Aromatic character of the molecule*: It has been observed that naphthalene like benzene undergoes nitration, sulphonation and halogenation reactions suggesting the aromatic nature of naphthalene molecule. So it is reasonable to assume that naphthalene contains at least one benzene ring in its molecule and in fact, it has been found to be so. On oxidation with air in presence of vanadium pentoxide naphthalene affords phthalic acid, i.e.,

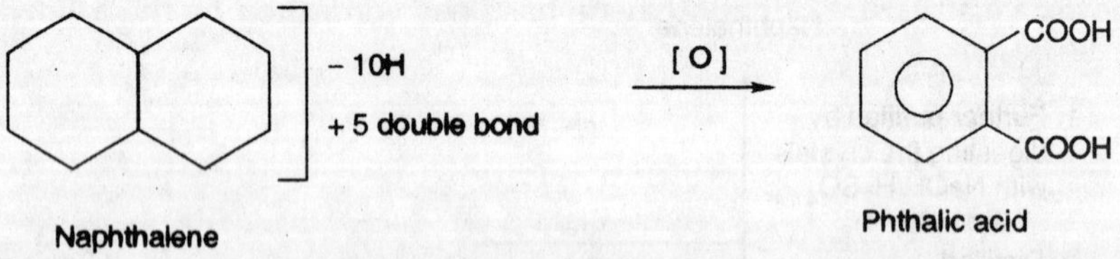

Naphthalene   Phthalic acid

On the basis of the evidences discussed above a part structure of naphthalene may be represented as

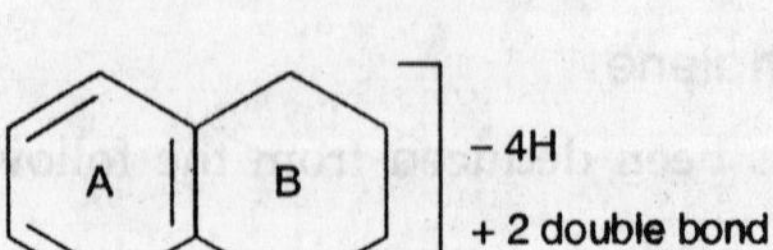

Naphthalene

v. *Both the rings are benzenoid*: That both the rings in naphthalene are benzenoid in character has been established from the experimental evidence as depicted below:

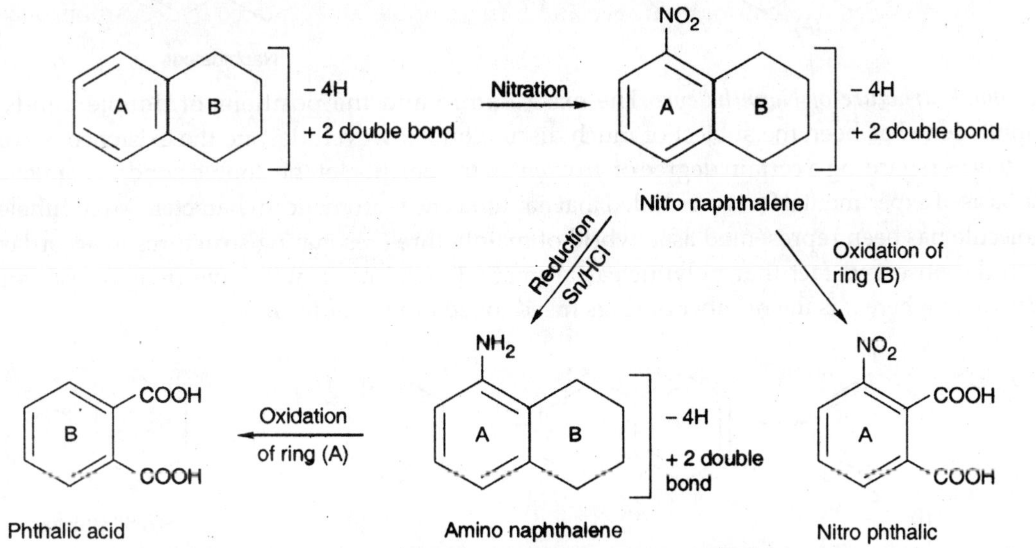

The above experiment unambiguously establishes that both the rings in naphthalene are benzenoid in character. It is known that aromatic ring containing electron withdrawing group resists oxidation while aromatic ring having electron releasing group is highly susceptible to oxidation. Thus, the provisional structure of naphthalene may be represented as under:

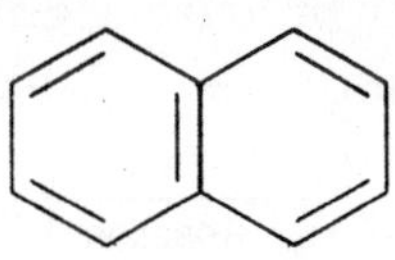

Naphthalene

vi. The above structure of naphthalene has been confirmed by the following synthesis due to *Haworth*.

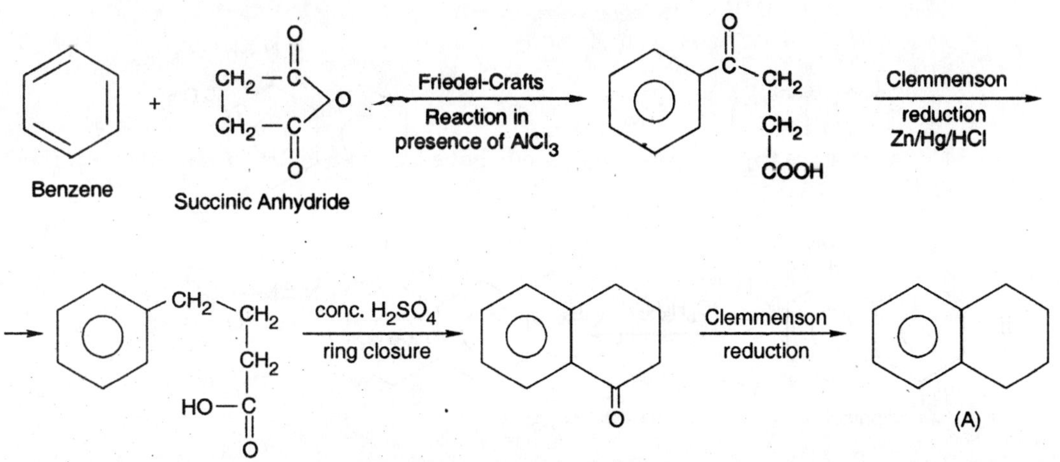

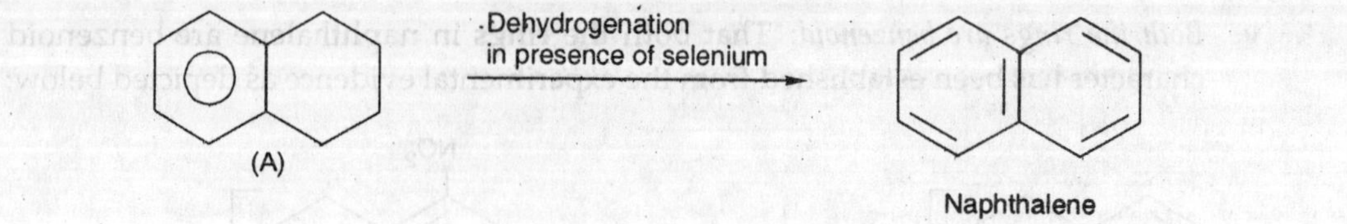

Bond structure of Naphthalene: The exact nature and the positions of double bonds in naphthalene has been the subject of much discussion. However, despite the existence of some evidences regarding a certain degree of *'fixation'* in the position of the double bonds, chemists on the basis of experimental facts concluded that naphthalene is aromatic in character. So naphthalene molecule has been represented as a hybrid of mainly three resonating structures in accordance with the observed fact that polynuclear aromatic hydrocarbon will have $(n + 1)$ resonating structures where n is the number of rings fused together in a molecule.

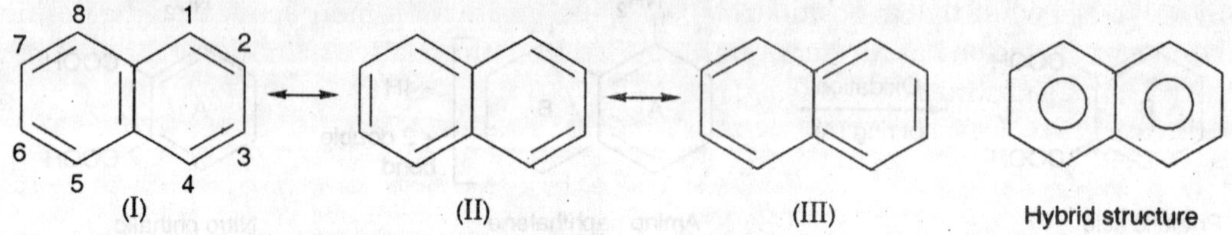

Among these, structure (I) has predominant contribution according to Fries rule— "the most stable arrangement of a polynuclear compound is that form which has the maximum number of rings in benzenoid condition."

Nature of the bonds in Naphthalene (Aromaticity) : It has been observed that 1, 2-bond is more active than 2, 3-bond from the coupling reactions as noted below:

i.

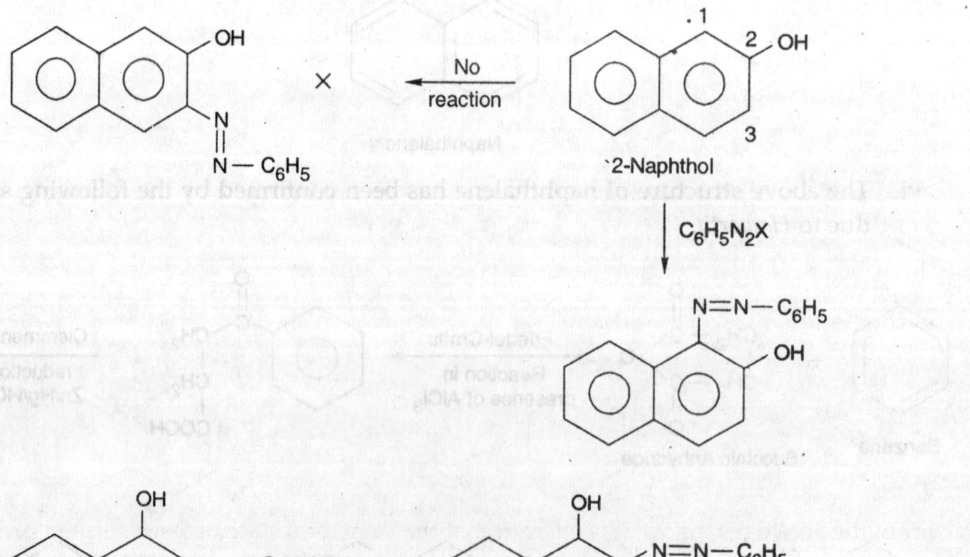

ii.

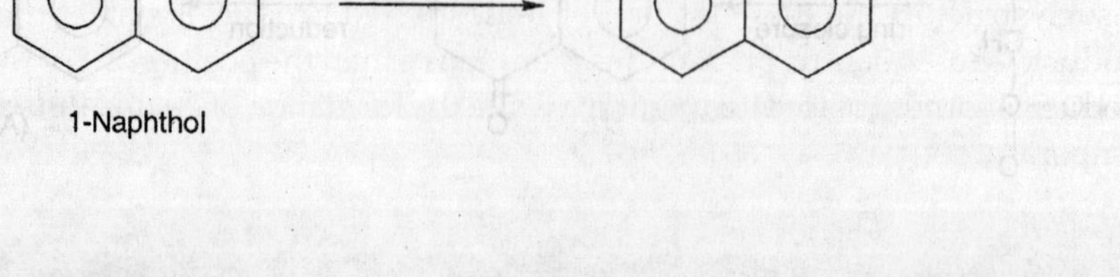

iii. 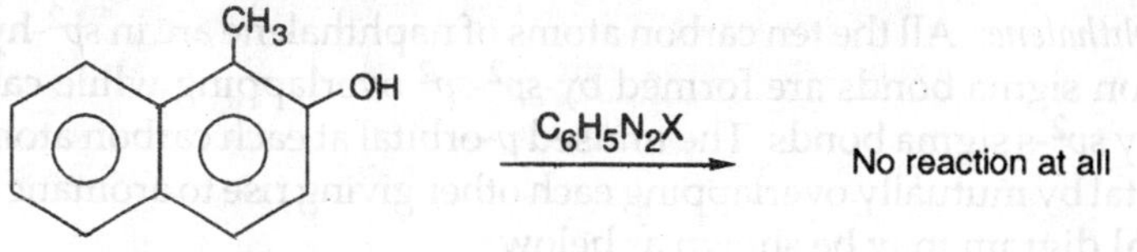

1-Methyl-2-naphthol

From the above experiments it may also be concluded that all the positions in naphthalene are not equally electron dense. Or in other words, double bonds in naphthalene are to some extent fixed. This has been supported by bond distance measurement which reveals that 1, 2-bond distance is 1.36Å while that of 2, 3 is 1.39Å. Hence it may be concluded that naphthalene is less aromatic than benzene.

Now the question arises which one position 1 or 2 is more active? Answer to this question has been secured from charge density calculations. Such calculation shows that charge density at position 1 is 0.44 while that at position 2 is 0.41. Thus, position 1 is more active than the position 2. The above conclusion has further been supported from the relative stabilities of the transition states of 1 and 2-substituted products. Thus,

Transition state of 1-substituted product:

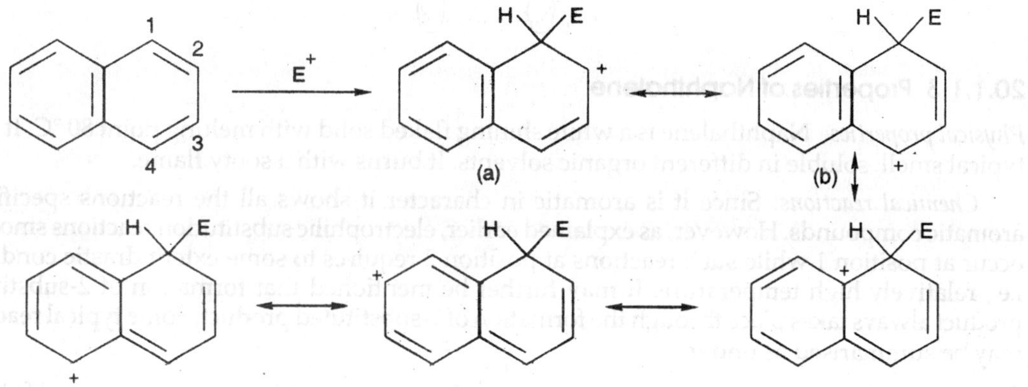

Transition state of 2-substituted product:

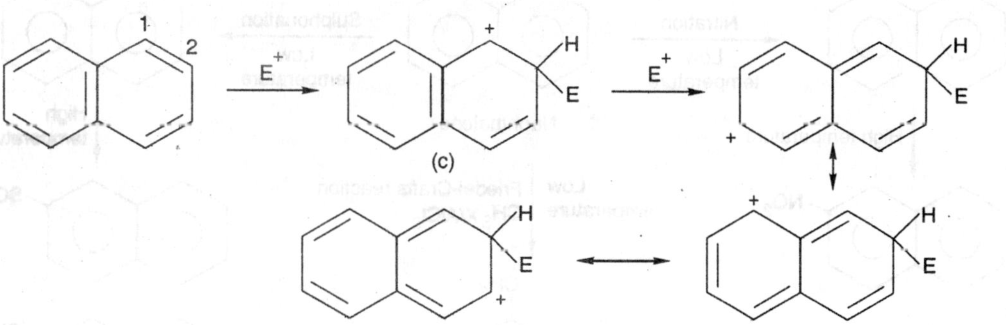

From the above resonance it is evident that the transition state of 1-substituted product has two contributing structures (a and b) in benzenoid condition while that of 2-substituted product has only one (c) such structure. So the transition of 1-substituted product is stabler than that of 2-substituted product. Consequently, position 1 is more active than the position 2. For this reason 1-substituted product is formed at low temperature while the formation of 2-substituted product requires high temperature.

Orbital structure of Naphthalene: All the ten carbon atoms of naphthalene are in sp^2-hybridised state and the carbon-carbon sigma bonds are formed by sp^2-sp^2 overlapping while carbon and hydrogen are connected by sp^2-s sigma bonds. The unused *p*-orbital at each carbon atom forms a continuous molecular orbital by mutually overlapping each other giving rise to aromatic character in naphthalene. The orbital digram may be shown as below.

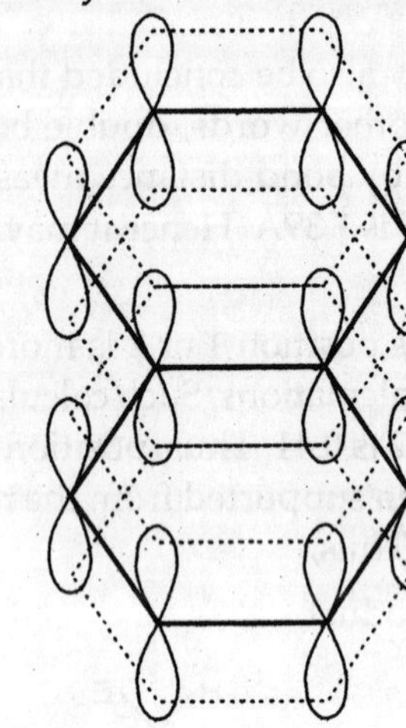

20.1.1.3 Properties of Naphthalene

Physical properties: Naphthalene is a white shining flaked solid with melting point 80 °C. It has a typical smell, soluble in different organic solvents. It burns with a sooty flame.

Chemical reactions: Since it is aromatic in character it shows all the reactions specific for aromatic compounds. However, as explained earlier, electrophilic substitution reactions smoothly occur at position 1 while such reactions at position 2 requires to some extent drastic condition, i.e., relatively high temperature. It may further be mentioned that formation of 2-substituted product always takes place through the formation of 1-substituted product. Some typical reactions may be summarised as under:

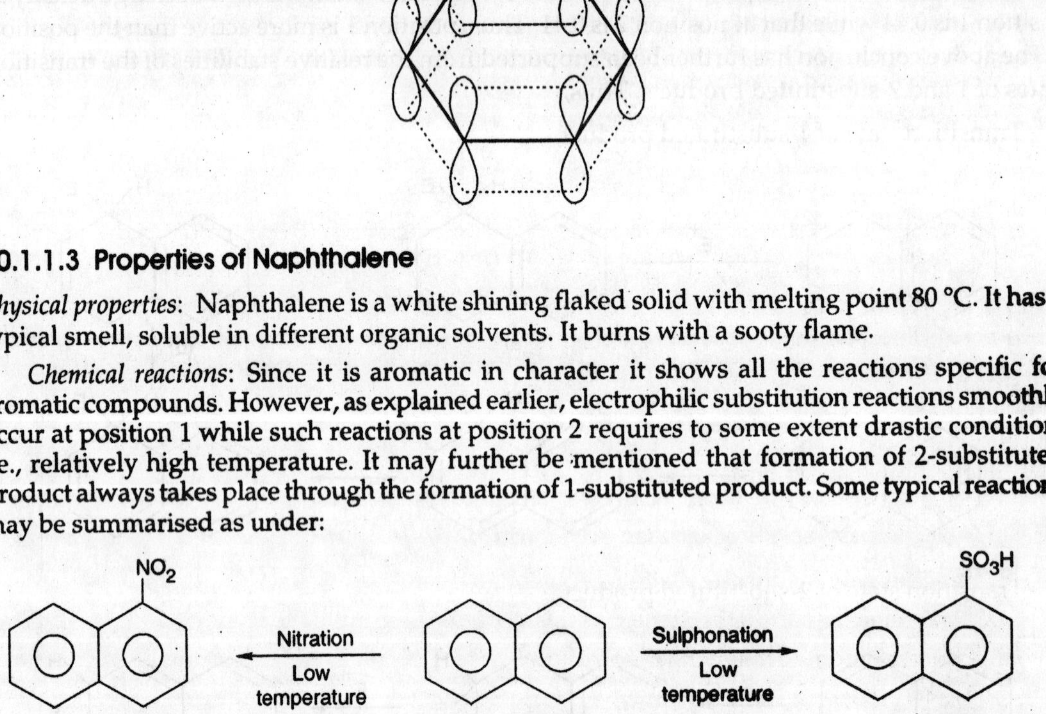

It may be mentioned that as the sulphonation and Friedel-Crafts reaction is carried out at high temperature, 2-substituted product is the main product in these two reactions.

Two most important derivatives of naphthalene are naphthols and naphthylamines. They are prepared by following the same general methods of preparation of such derivatives of benzene.

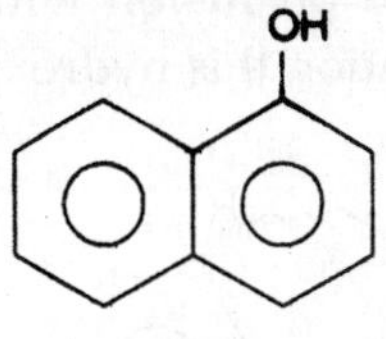
α-Naphthol

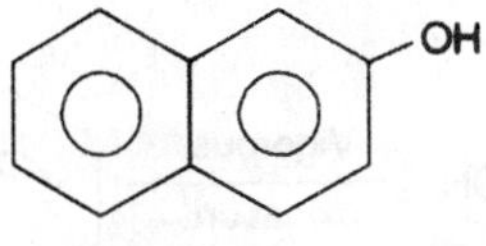
β-Naphthol

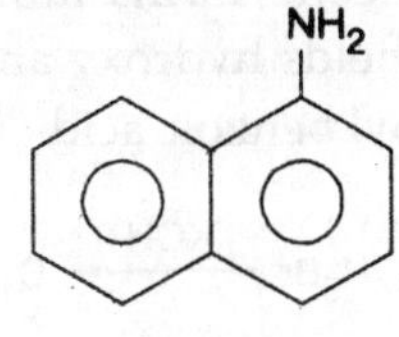
α-Naphthyl amine

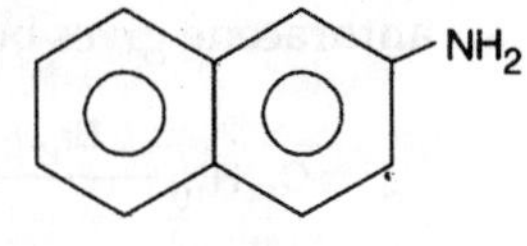
β-Naphthyl amine

Both these types of naphthalene derivatives are used in the manufacture of dyes.

PROBLEM 20.1

i. **Show that naphthalene is a bicyclic compound.**

ii. **Suggest the** product

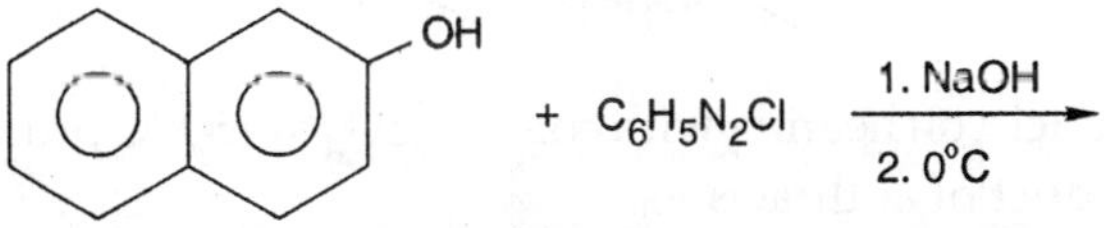

20.1.2 Anthracene

Anthracene, another member of polynuclear aromatic hydrocarbon is a constituent of coal tar. It is isolated from anthracene oil fraction of coal tar from which crude anthracene crystals are separated. Finally these crude crystals are purified to get pure crystals of anthracene having melting point 216 °C. It is used in the manufacture of alizarin dye and anthraquinone. It is a tricyclic fused aromatic hydrocarbon.

20.1.2.1 Structure of Anthracene

Its structure has been deduced from the following evidences:

i. **Analytical data indicate that it has the molecular formula, $C_{14}H_{10}$.**

ii. **On catalytic hydrogenation anthracene froms a completely saturated hydrocarbon, $C_{14}H_{24}$.**

$$C_{14}H_{10} \xrightarrow[14\,H]{\text{Cat [H]}} C_{14}H_{24}$$

This suggests the presence of seven double bonds in anthracene.

Again, the saturated hydrocarbon, $C_{14}H_{24}$, formed can be expressed as C_nH_{2n-4}. This reveals that saturated anthracene and hence anthracene is a tricyclic molecule and so its part structure may be represented as indicated below:

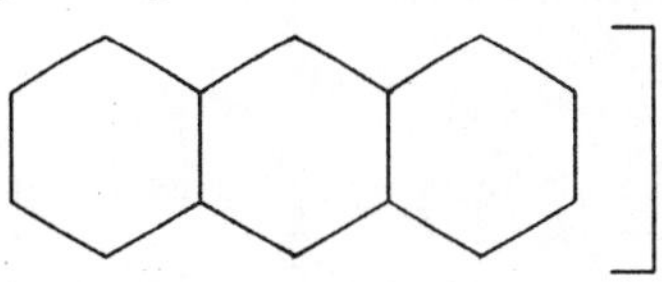
– 14H
+ 7 double bonds

iii. **It shows striking similarities with benzene and naphthalene and like them undergoes typical reactions of aromatic compounds. So it may be concluded that anthracene is aromatic in nature.**

iv. The conclusive evidence regarding its aromatic character has been secured from the following experiment:

Bromination of anthracene forms mono-bromo anthracene which on fusion with potassium hydroxide yields hydroxy anthracene. On vigorous oxidation this hydroxy anthracene gives benzoyl benzoic acid.

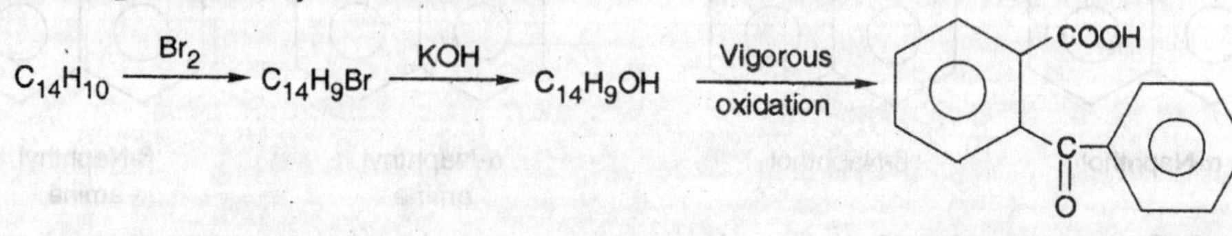

o-benzoyl benzoic acid

This experiment indicates that anthracene contains at least two benzene rings in its molecule and hence its part structure may be extended as under:

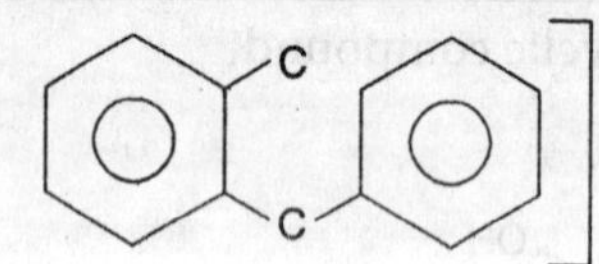

v. *o*-benzoyl benzoic acid on heating with conc. H_2SO_4 at 150 °C produces anthraquinone—the oxidation product of anthracene.

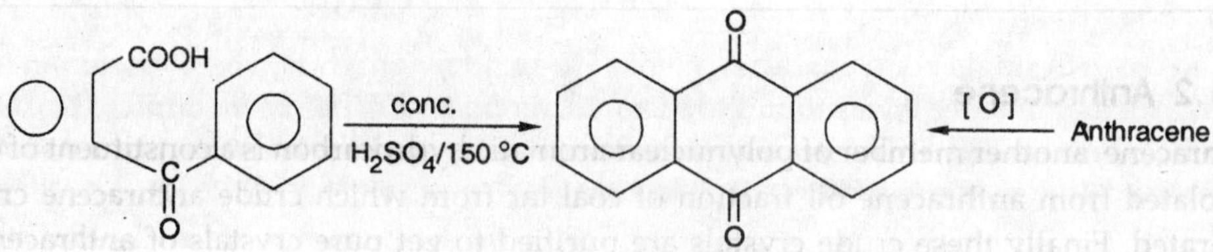

Anthraquinone

vi. Anthraquinone on reduction with Zn-dust yields anthracene. So the structure of anthracene may provisionally be expressed as

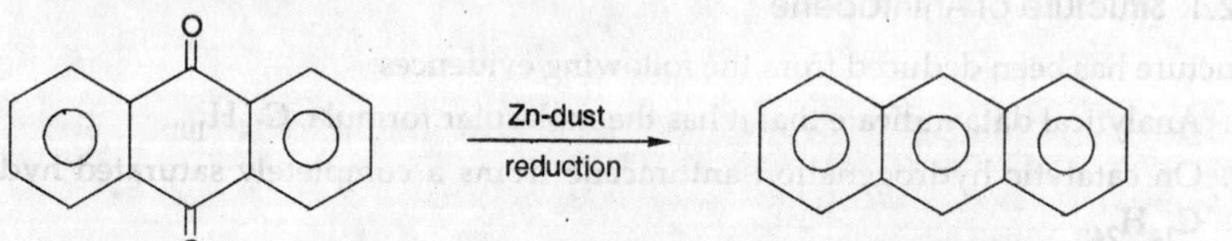

Anthracene

vii. The above provisional structure has been confirmed by the following synthesis.

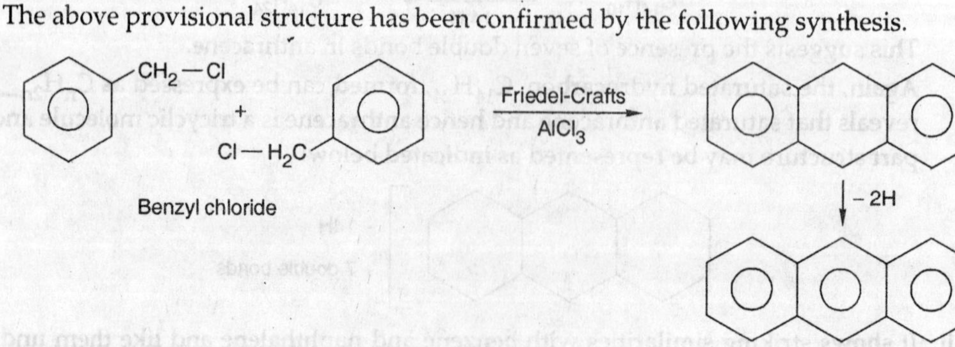

Anthracene

Bond structure of Anthracene: As mentioned anthracene is aromatic in nature, X-ray analysis reveals that it is a planar molecule. So it is assumed that anthracene is a resonationg molecule and exists as a resonance hybrid of the following structures.

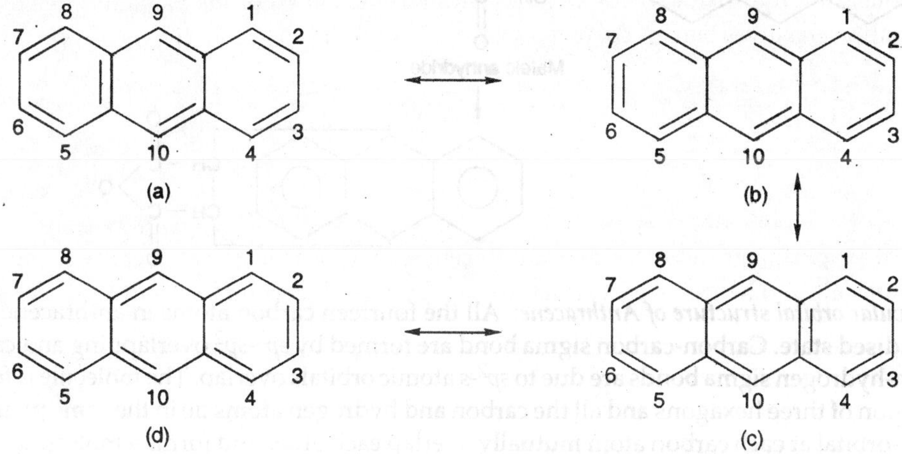

A careful analysis of the above structures indicates that out of four structures in three structures (a, b, c) there is a double bond at 1, 2-position and a single bond at 2, 3-positions. Hence it may be concluded that 1, 2-bond in anthracene has ¾ th double bond character while 2, 3-bond has ¾ th single bond character. Hence 1, 2-bond length should be shorter than that of 2, 3-bond. In actual practice it was found to be so. 1, 2-bond length has been found to be 1.37Å, while that of 2, 3 bond is 1.42Å. Thus, it may be concluded that double bonds in anthracene are to some extent fixed and so it is less aromatic than benzene.

Further, it is seen that in all the four structures there is a double bond at 9, 10 positions and since double bonds in anthracene are to some extent fixed, it is expected that 9, 10 positions should be highly active. In fact, it has been found to be so. These positions in reality resemble olefinic double bond and readily undergo addition reactions which is evidenced from the following reactions.

i.

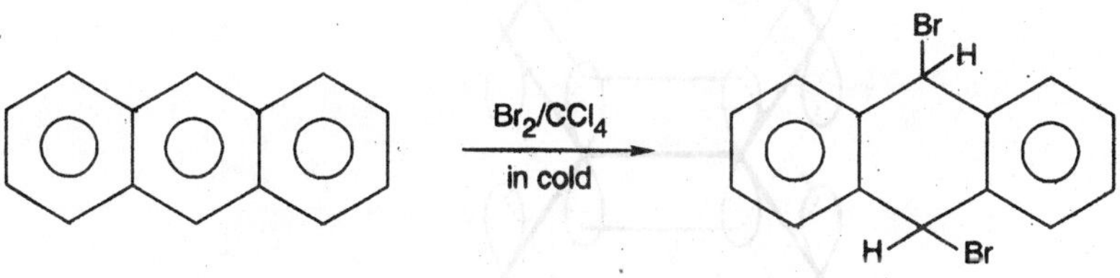

ii.

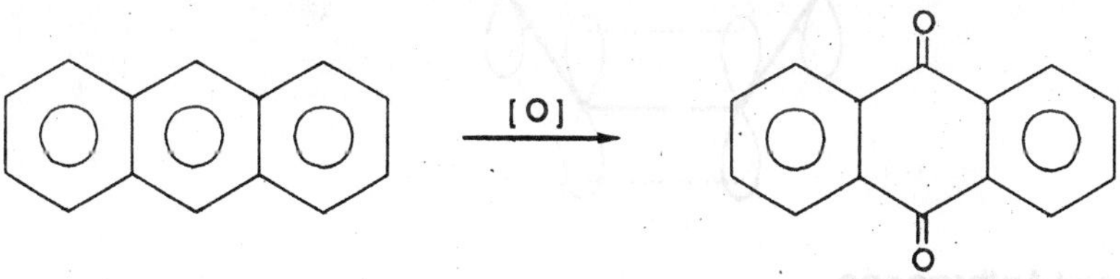

Anthraquinone

iii. 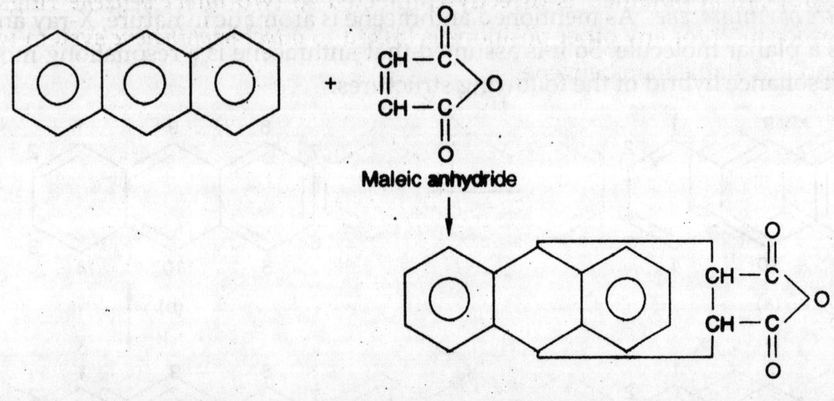

Molecular orbital structure of Anthracene: All the fourteen carbon atoms in anthracene are in sp^2-hybridised state. Carbon-carbon sigma bond are formed by sp^2-sp^2 overlapping and carbon-hydrogen-hydrogen sigma bonds are due to sp^2-s atomic orbitals overlap. The molecule is formed by the fusion of three hexagons and all the carbon and hydrogen atoms lie in the same plane. The unused *p*-orbital at each carbon atom mutually overlap each other and forms a molecular orbital which is continuous throughout the whole molecule and is spread over above and below the plane of the molecule resulting in the aromatic character of anthracene. The orbital diagram may be shown as below:

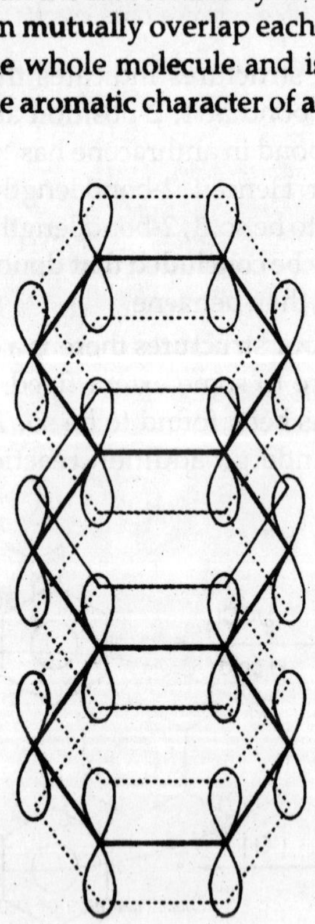

20.1.2.2 Properties of Anthracene

As mentioned, anthracene is an aromatic hydrocarbon and undergoes typical reactions of aromatic compounds such as nitration, sulphonation, halogenation, Friedel-Crafts reactions, etc. However, as pointed out during structure elucidation that 9, 10 positions are highly active so reaction primarily occurs at these positions. But, under certain conditions electrophilic substitution can take place at 1 and 2 positions. The higher activity at 9 and 10 positions is due to the fact that the intermediate carbocation obtained is directly connected to two *intact benzene* rings while intermediate carbocation for any other positions is linked to *intact naphthalene* system which is less aromatic and less stable than benzene.

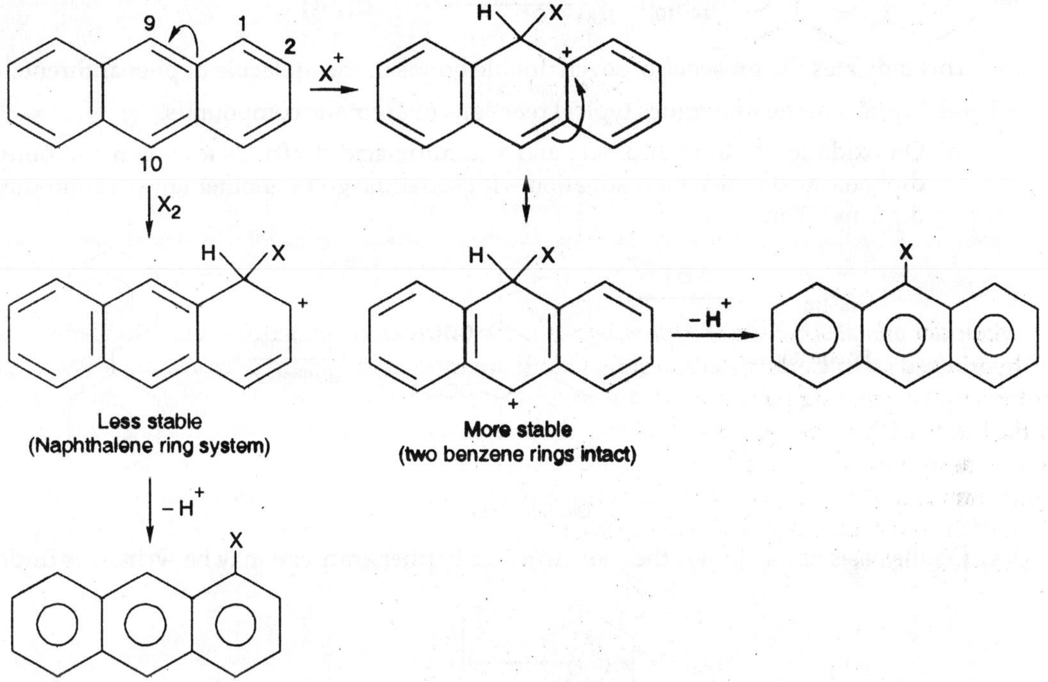

Dimerisation: An interesting reaction of anthracene is its dimerisation. On exposure of its saturated solution in xylene to sunlight it readily dimerises to form crystals of dimeric product known as dianthracene or para anthracene.

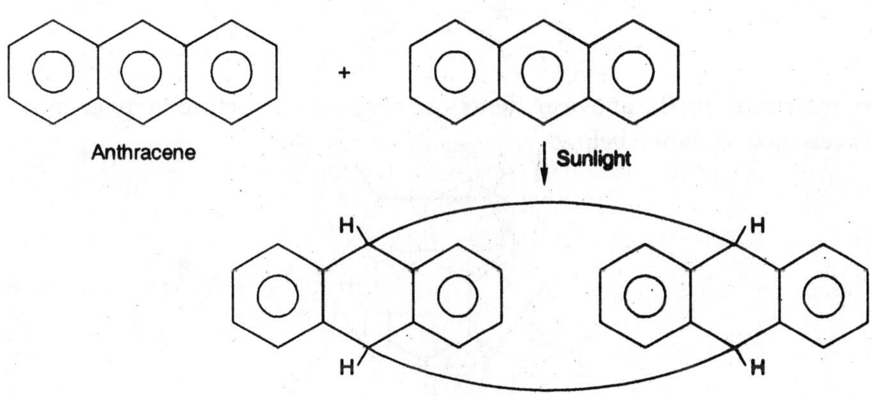

Dianthracene or *para* anthracene

20.1.3 Phenanthrene ($C_{14}H_{10}$)

Phenanthrene, an isomer of anthracene is also an ingredient of coal tar. Its structure has been deduced from various chemical experiments and logical arguments as presented below.

1. Analytical data and molecular weight determination establish its molecular formula as $C_{14}H_{10}$.

2. On catalytic hydrogenation phenanthrene furnishes perhydro compound having molecular formula, $C_{14}H_{24}$, i.e.,

$$C_{14}H_{10} \xrightarrow{\text{Cat [H]}} C_{14}H_{24}$$

This indicates the presence of seven double bonds in the molecule of phenanthrene.

3. (a) Phenanthrene undergoes typical reactions of aromatic compounds.

   (b) On oxidation with dichromate and sulphuric acid it affords a known compound, diphenic acid which on distillation with sodalime gives another known compound, diphenyl. Thus,

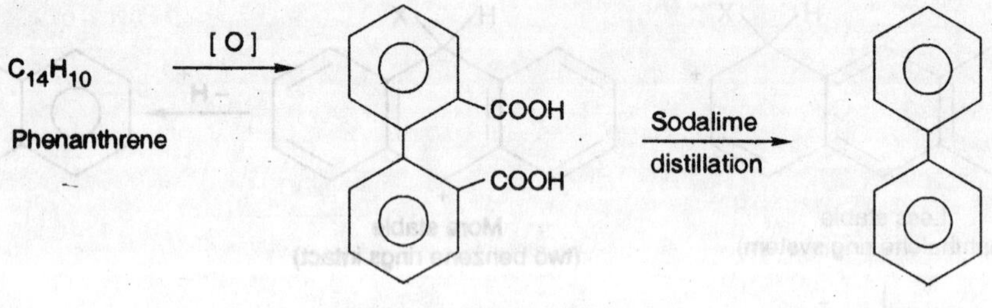

Dipheric acid Diphenyl

4. On the basis of the above, the part structure of phenanthrene may be written as under:

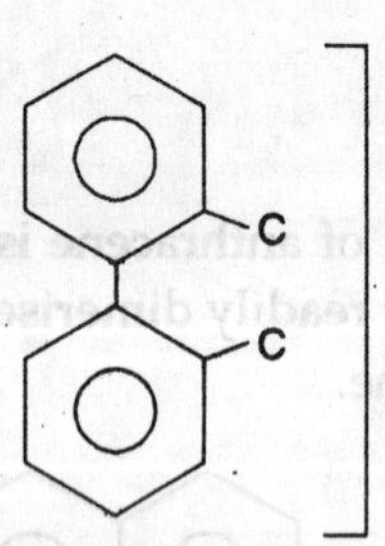

5. After scrutinising the above evidences a provisional structure for phenanthrene may be represented as shown below:

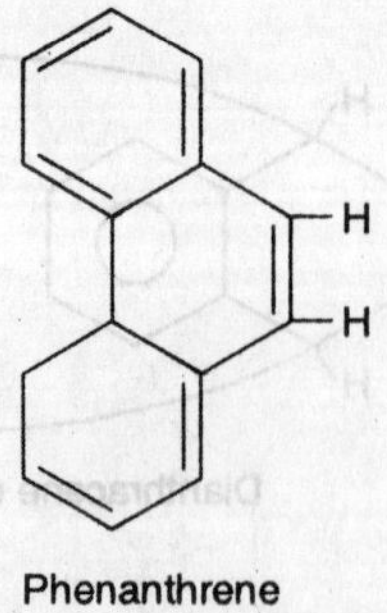

Phenanthrene

6. The above provisional structure has been confirmed by the following synthesis by Bardhan and Sengupta.

Step 1:

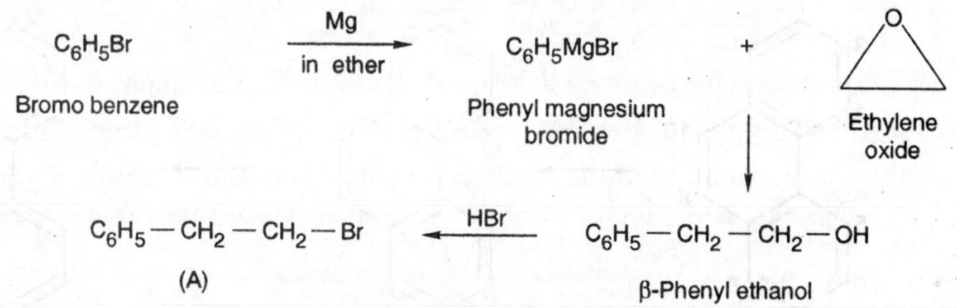

Step 2:

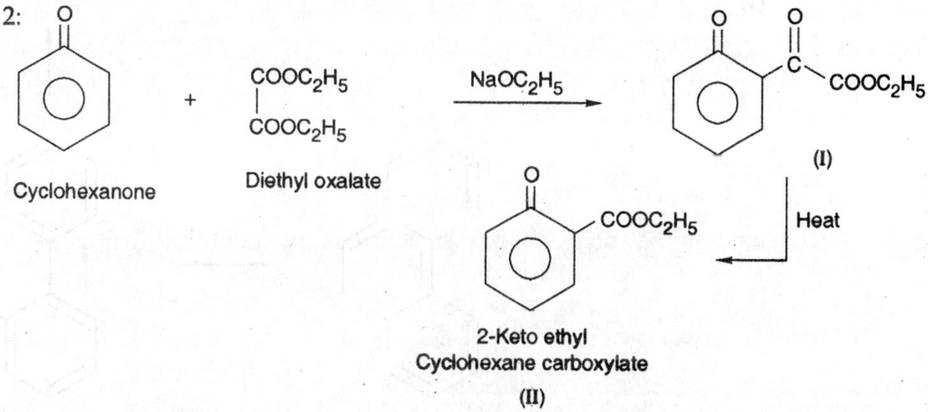

Step 3:

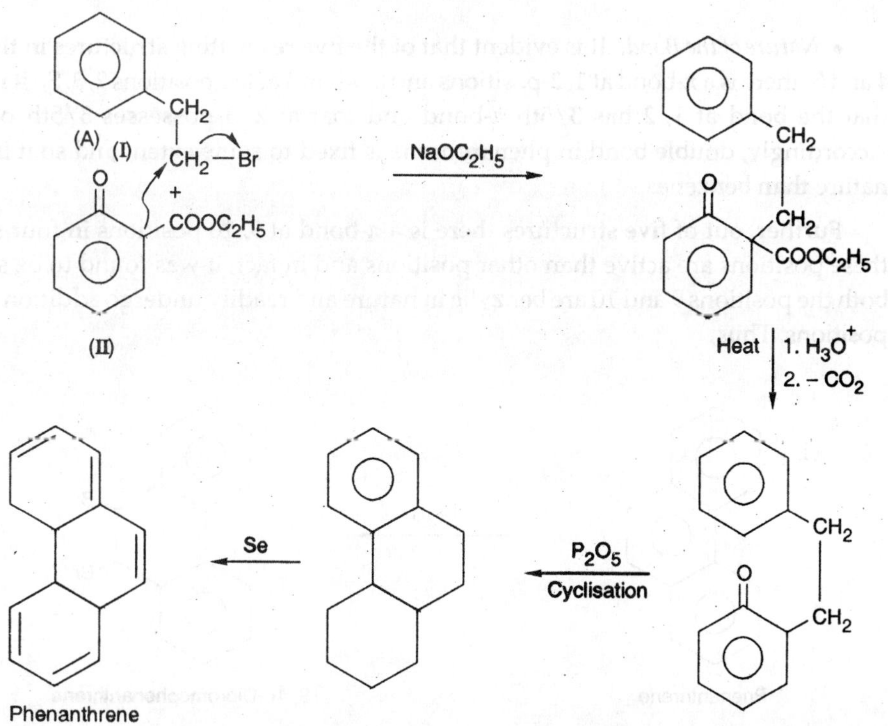

• *Bond structure of Phenanthrene*: Like anthracene phenanthrene was found to exist in resonance hybrid of the following structures.

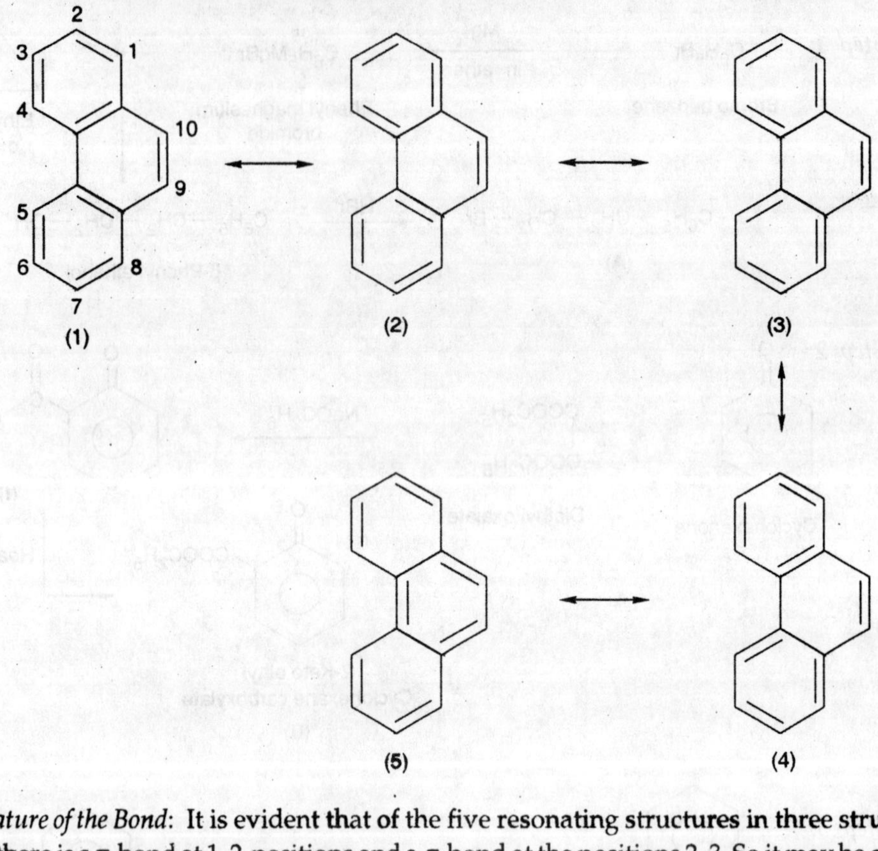

• *Nature of the Bond*: It is evident that of the five resonating structures in three structures (1, 4 and 5) there is a π-bond at 1, 2-positions and a σ-bond at the positions 2, 3. So it may be concluded that the bond at 1, 2 has 3/5th π-bond and that at 2, 3 possesses 3/5th σ-bond character. Accordingly, double bond in phenanthrene is fixed to some extent and so it is less aromatic in nature than benzene.

Further, out of five structures there is a π-bond at 9, 10 positions in four structures and so these positions are active than other positions and in fact, it was found to be so by the fact that both the positions 9 and 10 are benzylic in nature and readily undergo addition reactions at these positions. Thus,

i.

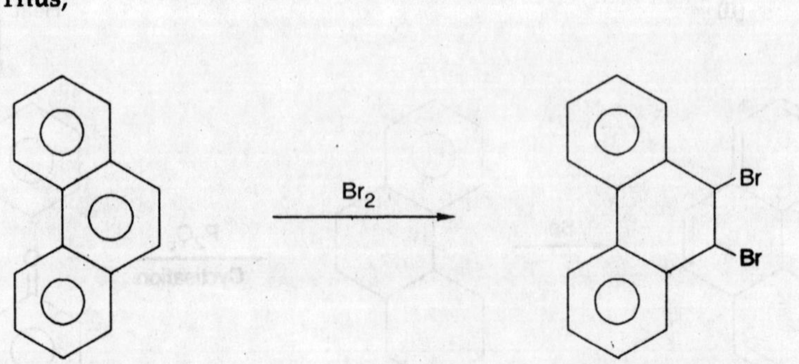

ii.

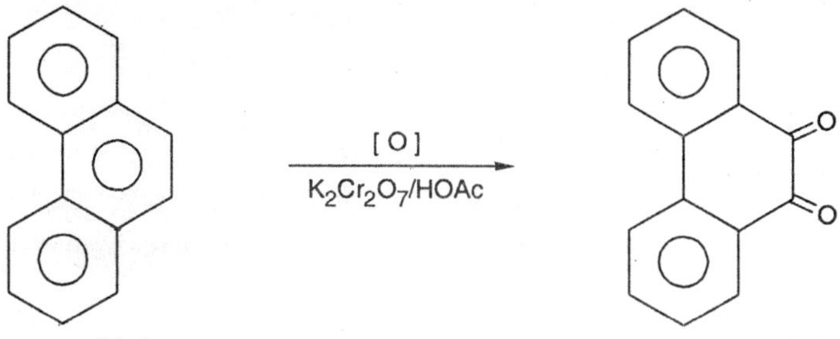

Phenanthra quinone

• *Orbital structure of Phenanthrene*: All the fourteen carbon atoms in phenanthrene are in the sp^2-hybridised state. Carbon-carbon sigma-bonds are due to sp^2-sp^2 overlap. All the three benzene rings along with their carbon and hydrogen atoms lie in the same plane. The unhybridised *p*-orbitals at each carbon atom mutually overlap each other to form a continuous molecular orbital spreading over above and below the plane of the molecule. This closed molecular orbital imparts aromatic character to phenanthrene. The orbital diagram may be represented as drawn below:

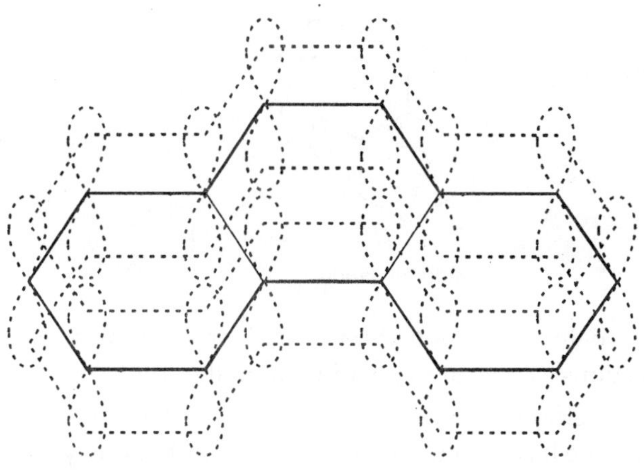

Orbital diagram of phenanthrene

20.1.3.1 Properties of Phenanthrene

Most of the reactivities of phenanthrene are confined around the positions 9 and 10. These two positions are relatively active than other positions. The reason behind the higher activities at these positions may be rationalised on the basis of greater stability of intermediate carbocations formed at these positions compared to intermediate carbocations resulting from other positions. The greater stability of carbocations at these positions is due to their direct attachment with intact benzene rings, or in other words, these two positions are benzylic in nature and so more stabilisation of carbocations occurs due to extended resonance. So both addition and substitution reactions (electrophilic) take place at these positions. Thus,

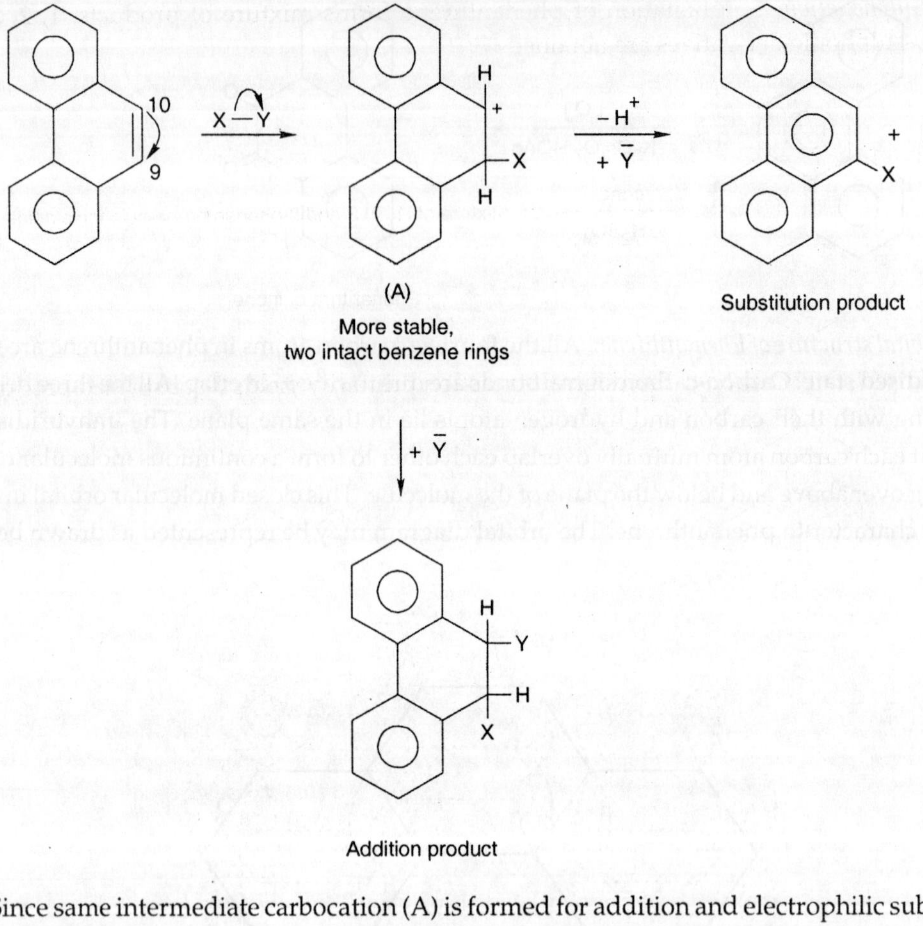

Since same intermediate carbocation (A) is formed for addition and electrophilic substitution reactions both the reactions can occur depending upon the conditions of the reactions.

Besides these two positions, electrophilic substitution can occur at 1, 2 and 3 positions to some extent. Phenanthrene has been found to undergo most of the typical reactions of aromatic compounds at these positions at different ease as expected. Thus,

i. *Nitration*: On nitration mixture of 1, 2 and 3-mononitro derivatives are formed of which 3-nitro derivative is the major product.

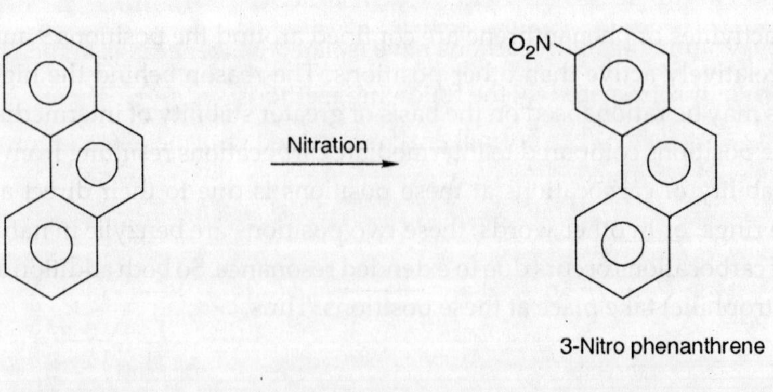

ii. *Sulphonation*: Sulphonation of phenanthrene forms mixture of products. 1, 2, 3, and 9-sulphonic derivatives are obtained.

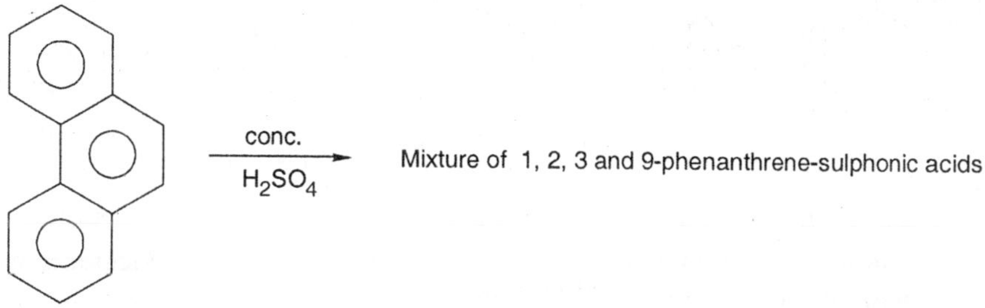

iii. *Friedel-Crafts reaction*: Friedel crafts reaction primarily yields 3-substituted product.

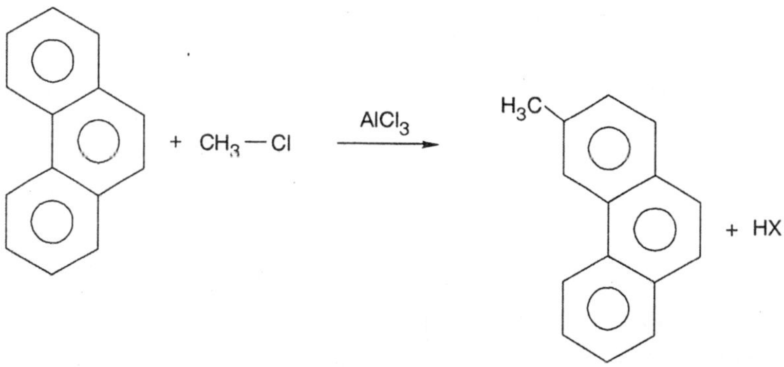

3-Methyl phenanthrene

PROBLEM 20.2

i. How will you prove that phenanthrene is an angularly oriented tricyclic compound?
ii. What happens in the following case?

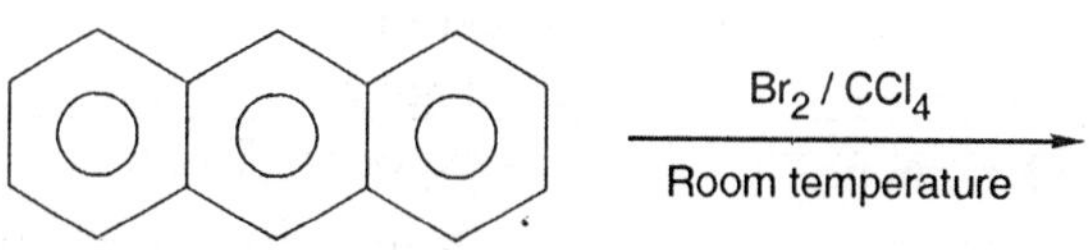

20.2 Simple Polynuclear Aromatic Hydrocarbons

These polynuclear aromatic hydrocarbons have isolated benzene rings in their molecules.

(a) **Diphenyl:** It is prepared by the following methods:

i. *Fittig's reaction*: When bromobenzene is treated with metallic sodium in ether solution diphenyl is formed.

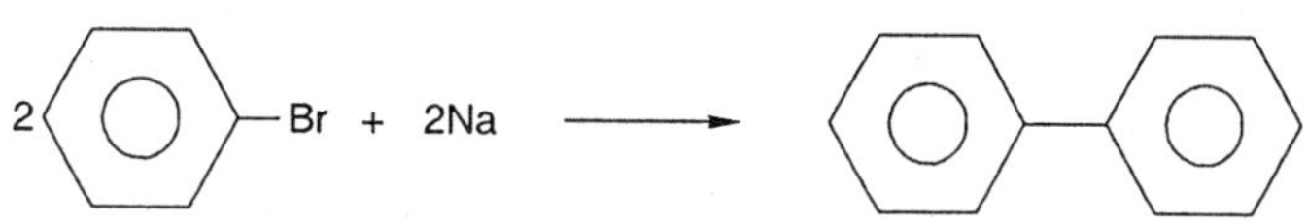

Bromobenzene Diphenyl

ii. *Ullmann synthesis*: In this synthesis iodobenzene is heated with copper powder in a sealed tube to yield diphenyl.

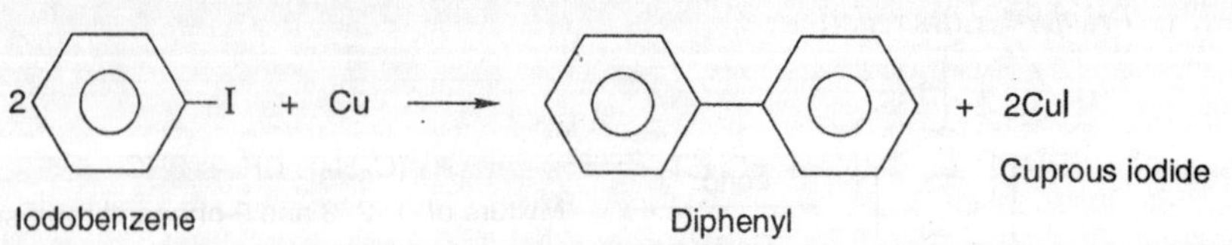

iii. *By diazotisation reaction*: When benzidine is diazotised, corresponding diazonium salt is obtained. When this diazo salt is allowed to stand in contact with hypophosphoric acid, diphenyl is obtained.

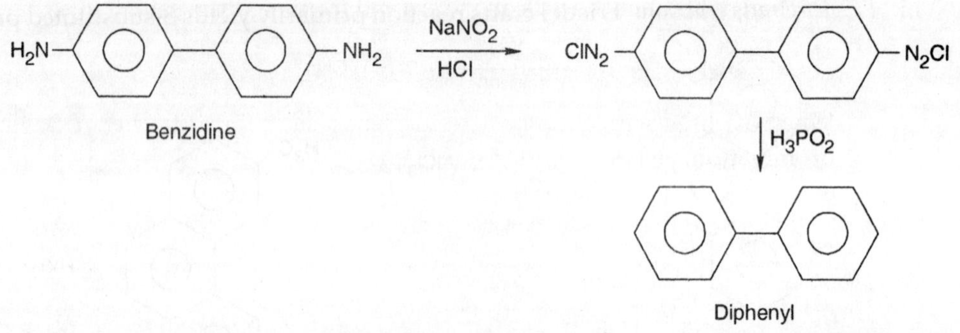

Diphenyl is a colourless solid having melting point at 70 °C. It undergoes all the characteristic reactions of aromatic compounds and behaves as phenyl substituted benzene in which phenyl substituent acts as electron releasing group and activates the benzene ring, particularly at *ortho* and *para* positions. When substituents are present at *ortho* positions in diphenyl, the molecule becomes dissymmetric and hence optically active.

(b) **Diphenyl methane:** It is a colourless crystalline solid and melts at 25 °C. It behaves chemically like diphenyl. It is prepared in the following way:

i. *Friedel-Crafts reaction*: Friedel-Crafts reaction between benzyl chloride and benzene forms diphenyl methane.

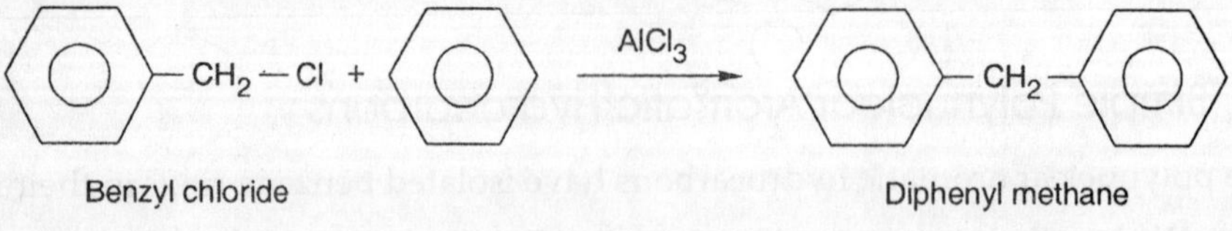

ii. *Reduction of benzophenone*: Benzophenone when reduced with hydroiodic acid in presence of red phosphorous, diphenyl methane is obtained.

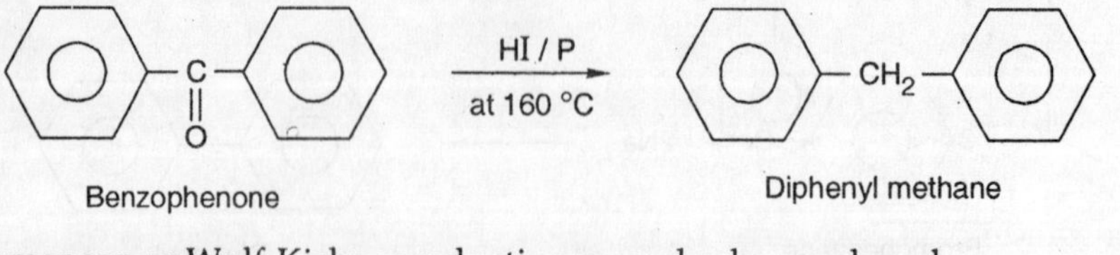

Clemmenson or Wolf-Kishner reduction may also be employed.

(c) **Triphenyl methane:** It is a colourless crystalline solid and melts at 94 °C. It is normally prepared by the following methods:

i. *Friedel-Crafts reaction:*

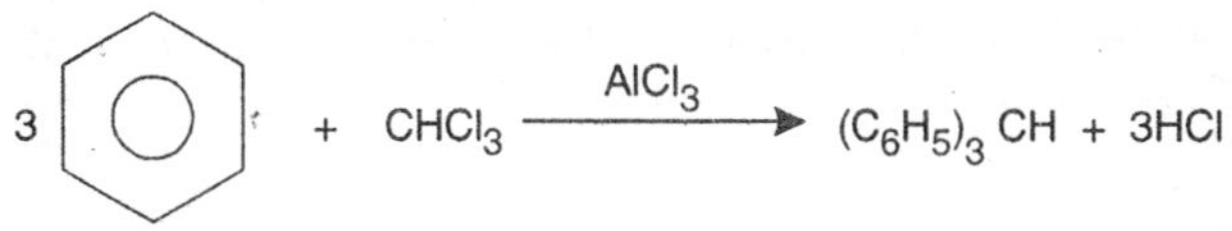

ii. Condensation of benzaldehyde with benzene may also yield triphenyl methane.

$$C_6H_5CHO + C_6H_6 \xrightarrow{ZnCl_2} (C_6H_5)_3\,CH + H_2O$$

Triphenyl methane is acidic in nature and forms sodium salt.

$$(C_6H_5)_3\,CH + Na \xrightarrow[\text{solution}]{\text{In ether}} (C_6H_5)_3\,\bar{C}\overset{+}{Na}$$

When oxidised with chromic acid in acetic acid, it forms triphenyl carbinol, and on bromination, yields bromide.

$$(C_6H_5)_3\,CH \xrightarrow{[\,O\,]} (C_6H_5)_3\,C{-}OH$$

Triphenyl carbinol

$$(C_6H_5)_3\,CH + Br_2 \longrightarrow (C_6H_5)_3\,C{-}Br$$

Triphenyl bromide

20.3 Carcinogenic Hydrocarbons

Recently there has been a considerable interest in the chemistry of complex polynuclear aromatic hydrocarbons as they are carcinogenic in nature, i.e., cancer producing. The hydrocarbon first shown to have carcinogenic activity is 1, 2, 5, 6-dibenzanthracene. Later other polynuclear aromatic hydrocarbons have been either isolated from coal tar or obtained by synthetic means to have strong carcinogenic activity. Some of the most powerful carcinogenic hydrocarbons are mentioned below:

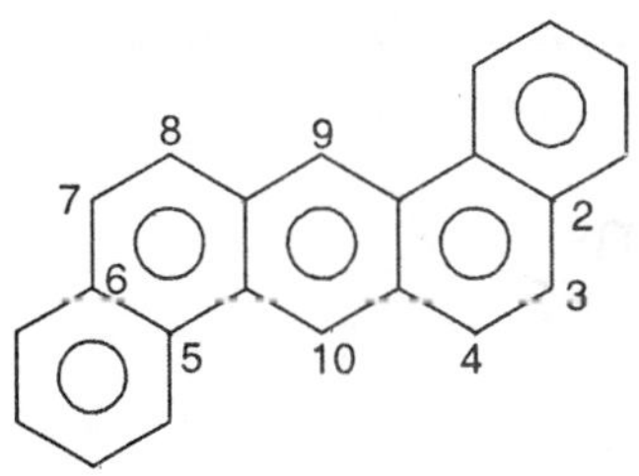

1, 2, 5, 6-Dibenzanthracene

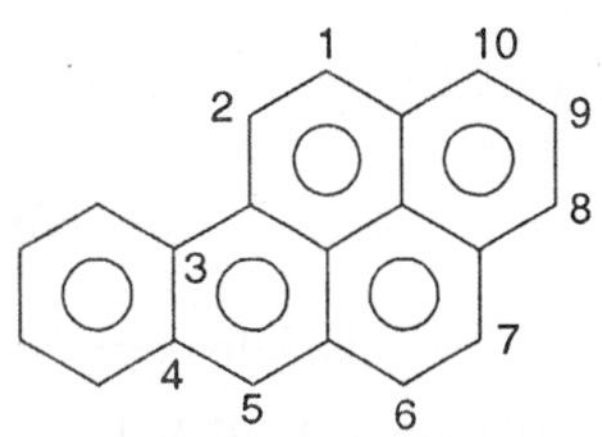

3, 4-Benzpyrene

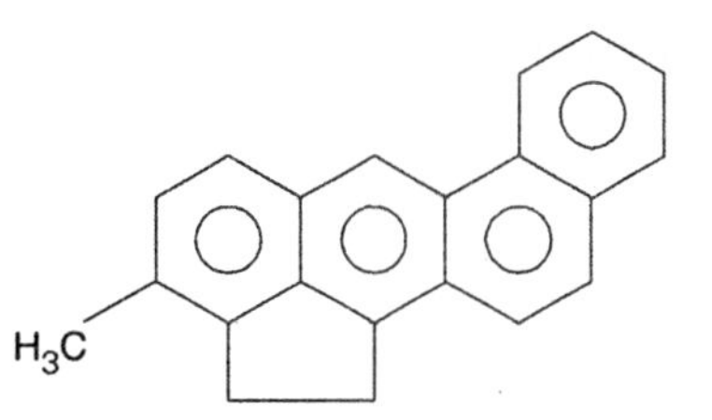

Methyl cholanthrene

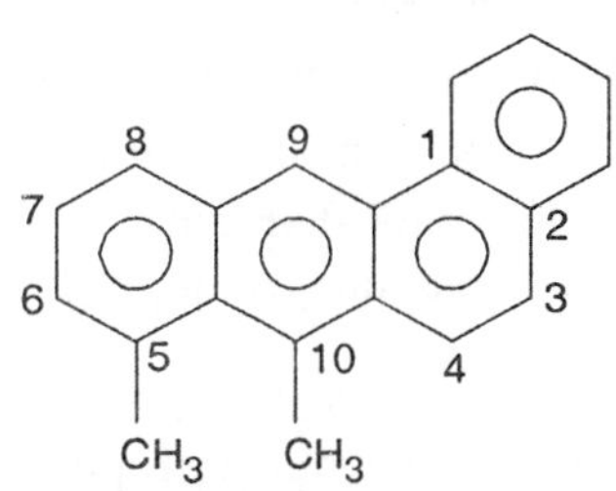

5, 10-Dimethyl-1, 2 benzanthracene

20.4 Uses of Polynuclear Aromatic Hydrocarbons

Polynuclear aromatic hydrocarbons are in use for variety of purposes as noted below:

1. Naphthalene is used as a valuable insect-repellant for preventing moths in clothes. Naphthalene is also used as the starting material for the preparation of many dyes. Some derivatives of naphthalene are of high therapeutic importance. Thus, (i) menadione (2-methyl-1,4-naphthaquinone, 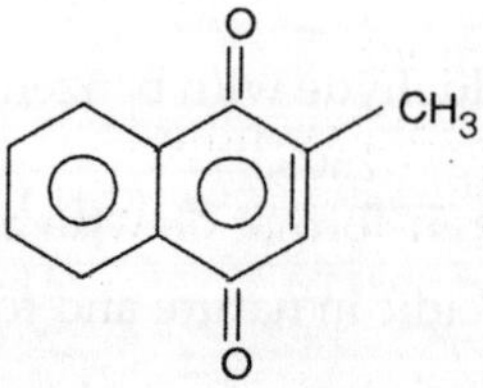) is a powerful blood clotting agent and is more potent than natural vitamin K (ii) propranolol [1-isopropyl-3-(I-naphyloxy)-propan-2-ol, 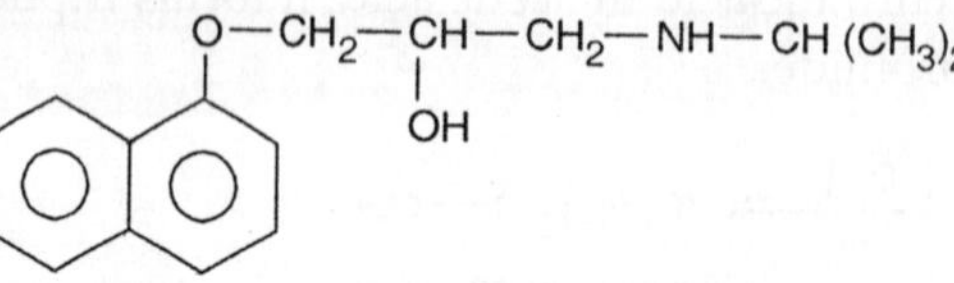] is used in treatment of angina pectoris, myocardial infraction, hypertension and cardiac arrhythmias. (iii) naphazoline [2-(1-naphthyl methyl)-2-imidazoline] is used for the symptomatic relief of rhinitis and sinuşitis.
2. Anthracene is used as the starting material for anthraquinone and anthraquinone dyes. Some derivatives of anthracene such as anthrone, anthraquinone and anthrol serve as ingredients of purgatives while 1, 8-dihydroxy-anthranquinone (dithranol) is used in the ointment for skin infections.
3. Phenanthrene is an important skeletal nucleus in bile acids, sex hormones and in cardiac glycosides. A few phenanthrene derivatives and codeine are used as analgesics. Codeine is also used as cough suppressants.

Model Questions

1. How would you isolate naphthalene from coal tar?
2. How would you establish the structure of naphthalene?
3. Describe the general reactions of naphthalene.
4. (a) Give the electrophilic substitution reaction of naphthalene.
   (b) Electrophilic substitution in naphthalene is faster at α-position compared to that at β-position.—Explain.
   (c) Described the orientation of sulphonation of naphthalene.
5. (a) Discuss the structure of anthracene.
   (b) Describe chemical properties of anthracene.

6. (a) Elucidate the structure of phenanthrene.
   (b) Describe the properties of phenanthrene.
   (c) What are the reactive positions of phenanthrene towards electrophiles.
7. Justify:
   (a) 1-position of naphthalene is more active than other.
   (b) Condensation of 2-phenyl ethyl bromide and cyclo-hexanone-2-carboxylate result in the formation of phenanthrene.
   Hints: (b) Bardhan-Sengupta's synthesis.
8. (a) Complete the following transformation with appropriate reagents and give structure of (A).

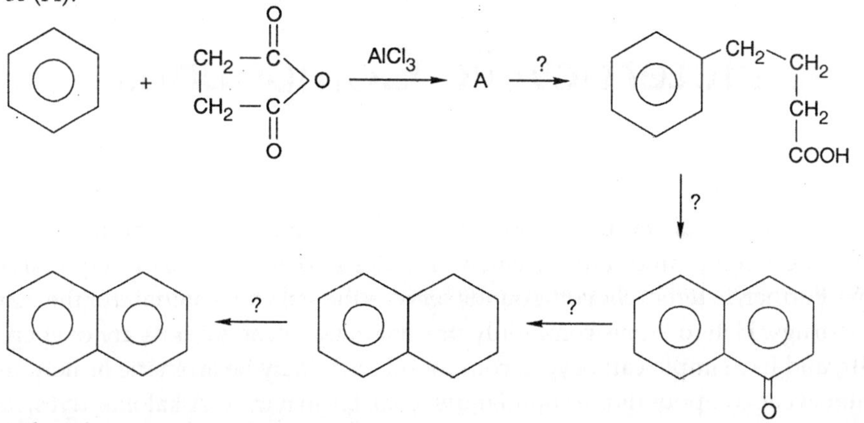

   (b) Why does naphthalene give 2-sulphonic acid derivative although it prefers 1-position for electrophilic substitution.
   (c) 2-Naphthol prefers coupling at α-position with diazonium salt rather than other positions.—Explain.
   (d) How would you prove that naphthalene contains two benzene rings?

CHAPTER TWENTY-ONE

Heterocyclic Compounds

Heterocyclic compounds are cyclic compounds having dissimilar atom or atoms in the molecule as ring atom. These compounds are extremely significant to life and are present in living cell in varied forms. Further, heterocyclic compounds serve as the starting materials for the manufacture of variety of drugs. Hetero atoms commonly present in these compounds are oxygen, nitrogen and sulphur, and like simple carbocyclic compounds they may be aromatic or non-aromatic in nature. Heterocyclic compounds are abundandly avialable in nature. Alkaloids, dyes, flavonoids, proteins, conmarins, enzymes, etc. belong to this category of compounds.

21.1 Classification of Heterocyclic Compounds

Like homocyclic compounds heterocyclic compounds may be classified into different categories of which following are important:

1. *Five-membered heterocyclic compounds*: Five-membered heterocycles may be looked upon as being derived from benzene by the replacement of C=C bond by hetero atom containing lone pair of electrons. They may contain one or more than one hetero atoms.

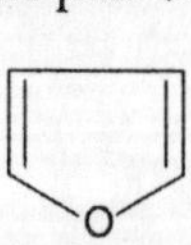

Furan

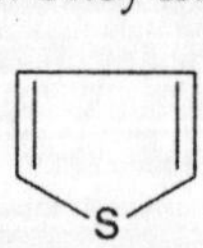

Thiophene

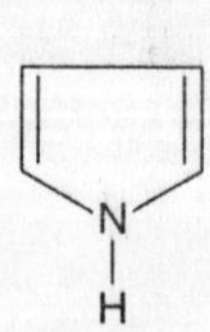

Pyrrole

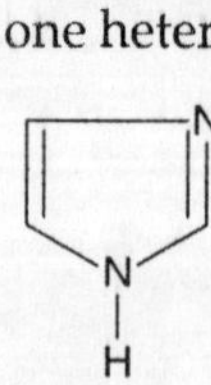

Imidazole

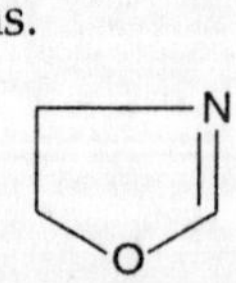

Oxazole

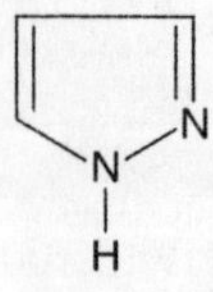

Pyrazole

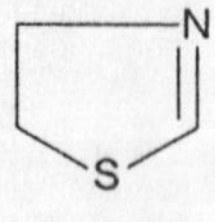

Thiazole

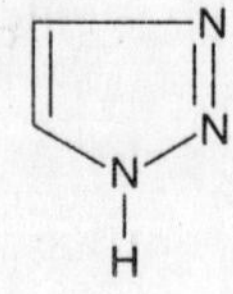

Triazole

2. *Six-membered heterocyclic compounds*: These are considered as being a derivative of benzene by replacing carbon atom or atoms by isoelectronic hetero atom or atoms.

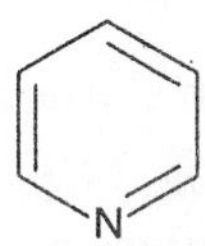
Pyridine

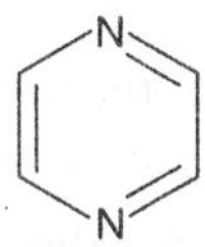
Pyrazine

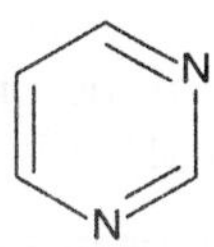
Pyrimidine

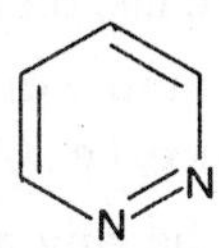
Pyridiazine

3. *Condensed heterocyclic compounds*: This heterocyclic system contains two or more rings fused together which may be partly carbocyclic and partly heterocyclic.

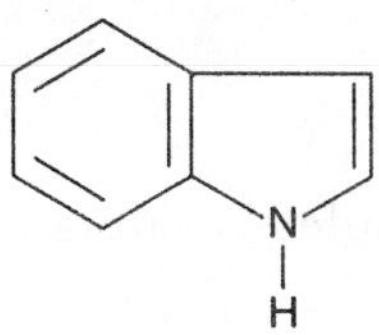
Indole

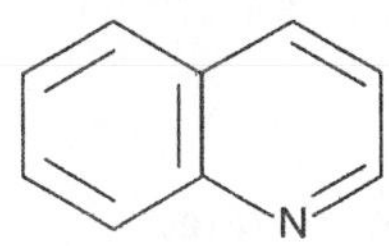
Quinoline

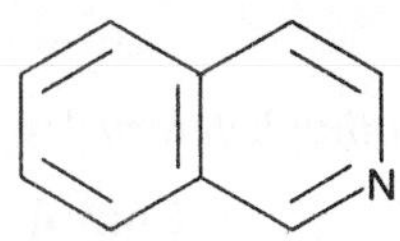
Isoquinoline

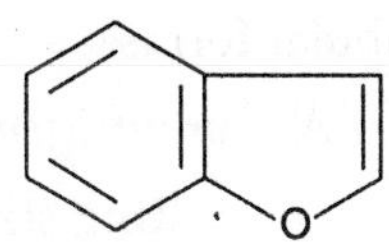
Benzofuran

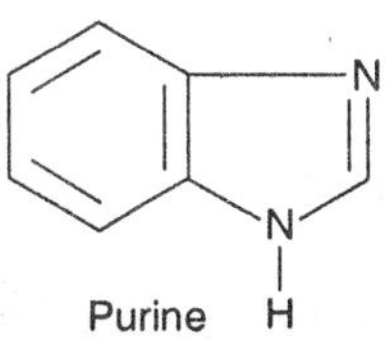
Purine

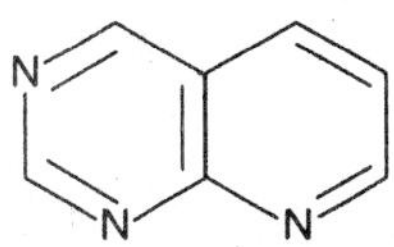
Pteridine

21.1.1 Numbering of the Positions of the Ring Atoms

Normally, in the case of heterocyclic system with single hetero atom, the position of the hetero atom is numbered as 1 and subsequent atoms (generally anticlockwise) are numbered in increasing succession. Relative positions are indicated by α, β, γ, etc.

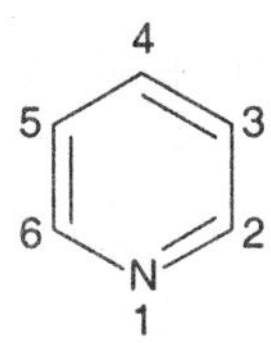
Pyridine

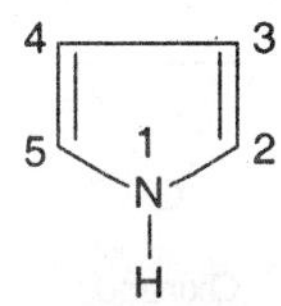
Pyrrole

In the case of polyheteroatomic system, that hetero atom is numbered 1 from which another hetero atom may be numbered by smallest number. Thus,

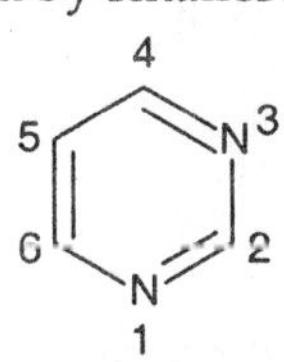
Pyrimidine

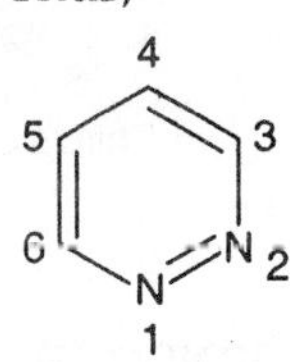
Pyridiazine

21.1.2 Nomenclature of Heterocyclic Compounds

Heterocyclic compounds are generally known by their trivial name. However, IUPAC nomenclature is available for these compounds. For such nomenclature some guidelines are followed as discussed in the sequel:

i. Prefixes oxa, thia and aza are used for oxygen, sulphur and nitrogen respectively.
ii. When two or more similar hetero atoms are present in the ring prefixes di, tri, tetra, etc are used, i.e., dioxa, triaza.
iii. If two or more different atoms occur in the ring, then their citation starts in the order of preference, i.e., O, S, O and N.
iv. Size of the ring and degree of unsaturation are indicated by suffixes as shown in the table.

According to this system three to six-membered heterocyclic compounds containing single hetro atom are named by combining the appropriate prefix or prefixes as shown in the following tabular forms.

A. *For nitrogen containing heterocycles*:

Ring size	Completely unsaturated	Completely saturated
3	— irine	—iridine
4	— ete	— etidine
5	—ole	—olidine
6	— in (ine)	— inane

B. *Non-nitrogeneous heterocyclic compounds*:

Ring size	Completely unsaturated	Completely saturated
3	— irene	—irane
4	— ete	— etane
5	—ole	—olane
6	— in	— ane

Some examples may be cited to elaborate the above system.

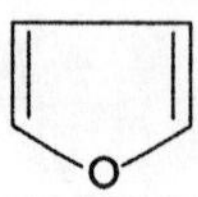
Oxole

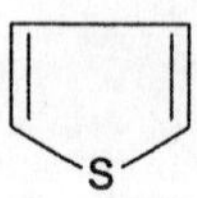
Thiole

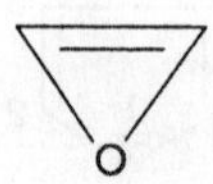
Oxirene

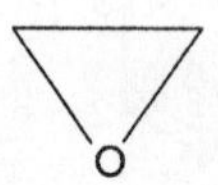
Oxirane

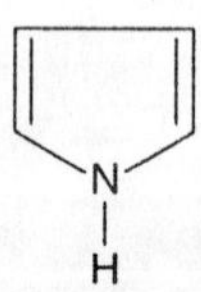
Azole

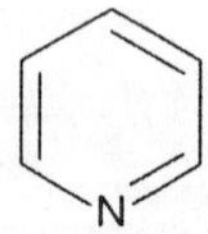
Azin

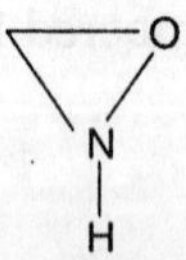
Oxaziridine

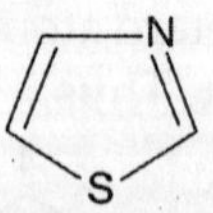
Thiazole

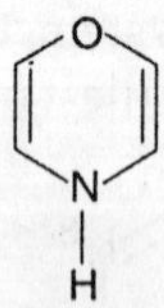
Oxazine

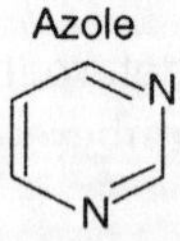
Diazine

21.2 Basic Principles Regarding the Reactivities of Heterocyclic Compounds

It has been observed that the reactivities of heterocyclic compounds are governed by some basic considerations as noted below:

(a) Lone pair of electrons on hetero atom has a significant role in controlling the reactivity.
(b) When heterocyclic compound is aromatic and the hetero atom is connected by a π-bond, the heterocyclic ring becomes electron deficient due to the electron withdrawing effect of C=X, where X is a hetero atom. So nucleophilic substitution reaction can easily occur.

(c) If hetero atom is joined by σ-bond and the heterocyclic compound is aromatic, the ring becomes rich in electrons. This is because sigma bonded hetero atom acts as electron releasing group and so the heterocyclic ring becomes susceptible to electrophilic attack.

21.3 Heterocyclic Compounds with One Hetero Atom

Heterocyclic compounds containing one hetero atom may be of different types as discussed below:

21.4 Five-membered Heterocyclic Compounds Containing One Hetero Atom

21.4.1 Aromaticity of Five-membered Heterocyclic Compounds

Most common members containing single hetero atom of this category of heterocyclic compounds are furan, pyrrole and thiophene. All of them are *aromatic* in nature. Their aromaticity originates from the generation of closed circuit of six π-electrons (sextet) — four being contributed by four carbon atoms and a paired electrons donated by the hetero atom. The molecular orbital diagram of this sextet may be represented by the following figure.

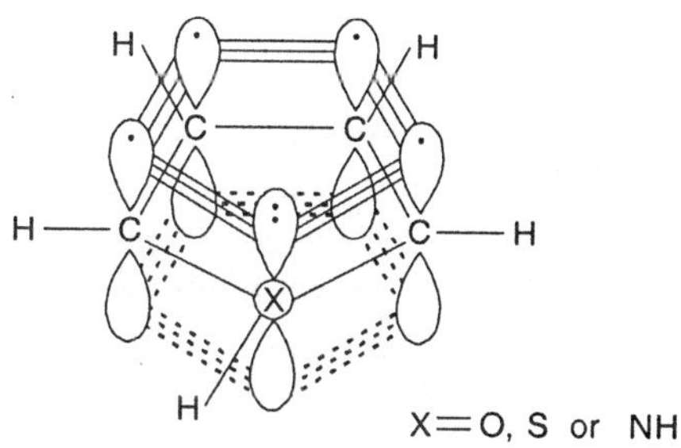

Overlap of *p*-orbitals in furan and pyrrole, thiophene

Aromatic character of these compounds is also revealed from their structures. Structurally, these heterocycles are represented as a resonance hybrid of the following structural units:

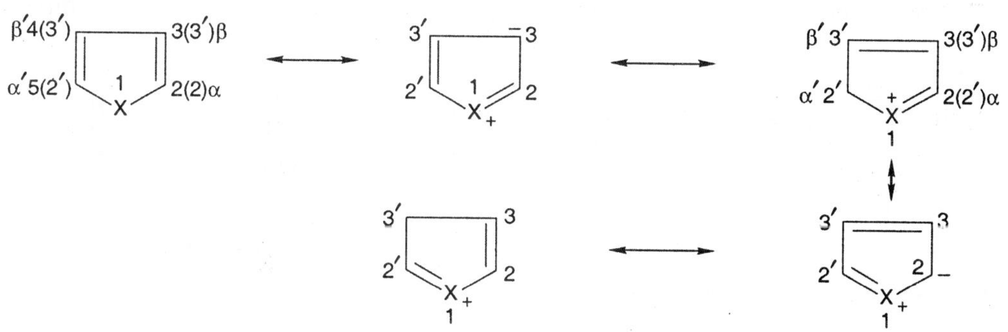

where X=O, S and NH for furan, thiophene and pyrrole respectively.

It may be mentioned that all these three members are not equally aromatic. It has been observed that their order of aromaticity is as indicated below:

Thiophene > Pyrrole > Furan

This order of aromaticity is in accord with the order of electronegativities of hetero atoms which stands as

O > N > S, i.e.,

oxygen is more electronegative than nitrogen and sulphur. Higher electronegativity makes an atom reluctant to release electrons and since oxygen is more electronegative than other it is very much reluctant to release its electron pair towards the formation of aromatic sextet and hence it is least aromatic.

Again, due to the presence of electronegative atom in the ring in general, they are less aromatic than benzene or in other words, they are more active than benzene.

21.4.2 Basicity of Five-membered Heterocyclic Compounds

All these heterocyclic compounds are weakly basic due to the contribution of lone pair of electrons on hetero atom towards the formation of aromatic sextet. The order of the basicity has been found to be furan > thiophene > pyrrole.

This order of basicity may be explained on the basis of dipole moment measurement. Dipole moment measurement reveals the dipole monent values of these three compounds as

Pyrrole → 1.81D

Furan → 0.70D

Thiophene → 0.51D

Recent nuclear magnetic resonance spectroscopic study indicates that in furan and thiophene the negative end of the dipole is towards the hetero atom but the negative end of the dipole is away from nitrogen atom in pyrrole. This suggests that oxygen and sulphur induce some inductive effect during its exhibition of aromatic character and so some electron density remains on hetero atoms—oxygen and sulphur; but the lone pair of electrons on nitrogen mainly lies over the aromatic ring and is less available on nitrogen atom. So pyrrole is least basic.

21.4.3 Chemical Reactivities of Five-membered Heterocyclic Compounds

The aromatic nature of these heterocycles indicates that they are rich in electrons and so are susceptible to undergo electrophilic substitution reactions. Although resonance susggests that all the positions (C_2—C_5) are electron rich and so electrophilic substitution can occur at all these positions but in actual practice it has been observed that the positions 2 and 5(2′) or α and α′ are more active than 3 and 4(3′) or β and β′ positions. This may be explained on the basis of comparison of relative stabilities of transition states of 2 and 3-substituted products. Thus,

Transition states of 3-substituted product:

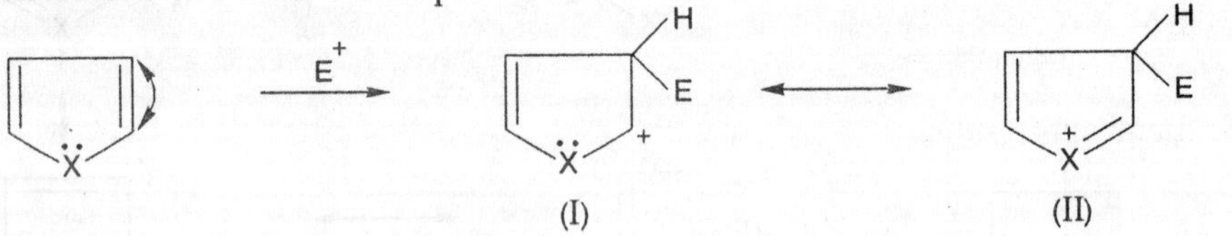

Transition state of 2-substituted product:

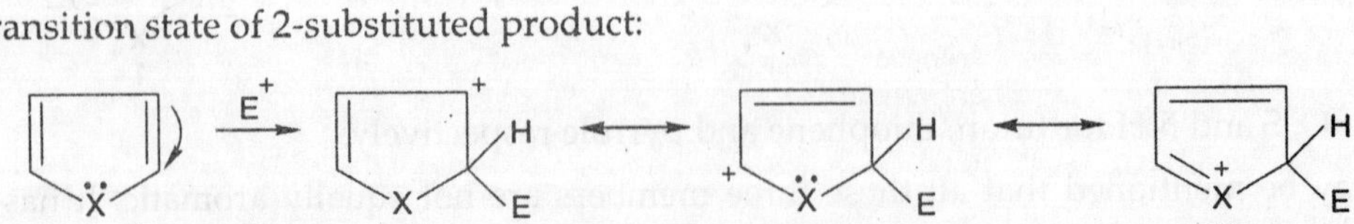

From the above it is seen that the transition state of 2-substituted product has three resonating structures whereas that of 3-substituted product has only two such structures. Hence, the transition state of 2-substituted product is stabler than that of 3-substituted product. Some common electrophilic substitution reactions exhibited by these compounds are illustrated with reference to pyrrole.

(a) *Reimer-Tiemann reaction*

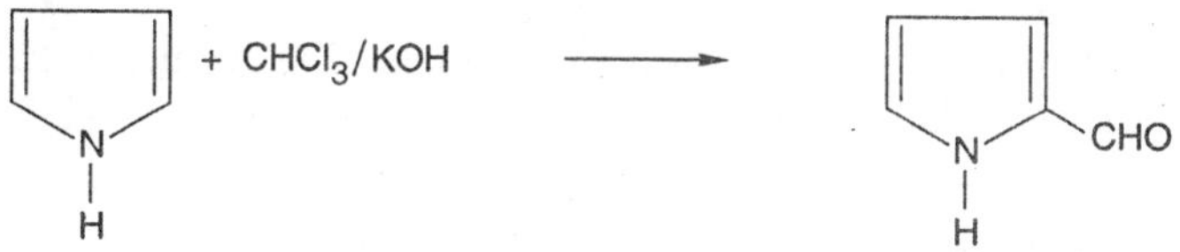

Pyrrole — Pyrrole-2-aldehyde

(b) *Nitration*

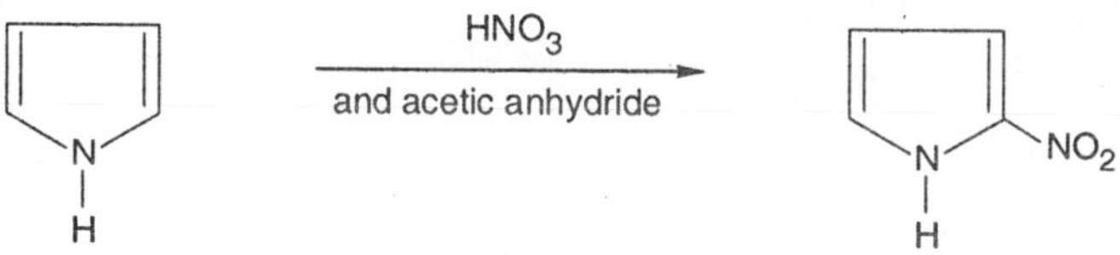

Pyrrole — 2-Nitro pyrrole

H_2SO_4 is not used because in presence of such acid decomposition of ring occurs.

(c) *Halogenation*: With iodine solution it forms iodo compound and with excess of iodine tetra iodopyrrole is formed which is used as a substitute for iodoform.

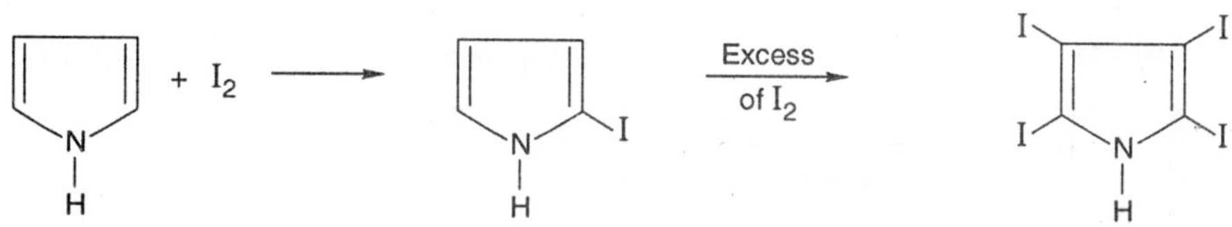

Pyrrole — 2-Iodopyrrole — Tetra-Iodopyrrole

(d) *Sulphonation*

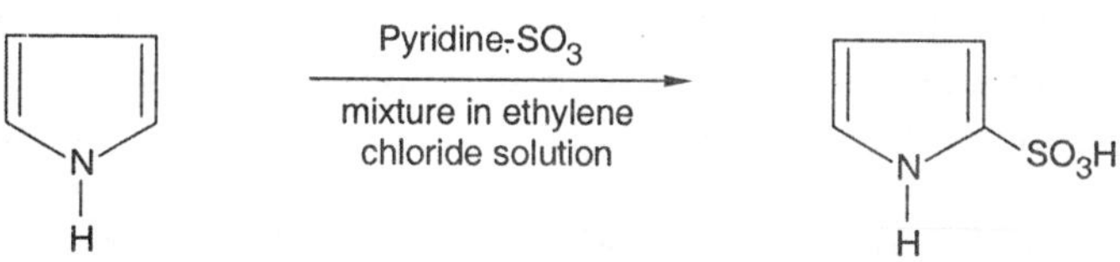

Pyrrole — Pyrrole-2-sulphonic acid

(e) *Friedel-Crafts reaction*

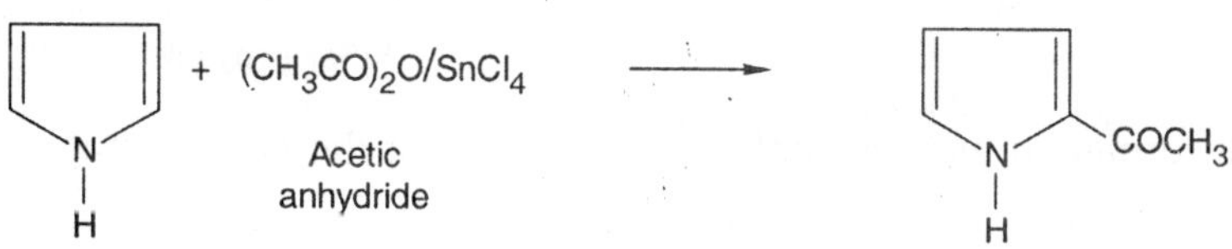

Pyrrole — 2-Acetyl pyrrole

- *Other Reactions:*

(a) *Ring expansion*: During Reimer-Tiemann reaction ring expansion may occur. Thus,

$$H-CCl_3 \xrightarrow{NaOH} CCl_2$$

Chloroform — Dichloro carbene

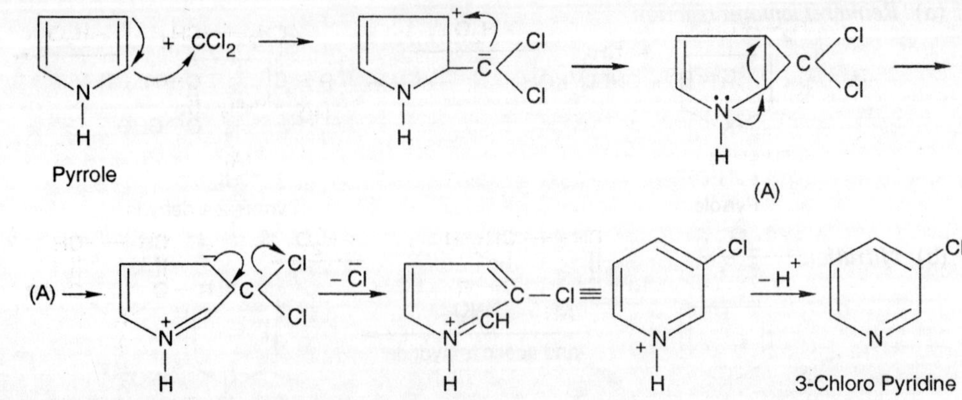

(b) On reduction pyrrole affords the following products:

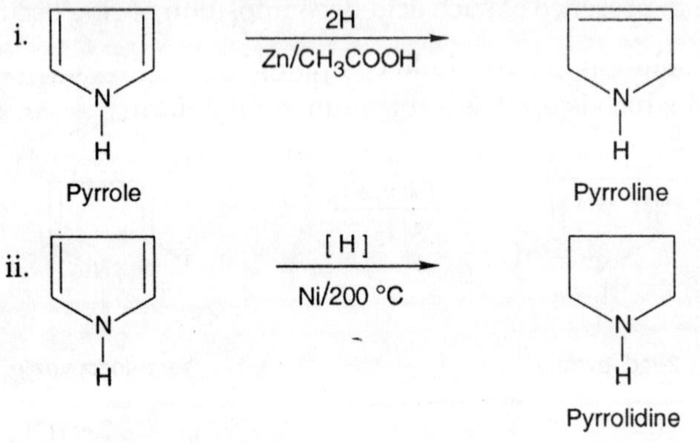

(c) *Acidic character*: As mentioned due to the contribution of lone pair of electrons towards the formation of aromatic sextet, these compounds are weakly basic and in some cases they show acidic character. For example,

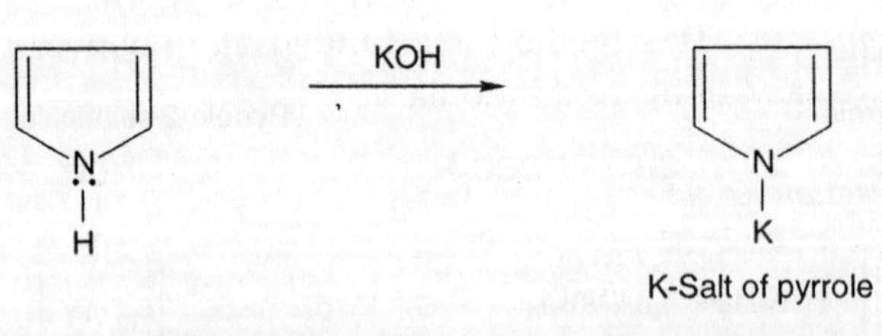

The salt formation may be explained by assuming the fact that the anion 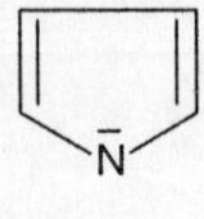 is stabilised by resonance as is observed in the case of phenoxide anion.

21.4.4 Preparation of Five-membered Heterocyclic Compounds

A. *Pyrrole*: Pyrrole may be synthesised by the following methods:

i. *Paal-Knorr synthesis*: This synthetic process involves the heating of 1, 4-diketones with ammonia or a primary amine, hydrazine, etc.

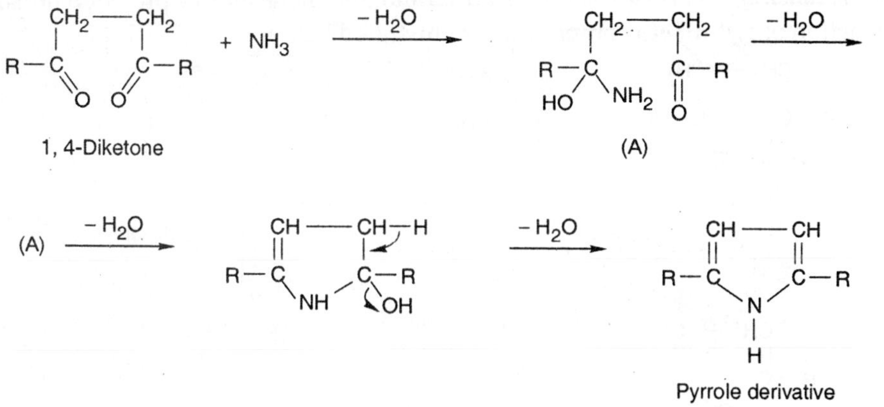

ii. *Knorr Pyrrole synthesis*: This method is considered as the most general and is carried out by condensing an amino-ketone and α, β-diketone or β-keto ester.

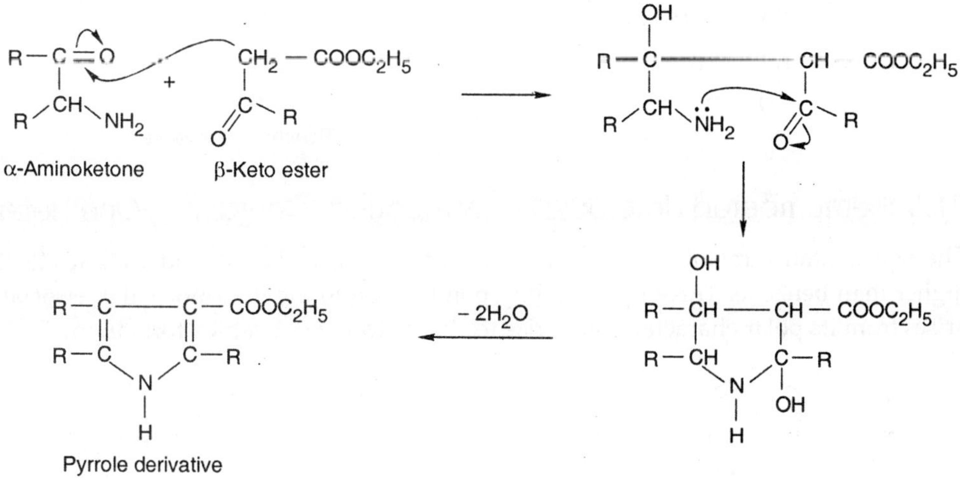

iii. *Hantzsch synthesis*: This method is a condensation between α-halo ketone, β-keto ester and primary amine or ammonia.

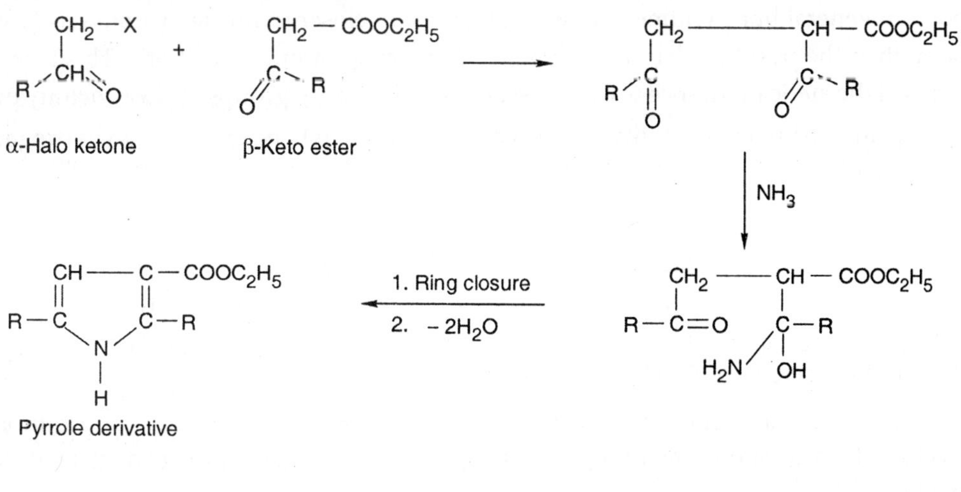

B. *Preparation of Furan and Thiophene*: Furan and thiophene may be prepared utilising similar reaction of 1, 4-diketo compounds as illustrated below:

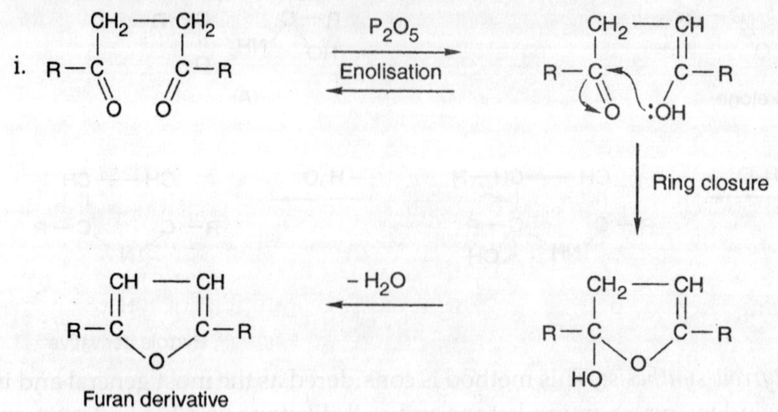

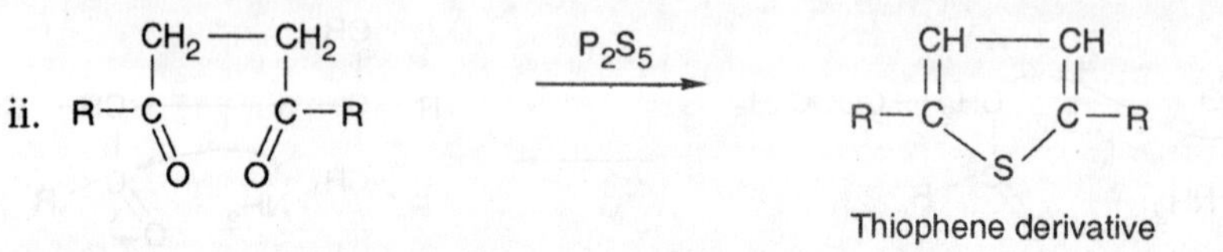

21.5 Six-membered Heterocyclic Compounds Containing One Hetero Atom

The representative member of this group is pyridine. It is a liquid, and boils at 115 °C which is higher than benzene. This higher boiling point is due to the intermolecular association which arises from its polar character giving rise to charge transfer complex formation.

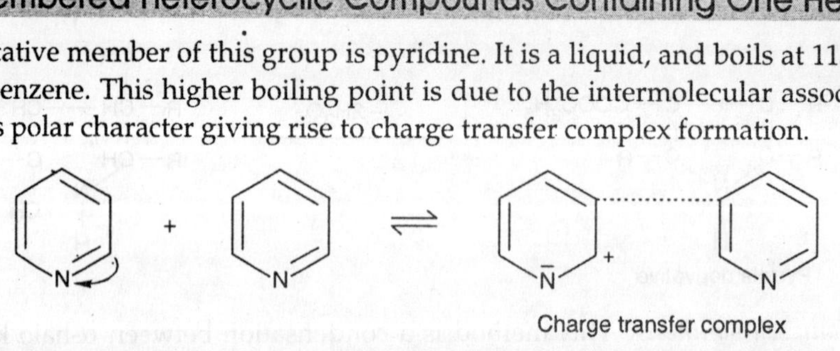

It has been observed that the presence of alkyl substituents in the ring increases the boiling point in general but pyridine ring with alkyl group closer to nitrogen atom has lower boiling point than the pyridine derivative having alkyl group at other positions. This is explained in terms of the steric hindrance towards association due to the groups at close vicinity of nitrogen.

Again, the higher solubility of pyridine in water than benzene is due to hydrogen bonding with water.

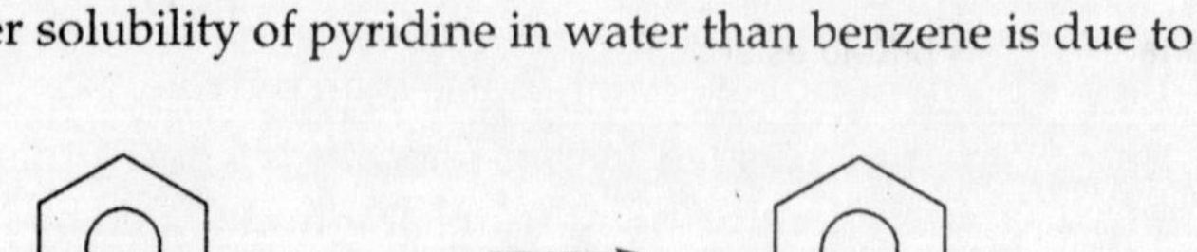

21.5.1 Aromaticity of Pyridine

Pyridine is aromatic in character and the aromatic sextet is formed by contribution of six π-electrons from six atoms including the nitrogen atom. The orbital picture may be represented as follows:

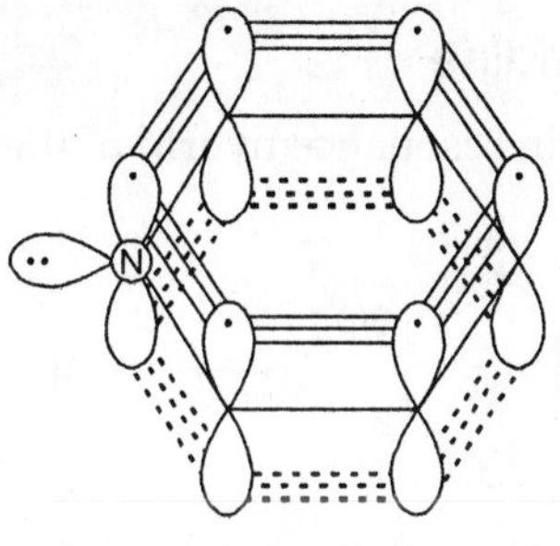

Overlap of *p*-orbitals in pyridine

Basicity of Pyridine: The lone pair of electrons on nitrogen atom is located in an sp^2 orbital which is perpendicular to the π-system of the ring. So lone pair of electrons on nitrogen atom is not utilised for the formation of aromatic sextet and is available for protonation. Pyridine, thus, behaves as a tertiary base with pk_b of 5.17. The basicity of pyridine is manifested by its formation of salt with acid and alkyl halide.

i. 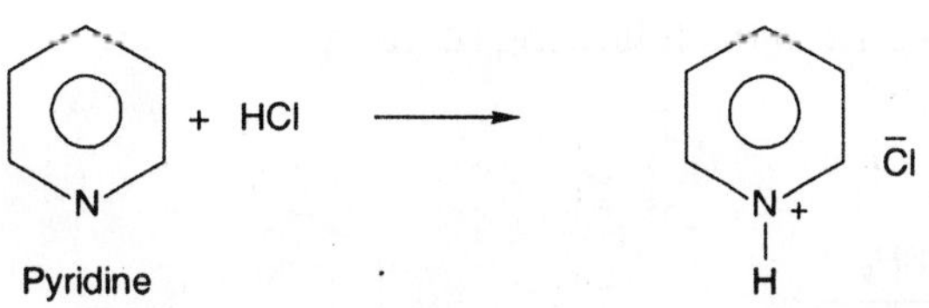

ii. 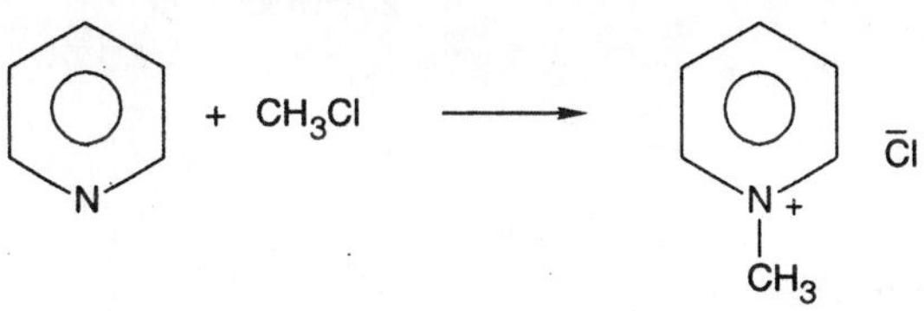

It may be mentioned that pyridine is more basic than pyrrole but less than an aliphatic amine. This is due to the following reasons:

i. Lone pair of electrons on nitrogen atom has not been utilised for the generation of sextet and hence available for protonation. On the other hand, in pyrrole lone pair of electrons on nitrogen has been used up for the formation of sextet and so is not available for protonation. Accordingly pyridine is more basic than pyrrole.
ii. In pyridine nitrogen atom is bonded by a π-bond. It is known that when lone pair of electrons on multiply bonded nitrogen atom are accommodated by an orbital which has more s-character would be less basic than the lone pair of electrons of nitrogen atom present in an orbital having less s-character. In aliphatic amine, lone pair of electrons is present on sp^3 hybridised orbital having less s-character than sp^2-hybridised orbital on which lone pair of electrons of nitrogen is present in pyridine. So pyridine is less basic than an aliphatic amine.

21.5.2 Chemical Activity of Pyridine

Since pyridine is aromatic it exists in resonance hybrid of the following structures:

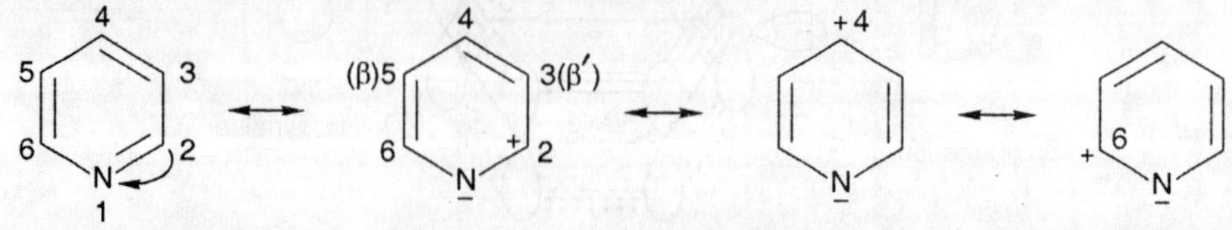

From the resonance, it is evident that the double bonded nitrogen atom behaves as an electron withdrawing group. So pyridine may be looked upon as benzene ring having electron withdrawing group. Accordingly, pyridine is deactivated as a whole, particularly at positions 2, 4 and 6. So it is expected that pyridine ring favours nucleophilic substitution reactions preferably at 2, 4 and 6 positions. Again, positions 3(β) and 5(β′) remain unaffected by the electron withdrawing effect by double bonded nitrogen atom and are relatively electron rich. Hence, electrophilic substitution reactions can take palce at these positions. In fact, above assumptions have been found to be true as is evidenced from the following reactions:

A. *Nucleophilic Substitution Reactions:*

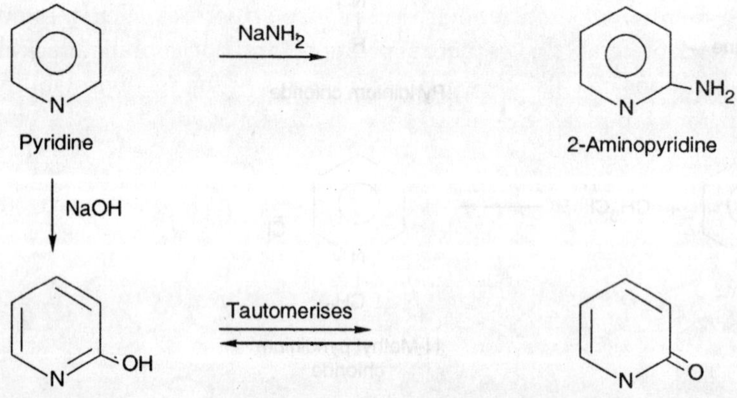

Mechanistically, the above reactions may be explained as

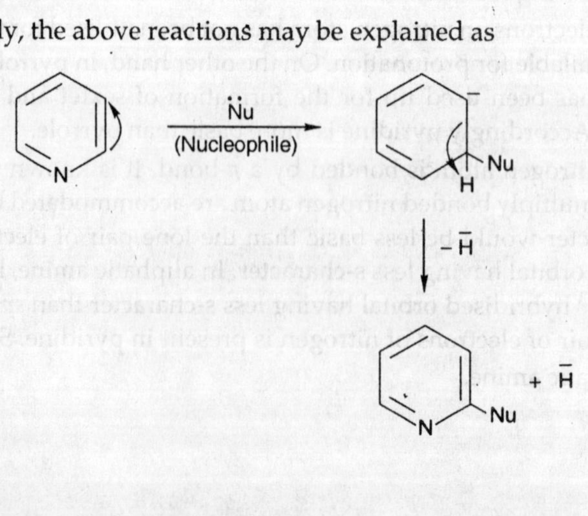

B. *Electrophilic Substitution Reaction:*

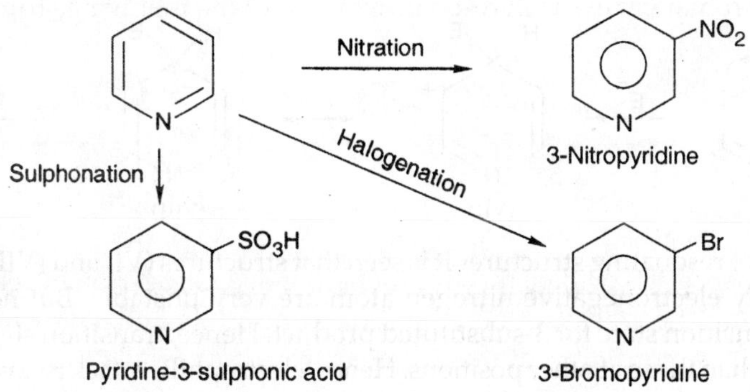

Mechanism of electrophilic substitution may be shown as under:

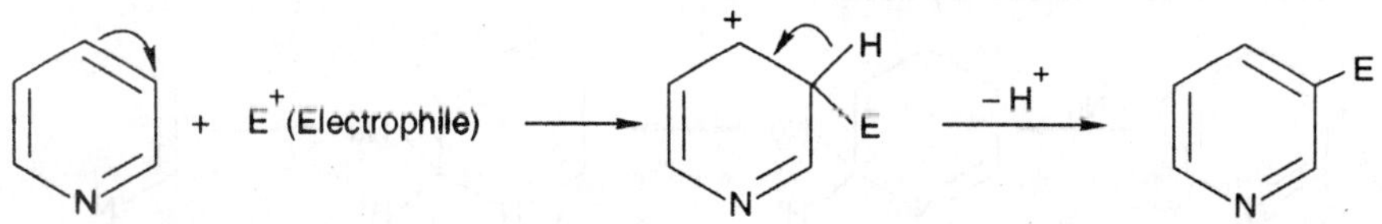

It may be mentioned that although resonance structures clearly establish the fact that electrophilic attack preferably takes place at position 3 and nucleophilic attack at 2 and 4 positions, but these observations can also be explained in terms of the relative stability of the transition states formed. For example,

i. *Electrophilic Substitution:*

(a) Attack at 3-position.

Transition state

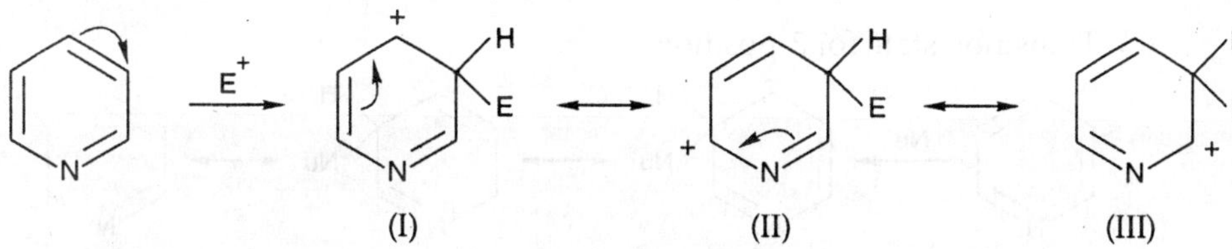

(I) (II) (III)

(b) Attack at 2-position.

Transition state

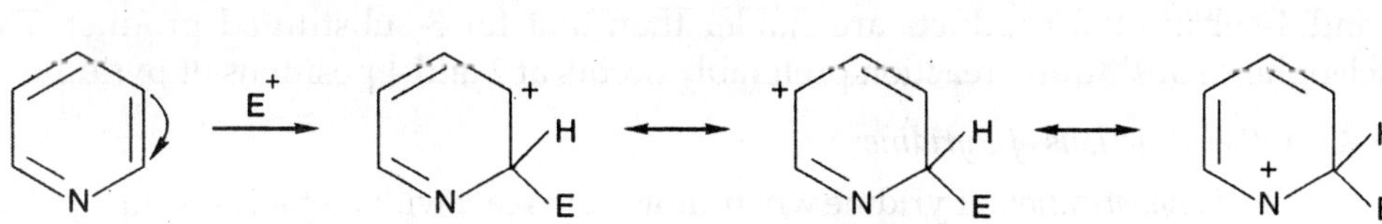

(IV) (V) (VI)

(c) Attack at 4-position.

Transition state

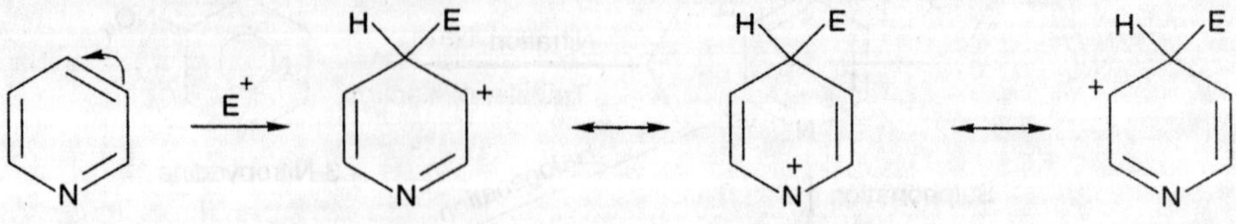

(VII) (VIII) (IX)

From the above resonating structures it is seen that structures (VI) and (VIII) carrying positive charge on strongly electronegative nitrogen atom are very unstable. But no such structure is present for the transition state for 3-substituted product. Hence, transition state for 3-substituted product is stabler than those at other positions. Hence, electrophilic attack is favoured at 3-position.

ii. *Nucleophilic Substitution:*

(a) Transition state for 2-position.

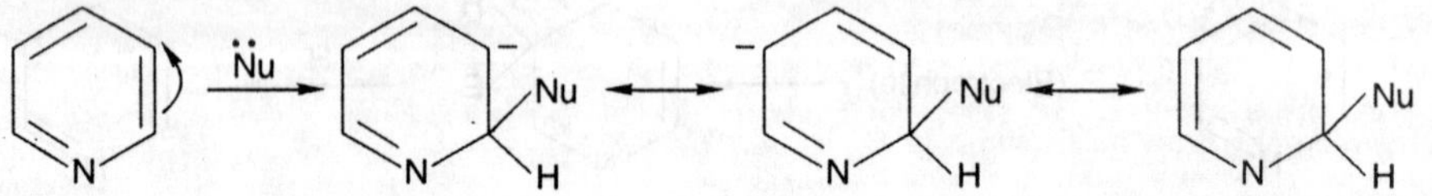

(X) (XI) (XII)

(b) Transition state for 4-position.

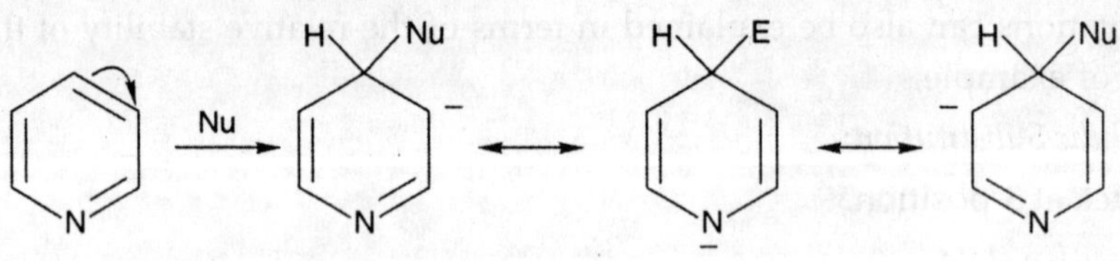

(XIII) (XIV) (XV)

(c) Transition state for 3-position.

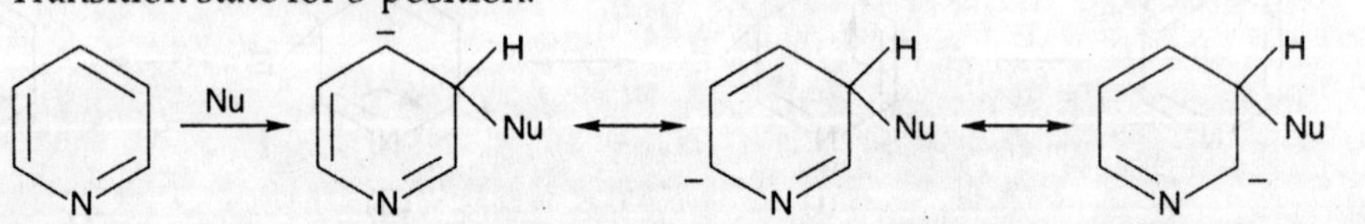

Resonating structures reveal that for 2- and 4-substituted products transition states have very stable structures (XII) and (XIV) bearing negative charge on nitrogen but similar structure is not available for the transition state of 3-substituted product. Accordingly transition states for 2- and 4-substituted products are stabler than that for 3-substituted product. That is why nucleophilic substitution reaction preferably occurs at 2 and 4 positions of pyridine.

C. *Other Reactions of Pyridine:*

1. *Polymerisation*: Pyridine when allowed to react with metallic sodium, polymerisation occurs.

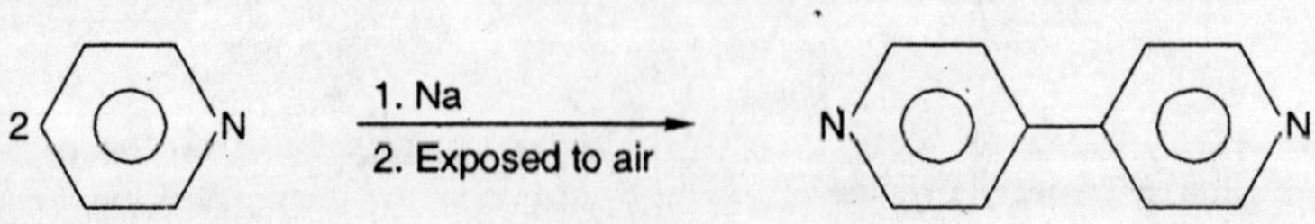

This may be explained as

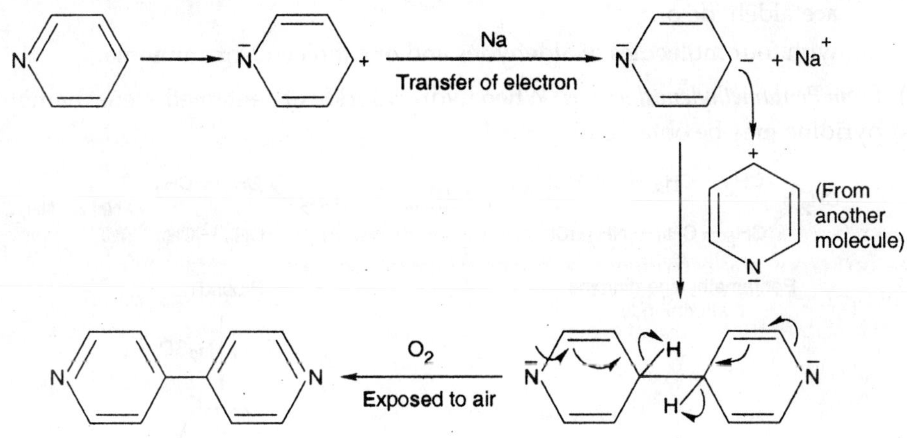

4, 4′-Dipirydyl

21.5.3 Preparation of Pyridine

Pyridine is prepared by the following methods:

(a) When mixture of acetylene and hydrogen cyanide is passed through a red-hot tube, pyridine is formed.

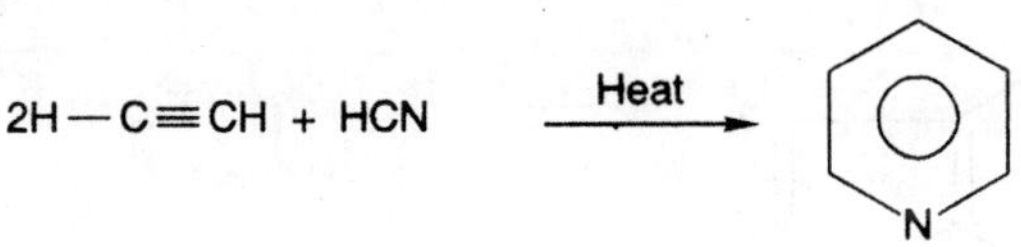

(b) *Hantzsch Synthesis*: This synthesis consists of condensation of β-dicarbonyl compound with an aldehyde and ammonia. Initially dihydro pyridine derivative is obtained which on oxidation furnishes pyridine.

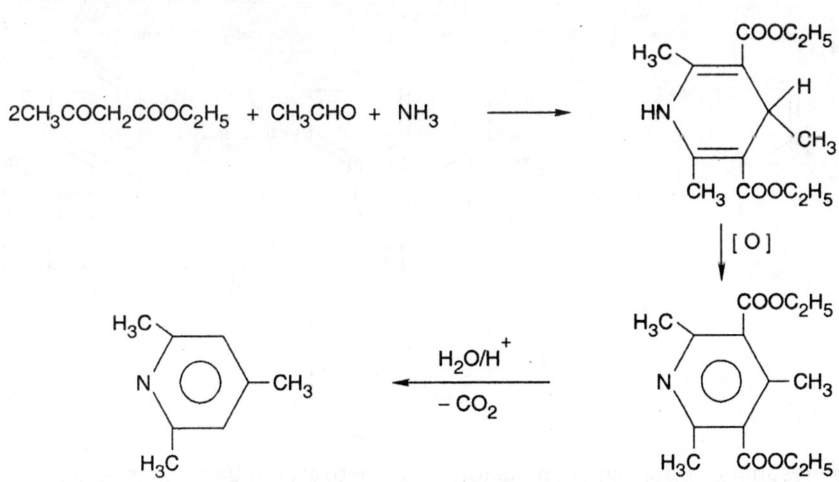

2, 4, 6-Trimethyl pyridine

- *Comments:*
  - i. Reaction may be carried out with one molecule of ester and two molecules of acetaldehyde or
  - ii. with four molecules of aldehydes and one molecule of ammonia.

(c) *From Pentamethylene diamine:* When hydrochloride of pentamethylene diamine is heated, pyridine may be obtained.

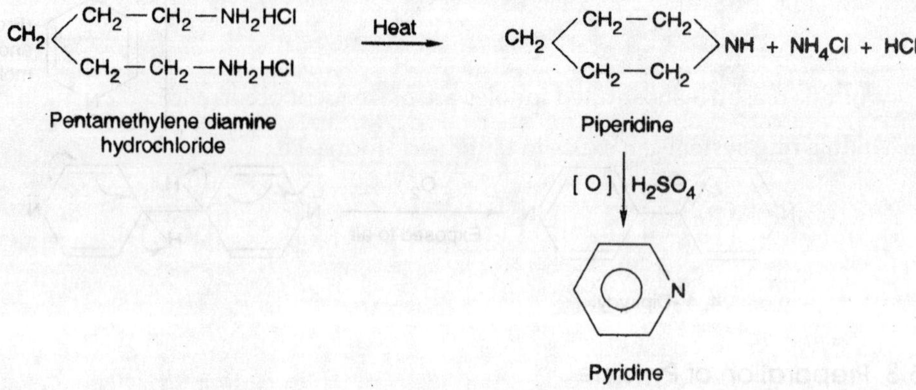

21.6 Condensed Heterocyclic Compounds Containing One Hetero Atom

Two most important classes of condensed heterocyclic system are (i) Indole and (ii) Quinoline.

21.6.1 Indole

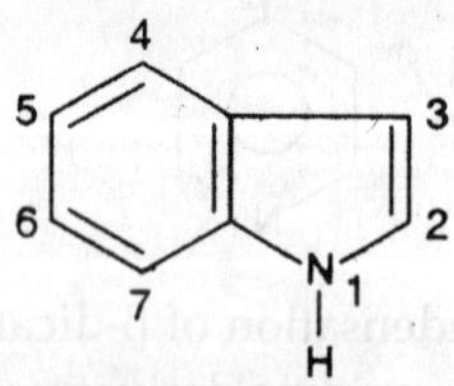

Structurally indole is benzopyrrole. It is aromatic and exists in resonance hybrid of the following structures.

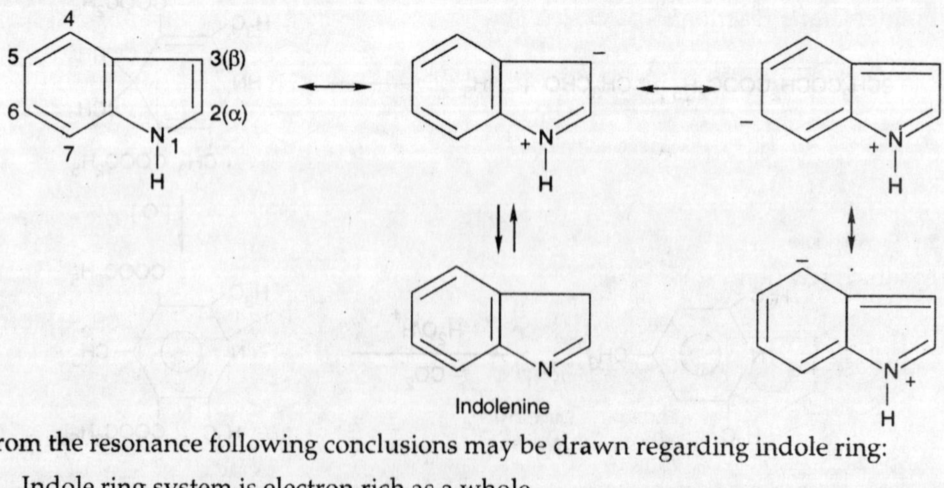

From the resonance following conclusions may be drawn regarding indole ring:

i. Indole ring system is electron rich as a whole.

ii. Positions 3, 4 and 6 are highly rich in electrons. Hence electrophilic substitution reaction can occur at these positions. Further, out of all these three positions 3-position is highly rich in electron, because as seen from the resonating structures, in the transition state for reaction at this position benzenoid ring remains intact, i.e.,

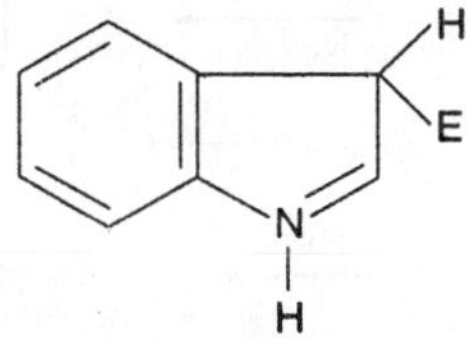

For this reason 3-substituted indoles are of frequent occurrence.

iii. Indole ring system can exists in tautomeric forms, i.e.,

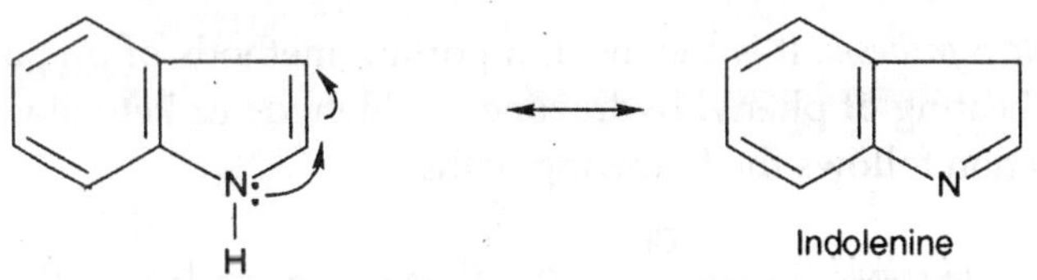

Indole

In fact, in nature some compounds are known having indolenine system.

21.6.1.1 Reactions of Indole

Most common reactions of indole are discussed in sequel:

i. Reimer-Tiemann reaction:

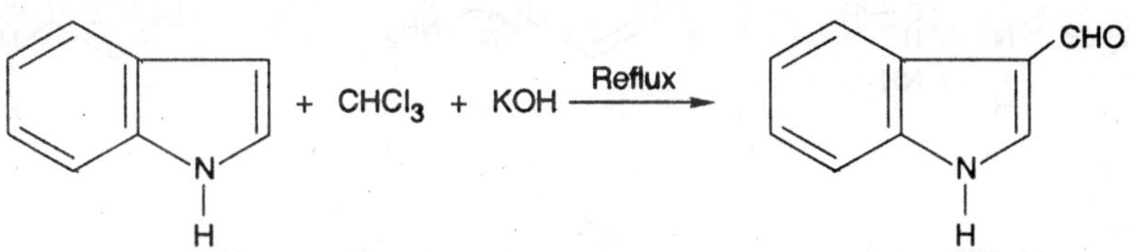

Indole 3-Aldehyde indole

ii. Freidel-Crafts reaction:

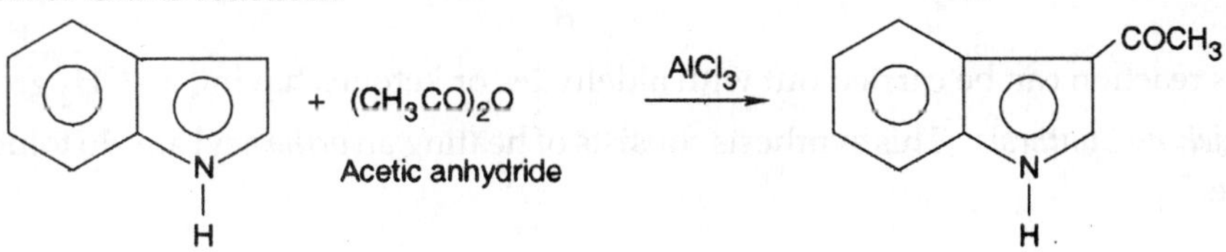

Indole

iii. Mannich reaction:

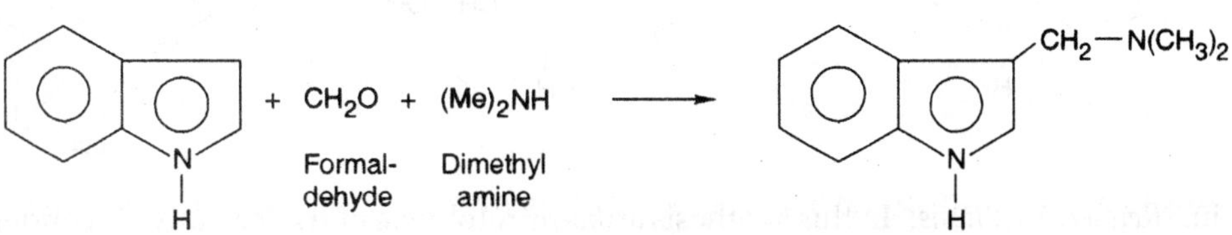

Indole Grammine

iv. *Reduction*: Indole can be reduced electrolytically or by tin and hydrochloride acid to 2, 3-dihydro indole.

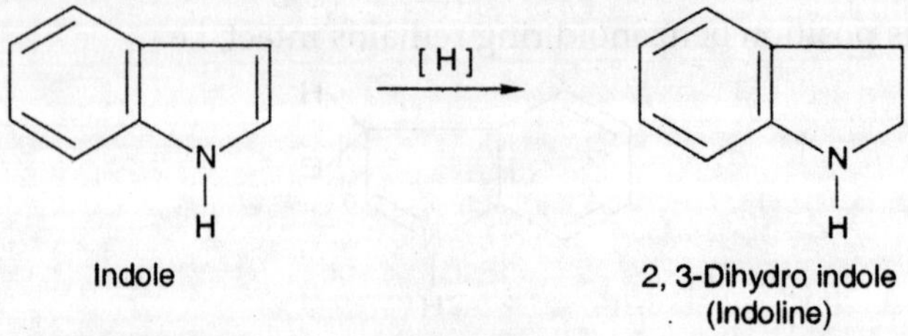

21.6.1.2 Preparation of Indole

Indole may be prepared by various methods.

i. *Fischer's Indole Synthesis*: It is the most important methods of preparation for indole. It involves the heating of phenyl hydrazone of aldehyde or ketone with polyphosphoric acid. The reaction follows the following paths:

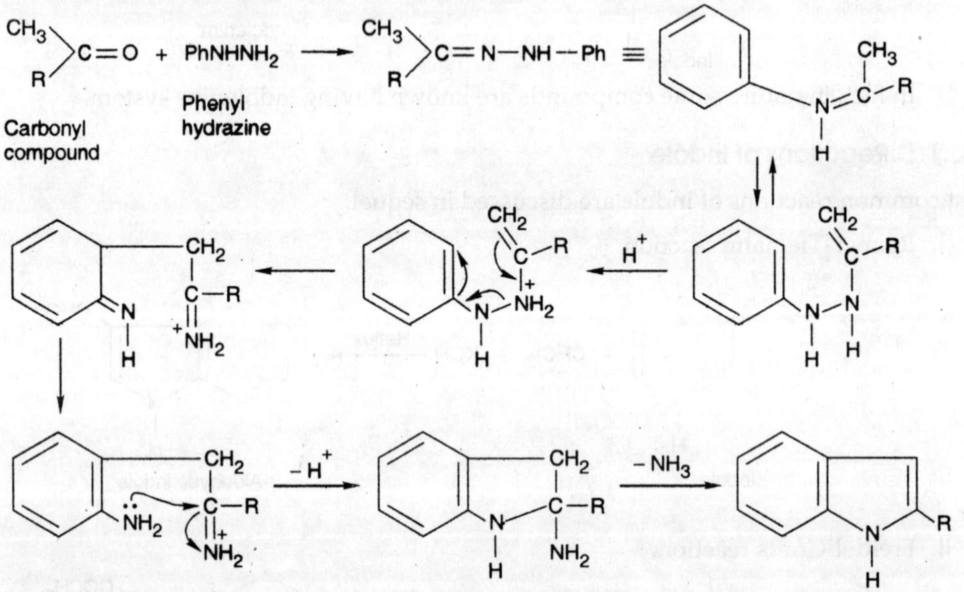

This reaction can be carried out with aldehydes or ketones having a - CH_2 group.

ii. *Madelung Synthesis*: This synthesis consists of heating an *ortho* acyl amido toluene with a base.

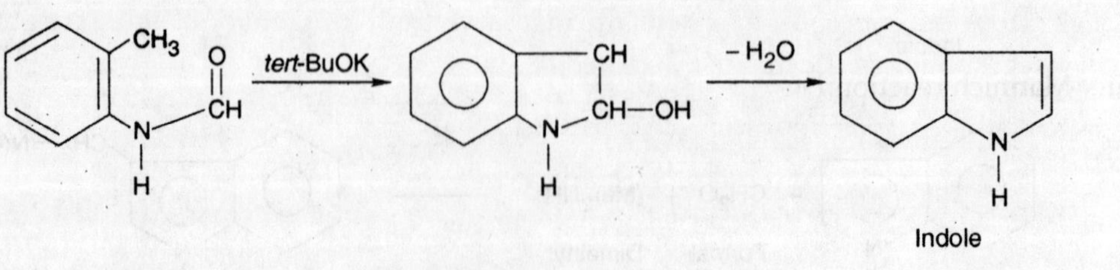

iii. *Reissert Synthesis*: In this synthesis *ortho*-nitrotoluene or its derivative is condensed with ethyloxalate in presence of alkoxide.

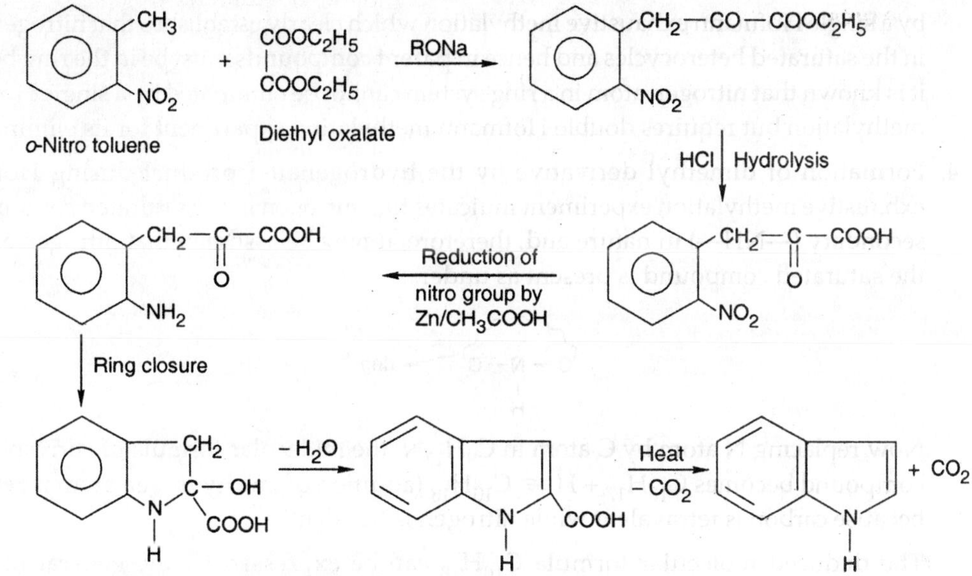

An important derivative of indole is the dye—*indigo.*

21.6.2 Quinoline and Isoquinoline

Quinoline and isoquinoline are the two isomeric heterocyclic compounds belonging to condensed ring systems. Both these isomeric heterocycles may be considered as the derivatives of six-membered heterocyclic compound, pyridine and in fact, they are benzopyridines. The structures of these two isomeric compounds have been derived from chemical evidences and logical arguments as presented below.

21.6.2.1 Structures of Quinoline and Isoquinoline

1. Both quinoline and isoquinoline have been found to have the same molecular formula, C_9H_7N.
2. On catalytic hydrogenation both of them furnish the same completely saturated molecule, $C_9H_{17}N$, i.e,

$$C_9H_7N \xrightarrow{\text{Cat [H]}} \underset{\text{Decahydro compound}}{C_9H_{17}N}$$

   This suggests that both these isomers possess five double bonds in their molecule.
3. Saturated compound formed during catalytic hydrogenation undergoes Hofmann degradation in the manner depicted below:

$$C_9H_{17}N \xrightarrow{2\,CH_3I} \underset{\text{Dimethyl derivative}}{C_9H_{16}N(CH_3)_2I} \xrightarrow{AgOH} C_9H_{16}N(CH_3)_2-OH \xrightarrow{-H_2O} C_9H_{15}N(CH_3)_2 + H_2O$$

$$C_9H_{15}N(CH_3)_2 \xrightarrow{\text{Further Hofmann}} C_9H_{15}N(CH_3)_3I \xrightarrow{\text{1. AgOH; 2. Heat; 3. } -H_2O} N(CH_3)_3 + C_9H_{14}$$

From the above, it is seen that nitrogen atom of the saturated compound is not eliminated by a single Hofmann exhaustive methylation which clearly establishes that nitrogen atom in the saturated heterocycles and hence in parent compounds must be in the ring because it is known that nitrogen atom in a ring system cannot be eliminated by a single Hofmann methylation but requires double Hofmann methylation experiment for its elimination.

4. Formation of dimethyl derivative by the hydrogenated product during Hofmann exhaustive methylation experiment indicates that nitrogen in the saturated compound is secondary (—NH—) in nature and, therefore, it may be assumed that nitrogen atom in the saturated compound is present as under:

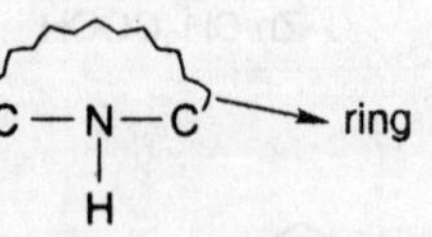

Now replacing N atom by C atom in $C_9H_{17}N$, the molecular formula of corresponding compound becomes $C_{10}H_{17} + H \equiv C_{10}H_{18}$ (addition of one hydrogen atom is required because carbon is tetravalent while nitrogen is trivalent).

The deduced molecular formula $C_{10}H_{18}$ can be expressed by the general formula, C_nH_{2n-2}, which unambiguously establishes its bicyclic nature and hence, it may be concluded that both quinoline and isoquinoline are bicyclic compounds and may be represented by the following structures (I) and (II):

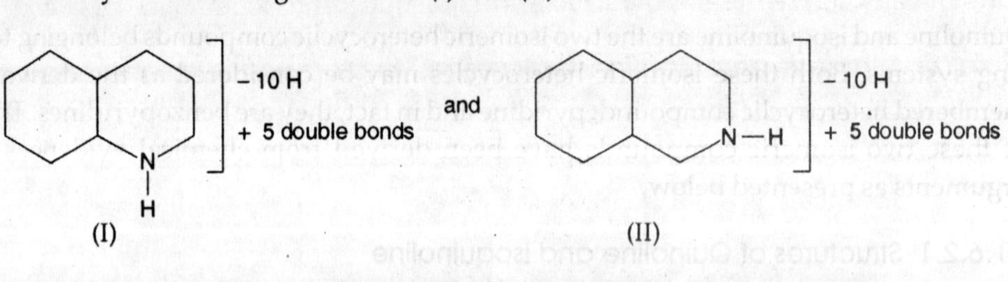

(I) (II)

5. It has been observed that both quinoline and isoquinoline undergo typical reactions of aromatic compounds such as nitration, sulphonation, halogenation, etc. So it is expected that these heterocycles are aromatic in nature and thus above part structures (I) and (II) may be extended to I(a) and II(a).

I(a) II(a)

6. Now the question arises, which structure represents quinoline and which one is isoquinoline? Answer to this question has been secured from the alkaline potassium permanganate oxidation. It has been observed that quinoline on oxidation gives pyridine 2, 3-dicarboxylic acid, while pyridine 3, 4-dicarboxylic acid (cinchomeronic acid) is obtained from isoquinoline. Thus,

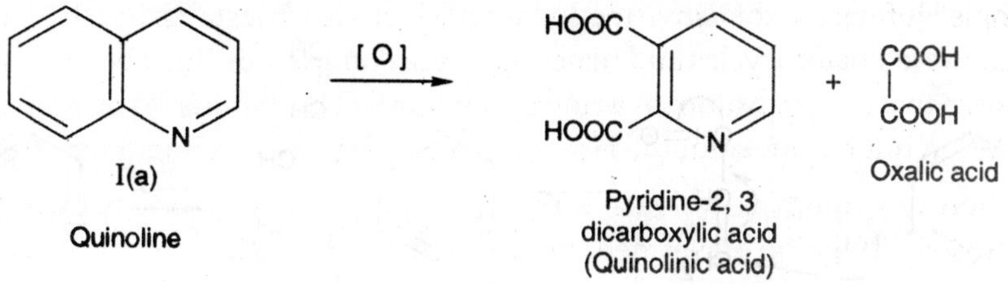

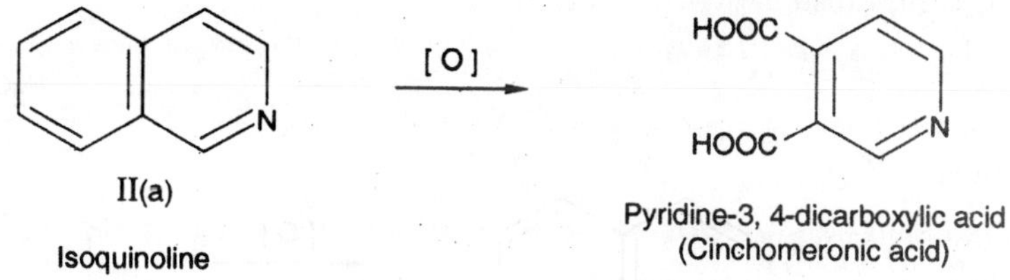

From the above experiment it is evident that in both the cases benzene ring undergoes cleavage and pyridine ring survives during oxidation. This is in accord with the observed fact that aromatic ring with electron withdrawing substituent (C=N—, can withdraw electrons), resists oxidative cleavage. Analysis of the products of oxidation further reveals that in quinoline benzene ring is fused at 2, 3 positions while the benzene ring is fused at 3, 4 positions in isoquinoline. Consequently, I(a) represents the structure of quinoline, and isoquinoline has the structure II(a).

21.6.2.2 Synthesis and Confirmation of the Structures of Quinoline and Isoquinoline

1. *Synthesis of Quinoline*

   (a) *Skraup Synthesis*: The most important synthesis of quinoline is due to Skraup. This synthetic process involves the heating a mixture of aniline and glycerol in nitro benzene using concentrated sulphuric acid and ferrous sulphate as catalysts. The reaction follows the paths as indicated below:

Stage 1:

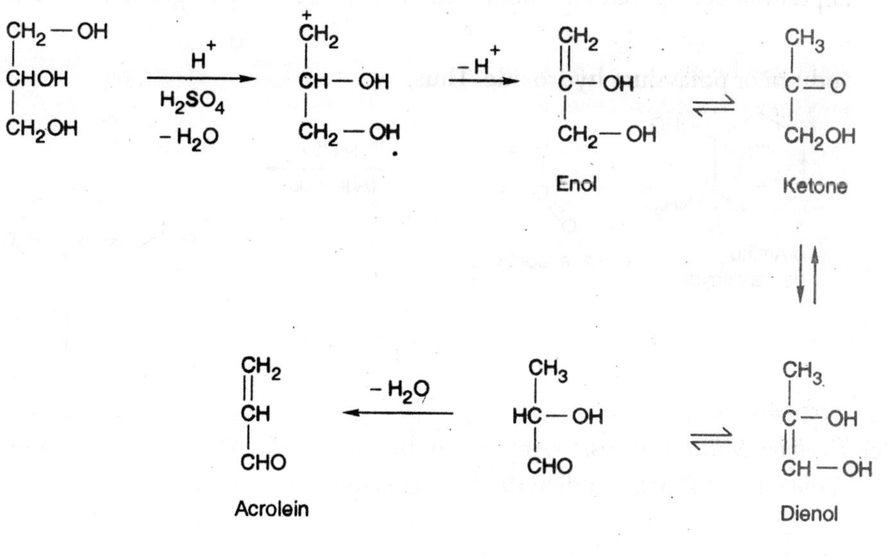

Stage 2:

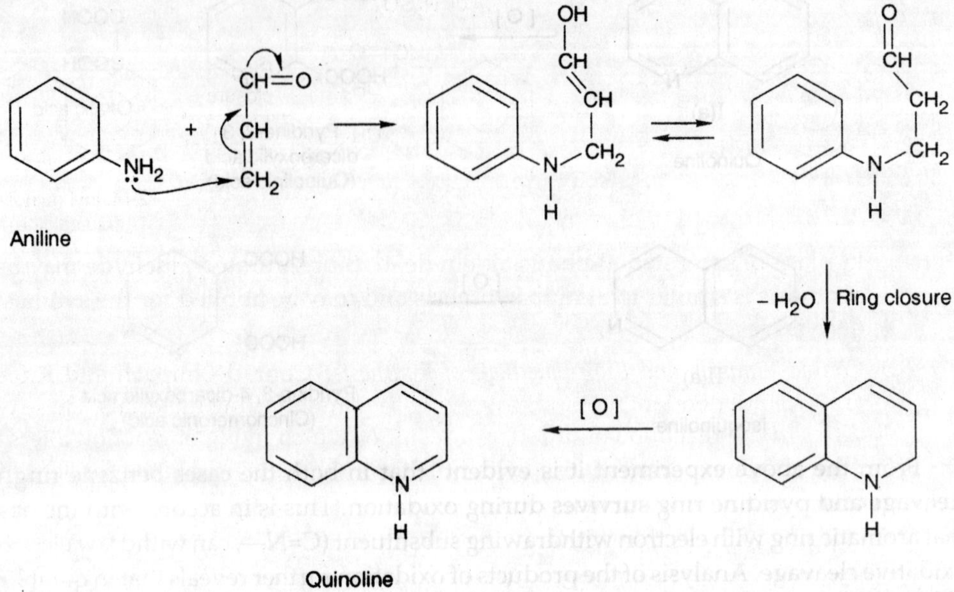

• *Comments*: (i) It is a general method for the synthesis of quoline and its derivatives. In place of aniline any primary aromatic amine having at least one vacant ortho position may be used. (ii) Nitrobenzene functions as oxidising agent while ferrous sulphate controls the reaction. (iii) Better yield may be obtained by using arsenic acid as oxidising agent as in this medium reaction becomes less vigorous.

(b) *Friedlander's synthesis*: This synthesis is also a general method for preparing quinoline derivatives. It consists of condensation between ortho amino aryl aldehyde with an aliphatic aldehyde having a keto methylene ($—CH_2—\overset{\overset{O}{\|}}{C}—$) group in presence of aqueous sodium or potassium hydroxide. Thus,

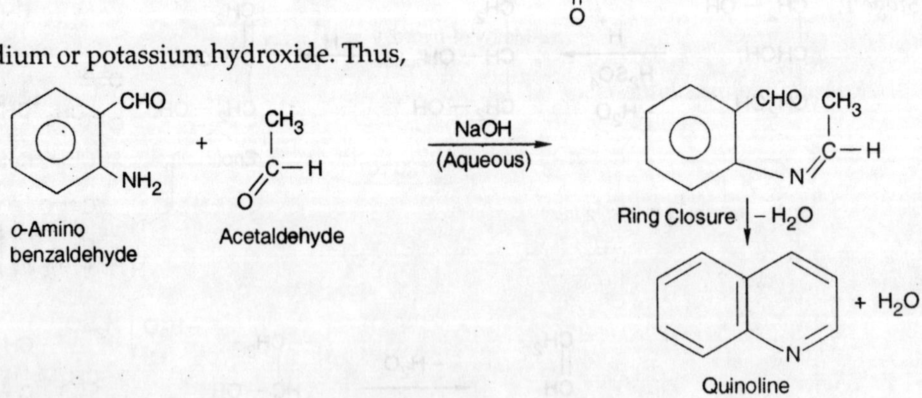

(c) *Doebner-Miller synthesis*: Any aromatic amine when allowed to condense with two molecules of aliphatic aldehydes having keto-methylene group ($—CH_2—\overset{\overset{O}{\|}}{C}—$) in presence of sulphuric acid, quinoline derivative may be obtained. For example,

$$CH_3-CHO + CH_3-CHO \xrightarrow[\text{dil. } H_2SO_4]{\text{Aldol}} CH_3-CH=CH-CHO$$

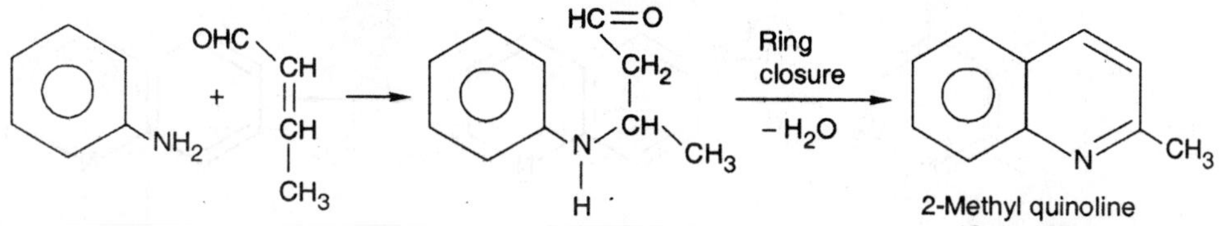

2-Methyl quinoline
(Quinaldine)

In place of saturated aliphatic aldehyde, α, β unsaturated aldehyde may be used. This synthesis is similar to Skraup synthesis and may be applied for the synthesis quinoline derivatives.

(d) *Conrad-Limpach and Knorr methods of Synthesis*: Conrad-Limpach and Knorr processes are two independent methods involving the same starting materials. These two methods differ in the reaction condition as a result of which mode of reaction alters resulting in the formation of different products. Both the methods consist of the condensation between aromatic amine and β-keto ester.

Conrad-Limpach synthesis:

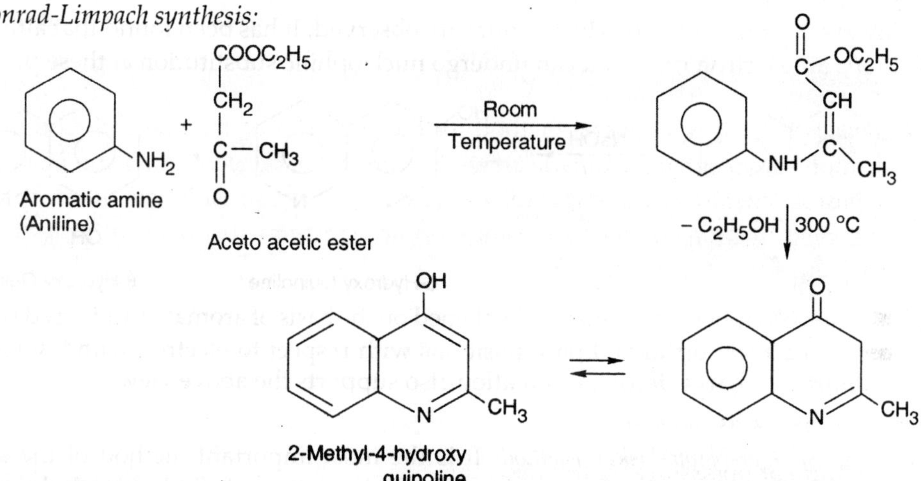

Knorr quinoline synthesis:

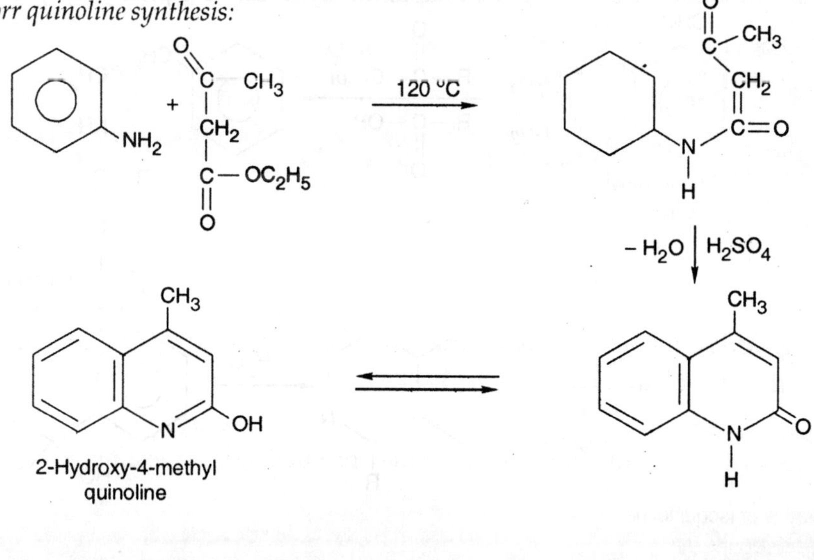

21.6.2.3 Activities of Quinoline Ring System

Quinoline is an aromatic compound and exists in resonance hybrid of the following structures:

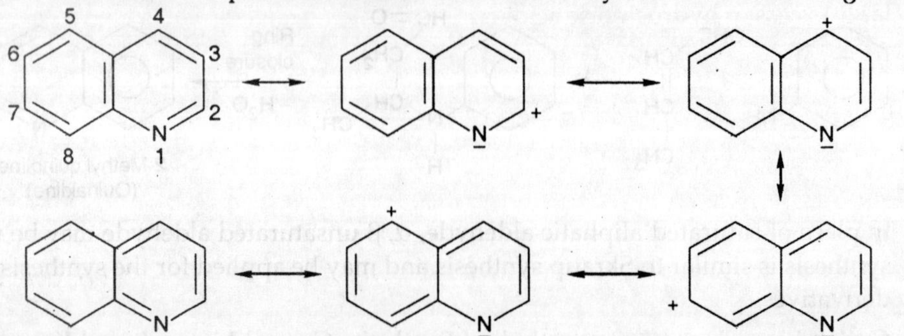

From the resonating structures following conclusions may be drawn regarding the activities of quinoline.

i. Quinoline ring is highly deactivated due to electron withdrawing effect of C=N system.
ii. It favours nucleophilic substitution reaction preferably at 2, 4, 5 and 7 positions.
iii. If electrophilic substitution occurs, it takes place at 3, 6 and 8 positions.

However, some anomalous behaviours are observed. It has been found that although 6 and 8 positions are electron rich yet it can undergo nucleophilic substitution at these positions, i.e.,

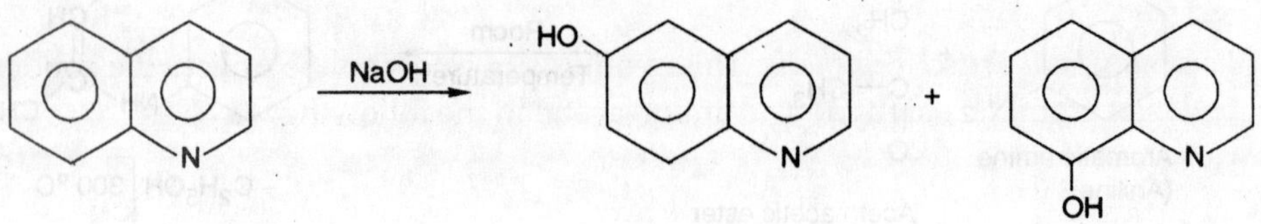

6-Hydroxy Quinoline 8-Hydroxy Quinoline

This anomalous behaviour may be explained on the basis of aromaticity of fused ring systems. Positions 8 and 6 are ortho and para positions with respect to electron withdrawing pyridine nucleus. Further, charge density calculation also supports the above view.

2. *Synthesis of Isoquinoline*
   i. *Bischler-Napierlaski's Method*: It is the most important method of the synthesis of isoquinoline. The starting material of this synthesis is β-phenyl ethyl amine.

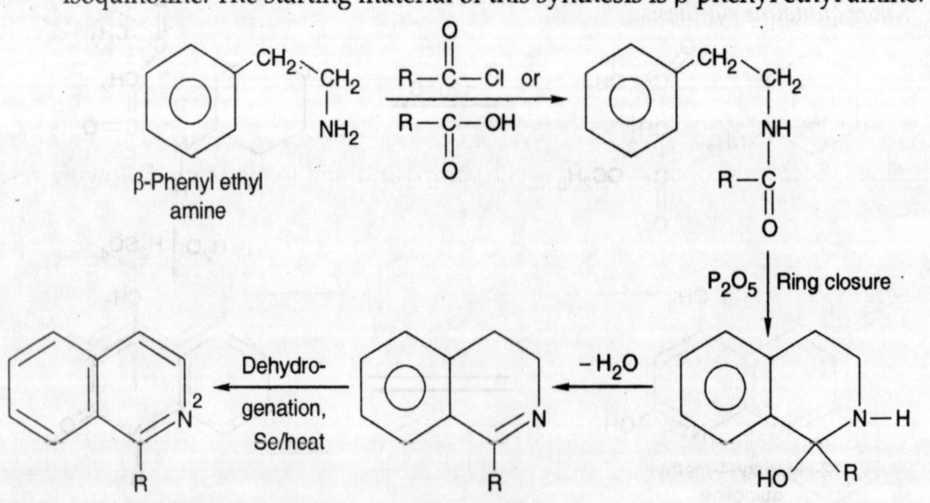

Derivative of Isoquinoline

ii. *Pictet and Spengler Synthesis*: In this synthesis condensation is carried out between a β-phenyl ethyl amine derivative and an aldehyde at a temperature of 100 °C in presence of large excess of hydrochloric acid.

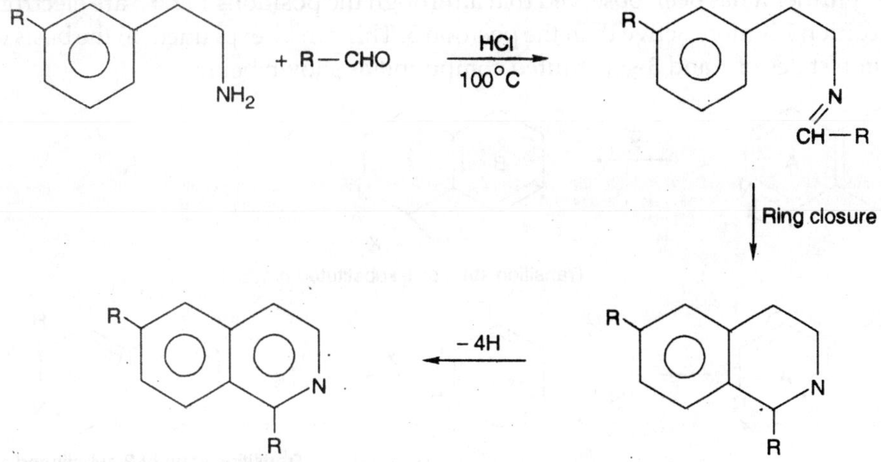

Isoquinoline derivative

iii. *Pomerantz and Fritsch Synthesis*: This synthesis of isoquinoline utilises the condensation between aromatic aldehyde and amino acetal in the following way:

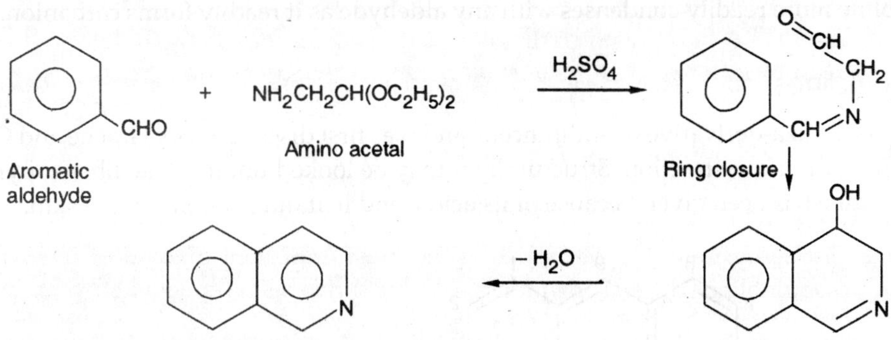

Isoquinoline

21.6.2.4 Activities of Isoquinoline Ring System

Isoquinoline is also an aromatic heterocyclic compound and exhibits the following resonating structures:

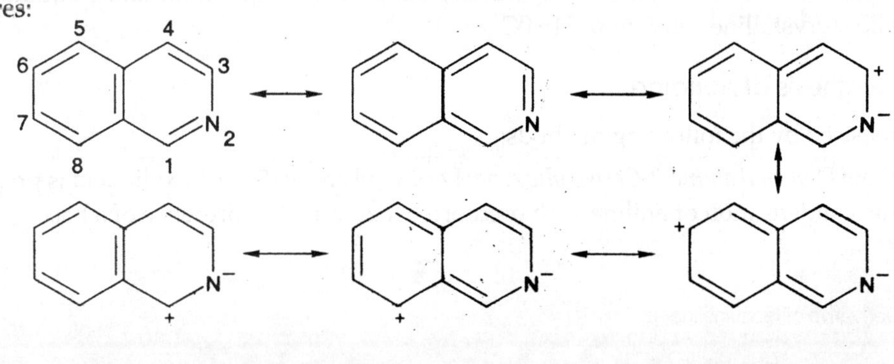

From the above resonance it is evident that like quinoline, isoquinoline ring is also deactivated due to the presence of C=N system and positions 1, 3, 6 and 8 are electron deficient and 4, 5 and 7 positions are relatively electron rich. So electrophilic substitution reactions may occur at 4, 5 and 7 positions, while positions 1, 3, 6 and 8 are highly favourable for nucleophilic substitution reactions. Further it has been observed that althrough the positions 1 and 3 are electron deficient yet the position 1 is more active than the position 3. This can be explained on the basis of stability of transition states of 1 and 3-substituted compound as shown below:

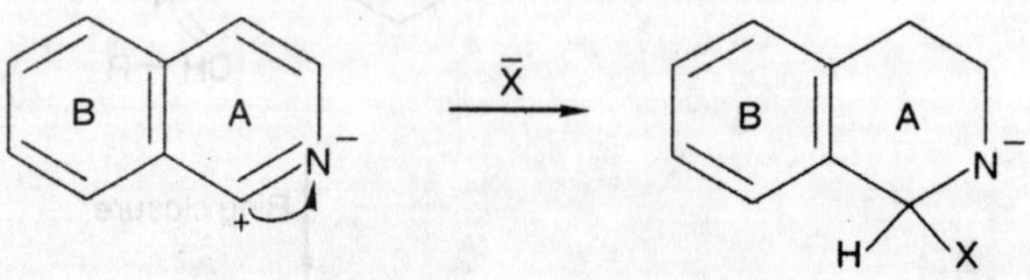

Transition state of 1-substituted product

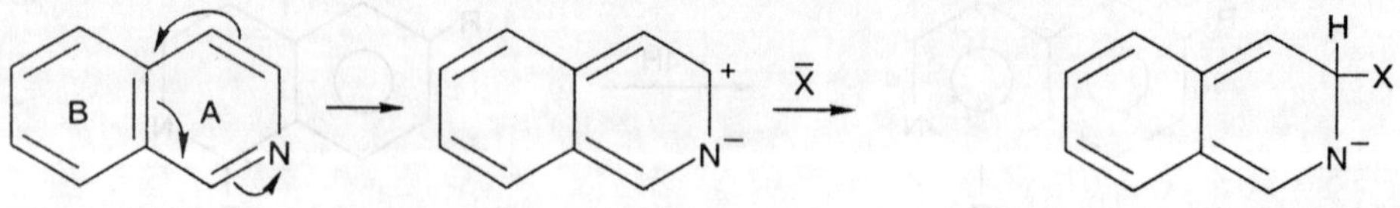

Transition state of 3-substituted product

It is seen that in the case of transition state for 1-substituted product benzene ring (B) remains intact but in the case of 3-substituted product, transition state does not have any such intact benzene ring. Hence, transition state for 1-substituted product is stabler than that of 3-substituted product. So 1-position is more electron deficient than position 3. For this reason, 1-methyl isoquinoline more readily condenses with any aldehyde as it readily forms carbanion.

21.7 Acridines

Acridine is the aza-derivative of anthrancene and was first discovered by Grache and Caro from coal tar in anthrancene fraction. Structurally it may be looked upon as the dibenzopyridine. Its name acridine has been given because of its acidic and irritating actions on the skin.

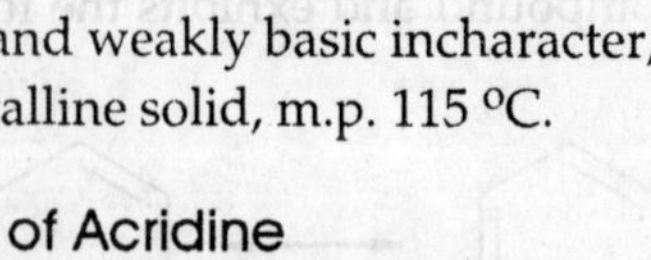

Acridine

It is aromatic and weakly basic incharacter, comparable to quinoline and isoquinoline. It is a pale yellow crystalline solid, m.p. 115 °C.

21.7.1 Synthesis of Acridine

It is synthesised by the following methods:

i. *From Diphenyl amine-2-Carboxylic Acid:* Diphenyl amine-2-Carboxylic acid is prepared by the condensation of aniline with α-chloro benzoic acid in presence of a base

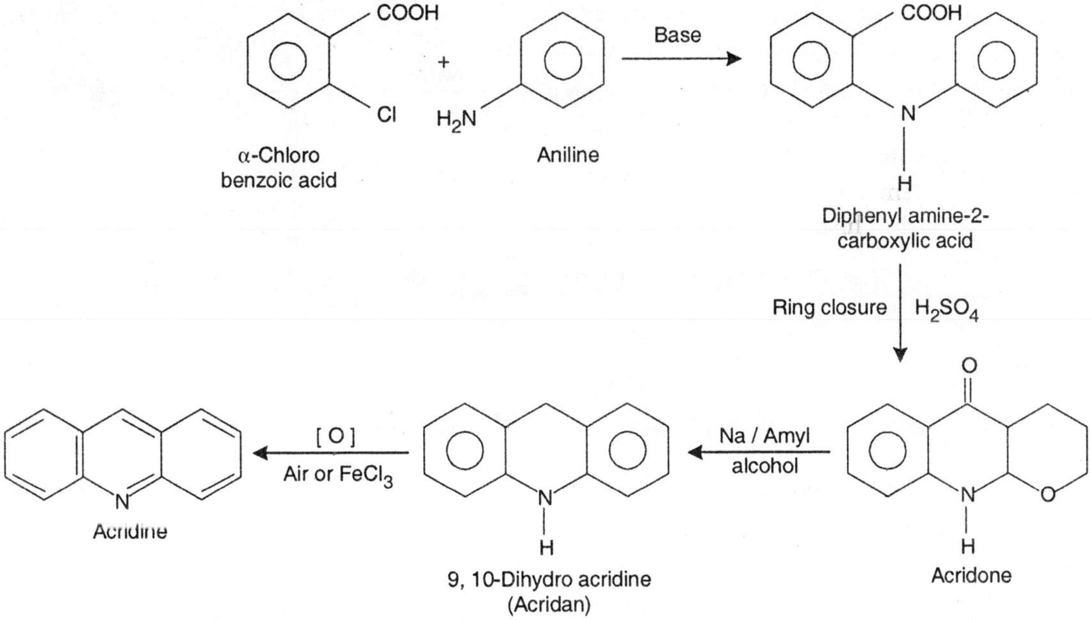

ii. *Pyrolysis of o-Hydroxy methyl diphenyl amines:*

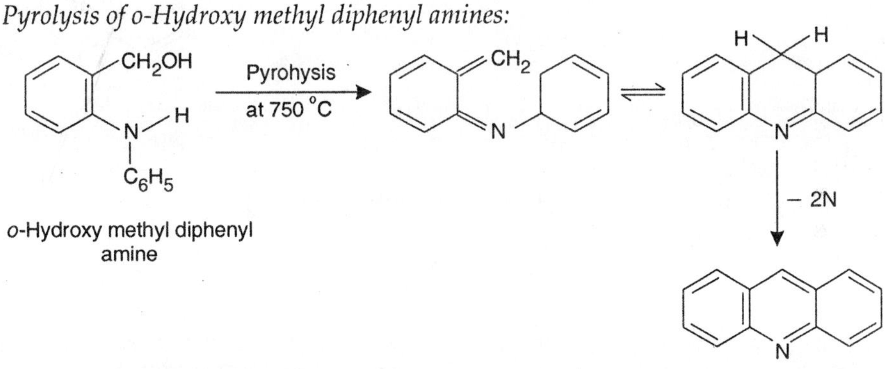

Acridine

Acridine ring system is an important skeleton found in many naturally occurring alkaloids, number of dyes and medicinally important substances. Some of such compounds are mentioned below:

(a) *Aminacrine:* It is I-amino acridine and it is highly active against many Gram-positive bacteria.

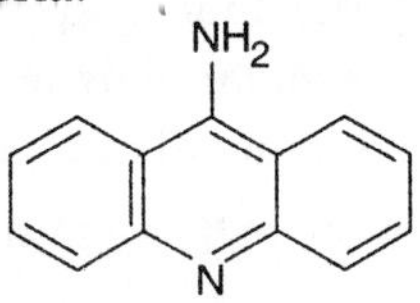

It is used as a disinfectant and antiseptic.

(b) Mepacrine (Quinacrine or Atebrin): It is 3-chloro-I-(-4′-diethylamino-3′-methyl-butylamino)-7-methoxy-acridine. It is prepared as follows:

Step-I

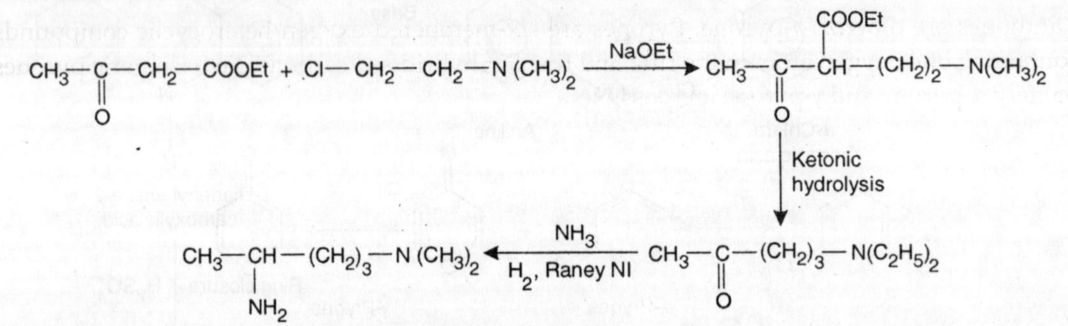

Step-II

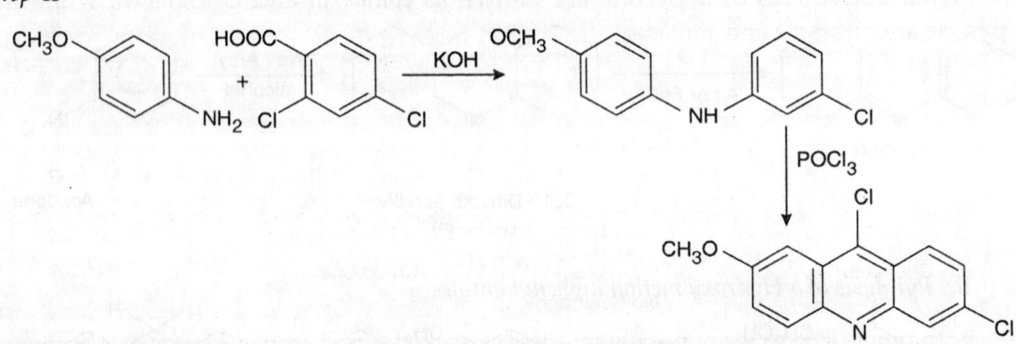

Step-III

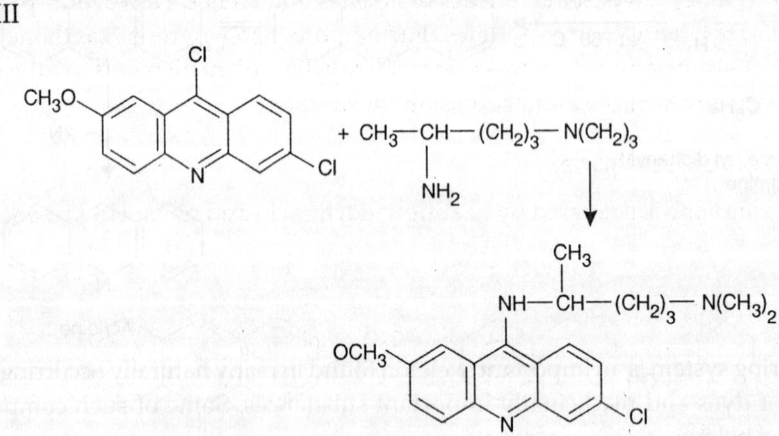

Mepacrine

Mepacrine has strong antimalarial property and is better than quinine. But due to its unpleasant side-effects it has been replaced by other antimalarial drug like chloroquine. It is now used in the treatment of giardiasis and for the removal of tape-worms.

(c) *Proflavine:* It is 3, 6-diamino acridine. It is also found to be active against Gram-positive bacteria and so is used as a disinfectant and antiseptic.

Acridine containing alkaloids have been isolated from the bark and leaves of several plants, for example, *Melicope farena* and *Evodia Xanthoxyloids* which are found in the forests of Queenland and Australia.

21.8 Xanthones

Xanthones are dibenzo-γ-pyrone. Pyrones are six-membered oxygen heterocyclic compounds containing one oxygen atom in the ring and five Sp^2 hybridised carbons. Two isomeric pyrones namely α-pyrone and γ-pyrone are possible.

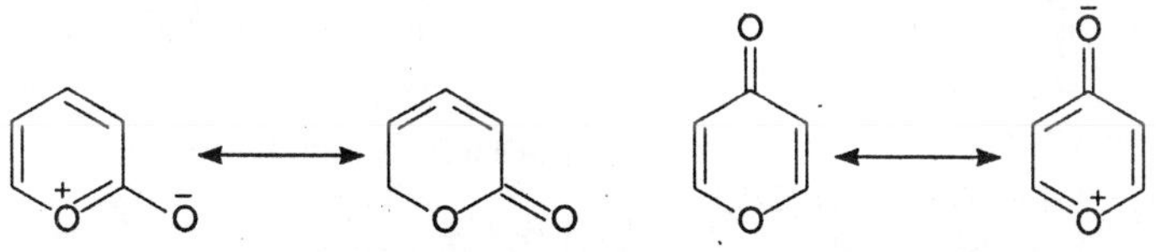

α-Pryone γ-Pryone

Benzo derivatives of α-pyrone are known as *coumarin* and *isocoumarin* while that of γ-pyrone are *chromone* and *xanthone.*

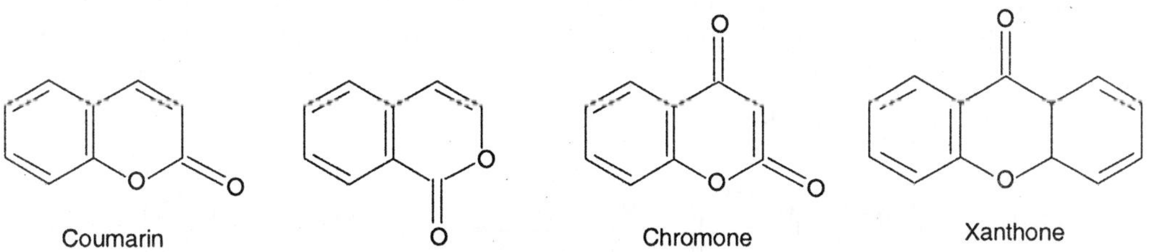

Coumarin *Iso*-Coumarin Chromone Xanthone

Both types of pyrones have characteristics of alkenes and arenes. However, γ-pyrone has a greater degree of aromaticity than α-pyrones. Further, dibenzo-γ-pyrone (xanthone) is highly stable and widely occurs in nature. Xanthones, in fact, are yellow plant pigments. All the xanthones are the hydroxy derivatives of the parent compound, xanthone.

21.8.1 Preparation of Xanthones

The first member xanthone is prepared by heating salicylic acid and phenol in presence of acetic anhydride.

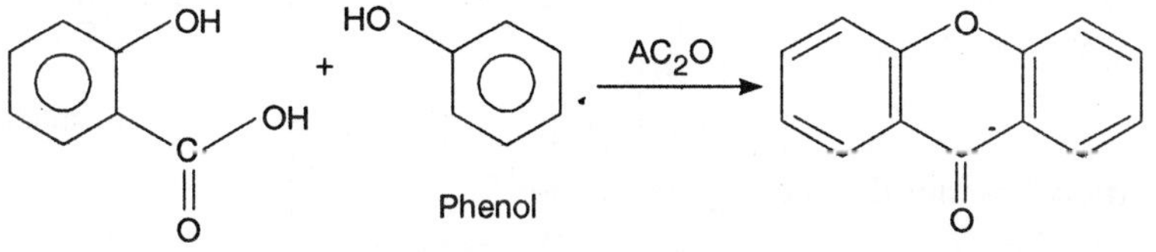

Salicylic acid Phenol

It is a solid substance metting at 175 °C and on reduction with hydrolodic acid it is converted to xanthene.

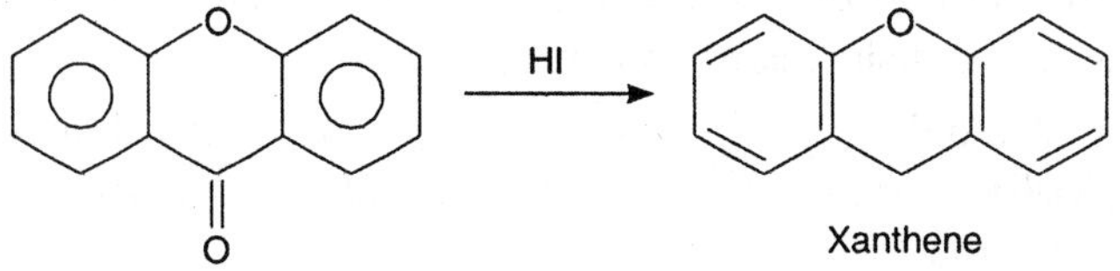

Xanthone Xanthene

On fusion with KOH it produces 2, 2′-dihydroxy benzophenone which establishes the structure of xanthone.

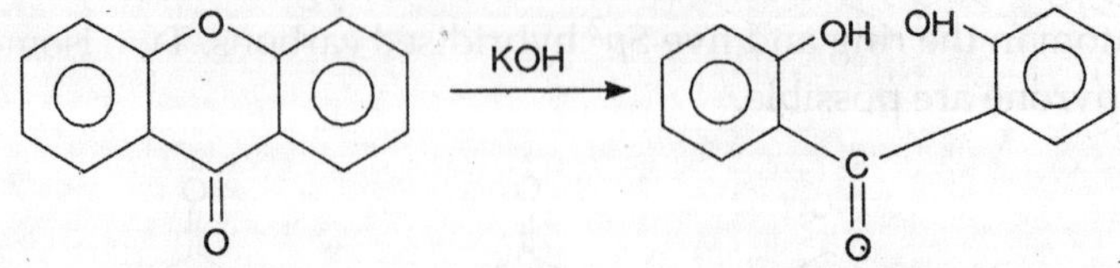

Xanthone 2, 2′-Dihydroxy benzophenone

21.8.2 Some Important Naturally Occurring Xanthones

Most important and common yellow vegetable dyes belonging to xanthone group are euxanthone, gentisin and gentisein.

(a) *Euxanthone:* It occurs as calcium or magnesium salt of glucuronic acid, euxanthic acid, in the Indian yellow. It is obtained from the urine of cows fed on mango leaves. On fusion with potassium hydroxide it yields 2, 6, 2′, 5′-tetra-hydroxy benzophenone which settles its structure as 1, 7-dihydroxy xanthone.

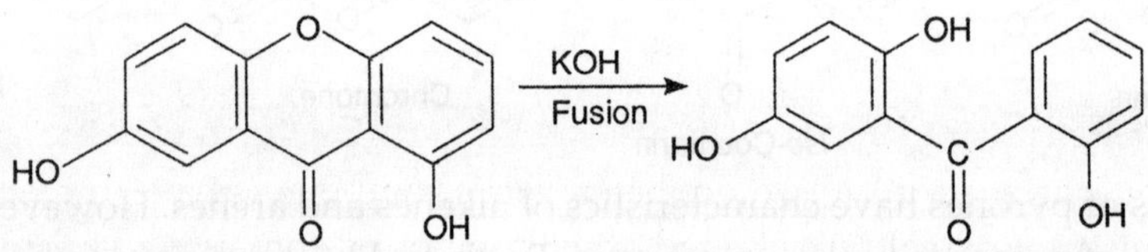

Euxanthone 2, 6, 2′, 5′,- Dihydroxy benzophenone

Its structure has further been confirmed by its synthesis

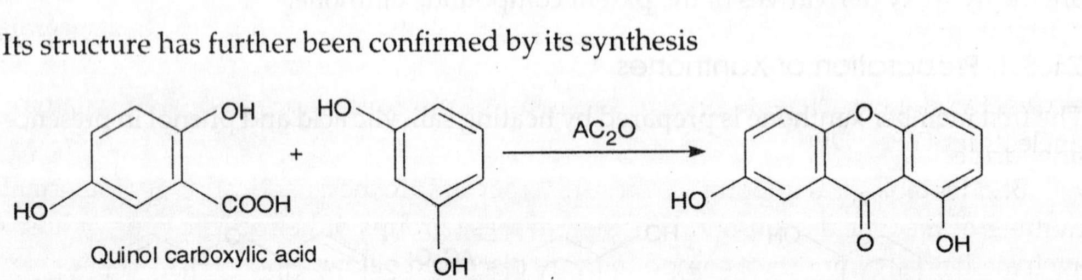

Quinol carboxylic acid Resorcinol Euxanthone

(b) *Gentisin:* It occurs mainly in the gentian root.

It has also been synthesised as below:

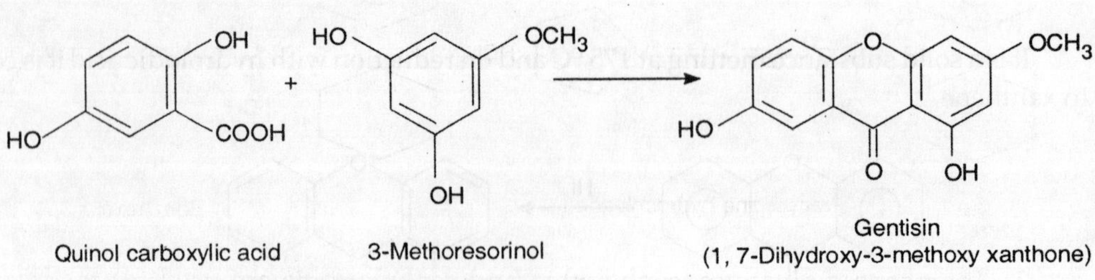

Quinol carboxylic acid 3-Methoresorinol Gentisin (1, 7-Dihydroxy-3-methoxy xanthone)

(c) *Gentisein:* It also occurs in gentian root. It has been assigned the structure, 1, 3, 7-trihydroxy xanthone.

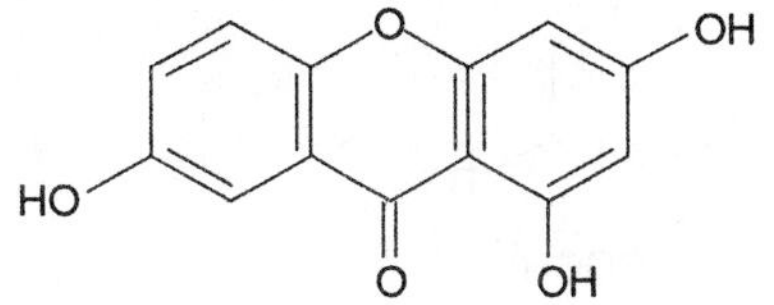

Gentisein
(1, 3, 7-Trihydroxy-xanthone)

It can be synthesised similarly by the condensation of quinol carboxylic acid and phloroglucinol.

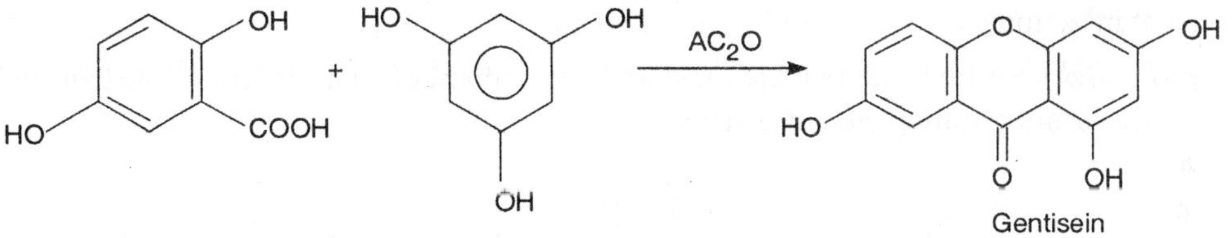

21.9 Uses of Heterocyclic Compounds with One Hetero Atom

Biologically and pharmaceutically monoheterocyclic compounds have immense significances. Thus prophyrin, a completely conjugated cyclic compound containing four pyrrole rings does not itself occur in nature but this frame work is present in *haemoglobin* (present in red blood corpuscles and carries oxygen from lungs to the body tissue), chlorophyll (the green colouring matter of plants essential for *photosynthesis*), and vitamin B_{12} (anti-pernicious anaemia factor). The indole ring system is present in essential amino acid, *tryptophan,* and plant-growth hormones, *auxins.* Pyridone nucleus is present in vitamins, nicotinic acid, pyridoxine (vitamin B_6), and nucleotides (TPN, DPN).

Besides biological importance these heterocycles are therapeutically very important. A large number of medicinal compounds belong to these groups of hetrocyclic compounds. A few of such medicinally important compounds are discussed below:

1. Procyclidine hydrochloride and benzhexol are potent antiperkinsonism drugs.

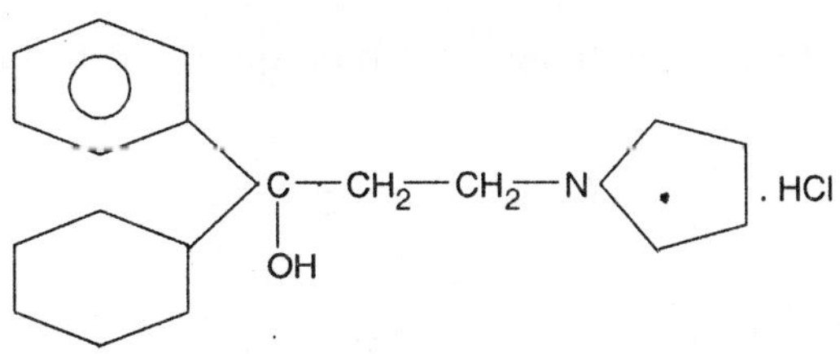

Procyclidine hydrochloride

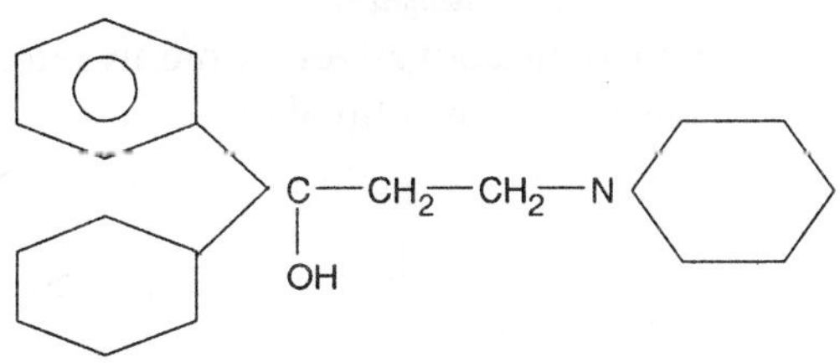

Benzhexol

2. Thiophene derivatives, cephalothin and cephaloridine are used for the treatment of staphylococcal infections.

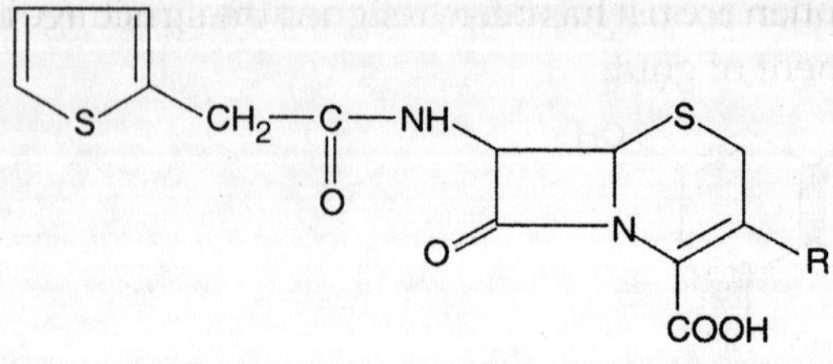

$R = O—CH_2—OCOCH_3$, Cephalothin

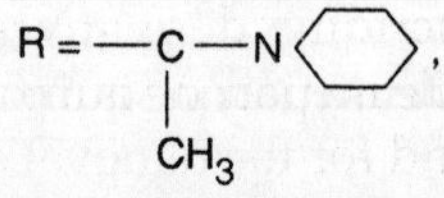
, Cephaloridine

3. Nitrofurazone, is a broad spectrum antibacterial agent. It is also useful in the treatment of infections of ear, eye, nose and vagina.
4. *Ranitidine,* is now extensively used in the treatment of gastric ulcer while frusemide is an important antihypertensive drug.

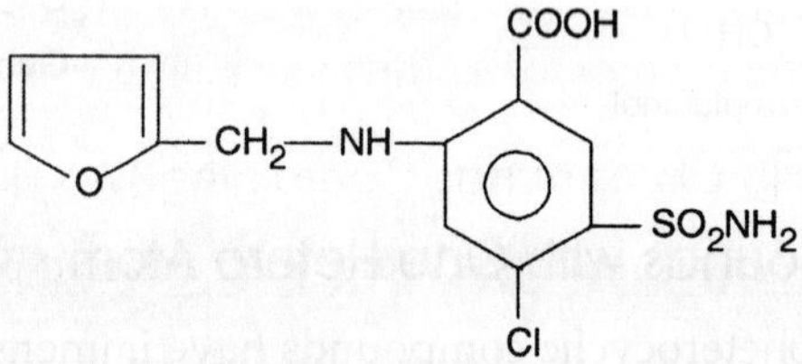

Frusemide

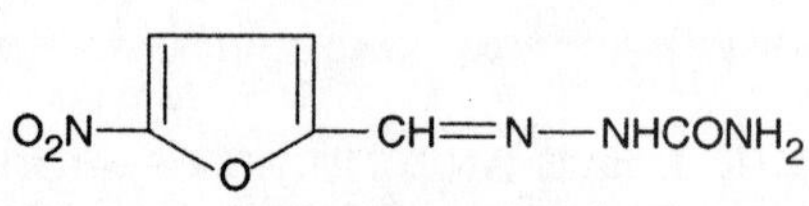

Nitrofurazone

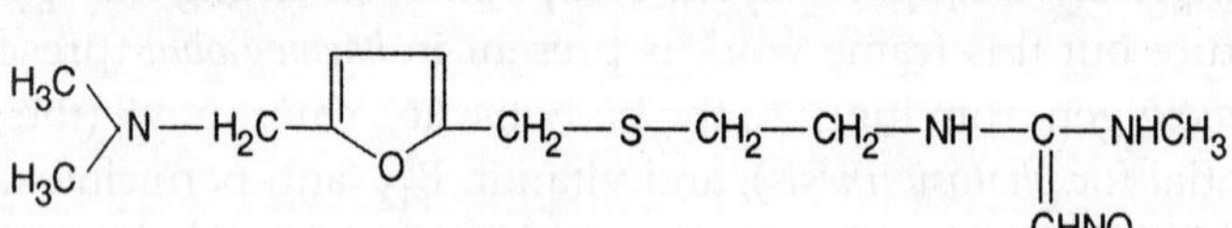

Ranitidine

5. *Isoniazid,* a pyridine derivative is highly effective medicine for pulmonary tuberculosis.

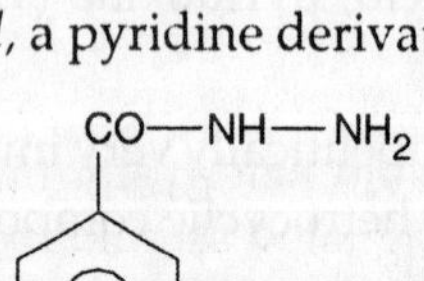

Isoniazid

6. Quinoline derivatives are highly important therapeutic agents. Chloroquine, primaquine are important antimalarial drugs.

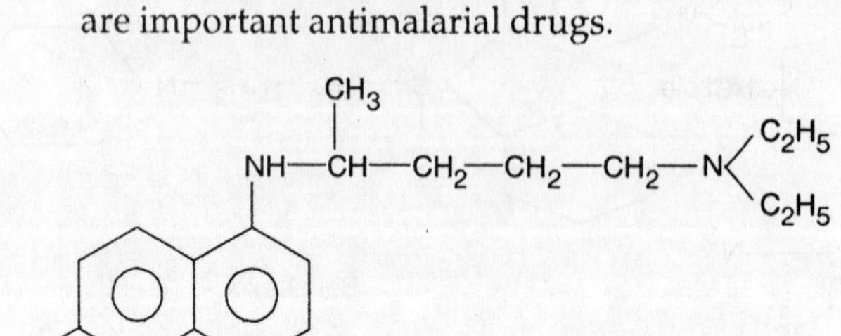

Chloroquine

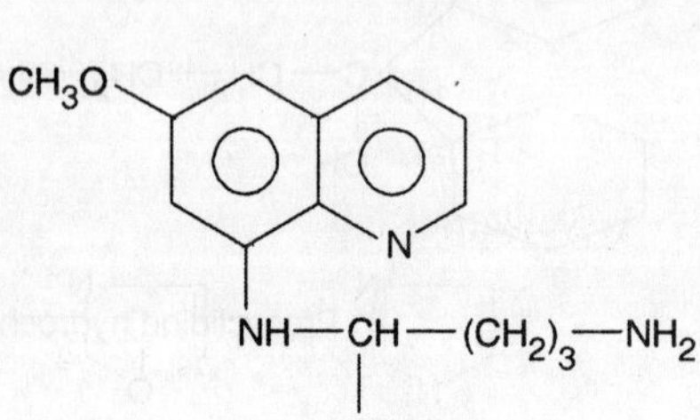

Primaquine

Cinchophen and neocinchophen are useful antipyretic and analgesic agents. Cincehophen is mainly used in the treatment of gout.

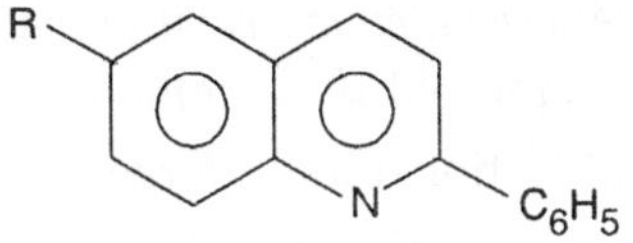

R = H, Cinchophen
R = CH_3, Neocinchophen

7. Amacrine, mepacrine and proflavine are acridine derivatives and are medicinally important as disinfectants and antiseptics while mepacrine is a potent antimalarial drug. It is also used in the treatment of giardiasis and for the removal of tapeworms.

   In addition to the above thereapeutic uses, these mono-heterocyclic compounds are important as chemical reagents and dyes.

21.10 Heterocyclic Compounds Containing Two Hetero Atoms

Among wide variety of heterocyclic compounds containing two hetero atoms in the ring, five and six-membered compounds are extremely common and widely studied.

21.10.1 Five-membered Heterocyclic Compounds Containing Two Hetero Atoms

When two hetero atoms are present in a five-membered ring, their relative positions may be either 1, 2 or 1, 3 as shown below:

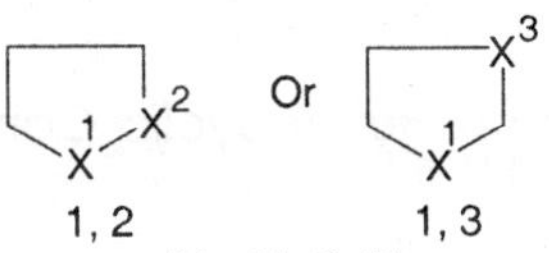

(X = N, O, S)

Of the two hetero atoms one is always nitrogen while second one may be nitrogen, oxygen or sulphur, consequently these heterocycles are termed as *azoles*. Thus heterocyclic compounds having two hetero atoms at 1, 2-positions are named as pyrazole, isoxazole and isothiazole respectively, nitrogen, oxygen and sulphur being the second hetero atom.

Similarly, the heterocyclic compounds in which the second hetero atom is present in 1, 3 relationship with respect to nitrogen already present are designated as imidazole, oxazole and thiazole for nitrogen, oxygen and sulphur.

Thus,

1, 2-*relationship*

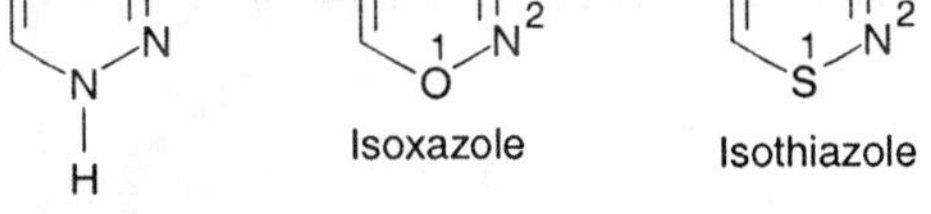

Pyrazole Isoxazole Isothiazole

1, 3-*relationship*

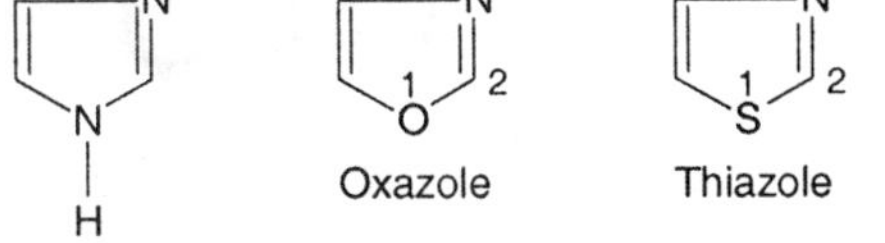

Imidazole Oxazole Thiazole

It is known that in heterocyclic compounds numbering by convention starts from the hetero atom. But when two different hetero atoms are present, the hetero atom which belongs to the highest group in the periodic table and the element of *least atomic weight in that group is* usually given preference. Thus the order of preference among these three common elements is oxygen > sulphur > nitrogen, i.e., oxygen atom is assigned position-1 in preference to other.

It may be mentioned that a large number of natural and synthetic compounds containing azole ring system are known which have immense pharmaceutical and biological importance such as antipyrine, histidine, histamine, allantoin, etc.

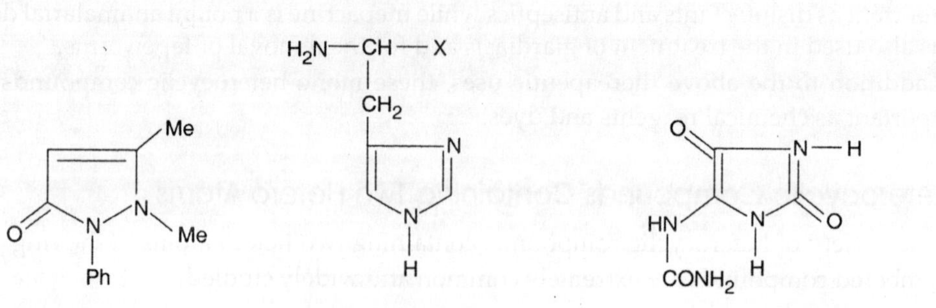

Antipyrine (antipyretic and analgesic)

X = COOH, Histidine, essential amino acid
X = H, Histamine, an 'antihistamine'

Allantoin (End product of nitrogen metabolisim in some animals)

21.10.1.1 Activity of Five-membered Heterocyclic Compounds Containing Two Hetero Atoms

All azoles are aromatic in character in which lone pair of electrons on the hetero atoms contribute towards the formation of aromatic sextet. Each of the three carbon atoms contributes one p_z electron, fourth electron is obtained from nitrogen while the second hetero atom (N, O or S as the case may be) provides two electrons for constructing aromatic sextets. The molecular orbital structures of 1, 2 and 1, 3 azoles may be shown as below:

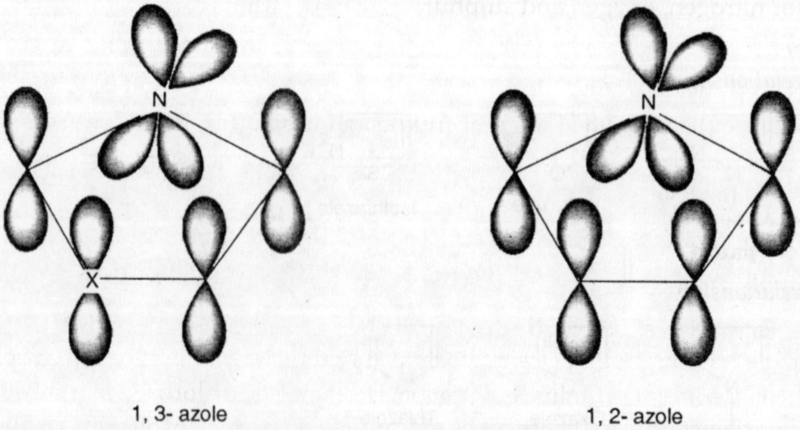

1, 3- azole

1, 2- azole

Like all other aromatic compounds these heterocycles exist in a resonance hybrid of the following structures:

1, 2-azoles:

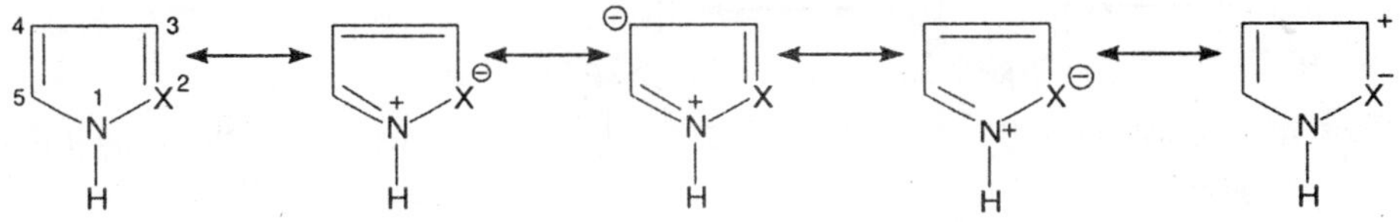

1, 3-azoles:

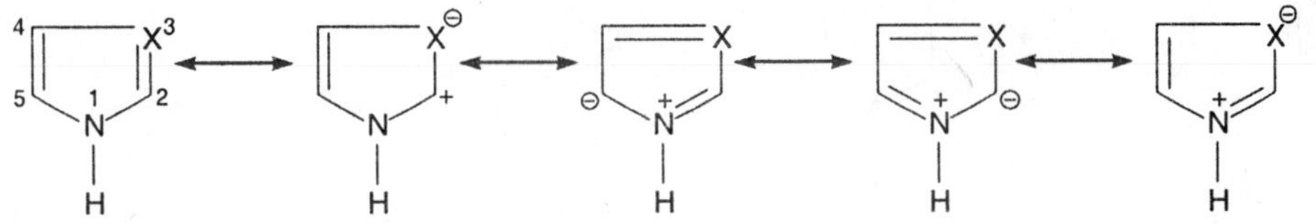

21.10.2 Pyrazole and Imidazole

Pyrazole: As stated before pyrazole is that type of heterocyclic compounds in which two nitrogen atoms are in 1, 2 positions. These heterocycles are most commonly prepared by the condensation between 1, 3-dicarbonyl compound and hydrazine or its derivatives.

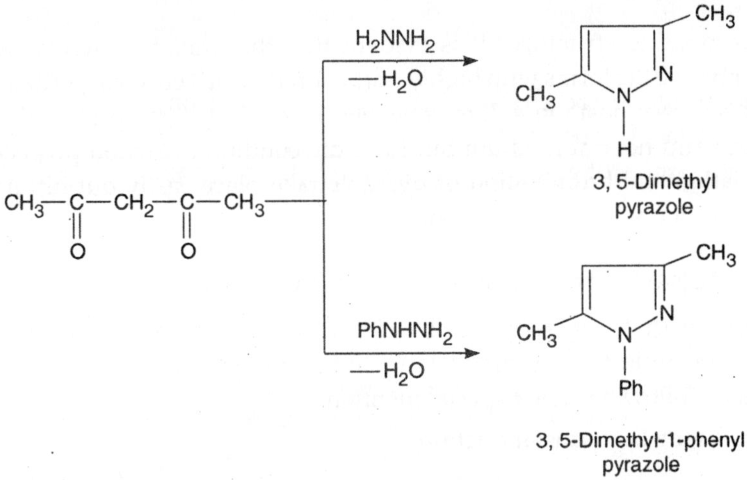

21.10.2.1 Properties of Pyrazole

Pyrazole is a colourless solid, m.p. 70 °C, and is soluble in water. It possesses a pungent smell and is a tautomeric substance with the following forms

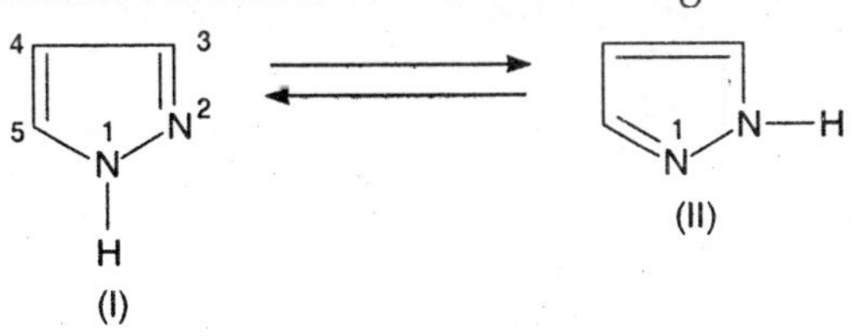

Pyrazole exhibits aromatic character and as such readily undergoes **electrophilic substitution** like halogenation, nitration and sulphonation, etc. It may be mentioned that **substitution preferably** takes place at position-4, which may be explained on the basis of relative **stabilities of transition** states.

Transition states for

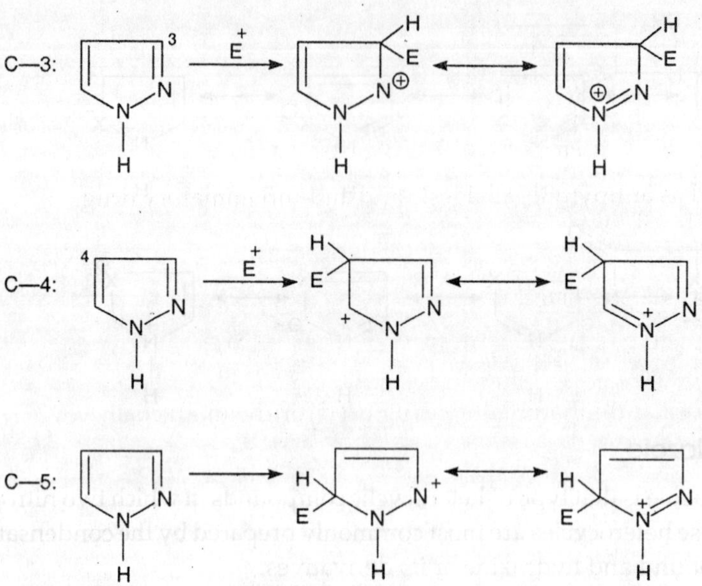

From the above resonating structures it is evident that the transition states for 3 and 5-substituted products involve the forms with highly unfavoured positively charged azomethine nitrogen. Hence attack occurs at position-4. It may be mentioned that electrophilic substitution smoothly occurs in basic and neutral medium but in acidic condition reaction proceeds with difficulty. Thus chlorination and bromination of pyrazole take place easily but nitration and sulphonation occurs under more drastic condition.

21.10.2.2 Biologically Active Pyrazole Derivatives and Their Uses

It is important to mention that pyrazole ring has attracted considerable attention of the physiologists and clinicians in last few years. A large number of medicinal compounds have been synthesised of which followings need special mention.

i. *Orisul* possesses a long bacteriostatic action.

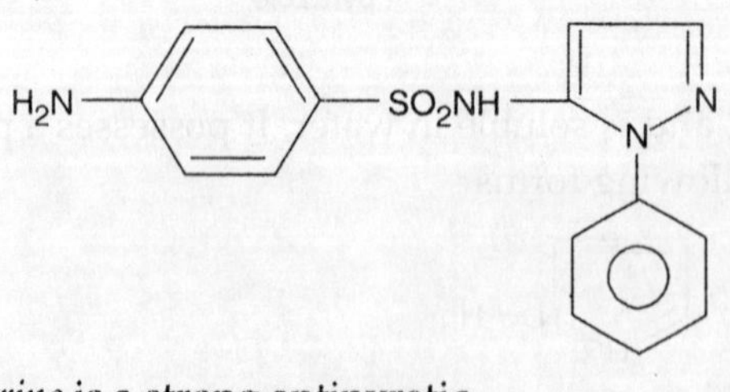

ii. *Antipyrine* is a strong antipyretic.

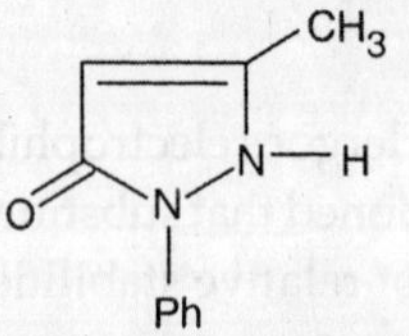

iii. *Analgin* is an important analgesic.

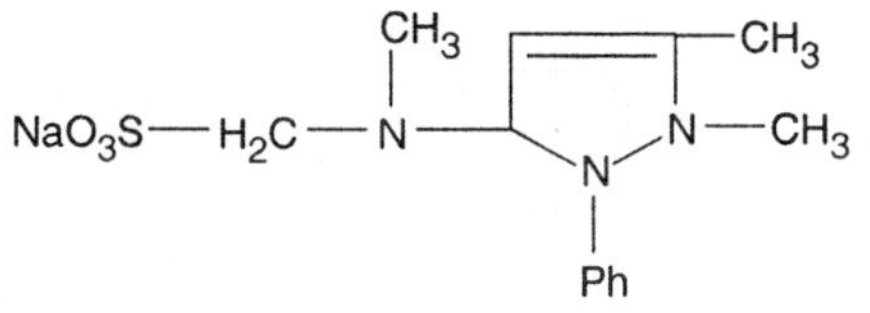

iv. *Phenyl butazone* is used as antipyretic, analgesic and anti-inflammatory drug.

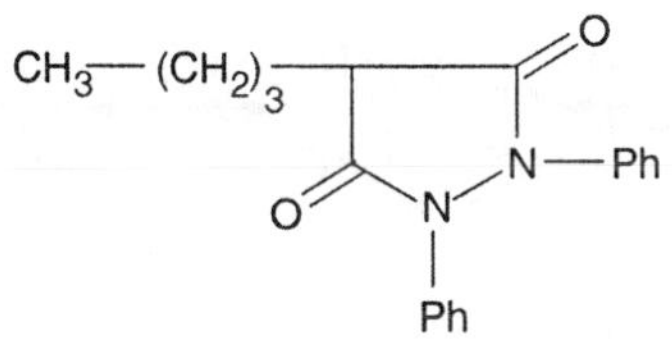

v. *Butazolidine* is a powerful anti-inflammatory drug used for rheumatic pain.

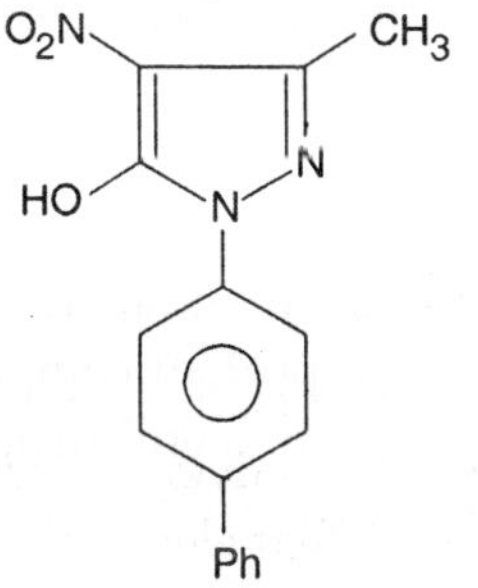

vi. *Phenazone* is an antipyretic. It also possesses local anaesthetic action and its solution (5%) is used as ear drop.

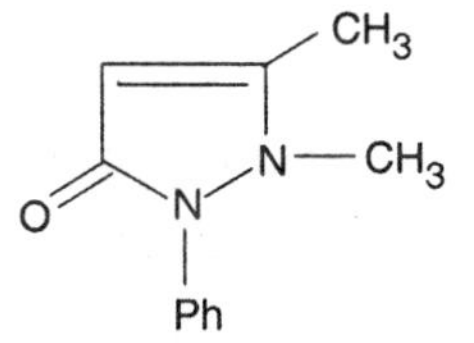

vii. *Sulphin pyrazone* is a uricosuric agent and is normally employed for the term treatment of chronic gout

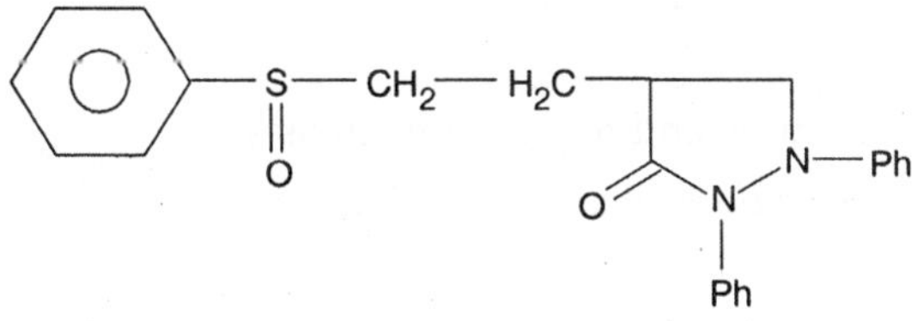

21.10.3 Imidazole

In imidazole ring system two nitrogen atoms are situated in 1, 3 positions. The most important method of synthesis of this ring system is due to *Radiszewski*. This method involves the condensation of 1, 2-dicarbonyl compound with an aldehyde in the presence of ammonia.

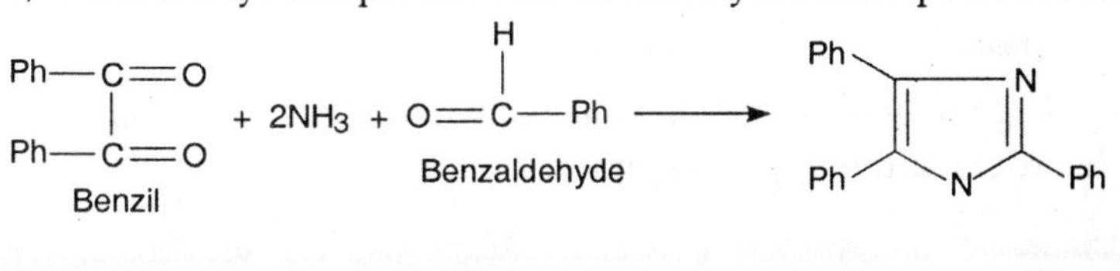

Imidazole is a colourless solid, m.p. 90 °C. It is more basic than pyrazole. It is a tautomeric substance and exists in two equilibrium forms

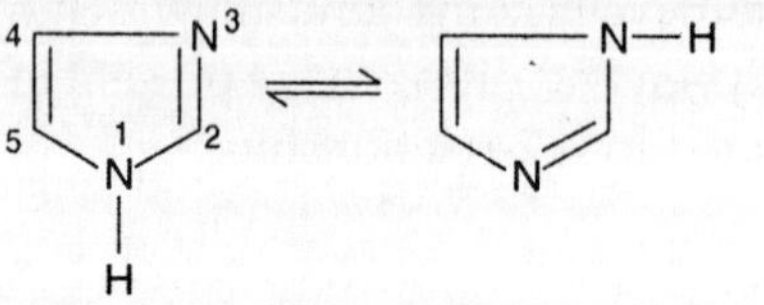

It exhibits aromatic character and is a resonance hybrid of the following structures

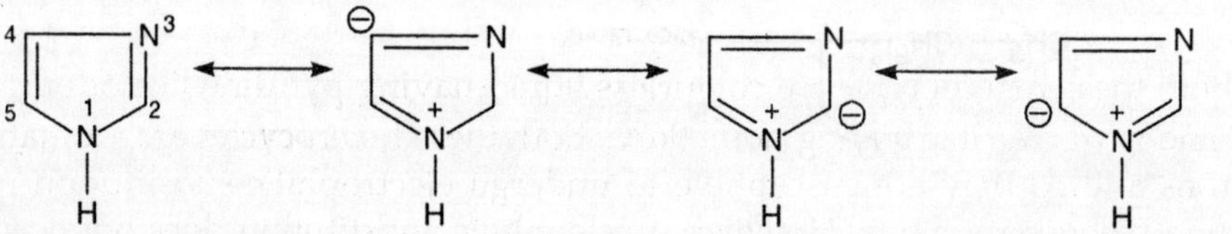

From the above resonance it is evident that it possesses increased activity toward electrophilic attack. Electrophilic substitution normally occurs at 4 and 5 position. If, however, 4 and 5 positions are blocked, 2-substituion may occur.

21.10.3.1 Biologically Active Imidazoles and Their Uses

Imidazole ring system is very important in living systems. Biofin, an imidazole derivative is an essential growth factor. This ring system forms a part of some important compounds such as purines, xanthine, co-enzyme-A, etc. A number of imidazoles are useful drugs used in the treatment of various ailments, a few of which are mentioned below:

i. *Histamine* stimulates the lacrimal and secretory glands.

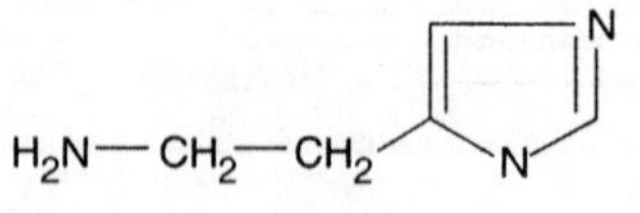

ii. *Metronidazole* is a potent amoebicide and may be used in all clinical forms of amoebiasis

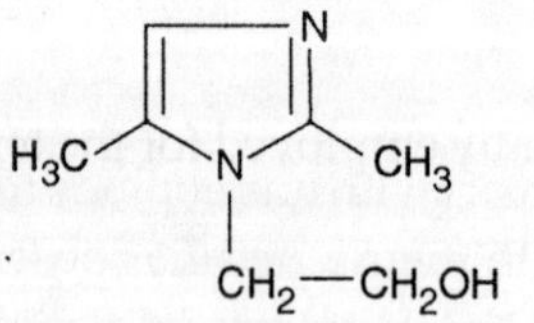

iii. *Nitridazole* is useful in both intestinal and hepatic amoebiasis.

iv. *Carbimazole and methimazole* are important antithyroid drugs.

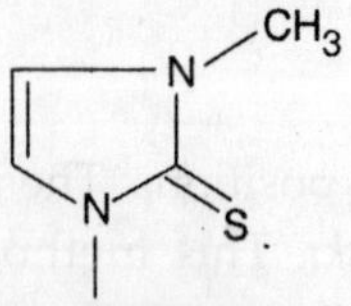

Carbimazole

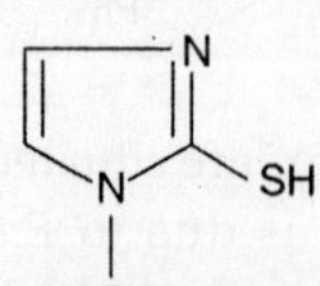

Methimazole

v. *Naphazoline hydrochloride* is a potent vasoconstrictor. It is very useful in the symptomatic relief of disorders of the upper respiratory tract.

21.10.4 Oxazoles and Isoxazoles

Oxazole and isoxazole are five-membered heterocyclic compounds in which two hetero atoms, oxygen and nitrogen are present. In oxzole, oxygen and nitrogen are present in 1, 3-relationship while in isoxazoles these hetro atoms are situated in 1, 2-relationship.

Oxazole Isoxazole

Both these heterocycles are colourless liquid having pyridine like odour. Oxazole boils at 69°C and isoxazole has boiling point 96°C. Both these heterocycles are aromatic and are rich in electrons and so they are susceptible to undergo electrophilic substitution reactions such as nitration halogenation, etc. However, nucleophilic substitution does not occur under normal condition.

Both these compounds are basic in nature but isoxazole is less basic than oxazole. This is because in isoxzaole both these electronegative atoms are present at consecutive positions. Again, due to the presence of both oxygen and nitrogen atoms at consecutive positions, isoxazole ring system becomes less stable than oxazole and infact on thermolysis isoxazole is readily converted to oxazole. This conversion may be explained as below:

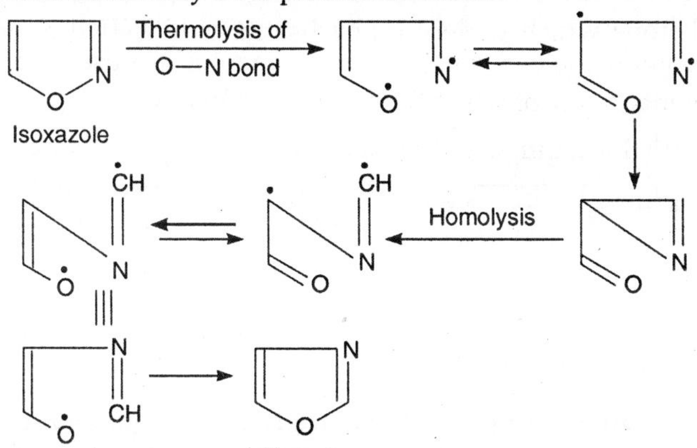

As mentioned before, these two ring systems do not react with nucleophilic reagent. However, when strong nucleophilic reagent is allowed to react with them a peculiar observation has been noted. Thus oxazole on treatment with strong base like $NaNH_2$ forms imidazole while isoxzole yields a ketonitrile under the same condition.

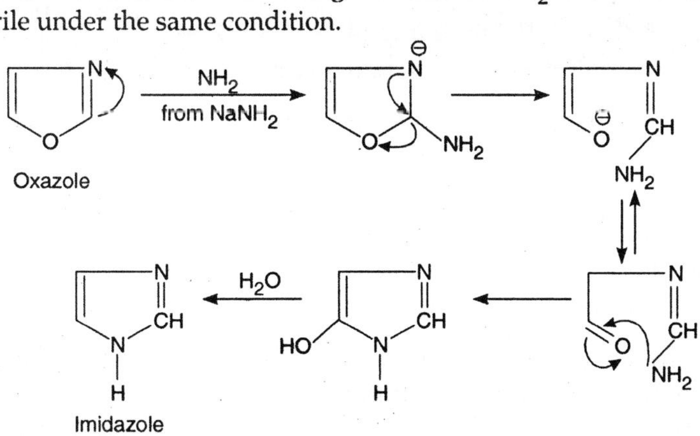

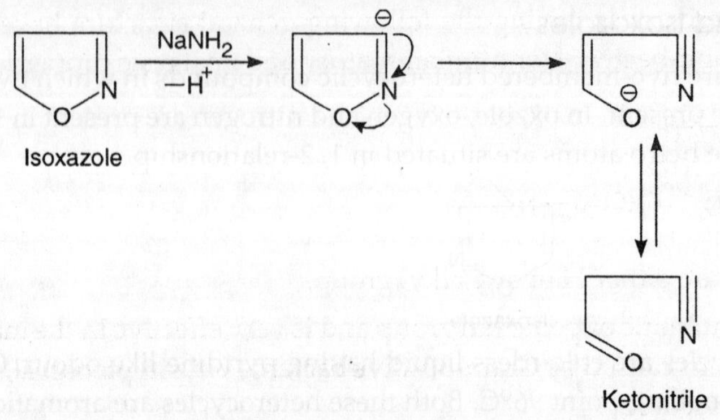

Isoxazole is prepared by the condensation and cyclisation reaction of α, β-diketone with hydroxylamine.

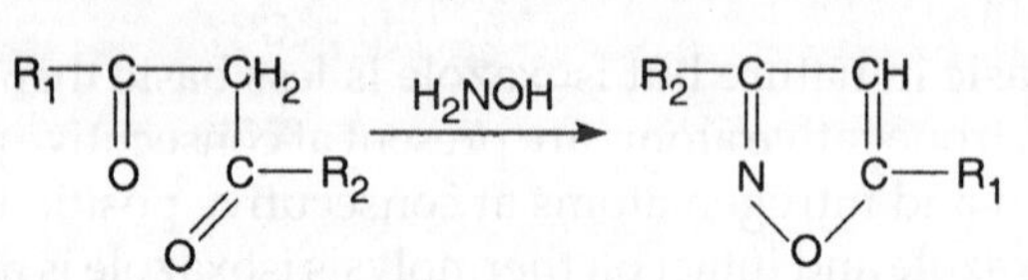

Oxazole is prepared by the most common method due to Robinson and Gabriel. This method involves an acylamino ketone which undergoes cyclisation and dehydration in presence of phosphorous pentoxide.

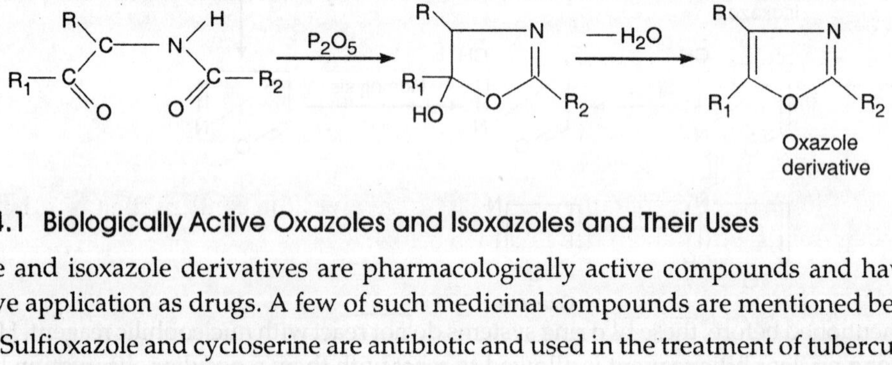

Oxazole derivative

21.10.4.1 Biologically Active Oxazoles and Isoxazoles and Their Uses

Oxazole and isoxazole derivatives are pharmacologically active compounds and have found extensive application as drugs. A few of such medicinal compounds are mentioned below:

i. Sulfioxazole and cycloserine are antibiotic and used in the treatment of tuberculosis and in urinary tract infections.

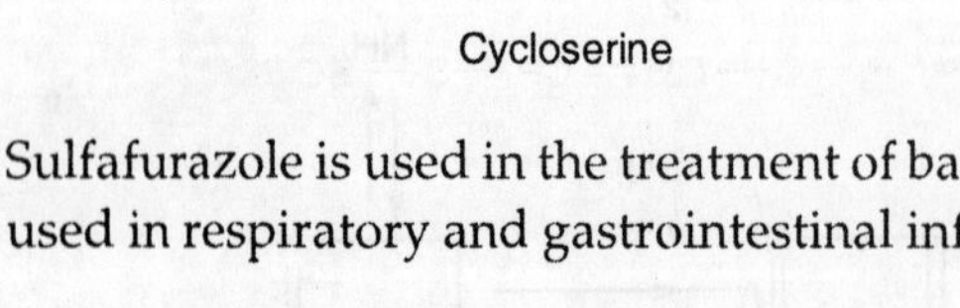

Cycloserine

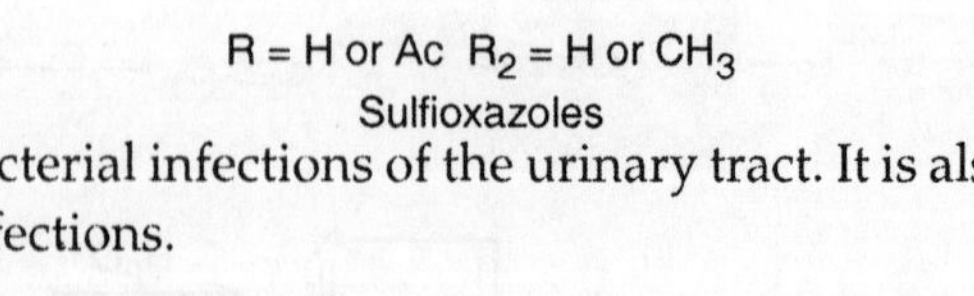

R = H or Ac R_2 = H or CH_3

Sulfioxazoles

ii. Sulfafurazole is used in the treatment of bacterial infections of the urinary tract. It is also used in respiratory and gastrointestinal infections.

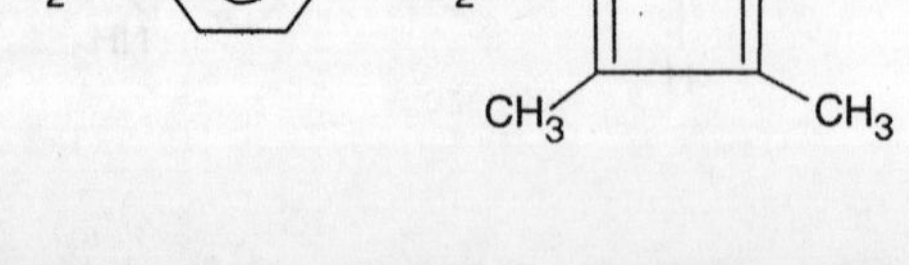

iii. Some oxazole derivatives having the following general structure have been found to have anti-viral, anti-bacterial, anti-inflammatory and analgesic properties.

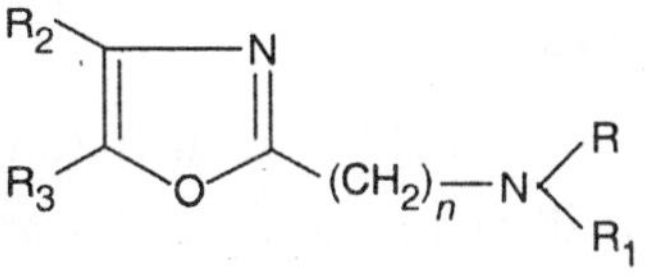

R, R_1, R_2 and R_3 are either H or any alkyl group.

iv. Cloxallin is an antibiotic of penicillin group and is very effective in the management and control of infections caused by Gram-positive bacteria, viz, streptococcal, staphylococcal, preumococcal infections.

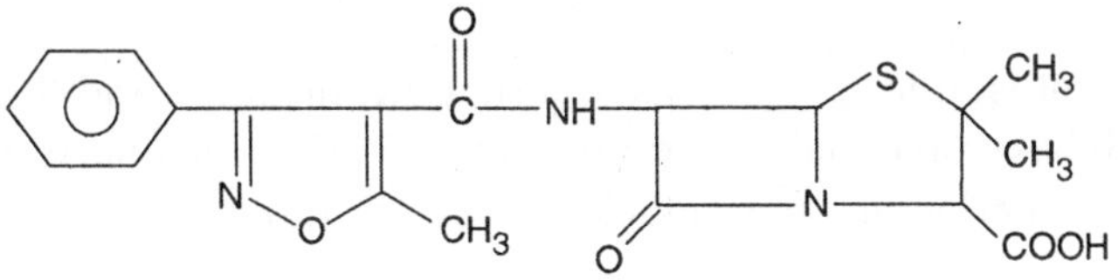

21.10.5 Thiazoles

As stated thiazoles are five-membered heterocyclic compounds having nitrogen and sulphur atoms in the ring. The relative positions may be either 1, 2 or 1, 3. When these two hetro atoms are present in 1, 3 positions such heterocyclic compounds are known as thiazoles while isothiazoles are those when these atoms are in 1, 2 positions. Structurally these two types of heterocycles may be represented as

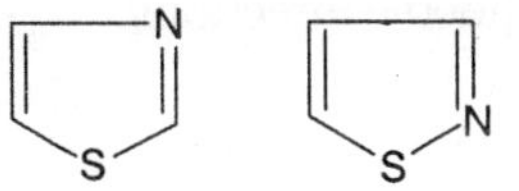

Thiazole Isothiazole

A general method of preparation of thiazoles involves the condensation of α-halogeno-carbonyl compounds with thioamides as shown below:

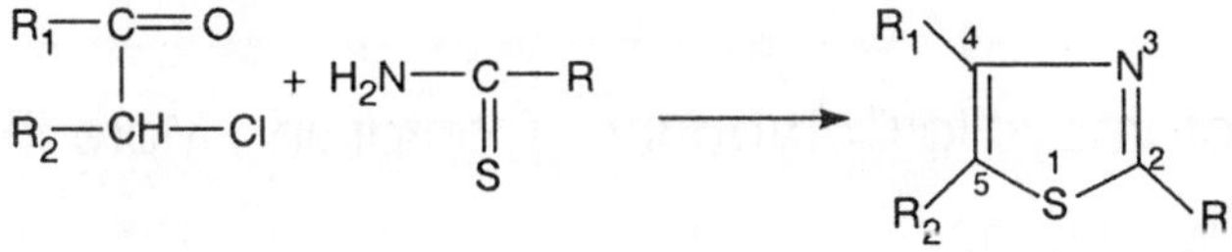

Thiazole derivative

Isothiazoles are normally prepared by the reaction between acetylene derivatives and sodium thiosulphate.

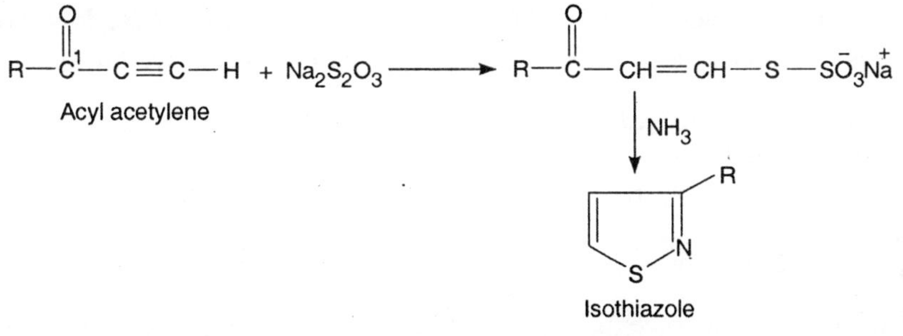

Isothiazole

Both these hetrocycles are aromatic in character and undergo usual electrophilic reactions. The substitution preferably takes place at the position-4 in isothiazole and at position-5 in thiazole.

21.10.5.1 Biologically Active Thiazoles and Their Uses

These hetrocyclic compounds are highly important in the field of medicine and agriculture.

i. Sulphasomizole is an antibiotic and has a medium duration of action against organisms.

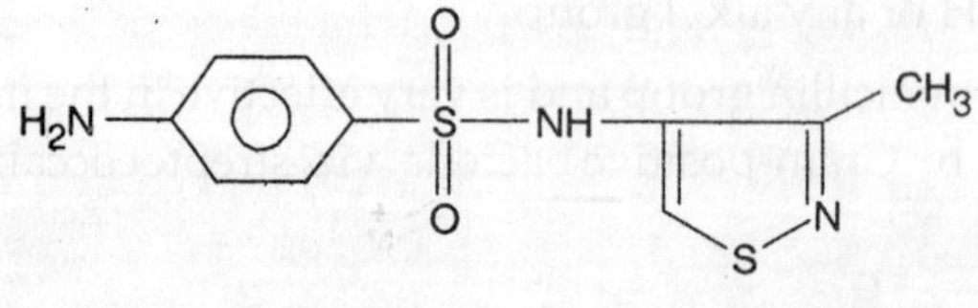

A large number of isothiazole analogs of histamine, histidine and thiamine have been prepared which have potential biological activity. Various isothiazole derivatives have been employed as herbicides and fungcides in agriculture.

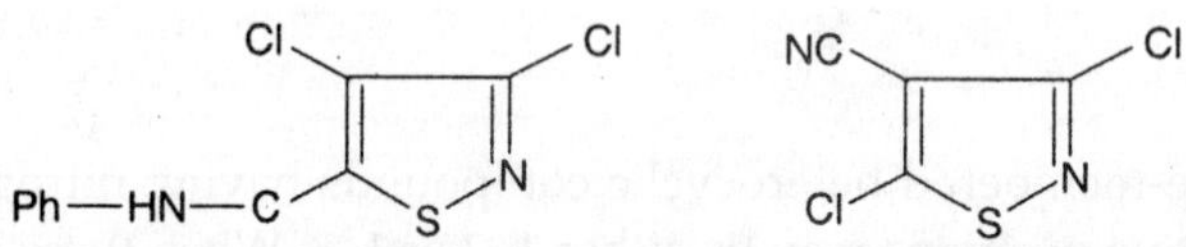

Thiazoles are structural component of peptide derived natural product, among them are antibiotics, siomycin, micrococin, antitumor antibiotics phleonycin and bleomycin. In addition, sulphathiazole is used for topical treatment of vaginal infection, and niridazole is used for the treatment of guinea-worm and amoebic infections.

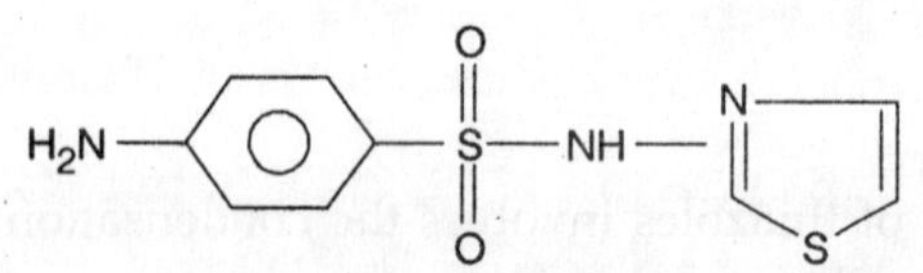

Sulphathiazole

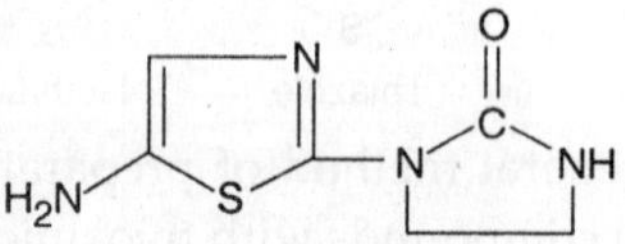

Niridazole

21.11 Five-membered Heterocyclic Compounds Containing More than Two Hetero Atoms

Triazole and tetrazoles are two important groups of five-membered heterocycles containing three and four nitrogen atoms in the ring. Structurally two isomeric triazoles are known while tetrazole exists in two tautomeric forms.

Out of two isomeric triazoles one is 1, 2, 3(1, 2, 5) isomer known as *osotriazole* and other is 1, 2, 4(1, 3, 4) isomer is termed as *triazole.* Each isomer once again exists in two tautomeric forms.

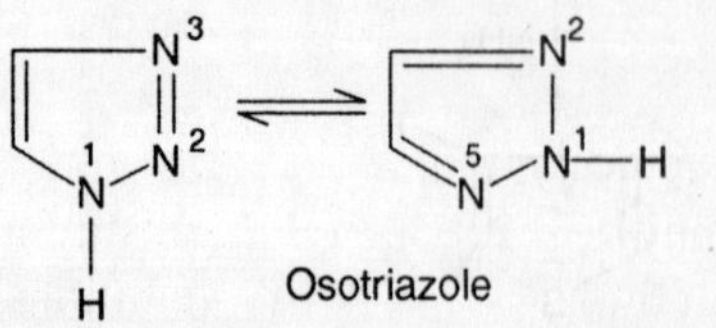

Osotriazole

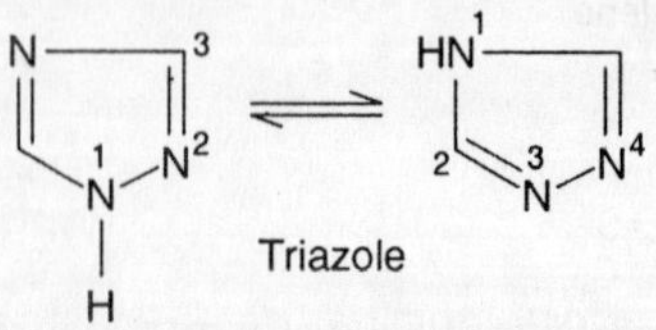

Triazole

Osotriazole is prepared by the reaction between hydrazoic acid and acetylene

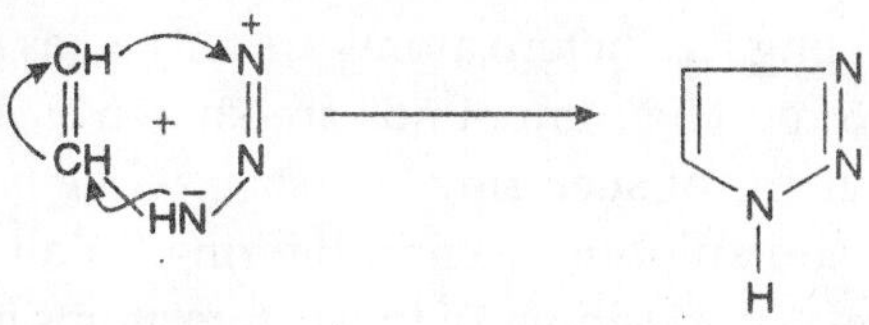

This reaction is 1, 3-dipolar addition reaction.

The derivatives of osotriazoles are conveniently prepared by the oxidation of osazone with potassium dichromate in presence of conc. H_2SO_4. Thus,

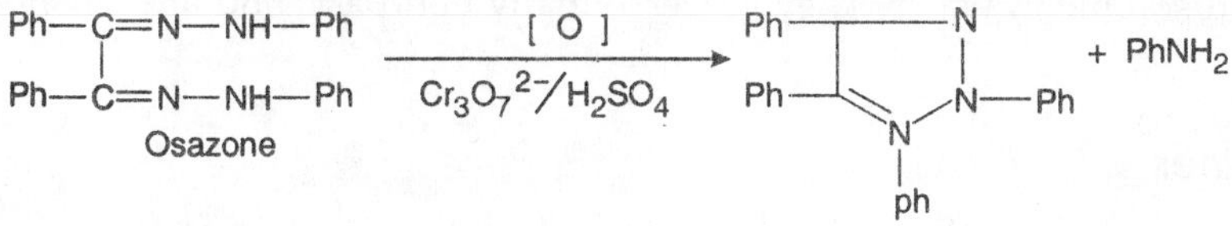

Triazoles are generally prepared by the reaction between hydrazides and amides under heating condition.

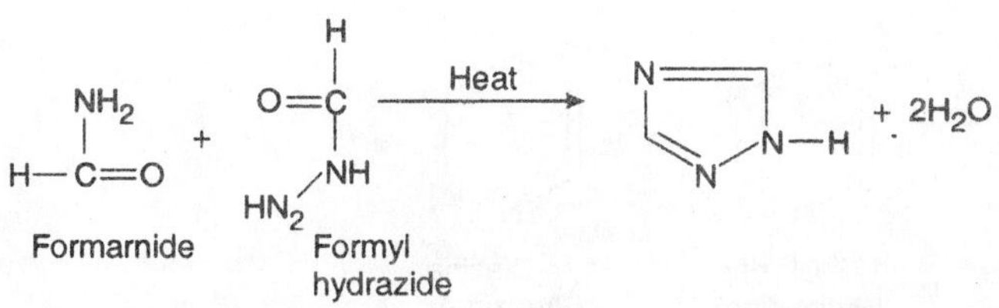

Both osotriazole and triazole are very stable compounds and weakly basic in nature.

Tetrazole contains four nitrigen and one carbon atoms in its nucleus. It exists in two tautomeric forms as shown below:

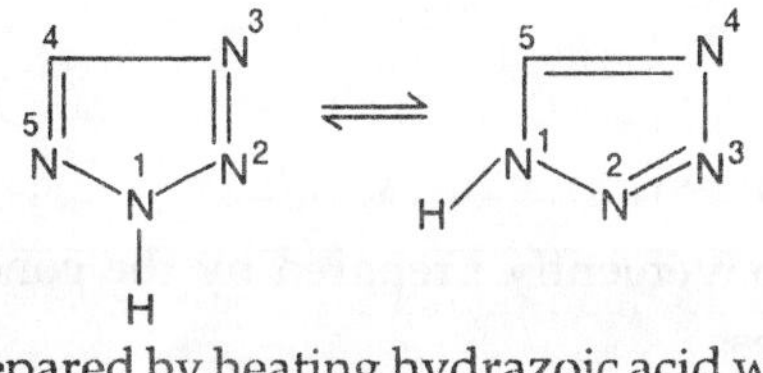

It is prepared by heating hydrazoic acid with hydrogen cyanide in benzene solution at 100°C. It is also a 1, 3-dipolar addition reaction.

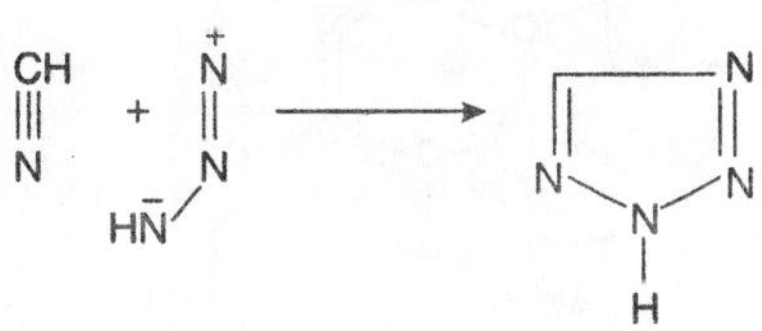

Tetrazole derivative may be prepared by the reaction between imidic chloride and sodiumazide

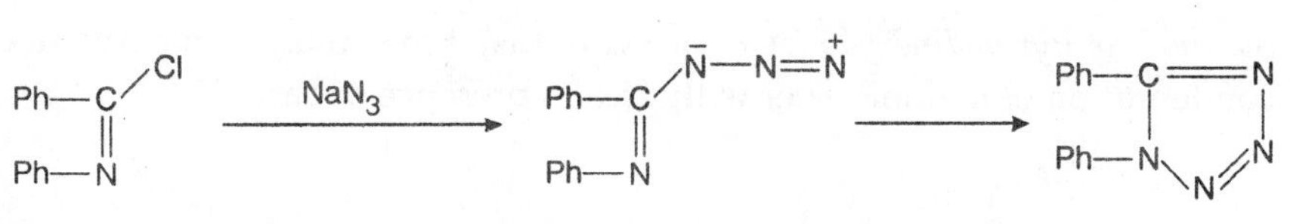

Tetrazole is colourless solid having no basic property.

21.12 Six-membered Heterocyclic Compounds Containing Two Hetero Atoms

Six-membered hetrocyclic compounds containing two hetero atoms are termed as *azines.* When both these hetero atoms are nitrogen, the heterocyclic compounds are known as *diazine.* But if nitrogen and oxygen atoms are present, the name of such ring is *oxazine* while *thiazine* is that heterocyclic system which contain nitrogen and sulphur atom in the ring. In all these *azines,* three isomeric forms are possible due to the relative positions of two hetero atoms in the ring i.e. 1, 2; 1, 3 and 1, 4. It may be mentioned that diazine are aromatic but oxazines and thiazines cannot be aromatic unless they carry positive charge.

Among all, these types of azines, diazines are most widely studied. Diazines are colourless compounds and soluble in water. They are, essentially non-basic and are much weaker bases than pyridine.

21.12.1 Diazines

As stated before diazines are those heterocycles in which two nitrogen atoms are present. Three isomeric diazines are possible depending upon the relative positions of two nitrigen atoms and all three are known.

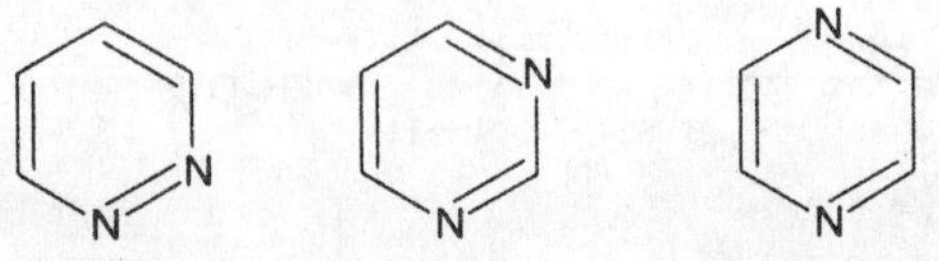

1, 2-Diazine (Pyridiazine) 1, 3-Diazine (Pyrimidine) 1, 4-Diazine (Pyrazine)

Among these three isomeric diazines, pyrimidines, are extensively studied because this ring system occurs in many compounds vital to living organism (present in nucleic acid).

21.12.1.1 Synthesis of Diazines

These diazines are commonly prepared by the following methods:

i. *Synthesis of Pyridiazine:* Pyridiazine is conveniently prepared by the condensation of hydrazine with unsaturated 1, 4-diketones.

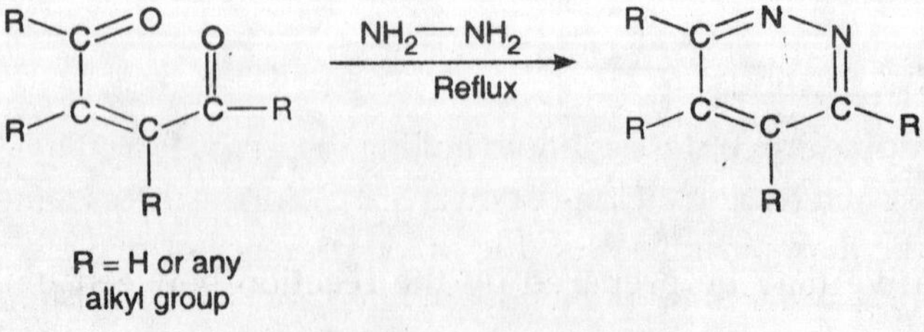

ii. *Synthesis of Pyrimidine:* Most simple synthesis of pyrimidine ring system consists of the condensation of malonic ester with urea in presence of base.

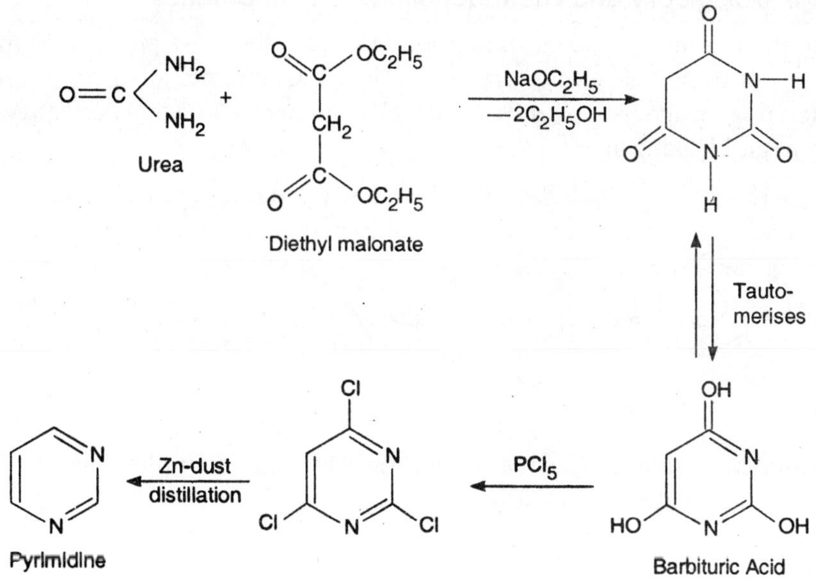

iii. *Synthesis of Pyrazine:* A very convenient and simple method of preparation of pyrazine ring system is the condensation between α-dicarbonyl compound and α-diamino compound.

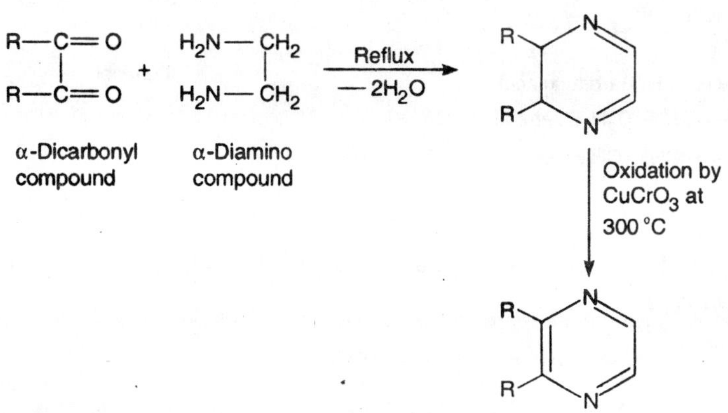

21.12.1.2 Properties of Diazines

Pyridiazine and pyrimidine are colourless liquid boiling respectively at 208 °C and 124 °C while pyrazine is a colourless solid having melting point at 55 °C. All the three isomers are aromatic in nature but less aromatic than pyridine. But due to the presence of two electron withdrawing nitrogen atoms these ring systems are highly deactivated and so electrophilic substitutions do not occur smoothly. However, as two nitrogen atoms are in meta relation in pyrimidine electron withdrawing effect is comparatively less in this ring system than other two isomers. For this reason and also due to the fact pyrimidine ring system is associated with living organisim, pyrimidine ring system has been studied to some extent.

21.12.1.3 Biologically and Pharmaceutically Active Diazines

All these three isomeric diazines are important from the view point of pharmacy and many derivatives of these hetrocycles are useful drugs. Cinnoline, a benzopyridiazine is used as antibacterial agent against *Escherichia Coli* while another pyridiazine derivative prizidilol acts as a β-adrenergic blocking agent.

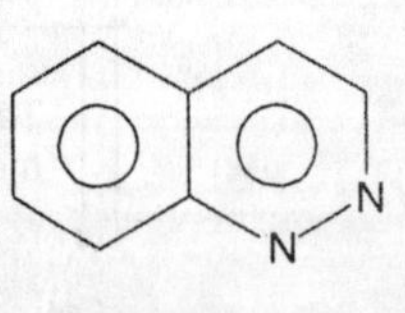

Cinnoline

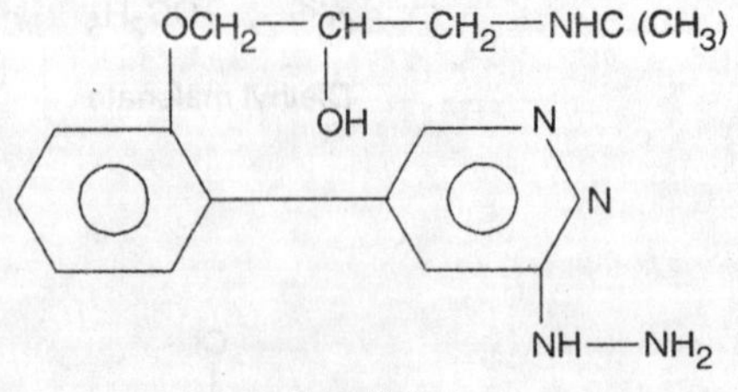

Prizidilol

Pyrimidine derivatives such as barbituric acid, veronal, luminol are very good hypnotics while pentothiol is used as an antiseptic

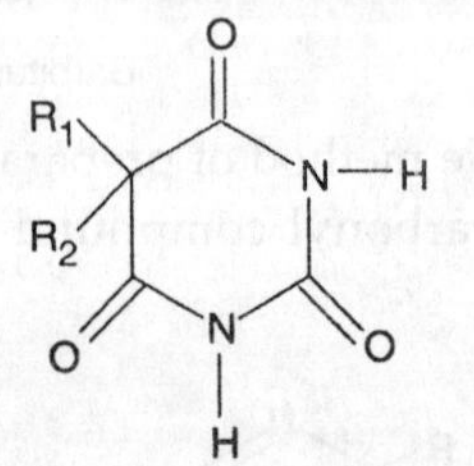

$R_1 = R_2 = H$, Barbituric acid

$R_1 = R_2 = —C_2H_5$, Veronal

$R_1 = —CH(CH_3)—CH_2—CH_2—CH_3$, Pentothiol

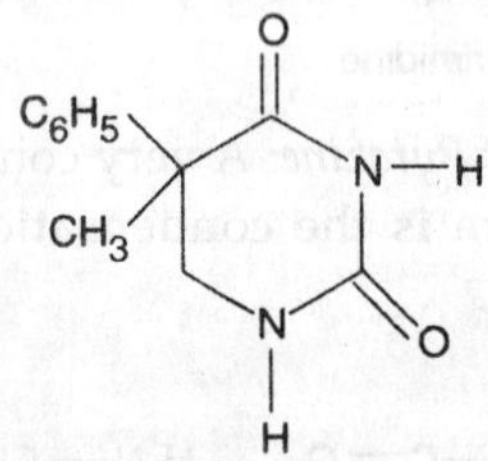

Luminol

Several sulpha drugs such as sulphadiazine sulphamerazine, and sulphamethazine are pyrimidine derivatives.

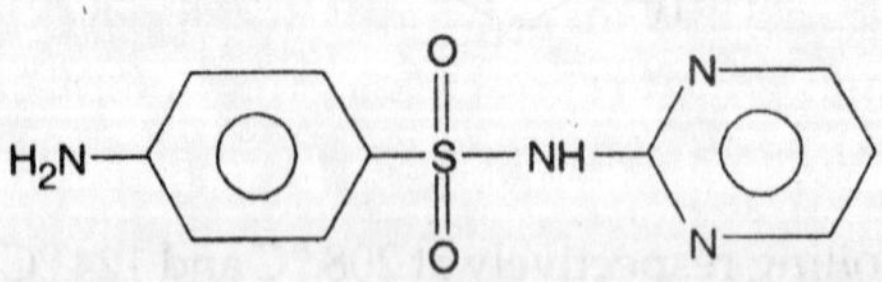

Sulphadiazine

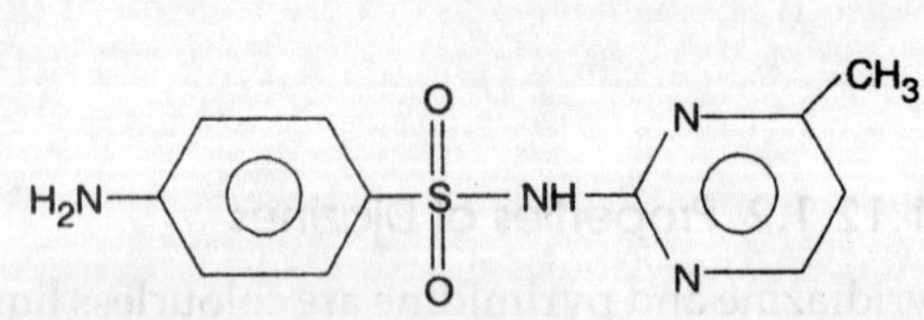

Sulphamerazine

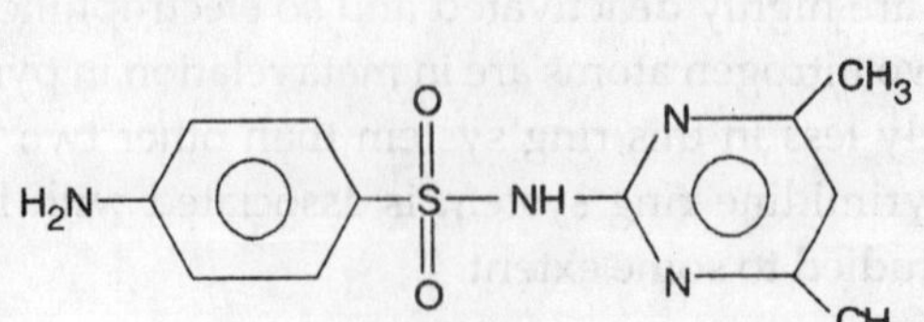

Sulphamethazine

Pyrimethamine is a substituted pyrimidine and is used as an antimalarial drug and **trimethoprim** which is another important compound having pyrimidine nucleus is an useful **antibacterial** agent and is used in the treatment of urinary and respiratory tract infections.

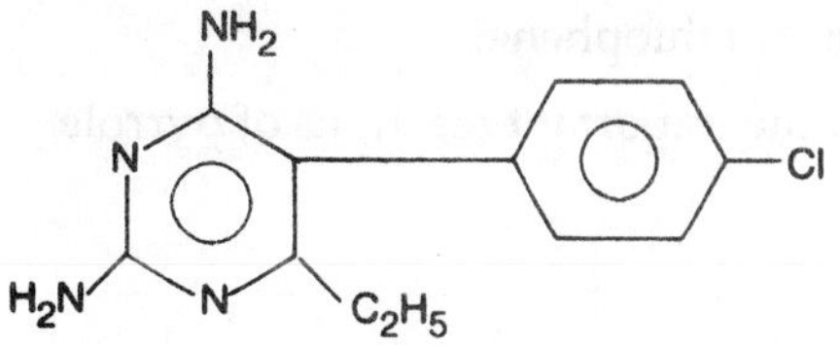

Pyrimethamine

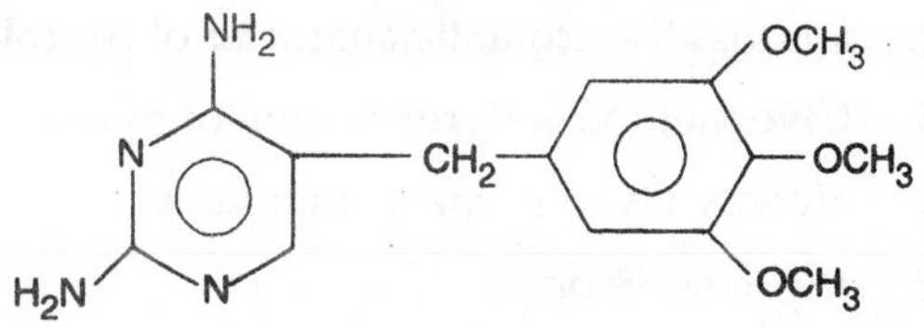

Trimethoprim

Three pyrimidines derivatives have biological significance. These are uracil, thymine and cytosine. Again adenine and guanine which are purine derivatives may be looked upon as pyrimidine derivatives. These purine derivatives are the building blocks of RNA and DNA.

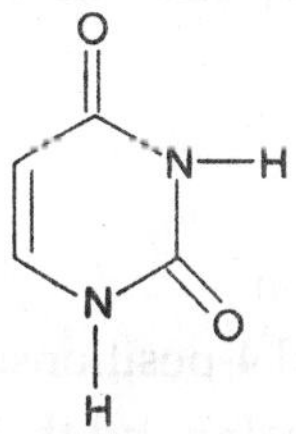

Uracil

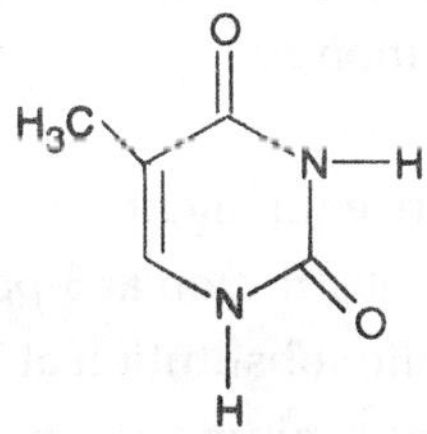

Thymine

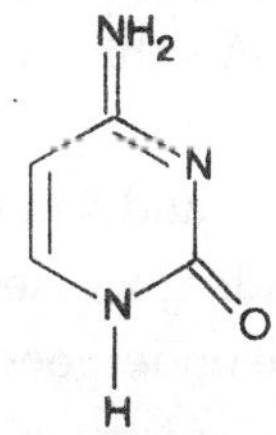

Cytosine

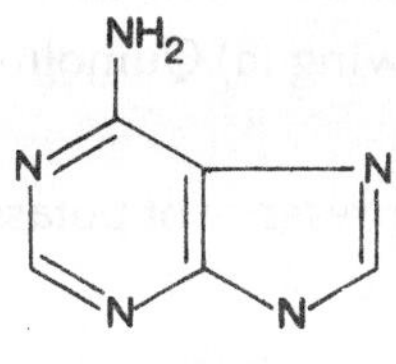

Adenine

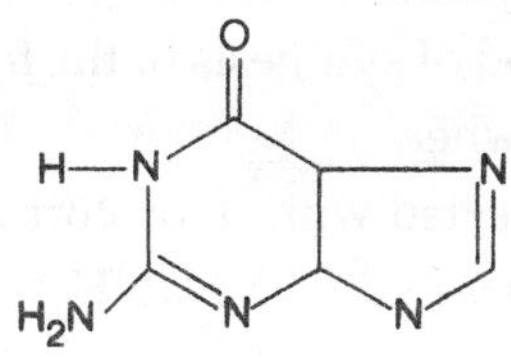

Guanine

Pyrazine derivatives have also find useful application as medicine. Diethyl carbamazine citrate is used in the treatment of filariasis particularly when caused by *Wuchereria bancrofti.* or *Loa loa*. It is specially used in the treatment of tropical eosinophila. Piperizine hydrate has been found to be very effective against roundworms (Ascaris) and threadworms. Rifampin (Rifadin) is a semisynthetic antibiotic obtained from rifamycin which represents a group of chemically related antibiotics obtained from *Streptomyces mediterrani.* Rifampin is a complex molecule containing naphthalene, furan, pyrazine and other nuclei. It has been found to be highly effective against *Mycobacterium tuberculosis* and is of great value in patients with drug resistant infection.

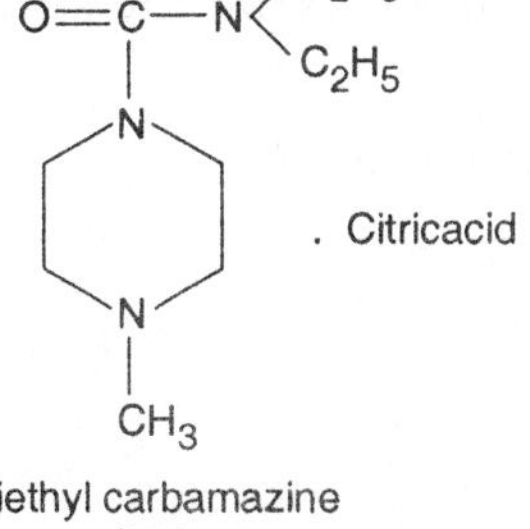

Diethyl carbamazine citrate

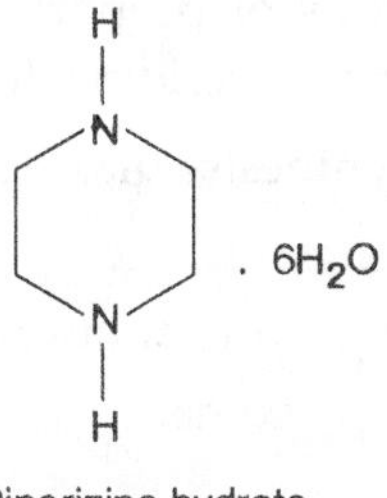

Piperizine hydrate

Model Questions

1. What are heterocyclic compounds? Give the classification and nomenclature of heterocyclic compounds.
2. Discuss the aromatic character of pyrrole, furan and thiophene.
3. Give methods of preparation of pyrrole. Give some important reactions of pyrrole.
4. How will you prepare thiophene?
5. Write notes on:
   (a) Skraup synthesis of quinoline
   (b) Fischer-Indole synthesis
   (c) Uses of heterocyclic compounds containing one hetero-atom.
6. Explan:
   (a) Position of 2 of pyrrole is more active towards electrophilic substituion while such reaction smoothly occurs at position 3.
   (b) Pyridine is more basic than pyrrole.
   (c) Positions -3 and 5 in pyrazole are equivalent
   (d) Indole undergoes electrophilic substitution at 3-position.
   (e) Quinoline undergoes nucleophilic substitution at 2 and 4-positions.
7. Discuss the chemistry of pyrazine, pyrimidine and pyridiazine and their uses.
8. How will you synthesise imidazole? What are are its uses?
9. Give one method of synthesis of the following (a) Quinoline (b) Isoquinoline (c) Diazine.
10. What happens when:
    (a) Pyrrole is treated with chloroform in presence of potassium hydroxide.
    (b) Pyridine is treated with $NaNH_2$.
11. How would you convert:
    (a) Pyrrole to 3-chloropyridine.
    (b) Pyridine to dipyridyl.
12. Give structures and uses of the followings:
    (a) Nitrofurazone (b) Piperizine
    (c) Chloroquine (d) Benzehexol
    (e) Primaquine (f) Isoniazid
    (g) Ranitidine (h) Cephalothin
    (i) Nitrofurazone.
13. Discuss the methods of preparation of acridines. Write the structures and uses of medicinally important aceridine derivatives.
14. How would you synthesise diazines? What are the uses?
15. Discuss the followings:
    (a) Aromaticity of pyrrole, furan and thiophene.
    (b) Aromaticity of pyridine.
    (c) Xanthones.

CHAPTER TWENTY-TWO

Drugs

INTRODUCTION

The word *'drug'* has been derived from the French word *drogue* which means a dry herb. In a general sense, a drug may be defined as a substance usually chemical compound used in the diagnosis, mitigation, treatment, cure or prevention of disease in man or other animals. According to WHO, a drug is any substance or product which is used or intended to be used to modify or explore physiological systems or pathological states for the benefit of the recipient.

An ideal drug should fulfil the following requirements.

i. When administered to the patient its action should be localised at the desired site.

ii. It should act on the system safely and efficiently.

iii. It should have least side effects.

iv. It should not affect physiological process.

v. The cells should acquire minimum resistance or tolerance.

- **Structure Activity Relationship (SAR) of Drugs**

It is known that activity of a drug is intimately associated with its structure. The various functional groups present in the drug molecule are responsible for the drug-receptor interaction. Thus, drugs with amino or hydroxyl functions normally bind with receptor through hydrogen bond. It has further been observed that any change in the functional groups in a drug can change the activity and toxicity significantly and in fact this is the basis of any structure-activity-relationship (SAR) analysis of the drug molecules. The SAR study involves pharmacological response, binding, toxicity or any other quantifiable parameters. In this study the essential structural features of the drug are identified. These essential structural features or functional groups are termed as *pharmacophores.* By changing the pharmacophores of any drug analogues are prepared to improve the pharmacological activity and to reduce toxicity. In this connection it may be mentioned that toxicity is an important factor in determining the activity of drugs. Toxicity prevents many compounds from their use as medicines. A large number of drugs have been withdrawn from the market for their toxicities. The drug industries expend considerable time and effort to avoid or minimise toxic effects by characterising and altering the groups responsible for toxicity.

It may be mentioned that functional groups have also an important role in determining the stability of the drug. Certain functional groups in drug molecules are suscesptible to chemical degradation. Thus, ester group when present in a drug can undergo smooth hydrolysis as for example aspirin which is hydrolysed to sabcylic acid. Again, insulin, a protein contains amide linkage and so unstable in acid medium and hence unsuitable for oral administration.

Another important point which needs mention is that the stereoisomeric nature of the drug has significant role in determining the activity. It has been observed that out of several enantiomeric forms of a particular drug only one may be active and others are inactive and sometimes may be fatal.

22.1 Sources of Drugs

The most important sources of drugs are:

i. Chemical synthesis
ii. Micro-organisms
iii. Minerals
iv. Plants
v. Animals.

22.2 Classification of Drugs

Drugs may be calssified in a various ways. However, classification on the basis of combination of both therapeutic actions and chemical structures is most popular. Some of the important classes of drugs are as enlisted below:

1. Hypnotics and Sedatives
2. Tranquillizers
3. Central Nervous Systems Stimulants
4. Cholinergic and Anticholinergic Agents
5. Adrenergic Stimulants and Blocking Agents
6. Histamine and Antihistamine Agents
7. Anaesthetics
8. Cardiovascular Agents
9. Haematological Agents (Coagulants and Anticoagulants)
10. Diuretics
11. Organometallic Therapeutic Agents
12. Antipyretic and Analgesic Drugs
13. Anthelmintics
14. Antimalarial Drugs
15. Antiprotozoal Agents
16. Antiseptics and Disinfectants

17. Antifungal Agents
18. Sulphonamides
19. Steroid Drugs
20. Antibiotics
21. Thyroid and Antithyroid Drugs
22. Antiparkinsonism Drugs
23. Muscle Relaxants
24. Antineoplastic Drugs
25. Expectorants and Antitussives
26. Anticonvulsant (Antileprosy Drugs).
27. Antitubercular Drugs
28. Antiviral Agents
29. Antifilarial Agents
30. Vitamins
31. Miscellaneous Drugs.

A few of the above classified drugs are discussed below with special reference to their synthesis, uses, structure-activity relation and mode of action.

22.2.1 Hypnotics and Sedatives

Hypnotics are central nervous system depressants that induce sleep to reduce emotional tension and restlessness while *sedatives* although are central nervous system depressants that reduce restlessness and emotional tension but do not produce sleep. Both hypnotic and sedative properties usually reside in the same drug—a large dose of the drug may act as hypnotic whereas a small dose of the same drug acts as a sedative. It may be mentioned that hypnotics when used in very large doses may produce anaesthesia, poisoning and even death in some cases. These progressive effects may be depicted as below:

$$\text{Sedation} \rightleftharpoons \text{Hypnosis} \rightleftharpoons \text{Anaesthesia} \rightleftharpoons \text{Coma} \longrightarrow \text{Death.}$$

It is pertinent to mention here that in a few cases a particular compound exerts only the specific effect, as for examples, potassium bromide acts only as a very good sedative, thiopentone sodium is a powerful hypnotic without having any sedative action.

22.2.1.1 Classification of Hypnotics and Sedatives

Hypnotics and sedatives are broadly classified into two categories; viz.

(i) Barbiturates,

(ii) Non-barbiturates.

22.2.1.2 Barbiturates

Barbiturates are cyclic *ureides* and are generally formed by the action of a dicarboxylic acid or its salt with urea in presence of sodium ethoxide. Thus,

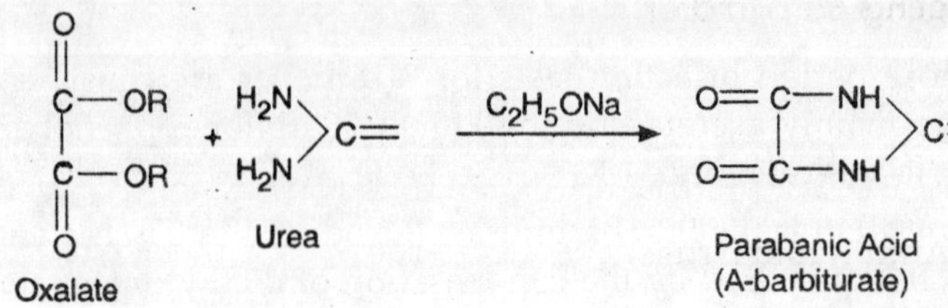

In general, barbiturates exert significant depressant action on the cerebrospinal axis. The degrees of depression, sedation, hypnosis or anaesthesia exclusively depend on the nature of barbiturate, its dose and route of administration.

22.2.1.2.1 Classification of Barbiturates

Barbiturates are classified arbitrarily on the basis of the duration of their clinical effects. A large number of barbiturates are in use, the most commonly used such barbiturates are tabulated below:

Commonly used Barbiturates

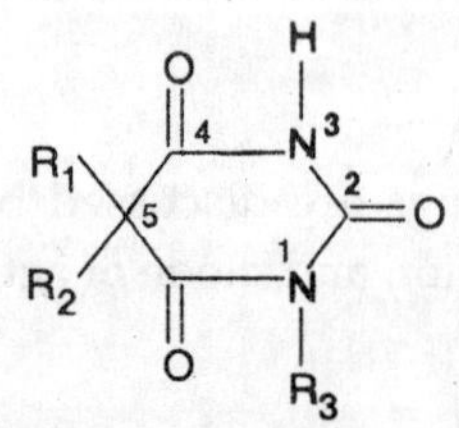

Sl. No.	Name of the Drug	Chemical Name (— barbituric acid)	Substitution			Duration of Action (Hour)
			R_1	R_2	R_3	
1.	Barbitone (Veronal)	5, 5-Diethyl —	C_2H_5—	C_2H_5	H	4-12
2.	Phenobarbitone	5-Ethyl-5-phenyl —	C_2H_5—	C_6H_5	H	4-12
3.	Methylpheno-barbitone	5-Ethyl-l-methyl-5 -phenyl —	C_2H_5—	C_6H_5	CH_3	1-4
4.	Allobarbital (Dial)	5, 5-Diallyl —	CH_2= CH — CH_2—	CH_2= CH — CH_2—		2-8
5.	Amobarbital (Amytal)	5-Ethyl-5-isopentyl—	C_2H_5	$(CH_3)_2$ — CH— CH_2— CH_2—		2-6
6.	Butobarbitone (Soneryl)	5-Ethyl-5-*n*-butly—	C_2H_5	CH_3— CH_2— CH_2— CH_2		2-6
7.	Hexobarbitone (Evipal)	5-Δ-Cyclihexenyl— 5-methyl-l-methyl—	CH_3	$(CH_2)_4$ — CH = C — (ring)	CH_3	
8.	Pentobarbitone (Nembutal)	5-Ethyl-5(l-methyl— butyl)—	C_2H_5	CH_3— $(CH_2)_2$ — CH — (with CH_3 branch)		2-4
9.	Thiopentone (Pentothal)	5-Ethyl-5-(l-methyl butly)-2-thio—	C_2H_5	CH_3— $(CH_2)_2$ — CH — CH_3	2-S	1-4

22.2.1.2.1.1 Long-Acting Barbiturates

The barbiturates whose period of action lasts for 8-16 hours are considered as long acting barbiturates. They are mainly excreted by the kidney. Barbitone, phenobarbital and methyl phenobarbital belong to this category.

(a) *Barbitone (Veronal):* It is the first barbiturate introduced by Fischer and Merling in 1903 into therapy. It is prepared by the condensation of diethyl malonate with urea in the presence of sodium ethoxide.

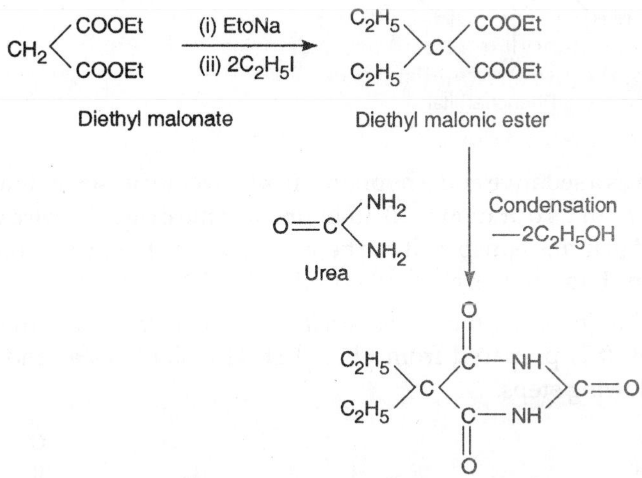

Barbitone (Veronal)

It is a powerful hypnotic and causes natural and dreamless sleep within 15-30 minutes after administration and lasts for 8-12 hours. However, its therapeutic index is low, i.e., a small dose can be poisonous. It is generally used in the treatment of epileptic seizure. Its dose is 0.3 to 0.6 g. It is also known as *barbital*.

(b) *Phenobarbital or Phenobarbitone (Luminal):* It is synthesised by the condensation of benzyl cyanide with ethyl carbamate followed by hydrolysis and ethylation when ethyl phenyl malonate is formed. This compound on treatment with sodium followed by ethyl chloride yields corresponding C-ethyl derivative. This product on condensation with urea furnishes phenobarbital.

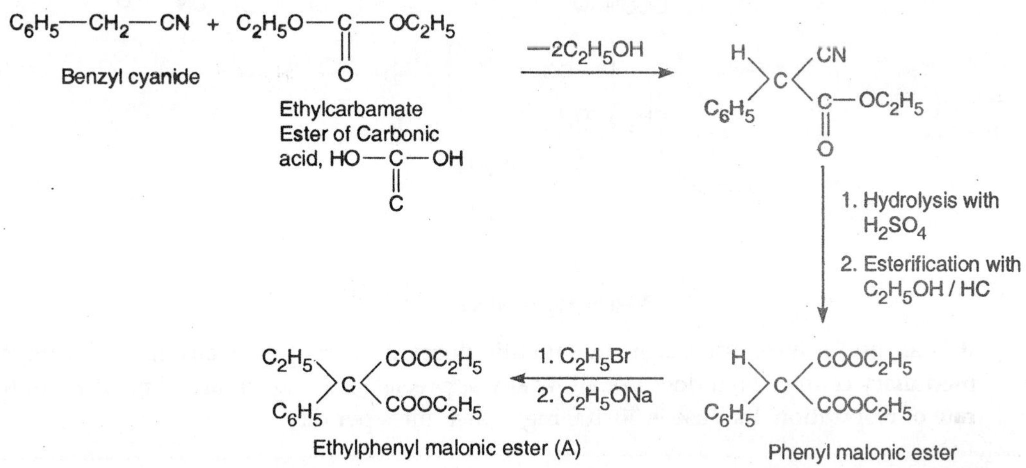

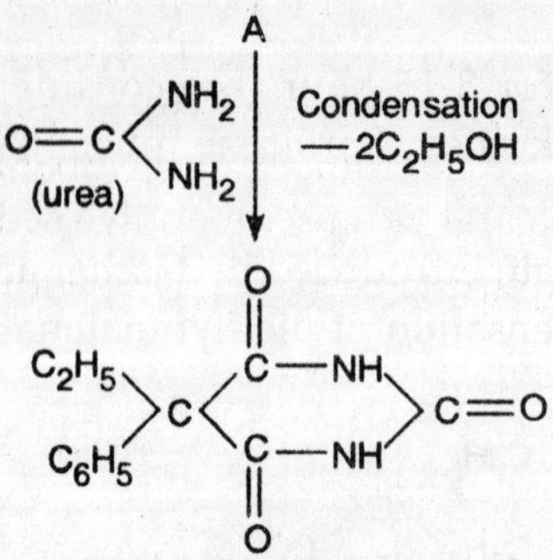

Phenobarbital

It is used both as a sedative and a hypnotic. It is slower in on-set of its action and requires about the hour but its duration is 10-16-hours. It is the drug of choice in the treatment of grandmal and petitmal epilepsy. It can be safely used for the treatment of cases of general convulsions in children. It is generally used in 30-129 mg dose.

(c) *Methyl Phenobarbital or Methyl Phenobarbitone (Prominal):* It is N-methyl derivative of phenobarbital. It is prepared from phenyl ethyl malonic ester and dicyandimide by involving following steps.

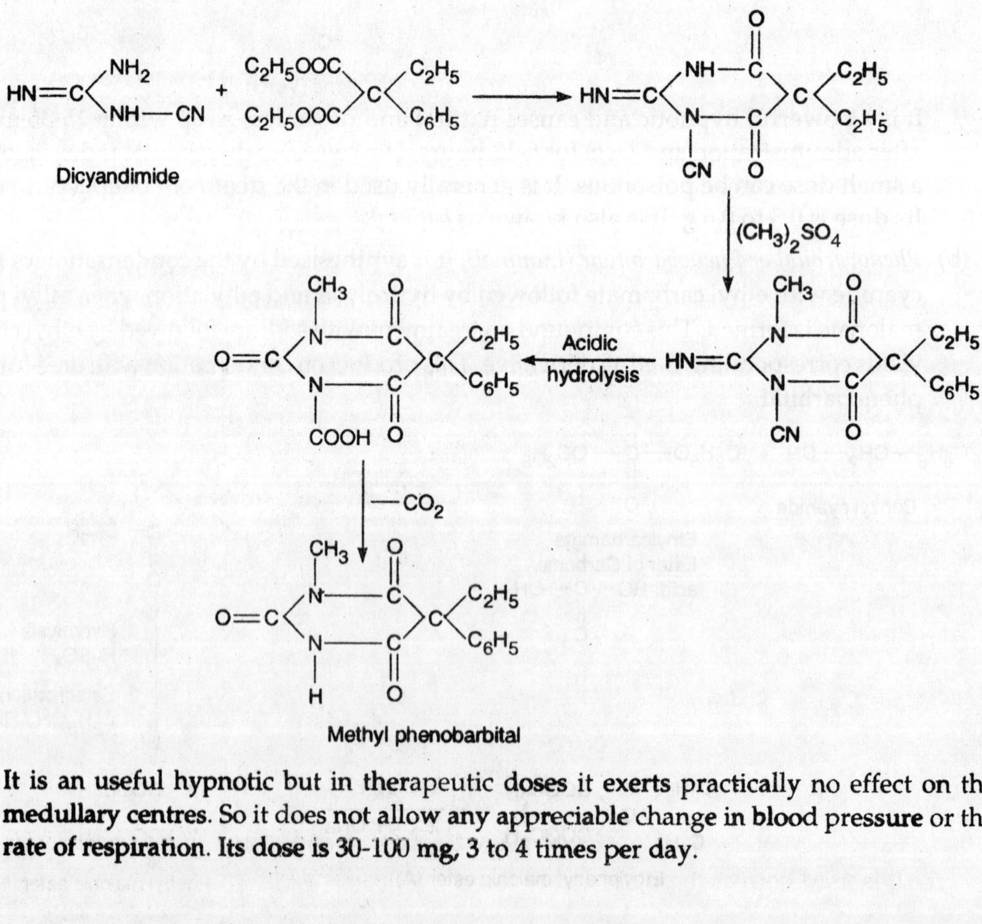

Methyl phenobarbital

It is an useful hypnotic but in therapeutic doses it exerts practically no effect on the medullary centres. So it does not allow any appreciable change in blood pressure or the rate of respiration. Its dose is 30-100 mg, 3 to 4 times per day.

22.2.1.2.1.2 Moderately-Acting Barbiturates

The on-set action of this type of barbiturate is 30 minutes and their hypnotic action lasts for 2-6 hours. Most of them are degraded first in the liver and subsequently excreted by kidney. Allobarbitone, butobarbitone and amobarbital are the important members of this category of barbiturate. They are generally used in insomnia and as a pre-operative sedative.

(a) *Allobarbitone (Dial):* It is obtained by condensing barbituric acid with allylbromide in the presence If sodium ethoxide.

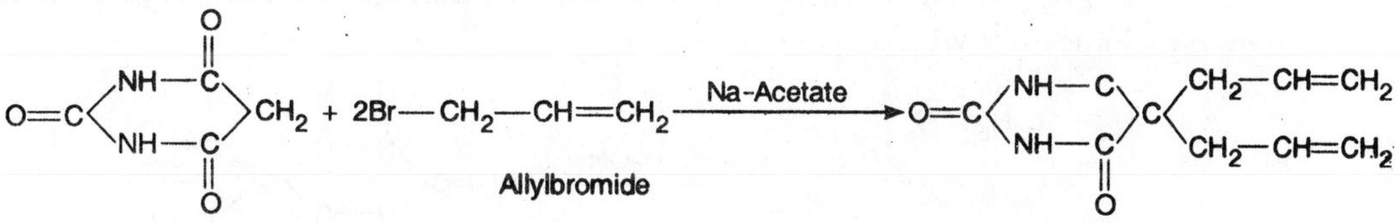

Barbituric acid Dial

It can be used both as sedative and hypnotic. Its dose is 30 mg, 3 to 4 times a day as a sedative and as a hypnotic 100 to 200 mg at night.

(b) *Butobarbitone:* It is synthesised by the reaction between urea and diethyl butylethyl malonate in presence of sodium ethoxide.

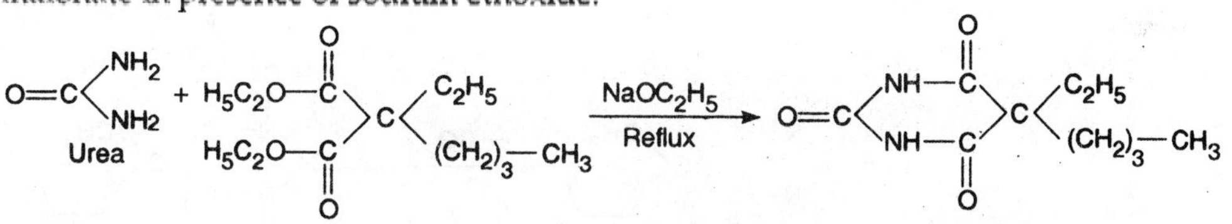

Butobarbitone

It is used both as hypnotic and sedative. It is used in 30-120 mg dose as a sedative and 100-200 mg at night as hypnotic.

(c) *Amobarbitone (Amytal):* It is prepared through following steps.

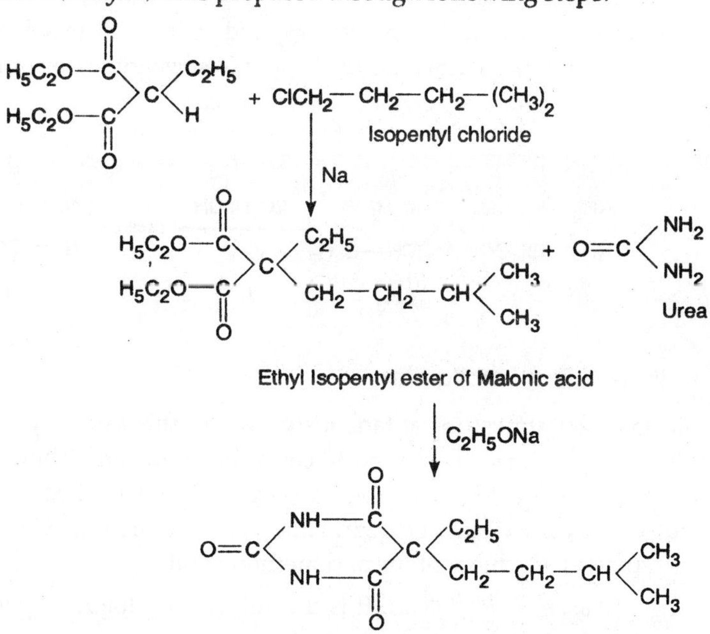

Amobarbitone (Amytal)

It is used both as hypnotic and sedative. Its dose is 300 mg.

22.2.1.2.1.3 Short-Acting Barbiturates

Those barbiturates have been considered as short-acting whose on-set of action falls within 15-20 minutes and their action last for 1-2 hours. These barburates are generally metabolised in the liver and are specially used in the treatment of insomnia and pre-operative medication. Hexabarbital and pentobarbital sodium are the most commonly used barbiturates of this group.

(a) *Hexobarbital or Hexobarbitone (Evipan):* It is prepared by the condensation of cyclohexenyl methyl malonic ester with dicyandimide.

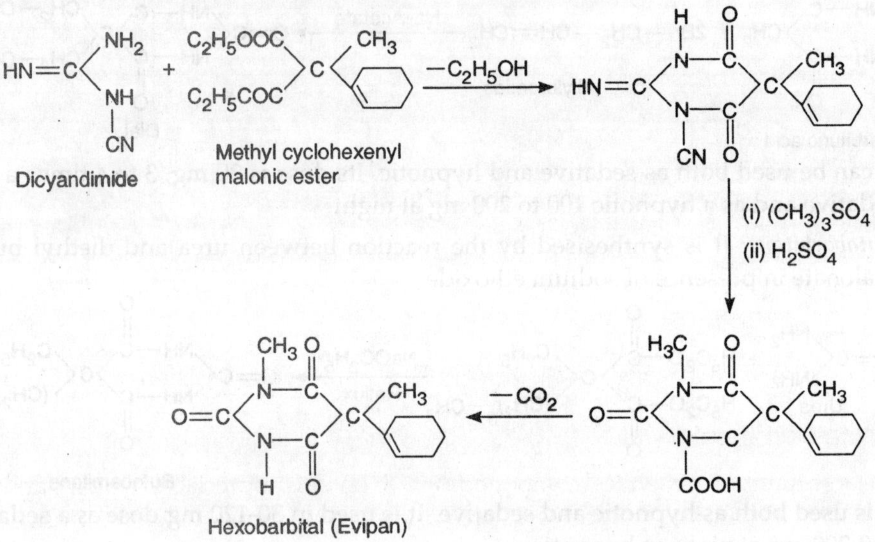

It is generally applied as hypnotic in doses of 250 to 500 mg orally for an adult patient.

(b) *Pentobarbitone or Pentobarbital:* It is mostly applied as its sodium salt and is used in the treatment of insomnia, as a basal anaesthetic and in strychnine poisoning. It is prepared by condensing ethyl-(I-methyl)-butyl ester with urea.

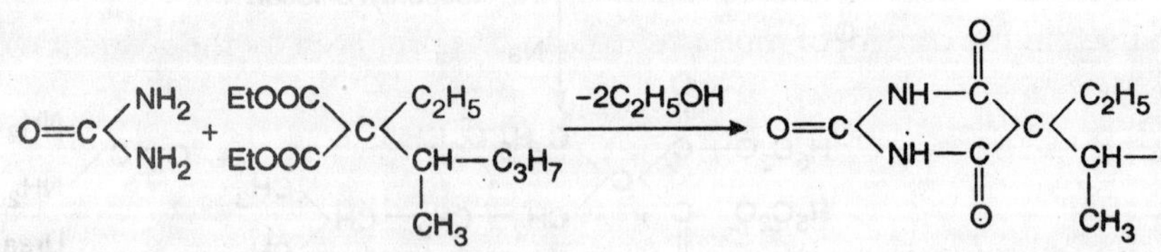

22.2.1.2.1.4 Ultra-Short-Acting Barbiturates

This type of barbiturates act almost instantaneously. Due to this property these are generally employed to produce general anaesthesia and to control convulsions. They may be employed alone or in conjunction with inhalation anaesthesia. They are first deposited in adipose but finally in the liver and kidney for their metabolic degredation and elimination. Common examples of this category of barbiturates are thiopentone and methohexital.

(a) *Thiopentone or Thiopental (Pentothal):* It is the sulphur analogue of pentobarbitone. It is prepared as indicated:

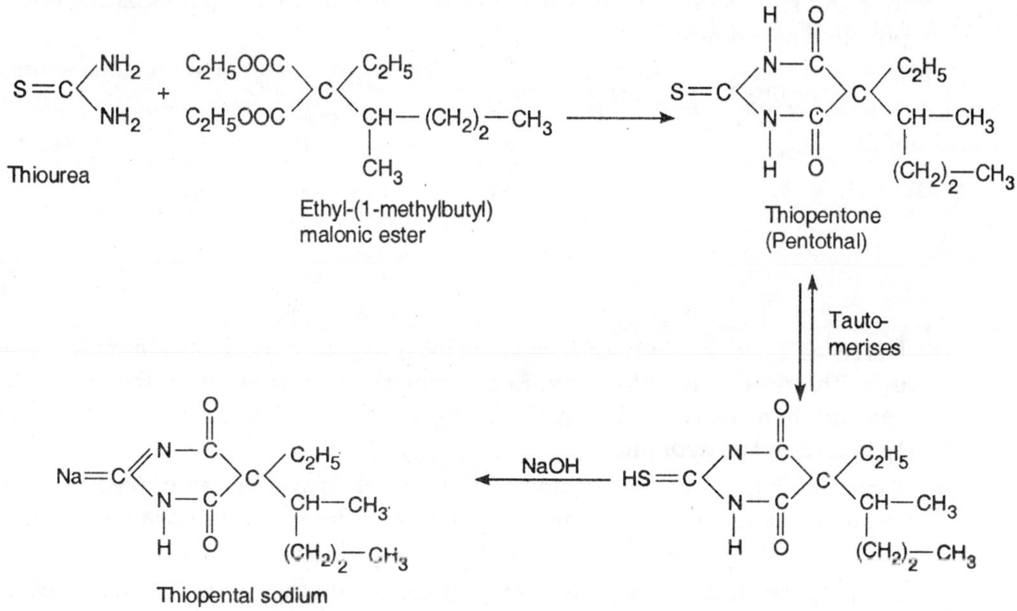

It is used as its sodium salt and is employed as intravenous injection of 100-150 mg doses.

22.2.1.3 Non-barbiturates

There are a large number of chemical compounds which possess appreciable hypnotic and sedative action but do not barbiturate structures. Like barbiturates they are also habit-forming of varied degrees. Structurally they belong to different types of compounds. A few of selected drugs of this category are discussed below:

(a) *Alcohols:* (i) Ethanol has played a prominent role as a sedative and hypnotic for centuries. But due to different problems associated with the use of alcohols such as the development of *Chronic alcoholism* on continued use, the use of other drugs have been recommended. However, a few alcohol derivatives like (i) trichloroethanol, CCl_3CH_2OH, m.p. 180 °C is used in the control of motion sickness. It is prepared by the reduction of chloral.

$$\underset{\text{Chloral}}{CCl_3{-}CHO} + 2H \xrightarrow{\text{Al-ethylate}} \underset{\text{Trichloro ethanol}}{CCl_3CHO}$$

(ii) Tribromoethanol, $CBr_3 — CH_2OH$, m.p. 80 °C has a very favourable hypnotic action as it induces sleep with a rapid on-set and lasts for 5 hours. A clear advantage over barbiturate is that it induces no addiction. It is prepared by the reduction of bromal as shown below:

$$\underset{\text{Bromal}}{CBr_3{-}CHO} + 2H \xrightarrow{\text{Al-ethylate}} \underset{\text{Tribromoethanol}}{CBr_3{-}CH_2OH}$$

It is also used as a general anaesthetic.

(b) *Aldehydes:* Members of this group are among the first of organic hypnotics.

i. *Chloral hydrate:* It was introduced in 1869 in the mistaken belief that it would be converted to anaesthetic chloroform in the body. However, it is reduced in the body to trichloro ethanol which is actually responsible for its depressant action. It is prepared as follows:

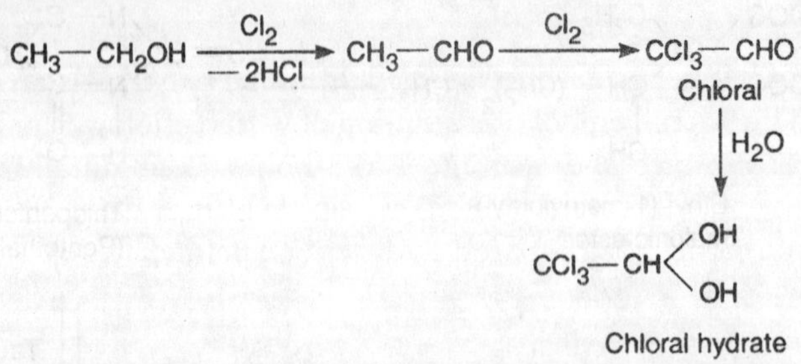

It is reliable and safe hypnotic, useful in inducing sleep where insomnia is not due to *pain*. The toxicity of chloral hydrate is remarkably increased by the simultaneous consumption of alcohol. Its dose is 250 mg, 3 times per day as sedative and 500 mg to 1g before bed as hypnotic.

ii. *Paraldehyde:* It is one of the oldest hypnotics. It is usually employed in delirium tremens, status epilepticus and in patients undergoing withdrawal therapy for alcohalism. A portion of the drug is excreted through the lungs.

It is prepared from acetaldehyde by polymerisation in presence of an acid catalyst.

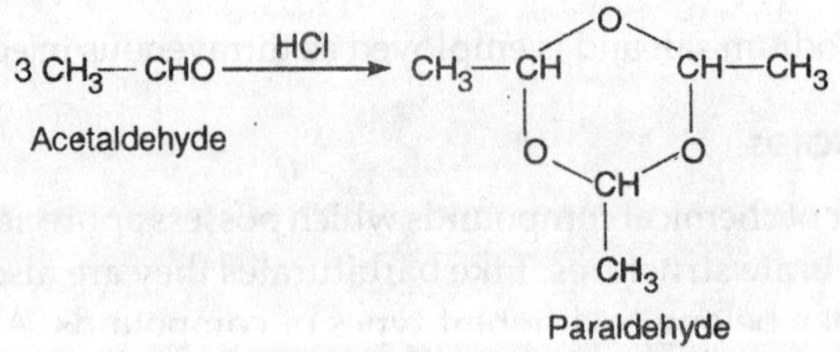

Its dose is 5 to 10 ml orally as sedative and 10-30 ml orally as hypnotic for adult patients.

(c) *Heterocycles:* An appreciable number of heterocycles have been found to possess significant hypnotic and sedative activity and have gained recognition in the therapeutic field. The most important member of this group is glutethimide. It is prepared by the Michael condensation of phenyl ethyl acetonitrile with acrylonitrile followed by saponification. After ring closure glutethimide is obtained.

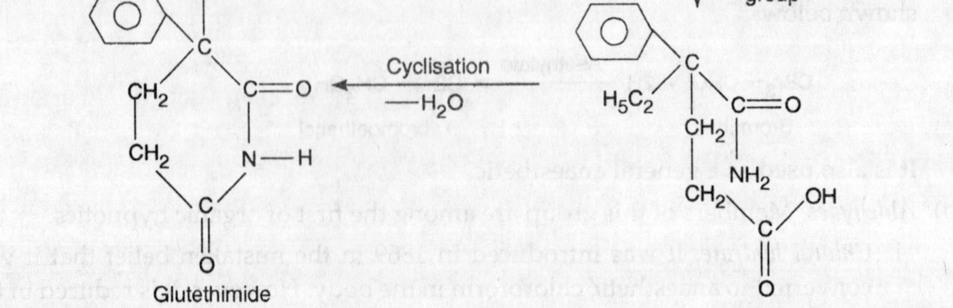

It is safely used for inducing sleep in all types of insomnia without causing depression of respiration. Its hypnotic action is parallel to moderately acting barbiturates. It is used in 250-500 mg doses.

Another member of heterocycle is *methyprylon* or *methyprylone*..It is an useful hypnotic agent employed in the management of insominia of varied etiology. It may induce sleep within a span of 45 minutes and lasts for 5 to 8 hours. Like glutethimide it is also a piperidine derivative. Its doses are 125-250 mg up to 3 times daily as sedative and 500 mg to 1g daily as hypnotic. It is prepared as described below:

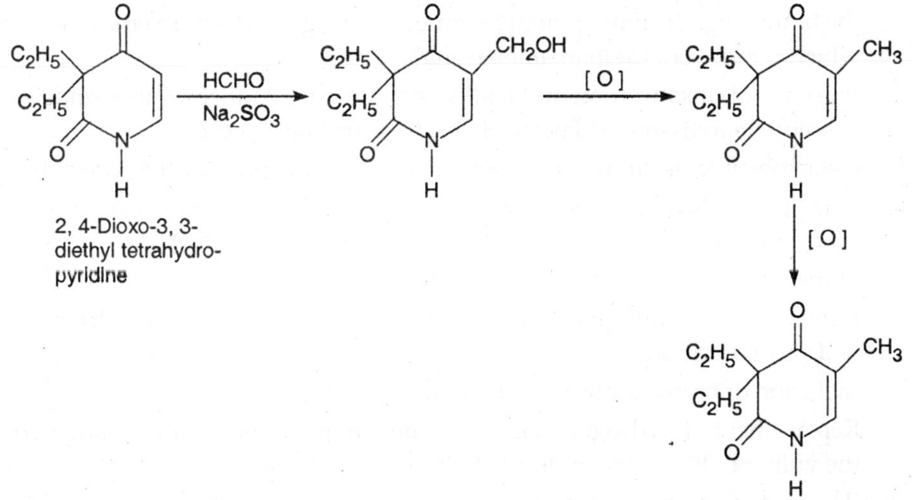

2, 4-Dioxo-3, 3-diethyl tetrahydropyridine

3, 3-Diethyl-5-methyl-2; 4-piperidine dione (Methyprylon)

(d) *Alkyl Substituted Ureas:* Alkyl substituted ureas are somewhat stronger in sedative action than amides. In the state of anxiety and insomnia this class of drugs are still preferred. Carbromal or diethylbromo acetyl urea is an important member of this class. It is used mainly as sedative and its usual dose is 500 mg orally per day.

$$H_2N—CONHCO—C(Br)(C_2H_5)_2 \text{ (Carbromal)}$$

22.2.1.4 Mode of Action of Hypnotics and Sedatives

In general the hypnotics act in two different ways, viz., (i) First they exert their action on sensory cortex as a result entry point (threshold) is raised when such sensory cortex becomes internally stimulated and in the second phase they interfere with the passage of impulses from the subsidiary centres in the hypothalamus to the cortex.

In normal human system, the cerebral electrical activity is directly dependent upon anxiety, emotional excitement and administration of certain potent CNS stimulant. At this stage, the administration of a reasonably overdose of hypnotics and sedatives is measurable by an electroencephalogram. Thus, this type of drugs specially, barbiturates depress the reticular activating system by weakening the synaptic transmission process.

22.2.1.4.1 Structure-Activity Relationship of Hypnotics and Sedatives

It has been observed that barbituric acid itself does not possess any hypnotic or sedative property. But if the two active hydrogen atoms at 5-position are replaced by appropriate substituents like-alkyl or aryl "hypnotic property" becomes prominent. During the assay of structure-activity relationship in barbiturates following interesting and significant facts have been observed.

i. Total number of carbon atoms in the two groups at 5-position should be between 4 to 10 for the optimal therapeutic results.
ii. The branched chain substituent shows more activity and shorter duration. The greater the branching, the more potent becomes the drug as is found in the case of pentobarbital which is more potent than amobarbital.
iii. Presence of unsaturation in the alkyl substituent produces compounds which are very susceptible to tissue oxidation. Hence they are short acting.
iv. Cylic substituents (aromatic or alicyclic) exert greater potency than open chain substituent.
v. Small chain alkyl substituents are resistant to oxidation and hence are long-acting.
vi. Presence of polar groups like —OH, —NH_2, $>C{=}O$, —COOH, etc. decreases the potency of the drug.
vii. Replacement of carbonyl oxygen by sulphur at the position 2 results in the rapid on-set and short duration.
viii. Inclusion of more sulphur decreases the activity.
ix. Replacement of hydrogen atoms at carbon atoms 1 and 3 with an alkyl group increases the vulnerability of the molecule to tissue oxidation.
x. Presence of halogen in 5-alkyl group increases the activity.

22.2.2 Coagulant and Anticoagulant Agents

Coagulant and anticoagulant agents are the drugs which act on the blood and the blood forming organs. In the normal condition the blood exists in liquid state, as a result it can safely and readily circulate through the blood vessels. However, under certain unusual condition there may be clotting of the blood in the vascular system. In such condition, clotting or coagulation of blood interferes in the circulation of blood which leads to serious results like *thromobosis*, even death in some cases.

It may be remembered that in some cases coagulation or clotting of blood becomes an important and essential defensive mechanism for arresting the undesirable bleeding (haemorrhage) caused by injury.

22.2.2.1 Mechanism of Clotting of Blood

From the above discussion it is thus evident that both the processes of clotting and anticlotting of blood are important biochemical processes. So it is desirable to know the mechanistic aspect of these important biochemical processes. Morawitz, in 1905 proposed a theory to explain these phenomena. According to his theory normal blood contains some ingredients such as (i) fibrinogen, a protein which forms insoluble protein fibrin (ii) prothrombin, another protein component, (iii) ionised calcium (iv) platelets (v) thromboplastin and (vi) some other factors. It has been suggested that the formation of fibrin—the solid material is responsible for the clotting of blood. This solid clotting matterial has been assumed to be formed by a series of reactions as depicted:

Tissue damage ⟶ Thromboplastin, a lipoprotein with molecular weight 168,000 found in tissues, blood and saliva.

The thromboplastin, thus formed and ionised calcium as well as other factors present in blood react with another protein component, prothrombin to form thrombin which is also a protein. Prothrombin is a glyco-protein having molecular weight 68,900 and requires vitamin K for its synthesis in liver while thrombin is a globulin protein whose molecular weight is 33,600. Finally thrombin formed reacts with globular protein component of the blood to generate both monomer and polymer of fibrin. Thus the complete process of formation of fibrin may be shown by the following flow-chart:

Tissue damage ⟶ Thromboplastin

↓ + Prothrombin + Ca^{++} + Other factors

Thrombin

↓ + Fibrogen

Fibrin (Monomer) ⟶ Fibrin (Polymer) ⟶ Clot (fusion of cells, platelets and polymerised fibrin)

22.2.2.1.1 Prevention of Blood Clotting

It is thus, evident from the above mechanism of formation of blood clot in the blood vessel, that the clotting or declotting depends upon the formation of fibrin and its fusion with some factors present in blood. So in order to prevent blood clotting following methods may be employed.

i. Removal of Ca^{++} with oxalates, citrates, E.D.T.A. ion-exchange resin, etc.
ii. Inhibition of the conversion of prothrombin to thrombin by the use of some drugs.
iii. By the stabilisation of platelets through the use of some hydrophobic agents.
iv. Controlling the formation of prothrombin by using some drugs.

Under normal condition, the clotting or coagulation of blood in the vascular systemis prevented by an organic chemical *heparin* formed in liver. The heparin maintains the proper balance of all the factors present in blood so that it does not coagulate within the vascular system. But if under the influence of some substance fluidity of blood is disturbed and clotting occurs, some agents, called *anticoagulant drugs* are used to retard the clotting or the blood.

Again, if blood injury occurs which us a common phenomenon in the life, bleeding occurs and in most of the cases blood coagulates normally but in abnormal condition blood does not coagulate in its own way and an excessive bleeding (*haemophilia*) may occur. This haemophilic condition is cured by the treatment with the drugs known as *coagulant drugs*.

22.2.2.2 Anticoagulant Agents

As mentioned before, retardation of coagulation is an essential aspect of blood transfusion to avoid thrombosis after operation or from other causes, to prevent recurrent thrombosis in phlebitis and pulmonary embolism and to minimise the propagation of clots in coronary arteries. This retardation of coagulation may be achieved by the use of some agents. The main function of these agents is to inactivate thrombin and other substances which prevent the formation of prothrombin in liver. These agents which are known as anticoagulants must possess the following requirement to be an ideal anticoagulating agents.

i. It must be useful orally or as an intradermal injection.
ii. It must produce rapid on-set of action.
iii. It should have minimum side effect.
iv. It should not possess any toxic property.
v. It should be cheaper in price.

There are a large number of anticoagulants either natural or synthetic in character.

(a) *Natural Anticoagulant:* The most important natural anticoagulant is heparin. It is mucopoly saccharide with molecular weight in the range 6,000-20,000. It is isolated from the lungs and liver of mammal and a few invertebrates. Its exact structure, molecular weight and activity depend upon the species, and the nature of tissues from which it is isolated. It has been observed that the activity of heparin is due to the sulphonic group present in it and its activity increases with the increase in the number of sulphonic groups. A part structure of heparin may be expressed as below:

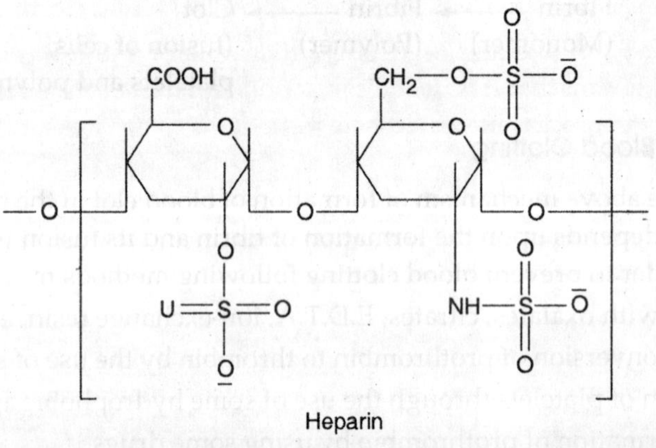

Heparin

Mode of action of Heparin: It has been assumed that the heparin inhibits the path of conversion of prothrombin to thrombin in the clotting process. It is nontoxic for short-term use. It is specially useful in maintaining the fluidity of the blood during heart surgery.

(b) *Synthetic Anti-coagulating Agents:* Various attempts have been made to find out synthetic substitutes of heparin by the sulphonation of large number of polysaccharides but none of them received wide acceptance due to their toxic nature. However, some other types of anticoagulants have been synthesised. Chemically, these anticoagulants belong to differ class of organic compounds of which coumarin and indanedione groups need special mention.

a. *Coumarin Group of Anticoagulants*

i. The most important member of this group is dicoumarol. It is synthesised from methyl salicylate through the following steps of reaction:

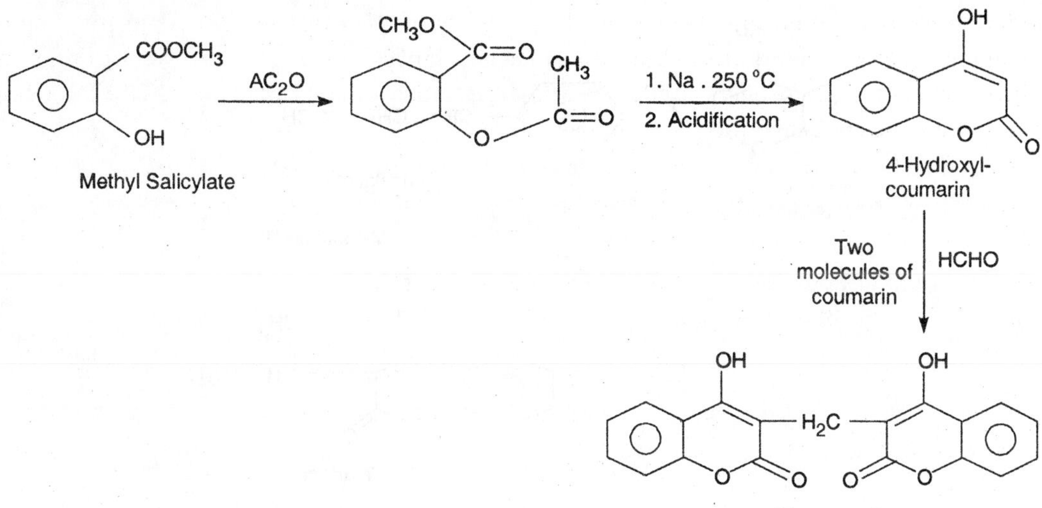

Dicoumarol

Dicoumarol can delay the rate of coagulation of blood probably by blocking the enzyme system responsible for the synthesis of prothrombin in liver. It is generally used as a prophylactic against post-operative thrombosis and embolism. It may be used alone or with heparin in the treatment of intravascular clotting

ii. *Tromexan or Pelentan:* It is also an useful anticoagulant and it has advantages over dicoumarol in the fact that it is quicker in action and more active but has some toxic property. It is prepared as indicated below:

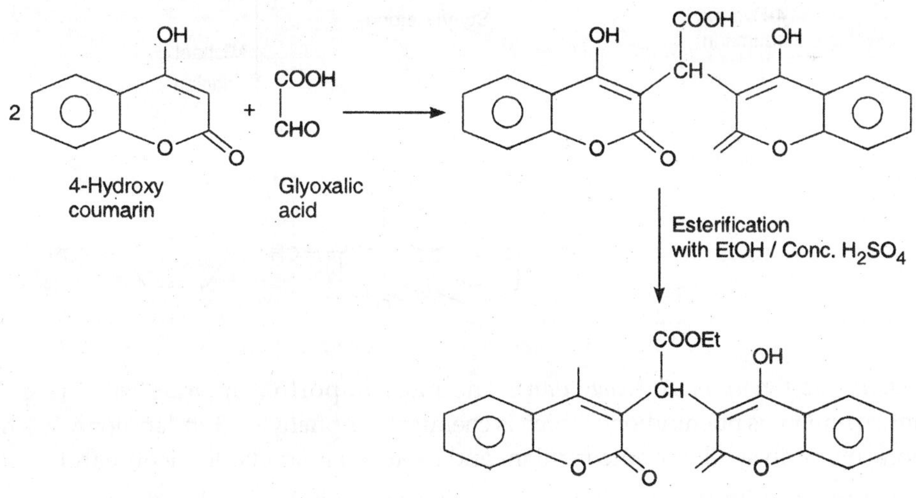

Tromexan

iii. *Warfarin:* Warfarin is also a synthetic anticoagulant of coumarin family. It may also be used as rodenticide.

It is prepared by the Michael condensation between 4-hydroxy coumarin and benzal acetone.

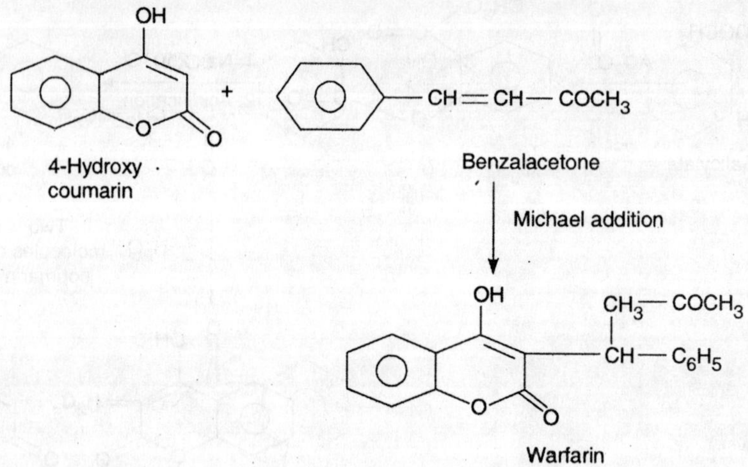

iv. *Nicoumalone:* It is similar in action to warfarin and may be used both as an anticoagulant and rodenticide. It is prepared by the Michael addition between 4-hydroxy coumarin and styryl ketone as shown below:

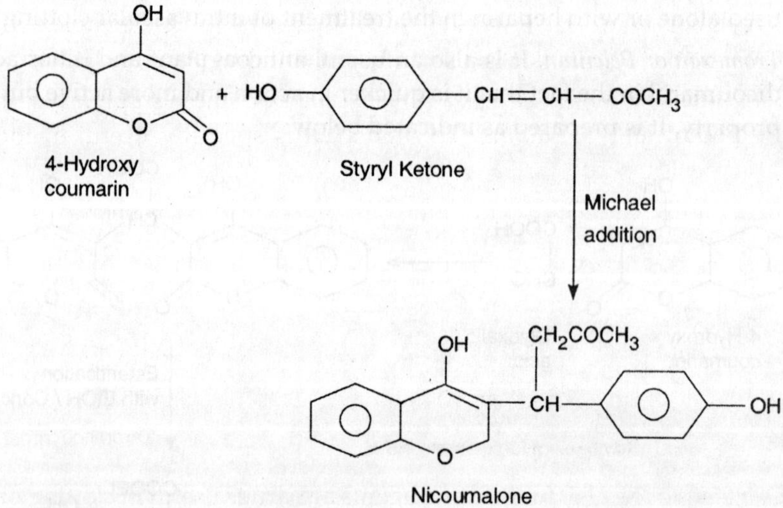

b. *Indandione Group of Anticoagulant:* The most importnat member of this group of anticoagulant is phenindione which is chemically 2-phenyl-1, 3-indandione. It is the first non-coumarin synthetic antcoagulant and its action is similar to dicoumarol.

It is prepared by the reaction between benzal-phthalide and sodium methoxide in methanol

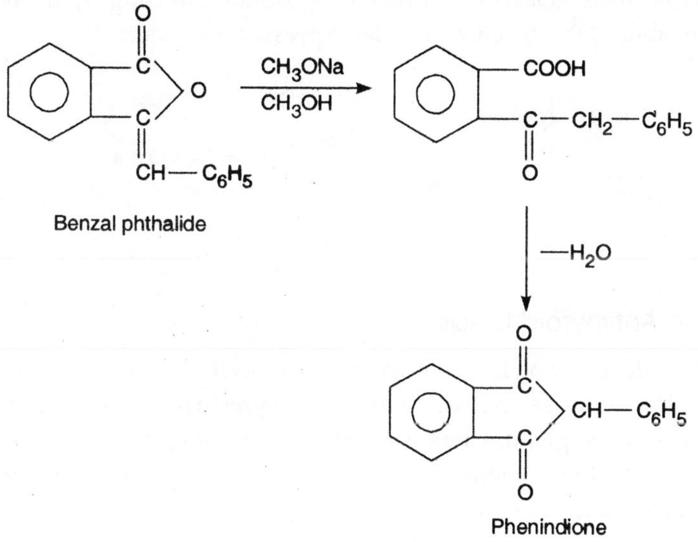

(b) *Miscellaneous Anticoagulants*

i. Sodium citrate may also be used as anticoagulant, Sodium citrate when taken orally is metabolised *in vivo* to citrate ion which forms soluble complex with calcium ion and it converts prothrombin to thrombin and thus prevents the formation of clot.

ii. *Sulphanilamido quinoxaline and Thrombodyn:* Both these sulphur bearing compounds are potent anticoagulants. Thrombodyn is specially useful in the treatment of thrombosis.

Structurally, these two compounds may be expressed as below:

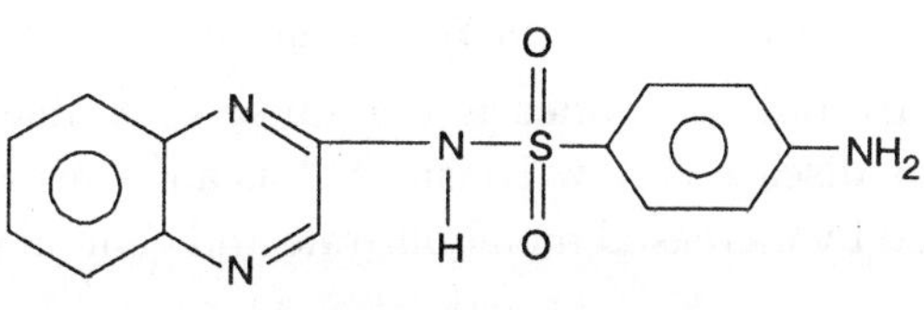

Sulphanilamido quinoxaline

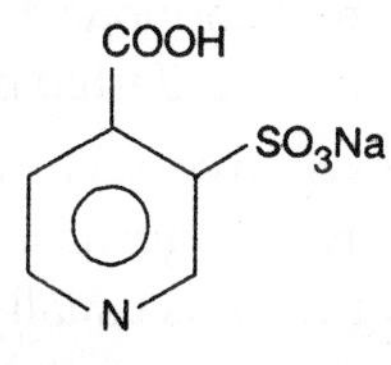

Thrombodyn

- *Coagulating Agents:* Coagulating agents are drugs useful in clotting of oozing blood. They are classified according to their structures as well as on the basis of their effect—systemic or local. There are large number of coagulants of which following groups are mentionable.

(a) *Vitamin K group:* Vitamin K_1 increases the time of blood clotting and vitamin K_2 which differs from vitamin K_1 in the structure of its side-chain but has the same effect as that of K_1.

(b) *Proteins and Amino Acids:* Proteins such as thrombin, fibrin and gelatin are used topically for clotting oozing blood. Amino caproic acid inhibits plasminogen, a precursor of thromboplastin.

(c) *Miscellaneous Coagulants*

i. Oxidised cellulose obtained by the oxidation of gauze or cotton forms an artificial clot and stops bleeding.

ii. *Carbazochrome salicylate:* It prevents systemic bleeding by decreasing capillary permeability. Its structure may be expressed as under:

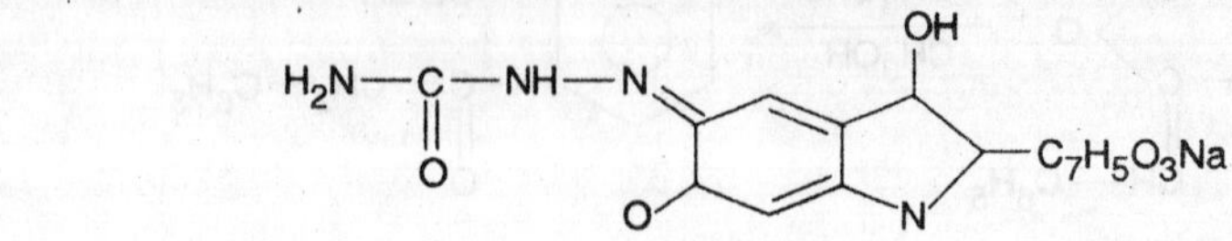

Carbazochrome salicylate

22.2.3 Thyroid and Antithyroid Drugs

Thyroid is a gland. Its chief function is to remove inorganic iodides from blood plasma. Its another important function is to synthesise thyroxine and liothyronine (tri-iodothyronine)—the two active hormonal constituents of the gland. Chemically these hormones are iodine containing amino acids. They are stored as protein constituents of the gland—thyroglobulin from which hormones are released after proteolysis.

22.2.3.1 Functions of Thyroid Hormones

The main function of thyroid hormones is to help in the growth, development and metabolic processes of the body. They also help to increase the total metabolic rate of the whole organism and in some tissues they also stimulate the rate of consumption of oxygen.

22.2.3.2 Diseases Caused by Thyroid Hormones

It has been observed that the *deficiency* of thyroid hormone secretion causes *Hypothyroidism*—a condition which is manifested by slowing down of all the metabolic processes of the body. The congenital thyroid hormone deficiency creates an irreversible clinical condition known as *cretinism*. This condition is manifested by stunted growth and mental retardation.

Again, excessive secretion of thyroid hormones is the cause of a disease termed as *Hyperthyroidism* or *Thyrotoxicosis.* This disease is now considered as a disease of the immune response disorder. It is usually marked by increased metabolic rate and general state of anxiety and restlessness.

22.2.3.2.1 Treatment of the above Diseases

The diseases caused by the deficiency of thyroid hormone secretion are treated by thyroid gland and thyroid hormonal drugs while antithyroid drugs are frequently used against hyperthyroidism—disease caused by excessive thyroid hormonal secretion.

(a) *Treatment of Thyroid Deficiency Disease (Hypothyroidism):* As stated above in this disease drugs from thyroid gland and thyroid hormones are used (i) The drug—thyroid is the cleaned dried and powdered thyroid glands of ox, pig or sheep free from connective tissues and any external fat. The powder is diluted with suitable diluent such as lactose to the required concentration. This powder is yellowish to buff coloured, amorphous powder with a faint meat-like smell and saline test. It is stored in tightly closed containers. It may be mentioned that this drug should not be prescribed to the patients having normal functioning gland. This is because administration of this drug may decrease the intrinsic secretion.

(ii) The drugs prepared from thyroid hormones are effectively applied for the treatment of thyroid deficiency disease. Commonly there are two thyroid hormones—thyroxine and liothyronine. Both of these hormones are the derivatives of thyronine which is a tyrosine derivative. Structurally, these two thyroid hormones may be expressed by the following structures.

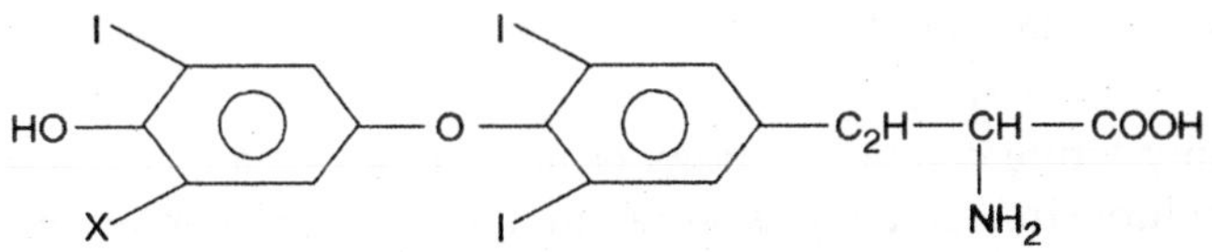

X = I, Thyroxine
X = H, Liothyronine

These two hormones are generally preferred over dried thyroid gland for the treatment of hypothyroidism. Sodium salt of the laevo isomer of thyroxine is normally used as thyroxine sodium. It is light yellow to buff-coloured finely crystalline powder. It is sparingly soluble in water. It should be stored in light resistant container as it becomes slightly pink on exposure to light. The sodium salt of another hormone, liothyronine sodium is a white to buff-coloured solid crystalline powder. It is insoluble in water. It is dextro-rotatory and is also stored in light-resistant container. it is generally used in thyroid deficiency when a rapid effect is required. Both thyroxine and liothyronine are qualitatively similar in their biological action but liothyronine is much more potent on molar basis.

(b) *Treatment of Hyperthyroidism:* It has already been mentioned that the disease, hyperthyroidism is caused by the excessive secretion of thyroid hormones. Such disease is treated with antithyroid drugs as they are capable of reducing the probability of synthesis of thyroxine and liothyronine.

- *Mode of Action of Drugs:* The antithyroid drugs used interfere in the process of incorporation of iodide ions into thyroglobulin, from which the thyroid hormones are synthesised. As a result, the process of synthesis of thyroid hormones is highly reduced. These drugs are applied before and after the surgical removal of thyroid glands and are generally given orally.

  Propyl thiouracil and carbimazole are the two main antithyroid drugs which are frequently used.

i. *Propylthiouracil:* It is the propyl derivative of thiouracil. Structurally it is 2, 3-dihydro-6-propyl-2-thioxo-4-pyrimidone as shown below:

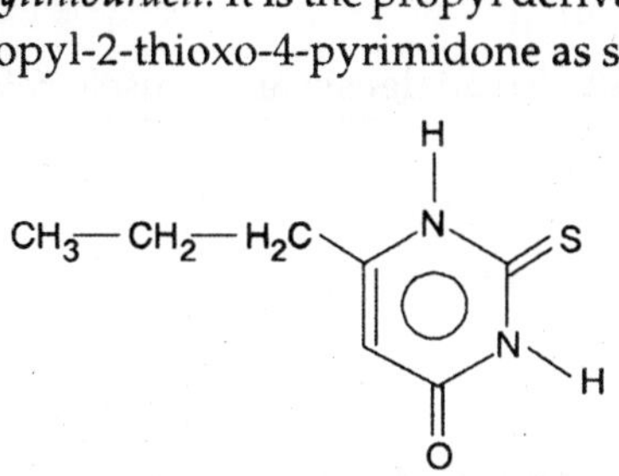

Propylthiouracil

It is white or pale cream coloured crystalline substance with a bitter taste. It is sparingly soluble in water and is kept in light-resistant container.

ii. *Carbimazole:* It is imidozoline derivative and its structure may be expressed as 3-methyl-2-thioxo-4-imidazoline-1-ethyl carboxylate as depicted below:

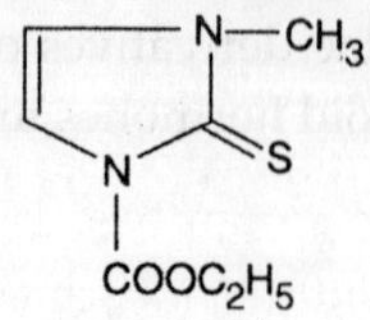

Carbimazole

It is a creamy white crystalline powder and possesses a characteristic odour. It is sparingly soluble in water and is stored in light-resistant container.

22.2.4 Anaesthetics

The term 'anaesthetic' has been deried from the Greek word *anaesthesia* which means insensitivity or lack of feeling. Thus anaesthetics may be defined as a group of drugs that produce loss of conciousness and, therefore, loss of all sensations. The effect of an anaesthetic is reversible which means that the effected organs return to normal condition as soon as the concentration of the anaesthetic is decreased. Thus, an anaesthetic produces temporary insensibility to pain feeling. either in the whole body or in a particular organ. These drugs are used in surgical operations to induce unconsciousness and, therefore, abolish the sensation of pain. Under anaesthesia, the patient does not feel any agony during operation and so the surgeon can work carefully and effectively. The advent of anaesthetics has created a stir in the field of surgery. In brief, anaesthetic should fulfil the following objectives:

i. A safe and pleasant insensibility for the patient.
ii. Sufficient relaxation so that surgery can be readily achieved.
iii. Prompt recovery of the patient to pre-operative physiological condition.

It may be mentioned that till to-day no such ideal anaesthetic is available which can provide the above objectives. However, by the application of combination of anaesthetic and ancillary drugs available in the hands of skilled person the above objectives can be achieved.

22.2.4.1 Characteristics of Ideal Anaesthetic

An ideal anaesthetic drug should have the following characteristics:

i. It should be economical
ii. It should be potent, inflammable and inert
iii. It should produce quick, and smooth induction
iv. It should produce not only anaesthesia but also analgesia and muscle relaxation
v. It should be non-toxic, nonirritating
vi. It should not produce nausea or vomiting
vii. It should be stable towards sodalime, light and heat.

22.2.4.2 Classification of Anaesthetic Drugs

Anaesthetic agents are classified broadly into two groups on the basis of their effect.

i. *General Anaesthetics:* These are those anaesthetics which can depress the central nervous system to such an extent that all the sensitivity to pain feeling is lost, i.e., these agents produce unconciousness all over the body.

ii. *Local Anaesthetics:* These anaesthetics do not affect the whole body but produce insensibility to pain feeling in a restricted area of the body.

22.2.4.2.1 General Anaesthetics

General anaesthetics have further been divided into three groups based solely on the method of administration. These are (i) inhalation anaesthetics, (ii) intravenous anaesthetics and (iii) basal anaesthetics.

Inhalation Anaesthetics: These are generally volatile liquids or gaseous in nature and are administered through inhalation process. A few typical members of this group of anaesthetic agents are discussed.

22.2.4.2.1.1 Nitrous Oxide

It is first anaesthetic. It is prepared by heating ammonium nitrate up to 200 °C.

$$\underset{\text{Ammonium Nitrate}}{NH_4NO_3} \xrightarrow{200\,°C} \underset{\text{Nitrons oxide}}{N_2O} + 2H_2O$$

It is the weakest but the safest inhalation general anaesthetic. It is usually administered in conjunction with other potent inhalation anesthetics such as halothane and methoxy fluorane. However, its anaesthetic action may be further broadened by the incorporation of neuromuscular blocking agents by which its muscle relaxant characteristics are enhanced to a considerable extent. Some patient often get an attack of *hysteria* and for this reason it is termed as *'laughing gas'*. Its main uses are as follows.

i. For short dental operation (ii) to provide a state of unconsciousness due to surgery under spinal anaesthesia.

22.2.4.2.1.2 Ether

It is the first compound to be used as an anaesthetic by American physician Crawford Long. It is prepared by Williamson's sysnthesis as depicated below.

$$\underset{\text{Ethanol}}{C_2H_5OH} + H_2SO_4 \longrightarrow \underset{\text{Ethyl hydrogen sulphate}}{C_2H_5HSO_4} + H_2O$$

$$C_2H_5HSO_4 + C_2H_5OH \longrightarrow \underset{\text{Ether}}{C_2H_5\text{—}O\text{—}C_2H_5} + H_2SO_4$$

Ether is a safe anaesthetic. Its principal site of action is central nervous system. It is cheap and if properly stored, it is comparatively stable. It is used for producing insensitivity to pain in surgical trauma. However, it is to some extent irritating to mucous membrane and its vapours are inflammable.

22.2.4.2.1.3 Divinyl Ether

It is prepared from ethylene chlorohydrin in the following manner.

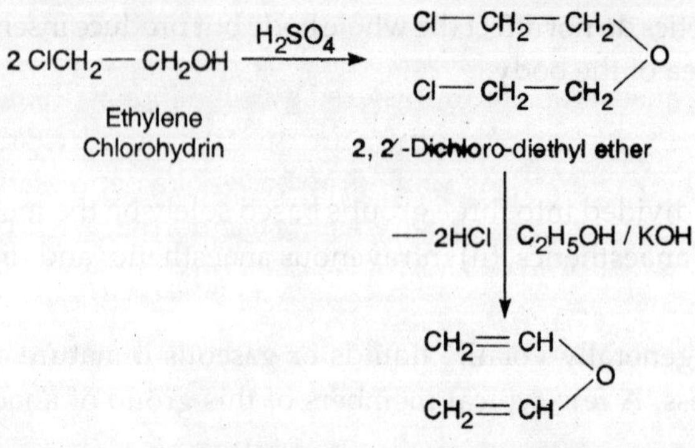

Divinyl ether

It is nearly seven times more potent than ether with a speedy recovery. It is used in the minor operations of short duration when rapid induction and recovery are required. It is especially useful for dental procedures.

22.2.4.2.1.4 Halothane (Fluothane)

Chemically it is 2-bromo-2-chloro-1, 1, 1,-triflouro-ethane.

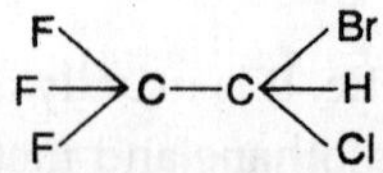

It is the most widely used anaesthetic agent at present. It is used in almost every type of surgical procedure. Anaesthesiologists prefer it because of the ease with which they can lighten or deepen the level of anaesthetic level. It is nearly four times active than ether with therapeutic index twice that of ether. It is administered by inhalation. It is prepared by bromination of 2-chloro-1,1,1-triflouro ethene followed by fractional distillation of the product formed.

22.2.4.2.1.5 Methoxy Flurane

Chemically it is 2, 2-dichloro-1, 1-difluoro ethyl methyl ether, 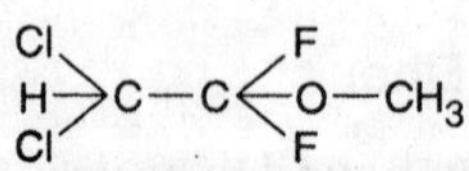.

It is one of the most potent anaesthetic agents frequently used today. In fact, it is employed to cause comparatively light anaesthesia with deep analgesic and muscle relaxation. It is useful for short surgical operations like obstetrics.

22.2.4.2.1.6 Chloroform

It is among the most widely used general anaesthetics. It is prepared from bleaching powder and ethyl alcohol or acetone as shown below:

$$CaOCl_2 + H_2O \longrightarrow Ca(OH)_2 + Cl_2$$

$$C_2H_5OH + Cl_2 \longrightarrow CH_3CHO + 2HCl$$

$$CH_3CHO + Cl_2 \longrightarrow CCl_3CHO + 3HCl$$

$$2\ CCl_3CHO + Ca(OH)_2 \longrightarrow \underset{\text{Chloroform}}{CHCl_3} + Ca(HCOO)_2$$

It is a potent anaesthetic administered by inhalation. It has both reasonably good muscle relaxant and analgesic properties. It has liver and kidney toxicity.

22.2.4.2.1.7 Cyclopropane

Cyclopropane is one of the most potent anaesthetics administered by inhalation with the help of a brass regulator. The chief merit of cyclopropane over others are due to its non-irritant nature and rapid recovery from anaesthesia. However, it has some drawbacks like depressant effects on respiration, tendency to induce cardiac arrhythmais and to enhance haemorrhage. It is prepared by the action of metal such as sodium, magnesium or zinc on 1, 3-dichloro propane.

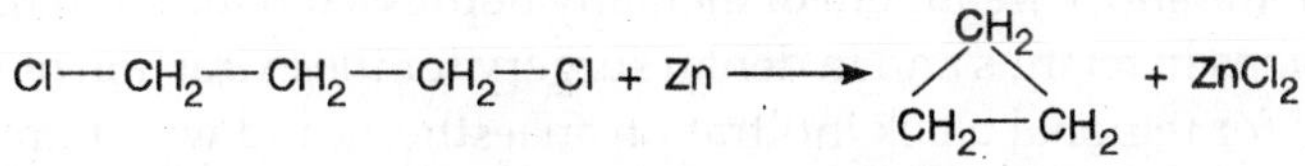

22.2.4.2.2 Intravenous Anaesthetics

Intravenous anaesthetics generally cause unconsciousness when administered parenterally. However, the duration of action can be safely monitored depending on the quantity of drug used.

A few representative members of this group of anaesthetics are discussed below:

22.2.4.2.2.1 Pentothal Sodium (Thiopental Sodium)

It is one of the most widely used non-volatile intravenous general anaesthetic drugs. It is generally prepared from malonic ester as shown below:

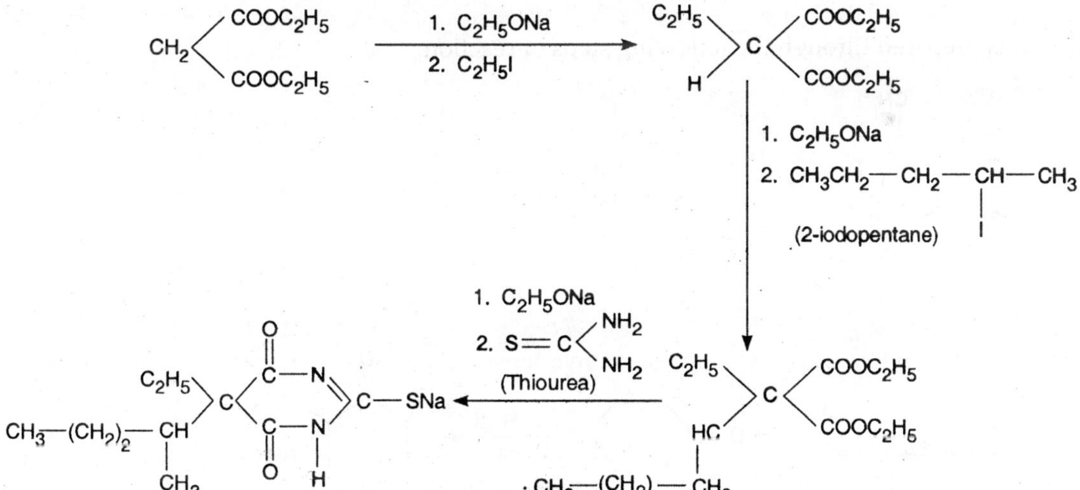

It is white to yellowish-white powder. It is dissolved in distilled water just prior to use. It is administered intravenously and to some extent rectally (containing a green dye) for the following surgical procedures:

i. Orthopaedic operations and manipulations.
ii. Obstetric repair procedures.
iii. Dilatition and Curettage.

However, it has some limitations as mentioned.

It can not be used for

i. the children below the age of 10 years
ii. the patients having potential respiratory block or depressed respiration
iii. the patients having advanced myocardial disease
iv. the patients having impending shock or having haemorrhage.

It is also used as a basal anaesthetic in many procedures of surgery. It is also used to produce muscular relaxation in the shock treatment of mentally depressed patients. It has also been used to control the convulsions in tetanus and in dental surgery for the extraction of tooth. It may also be used with procaine for regional block infiltration anaesthesia and with tetracaine for general anaesthesia.

22.2.4.2.2.2 Ketamine Hydrochloride

Structurally it is cyclohexanone-2 (2-chlorophenyl)-2-(methylamino) hydrochloride.

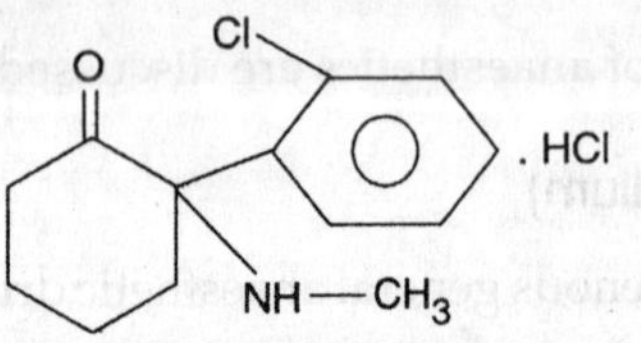

Ketamine Hydrochloride

It is prepared through the following steps of reaction:

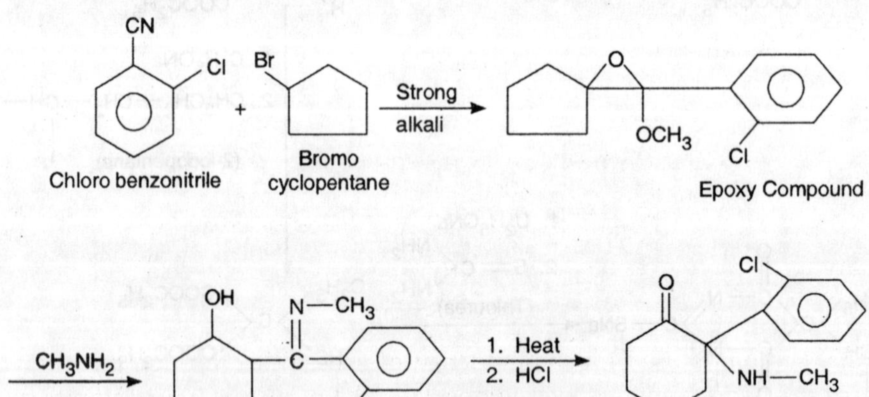

It is a rapid-acting general anaesthetic agent which causes anaesthesia accompanied by deep analgesia. It is an intravenous anaesthetic agent of choice for surgical operations of short duration.

22.2.4.2.2.3 Methohexital Sodium (Methohexitone Sodium)

Its synthesis involves the following steps of reactions as discussed in sequel:

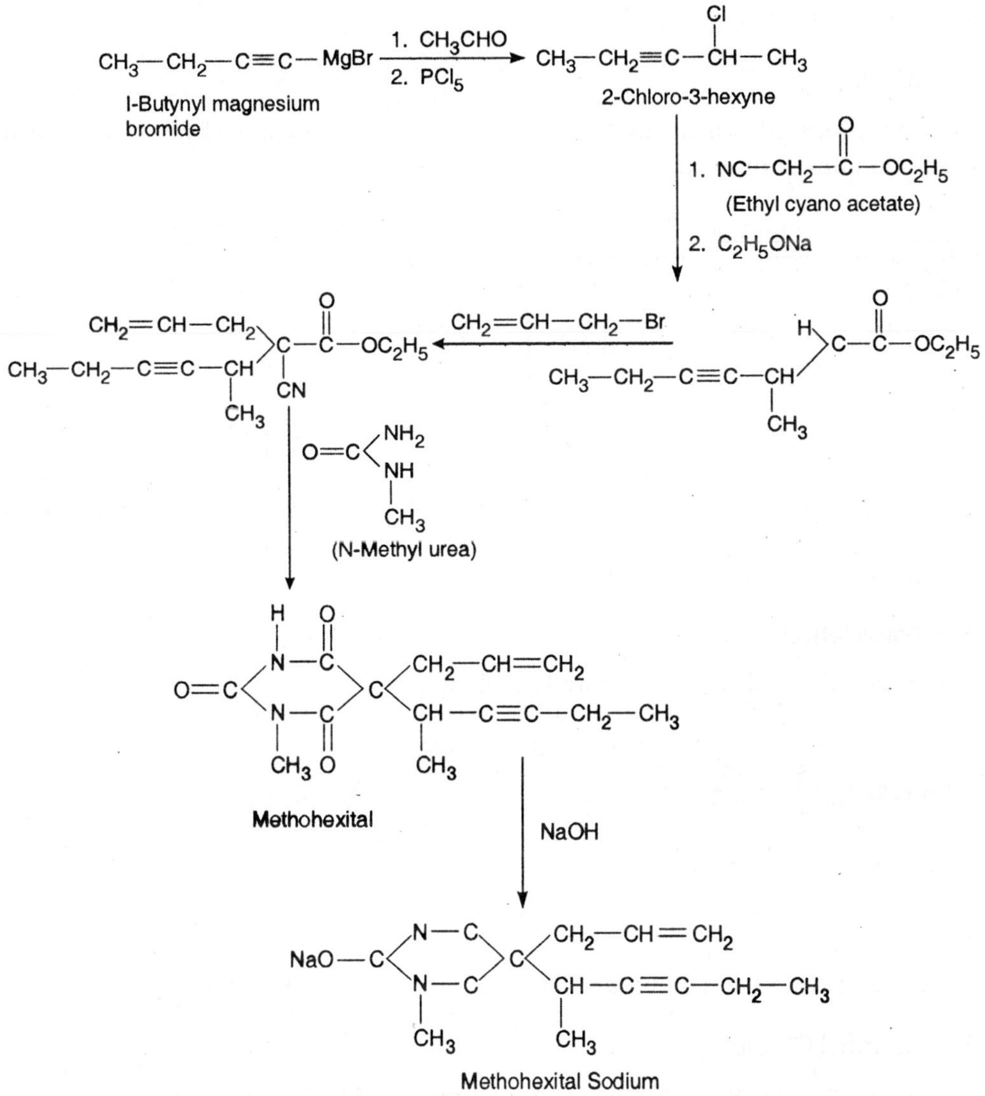

Methohexital sodium is used for the induction of anaesthesia through the intravenous administration. It has two advantages over thiopental sodium, such as (i) less affinity towards fatty tissues and (ii) greater potency. Its on-set of action is quite rapid and its recovery is also rapid. For this reason it is useful for short surgical operations like oral surgery, gynaecological investigation, genitourinary procedures and electroconvulsive therapy.

22.2.4.2.3 Basal Anaesthetics

Basal anaesthetic agents are those which can induce unconsciousness but the depth of unconsciousness is not enough for any surgical procedure. They are frequently used before the administration of inhalation anaesthetics. They are also used for repeated short term procedures in children, like the changing of painful dressings. These anaesthetic agents have three significant merit points, viz., (i) devoid of mental distress (ii) pleasant induction and (iii) lesser respiratory irritation. They are generally administered through rectum. A few representative members are cited below.

22.2.4.2.3.1 Avertin

It is a solution of tribromoethanol in amylene hydrate. It is usually prepared by the reduction of bromal with aluminium isopropoxide.

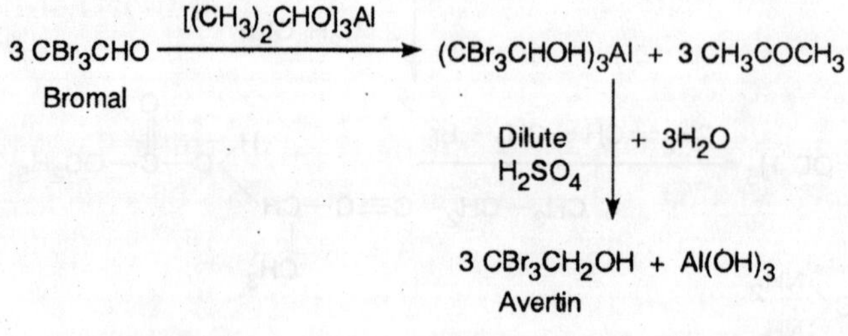

It is administered rectally. It is generally used for inducing short sleep and then full surgical anaesthesia is completed by one of the volatile anaesthetics. The main advantage of this anaesthesia being its pleasant induction without any irritation.

22.2.4.2.3.2 Paraldehyde

It is the trimer of acetaldehyde and is prepared as follows:

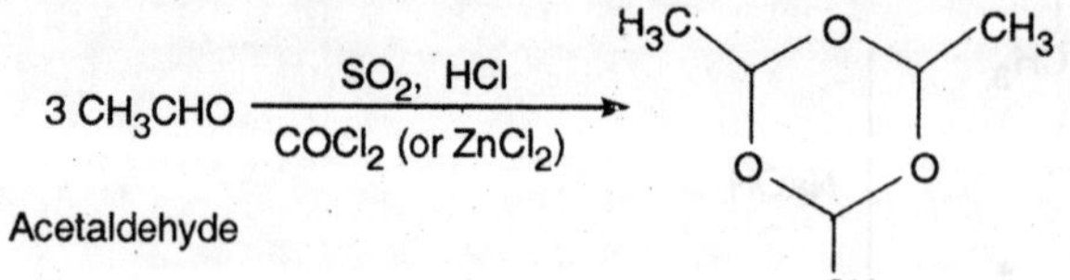

It is one of the oldest and best hypnotics having anti-convulsant effects. It is sometimes used as obstetrical analgesic where it is administered in large doses through rectum.

22.2.4.2.3.3 Fentanyl Citrate

Chemically, it is N-phenyl—N—[1-(2-phenylethyl)-4-piperidinyl]-2-hydroxy-1, 2, 3-propane-tricarboxylate.

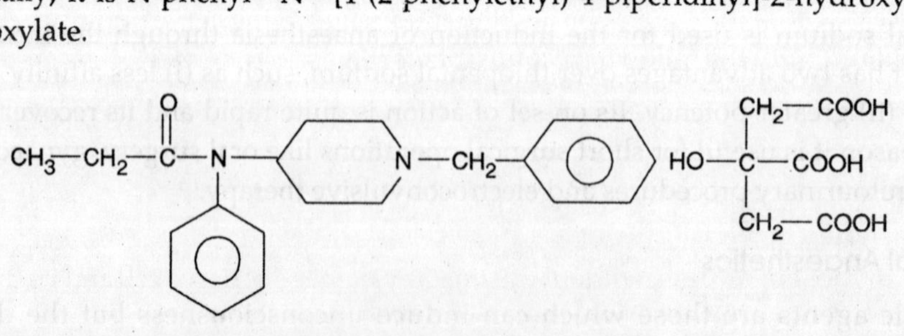

It is normally used as an analgesic for the control of pain associated with all kinds of surgery. It is used as an adjunct anaesthetic agent. It is one of the components in 'Fentanyl citrate and Droperidol Injection' which is generally used as premedication for anaesthesia and also as a supplement for induction and maintenance of anaesthesia.

22.2.4.3 Mode of Action of General Anaesthetics

A large number of theories have been put forward to explain the mode of action of general anaesthetics. Some important theories are discussed below.

22.2.4.3.1 Lipid Theory

According to this theory the site of action of anaesthetics is usually hydrophobic in nature. It has been assumed that greater the lipid solubility of an anaesthetic agent higher is its potency.

22.2.4.3.2 Biochemical Theory

It has been observed that barbiturates normally interfere with the creation of high energy products by decoupling oxidative phosphorylation. It has been suggested that the cerebral oxygen consumption is considerably decreased in human body when treated with anaesthetic drugs. This is expatiated by the fact that anaesthesia invariably retards the central nervous system activity as a result of which oxygen intake is considerably decreased.

22.2.4.3.3 Physical Theory

According to this theory, the size of anaesthetic molecule is the determining factor for their ability to reach the site of action. It has also been suggested that the anaesthetic agent starts functioning when the critical space within the membrane is charged with the anaesthetic molecule.

22.2.4.3.4 Miscellaneous Theory

One of the suggestions put forward is that the decrease in surface tension caused by an anaesthetic agent is directly related to its activity. Another possible explanation is that there is direct relation between the structure of the membrane and the mode of action of anaesthetic agent. However, the most important fact is that the lipid portion of the membrane is the site of action of anaesthetic agent.

22.2.4.4 Local Anaesthetics

Introduction: Local anaesthetics are chemical compounds which are applied topically or by localised injection to reduce or block pain sensation. These anaesthetics when directly employed to the peripheral nervous tissues block nerve-conduction and abolish all sensations in the part applied. It tends to block both the generation and the conduction of the nerve impulses. An ideal local anaesthetic should fulfil the following requirements.

i. It should be non-irritating.
ii. It should not be painful.
iii. It should be stable.
iv. Its toxicity should be very low.
v. It should produce anaesthesia without causing any damage of nerve cell and its duration of action should be sufficient for carrying out operation.

22.2.4.4.1 Classification of Local Anaesthetics

Local anaesthetics are broadly classified into two groups—(i) Natural and (ii) Synthetic. However, synthetic agents are available in larger number than its natural counter-part.

22.2.4.4.1.1 Natural Local Anaesthetics

Cocaine: It is the first chemical compound to be used as a local anaesthetic. It was introduced by Koller in 1884 as local anaesthetic in eye surgery. This application represented the beginning of the development of anaesthetic drug in medicinal practice. Halsted in 1885 showed that cocaine could be used to induce nerve block. This work of Halsted in America became the basis of block anaesthesia in surgery. The clinical application of cocaine in the spinal anaesthesia occurred in the beginning of 20th century.

Cocaine is an alkaloid isolated from the leaves of *Erythroxylum coca*. Chemically it is methyl benzoylecgonine.

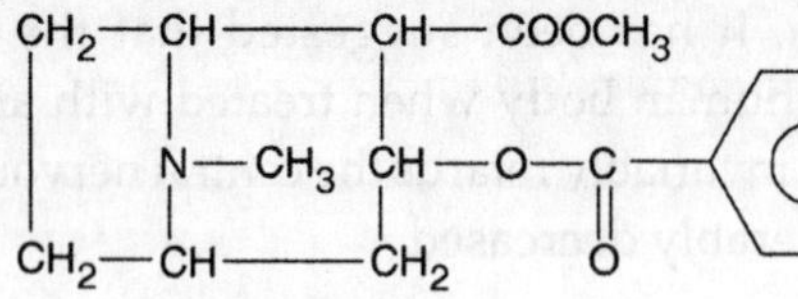

Cocaine

Its chloride is generally used. This salt occurs as colourless crystals. It is soluble in water, alcohol, chloroform and in glycerine. Generally 2-4 per cent solution is used in ophthalmic practice.

It has been observed that the *"anaesthesiophoric"* moiety of cocaine is its hydrolytic products, i.e., Benzoyl ecgonine and tropocaine as shown below:

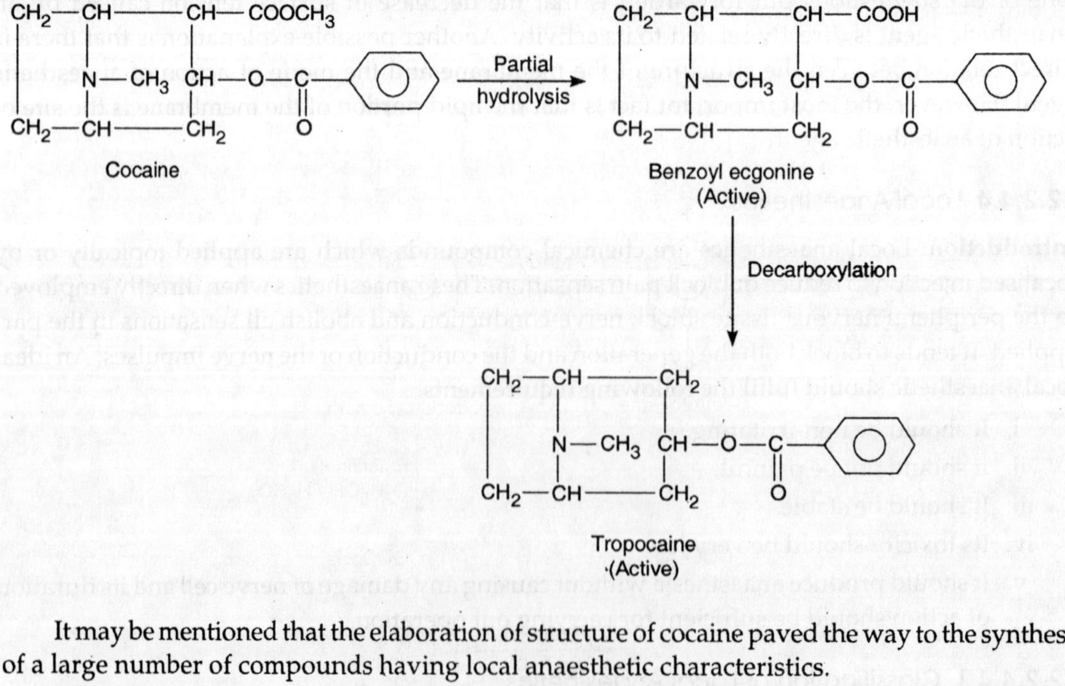

It may be mentioned that the elaboration of structure of cocaine paved the way to the synthesis of a large number of compounds having local anaesthetic characteristics.

However, cocaine is not free from drawbacks. It is harmful to the cornea and it may cause mydriasis. In fact, these drawbacks have resulted in extensive research aimed at the preparation of more desirable local anaesthetics.

22.2.4.4.1.2 Synthetic Local Anaesthetics

Einhorn in 1905 recognised that the presence of basic nitrogen atom in the esterified alcohol is the primary requirement of a compound to have local anaesthetic property. So he generalised that all aromatic esters may possess the ability to cause anaesthesia and he prepared two types of esters, viz.,

i. Methyl ester of *p*-amino-m-hydroxy benzoic acid.

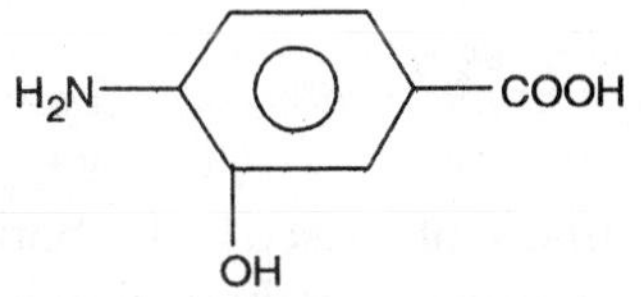

ii. Methyl ester of *m*-amino-*p*-hydroxy benzoic acid.

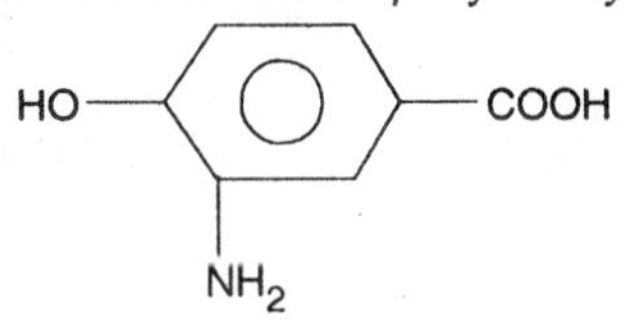

This generalisation led to the preparation of a large number of analogous esters. It was, however, observed that higher alkyl groups and those with normal chains are most active. A few of the most important compounds are mentioned below.

22.2.4.4.1.2.1 Benzocaine

Chemically it is ethyl-*p*-amino benzoate, i.e.,

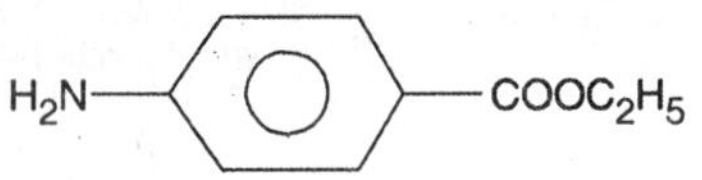

Its synthesis involves the following steps:

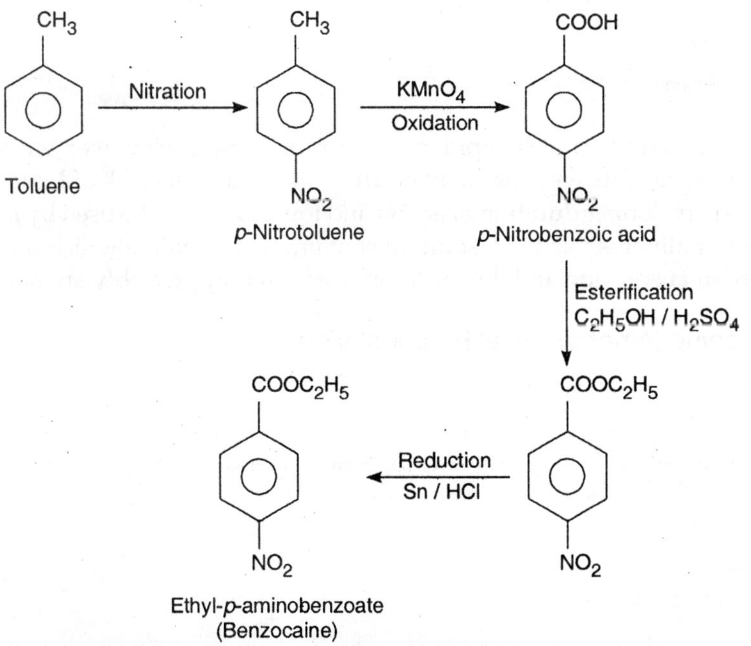

Since it is insoluble is water, it is used as an ointment to get rid of pain due to wounds, ulcers and mucous surfaces. It forms an ingredient in various creams, ointment, powders, aerosol sprays for the relieve of the pain of naked surfaces and severely inflamed mucous membranes.

22.2.4.4.1.2.2 Procaine (Ethocaine Hydrochloride, Novocaine or Scurocaine)

Chemically it is 2-(diethylamine)-ethyl-*p*-amino benzoate monohydrochloride.

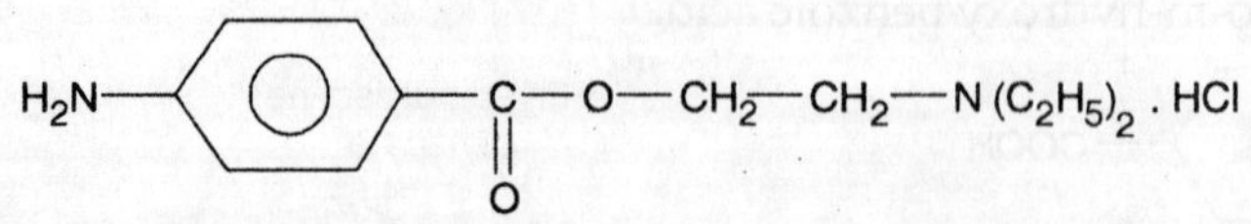

It is most widely used local anaesthetics. It was first synthesised by Einhorn in 1905. Several methods are available for its synthesis. One of the common methods involves the following steps.

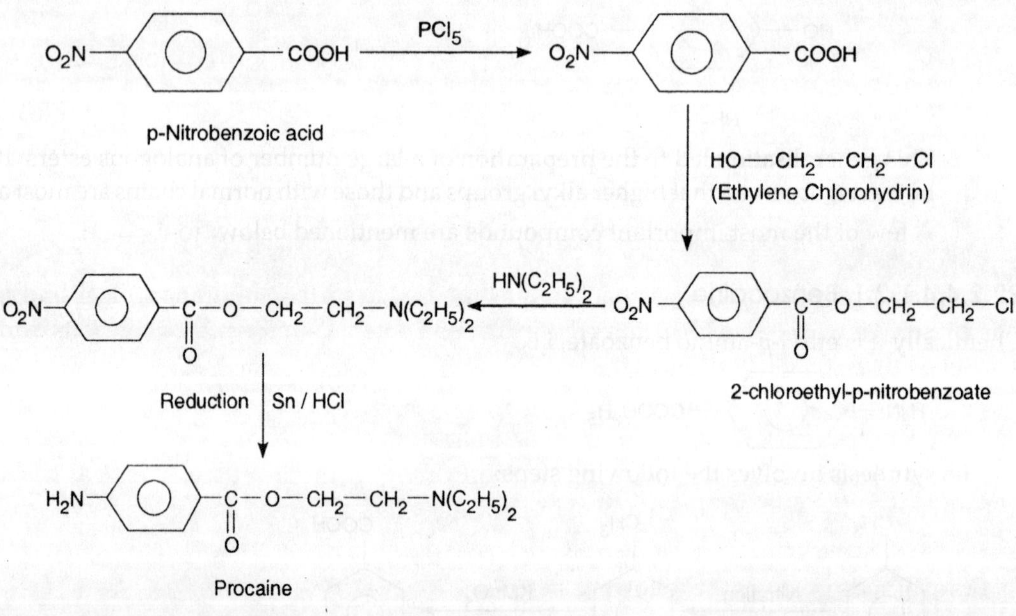

It is a powerful anaesthetic but not so rapid in its action as cocaine. However, it is least toxic in nature. The salient feature of its wide use may be attributed due to its lack of local irritation, minimal systematic toxicity, longer duration of action and low cost. It can be used by infiltration for effective action. Normally it is used in a solution containing adrenaline which modifies the activity through retarded absorption and the duration of action is appreciably enhanced.

22.2.4.4.1.2.3 Tetracaine (Amethocaine) Hydrochloride

Structurally, it may be expressed as under

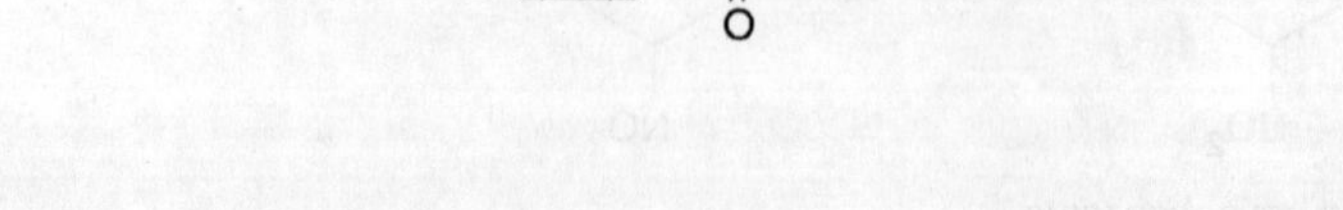

It is prepared through the following steps of reactions

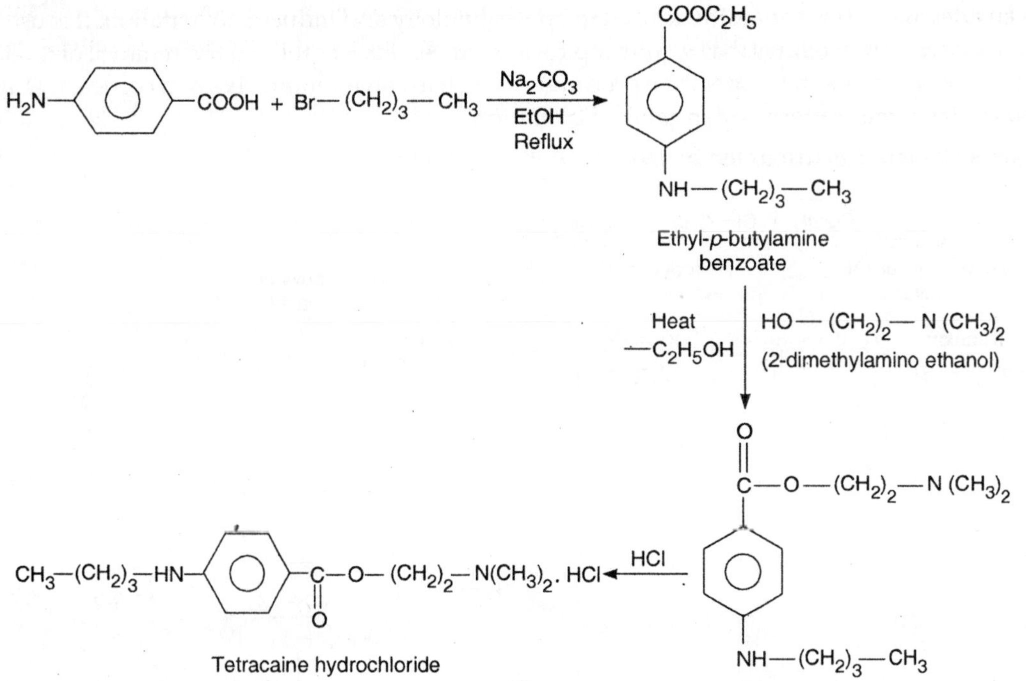

It is an all-purpose local anaesthetic frequently used in surface infiltration, block and spinal anaesthesia. It is reported to be 10 times more toxic and potent than procaine whereas its duration of action is twice than that of procaine.

22.2.4.4.1.2.4 Cyclomethycaine Sulphate (Cyclomethycaine)

It is widely used as an effective topical anaesthetic in thermal and chemical burns, in dermatological lesions, sun burn and skin abrasions. It is also used in urology, gynaecology, obstetrics procedure.

Its synthesis involves the following steps:

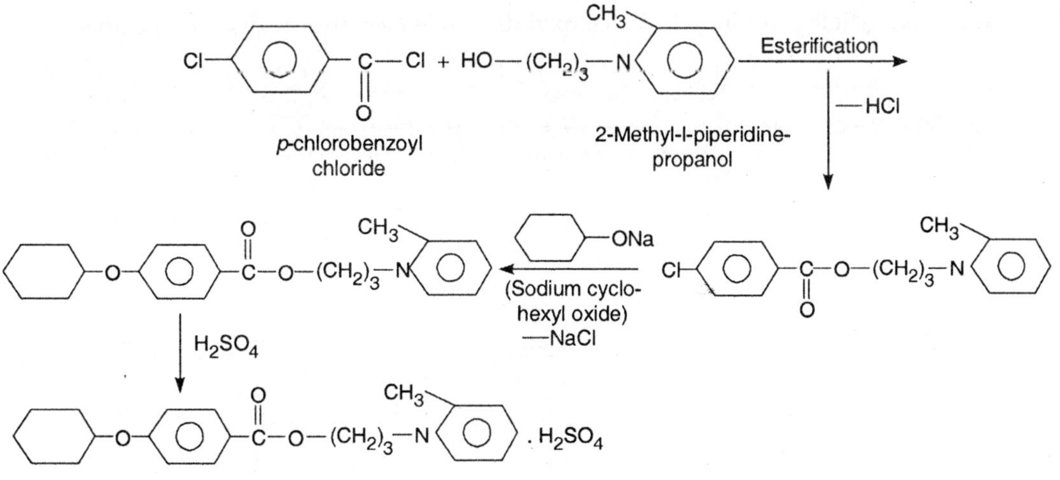

22.2.4.4.1.2.5 Proxymetacaine Hydrochloride (Proparacaine Hydrochloride)

It is an effective surface anaesthetic used in ophthalinology and induces no irritation. It is useful for most occular procedures that require topical anaesthesia such as tonometry, removal of foreign particles and various short operative procedure, which involve conjunctiva and cornea. It is also used in glaucoma surgery and in cataract operation.

It is prepared as discussed below:

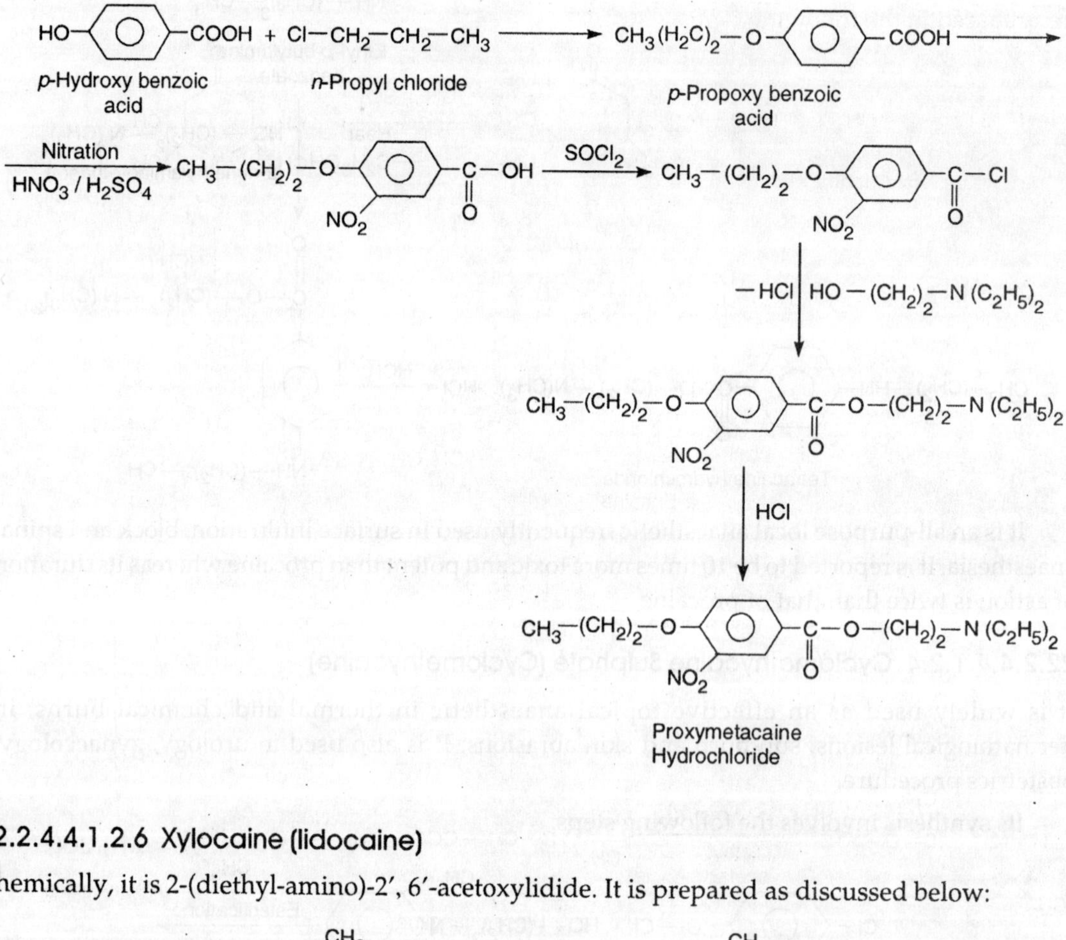

Proxymetacaine Hydrochloride

22.2.4.4.1.2.6 Xylocaine (lidocaine)

Chemically, it is 2-(diethyl-amino)-2′, 6′-acetoxylidide. It is prepared as discussed below:

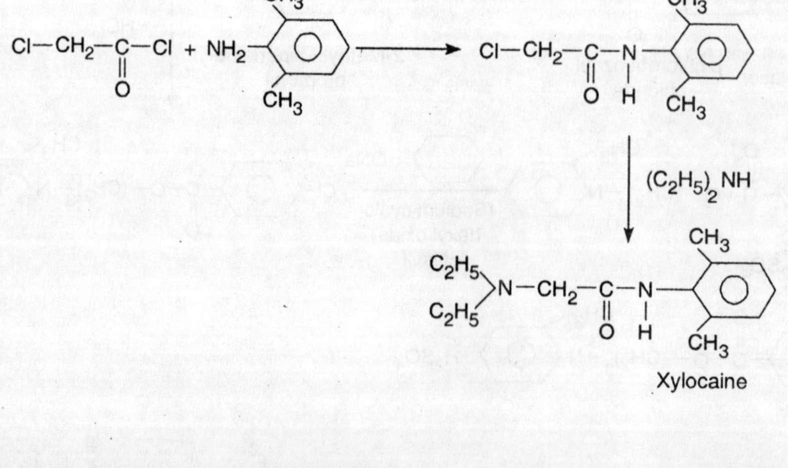

Xylocaine

Hydrochloride of xylocaine is used as local anaesthetic. It produces more prompt, intense and extensive anaestheria than procaine hydrochloride. It is useful for infiltration and block anaesthesia. An ointment containing 5% xylocaine in water-soluble polyethylene glycols is used in dental procedure.

22.2.4.4.1.2.7 α- and β-Eucaine

These two anaesthetics belong to piperidine group of chemical compounds. These two compounds are prepared in the following way:

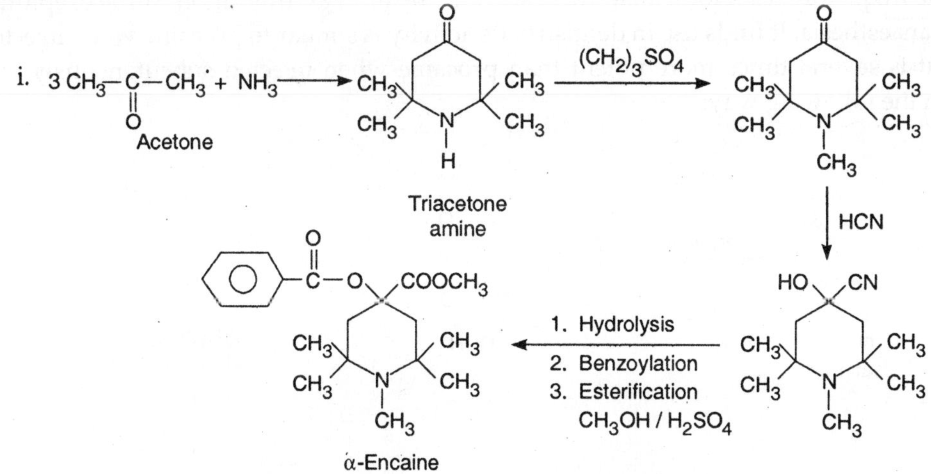

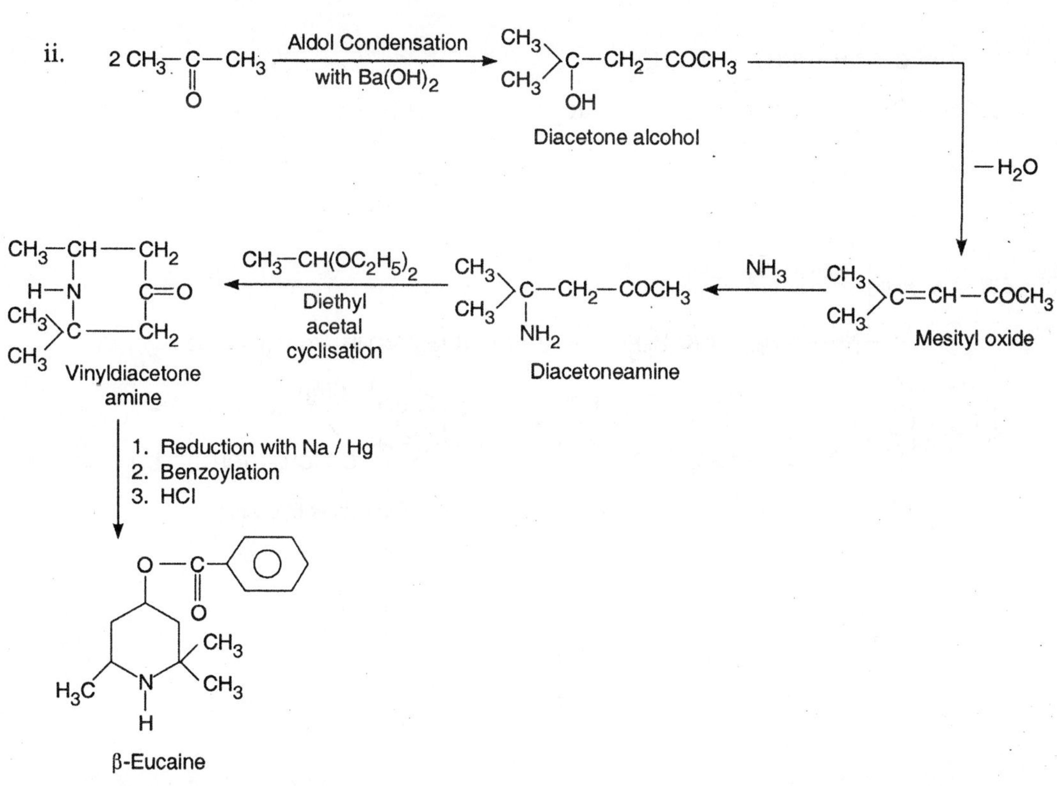

α-Eucaine is a cheap substitute of cocaine. It is less toxic than cocaine. Its main drawback is that it is painful and irritant when injected. That is why it has been replaced by β-eucaine. β-Eucaine is used as a local enaesthetic in many surgical procedures. It is less toxic than α-eucaine.

22.2.4.4.1.2.8 Dibucaine Hydrochloride (Cinchocaine Hydrochloride)

Structurally, it belongs to quinoline ring system. It is one of the most toxic, potent and longest acting of the frequently used local anaesthetics. It may be used as infiltration, surface, epidural and spinal anaesthesia. It finds use in dentistry. Its activity is similar to procaine when injected. However, it is several times more potent than procaine when injected subcutaneously. It is prepared in the following way:

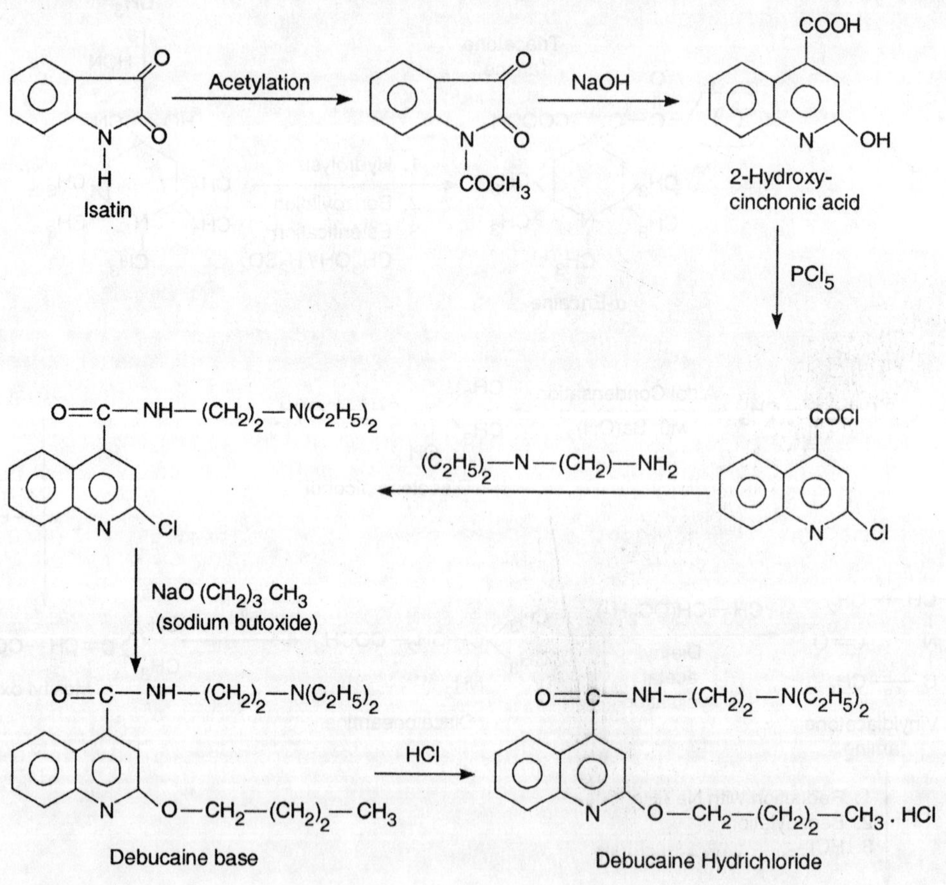

22.2.4.4.1.2.9 Phenacaine Hydrochloride (Holocaine Hydrochloride)

It is synthesised from *p*-phenetidine as shown below:

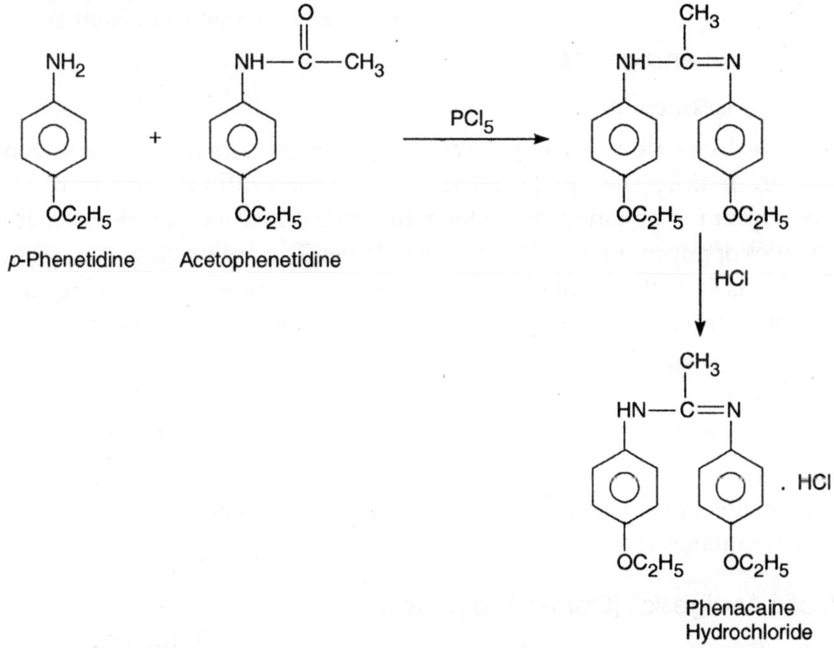

It is one of the oldest synthetic local anaesthetics. It is primarily used as 1% solution for effecting anaesthesia of the eye.

22.2.4.4.1.2.10 Eugenol

It is a phenolic compound having the structure as indicated below:

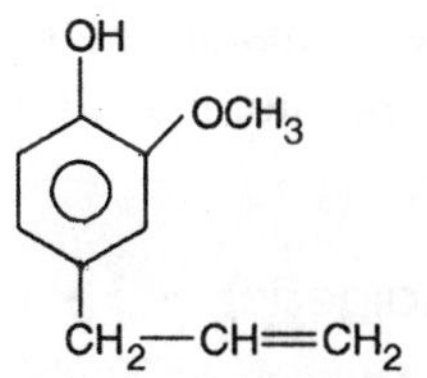

It is a naturally occurring phenolic ether and occurs in clove oil and many other essential oils. It is frequently used in dental procedures as an obtudent for hypersensitive dentine, caries or exposed pulp and as a temporary anodyne dental filling.

22.2.4.4.2 Mode of Action of Local Anaesthetics

Local anaesthetics reversibly prevent the generation and the propagation of active potentials in all excitable membranes including nerve fibres by stabilising the membrane. They achieve this by preventing the transient increase in sodium permeability of the excitable membrane. Generally small diameter cells are more sensitive to their action than larger diameter cells. It has also been observed that small diameter nerve fibres are more susceptible to the action of local anaesthetics than larger diameter ones. However, it may be remembered that fibre diameter though very important but is not always the only factor that determines the relative sensitivity of the nerve fibres to the action of the local anaesthetics.

22.2.5 Analgesics

Analgesics are remedial agents which by virtue of their action on central nervous system lower the sensation of pain.

22.2.5.1 Classification of Analgesics

Analgesics are broadly classified into two groups:

(a) *Narcotics:* These drugs produce analgesia and sleep, and in high doses cause unconsciousness. They are mainly the opium alkaloids or their synthetic and semi-synthetic derivatives. Opium is obtained by making superficial incisions on the immature and unripe capsules of poppy-plant—*Papaver somniferum.* The opium class of narcotic drugs are considered as very strong analgesics. They are also very potent and clinically useful agents causing depression of central nervous system. Morphine, codeine, phethidine, etc. belong to this category of analgesics. They are generally referred to as *Opioid or Opiate group* of *analgesics.*

It may be mentioned that the chronic use of these analgesics leads to addiction.

(b) *Non-narcotics:* These are weak analgesics but do not cause addiction. They usually produce an antipyretic effect also. Aspirin, analgin, phenacetin, cinchophen, etc. constitute the examples of non-narcotic analgesics.

22.2.5.1.1 Narcotic Analgesics (Opioid Analgesics)

As mentioned earlier these analgesics produce drowsiness and analgesia. The term 'narcotic' is derived from the Greek word *"narcotue"* which means drowsiness. The term narcotic is now used to refer to dependence producing drugs.

Narcotic analgesics produce euphoria which is an important factor in their addictive property. This property of these drugs limits their use. Besides this property, these drugs have other limitations such as respiratory depression, decreased gastrointestinal motility which causes constipation, increase billiary tract pressure and pruritus due to histamine release. These drawbacks of narcotic drugs led to develop other analgesics having minimal addictive actions and fewer side-effects.

22.2.5.1.1.1 Classification of Narcotic Analgesic (Opioid Analgesic)

Narcotics or opioid analgesics are generally classified on the basis of their basic chemical structures as depicted below:

22.2.5.1.1.2 Morphine Group

These opioid analgesics are structurally related to naturally occurring opium alkaloid, morphine. They are potent analgesics. A few most important member of this group of opioid analgesics are discussed below:

1. *Morphine Sulphate:* Morphine is the major constituent of the poppy plant. Although it has been synthesised yet even today the main bulk of morphine is obtained from natural source:

   Isolation: It can be isolated by following any of the common methods. Most frequently used method of isolation of morphine involves concentration of aqueous extract of powdered plant materials followed by its neutralisation with calcium chloride solution. The neutralised solution is filtered and is further concentrated. The crude morphine hydrochloride separates out. It is purified by precipitation with ammonia and crystallised as sulphate. Structurally it is be expressed as

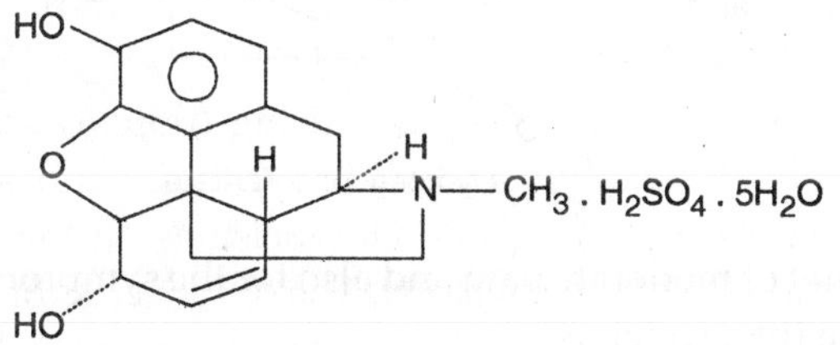

It is employed as analgesic, antitussive, adjunct to anaesthesia and nonspecific antidiarrheal agent. In lower dose it alleviates continued dull pain but in higher dose it relieves acute pain of traumatic or visceral origin. It is specifically used in the management of post-operative pain and pre-operative apprehension.

2. *Diamorphine Hydrochloride:* Structurally, it is hydrochloride of diacetyl derivative of morphine and prepared as under:

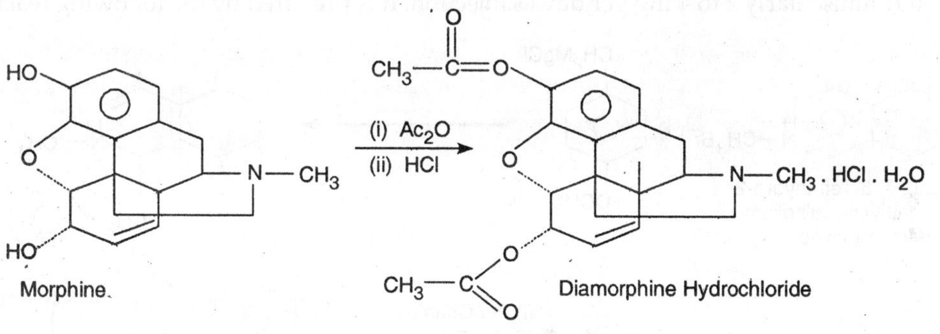

It is found to be more potent analgesic than morphine but has a shorter duration. It is normally used for the relief of severe pain particularly in terminal illness. It can be used in pre- and post-operative stages but as it is habit-forming in nature its use is rigidly controlled.

3. *Codeine:* It is monomethyl ether of morphine and is the congener of morphine, i.e.,

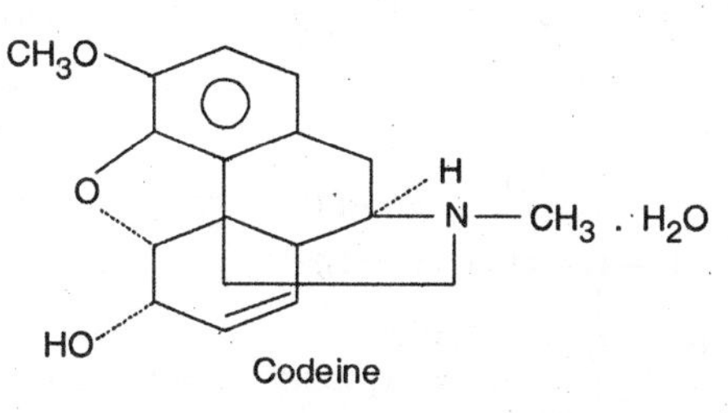

Its action is similar to morphine but its analgesic activity is much less.

4. *Hydrocodone Tartrate:* It is prepared from codeine as shown below:

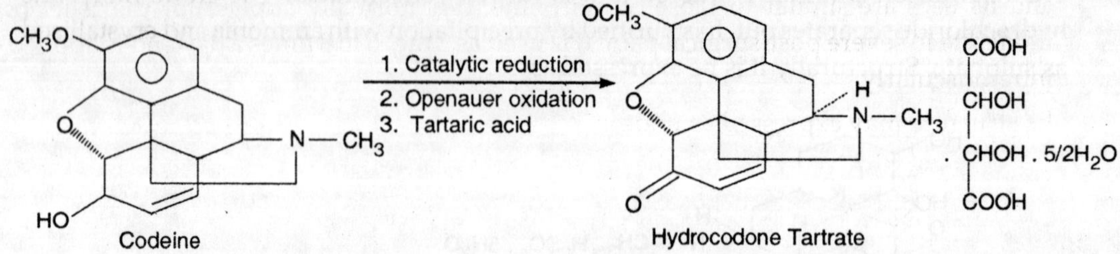

It is generally used for the relief of moderate pain and also for the symptomatic treatment of cough. It is more addictive than codeine.

22.2.5.1.1.3 Morphinan Group

Morphinan group of compounds conain a modified morphine nucleus in their molecules. These type of chemicals were found to be potent analgesics. Two classical examples of this group are considered below:

1. *Levorphanol Tartrate (Levorphanol):* It is a potent narcotic analgesic. It is used effectively for the management of both moderate and severe pain. At lower dose it produces anaesthesia. It is generally employed 1.5-4.5 mg twice orally per day for severe pain while as intramuscularly 2 to 4 mg per day as injection. It is prepared by the following reactions.

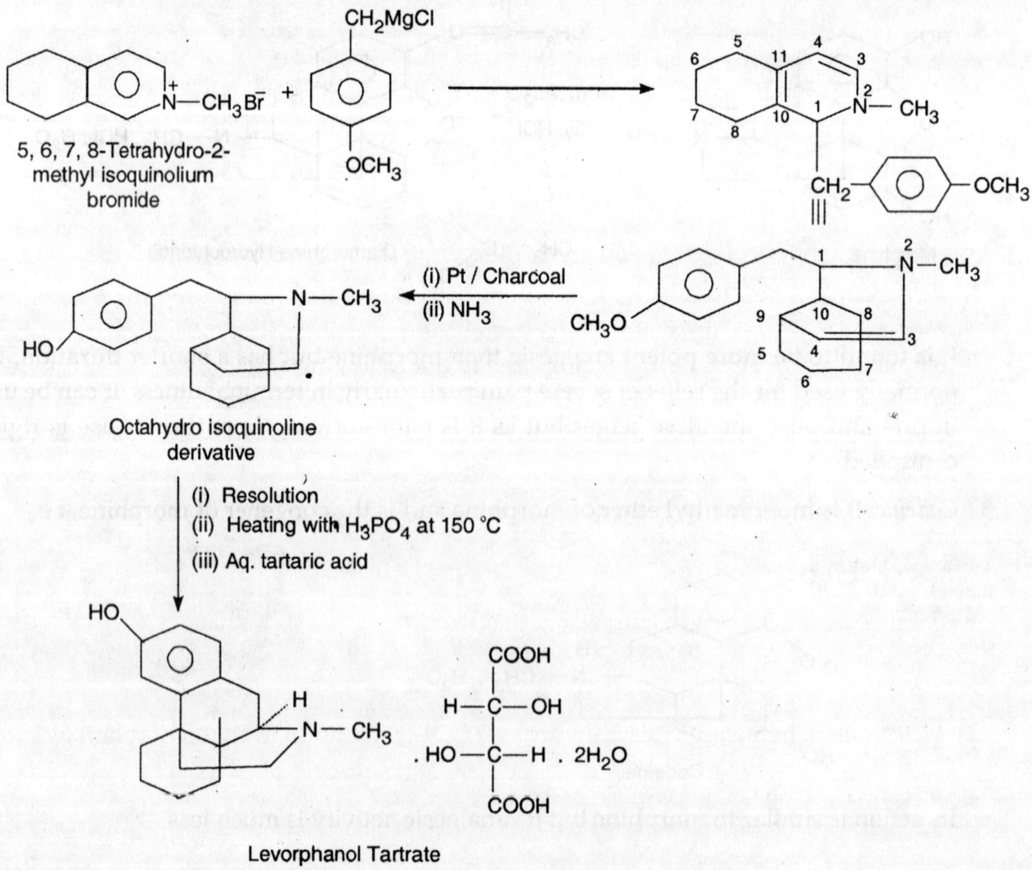

2. *Butrophanol Tartrate (Butrophanol):* It is a synthetic opiod parenteral analgesic with actions and its uses are similar to those of morphine. It is normally applied for the relief of moderate to severe post-surgical pain. It is used as 2 mg, 6 to 8 times a day and is applied intramuscularly.

   Its structure may expressed as under:

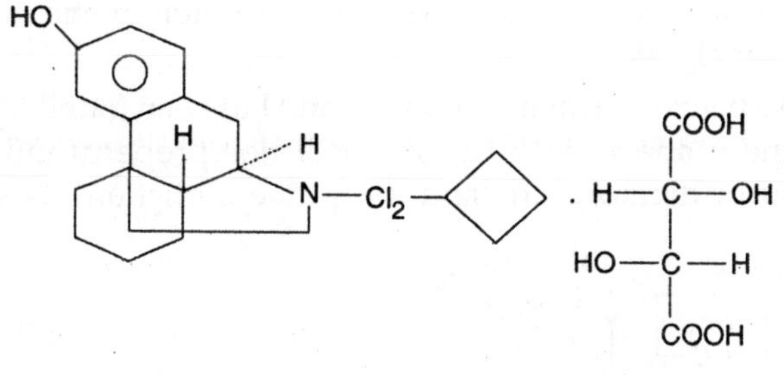

It is prepared from 5, 6, 7, 8-tetrahydro-2-cyclo-butyl methyl-isoquinolium bromide following the similar pathways as applied in the case of levorphanol tartrate.

22.2.5.1.1.4 Morphan Group

Morphan nucleus is a bridged perhydroazocine skeleton containing compound as shown below:

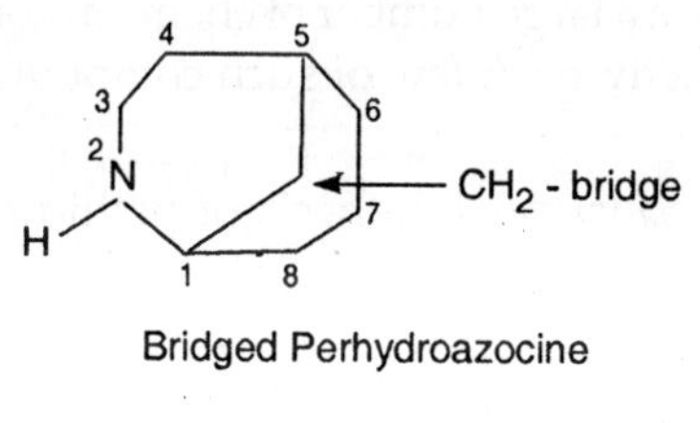

Bridged Perhydroazocine

Important members of this group are pentazocine, cyclazocine and metazocine.

1. *Pentazocine:* It is 3 to 4 times less potent than morphine and is used for the control of moderate to acute pain. It also exerts some sedative actions. Its dose is 20-60 mg as lactate, 6-8 times a day. Pentazocine is prepared in the following way:

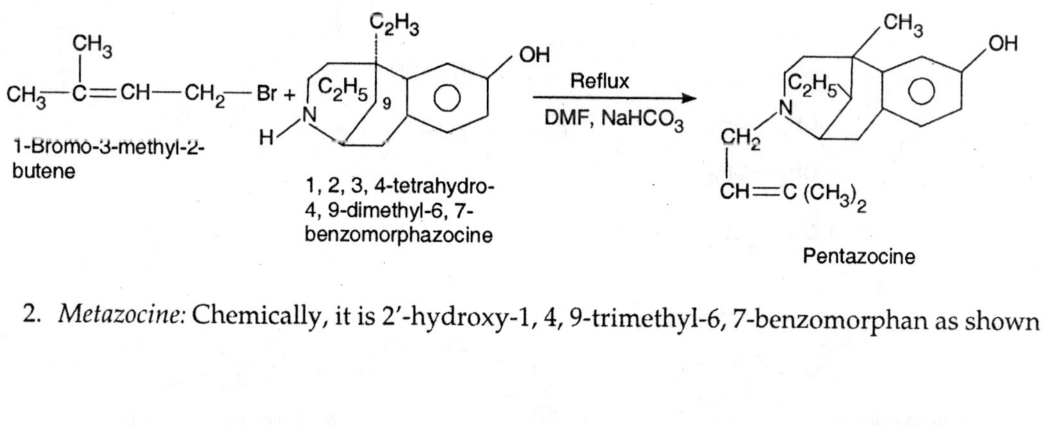

2. *Metazocine:* Chemically, it is 2'-hydroxy-1, 4, 9-trimethyl-6, 7-benzomorphan as shown:

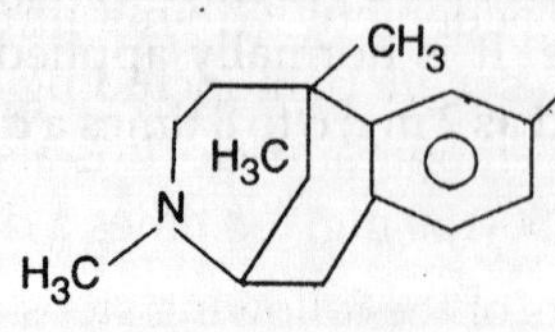

It has strong analgesic action. But due to its high psychotomimetic side-effects it is not generally used as an analgesic.

3. *Cyclazocine:* It is also a benzomorphan derivative and has been found to be 40 times more potent than morphine as analgesic. It has less addiction property and is used clinically for the management of diamorphine and morphine addiction. Its structure may be expressed as under.

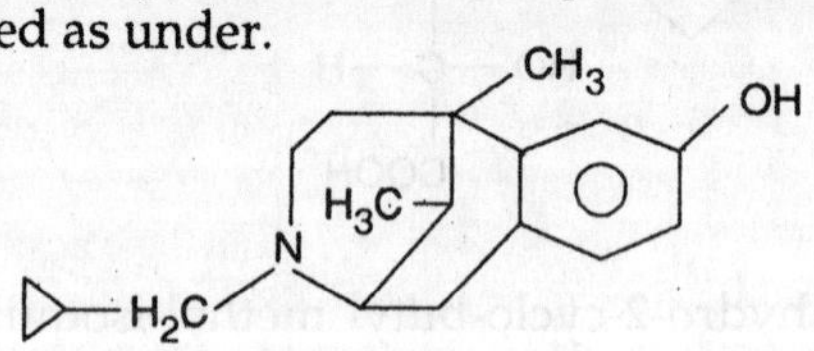

22.2.5.1.1.5 Phenylpiperidine Group

The discovery of narcotic analgesic activity in 4-phenylpiperidine class of compounds is to some extent accidental. During the search for anticholinergic drug structurally analogous to atropine it was observed that meperidine (phethidine), a 4-phenylpiperidine derivative is a potent narcotic analgesic. This discovery ultimately led to prepare a large number of chemical compounds having 4-phenylpiperidine skeleton having analgesic activity. A few of such compounds are discussed below:

1. *Pethidine hydrochloride (Meperidine hydrochloride):* Synthesis of pethidine hydrochloride involves the following steps:

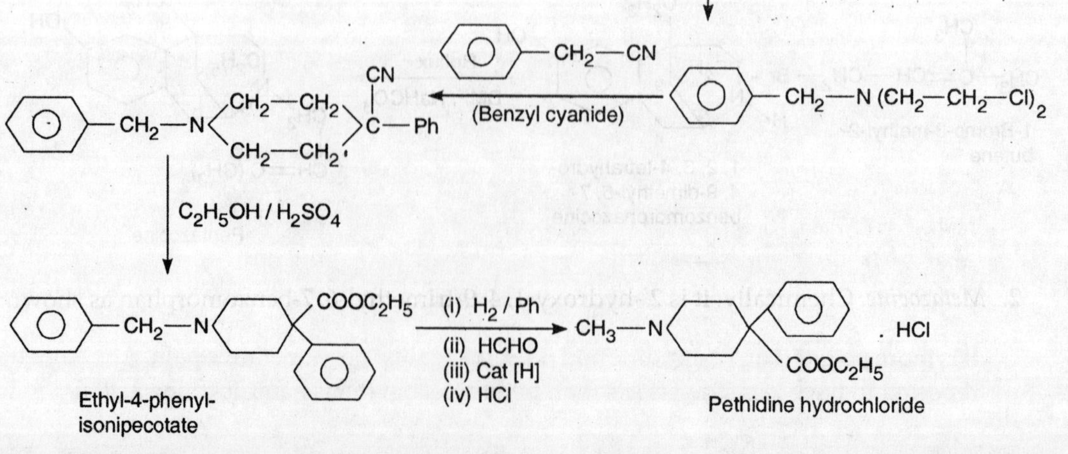

Phethidine is an analgesic with morphine-like action but with minimum habit forming nature. It is used for the relief of moderate to severe pain including labour and post-operative pain. It has atrophine-like action on smooth muscle. It is also used to induce both sedative and analgesic action. Its dose is 50-150 mg, 6-8 times a day orally.

2. *Fentanyl Citrate (Fentanyl):* Its synthesis consists of the following steps of reactions:

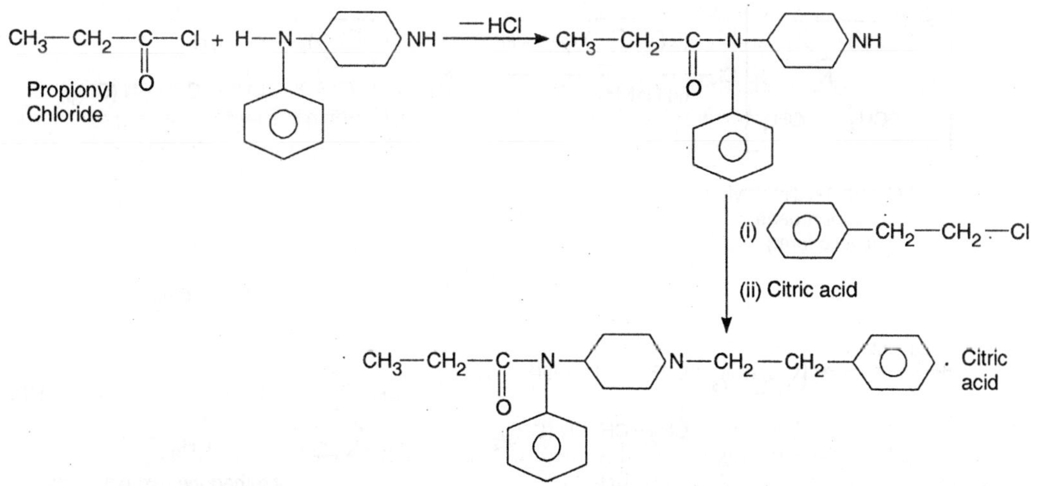

It is a potent narcotic analgesic generally used for the arrest of all types of post-operative pain. It has rapid on-set and short duration of action. Its doses are 0.05 to 1 mg, 30-60 minutes before surgical procedure (intramuscular) and 0.05 to 0.1 mg intravenously for rapid analgesic action.

3. *Anileridine (Leridine):* It is obtained by the condensation of 4-aminophenylethyl chloride hydrochloride with ethyl ester of 4-phenyl hexahydro isonicotinic acid carbamate.

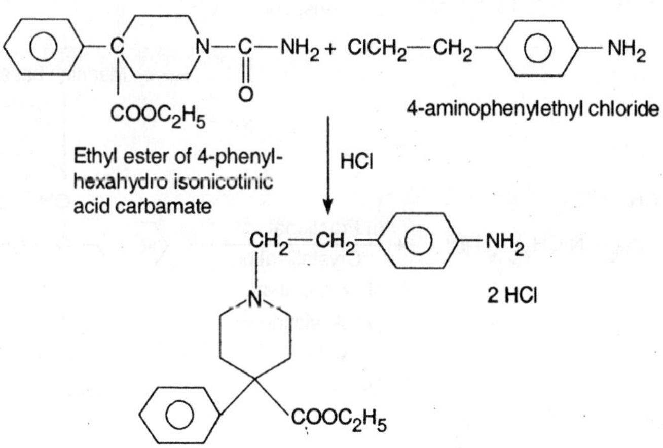

Anileridine hydrochloride

It is more potent than phethidine and is useful against post-operative pain. Although it is reported to have less side-effects than pethidine, but it has habit-forming action.

22.2.5.1.1.6 Phenylpropylamine Group

It is an important class of analgesics belonging to opioid group. These are considered to be extremely flexible among most analgesics conformationally. A few important members are considered below:

1. *Methadone hydrochloride (Amidine or adanone):* It is prepared as below:

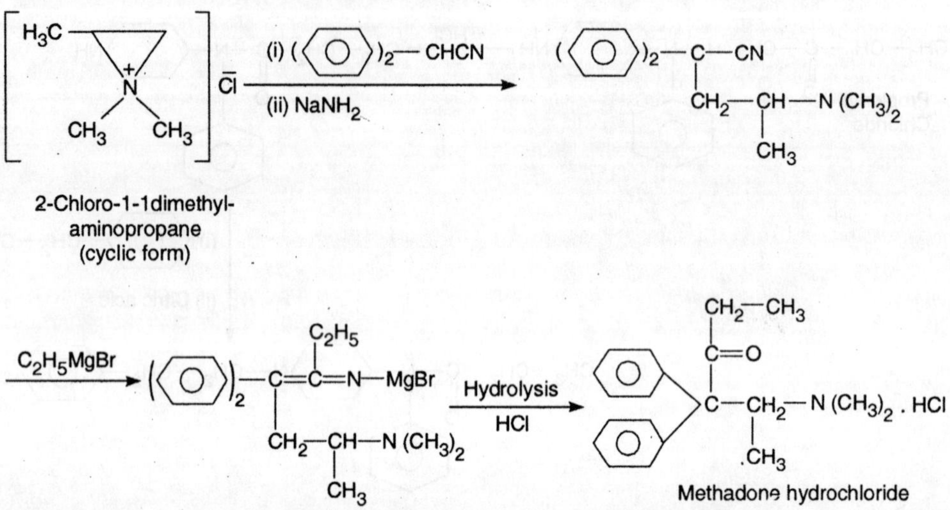

It is an active opioid analgesic having actions similar to morphine but it is less potent than morphine. It has also sedative and antitussive properties. It helps in the temporary maintenance and treatment on dependence on narcotic drugs.

2. *Dextro protoxyphene hydrochloride (Propoxyphene hydrochloride):* Synthesis of this opioid analgesic involves the following steps:

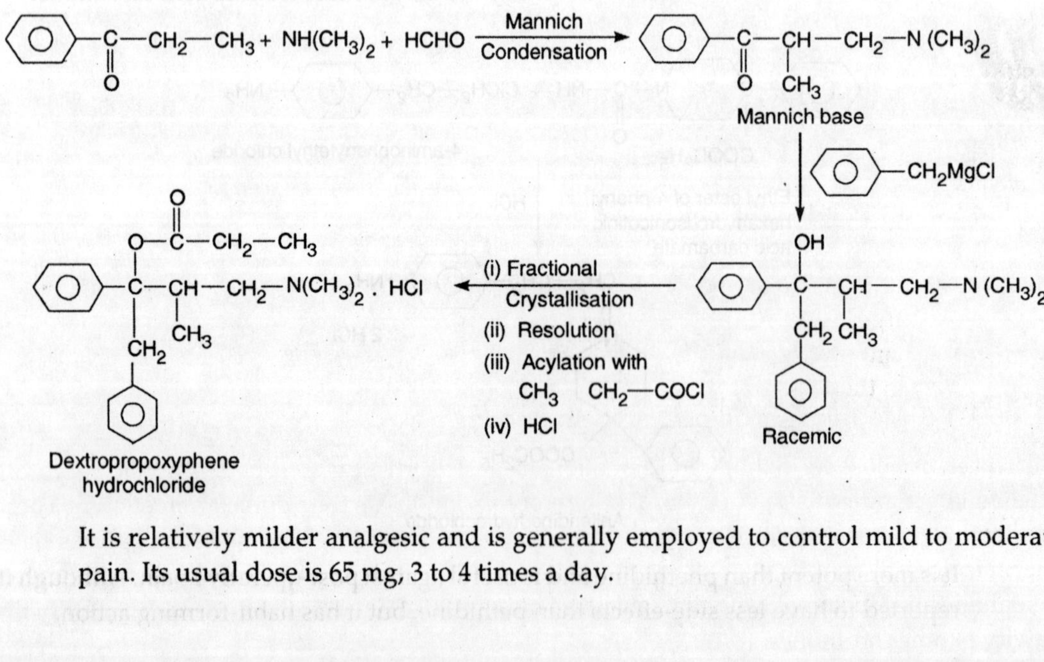

It is relatively milder analgesic and is generally employed to control mild to moderate pain. Its usual dose is 65 mg, 3 to 4 times a day.

22.2.5.1.1.7 Miscellaneous Group of Opioid Analgesics

Search has been made to prepare narcotic analgesics belonging to different structural pattern of chemical compounds. A few examples of such analgesics with their uses are mentioned below:

1. *Tildate hydrochloride (Tilidine, Tilidine hydrochloride):* Structure of this analgesic may be expressed as below:

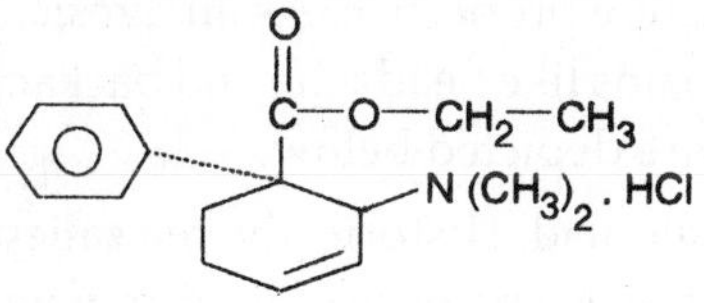

   It is usually used in the treatment of moderate to severe pain. Its normal dose is 50-100 mg, 4 times per day.

2. *Dezocine:* It possess analgesic as well as narcotic antagonist properties and is normally administered by injection (dose 10-15 mg) for the relief of severe pain. It is represented by the following structure:

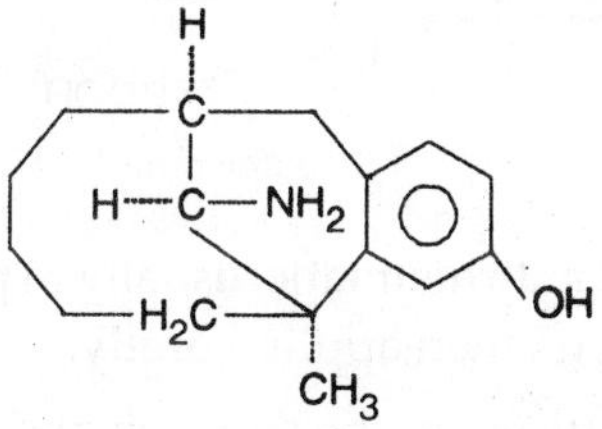

3. *Sufentanil* and 4. *Nexeridine hydrochloride:* These are the two other narcotic analgesics. They are expressed by the structures below:

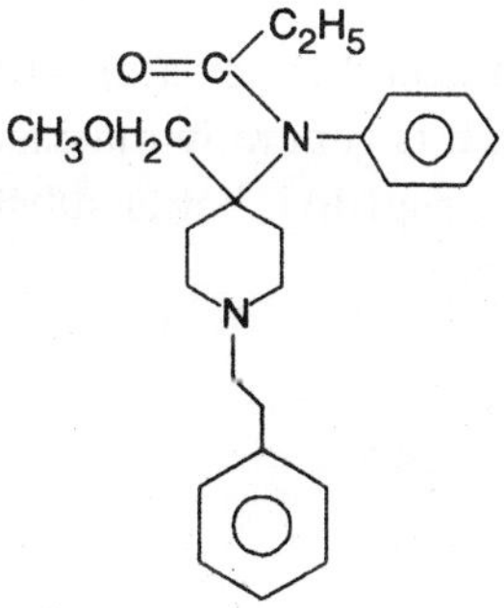

Sufentanil

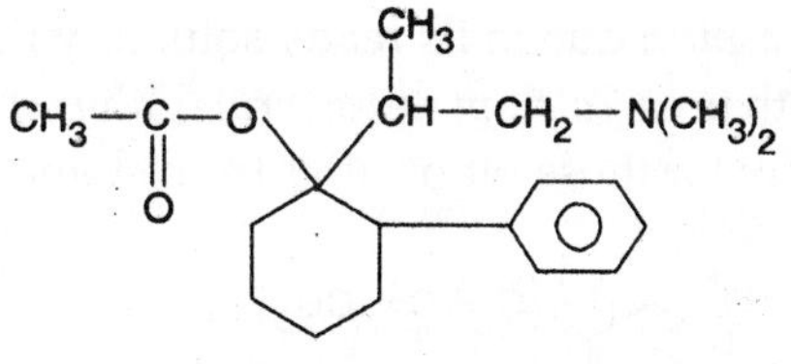

Nexeridine hydrochloride

22.2.5.1.1.8 Mode of Action of Opioid Analgesics

It has been established that opioid (narcotic) analgesic activate stereospecific opioid receptors situated in certain parts of the CNS. These receptors modulate the appreciation of pain. These receptors have been identified as endorphins type of peptides. This type of peptides have pharmacological actions on opioids. Two important members of endorphins, methionine-enkephalin and leucine-enkephalin, which are most probably neurotransmitters, can modify the activity of other hormones.

22.2.5.1.2 Non-narcotic (Non-opioid) Analgesics

Non-narcotic analgesics are primarily antipyretics or febrifuges and are normally used as remedial agents for lowering the body temperature in pyrexia. However, they have mild analgesic activity. For this reason they are also known as *antipyretic-analgesics.* The most commonly used analgesic of this category are paracetamol, aspirin, analgin pyrozolones and quinoline derivatives. It may be mentioned that these analgesics have no addictive properties. As analgesic, their use is very limited. They are usually used in mild aches and pains like headache and backache. Preparations and uses of some of the analgesics of this gruop are depicted below:

1. *Aspirin:* It is the acetyl derivative of salicylic acid. Historically, the salicylates are among the first of this group to achieve recognition as analgesics. Aspirin was introduced into medicine by Drester in 1899. It is prepared by refluxing salicylic acid with either a mixture of acetic anhydride and acetic acid in presence of concentrated H_2SO_4 or with acetic anhydride in presence of pyridine.

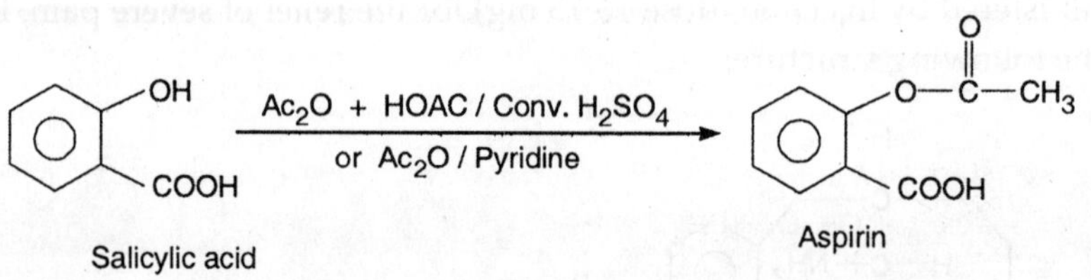

   Aspirin is used as an antipyretic, analgesic and antirheumatic, usually in powder, capsule or in tablet form. It has some anaesthetic action when applied orally.

   It has some side-effects. It may cause minute ulcers in the stomach and cause bleeding. Some persons are allergic to aspirin. The normal allergic reaction is rashes on skin, lowering of blood pressure, bronchial spasm, profuse sweating, intense thirst, neusia and vomitting.

   Aspirin is also used as its calcium salt (calcium acetyl salicylate) which is known as *soluble aspirin* due to its ready solubility in water. It is generally marketed as a complex salt with urea, *calcium carbaspirin (Calurin).* Soluble aspirin is better substitute for aspirin specially for those who suffer from stomach ulcers.

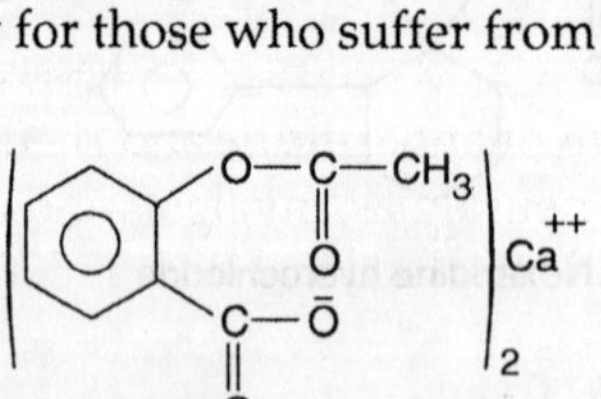

Soluble aspirin

   Aspirin is regarded as the drug of choice in the reduction of fever due to its high degree of effectiveness and wide safety margin. As aspirin inhibits platelet function, it has been employed prophylactically to minimise the incidence of myocardial infraction and transient ischemic attacks. Its usual dose is 300-650 mg every 3 or 4 hours orally.

2. *Salol and Oil of Wintergreen:* Salol is phenyl salicylate and is prepared by heating salicylic acid and phenol at 120 °C in presence of $POCl_3$. It was first introduced as a drug by Nencki.

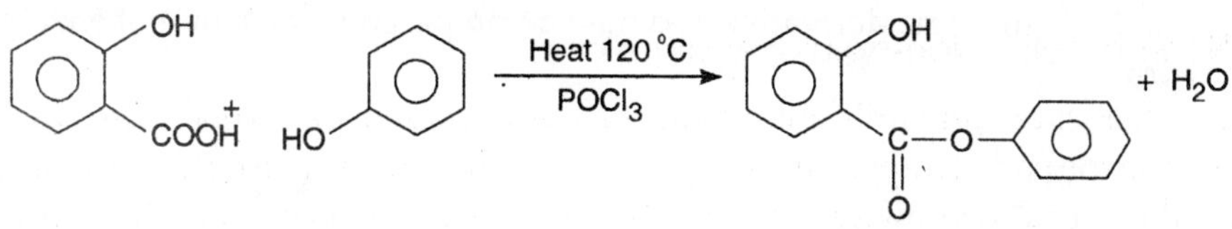

Salol

It is used as antipyretic and also as external antiseptic and mild analgesic. When it is taken by a patient, it passes unhydrolysed in the stomach but undergoes hydrolysis slowly in the intestine into phenol and salicylic acid which are active components. Since its biological hydrolysis is very slow, its toxic effects (due to active components) remain hidden and only its analgesic and antipyretic effects are shown. This principle is known as *salol principle or Nencki principle.* There are two types of salol—true and partial. True salols are those in which both salicylic acid and phenol are active pharmacologically. Salol itself and betol (β-naphthyl salicylate) belong to true salol group while partial salols are those in which either acid or the phenolic hydroxyl is pharmacologically active. Methyl salicylate (oil of wintergreen) which is marketed as *Iodex* is the most important member of partial salol group.

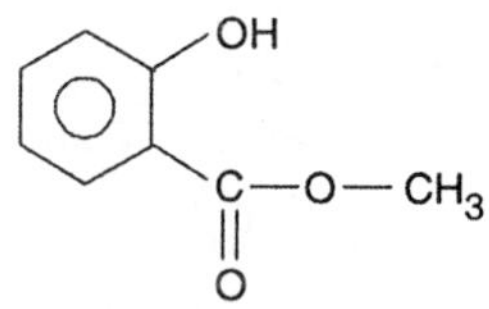

Methyl salicylate
(Oil of wintergreen)

3. *Paracetamol:* Paracetamol is the acetyl derivative of *p*-aminophenol and is prepared as below:

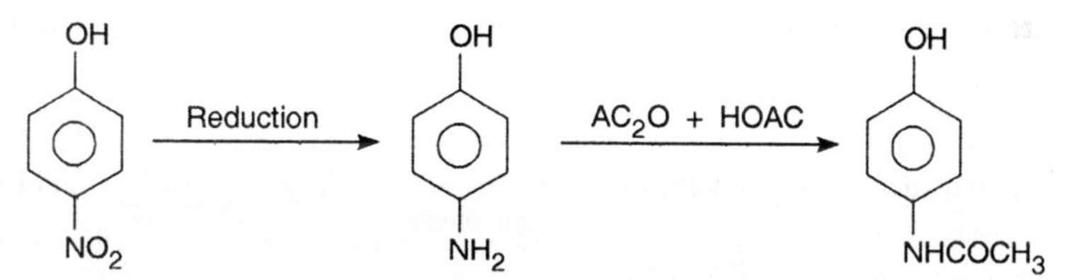

p-Nitrophenol *p*-Aminophenol Paracetamol

It may be effectively used in a broad spectrum of antiarthritic and rheumatic conditions linked with musculoskeletal pain, headache, neuralgias, myalgias and dysmenorrhea. It is particularly useful for aspirin-sensitive patients. Its usual dose is 500 mg to 1 g, 3 to 4 times a day.

4. *Phenacetin:* Chemically, it is *p*-ethoxy acetanilide and is prepared from phenol as shown below:

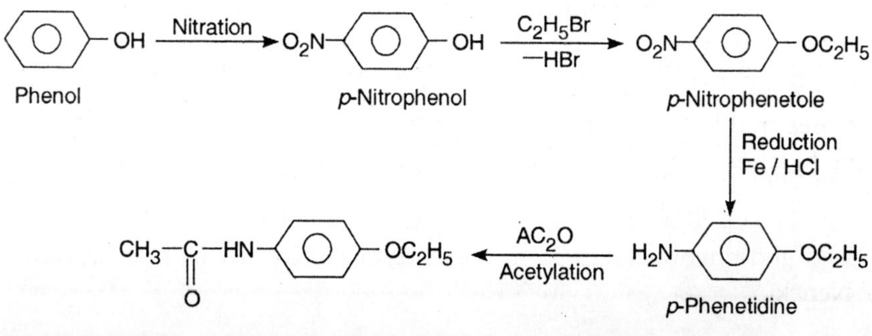

5. *Cinchophen:* It is quinoline derivative and may be prepared from *o*-aminobenzaldehyde cyanohydrin

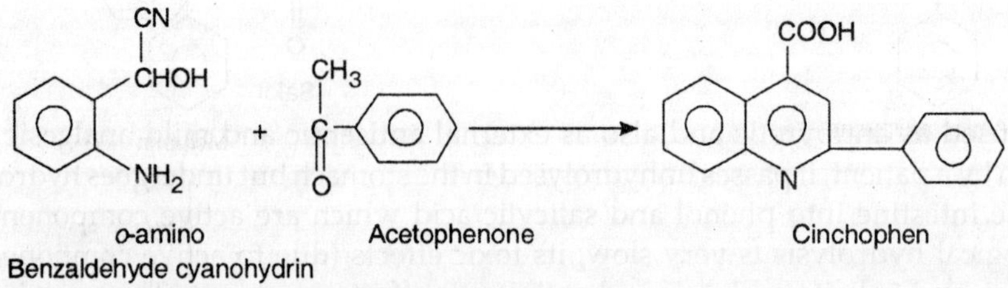

Cinchophen has similar action as salicylates. It is mainly used in the treatment of gout. It has limited use because of its tendency to cause jaundice and other toxic symtoms. It has now been replaced by safer drugs. It is used in 300-600 mg dose per day.

6. *Aminopyrine (Amidopyrine):* It is pyrazoline derivative. It is prepared from antipyrine in the following manner.

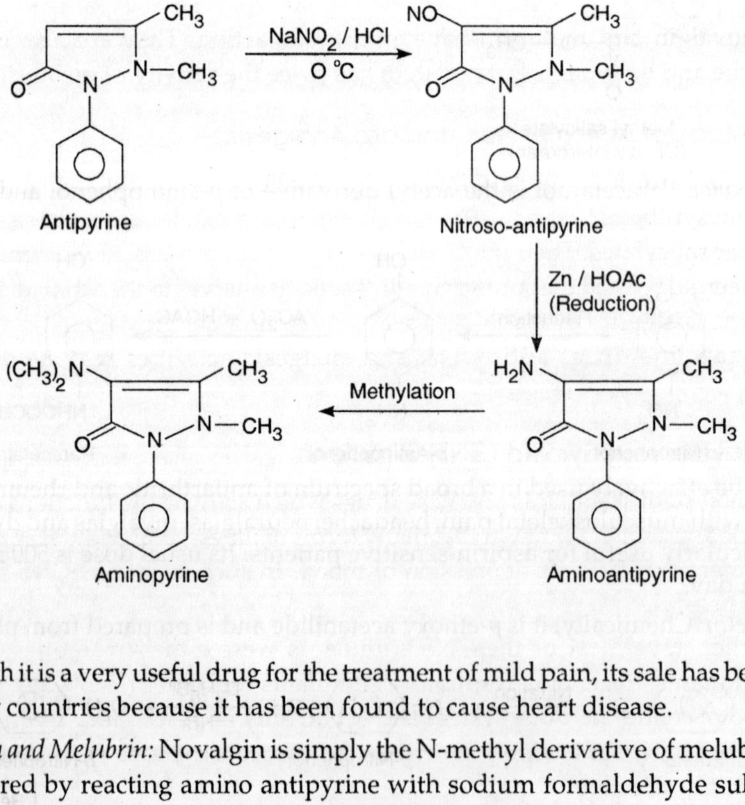

Although it is a very useful drug for the treatment of mild pain, its sale has been prohibited in many countries because it has been found to cause heart disease.

7. *Novalgin and Melubrin:* Novalgin is simply the N-methyl derivative of melubrin. Melubrin is prepared by reacting amino antipyrine with sodium formaldehyde sulphoxide, and methylation of melubrin with dimethyl sulphate gives novalgin.

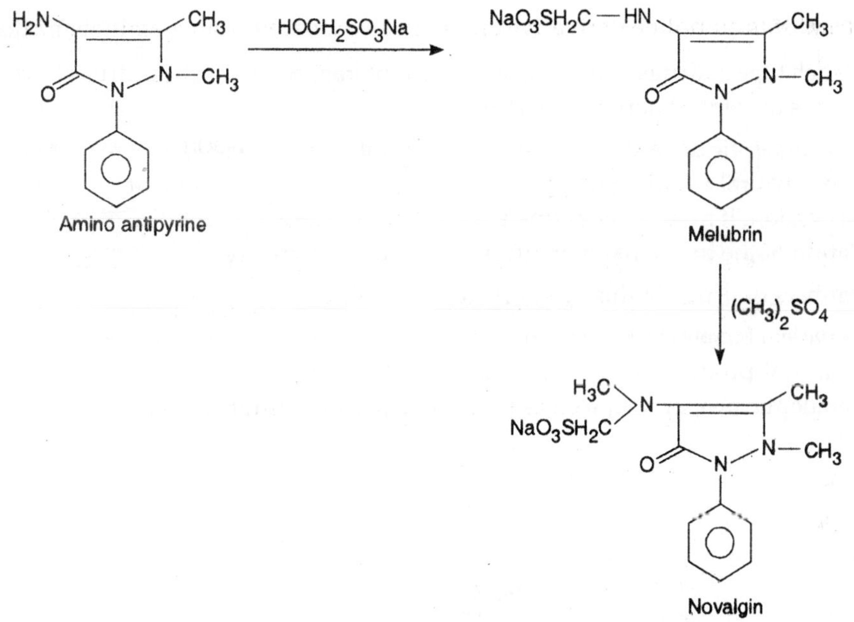

Both novalgin and melubrin have antipyretic action. They are also used to subside headache and bodypains but novalgin has twice the activity of melubrin.

22.2.5.1.2.1 Mode of Action of Non-narcotic Analgesics

The antipyretic and anti-inflammatory properties of salicylates are due to their inhibitory effect on prostaglandin synthesis. Vane in 1951 has shown that prostglandin synthesis is inhibited by aspirin and other salicylates. Their inhibitory activity is proportional to their anti-inflammatory actions. It has been suggested that prostaglandins sensitise nerves to the action of pain stimulants. Other antipyretic analgesics probably also act by inhibiting the prostaglandin synthesis. But in the case of pyrazoline drugs antipyretic and analgesic activities may be due to different mechanism.

22.2.6 Central Nervous System (CNS) Stimulants

Central nervous system stimulants are those drugs which activate the functions of various parts of central nervous system. It is known that many forms of illness, both mental and physical cause depression of mental activity or depression of mood. In such situations CNS stimulant drugs become highly helpful.

In the earlier days most of the CNS stimulants were either analeptics (restorative) or respiratory stimulants. In general, respiratory stimulants function in two ways, viz., change the pH in the blood of central nervous system and act directly on respiratory centre of the nervous system. In most of the cases analeptics increase the vasoconstrictions of the blood vessel walls which are primarily affected.

22.2.6.1 Classification of Central Nervous System Stimulants

CNS stimulants are broadly classified into three groups: (i) analeptics (ii) xanthine derivatives and (iii) miscellaneous CNS stimulants:

22.2.6.1.1 Analeptics

Analeptics are such type of drugs which are used to counteract narcosis. These drugs have specific stimulating actions on central nervous system.

An effective analeptic drug should stimulate respiration producing an increased ventilation and improved peripheral circulation. These drugs are mainly used to combat the drug-induced respiratory depression. It may be mentioned that excessive dose of analeptics may result a wide spread stimulation of the brain that may ultimately cause convulsions.

A few members of drugs of this category are discussed.

(a) *Strychnine and Picrotoxin:* Strychnine is the first member to be used as analeptic stimulant. It is a natural product and has been isolated from *strychnos nux vomica.* But due to its weak analeptic property as well as poisonous nature it is rarely used.

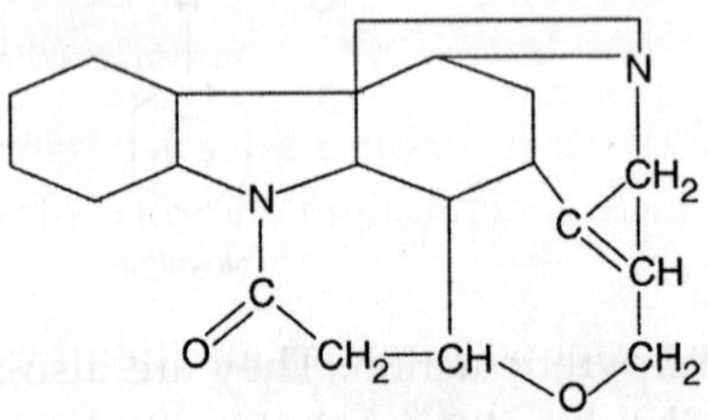

Strychnine

Picrotoxin is also a naturally occurring analeptic agent. It is isolated from the seeds of the shrub *anamirta cocculus.* It is a powerful central nervous system stimulant commonly used to combat the adverse effect caused from overdose of barbiturates and other drugs.

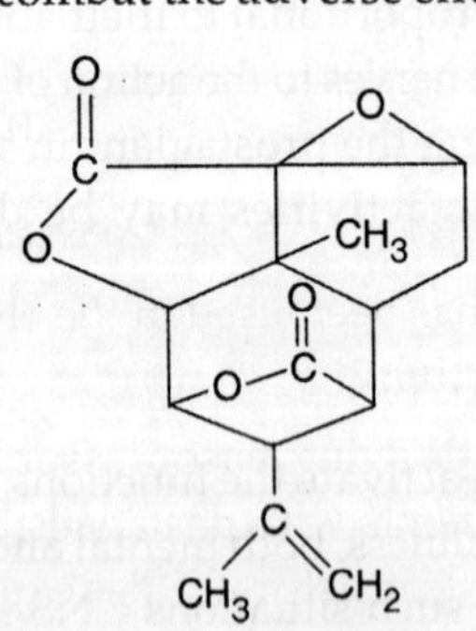

Picrotoxin

(b) *Nikethamide (Coramine):* It is a respiratory stimulant. It has an intermediate central stimulant effect. It is prepared as shown below:

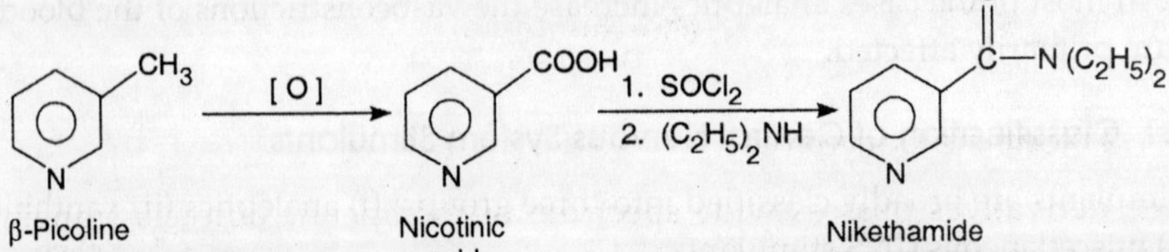

It is a cardiovascular drug having a direct action on heart. It is used to promote coronary flow in myocardial infraction. It is also used as a respiratory stimulant.

(c) *Ethamivan (Etamivan):* Ethamivan is prepared from vanillin as discussed below:

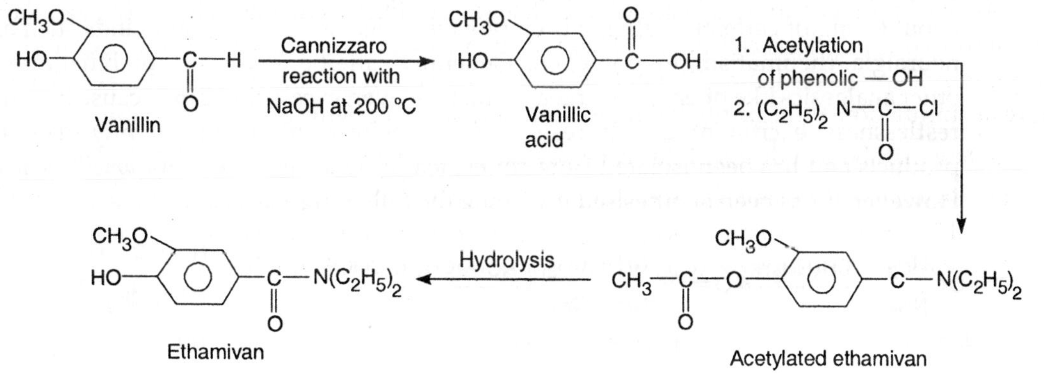

Ethamivan is a respiratory stimulant and is useful as an adjunctive agent in the treatment of severe respiratory depression. It produces general stimulation of central nervous system but its high dose may lead to convulsions.

(d) *Pentetrazol (Metrazole):* Formerly pentetrazol was used as injection for the treatment of drug-induced coma and as a convulsant for shock-therapy. But due to unfavourable therapentic index it has now been replaced by more effective and less hazardous drugs. Its preparation involves the following reactions.

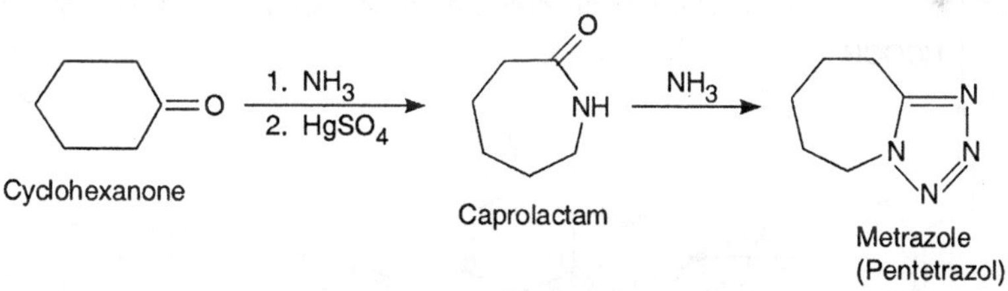

It is now used to induce convulsion in animal. It has been used in the elderly subjects to alleviate the symptoms of mental and physical activity.

(e) *Doxapram (Dopram):* It is a respiratory stimulant having vasopressor properties. It is frequently used to stimulate respiration in the patients with postanaesthetic respiratory depression and to hasten arousal during this period. Structurally, it is expressed as below:

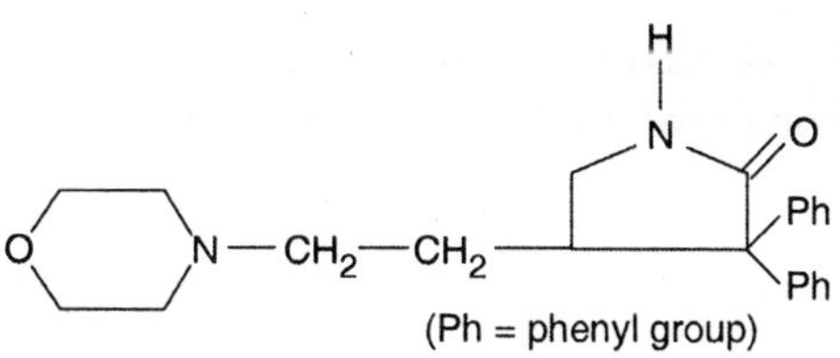

(Ph = phenyl group)
Doxapram

22.2.6.1.2 Xanthine Derivatives

Xanthine derivatives possess wide spectrum of therapeutic efficacies ranging from their stimulation of cardiac muscle and central nervous system, enhanced diuresis and a soothing relaxation of bronchi and the coronary arteries. Most of these derivatives are naturally occurring compounds. Illustrative members of this class of compounds are caffeine, theobromine, theophylline, aminophylline and proxyphylline.

(a) *Caffeine:* It is the most important member of this group. A cup of tea or coffee contains about 60 mg of caffeine. Caffeine is employed in headaches of certain kinds such as in neuralgia, rheumatism, migraine, etc. Generally caffeine is used in combination with other analgesics like phenacetin and aspirin. However, excess doses may cause insomnia, restlessness, excitment and diuresis. Caffeine belongs to alkaloid family of natural products and has been isolated from coffee, tea or the dried leaves of *Camellia sinensis.* However, it has been synthesised involving the following reactions:

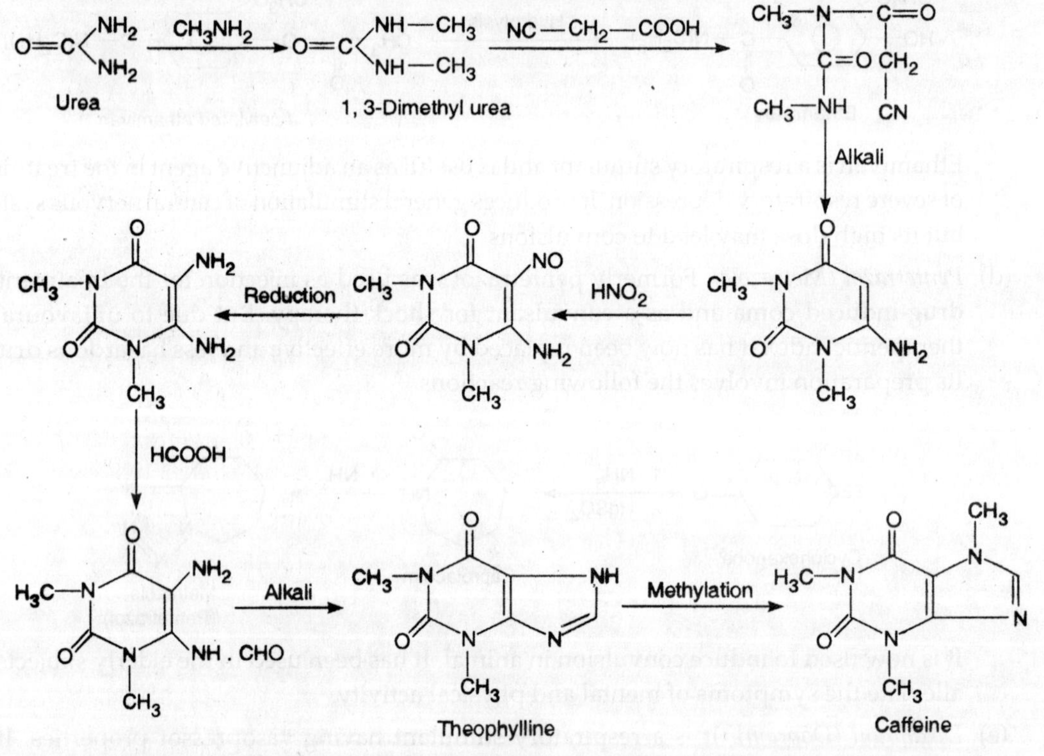

(b) ***Theophylline:*** **Theophylline is often used in the treatment and symptomatic relief of acute and chronic bronchial asthma, bronchospasm, cardiac dyspnea and angina pectoris.**

Theophylline is also a naturally occurring compound; however, it can be prepared as described during the preparation of caffeine. Its structure may be expressed as below:

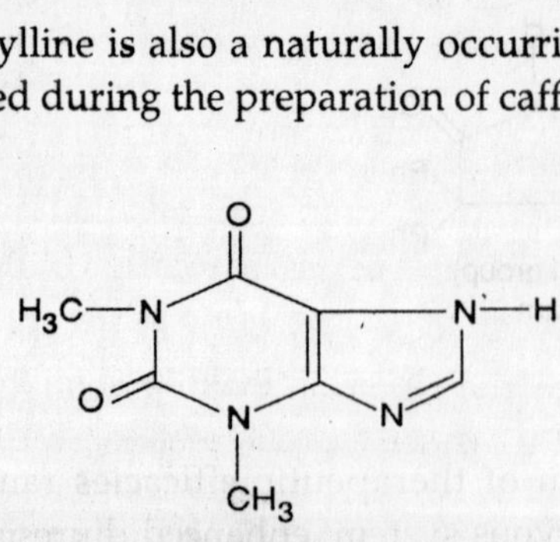

Theophylline

(c) *Theobromine:* Theobromine is also a xanthine derivative. It is the main component of cocoa. It is, however, prepared from N-methyl urea as depicted below:

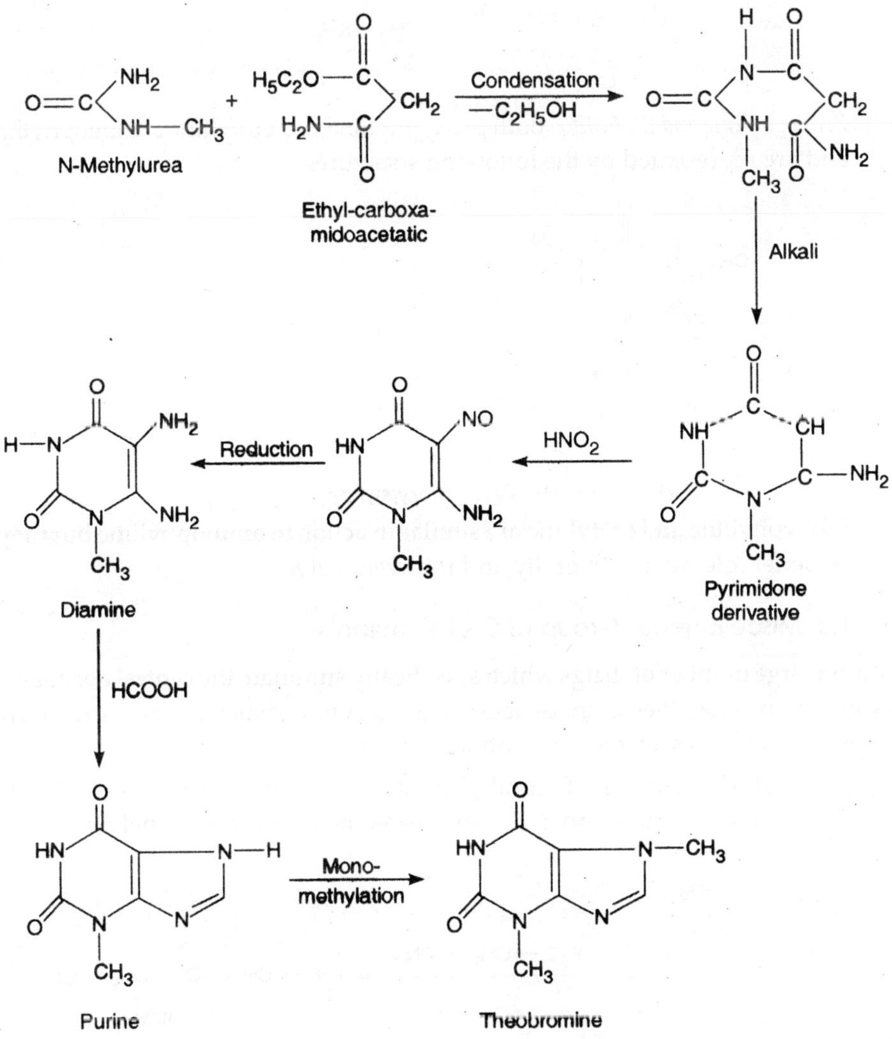

The action of theobromine on central nervous system is minimum and so it is used for other effects like diuretic effect on the coronary arteries without showing any significant side-action of central stimulation.

(d) *Aminophylline:* It is often used for the treatment and control of congestive heart failure, bronchial asthma, Cheyne-Stokes respiration, cardiac paroxymal dyspnea. It is a vital ingredients of many cough syrup used to reduce the cough reflexes and to cause expectoration.

Aminophylline is usually prepared by the vigorous shaking of mixture of theophylline and ethylene diamine in the ratio 2 : 1 in anhydrous ethanol. Structurally it may be represented as shown:

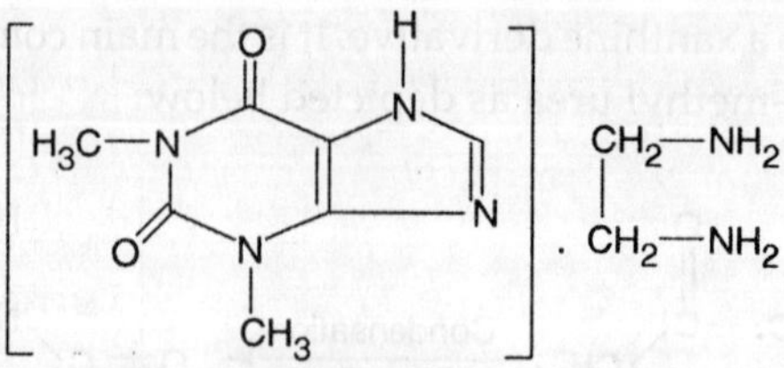

(e) *Proxyphylline and Etofylline:* Both proxyphylline and etofylline are theophylline derivatives and are represented by the following structures:

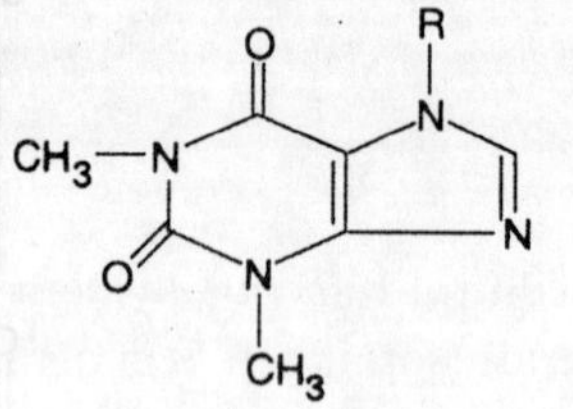

$R = —CH_2—CH_2—OH$ Etofylline

$R = —CH_2—CH(OH)—CH_3$ Proxyphylline

Proxyphylline and etofylline are similar in action to aminophylline but they are found to be better tolerated both orally and intravenously.

22.2.6.1.3 Miscellaneous Group of CNS Stimulants

There are a large number of drugs which specifically stimulate the central nervous system. These drugs are grouped together as anorexigenic agents. A few of such drugs, particularly those which act on central nervous system, are mentioned below:

(a) *Flurothyl:* The synthesis of flurothyl involves the interaction between 2, 2,2-trifluoro-ethyl-*p*-toluene sulphonate and 2, 2, 2-trifluoro-ethoxide as shown below:

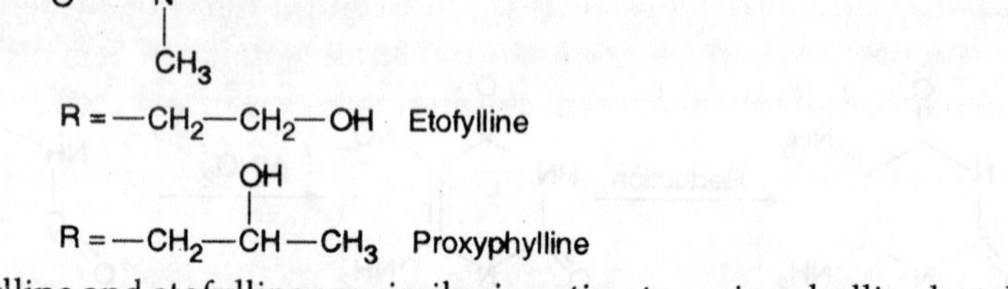

2, 2, 2-Trifluro-ethyl-*p*-toluene sulphonate

Flurothyl is capable of producing both tonic and clonic convulsions in experimental laboratory animals. It is frequently used as an alternative for electro convulsive therapy in the treatment of mental disorders. The on-set of action of this stimulant requires 15-20 seconds. Initially myoclonic convulsions occur which turn to violent tonic phase and it lasts for 30-90 seconds.

(b) *Amphetamine (Benzedrine):* It is a psychomotor stimulant and is generally used to improve the outlook of the patients with mental depression. It exerts a significant stimulating effect on the central nervous system. Its main use is to suppress appetite but its euphoriant qualities are a serious drawback. It is commonly prepared through following routes.

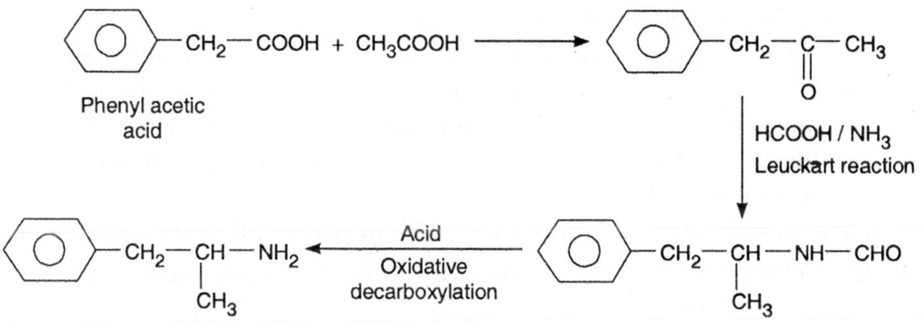

Amphetamine

(c) *Methylphenidate:* Methylphenidate is a mild central nervous system stimulant with therapeutic potency in between caffeine and amphetamine. It is generally employed in the treatment of brain dysfunction in children.

It is prepared as discussed below:

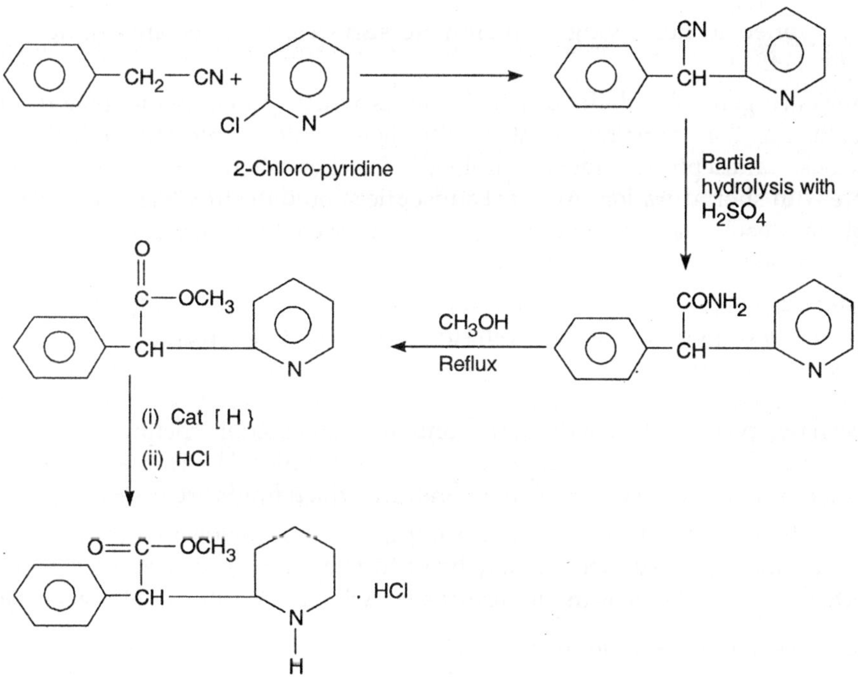

Methylphenidate hydrochloride

22.2.6.1.4 Mode of Action of CNS Stimulants

As mentioned before analeptics stimulate respiration giving an increased ventilation. They act as barbiturate antagonists as was observed in the case of nikethamide (coramine). Doxapram produces only a transient increase in respiration. Patients having depressed central activity may exhibit decreased pressor responses and ventilatory activity with doxapram.

Xanthine derivatives have been reported to afford cortical, medullary and spinal stimulation in large doses. They also produce stimulation of the medullary vasomotor centre. As a result peripheral resistance and blood pressure are increased. They can bring about vasoconstriction of cerebral arteries and that is why they are used in combination with ergot to relieve migraine headaches. In asthma they may be used to produce both relaxation of bronchial smooth muscle and respiratory stimulation. Xanthine derivatives have been reported to cause diuresis by increasing glomerular filtration and by blocking tubular reabsorption of sodium salts.

Fluoroethyl is normally used as a convulsant to produce electroshock like effects in the treatment of mental disorders.

22.2.7 Antiseptics, Disinfectants and Surfactants

The term 'septic' orignates from the Greek word 'septikos' meaning rotten or putrified. Medically, the term septic indicates a state infected by pus-forming organisms. The anti-infective agents which are directly applied to the skin wound etc. termed as *antiseptics* as well as *disinfectants*. However, the term 'anti-septic' is usually used to indicate those anti-infective agents which are applied to living tissues. Consequently, anti-septics are bacteriostatic in nature and generally do not sterilise the surface under treatment. On the other hand, disinfectants are bacterocides and are generally applied to non-living or inanimate surfaces. Disinfectants rapidly produce irreversible lethal effects.

Antiseptics are generally defined as substances which prevents the growth of micro-organisms as long as they remain in contact with them while disinfectants kill the organism outright. Obviously, antiseptic is milder but prolonged in action whereas the action of disinfectants are immediate with short duration. An ideal antiseptic should destroy bacteria, fungi, viruses, spores and other infective agents without causing any harm to the tissuses of the host. It may be mentioned that in medicine antiseptics are always applied locally due to their systematic toxicity.

A surfactant is a surface active agent and basically is a chemical compound which when dissolved in water or dispersed in liquid cleans the surface by removing oil, grease, etc., in which dust particles are dispersed. The cleansing action of a surfactant depends upon its surface activity. The surface activity is a special property which decreases the surface tension at the boundary surface between two phases. Most of the surfactants are water soluble chemical compounds and contain both hydrophobic and hydrophilic groups in their molecules. They are accumulated in the interfaces and act on the bacterial cell membrane in which lipids are present.

Surfactants are classified broadly into two groups, viz., ionic (ionogenic) and non-ionic (non-ionogenic) surfactants. Ionic surfactants may be of three types: (i) surfactants whose surface-active properties reside in anion as in the case of soap which in solution yields a simple cation, Na^+ and a surface-active carboxylate anion ($R-\underset{\underset{O}{\|}}{C}-\bar{O}$) are known as *anionic surfactants.* (ii) *cationic surfactants* are those in which the surface-active properties are the residents of a cation. Amine salts, quaternary ammonium compounds and nitrogenous and non-nitrogenous bases belong to this group. (iii) *amphoteric (ampholytic) surfactants* are those which contain both basic and acidic functions in their structures and can act as anionic or cationic depending on the pH range of the solution.

From the above discussion it is thus evident that antiseptic, disinfectant and surfactants are closely related substances and broadly speaking, all the three groups of substances are anti-infective agents and are complimentary to each other.

22.2.7.1 Standardisation of Antiseptic Property (Disinfecting Property)

Antiseptic action of a substance is standardised by *Rideal Walker method*. In this process at first the time required to kill a 24-hour culture of *B. typhos* by the minimum concentration of phenol is determined. In the next step the minimum concentration of the unknown substance which produce the same effect under identical conditions is determined. This relation is termed as Phenol coefficient or Rideal-Walker coefficient. It may be mentioned that this coefficient gives a rough idea of the value of an antiseptic.

22.2.7.2 Some Important Members of Antiseptics

Antiseptics may belong to different classes of organic compounds. Most commonly used antiseptics may be discussed under the following headings:

1. *Alcohols and Aldehydes:* (a) Alcohols particularly ethyl alcohol and isopropyl alcohols are extensively used as antiseptics. Generally 70% aqueous solutions of alcohols are used for bactericidal action. In some cases absolute alcohol may be used for the relief of carcinoma and in other conditions where pain is local. It has been observed that isopropyl alcohol has better antiseptic action than ethyl alcohal. Isopropyl alcohol is generally used to remove creosote from the skin and as a disinfectant for the skin and surgical instruments.

   (b) *Carboxide:* Commercially available product is a mixture of ethylene oxide (10%) and CO_2 (90%) and is usually used for the sterilisation of medical equipments.

   (c) *Formaldehyde:* Formaldehyde is used as an excellent germicide. Formaldehyde in gas form is used to disinfect rooms, clothing, instruments, etc. Its 40% solution in alcohol or water is used to harden skin to prevent excessive perspiration and to disinfect hands.

   Other aldehydic compounds which are used as antiseptics are paraformaldehyde, glutaraldehyde (Cidex).

   (d) *Urotropine:* Urotropine which is a condensation product of formaldehyde and ammonia is genrally used as urinary disinfectant. It is also used for disinfection of gall bladder, meninges, etc.

2. *Metal Containing Antiseptics:* The most important compounds of this type of antiseptics is the mercury compounds. The antibacterial action of these compounds is assumed to originate from their interference with SH (sulphydryl) compounds which are the essential cellular metabolites. Most commonly used mercury compound is mercurochrome. It is usually prepared by the mercuration of dibromo-fluorescein with mercuric acetate in an alkaline solution. Its structure may be expressed as shown below:

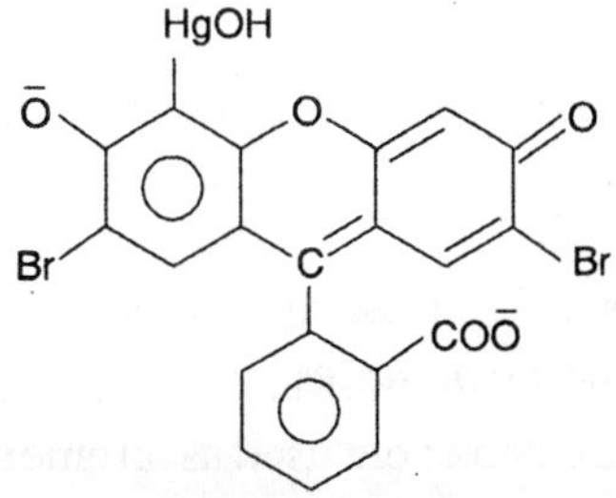

Mercurochrome

It is used as 2% aqueous solution. It is non-irritating and is used on wounds, skin and mucous surfaces.

3. *Halogens and Halogenated Compounds:* Halogens and halogenated compounds are an important group of antiseptics known since a ling time. The simple halogen, chlorine is a potent germicide. 0.10 to 0.25 parts per million is the usual concentration of chlorine to kill most of the organisms within 20 seconds. It is now-a-days widely used as a disinfectant for drinking water. Chlorine is generally used either as bleaching powder (Calx chlorinata), as Dakin's solution or as chloramine-T.

It is known that when chlorine comes in contact with water forms hypochlorous acid which chlorinate amide nitrogen of bacterial protein as shown below:

$$Cl_2 + H_2O \longrightarrow \underset{\text{Hypochlorous acid}}{HOCl} + HCl$$

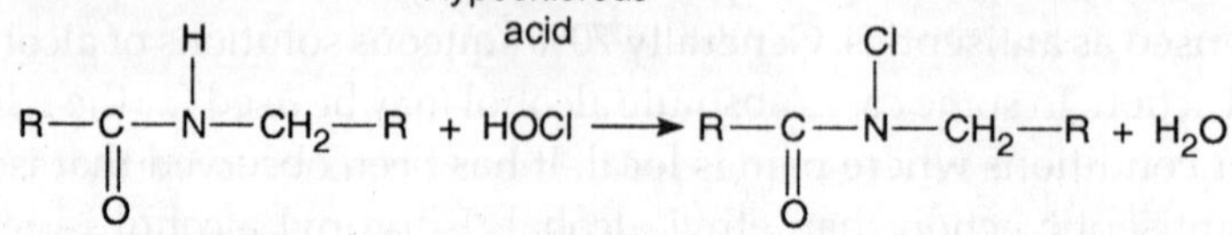

Protein

It may be mentioned that bleaching powder which contains 30-35% available chlorine is too irritating to be used on tissue but *Dakin's Solution* which is prepared by reacting bleaching powder with sodium carbonate followed by buffering the filtrate with boric acid is used for washing of wounds. The reactions taking place in Dakin's solution are as under:

$$Ca(OCl)_2 + Na_2CO_3 \longrightarrow 2NaOCl + CaCO_3$$

$$CaCl_2 + Na_2CO_3 \longrightarrow 2NaCl + CaCO_3$$

$$Ca(OH)_2 + Na_2CO_3 \longrightarrow 2NaOH + CaCO_3$$

$$2\ NaOH + 4\ H_3BO_3 \longrightarrow Na_2B_4O_7 + 7H_2O$$

Chloramines which are prepared by the action of hypochlorite solution on organic imino or amino compound is less irritant, stable solid and are better therapeutic agents. *Chloramine-T* or *chlorozone* is an aromatic chloramine. Chemically, it is sodium *p*-toluene sulphone-chloramide as shown below:

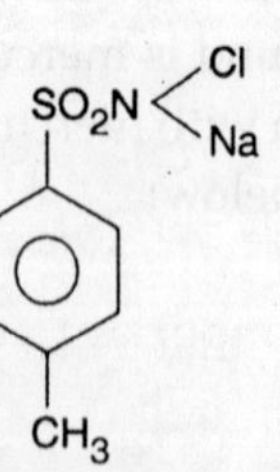

Chloramine-T

0.1% aqueous solution of caloramine-T is used for dressing wounds. It is also used as a disinfectant lotion in some infections diseases like measles.

Iodine is an important antiseptic chemical. It is extensively used as an emergency antiseptic under the name of *tincture iodine*. Some iodine compounds such as iodoform, vioform are frequently used as antiseptic. Iodoform (CHI_3) prepared by the action of free iodine on acetone or alcohol under warm condition is mainly used in dressing wounds.

$$C_2H_5OH + 4I_2 + 3Na_2CO_3 \longrightarrow CHI_3 + HCOONa + 5NaI + 3CO_2 + 2H_2O$$

$$CH_3COCH_3 + 3I_2 + 2Na_2CO_3 \longrightarrow CHI_3 + CH_3COONa + 3NaI + 2CO_2 + H_2O$$

Vioform is a non-poisonous, odourless substitute of iodoform. It is prepared by iodination of 8-hydroxy quinoline.

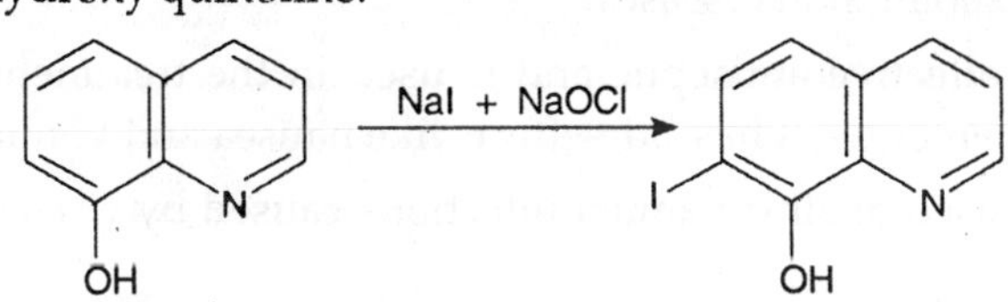

8-Hydroxy quinoline Vioform

It is used as a dusting powder for wounds and, ulcers.

4. *Phenolic Compounds:* Phenol, commonly known as carbolic acid was first introduced as an antiseptic in surgery by Lister in 1867. However, due its irritant action it has been replaced by more effective and less toxic phenolic derivatives. A few important phenolic derivatives which are commonly used are discussed below.

   (a) *Thymol:* It is naturally occurring antiseptic isolated from oil of thyme. It is disinfectant as well as anthelmintic. It is used as a flavouring agent in most of the mouth washes and gargles. It may be prepared from *m*-cresol as shown under:

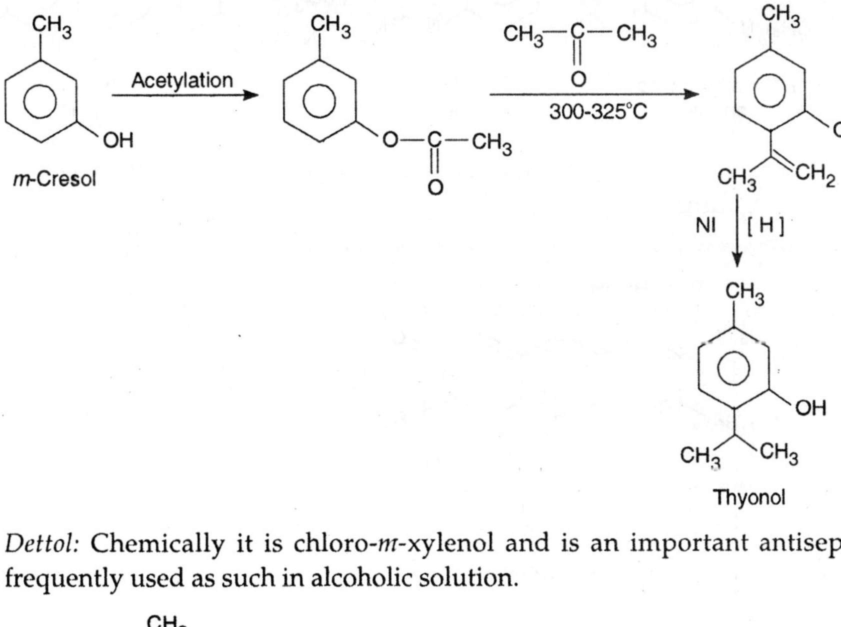

Thyonol

   (b) *Dettol:* Chemically it is chloro-*m*-xylenol and is an important antiseptic and is frequently used as such in alcoholic solution.

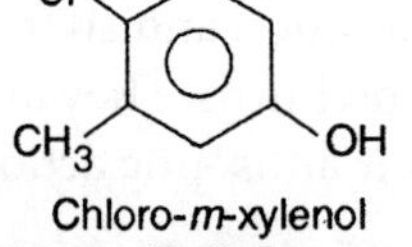

Chloro-*m*-xylenol
(Dettol)

Another chlorophenol compound is hexachlorophene. It is extensively used antiseptic. It is incorporated into creams and soaps.

5. *Nitrofuran Derivatives:* Nitrofuran derivatives have excellent antiseptic properties. Some important members of this series now in use include nitrofurazone, furazolidone and nifuroxime. Nitrofurazone is very effective against an wide range of both Gram-positive and Gram-negative organisms. It is normally used in cases of infections occurring due to burns, ulcers, wound and some skin diseases.

   Furazolidone is also an effective antiseptic and is used in the treatment of bacterial diarrhoeal disorders and enteritis. It has side-effects like nausea and vomiting.

   Nifuroxime is generally used against vaginal infections caused by *Candida albicaus* or *Trichomonas Vaginalis.*

6. *Synthetic Dyestuffs:* Certain dyes have been found to destroy the bacteria without damaging tissues. Extensively used dyes belong to acridine, thiazine, triphenyl, methane and azo groups of dyes. These dyes possess antiseptic and antiprotozoal actions and they can promote wound healing. They are slow acting and have remarkable specificity. Thus,

   (a) *Methylene blue, a thiazine dye,* is primarily used as an intestinal and urinary antiseptic. It is also used to test renal functions of kidneys for staining vital nerves. It is also used as an antidote of cyanide and nitrate poisoning. It is prepared as under:

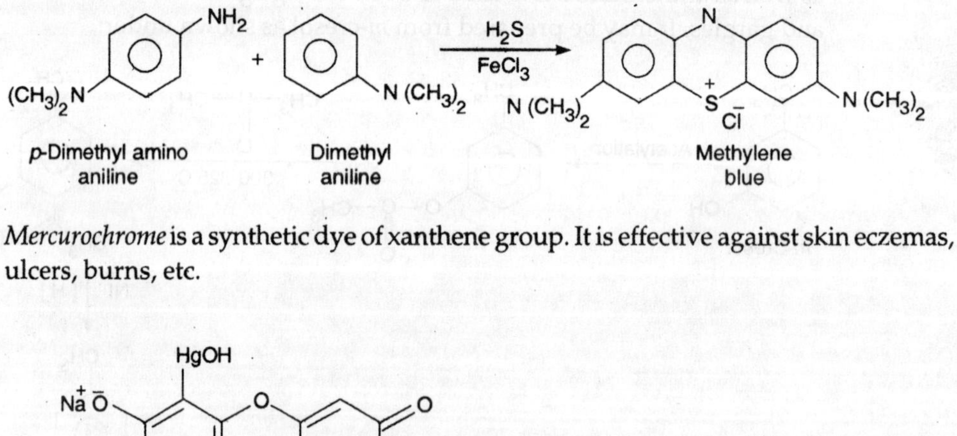

   (b) *Mercurochrome* is a synthetic dye of xanthene group. It is effective against skin eczemas, ulcers, burns, etc.

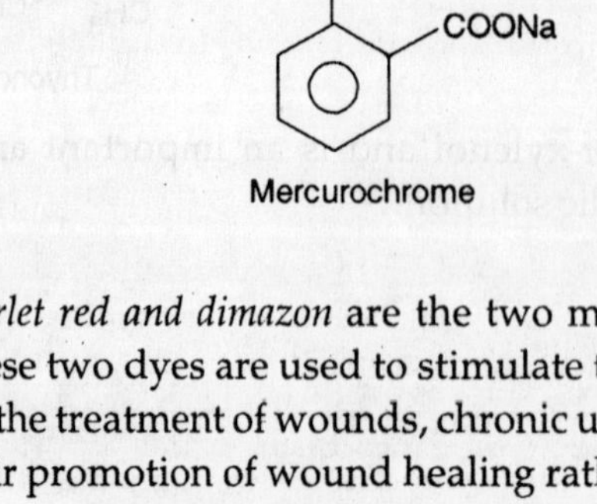

Mercurochrome

   (c) *Scarlet red and dimazon* are the two most common antiseptics of the *azo dye group.* These two dyes are used to stimulate tissue proliferation and so they are often used for the treatment of wounds, chronic ulcerations and burns. They are more useful for their promotion of wound healing rather than their antiseptic action.

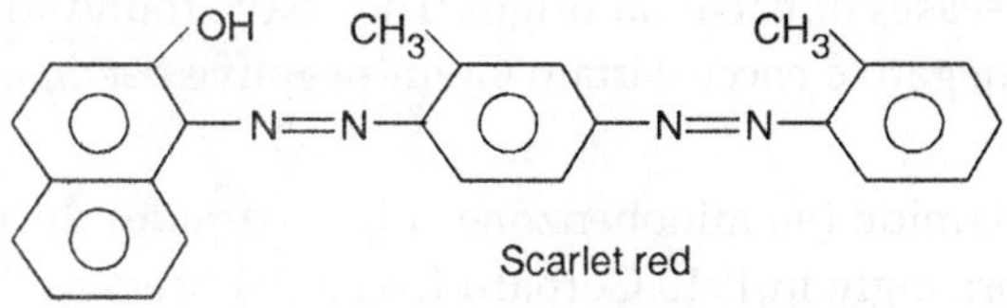

Scarlet red

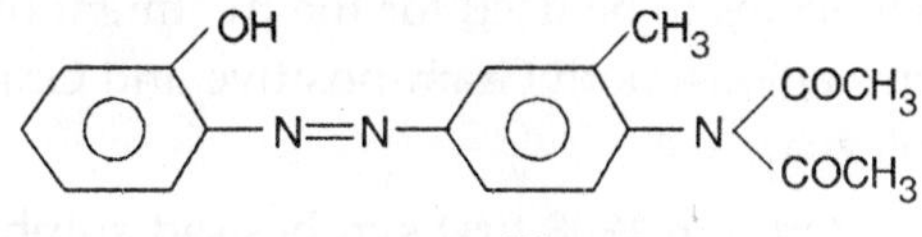

Dimazon

(d) *Salacrin, proflavin and acriflavin* are the most common and useful antiseptic dyes of *acridine group*. Due to their yellow colour they are known as flavins. They are active against Gram-positive organisms. They are used as anti-bacterial agents.

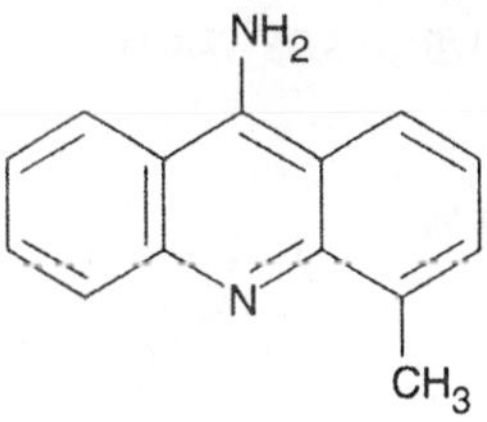

Salacrin

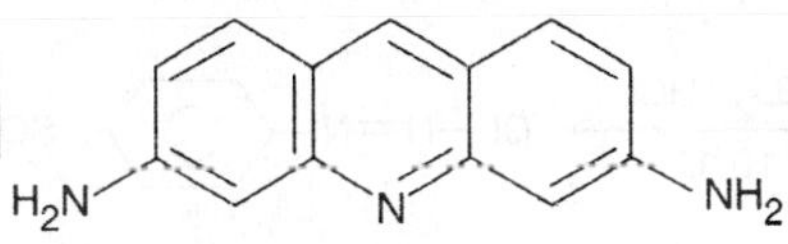

Proffavin

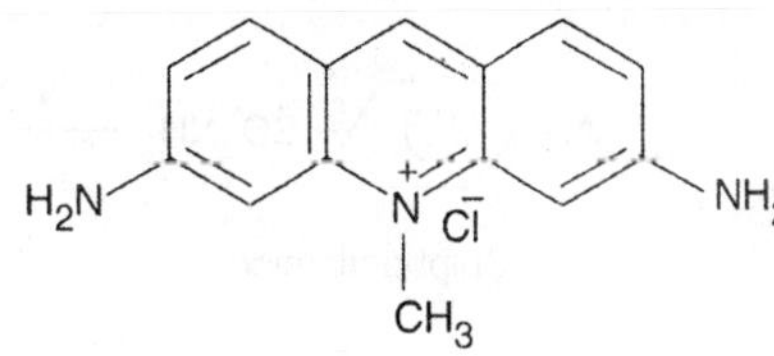

Acriflavin

7. *Surfactants:* As mentioned before that, surfactants may function as antiseptics. The anionic surfactants, i.e., soap, sodium, lauryl sulphate are antibacterial mainly against Gram-positive bacteria while the cationic surfactants such as benzalkonium chloride (zephiran), cetylpyridinium chloride (ceepryn), benzethoniun chloride (phenerol), cetyldimethyl benzyl ammonium chloride (Triton, K-12) are active against Gram-negative bacteria.

   Cationic surfactants are used as 10% solutions or tinctures in the concentrations of 1 : 200 to 1 : 1000. They are more potent at higher pH but their activity is decreased appreciably by soap, pus and organic matter.

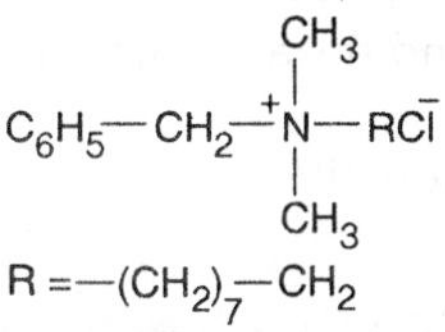

Benzalkonium Chloride (Zephiran)

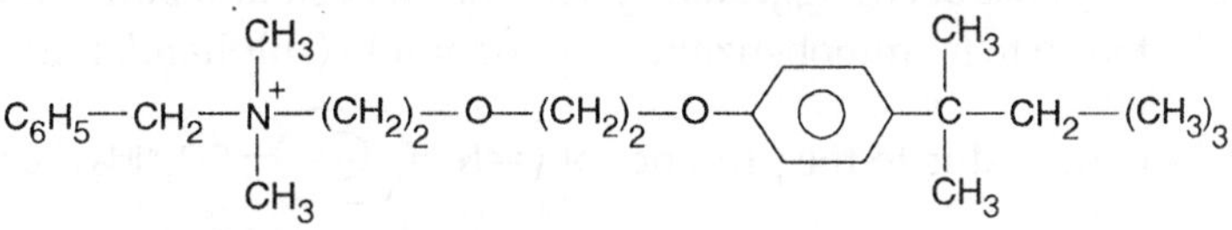

Benzthonium Chloride (Phenerol)

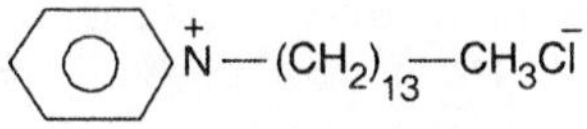

Ceepryn

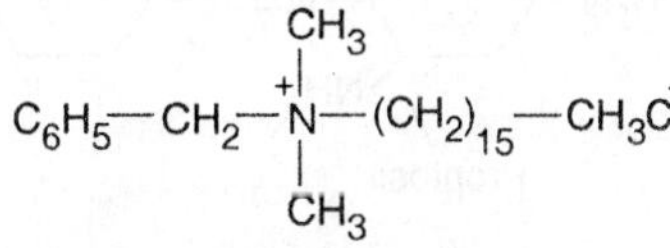

Triton, K-12

Sodium lauryl sarcosinate (Deriphat), an ampholytic surfactant is mainly used in toothpaste composition because it acts as enzyme inhibitor and is used to reduce dental caries.

$$CH_3(CH_2)_{10}-CH_2-NH-CH_2-CH_2-COONa$$

Sodium lauryl sarcosinate

22.2.8 Sulphonamides (Sulpha Drugs)

Sulphonamides or sulpha drugs are the synthetic chemotherapeutic agents which contain sulphonamide ($-\overset{O}{\underset{O}{\overset{\|}{\underset{\|}{S}}}}-NH_2$) functionality in their molecule. They are the first most active bactericides to be used for the treatment of diseases of bacterial origin. They have found to be active against both Gram-positive and Gram-negative cocci, certain Gram-negative bacilli and protozoa.

Glemo in 1908 first synthesised sulphanilamide (*p*-aminobenzone sulphonamide) during his study on the preparation of azodyes. Surprisingly in 1910 Gerhard Domagk observed that such azodyes containing sulphonamide functionality are active against *streptococci.* Domagk tested an azo-dye, 4-sulphonamide-2′, 4′-diaminobenzene and noticed its significant curative properties and named it *prontosit* which was found to be highly active against homolytic *streptococci.* It may be synthesised by diazotising sulphanilamide followed by coupling with *m*-phenylene diamine.

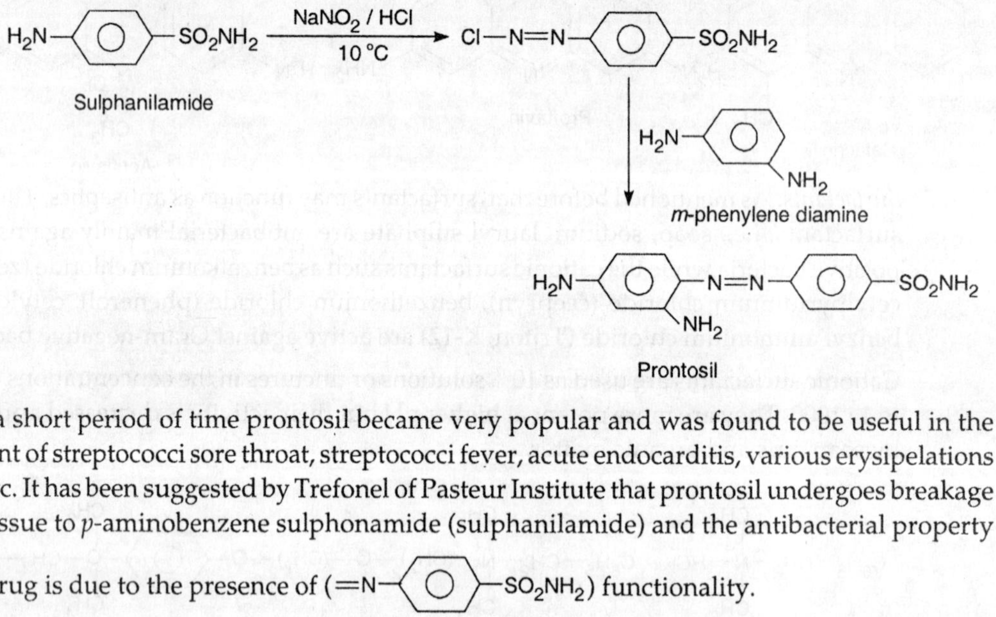

In a short period of time prontosil became very popular and was found to be useful in the treatment of streptococci sore throat, streptococci fever, acute endocarditis, various erysipelations cases, etc. It has been suggested by Trefonel of Pasteur Institute that prontosil undergoes breakage in the tissue to *p*-aminobenzene sulphonamide (sulphanilamide) and the antibacterial property of the drug is due to the presence of ($=N-C_6H_4-SO_2NH_2$) functionality.

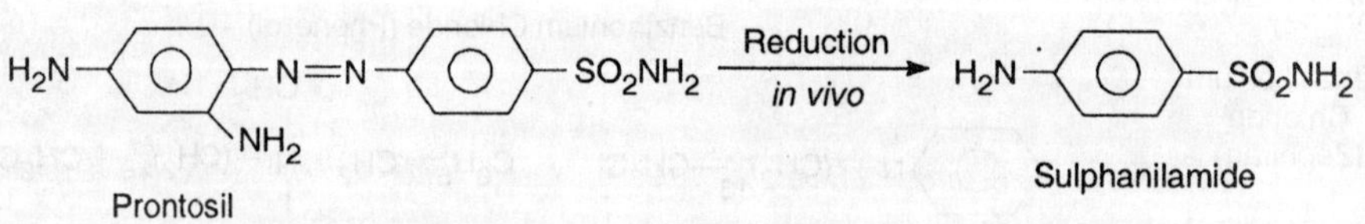

The above observation served as an impetus for the synthesis of a large number of sulphonamides by the substitution at N^1 ($H_2N^4-C_6H_4-SO_2N^1H_2$) and testing their antibacterial activity.

These drugs are widely used in the treatment of various diseases, viz., pneumonia, gonorrhoea, meningitis, dysentry, blood poisoning, scarlet fever, tonsilitis, sinus infections, etc. These drugs were found to be less toxic and highly effective.

22.2.8.1 Classification of Sulphonamides

Sulphonamides have been classified on the basis of their therapeutic utility as discussed in the next page.

22.2.8.1.1 Sulphonamides Used for General Infections

These are usually administered orally and employed against streptococcal, meningococcal, gonococcal, staphylococcal and pneumococcal infections. Sulphanilamides, sulphathiazole, sulphapyridine, sulphamerazine, sulphadiazine, sulphadimidine, etc. are the common members of this class of sulpha drugs.

(a) *Sulphanilamide (p-Aminobenzene sulphonamide):* It is synthesised through the following reactions:

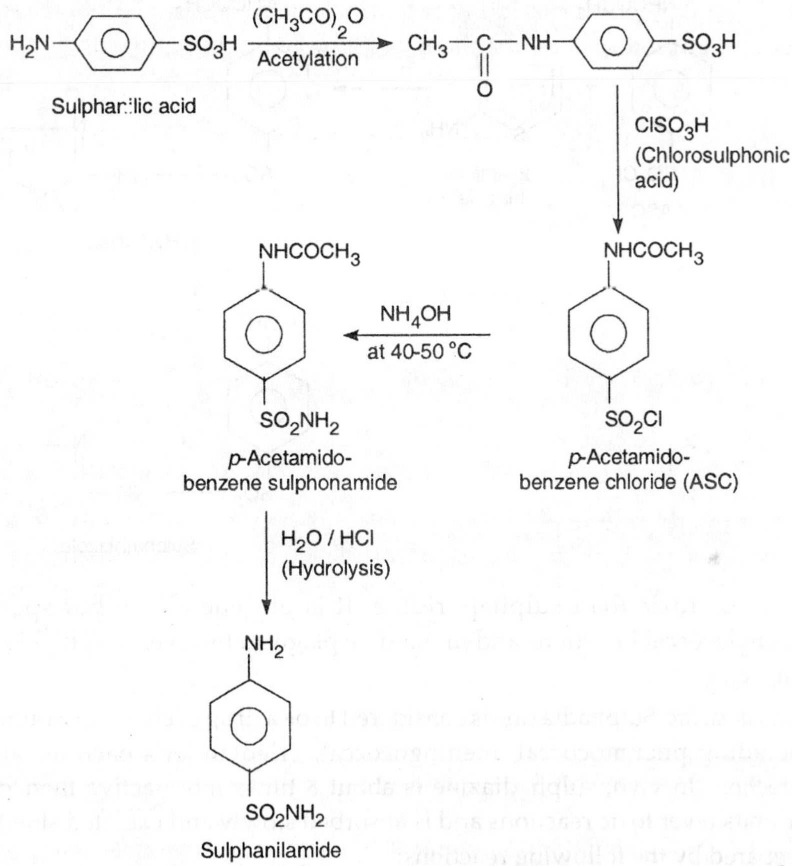

Due to its high toxicity it has now being replaced by other less toxic sulpha drugs. However, it is still used in veterinary medicine:

(b) *Sulphapyridine:* Its synthesis involves the following steps of reactions:

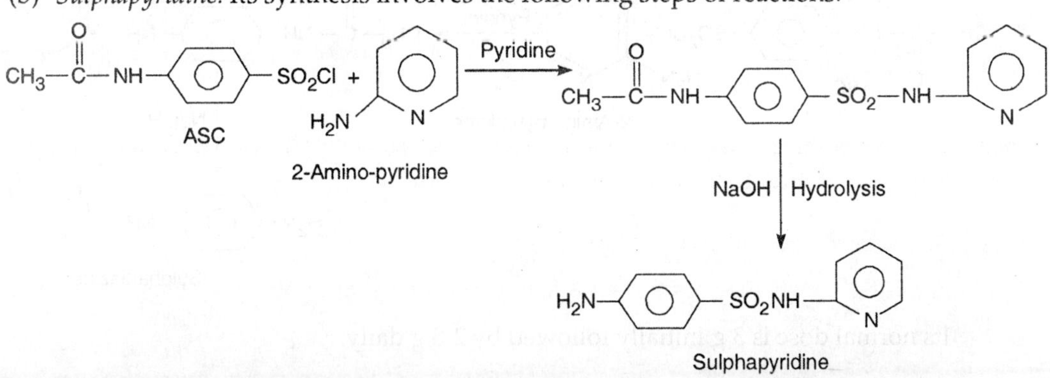

Sulphapyridine is the first drug to have an outstanding curative action on pneumonia. It is more potent than sulphanilamide in the treatment of streptococcal and gonococcal infections. It is mainly used in the treatment of dermatitis herpetiformis of such patients who do not give positive response to dapsone. It is employed as 0.5 to 3 g dose daily.

(c) *Sulphathiazole (Cibazole):* It is best prepared by the following reactions:

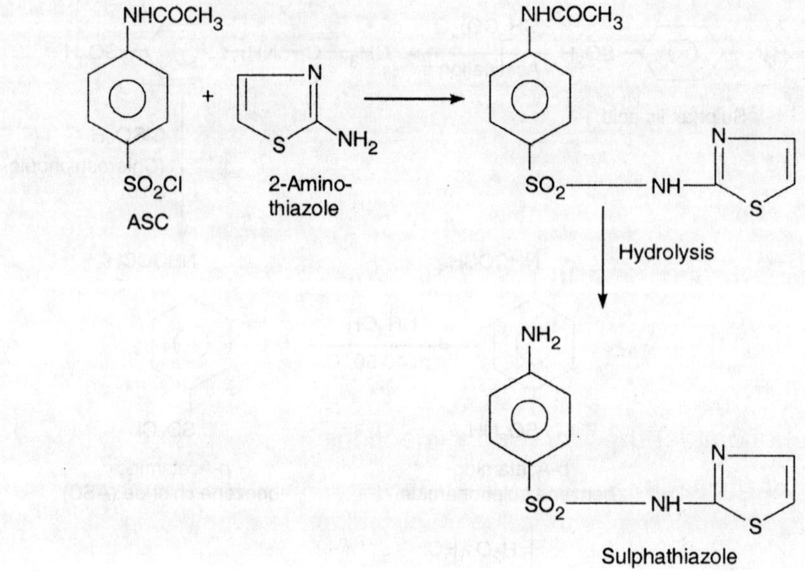

It is less toxic than sulphapyridine. It is of general use but specifically against staphylococcal infections and in bubonic plague. However, it is highly bacteriostatic in nature.

(d) *Sulphadiazine:* Sulphadiazine is considered to be a drug of choice in a number of infections, including pneumococcal, meningococcal, Friedlander's bacillus, and H. influenza infection. In vivo, sulphadiazine is about 8 times more active than sulphonamide. It exhibits fever toxic reactions and is absorbed slowly and excreted slowly. It is generally prepared by the following reactions:

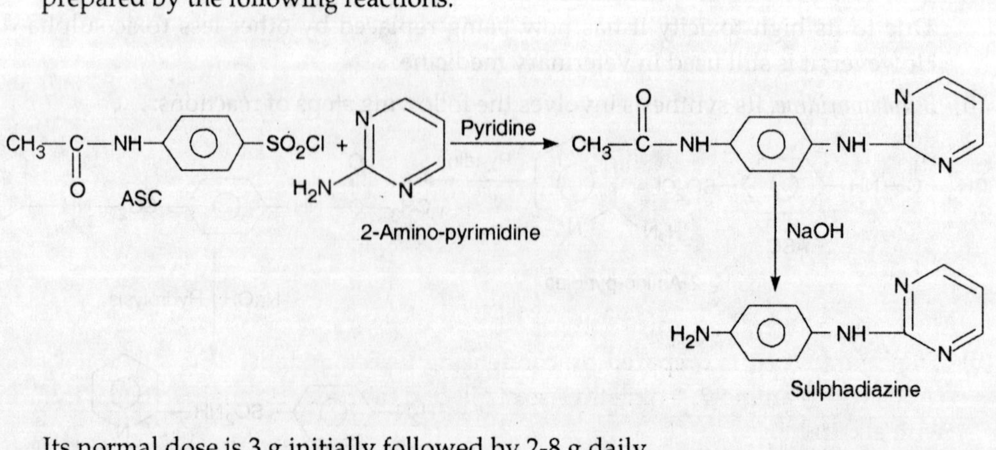

Its normal dose is 3 g initially followed by 2-8 g daily.

(e) *Sulphamerazine:* Sulphamerazine has the general properties of sulphonamides however it is more potent than sulphonamide in vivo. It is absorbed more rapidly but excreted more slowly. It is mostly used in conjunction with other sulphonamides. Its synthesis involves the following reactions.

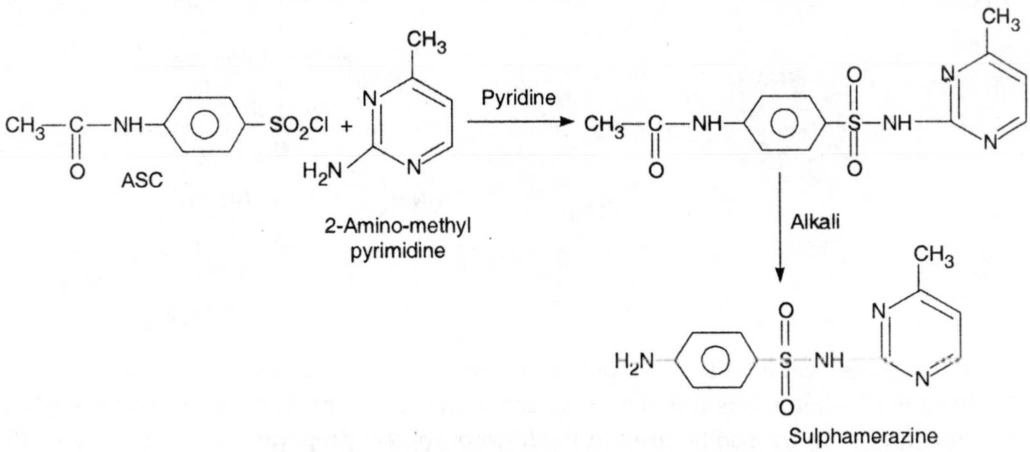

22.2.8.1.2 Sulphonamides Used for Urinary Infections

A large number of sulpha drugs are in use for the prevention and treatment of urinary tract infections. Sulphaectamide, sulphafurazole, sulphisomidine, etc. are the examples belonging to this category.

(a) *Sulphacetamide:* It is one of the highly soluble sulpha drug. It is excreted primarily in the urine. Due to its high solubility and ready elimination it has been found to be useful for the treatment of urinary infections. It is usually used in the dose of 4 g initially followed by 1 g every four hours.

It is prepared by careful hydrolysis of diacetyl derivative of sulphanilamide.

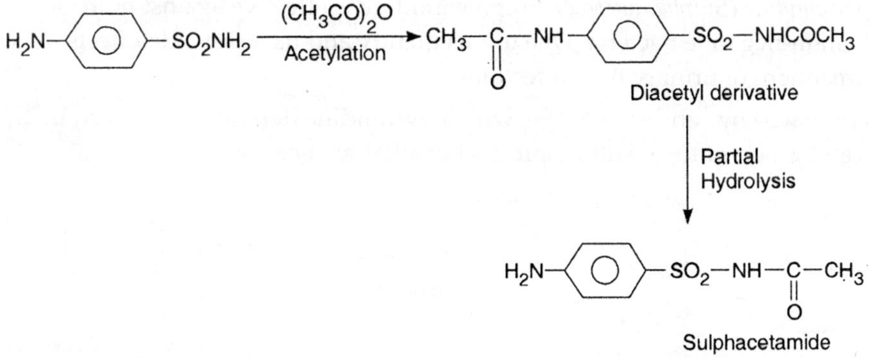

(b) *Sulphafurazole:* It is prepared by condensing *p*-acetomidobenzene sulphonyl chloride (ASC) with 5-amino-3, 4-dimethyl isoxazole and the product thus obtained is hydrolysed with alkali.

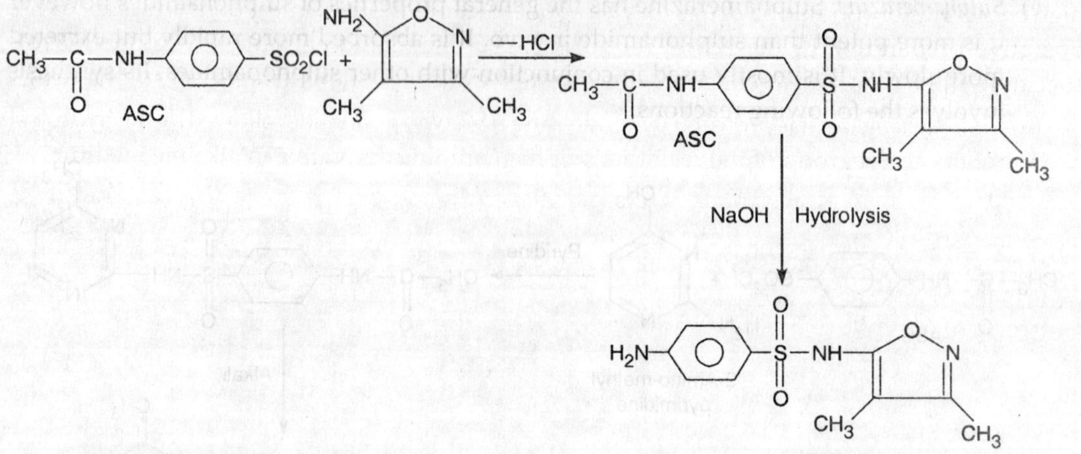

Sulphafurazole

It is soluble over a wide range of pH. It is used for infections involving sulphonamide-sensitive bacteria. It is found to be effective in the treatment of Gram-negative urinary infections. It may also be used in the form of topical preparations for the treatment of some infections such as vaginitis caused by *Homophilus Vaginalis*. Its required dose is 2 to 4 g initially followed by 4 to 8 g per day in 4-6 divided doses.

Sometimes its acetyl derivative sulphisoxazole acetyl is used. It is suitable for oral administration especially in liquid preparation of the drug. Its required dose is 2 to 4 g oral (adult) initially followed by 4 to 8 g per day.

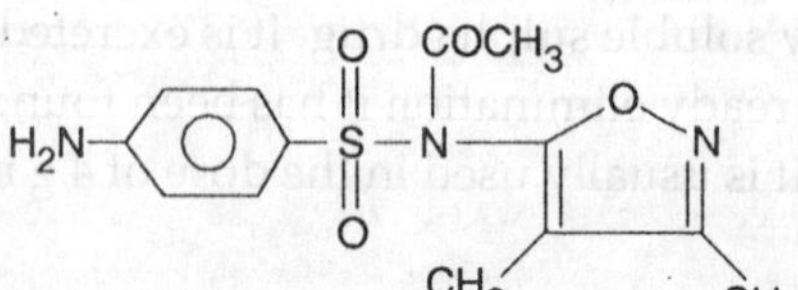

Sulphisoxazole acetyl

(c) *Sulphisomidine (Sulphadimetine)*: Sulphisomidine is effective against both Gram-positive and Gram-negative bacteria. Due to this quality and its lesser side-effects, it is used for the treatment of urinary tract infections.

It is prepared by condensing ASC with a pyrimidine derivative followed by hydrolysis of acetyl group of the resulting product in alkaline medium.

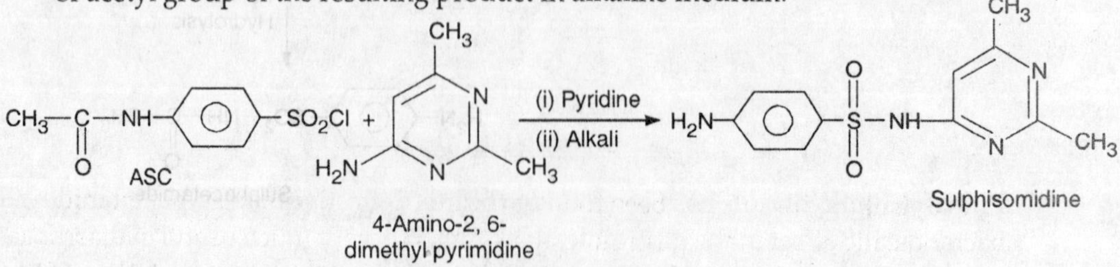

22.2.8.1.3 Sulphonamides Used for Intestinal Infections

A large number of insoluble sulphonamides, in general, are not readily absorbed from the gastrointestinal tract. But due to hydrolysis in large intestine active sulphonamide is released in high concentration. So sulpha drugs may be applicable for intestinal infeactions and also for pre-operative preparation of the bowel for surgery. Sulphaguanidine, phthalyl-sulphathiazole, succinyl sulpha thiazole etc. constitute the common examples of this category of sulpha drugs.

(a) *Sulphaguanidine:* It is prepared by condensing ASC with guanidine followed by the hydrolysis of the acetyl group of the resulting sulphaguanidine derivative in alkaline medium.

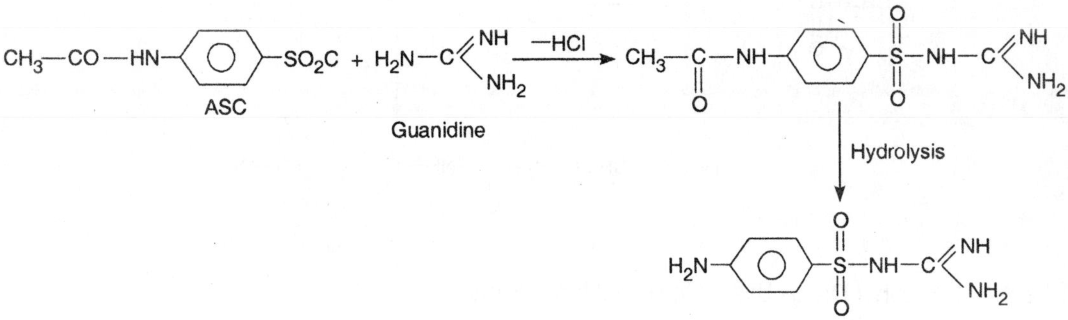

Sulphaguanidine

Sulphaguanidine constitutes one of the best drugs for the treatment of bacillary dysentery only. Slight toxic effects such as rashes and haematuria have been observed. It is usually used as 3 g, 3 to 4 times a day for three days doses.

(b) *Phthalyl sulphathiazole:* It is synthesised by the reaction between phthalic anhydride and sulphathiazole.

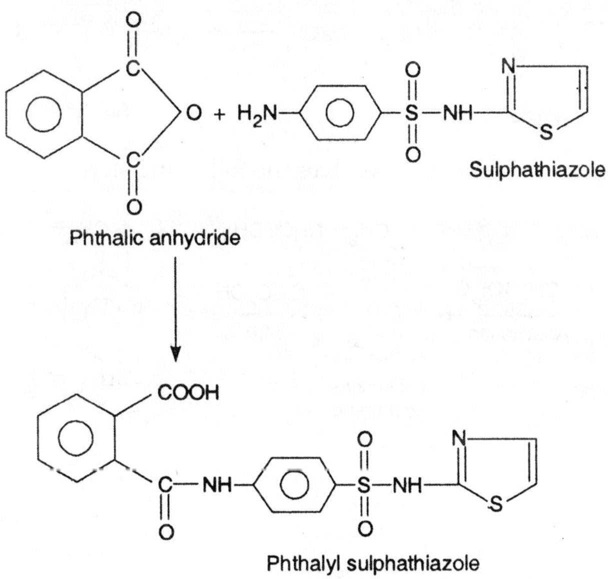

Phthalyl sulphathiazole

Phthalylsulphathiazole has been found to be more effective than sulphaguanidine. It has bacteriostatic effect in the gastrointestinal tract. It is very much useful in diarrhoeas and ulcerative colitis. It may also be employed in the pre-operative treatment of patients undergoing intestinal tract surgery. It is also useful in the treatment of bascillary dysentery of *Sonne, Flexner* and *Shiga species.* Its recommended dose is 5 to 10 g per day in several divided doses.

(c) *Succinyl sulphathiazole:* It is an important drug for intestinal infection. It is generally used in bascillary dysentry and cholera. It is used in 10 to 20 g per day in divided doses. Its preparation involves the condensation of succinic anhydride with sulphathiazole.

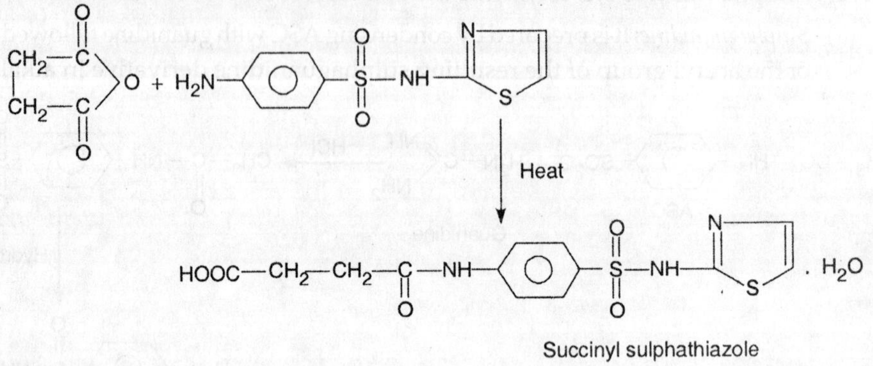

Succinyl sulphathiazole

22.2.8.1.4 Sulpha Drugs Used for Local Infections

There are a few sulpha drugs which are exclusively employed for local applications. Sulphacetamide sodium and maphenide are the examples of this category.

(a) *Sulphacetamide Sodium:* It is mainly used for local application in injuries or infections of the eyes such as conjunctivitis and prophylaxis of ocular infections after injuries or burns. It is used as 10%, 15%, 20% and 30% solution as eye-drops and 2.5% and 6% as ointment. It is prepared by the reaction between sodium hydroxide and sulphacetamide.

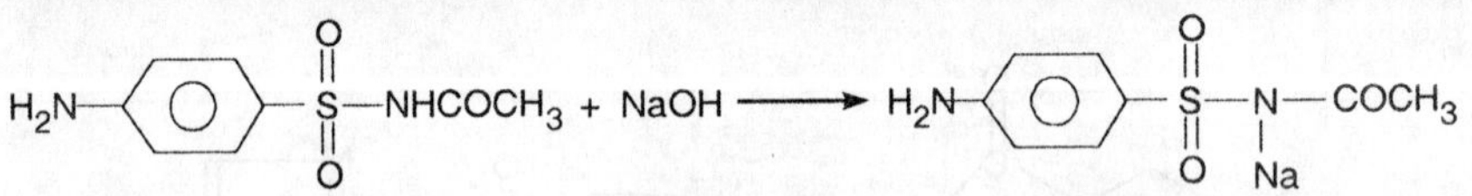

Sulphacetamide Sulphacetamide sodium

(b) *Mephenide:* Synthesis of mephenide involves the following steps:

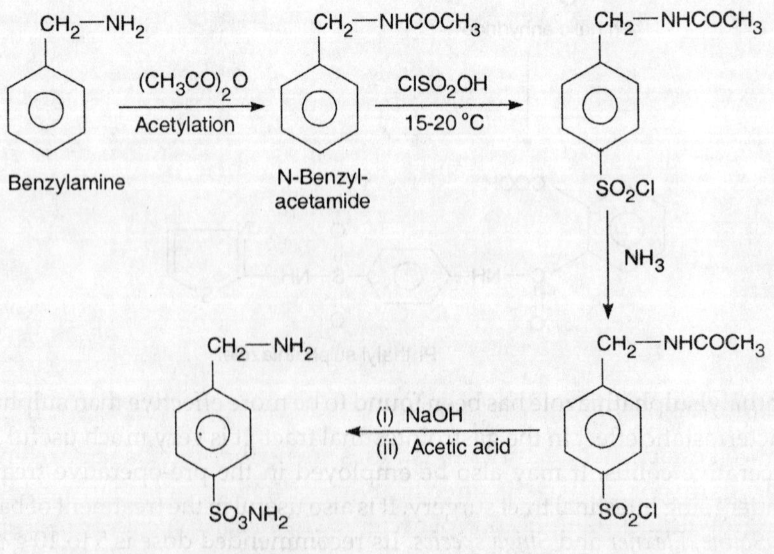

Mephenide

Mephenide is also known as marphanil or sulphamylon and is 500 times more bacteriostatic than sulphathiazole. It is also referred to as German penicillin. Mephenide is primarily used in the treatment of gas gangrene. It may also be used in the treatment of third-degree burns and infection due to *Pseudomonas acruginosa.* It is applied as 5% solution of its hydrochloride or propionate. Nowadays it is used with streptomycin for the treatment of slow-healing wounds.

22.2.8.1.5 Some Sulphonamide Related Drugs

There are some sulpha drugs which differ from the basic sulphonamide nucleus but possess anti-bacterial properties. Followings are the typical members of this group of drugs:

(a) *Dapsone:* It is prepared as indicated below:

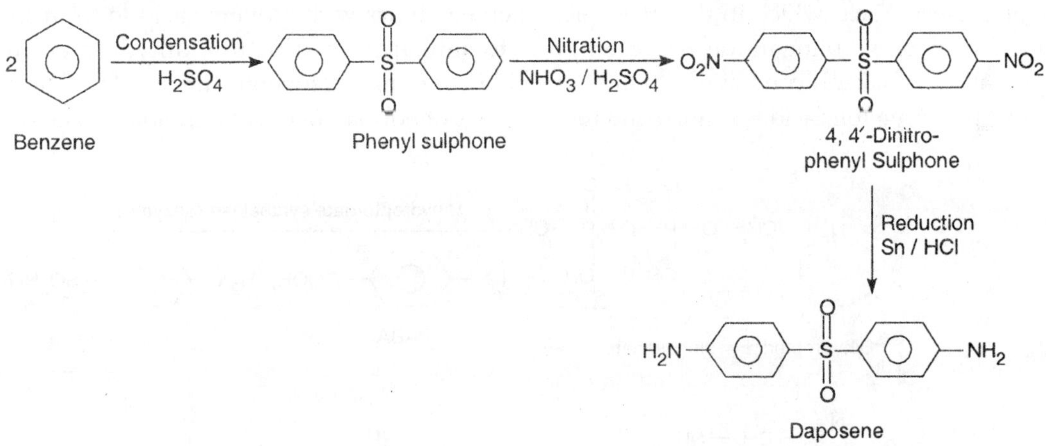

Dapsone behaves like sulphonamides and is the drug of choice in the chemotherapy of leprosy and nocardiosis. It is highly useful as a suppressant in the treatment of *Dermatitis herpetiformis.* Its recommended doses are 25 mg twice a week initially for one month followed by 25 mg per day each month as leprostatic; 100 to 200 mg per day as suppressant for dermatitis herpetiformis.

(b) *Nitrosulphathiazole:* It is specially used as a rectal injection as an adjunct in the local treatment of non-specific ulcerative colitis. It is employed in 10 ml of a 10% suspension after each stool and at bed time. It is expressed by the following structure:

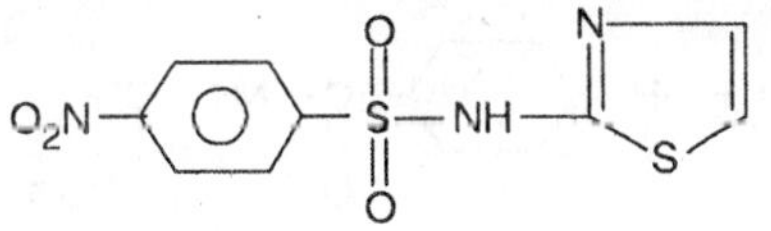

Nitrosulphathiazole

22.2.8.2 Mechanism of Action of Sulphonamides (Sulpha Drugs)

It has been well established that sulphonamides are not bactericide but bacteriostatic in nature, i.e., these drugs do not kill bacteria directly at the concentration in which they are used but they prevent the growth and multiplication of bacteria. The cause of such type of action (bacteriostatic) of these drugs originates from their similarity in structure with *p*-aminobenzoic acid (PABA). It is known that bacteria synthesise folic acid (Vitamin B_9) which is necessary for their growth and the key compound for the synthesis of folic acid is PABA. The drug, sulphonamide, is a structural analog of PABA.

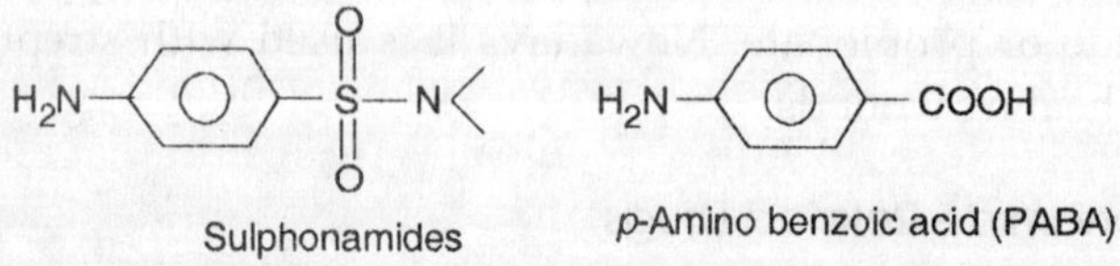

Bacteria cannot discriminate between these two compounds and hence uses sulphonamides instead of PABA (an example of mistaken identity). As a result, pseudofolic acid (wrong folic acid) is synthesised inhibiting the further growth of bacteria. In the normal course, the first step of the synthesis of folic acid involves the coupling of dihydropteridine diphosphate with PABA yielding pteroic acid which in the subsequent step combines with glutamic acid to form folic acid. But when sulphonamide is present, due to similarity in structure, dihydropteridine diphosphate mistakenly combines with sulphonamide and forms a compound different from pteroic acid. Thus wrong folic acid is formed and the synthesis of normal folic acid is inhibited. Thus,

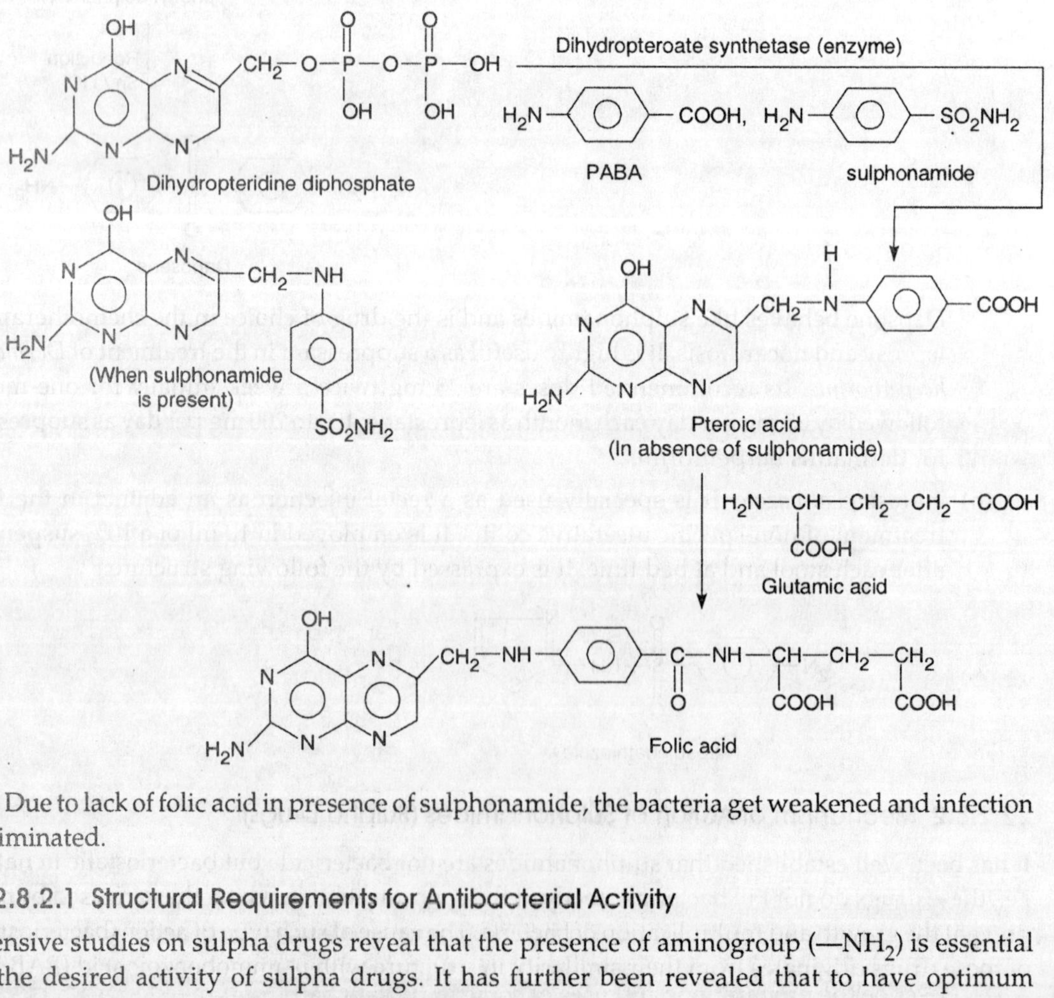

Due to lack of folic acid in presence of sulphonamide, the bacteria get weakened and infection is eliminated.

22.2.8.2.1 Structural Requirements for Antibacterial Activity

Extensive studies on sulpha drugs reveal that the presence of aminogroup (—NH_2) is essential for the desired activity of sulpha drugs. It has further been revealed that to have optimum antibacterial activity in addition to amino group the presence of the following structural features are also necessary.

i. Amino and sulphonyl groups must be para to each other i.e., para amino benzene sulphonic acid moiety is essential.

ii. For optimum activity $PhNH_2$ functionality must be unsubstituted as has been observed in the case of prontosil. The structure of prontosil is similar to that of sulphanilamide with substitution at —NH_2 group. As such it does not exhibit any antibacterial activity in *vitro* but in *vivo* —N=H-grouping is reduced to active metabolite sulphanilamide.

iii. Absence of benzene ring or the presence of additional benzene ring decreases the activity.

iv. Mon substitution on the nitrogen atom of SO_2NH_2 group with hetero atom increases the activity while disubstitution has reverse effect.

It has also been observed that N-heterocyclic derivatives of sulphonamides, viz, sulphadiazine, and sulphathiazole have broad spectrum antimicrobial activity. They are, in general, more soluble in water and hence better absorbed and retained better i.e., excreted showly,

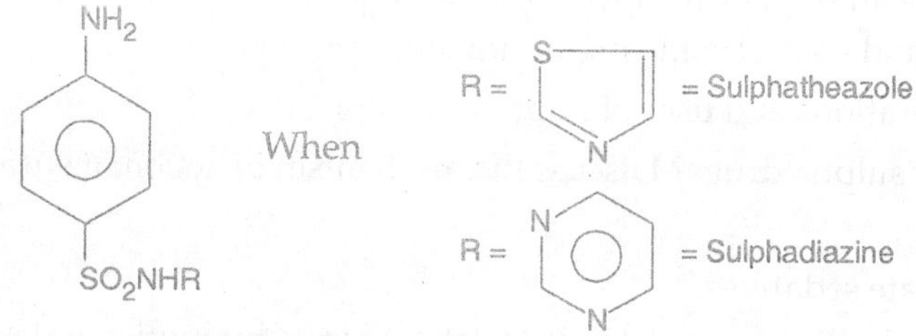

22.2.8.3 Therapeutic Aspects of Sulpha Drugs

Sulpha drugs, in general, *in vitro* is converted to N^4-acetyl analogues and a portion of this acetyl compound is excreted. It has been found that these acetyl derivatives have lower pK_a value and lower solubility than the corresponding sulphonamides. These N^4-acytylated products have the tendency to crystallise in the renal tubules and so they create some obstruction in the kidney which ultimately may lead to kidney damage. The formation of of crystalluria depends upon some cardinal factors such as solubility of sulphonamides in the urine, degree of acetylation, solubility of N^4-acetylated product, rate of excretion of sulphonamides and its metabolites and lastly the pH and volume of urine excreted.

The crystalluria formation may be minimised by different ways namely (i) increasing the intake of water during sulphonamide therapy (ii) alkalinisation of urine by administering sodium bicarbonate or other alkaline formulation and (iii) by administering mixture of sulphonamides of the same category in such quantities that none of the drugs may reach a renal concentration which may cause crystalluria.

Model Questions

1. What do you mean by the term drug? What are its sources? How are the drugs classified? Mention some important classes of drugs?
2. What are hypnotics and sedatives? How are they classified?
3. Describe the preparations and uses of some important barbiturates.

4. Explain the term coagulant and anti-coagulant agents. Discuss the mechanism of blood clotting. Discuss the synthesis and uses of some coagulant and anti-coagulant agents.
5. What are the functions of thyroid hormones? What types of diseases are commonly caused by thyroid hormones? How are these diseases treated? Mention some important drugs generally used.
6. What are anasthetics? What are the characteristics of an ideal anaerthetic? How are anasthetics classified? Mention the name of at least one drug of each class of anaesthetics and discuss their preparations and uses.
7. Discuss the preparation and uses of opiod analgesics. What is the mode of action of opiod analgesics.
8. Mention the name of some common non-opioid analgesics? Discuss their synthesis and uses. How are they act?
9. Write a short resume on CNS stimulant.
10. Explain the terms—antiseptics, disinfectant and surfactant. How are they classified? Discuss the preparations and uses of some important antiseptic agents.
11. Discuss the preparations and uses of important sulpha drugs.
12. What is meant by sulpha drugs? Discuss the mechanism of action of sulpha drugs.
13. Write notes on:
    (a) Non-barbiturate sedatives.
    (b) Mode of action and structure activity relationship of hypnotics and sedatives.
    (c) Mode of action of anaesthetics.
    (d) Standardisation of antiseptics.
14. Discuss in short the significance of functional groups in drug action.
15. What are requirements for an ideal drug? Discuss in short structure activity relationship of drugs.

Part II

Chemistry of Natural Products

Chemistry of Natural Products

INTRODUCTION

From the prehistoric age, man has an intrinsic dependence on nature for his survival. The nature has provided him essentials like food, clothes, shelters and medicines for his survival. This dependence of man on nature has invoked tremendous interest in the scientific world which ultimately led to the isolation of a vast number of organic chemicals from their natural sources usually plants. The commencement of the systematic study in the early part of nineteenth century has culminated in the isolation and purification of a large number of organic chemicals from natural sources and the study of their reactions afforded the main problems of organic chemistry and led the foundation stone of modern organic chemistry. In recent years, it has been possible to isolate numerous phytochemicals due to the introduction of sophisticated instrumentations like GC, GCMS, HPLC, ^{1}H and ^{13}CNMR spectroscopy, high resolution mass spectroscopy, ORD/CD, X-ray crystallography and in fact, at present, natural product chemistry has undergone an explosive, growth and has emerged as a distinct discipline. The diversity of structures and variety of reactions undergone by the phytochemicals have created a stir in the scientific world and have attracted a large number of chemists all over the world to undertake scientific research on plant chemistry. The study on the chemistry of diverse phytochemicals has brought to light many theories which are now fundamental to organic chemistry.

Besides academic importance, plant products possess significant therapeutic values. Phytochemicals are now being used directly or indirectly as medicines in the treatment of various ailments due to their unique curative properties. At present, the drugs, isolated from natural sources is about 50% of the marketable total drugs. Many phytochemicals have also been found to have pesticidal properties.

Among the vast number of natural products, those having cyclic-skeleton preferably polycyclic molecular architecture are being considered to be of greatest importance. Most commonly occurring natural products of this group of cyclic compounds having immense medicinal activity are the huge number of alkaloids, terpenoids, carbohydrates, glycosides, amino acids, proteins, lipids, phenolic compounds and purines. So in this part, chemistry of these types of natural products are dealt with in the subsequent chapters.

CHAPTER ONE

Carbohydrates

INTRODUCTION

Carbohydrates may be looked upon either as naturally occurring optically active polyhydroxy carbonyl compounds or as those naturally occurring organic substances which can yield optically active polyhydroxy carbonyl compounds on hydrolysis. A large number of carbohydrates can be represented by the general formula, $C_n(H_2O)_n$ such as glucose, $C_6H_{12}O_6$, $[C_6(H_2O)_6]$. For this reason in the primitive stage of carbohydrate chemistry, they were considered as the hydrates of carbon. However, subsequent development of the chemistry of carbohydrates reveals that a large number of carbohydrates are known such as rhamnose, $C_6H_{12}O_5$, rhamohexose, $C_7H_{14}O_6$ which do not conform to the above general formula. Again, an appreciable number of organic compounds are known having the general formula, $C_n(H_2O)_n$, i.e., formaldehyde, CH_2O, acetic acid, $C_2(H_2O)_2$, etc. are not carbohydrates. Once again, simple polyhydroxy carbonyl compounds, like dihydroxy acetone ($HO-CH_2-\underset{\underset{O}{\|}}{C}-CH_2-OH$) are not carbohydrates. Thus, the essential requirements for an organic compound to be carbohydrate are— they must be polyhydroxy carbonyl functionality containing substances with optical activity and must occur in nature as stated in the beginning.

1.1 Classification of Carbohydrates

Carbohydrates are broadly classified into two categories:

1. *Sugars*: These are crystalline solids soluble in water. They have sweet taste. That is why they are also known as *saccharides*.
2. *Polysaccharides*: These are complex carbohydrates and on hydrolysis furnish a large number of sugars.

Sugars are further classified into several categories as under:

(a) *Monosaccharides*: These sugars are simple and smallest unit, i.e., they cannot be further hydrolysed. Monosaccharides contain 3-10 carbon atoms in their molecules, i.e., glyceraldehyde, $C_3H_6O_3$, erythrose, $C_4H_8O_4$, arabinose, $C_5H_{10}O_5$, glucose, $C_6H_{12}O_6$, fructose, $C_6H_{12}O_6$ etc.

(b) *Disaccharides*: These are sugar type carbohydrates which on hydrolysis produce two units, like or different, of monosaccharides.

Similarly, on the basis of number of monosaccharides produced on hydrolysis, sugars have been grouped into tri, tetra, penta saccharides, etc.

It may be mentioned that sugars other than monosaccharides which yield 2-10 units of monosaccharides on hydrolysis, are known as *Oligosacchardies.*

From above discussion it is thus evident that the chemistry of carbohydrates is mainly controlled by the chemistry of monosacchardies because carbohydrates may be looked upon as the polymer of monosaccharides. It is, therefore, obvious that in carbohydrate chemistry, chemistry of monosaccharides has drawn the maximum attention of chemists and has been extensively studied.

1.2 Chemistry of Monosaccharides

As mentioned earlier monosaccharides are the smallest unit of sugar family. The carbonyl group present in these sugars may be an aldehydic (—CHO) or a keto (> C = O) group. Consequently, monosaccharides have been divided into two groups.

(a) Those containing aldehyde group are known as *aldose* and

(b) monosaccharides having keto function are termed as *ketose.*

1.2.1 Nomenclature of Monosaccharides

Monosaccharides whether aldose or ketose are named as triose, tetrose, pentose, hexose, etc. according to the number of carbon atoms present in their molecules and aldehyde or keto functionality is indicated by adding the word aldo or keto in the prefix. Thus aldotriose, ketotriose, aldotetrose, ketotetrose, etc.

1.2.2 Configurational Designations

From the definition of carbohydrates it is evident that the smallest member of this family must contain three carbon atoms. Again, as carbohydrates are optically active such a member should be aldotriose (ketotriose is optically inactive). Thus, the structure of the first member of monosaccharide may be written as

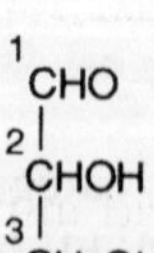

Glyceradehyde

Scrutiny of the above structure of glyceraldehyde reveals that its central carbon atom (C_2) is chiral in nature. Hence it must exist in two enantiomeric forms as shown below:

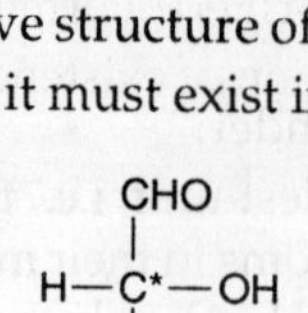

D-Configuration
(D-Glyceraldehyde)

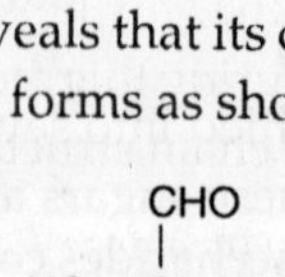

L-Configuration
(L-Glyceraldehyde)

The two enantiomers differ in the configuration of hydroxyl group at chiral centre (*). The one in which hydroxyl group is oriented at right-hand direction is designated as D-form while the other in which the hydroxyl is at left-hand direction is termed as L-form. These D and L letters indicate their absolute configuration. Further, it has been observed that the steric structure of monosaccharides is related to the two enantiomers of glyceraldehyde. Hence sugars, particularly monosaccharides, are named on the basis of absolute configurations of D- and L-Glyceraldehyde. The sugars having the same configuration as *D-Glyceraldehyde* at the highest numbered chiral carbon (the penultimate carbon atom) are designated as D-Monosaccharides and a sugar on which the penultimate chiral has the same configuration as L-Glyceraldehyde is designated as belonging to L-series. It may be mentioned that D and L configurations have no relation to signs (+) and (–). As mentioned earlier, D and L indicate only the absolute configurations.

It has been found that most of the members of naturally occurring sugars belong to D-series.

Among the monosaccharides the most abundant and extensively investigated member is D-Glucose, an aldohexose. In fact, the study on the chemistry of sugars is primarily confined within the chemistry of this abundant member.

1.2.3 General Properties of Monosaccharides

(a) *Properties common to aldose and ketose*

i. Since both aldose and ketose possess hydroxyl functions they form acetyl derivatives on treatment with acetic anhydride—the number of acetyl groups introduced depends upon the number of hydroxyl groups present, i.e., triose forms diacetyl derivatives, tetrose affords triacetyl derivatives, etc.

ii. In conformity with the presence of carbonyl group they respond to carbonylic tests, such as formation of oxime, cyanohydrin, etc.

iii. On simple heating they do not liberate molecule of water. This suggests that more than one hydroxyl groups are not present at a particular carbon atom [carbon atom containing more than one hydroxyl functions is very unstable and readily eliminates a molecule of water, i.e.,

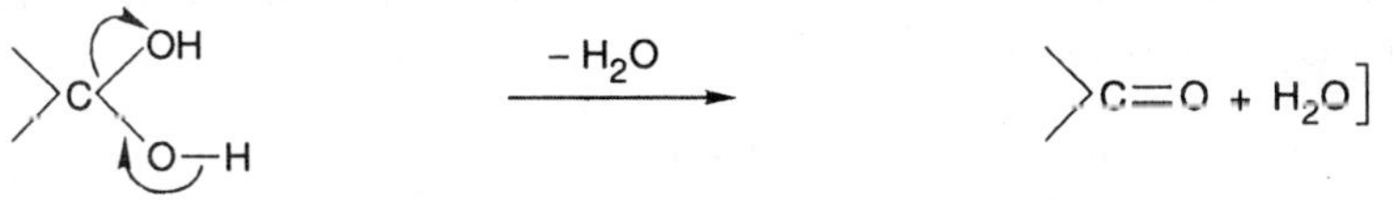

iv. On reduction with hydroiodic acid in presence of red phosphorous normal chain hydrocarbons are formed — the length of the chain depends on the number of carbon atoms present in monosaccharide, i.e., for triose *n*-propane, for tetrose *n*-butane, for pentose *n*-pentane, for hexose *n*-hexane are formed. Formation of normal chain hydrocarbons during this reduction is an indication of existence of monosaccharides in open straight chain structure.

(b) *Properties shown only by aldose*

i. Aldoses reduce Tollen's reagent and Fehling's solution.

ii. On oxidation with nitric acid, aldoses yield carboxylic acids without any loss of carbon atoms.

(c) *Properties exhibited only by ketose*

i. Ketoses also respond to Tollen's and Fehling's test.

ii. On oxidation with nitric acid, ketoses form carboxylic acids with lesser number of carbon atoms.

PROBLEM 1.1

Explain:

(a) Formaldehyde, CH_2O, and acetic acid, $C_2H_4O_2$, satisfy the general expression, $C_n(H_2O)_n$, yet they are not carbohydrates but glucose, $C_6(H_2O)_6$, belong to carbohydrate family.

(b) Aldotriose is sugar but ketotriose is not.

(c) On reduction with HI/P monosaccharides form corresponding normal chain hydrocarbons.

(d) Monosaccharides on simple heating do not eliminate water molecule.

1.2.4 Some Representative Members of Monosaccharides

On the basis of the general properties enumerated above structures of some of the representative members of sugar family may be written as under:

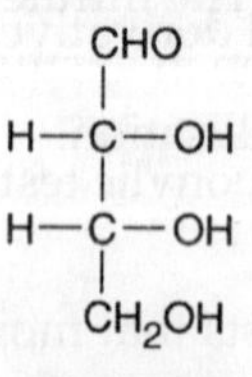

Aldotetrose
D-Erythrose

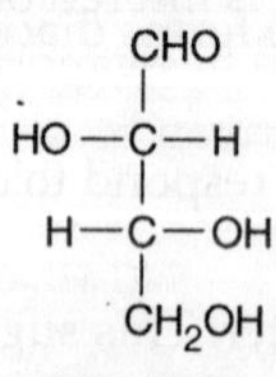

D-Threose

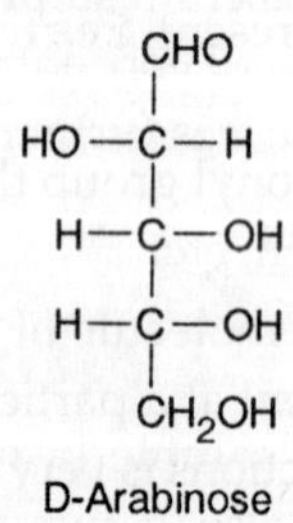

D-Arabinose

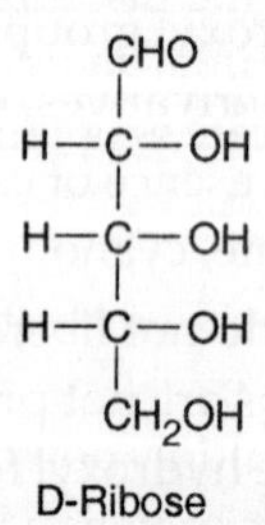

D-Ribose

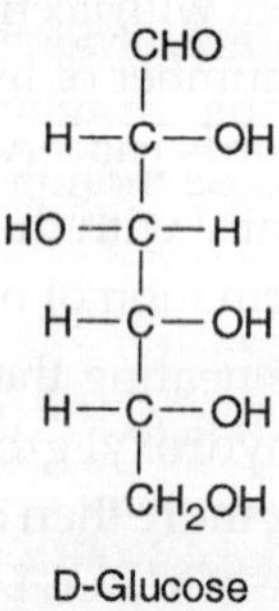

D-Glucose

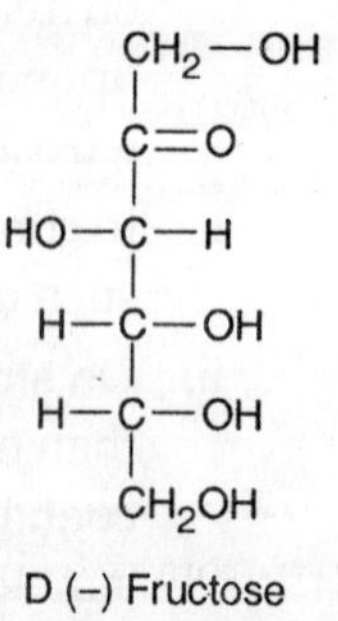

D (–) Fructose

1.2.5 Deoxy Sugars

Some carbohydrates have been isolated from natural source which contain one or more hydroxyl less than expected. Such carbohydrates are known as *deoxy sugars*. In naming these carbohydrates, the prefix, *deoxy*, is used with the name of original oxygen containing carbohydrate and indicating the position at which hydroxyl group (s) is absent by number. The most important member of deoxy sugar family is 2-Deoxy-D-ribose which is present in the living cells.

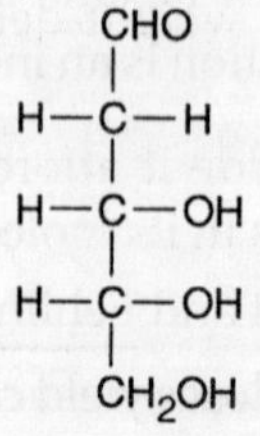

2-Deoxy-D-ribose

1.2.6 Chemistry of D (+)-Glucose

As mentioned earlier D(+)-Glucose is the most important member of monosaccharide abundantly occurring in nature. Not only the chemistry of monosaccharides but also the chemistry of whole carbohydrates has been developed centring the studies on the chemistry of one and this most important member. In fact, chemistry of D(+)-Glucose may be looked upon as the chemistry of the carbohydrates. It is, therefore, felt pertinent to present here the chemistry of D(+)-Glucose to some extent in detail.

Isolation of D(+)-Glucose: Glucose occurs in honey and various sweet fruits. It also occurs in grape juice. That is why it is also known as *grape sugar*. Glucose is a normal constituent of blood.

In the laboratory it is prepared from sucrose. Sucrose is dissolved in 90% alcohol and is warmed at about 50-60 °C with concentrated hydrochloric acid for nearly two to three hours with occasional strirring. Sucrose is hydrolysed to glucose and fructose.

$$\underset{\text{Sucrose}}{C_{12}H_{22}O_{11}} + H_2O \longrightarrow \underset{\text{Glucose}}{C_6H_{12}O_6} + \underset{\text{Fructose}}{C_6H_{12}O_6}$$

The reaction mixture is cooled when glucose crystallises out.

1.2.6.1 Manufacture of D (+)-Glucose

D (+)-Glucose is manufactured from starch. Starch from potato, rice, etc. is hydrolysed with dilute sulphuric acid under pressure for about two hours. The reaction mixture is cooled and neutralised with calcium carbonate, the insoluble calcium sulphate is filtered out. The filtrate is decolourised by filtering through animal charcoal and concentrated by evaporation in vacuum and cooled when glucose monohydrate is obtained. It is further purified by crystallisation.

$$\underset{\text{Starch}}{(C_6H_{10}O_5)_n} + nH_2O \xrightarrow[H_2SO_4]{\text{dil.}} n(C_6H_{12}O_6)$$

D (+)-Glucose is a white crystalline powder soluble in water. It is optically active and dextrorotatory and because of its dextrorotation it is also known as *dextrose*. Glucose is an essential constituent of metabolic processes of living organism. In the blood, a definite concentration is to be maintained because both excess and deficiency are fatal for organism. The concentration of glucose in the body is maintained by the action of a hormone called *insulin*.

1.2.6.2 Structure of D (+)-Glucose

The structure of D(+)-glucose has been settled from the evidences as narrated below:

Open chain structure

i. Elemental analysis and molecular weight determination reveal that it has molecular formula, $C_6H_{12}O_6$.

ii. On acetylation with acetic anhydride it affords penta acetyl derivative indicating the presence of five hydroxyl functions in its molecule.

$$C_6H_{12}O_6 + 5(CH_3CO)_2O \longrightarrow \underset{\text{Penta acetyl derivative}}{C_6H_7(OCOCH_3)_5O}$$

iii. When heated gently glucose does not eliminate any molecule of water. This is a clear indication that the glucose molecule is stable and not more than one hydroxyl group is attached to any one carbon atom. Hence its five hydroxyls must be attached to five different carbon atoms.

iv. On treatment with hydroxyl amine hydrochloride under usual condition it furnishes an oxime derivative suggesting thereby the presence of a carbonyl function in glucose molecule.

v. Oxidation by mild oxidising agent like bromine water, glucose yields a mono-carboxylic acid having the same number of carbon atoms. This reveals that the carbonylic function present in glucose is aldehydic in nature, i.e.,

$$\underset{\text{Glucose}}{C_6H_{12}O_6} \xrightarrow[Br_2 / H_2O]{[O]} \underset{\text{Gluconic acid}}{(C_5H_{11}O_5)COOH}$$

vi. Reduction of glucose with hydroiodic acid and red phosphorous yields *n*-hexane. This indicates that all the six carbon atoms in glucose are present in a straight chain.

Based on the evidences as described above it has been suggested that glucose is a straight chain molecule as represented below:

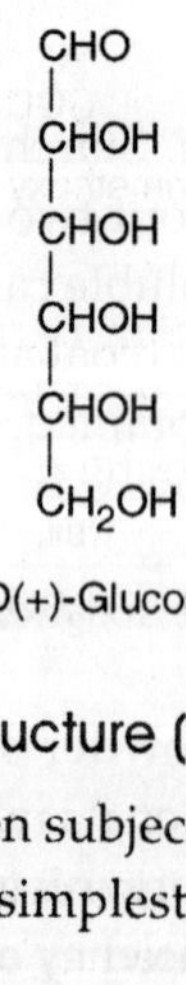

D(+)-Glucose

1.2.6.2.1 Drawbacks of Open Chain Structure (Backgrounds of Ring Structure)

The proposed open chain structure has been subjected to the following serious drawbacks:

(a) Glucose molecule fails to undergo simplest addition reaction with reagent like sodium bisulphite.

(b) It forms cyanohydrin with great difficulty.

(c) On treatment with absolute methanol in presence of dry hydrochloric acid it forms

  i. only monomethyl ether derivative.

  ii. two such isomeric monomethyl ether derivatives designated as α- and β-glucosides are formed, i.e.,

$$C_6H_{12}O_6 \xrightarrow{CH_3OH / HCl} \underset{\text{α- and β-monomethyl ether derivatives}}{C_6H_{11}O_5\,(OCH_3)}$$

  iii. Monomethyl ether derivatives fail to respond Tollen's and Fehling's tests.

(d) Although free glucose forms oxime derivative but its penta acetyl derivative does not afford any oxime derivative.

(e) Glucose exhibits mutarotation (spontaneous change of specific rotation of a freshly prepared solution of an optically active compound with time up to an equilibrium value).

In the basis of the above drawbacks it has been suggested that the aldehydic function and one of the hydroxyl groups are intramolecularly locked together in D(+)-glucose forming a cyclic hemiacetal, i.e., glucose has a ring structure.

1.2.6.2.2 Size of the Ring

Now the question arises which alcoholic hydroxyl function is involved in the formation of hemiacetal with aldehydic group. To have a meaningful answer of this question tetramethoxy glucose is subjected to oxidation with nitric acid when trimethoxy glutaric acid is formed as one of the major products.

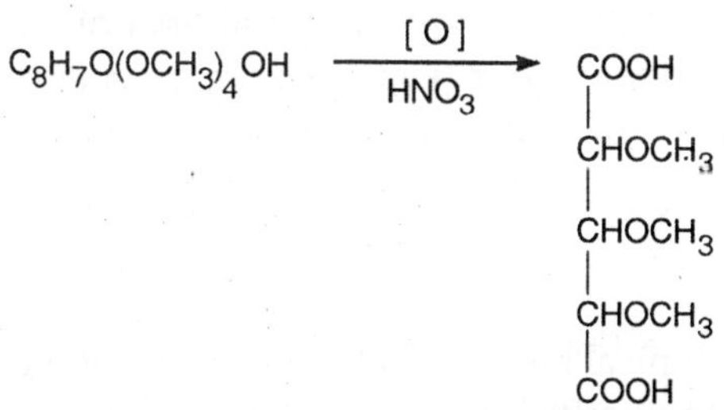

Trimethoxy glutaric acid

Formation of trimethoxy glutaric acid from tetramethyl glucose clearly suggests that only one methoxylated carbon atom is lost during oxidation and therefore, only one methoxylated carbon atom in tetramethyl glucose is outside the ring while other three such carbon atoms exist inside the ring. This is only possible if hemi-acetal formation in free glucose involves C_1.(—CHO group) and C_5—OH establishing thereby the six-membered cyclic structure for glucose.

1.2.6.2.3 α- and β-D(+)-Glucose

Formation of intramolecular hemiacetal creates a new chiral centre of C_1 and as the ring structure is rigid C_1—OH(hemi-acetal OH) must have two orientations generating two right structure, in one it is in the right -hand direction designated as α-D(+) glucose and in other it is in the left-hand direction known as β-D(+) glucose. In fact, two such different types of glucose have been isolated (Two different monomethyl derivatives are formed).

1.2.6.2.4 Ring-Chain Tautomerism

Glucose exhibits mutarotation which is a phenomenon of change of specific rotation with time up to an equilibrium value. In the case of glucose, this phenomenon of mutarotation can only be rationally interpreted (vide 1.3) if it is assumed that two forms (α and β) are interconvertible and their interconversion takes place via the open chain structure (I). Thus D(+)-glucose molecule constitutes an example of ring-chain tautomerism involving one open chain structure and two six-membered ring forms (II and III).

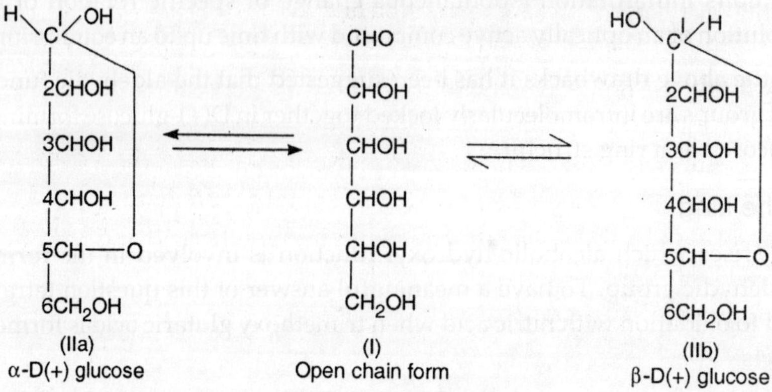

Before going into further discussion regarding the structural feature, particularly stereochemical aspect of glucose it is felt pertinent to present here the chemistry of fructose—an important member of ketose, phenomenon of mutarotation, some significant conversions and some special reactions of monosaccharides.

1.2.7 Chemistry of D (–)-Fructose

D (–) Fructose is the most common and typical member of ketose family of monosaccharides. It occurs along with glucose in many sweet fruits. It also occurs in sucrose. It is the major constituent of an important polysaccharide, *insulin*, the blood sugar controlling hormone in the body of living organism. It is laevorotatory in nature.

1.2.7.1 Preparation of D (–)-Fructose

In the laboratory it is prepared from sucrose. Aqueous solution of sucrose is hydrolysed with dilute sulphuric acid at a boiling temperature for an hour. The resulting reaction mixture is cooled and neutralised by adding barium carbonate when barium sulphate is precipitated. It is filtered and the filtrate is concentrated and lime water is added to it when sparingly soluble calcium fructoside is precipitated. It is filtered and carbon dioxide is passed through the suspension of fructoside in water when calcium carbonate is precipitated which is removed by filtration. Filtrate is concentrated to a syrupy liquid and cooled when fructose crystallises out gradually.

$$\underset{\text{Sucrose}}{C_{12}H_{22}O_{11}} + H_2O \longrightarrow \underset{\text{Glucose}}{C_6H_{12}O_6} + \underset{\text{Fructose}}{C_6H_{12}O_6}$$

Fructose is manufactured by the hydrolysis of *insulin*, a polysaccharide, with dilute sulphuric acid.

1.2.7.2 Properties of D (–)-Fructose

Fructose is a colourless crystalline solid, soluble in water. It exhibits the common properties of monosaccharides. It shows specific rotation of –133° which changes to a steady value of –92°.

1.2.7.3 Structure of D (–)-Fructose

D (—)-Fructose having the molecular formula, $C_6H_{12}O_6$ exhibits most of the characteristics of D (+)-glucose with minor exception. Thus,

i. it forms penta-acetyl derivative on acetylation and does not eliminate molecule of water on heating,

ii. it affords oxime but is not oxidised with bromine water indicating the ketonic nature of the carbonyl group present in its molecule.

iii. on reduction with hydroiodic acid and red phosphorous at a temperature of 100 °C it yields *n*-hexane as major product suggesting its straight chain nature.

iv. cyanohydrin of D (–) fructose on reduction with hydroiodic acid and red phosphorous yields 2-methyl hexanoic acid, i.e.,

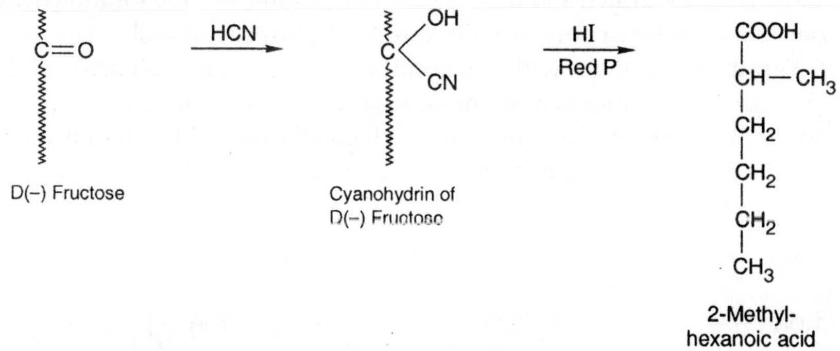

The formation of 2-methyl hexanoic acid suggests that the keto-group in fructose is at the position 2 and accordingly it is represented by the following straight chain structure.

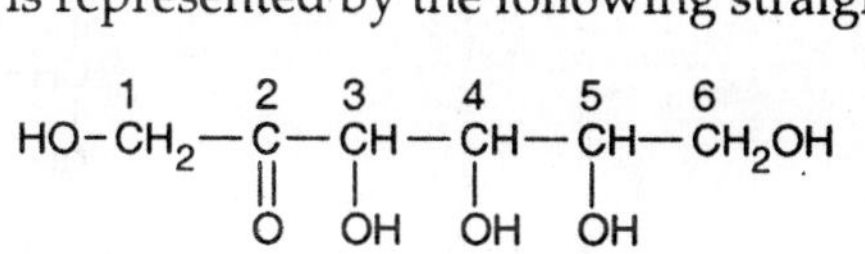

But this straight chain structure has been found to have same drawbacks as are observed for the open chain structure of D (+)-glucose, i.e., (i) its penta-acetyl derivative does not form oxime, (ii) but it forms two different mono-methyl derivatives on treatment with absolute methanol and dry hydrochloric acid, (iii) it exhibits *mutarotation*, etc., on the basis of which cyclic structure involving intramolecular ketal formation between keto carbonyl and one of the alcoholic hydroxyl functions has been assumed. Again, tetra-methyl D (–) fructose on oxidation with nitric acid furnishes trimethoxy glutaric acid. Thus D (–) fructose is a six-membered cyclic molecule and since it exhibits mutarotation there must be an equilibrium between cyclic froms and an open chain form similar to D (+) glucose. Based on these evidences the structure of D (–) fructose has been represented as the equilibrium of the following structures:

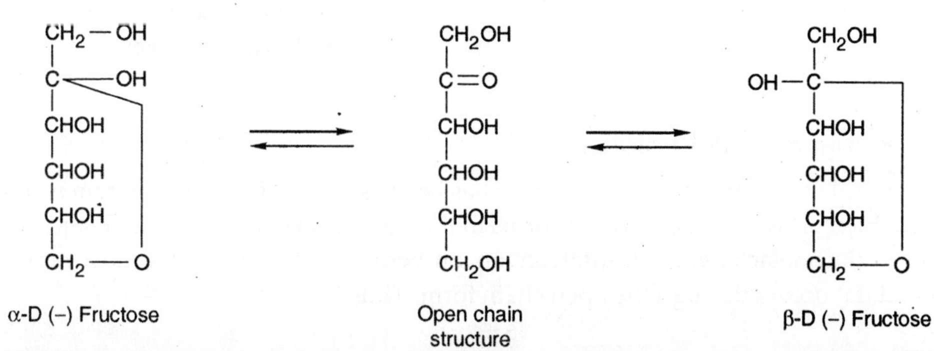

It may be mentioned in this connection that in association with other molecules, D (–) fructose can exist in *five-membered ring form* as has been observed in *sucrose and insulin* but in the free state five-membered ring structure is very unstable and so fructose having five memberd ring has not been isolated in free state.

1.3 Mutarotation

Mutarotation is a phenomenon which may be defined as the spontaneous change of specific rotation of a freshly prepared solution of an optically active compound with time up to an equilibrium value. The best known and widely illustrated example is the solution of D (+)-glucose. It has been observed that when a pure sample of α-D (+)-glucose is dissolved in water its specific rotation (+110°) gradually changes with time until it reaches to an equilibrium value of +52.5°. Similarly, in the case of β-isomer whose initial rotation of +19.5° ultimately changes to 52.5°. Another example that may be cited in this regard is gluconolactone. When its δ-isomer is dissolved in water its specific rotation (+63°) changes to +12° and γ-isomer (+67°) ultimately shows the same value (+12°). Thus,

i.

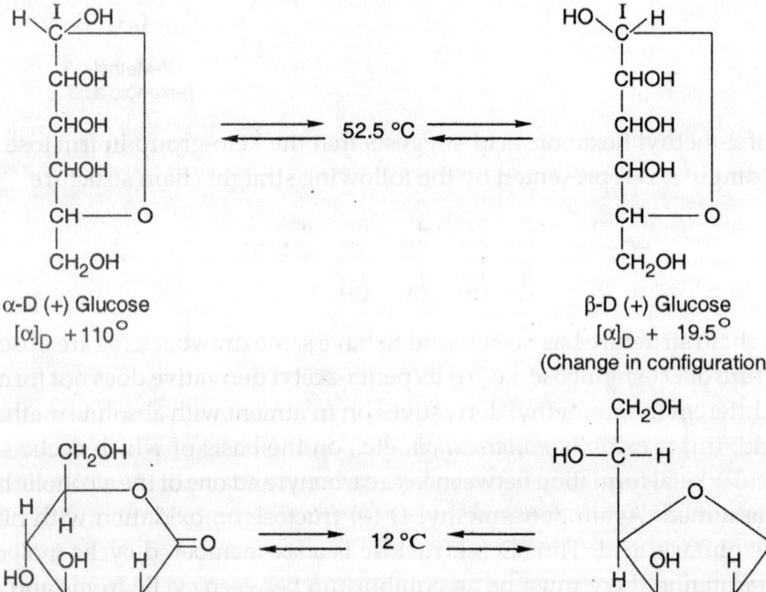

ii.

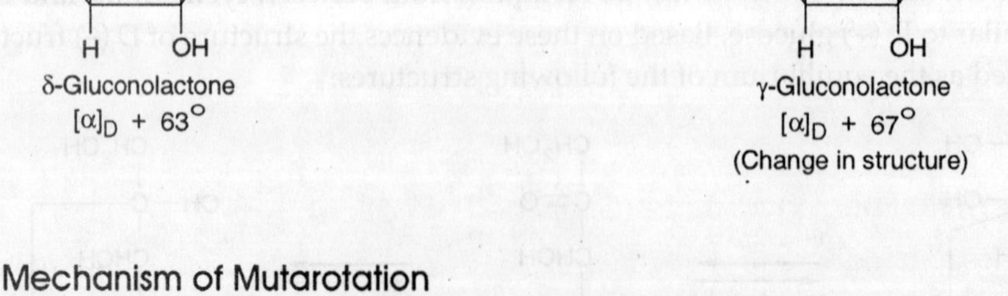

1.3.1 Mechanism of Mutarotation

In order to explain the above phenomenon it has been assumed that mutarotation is due to the interconversion of two forms, α- and β-forms in the case of D (+)-glucose and δ- and γ-forms in the case of gluconolactone. Such interconversion between the two forms most rationally be interpreted if it occurs through the open chain form. Thus,

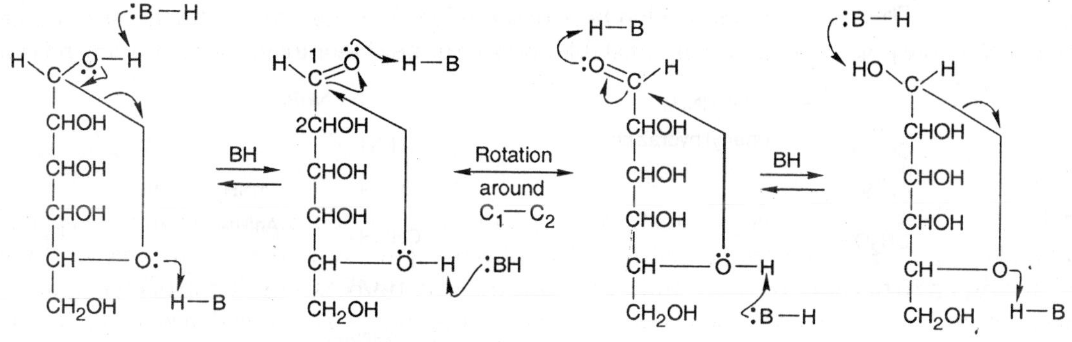

α-form of D (+) Glucose — Open chain — β-form of D (+) Glucose

From the above mechanistic path of mutarotation it is evident that interconversion of α- and β-forms of D (+)-glucose is possible if there is the formation of their open chain forms. Thus, when the solution of D (+)-glucose exhibits mutarotation, the equilibrium solution must contain two rings and one open chain form. Similar is the case with gluconolactone, i.e.,

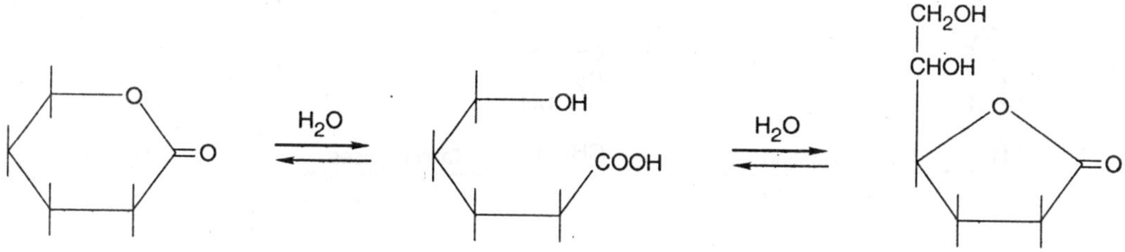

δ-form — Gluconic acid — γ-form

1.3.2 Nature of Catalyst

It is evident from the above mechanism that the interconversion occurring requires amphoteric catalysts. That is why mutarotation is observed in water solution. That the presence of amphoteric catalyst is essential has been supported by the fact that D (+)-glucose does not exhibit mutarotation when it is observed either in pyridine or in phenol solution but it exhibits mutarotation as usual in the equivalent mixture of phenol and pyridine solution.

1.4 Some Special Reactions of Monosaccharides

1.4.1 Reaction with Phenylhydrazine (Osazone Formation)

Reaction of monosaccharides with phenylhydrazine is very interesting and has drawn the keen interest of chemists working in the field of carbohydrate chemistry. Monosaccharides contain only one carbonyl function and so it is expected that stoichometrically only one molecule of phenylhydrazine should be involved in reaction with any monosaccharide with the formation of corresponding phenylhydrazone. Amazingly, three molecules of phenylhydrazine react with one molecule of monosaccharide and the product is osazone instead of phenylhydrazone. For example, D (+)-glucose on reaction with three molecules of phenylhydrazine yields glucosazone.

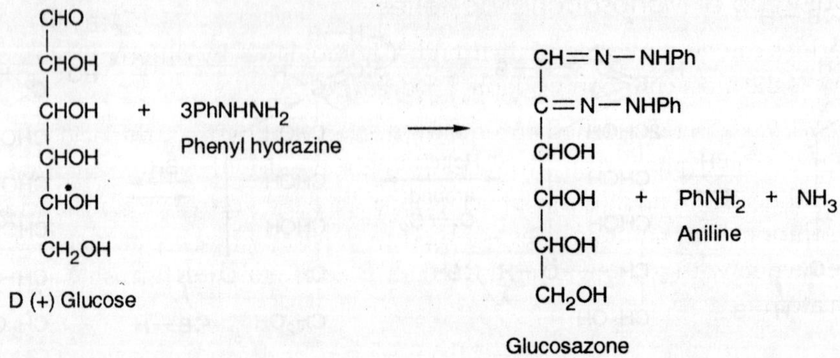

1.4.2 Action of Alkali

In dilute alkali monosaccharides undergo rearrangement to form a mixture of products. Thus, when D (+)-glucose is warmed with dilute alkali mixture of D (+)-mannose, D (+)-glucose and D (–)-fructose are formed and the mixture is almost optically inactive. Similar is the case with D (+)-mannose and D (–)-fructose. This reaction is known as *Lobry* de *Bruyan-van Ekenstein transformation*. Thus,

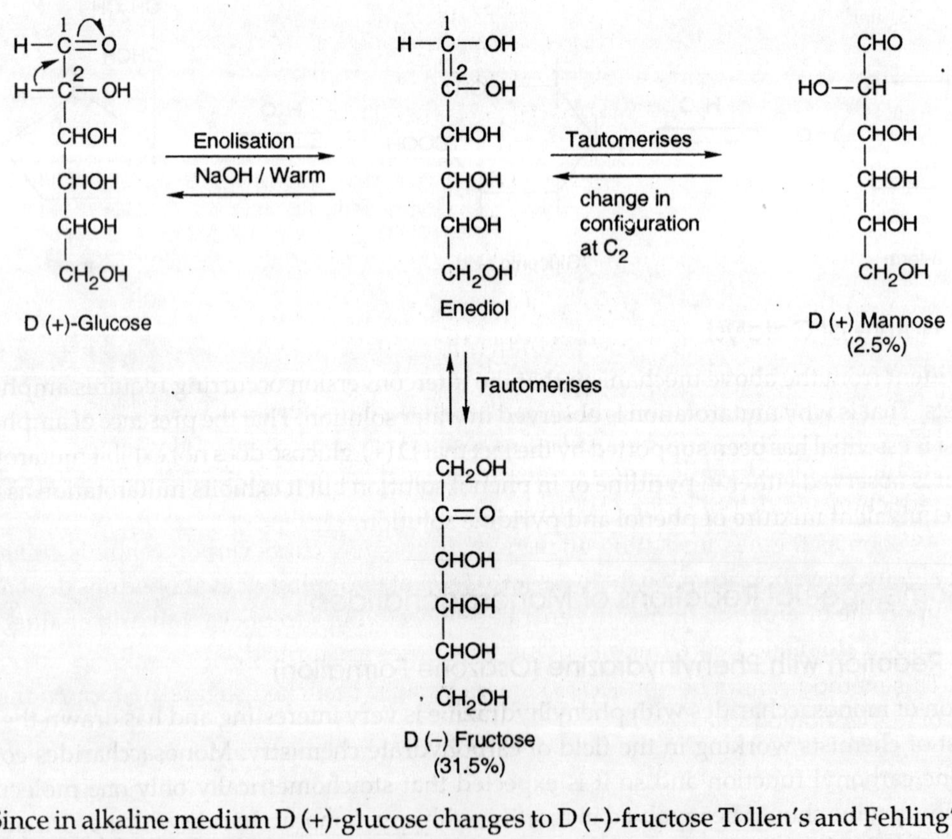

Since in alkaline medium D (+)-glucose changes to D (–)-fructose Tollen's and Fehling's tests which are also carried in alkaline condition cannot be reliably applied for the differentiation of aldoses and ketoses.

1.4.3 Stepping Up of Monosaccharide-series

Monosaccharides can be converted to their higher homologues by different methods of which following one is the most commonly adapted procedures.

- *Killiani Method*: In this method an aldose is treated with hydrocyanic acid when cyanohydrin is obtained. The cyanohydrin produced is hydrolysed with barium hydroxide solution followed by acidification with dilute sulphuric acid when polyhydroxy carboxylic acid is obtained in aqueous solution. This solution is evaporated to dryness when a γ-lactone is formed. This lactone on reduction with sodium amalgam in faintly acidic solution furnishes aldose with one more carbon atom.

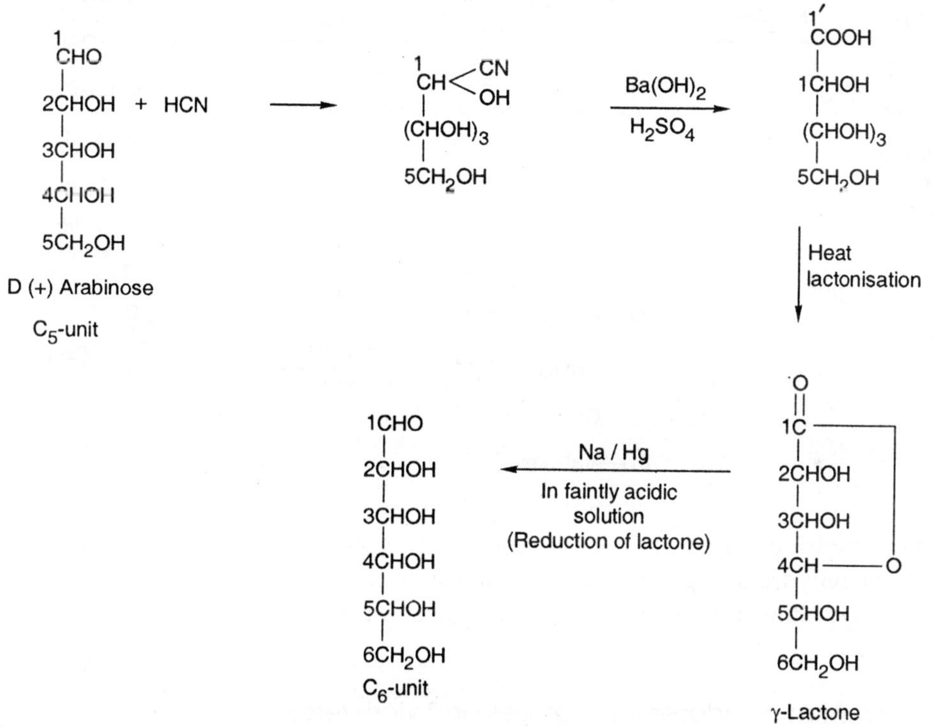

Note:

i. Reduction of aldehydic group is more easy than lactone ring. So in order to check the reduction at aldehydic stage faintly acidic solution is used.

ii. As soon as there is formation of cyanohydrin, a new chiral carbon centre is created at aldehydic carbon atom. So there are formation of two epimeric cyanohydrins depending upon the orientation of newly generated hydroxyl group of cyanohydrin at aldehydic carbon atom and hence mixture of higher aldoses are formed.

iii. This method cannot be applied to ketoses because branched sugars are formed instead of higher homologue, i.e.,

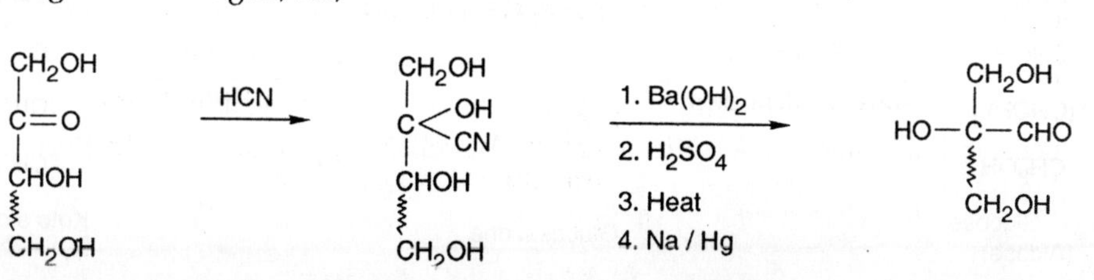

1.4.4 Stepping Down of Monosaccharide-series

Out of different methods known for stepping down the monosaccharide-series, method due to Wohl is frequently employed.

- *Wohl's Method*: This method involves the formation of oxime of an aldose which is converted to cyanoacetyl derivative in the subsequent step by the action of acetic anhydride. The cyanoacetyl derivative formed is warmed with ammoniacal silver nitrate solution when aldose having one carbon atom less is obtained.

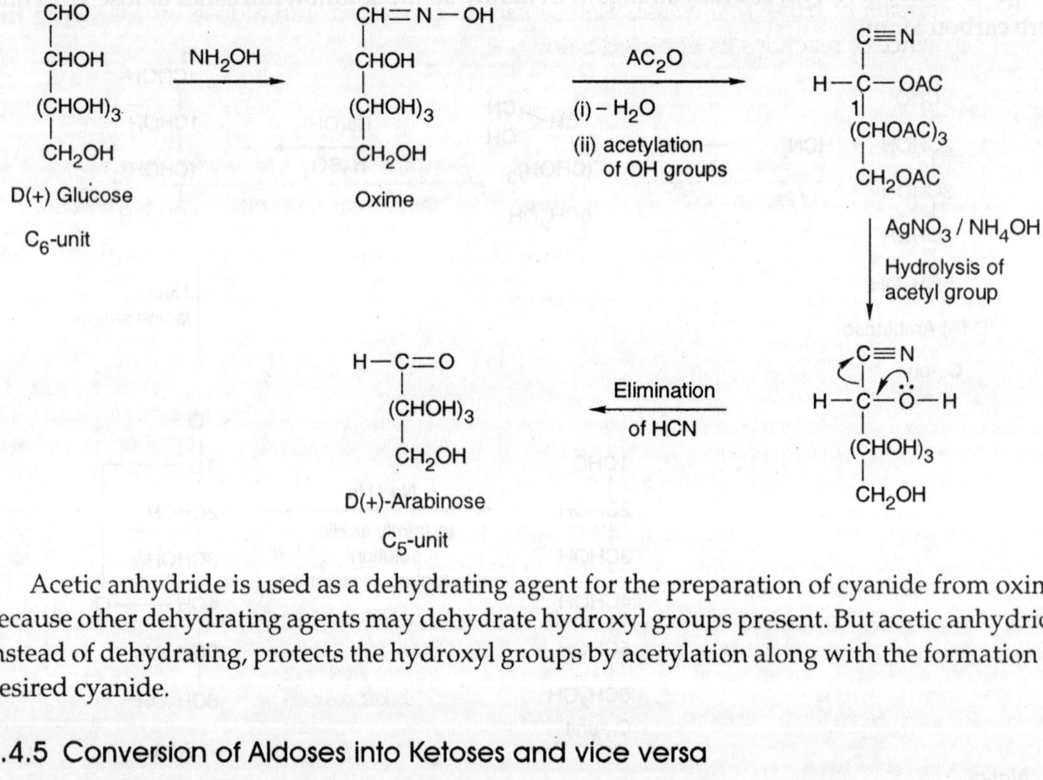

Acetic anhydride is used as a dehydrating agent for the preparation of cyanide from oxime because other dehydrating agents may dehydrate hydroxyl groups present. But acetic anhydride instead of dehydrating, protects the hydroxyl groups by acetylation along with the formation of desired cyanide.

1.4.5 Conversion of Aldoses into Ketoses and vice versa

Both aldoses and ketoses can be interconverted. This interconversion is very useful, particularly for ketoses in their stepping up and down of the series, because methods normally available for these purposes, as mentioned earlier, cannot be applied in the case of ketose. During ascending and descending of ketoses initially the starting ketose is converted into aldose having same number of carbon atoms. Such converted aldose is then stepped up or down to aldose following usual procedure. This changed aldose is now converted to the desired ketose.

(a) *Conversion of an aldose into a ketose*: Conversion of an aldose into a ketose having same number of carbon atoms proceeds through the following steps:

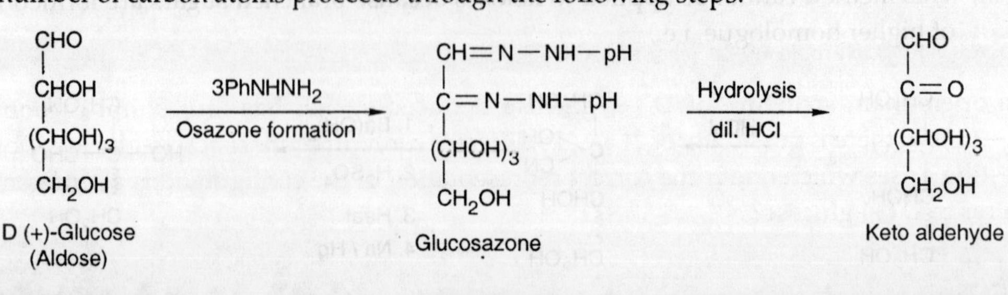

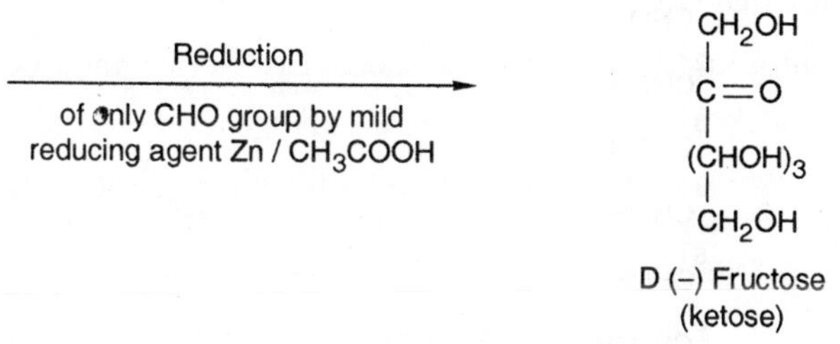

(b) *Conversion of ketose into aldose*: Ketose can be converted into aldose by following the sequence of reactions as depicted below:

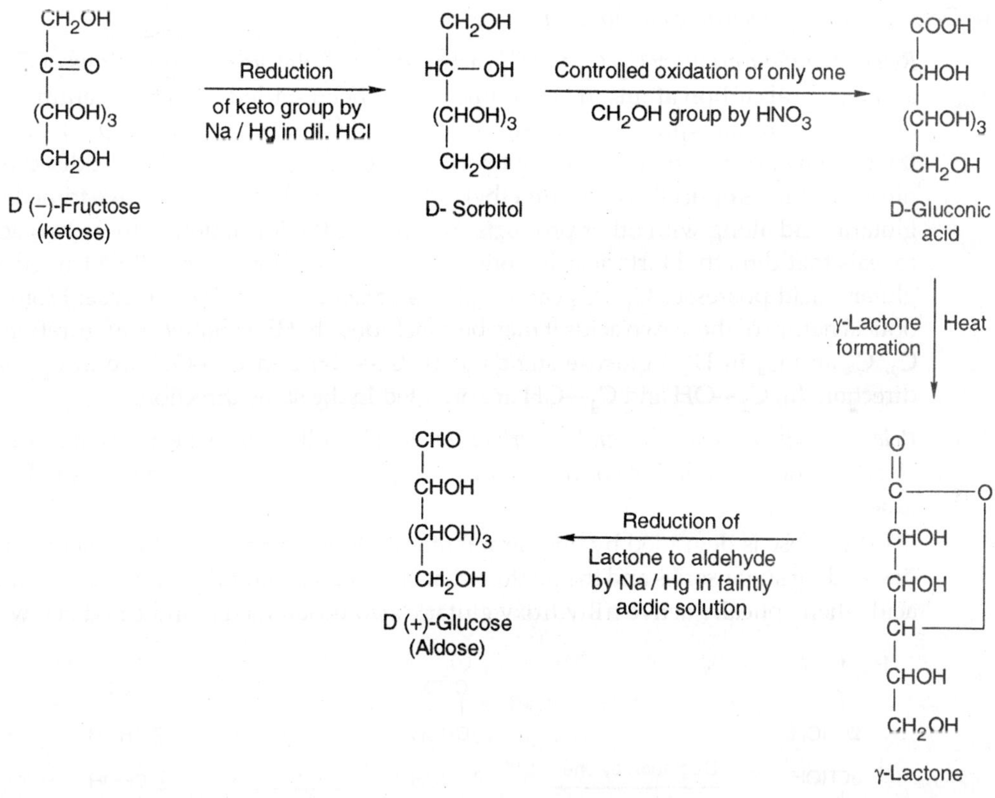

It may be remembered that during reduction of keto group a new chiral carbon atom is formed. So epimers will be formed and in fact, along with D-sorbitol, D-mannitol is also formed. Hence in the final stage mixture of D (+)-glucose and D (+)-mannose are formed which needs separation to get pure aldose.

1.5 Configuration of D (+)-Glucose

The open chain structure of D (+)-glucose deduced earlier has four chiral carbon atoms (C_2—C_5). So there is possibility of 2^4, i.e., 16 different configurations for D (+)-glucose. Obviously question arises which one is the correct representation of the configurations at different chiral centres in D (+)-glucose?

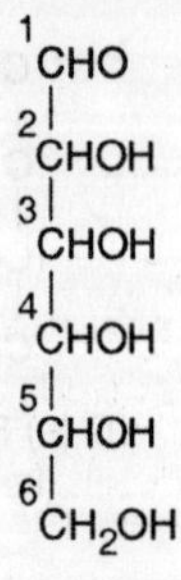

The configurations at different chiral carbon atoms in D (+)-glucose have been settled from the following experimental evidences:

(a) *Determination of Relative configurations*

i. *Relative configurations of C_2, C_3 and C_4-carbon atoms*: Relative configurations of C_2, C_3 and C_4 chiral carbon atoms in D (+)-glucose has been settled from the identification of different products produced during nitric acid oxidation of tetramethyl D (+)-glucose. It has been observed that tetramethyl derivative of D (+)-glucose when oxidised with nitric acid yields optically active dimethyl tartaric acid and optically inactive trimethoxy glutaric acid along with other products. Scrutiny of the formation of these two acids reveals that dimethyl tartaric acid contains C_1 to C_4 carbon atoms while trimethoxy glutaric acid possesses C_1—C_5 carbon atoms of tetramethyl D(+)-glucose. From the optical nature of these two acids it may be concluded that the relative configurations at C_2, C_3 and C_4 in D(+)-glucose stands as (i) C_2—OH and C_3—OH are in opposite direction, (ii) C_2—OH and C_4—OH are oriented in the same direction.

ii. *Relative configurations of C_3 and C_5 carbon atoms*: The following experimental evidence clearly settles the relative configurations of C_3 and C_5-chiral carbon atoms in D (+)-glucose.

D (+)-glucose is degraded by one carbon atom following any one of the methods for descending sugar series and the pentose that is formed is carefully oxidised with nitric acid when optically active trihydroxy glutaric acid is obtained as indicated below:

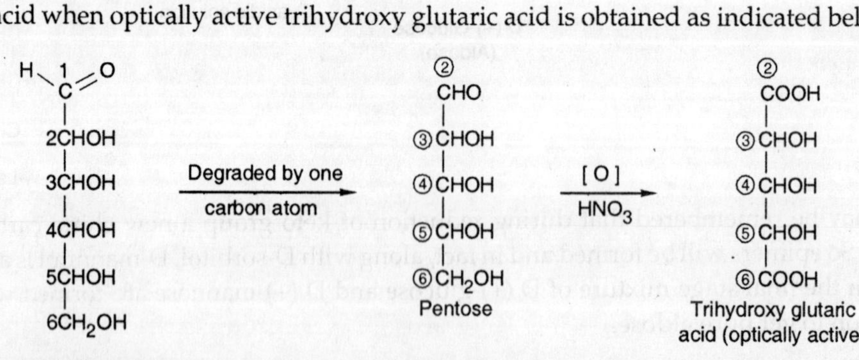

[Number in circle indicates the carbon atom number of D (+)-glucose]

From the above oxidation it is evident that trihydroxy glutaric obtained contains C_2 to C_6 carbon atoms of the parent D (+)-glucose. Since this glutaric acid is optically active C_3—OH and C_5—OH of D (+)-glucose must be in opposite direction to each other. Thus, relative configurations of different chiral carbon atoms stand as:

i. C_2—OH and C_3—OH are in opposite directions.

ii. C_2—OH and C_4—OH are in same diréctions.

iii. C_3—OH and C_5—OH are in opposite directions.

(b) *Fixation of the configuration of one of the carbon atoms* (Absolute configuration of D (+)-glucose): The configuration of C_5—carbon atom in D (+)-glucose has been absolutely settled by preparing D (+)-glucose starting from D (+)-glceraldehyde. It is known that D (+) glyceraldehyde has its hydroxyl function at C_2 atom oriented in right-hand direction. When it is subjected successively to Killiani method of stepping up of the monosacchardide series, a large number of isomeric aldohexoses are obtained all of which contains hydroxyl group at the penultimate carbon (C_5) directed towards right-hand direction. Of these large number of isomeric aldohexoses one of the isomers has been found to be completely identical in all respects with the naturally occurring D (+)-glucose. Accordingly, C_5-OH in (D (+)-glucose is located at the right direction, i.e.,

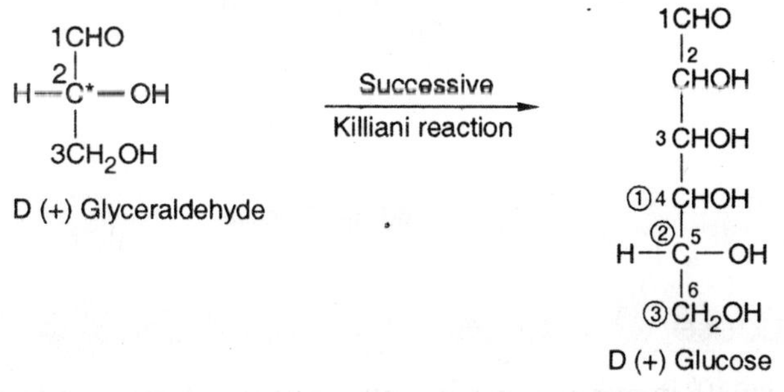

[Number in the circle is the number of D (+)-glyceraldehyde]

Based on the experimental evidences discussed above, the absolute configuration of different chiral carbon atoms exluding that of C_1 in D (+)-glucose may be represented as

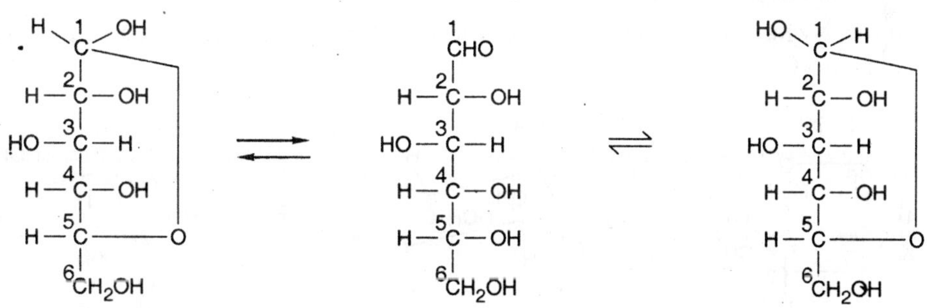

α-D (+)-Glucose D (+)-Glucose β-D (+)-Glucose

(c) *Configuration af C_1 of D (+)-glucose:* Fischer arbitrarily assigned the configuration at C_1 atom of D (+)-glucose. He assumed that in α-D (+)-glucose C_1-OH group is at the right-hand direction while in β-D (+)-glucose C_1-OH group exists in left-hand direction. Subsequently Boeseken secured experimental evidence in support of Fischer assumption. Boeseken observed that the conductivity of boric acid solution is changed towards higher direction when α-D (+)-glucose is added to this solution but on long standing decreases to a constant value. But the reverse effect is observed with β-D (+)-glucose, i.e., in this case low conductance value slowly increases to a constant value. This observation has been explained on the basis of formation of complex by *cis*-1, 2-glucol system with boric acid.

1.6 Haworth's Projection Formula

Haworth proposed a hexagonal formula based on pyran structure (six-membered ring containing an oxygen atom is known as *pyran ring* 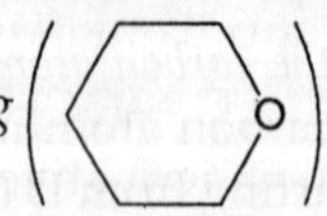). Fischer's projection formula may be changed to Haworth's projection formula by assuming that all the groups on the left-hand side of Fischer's formula are above the plane of the pyran ring and all those on right-hand side in Fischer's representation are below the plane of pyran ring. Thus,

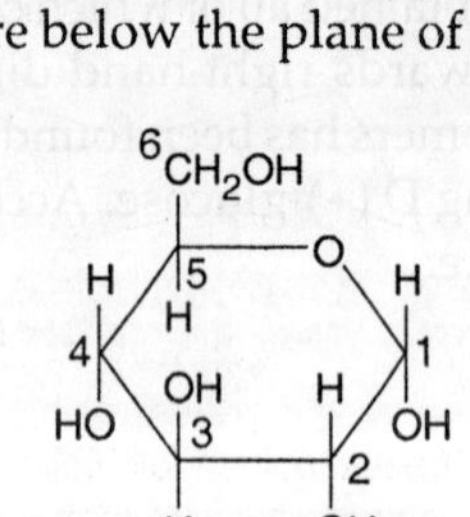

α-D (+)-Glucose

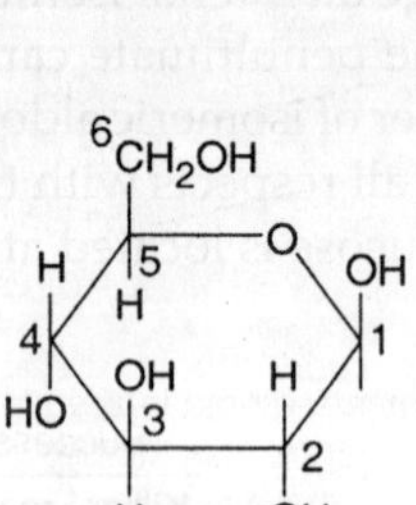

β-D (+)-Glucose

1.7 Conformation of D(+)-Glucose

It is known that C—O—C bond angle is 110⁶ in pyran which is very close to C—C—C— tetrahedral bond angle 109°28′. Hence it is expected that pyran ring should have similar behaviour like cyclohexane ring system.

On this background pyran structures for α- and β-D(+)-glucose can be represented as (III) and (IV) respectively.

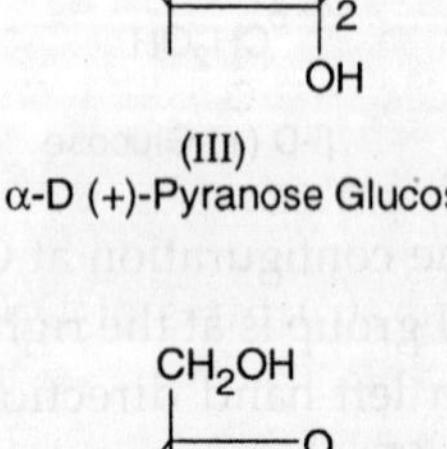

(III)
α-D (+)-Pyranose Glucose

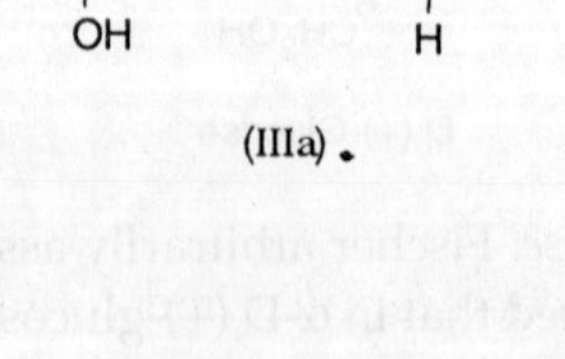

(IIIa)

⇌

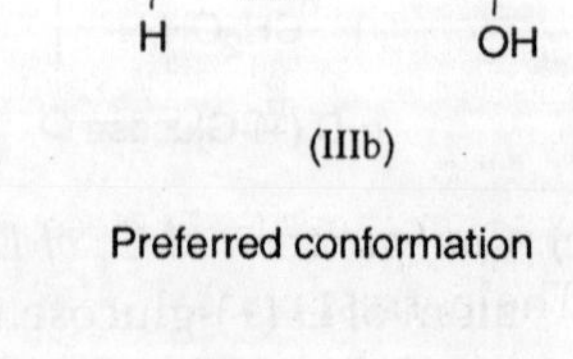

(IIIb)
Preferred conformation

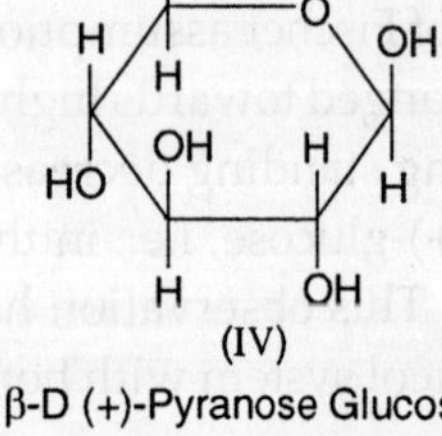

(IV)
β-D (+)-Pyranose Glucose

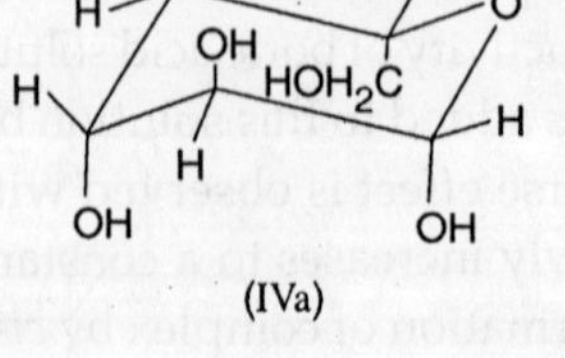

(IVa)

⇌

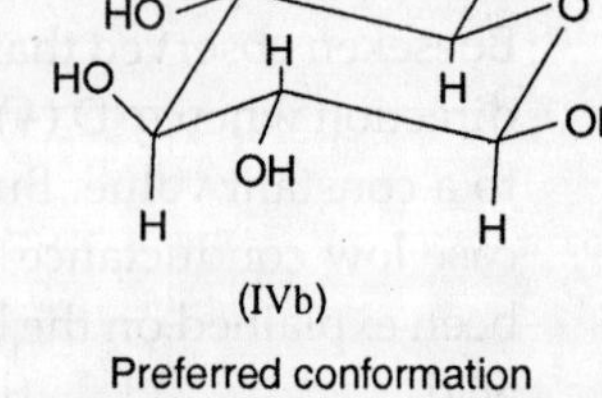

(IVb)
Preferred conformation

Out of (IIIa) and (IIIb), (IIIb) contains maximum number (four out of five) of hydroxyl groups in equatorial positions and so it is the stable conformer of α-form. Similarly, (IV) where all the substituents are in equatorial positions is the stable conformer of β-isomer. That is why in equilibrium solution, β-form predominates (approximately 64%).

In this connection it may be mentioned that C_1—OCH_3 derivative of β-D (+)-glucose is less stable, i.e., more reactive than the corresponding derivative of α-D (+)-glucose. This is because of the fact that the dipole-dipole interaction between oxygen atom of pyran ring and the oxygenated substituents like —OCH_3 and —$OCOCH_3$ at C_1 is greater when these groups are in equatorial positions than the such interaction when these groups are in axial positions as indicated below:

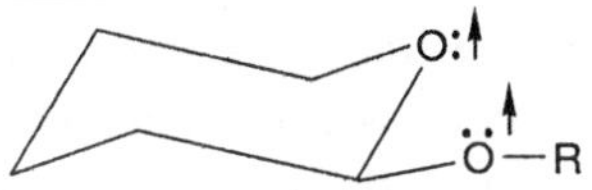

β-form
More dipole-dipole interaction
and hence less stable,
i.e., more reactive

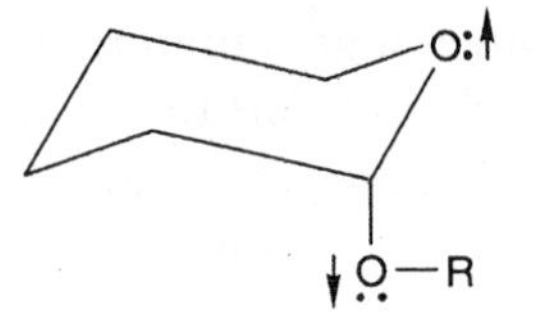

α-form
Less dipole-dipole interaction
and more stable than β-form

1.8 Stereoconfigurations at Different Chiral Carbon Atoms in D (-)-Fructose

The stereo configurations at different chiral centres in D(–) fructose has been settled from the osazone formation. It is known that osazone formation involves only C_1 and C_2 carbon atoms of both D(+)-glucose and D(–) fructose. It has been observed that the osazone of D(–) fructose is completely identical to that of D(+)-glucose. Thus it is unambiguously established that both D(+)-glucose and D(–) fructose must have identical stereo configurations at carbon atoms from C_3—C_5. C_1 and C_2 atoms of D(–) fructose are non-chiral and hence complete stereochemical representation of D(–) fructose may be expressed as below:

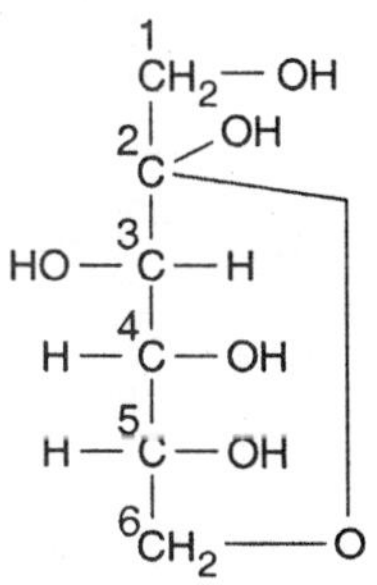

α-D (–)-Fructose

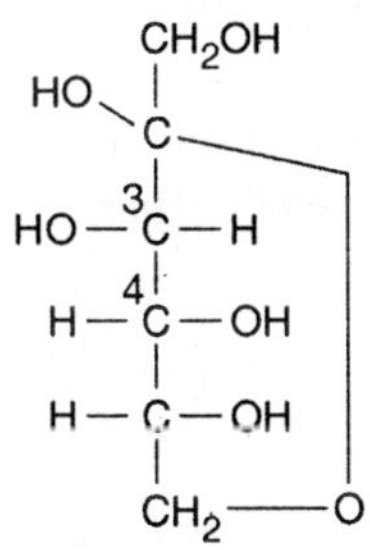

β-D (–)-Fructose

The corresponding Haworth projection formula and conformational structures of D (–)-fructose may be written as under:

Haworth Pyranose structure

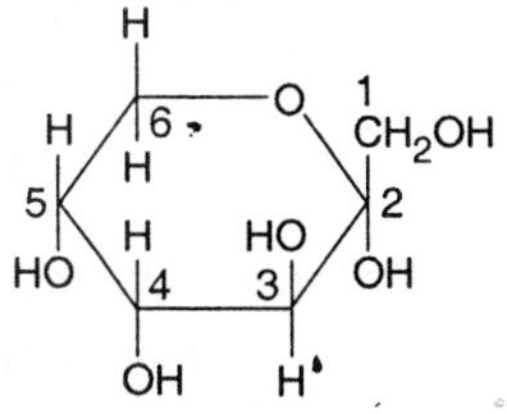

α-D (–)-Fructose

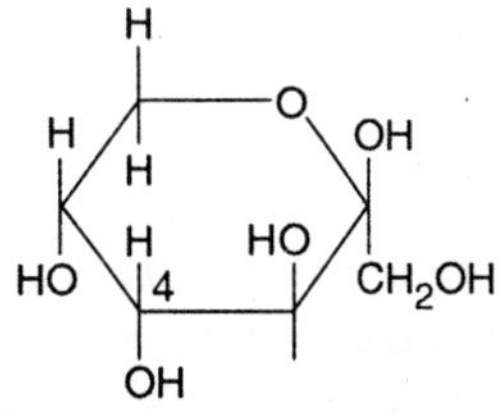

β-D (–)-Fructose

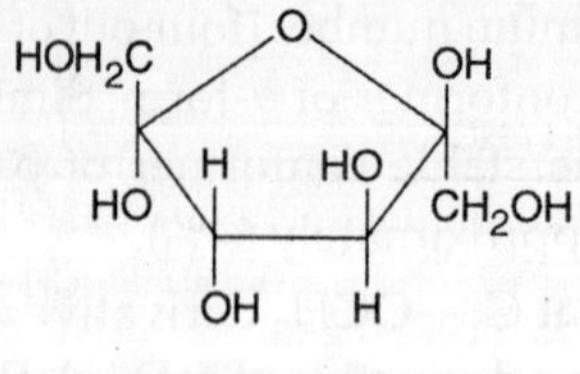

β-D (–)-Fructofuranose

1.9 Anomeric Carbon Atom and Anomers

Glucose and other sugars undergo intramolecular acetal or ketal formation by the interaction between carbonyl group and one of the alcoholic hydroxyl functions present in them. The resulting products are cyclic acetals or ketals. In this reaction the carbonyl carbon atom becomes asymmetric and two isomers are formed, i.e.,

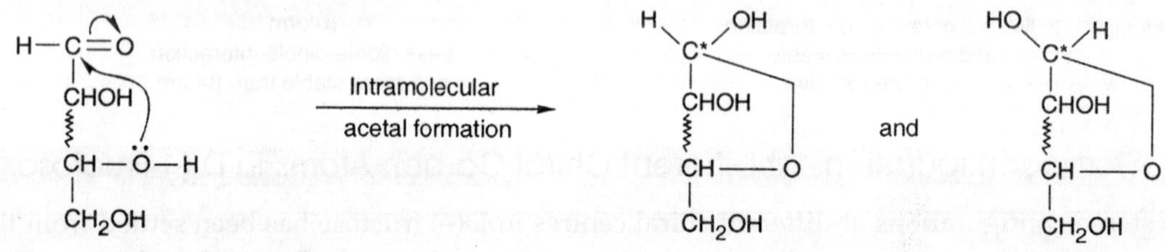

α-isomer β-isomer

During this reaction *marked C becomes asymmetric carbon and two isomers formed differ only in the configuration at newly generated asymmetric carbon atom. These isomers are termed as *anomers* and the newly generated asymmetric carbon atom is termed as *anomeric carbon*. Thus, anomers may be defined as sugars which have same configurations at all chiral carbon excepting at anomeric carbon atom. α-D (+)-glucose and β-D (+)-glucose are anomers. It may be remembered that anomers and epimers are not identical. Epimers are those which differ in configuration at only one chiral carbon atom excepting that at anomeric carbon. D (+)-glucose and D (+)-mannose are epimers to each other as they differ in configuration at C_2 only.

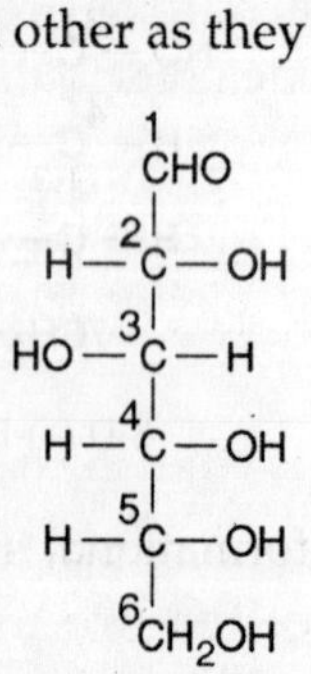

D (+)-Glucose

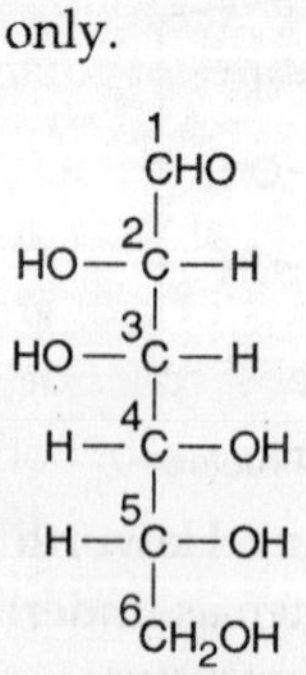

D (+)-Mannose

1.10 Glycosides

Glycosides are the organic derivatives of cyclic acetal or ketal of sugars in which hydrogen atom of acetal OH is replaced by alkyl or aryl group. Thus,

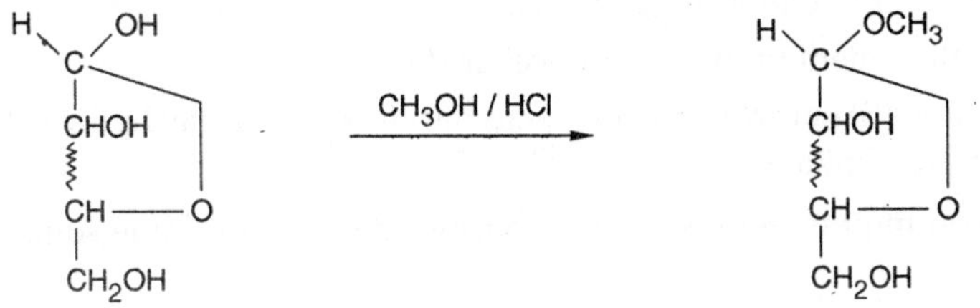

Methyl glycoside

Glycosides cannot reduce Tollen's and Fehling's solution due to the blocking of acetal hydroxyl (dormant carbonyl) by organic group. For this reason glycosides are called *non-reducing sugars.* The individual glycosides are named after the name of parent sugar. Thus, glycosides of glucose are known as glucosides. Similarly, fructosides are the glycosides of fructose. It may further be mentioned that glycosides do not exhibit mutarotation and hence cannot be present as equilibrium mixture but is present in only one form either as α- or as β-form.

Problem 1.2

Define the terms:

(a) Anomer (b) Epimer

(c) Reducing sugar (d) Non-reducing sugar

1.11 Chemistry of Disaccharides

Disaccharides are those sugars which on hydrolysis with dilute acids or enzymes form two monosaccharide units identical or different. Or in other words, disaccharides may be looked upon as the combination of two monosaccharides. Since in cyclic structure (monosaccharides mainly exist in cyclic structures with very minor contribution of open chain form) all the carbon atoms contain hydroxyl groups, it is obvious that their combination in disaccharides must involve two hydroxyl groups, one from each monosaccharide. Again, in every monosaccharide, there are two types of hydroxyl groups, viz., (i) alcoholic and, (ii) acetal hdroxyl groups. Consequently there may be three modes of combination of two monosaccharide units in disaccharides.

Combination may involve

i. acetal hydroxyl of both units, i.e., glycoside with respect to both the monosaccharides.
ii. acetal hydroxyl of one and alcoholic hydroxyl of other, i.e., glycoside with respect to only one monosaccharide and
iii. alcoholic hydroxyls of both the units, i.e., disaccharide is ether in character.

Now the question arises whether disaccharides are glycosides or ether. It has been observed that disaccharides are always glycosides in nature and hence the two monosaccharides in disaccharides are combined according to probabilities (i) or (ii) or in other words, since disaccharides are glycosidic in nature, the involvement of acetal hydroxyl of at least one of the units of monosaccharide is essential but acetal hydroxyl group of other monosaccharide may or may not be involved.

Again, the unit whose acetal hydroxyl function is involved must exist either in α- or in β-form. Accordingly, identification of any disaccharide necessitates the elaboration of following three points.

i. Identification of two monosaccharides.
ii. Points of attachment of two monosaccharides.
iii. Anomeric (α or β) nature of the monosaccharide whose acetal hydroxyl group is involved in disaccharide linkage.

Some of the common members of disaccharides are sucrose (cane sugar), maltose, lactose milibiose, etc.

1.11.1 Sucrose (Cane sugar)

Sucrose is our common table sugar and is obtained from sugar cane and sugar beets. It is found in all photosynthetic plants.

1.11.1.1 Manufacture of Sucrose

Sucrose is mainly extracted from sugar canes. Sugar canes are cut into small pieces and washed, and these small pieces are crushed to squeeze out the juice and the residual known as *bagasse* is left out.

The juice obtained is a dark brown liquid containing 15-20% sucrose along with other materials such as glucose, fructose, vegetable proteins and other organic materials. This juice is purified following different procedures and then concentrated. Finally, crystals of sucrose are separated by centrifugal machine from mother liquor known as *molasses*. The crystals are dissolved in water and is decolourised by filtering through animal charcoal or *norit* (activated coconut charcoal).

By-products of Sugar Industry

i. *Molasses*: It is the mother liquor left out after the separation of sugar cyrstals. It is mainly used in the manufacture of ethanol and also as a manure.

ii. *Bagasse*: It is the solid material left out after the extraction of juice from sugar cane. It is mainly used as fuel.

1.11.1.2 Properties of Sucrose

i. It is a crystalline solid, having melting point 186 °C, soluble in water and is dextrorotatory, $[\alpha]_D = + 66.50°$.

ii. On hydrolysis with mineral acid or by enzyme, *invertase* sucrose forms equimolecular mixture of D (+)-glucose and D (—)-fructose, i.e.,

$$C_{12}H_{22}O_{11} + H_2O \xrightarrow[\text{invertase}]{\overset{+}{H}\text{ or}} \underset{\text{D (+)-Glucose}}{C_6H_{12}O_6} + \underset{\text{D (–)-Fructose}}{C_6H_{12}O_6}$$

iii. When heated with concentrated sulphuric acid sucrose forms CO_2 and SO_2, i.e.,

$$C_{12}H_{22}O_{11} + H_2SO_4 \longrightarrow CO_2 + SO_2 + H_2O$$

iv. On fermentation with yeast it furnishes glucose and fructose due to hydrolysis by enzyme *invertase* and next another enzyme *zymase* converts glucose and fructose into ethyl alcohol.

$$C_{12}H_{22}O_{11} + H_2O \xrightarrow{\text{Invertase}} \underset{\text{D (+)-Glucose}}{C_6H_{12}O_6} + \underset{\text{D (–)-Fructose}}{C_6H_{12}O_6}$$

$$\text{Glucose and Fructose} \xrightarrow{\text{Zymase}} \underset{\text{Ethyl alcohol}}{C_2H_5OH} + CO_2$$

1.11.1.3 Structure of Sucrose (Cane sugar)

The structure of cane sugar has been settled from the following physical and chemical evidences as well as from the logical arguments.

1. Elemental analysis and molecular weight determination suggest the molecular formula $C_{12}H_{22}O_{11}$ for sucrose.
2. On acetylation with acetic anhydride it forms octa-acetyl derivative and on methylation with dimethyl sulphate and alkali it furnishes octamethyl derivative. These experiments indicate the presence of eight hydroxyl groups in sucrose.
3. (a). On hydrolysis with mineral acid cane sugar yields two fragments, (A) and (B), i.e.,

$$C_{12}H_{22}O_{11} + H_2O \xrightarrow[\text{HCl}]{\text{Dilute}} \underset{(A)}{C_6H_{12}O_6} + \underset{(B)}{C_6H_{12}O_6}$$

(b) Similarly, hydrolysis of octamethyl derivative under similar condition affords tetramethyl derivative of (A) and tetramethyl derivative of (B).

$$C_{12}H_{14}(OCH_3)_8O_3 \xrightarrow[\text{HCl}]{\text{Dilute}} \underset{\text{Tetramethyl -A}}{C_6H_8(OCH_3)_4O_2} + \underset{\text{Tetramethyl -B}}{C_6H_8(OCH_3)_4O_2}$$

• *Identification of Fragment (A)*: Fragment (A) obtained from cane sugar has been found to possess the following characteristic properties:

i. forms penta-acetyl derivative on acetylation.
ii. yields an oxime on treatment with hydroxylamine hydrochloride.
iii. on oxidation with bromine water yields a carboxylic acid without any loss of carbon atom.
iv. on treatment with absolute methanol in presence of dry hydrochloric acid furnishes monomethyl derivative.
v. does not produce any additive product with sodium bisulphite solution.
vi. exhibits mutarotation and
vii. its penta-acetyl derivative fails to form any oxime derivative.

A scrutiny of the above properties clearly suggests that fragment (A) is a monosaccharide molecule of the type aldohexose possessing cyclic oxide structure.

• *Size of the Ring*: The tetramethyl (A) obtained from the hydrolysis of octamethyl derivative of sucrose when oxidised with nitric acid furnishes optically inactive trimethoxy glutaric acid and optically active dimethyl tartaric acid, i.e.,

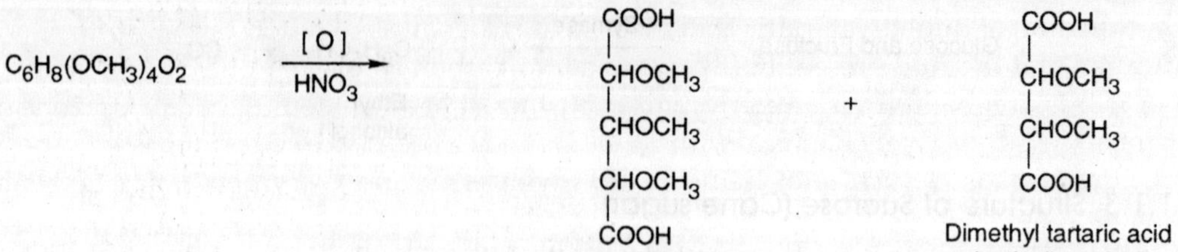

Dimethyl tartaric acid (optically active)

Trimethyoxy glutaric acid (optically inactive)

Formation of trimethoxy glutaric acid from tetramethyl (A) by the loss of one methoxylated carbon atom reveals the six-membered pyranose nature of (A) while optically inactive nature of this acid and optically active nature of other acid (dimethyl tartaric acid) remind of the similarity of the fragment (A) with D (+)-glucose and in actual practice, it was found to be so by the comparative study of (A) with the authentic specimen of D (+)-glucose. Thus, the structure of the fragment (A) may be written as

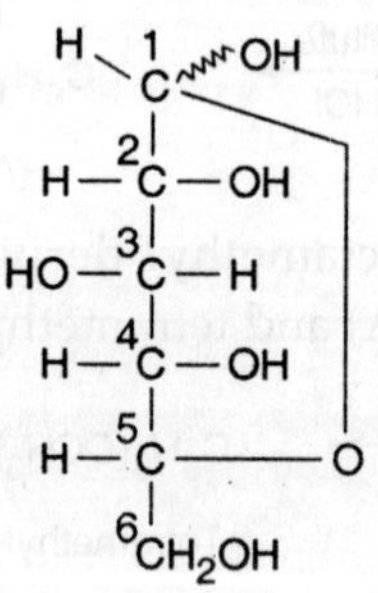

α- or β-D (+) Glucose (Fragment A)

- *Characterisation of the Fragment (B)*: Fragment (B) has been characterised from its following properties:

i. furnishes penta-acetyl derivative.
ii. forms oxime with hydroxyl amine hydrochloride but cannot be oxidised to carboxylic acid by bromine water.
iii. penta-acetyl derivative does not form oxime.
iv. like glucose it also exhibits mutarotation.

Careful analysis of all these properties reveals that fragment (B) is a ketohexose having cyclic oxide structure.

- *Size of the Ring*: The tetramethyl (B) produced during the hydrolysis of octamethyl derivative of the parent disaccharide yields dimethyl tartaric acid as the major product. Thus,

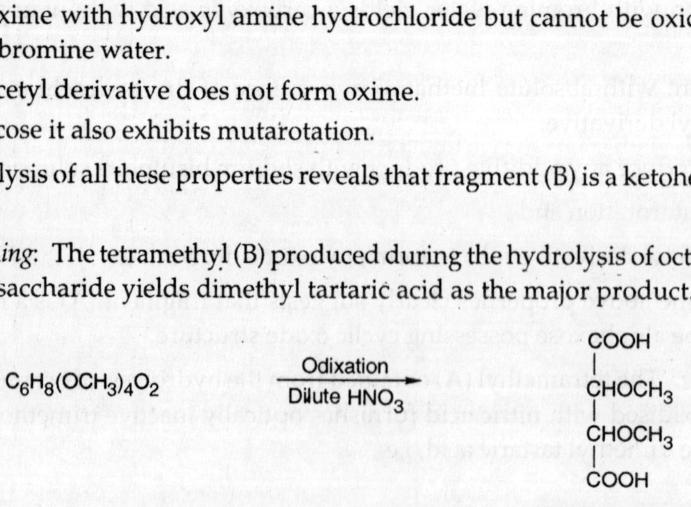

Dimethyl tartaric acid (optically active)

Formation of dimethyl tartaric acid by the loss of two methoxylated carbon atoms is a clear indication that the ring present in (B) contains four carbon atoms and one oxygen atom. Or in other words, fragment (B) is a keto-furanose. Further, it has been found that the osazone of the fragment (B) is completely identical with that of D (+)-glucose, hence keto group is at C_2-position. Thus, the furnaose structure of fragment (B) involves C_2 and C_5 carbon atoms for its cyclic structure.

Once again, comparison of physical and other properties of fragment (B) characterises it as D-fructose. However, foregoing evidences suggest that in sucrose, fructose is present in furanose form. Thus, the structure of the fragment (B) may be expressed as

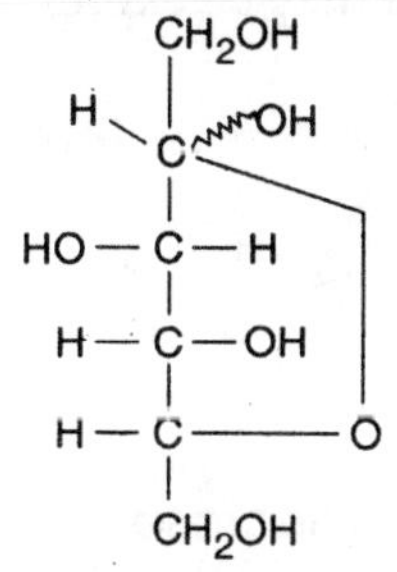

α- or β-D (–)-fructo-furanose

• *Point of Attachment of the Fragments (A) and (B)*: Which hydroxyl groups are involved in the attachment of the two monosaccharides identified as D (+)-pyrano-glucose and D (—)-fructo-furanose in sucrose have been settled from the observations that it neither exhibits mutarotation nor it can reduce Tollen's and Fehling's solutions. These observations unambiguouly settle that acetal hydroxyl of glucose portion and ketal hydroxyl of fructose are involved in linking these two monosaccharides in sucrose.

• *Stereochemical nature of Glycosidic Linkage*: Since reducing groups (acetal and ketal) are involved in both the monosaccharides, they must be present either as α- or as β-form. This issue has been settled by enzymatic hydrolysis. It is known that enzyme *maltase* hydrolyses only α-glycosides while β-glycosides are hydrolysed by the enzyme *emulsin*. Sucrose is hydrolysed by both the enzymes. Thus one of the monosaccharide in sucrose is present in α-form while the other exists in β-form. But question arises which one is which? The answer to this question has been secured from specific enzymatic hydrolysis experiments. Sucrose is hydrolysed by enzyme called *α-glycosidase* obtained from yeast which indicates the α-configuration at glucoside portion. Similarly, sucrose is also hydrolysed by the enzyme *sucrase*, a specific enzyme which hydrolyses only β-fructo-furnanosides. This settles the β-configuration at the fructoside portion.

On the basis of evidences thus deduced, structure of sucrose (cane sugar) stands as α-D (+) glucopyranosyl-β-D (–)-fructo-furnanoside as written below:

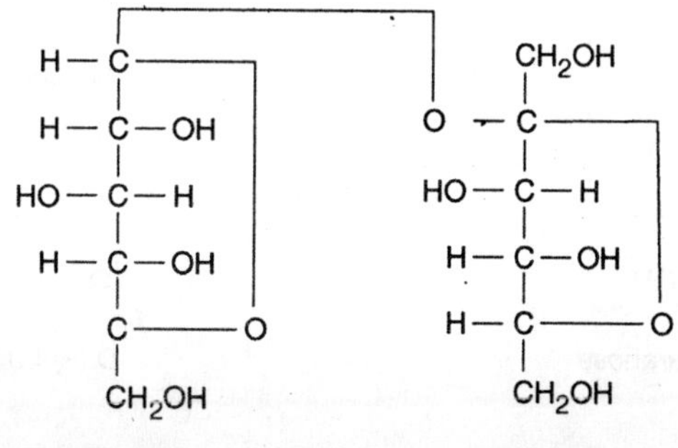

Haworth's structure may be expressed as below:

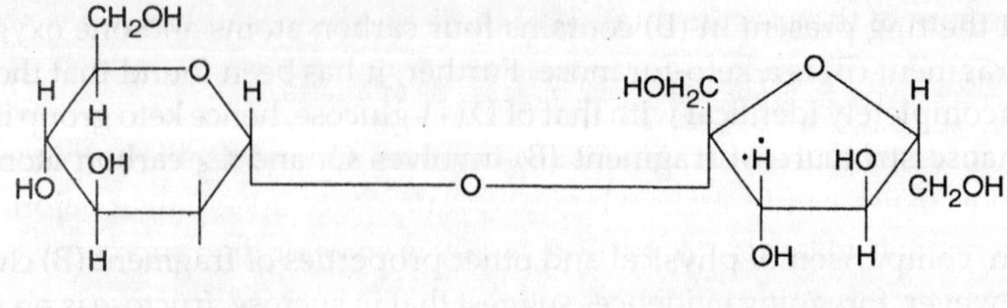

α-D (+)-Glucose portion β-D (–)-Fructose portion

Conformational structue of sucrose may be expressed as under:

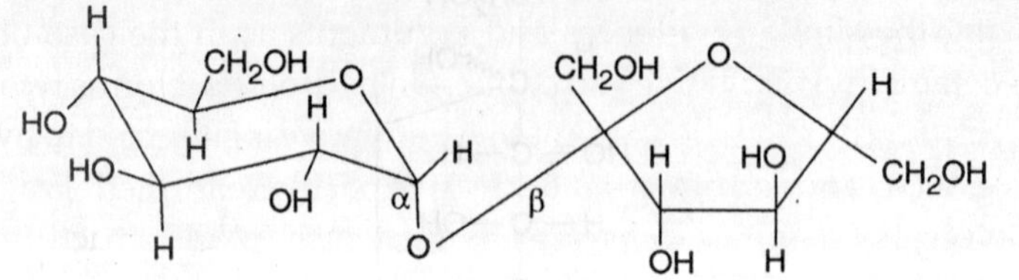

1.11.2 Invert Sugar and Inversion of Sucrose

When sucrose is hydrolysed by the treatment with dilute mineral acids it forms equimolecular mixture of D-glucose (specific rotation = +52.5° and D-fructose (specific rotation = –92°) and the specific rotation of sucrose (+ 66.5°) solution is changed. The solution of the mixture exhibits specific rotation of only –20°. As the optical rotation of sucrose solution changes from positive value (+66.5°) to negative value (–20°) during hydrolysis, this phenomenon is termed as *inversion of sucrose*, and mixture of glucose and fructose is known as *invert sugar*. The same hydrolysis can be achieved by the enzyme *invertase* found in yeast. Thus,

$$\underset{\substack{\text{Sucrose} \\ [\alpha]_D = +66.5^\circ}}{C_{12}H_{22}O_{11}} \xrightarrow{\text{Acid / invertase}} \underset{\substack{\text{D-Glucose} \\ [\alpha]_D = +52.5^\circ}}{C_6H_{12}O_6} + \underset{\substack{\text{D-Fructose} \\ [\alpha]_D = -92^\circ}}{C_6H_{12}O_6}$$

Mixture, $[\alpha]_D = -20^\circ$
(invert sugar)

The inversion of sucrose is due to the fact that during hydrolysis, initially there is formation of α-D (+)-glucopyranose and β-D(+)-fructofuranose. But β-D(+)-fructofuranose is very unstable and so it readily changes into the stable form D (—)-fructopyranose which is laevorotatory and its rotation is much greater than that of D (+)-glucopyranose. Thus,

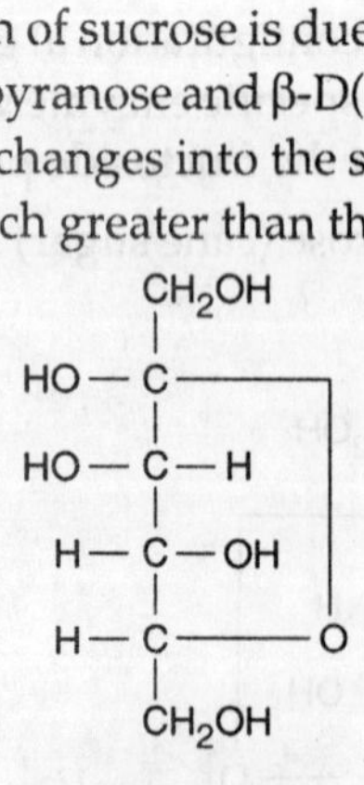

D (+)-fructofuranose

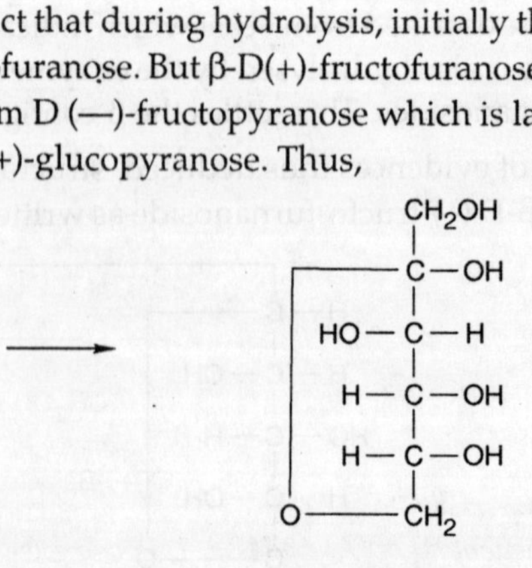

D (–)-fructopyranose

Since one mole of sucrose produces one mole each of glucose and fructose the specific rotation is one half of the sum of the specific rotation of these two monosaccharides,

$$\frac{1}{2}[52.5 + (-92^\circ)] = \frac{1}{2}(-39.5) = -19.75^\circ.$$

It may be mentioned that invert sugar is sweeter than sucrose itself. For this reason industrial users of sugar like bakers, candy-makers hydrolyse sucrose to invert sugar before use. Due to the presence of invert sugar in larger proportion, honey is sweeter than sucrose.

1.11.3 Lactose

Lactose is a disaccharide of mammalian origin and is found in milk. Its structure has been determined following the similar evidences and arguments as in the case of cane sugar. Like cane sugar it forms octamethyl derivative and oxime. On hydrolysis it forms two monosaccharides $C_6H_{12}O_6$ (A) and $C_6H_{12}O_6$ (B). But when octamethyl derivative is subjected to hydrolytic cleavage, trimethyl derivative of (A) and tertramethyl derivative of (B) are formed. Fragment (A) exhibits all the properties, typical of a monosaccharide having a cyclic oxide structure.

- *Size of the Ring*: The size of the ring present in (A) has been deduced as follows:

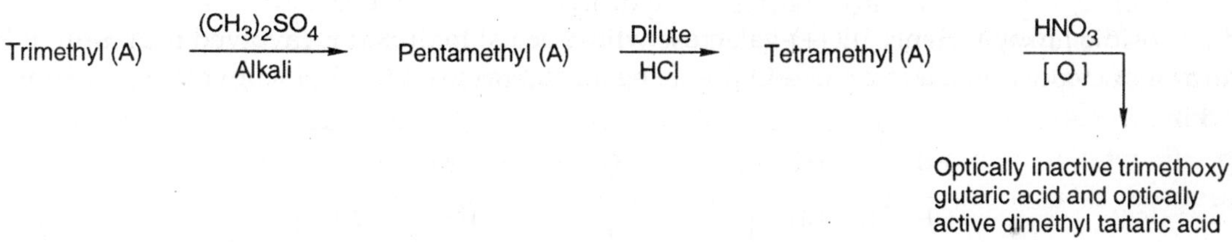

All the above characteristics discloses the similarity of (A) with D(+)-glucose and indeed it was found to be so by comparative study. Hence (A) is D(+)-glucopyranose.

Fragment (B) has similar properties like (A) *differing only in the fact* that on oxidation with nitric acid it forms optically active trimethoxy glutaric acid and optically active dimethyl tartaric acid. Formation of optically active trimethoxy glutaric acid from tetramethyl (B) suggests that both C_2—OCH_3 and C_4—OCH_3 as well as C_2—OCH_3 and C_3—OCH_3 are in opposite directions. Thus, fragment (B) is an epimer of D(+)-glucose. Survey of literature reveals the similarity of fragment (B) with D (+)-galactose and in fact, (B) has been identified as D (+)-galactose.

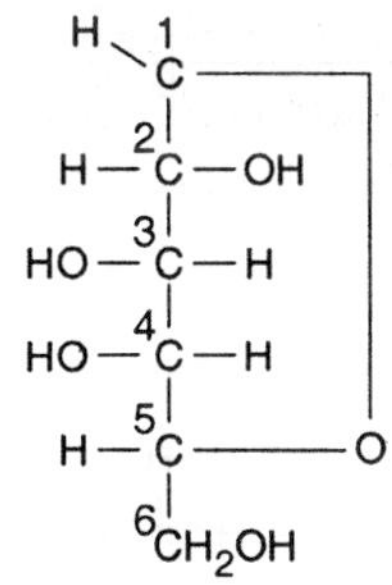

D (+)-Galactose

- *Point of Attachement of (A) and (B)*: Lactose exhibits mutarotation and reduces Tollen's and Fehling's solutions suggesting the fact that acetal hydroxyl of only one monosaccharide has been involved in the linkage and acetal hydroxyl of other is free. Formation of trimethyl (A) and tetramethyl (B) during hydrolysis of octamethyl derivative of lactose supports the above conclusion as well as establishes that acetal hydroxyl of (A) is free, i.e., one of the alcoholic hydroxyl groups of (A) is blocked in disaccharide linkage and hence, it forms trimethyl instead of tetramethyl derivative. Consequently acetal hydroxyl of (B), i.e., D-galactose is connected with one of the alcoholic hydroxyls of (A), i.e., D(+)-glucose.

• *Position of Alcoholic hydroxyl of (A) involved in the linkage*: The position of the alcoholic hydroxyl group of D(+)-glucose involved in disaccharide linkage has been settled as mentioned below:

Lactose readily forms an osazone on treatment with phenylhydrazine. This suggests that C_1- and C_2-hydroxyl groups are free in D-glucose unit.

Now lactose is degraded by one carbon atom and such degraded lactose once again forms osazone. This reveals that C_2- and C_3-hydroxyl groups are free in this unit. But when this degraded lactose is further degraded by one carbon more and is subjected to osazone formation, no such osazone is formed this time establishing thereby the fact that C_4-hydroxyl group of D-glucose unit is blocked. Accordingly, the disaccharide linkage involves C_1-hydroxyl (acetal hydroxyl) of D (+) galactose and C_4-hydroxyl (alcoholic) of D (+)-glucose.

Nature of Glycosidic linkage: Lactose is hydrolysed by enzyme lactase which is specific for β-glycosidic linkage. Hence, D (+)-galactose whose acetal hydroxyl is involved is present in B-form in lactose. Thus, lactose is 4-O-β-D (+)-galactopyranosyl-D(+)-glucopyranose as shown below:

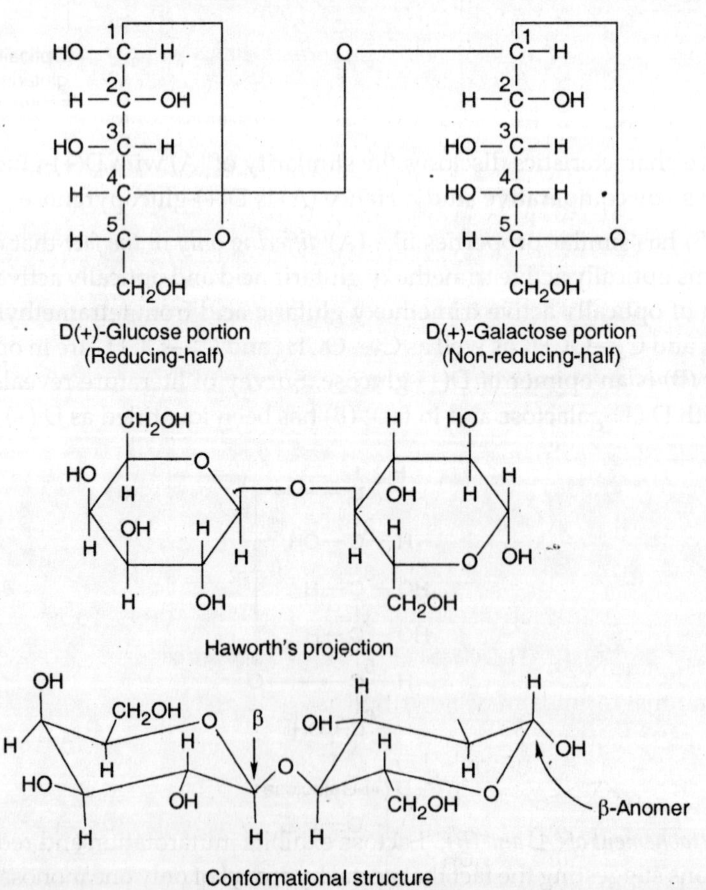

Conformational structure

1.11.4 Melibiose

It occurs in the free state in wild mallow. It is a disaccharide containing one molecule of D(+)-glucose and one molecule of D(+)-galactose, which were identified as usual and both these monosacchardides are present in pyranose form. However, melibiose was found to be a reducing sugar which means that acetal hydroxyl of one and alcoholic hydroxyl group of other are locked together in forming the disaccharide linkage.

Octamethyl derivative of melibiose on hydrolysis forms trimethyl D(+)-glucose and tetramethyl D(+)-galactose suggesting that alcoholic hydroxyl of glucose and acetal hydroxyl group of galactose are the points of combination of two monosaccharides.

The position of alcoholic hydroxyl group of D(+)-glucose involved in the linkage has been settled from the fact that during hydrolysis of octamethyl derivative of any disaccharide this hydroxyl group becomes free and present as free hydroxyl in the methylated derivative of monosaccharide. Thus, it may be concluded that trimethyl derivative of glucose obtained during hydrolysis of octamethyl derivative of melibiose possesses this free hydroxyl group. When this trimethyl D(+)-glucose derivative is treated with trityl chloride forms a solid trityl derivative. This test is specific for primary hydroxyl group. Hence C_6-primary hydroxyl group of D(+)-glucose is combined with C_1-hydroxyl (acetal hydroxyl) of D(+)-galactose in melibiose.

D(+)-Galactose is present in α- form as determined from the specific rotation of melibiose. Thus, melibiose is 6-O-α-D (+) galactopyranosyl-D(+)-glucopyranose which may be represented by the following structure:

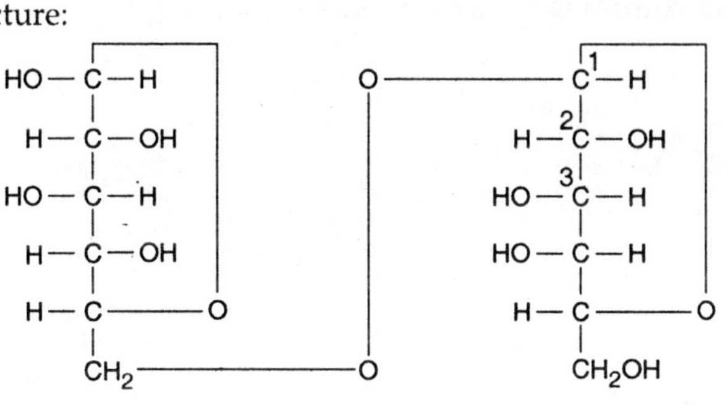

D(+)-Glucose portion
Reducing half

D(+)-Galactose portion
Non-reducing half

• *Haworth's projection structure*:

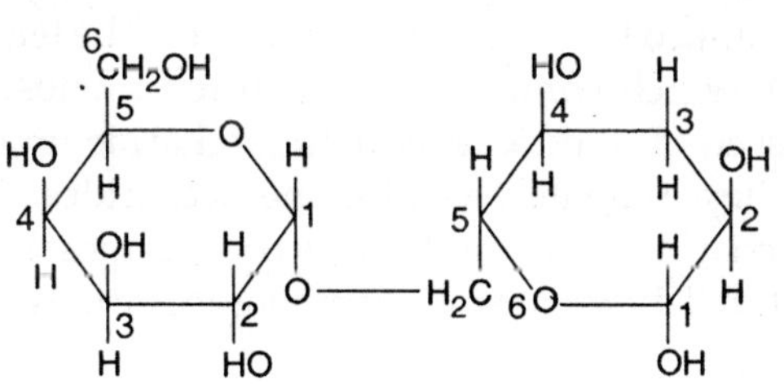

Galactose half

Glucose half

Its conformational formula may be written as

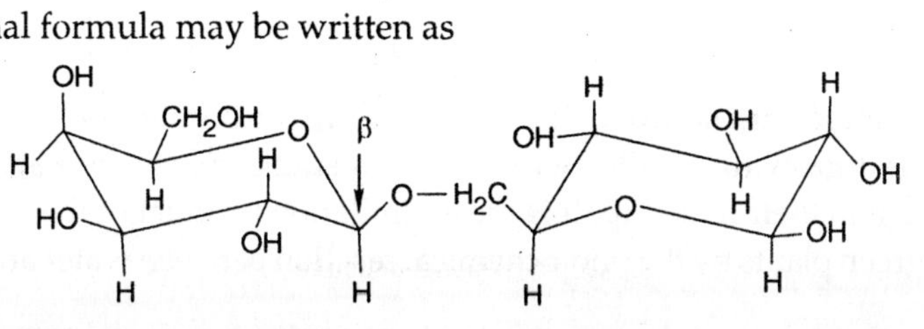

1.11.5 Maltose

Maltose is a disaccharide obtained by the hydrolysis of starch. It is also formed during fermentation. It consists of two molecules of D(+)-glucose and is a reducing sugar. It is linked through C_4-hydroxyl (alcoholic) and C_1-hydroxyl (acetal) groups of two glucose molecules and undergoes hydrolysis by the enzyme maltase specific for α-glucosidic linkage. Accordingly, maltose is 4-O-α-D (+)-glucopyranosyl-D-glucopyranose and can be represented by the following structures:

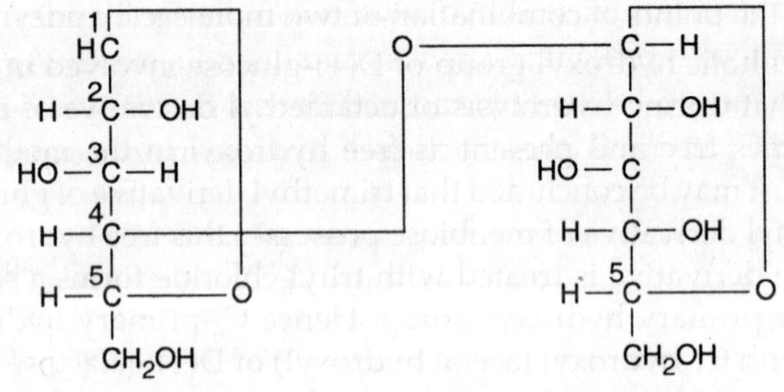

Reducing half   Non-reducing half

Conformationally its α-form may be expressed as:

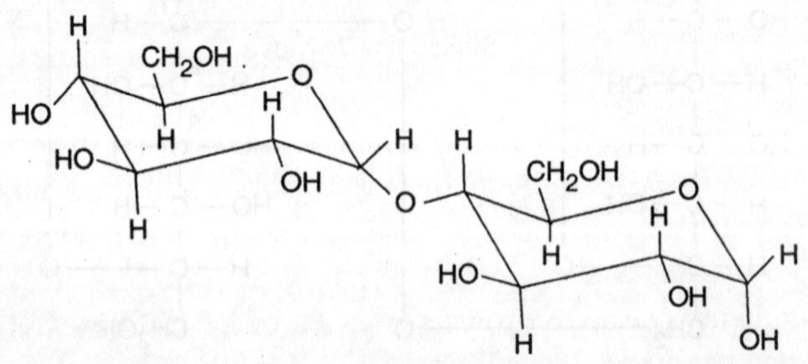

1.12 Polysaccharides

Polysaccharides are high molecular weight polymers formed by repeated condensation of monosaccharides which are linked by the glycosidic linkages. The term polysaccharide is usually applied to those polymers which contain more than ten monosaccharides but in practice polysaccharides are composed of hundreds of monosaccharide units. They are also known as "*Glycans*". On hydrolysis they ultimately yield monosaccharides. They may contain same or different kinds of monosaccharides. Polysaccharides containing same type of monosaccharides are known as *'homoglycan'*, but if different kinds of monosaccharides are present, polysaccharides are termed as *'heteroglycan'*.

Two most important polysaccharides are starch and cellulose.

1.12.1 Starch

Starch is the most important source of carbohydrates in the human diet and serve as the reserve food for a new and growing plants. Starch is not a single substance—starches from different sources are present in their make up. It is the assimilation product of the green cells of plants. It is formed in the green plants by the photochemical reaction between water and oxygen in presence of chlorophyll and sunlight. It occurs as reserve carbohydrate in potatoes, seeds, grains, many fruits and plants.

1.12.1.1 Structure of Starch

In general starch consists of two structurally different polysaccharides—a micro cystalline water soluble component known as amylose (20%) and an amorphous water insoluble part termed as amylopectin.

(a) *Structure of Amylose:* Amylose is hydrolysed completely by enzyme 'diastate' yielding maltose. So maltose is present in amylose and hence in starch. Again as maltose is 4-O-(α-D-gluco-pyranosyl)-D-glucopyranose, different glucose units in amylose are linked through C_1 and C_4 atoms. So the structure of amylose may be expressed as shown below:

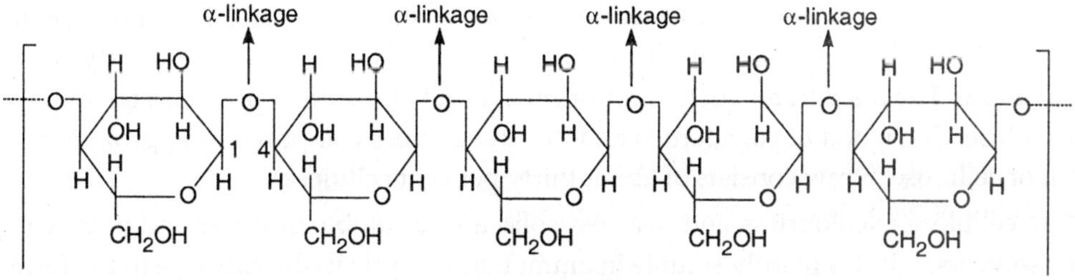

Structure of Amylose

(b) *Structure of Amylopectin*: Amylopectin when hydrolysed by the enzyme diastase forms 55% of maltose and a high molecular weight polysaccharides known as dextrin. This suggests that in addition to 1, 5 linkage (as in maltose) there is some other linkages which are not attacked by diastase.

Fully methylated amylose on hydrolysis gives 4% of 2, 3-di-O-methyl derivative of glucose along with other products. Formation of 2, 3-dimethyl derivative is a clear indication that amylopectin is a branched polymer and branched chain is linked through C_6 atom of glucose unit. On the basis of the above observations structure of amylopectin has been represented as below:

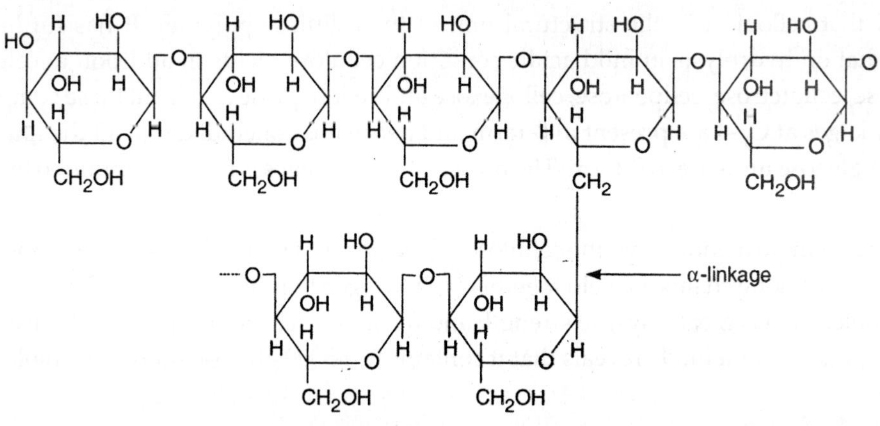

Amylopectin

From the evidence described above starch is expressed by the following structure in which all the glucose units are joined by α-linkage.

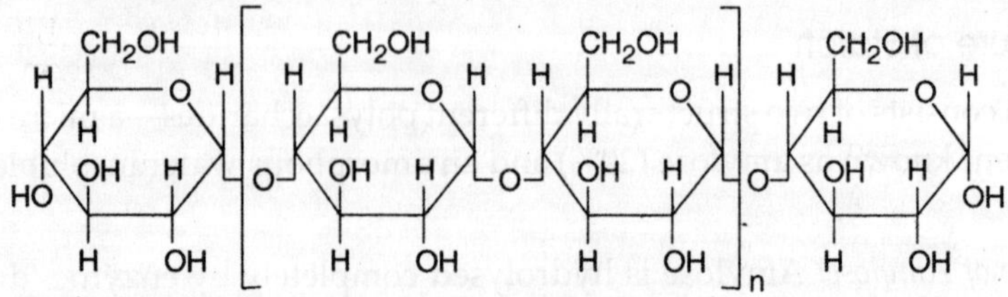

Structure of Starch

1.12.2 Cellulose

Cellulose is the actual skeletal constituent of the cell-wall of plants and is responsible for the texture, rigidity, shape and durability of the plants. It is the most abundantly occurring phytochemical. The plant fibres such as cotton, jute, flax, hemp and ramie consist of more or less pure cellulose. The wood of corniferons and deciduous trees composed of approximately fifty per cent of cellulose. Straw consists of about thirty per cent cellulose.

Pure cellulose is colourless and tasteless solid and insoluble in water and other common organic solvents, but it is readily soluble in ammoniacal cupric hydroxide due to the formation of a complex. It dissolves in strong hydrochloric acid but undergoes degradation to form the products of low molecular weight.

Cellulose is generally isolated from cotton and wood and is usually marketed as a *pulp*. Cellulose is available in three different forms, viz., α-, β- and γ-form is insoluble in both alkali and acid.

1.12.2.1 Structure of Cellulose

Elemental analysis reveals that cellulose has the molecular formula, $(C_6H_{10}O_5)_n$ and on hydrolysis with fuming hydrochloric acid it forms D-glucose in 96% yield indicating that it is a polymer of D-glucose only. When cellulose is dissolved in solvents in which glucose is soluble, colloidal solutions are obtained. This suggests that cellulose is a linear molecule which is further confirmed by X-ray analysis. Partial hydrolysis of cellulose yields the disaccharide, cellobiose. So it may be concluded that cellobiose is the structural unit of the cellulose polymer. It has further been observed that on hydrolysis in mild acidic condition cellulose yields in addition to cellobiose, cellotriptose, cellotetrose, cellpentose, cellohexose and celloheptose and in all these components glycidic linkages at C_1–4 are present in β-form and hence it is concluded that all the linkages of different D-glucose units are in β-form. The presence of β-linkages is further supported by kinetic study.

It is important to mention that the cellulose molecule is not planar but is a three-dimensional brick work. In this long chains are held together by hydrogen bonding. Due to hydrogen bonding cellulose molecule has great physical strength and flexibility. The molecular weight of cellulose obtained by different methods reveals that it contains 500-5000 glucose units in its molecule.

Based on the above evidences a possible structure of cellulose stands as shown below:

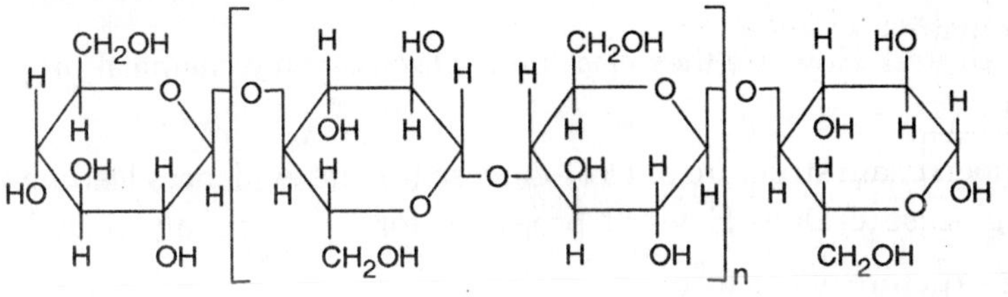

Cellulose

1.13 Usefulness of Carbohydrates in Human Life

Carbohydrates are very useful to human beings. They provide basic requirements for life, viz., food is obtained from starch, and cellulose is the source of clothes in the form of cotton, rayon linen, and shelter materials like wood is also obtained from cellulose. Glucose, the most fundamental member of carbohydrate family, serves as a source of instant energy, and is normally used as the starting material for the preparation of vitamin C. It finds extensive application in the pharmaceutical preparations as tonicity agents, tablet binder and diluent. It is also used in the manufacture of confectionery, Jams, syrups, etc. The disaccharide, sucrose, is the important source of sweetening agent and food. It is also used as a preservative for fruit products while another disaccharide, lactose, is an ingredient of foods specially for children and is also employed as a diluent, filter and excipient for compressed tablets and capsules. Maltose an important disaccharide present in germinating seeds is used in brewing, soft drinks, food industry, in pharmaceutical excipient. Starch in addition to providing food, is widely used in pharmacy as diluents, disintegrants, binders, adhesive, absorbent, suspending and emulsifying agents. Some of its derivatives have wide applications in pharmacy. Thus dextrin is used as an diluent for tablets and capsules and cyclodextrins are used in tablets to stabilise the drugs against oxidation or decomposition. *Sodium starch glycollate* commonly known as primojel is commonly used in the tablets and capsule formulation to improve the rate of tablet and capsule disintegration and hence to increase the rate of drug dissolution. *Hydroxyethyl derivative* of starch is also used in pharmaceutical formulations as diluent, disintegrant and dispersant. Cellulose, another member of polysaccharides has significant applications in variety of fields. As mentioned before. Cellulose itself serves as the source of basic needs of human life. Its different derivatives find extensive application in the field pharmacy. *Ethyl, methyl* and *hydroxypropyl methyl derivatives of cellulose* are used as tablet binders, coating materials for micro-capsules, as thickening agents in creams, lotions, gels and ointments. *Cellulose xanthate* is used to prepare *viscose rayon,* and *cellophane, Carboxymethyl cellulose* (C.M.C.) is employed as a thickening agent in glues and as a binder for synthetic reagents and in textile. *Cellulose triacetate* has been used in the manufacture of photographic film and textile fibres under the trade name *tricel* or *aranel. Cellulose acetate phthalate* is employed as an enteric coating material for tablets and capsules which resist stimulated gastric fluid and dissolve in intestinal fluid.

Model Questions

1. What are carbohydrates? How are they classified? Discuss some chemical properties of monosaccharides.
2. (a) Establish the open chain structure of D(+)-glucose (b) Site evidences leading to cyclic structure of D(+)-glucose (c) Draw Haworth projection formulae of α- and β-D(+)-glucose.
3. Establish the ring structure of fructose.
4. How will you bring about the following conversions?
   (a) Aldopentose to aldohexose.
   (b) Ketose into aldose and vice versa.
5. Write notes on:
   (a) Killiani synthesis
   (b) Wohl's degradation for chain shortening in aldose
   (c) Mutarotation
   (d) Pharmaceutical uses of carbohydrates
   (e) Glycosides
   (f) Invertsugar.
6. Explain:
   i. Glucose and fructose form same osazone.
   ii. In solution β-D(+)-glucose predominates.
   iii. α and β-methyl glucoside do not reduce Tollen's and Fehling's solutions.
   iv. Ketose cannot be directly stepped up and down by common methods.
7. (a) Discuss the essential points to be elaborated for identification of a disaccharide (b) How will you establish the structure of sucrose.
8. (a) How are α-amylose and amyl pectin separated from starch?
   (b) Discuss the modern views regarding the structure of α-amylose and amyl pectin.
9. How is pure cellulose obtained from natural sources? Discuss the present views regarding the structure of cellulose.
10. (a) Discuss the pharmaceutical uses of starch and cellulose.
    (b) Write notes on derivatives of starch and cellulose.
11. Discuss the structure of the following:
    (a) Maltose
    (b) Lactose
    (c) Cane-sugar.

CHAPTER TWO

Glycosides

2.1 Introduction

As mentioned before (vide chapter **one**) that the glycosides are the organic derivatives of cyclic acetal or ketal of sugars derived by the replacement of hydrogen atom of acetal OH group by alkyl or aryl group. Thus,

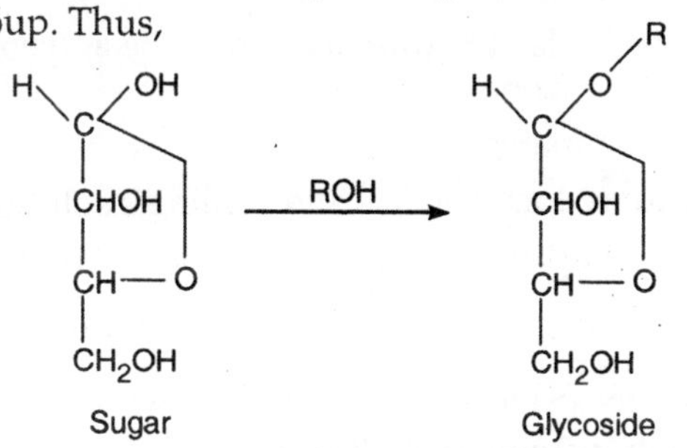

Glycoside is the general name. The individual glycoside is named on the basis of the sugar form which it is derived. For example, glycosides of glucose are known as *glucosides* while those derived from fructose are termed as *fructosides.* It may be mentioned that glycosides are non-reducing sugars due to the blocking of acetal hydroxyl by organic group and so cannot reduce Fehling's and Tollen's reagents. They do not exhibit mutarotation also and hence cannot be present in equilibrium mixture but are present in only one form, either as α- or as β-form. i.e.,

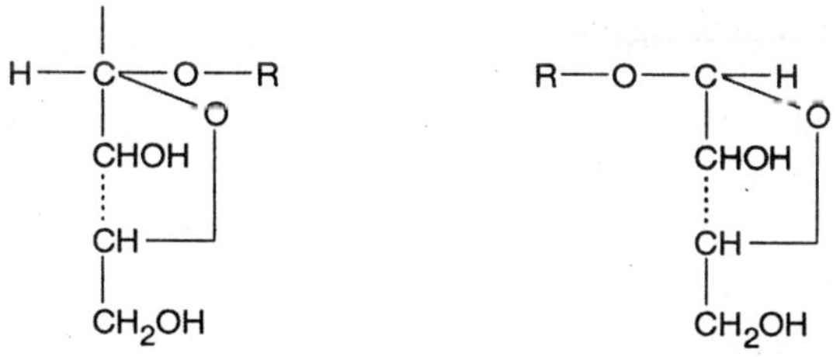

α-Glycoside (-OR in the right-hand direction)

β-Glycoside (-OR in the left-hand direction)

Glycosides are natural products and in nature almost all the glycosides exist in β-configuration at anomeric centre. However, two execeptions are known, O—ethyl—α—D—galactopyranoside isolated from lupin and glyceryl—α—D—galactoside extracted from some seaweed. Glycosides on hydrolysis by enzyme or acid yield two fragments—(i) carbohydrate fragment and non-carbohydrate fragment. The carbohydrate fragment is called *glycone* and the non-carbohydrate fragment is referred to as *aglycone*, Thus,

$$\text{Glycosides} \xrightarrow[\text{Enzyme or Acid}]{\text{Hydrolysis}} \underset{\text{(Sugar portion)}}{\text{Glycone}} + \underset{\text{(Non-sugar part)}}{\text{Aglycone}}$$

It may be remembered that disaccharides, trisaccharides and polysaccharides also belong to glycoside family. The sugar component of glycoside is generally D-glucose, although in some cases other monosaccharides such as D-fructose, D-mannose, D- and L-galactose, L-rhamnose, D-ribose and D- and L-arabinose. In rare cases, the sugar moiety may be di- or trisaccharides. The aglycone, in most of the cases, contains at least one hydroxyl group (alcoholic or phenolic) to which the glycosidic hydroxyl function of sugar component is joined. Such linkage as we know is known as *glycosidic linkage.* In addition, in some cases sugar portion may be linked with N, C and S atoms of the aglycone part.

2.2 Classification of Glycosides

In general, glycosides are classified on the basis of nature of atom of the aglycone to which the sugar portion is connected.

i. O - glycosides
ii. N - glycosides
iii. C - glycosides
iv. S - glycosides

However, each of the above classifed glycosides has further been divided into several groups according to the nature of aglycone moiety as mentioned below:

i. Phenolic glycosides
ii. Flavonoid glycosides
iii. Steroidal glycosides or cardiac glycosides
iv. Anthraquinone glycosides, etc.

2.3 Biological and Pharmaceutical Significance of Glycosides

Glycosides are present in most of the plants and animals and play a vital role in the life of plants and are closely associated with protective, regulatory and sanitary functions. They may serve as sugar reserves, as waste products of plant metabolism. In some cases glycosides are used to remove harmful substances such as phenols by detoxication mechanism. Some glycosides such as glycosides of anthocyanin pigments are found to increase the rate of photosynthesis.

Many glycosides have been found to have pharmaceutical activity. For examples, cardiac glucosides, anthraquinone glycosides, phenolic glycosides are medicinally very important.

Many natural glycosides serve as the source of dyes and pigments. Thus, Indican is the main source of natural blue dye *indigo.*

2.4 Isolation of Glycosides

Glycosides are normally isolated by adapting the following method:

The crude plant material is dried and finely powdered. The finely powdered plant material is extracted with alcohol in a soxlett apparatus. The concentrated extract so obtained is treated with lead acetate to precipitate proteins and tannius. It is then filtered and lead is removed as lead sulphide by passing a current of hydrogen sulphide. It is once again filtered and the filtrate is heated at a temperature of 60 °C to destroy the enzymes present and finally concentrated when crude glycosides obtained which is then purified by using usual methods like fractional solubility, fractional crystallisation and different chromatographic techniques.

• *Properties of Glycosides:* Glycosides as a class, in general, are colourless, crystalline compounds, soluble in water. They are optically active and are non-reducing in character. Neither α- nor β-glycosides exhibit mutarotation. Glycosides are readily hydrolysed to parent sugar and aglycone. They are also hydrolysed by enzymes. Enzyme, *emulsin,* hydrolyses only β-glycosides while α-glycosides are specifically hydrolysed by the enzyme *maltase.* For this reason, enzymatic hydrolysis is used to settle the nature of linkage in glycosides.

2.5 General Method for the Determination of the Structure of Glycosides

The general method for the determination of the structure of glycosides involves the following steps.

2.5.1 Degradation of Glycosides

The first step for the determination of the structure of glycoside is the hydrolytic cleavage by mild acid hydrolysis. During this hydrolysis glycosidic linkage undergoes cleavage and the glycoside is degraded to sugar and non-sugar components.

$$\text{Glycosides} \xrightarrow[\text{(acid)}]{\text{Mild hydrolysis}} \text{Sugar} + \underset{\text{(Aglycone)}}{\text{Non-sugar}}$$

These components are separated by chromatographic resolution and the components are characterised by usual procedures.

2.5.2 Nature of Glycosidic Linkage

The second step is to settle the nature of glycosidic linkage. For this purpose enzymatic hydrolysis is employed. As mentioned before enzyme *emulsin* hydrolyses only β-glycosidic linkage and the enzyme *maltase* can only hydrolyse α-glycosidic linkage.

It may be mentioned that when the sugar portion is di- or tri-saccharide, specific enzymes are used to effect only the partial hydrolysis of glycosides. Further, if more than one hydroxyl functions are present in aglycone, some special methods are employed depending upon the nature of aglycone to ascertain which one hydroxyl function has been involved in the glycosidic linkage.

2.5.3 Synthesis

The last step is the confirmation of the structure by its synthesis. The synthesis of glycosides, in general, involves the reaction between *acetobromohexose* and an alcohol or phenol (aglycone).

2.5.4 Spectral Measurements

Different physico-chemical techniques such as IR, UV, H^1NMR, mass spectrometry and X-ray analysis are also suitably employed to ascertain the structures of glycosides.

2.6 Synthesis of Glycosides

As mentioned before, synthesis of glycosides consists of two distinct steps.

- *Step I: Synthesis of Acetobromohexose:* Acetobromohexose to be synthesised is tetra-O-acetyl-α-D-glucopyranose-I-bromide. There are a large number of methods for its synthesis, the most commonly followed method is described below:

Glucose penta-O-acetyl derivative is prepared by the treatment of acetic anhydride with D-glucose either in the presence $ZnCl_2$ or in presence of sodium acetate. However, in presence of $ZnCl_2$, the product formed is α-isomer while β-isomer is formed in presence of sodium acetate. Further, β-isomer may be converted into the α-isomer by heating it with acetic anhydride at 110 °C in presence of Zinc chloride.

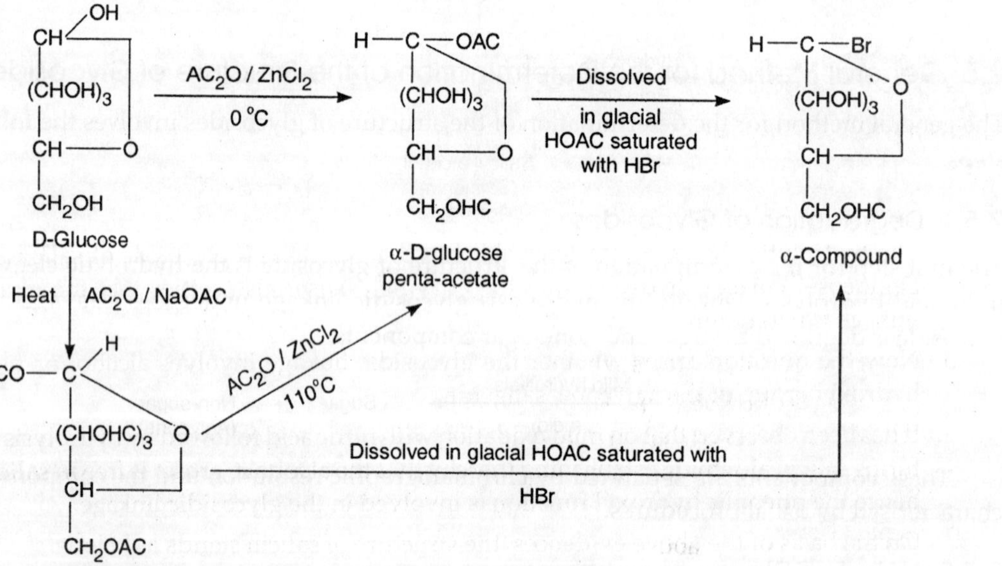

It may be mentioned that always α-isomer is obtained whether penta-acetate used is the α- or β. compound,.

- *Step II:* In the second step acetobromohexose is converted into glycosides. The bromine atom in acetobromohexose and is readily replaced by hydroxyl group (alcoholic or phenolic).

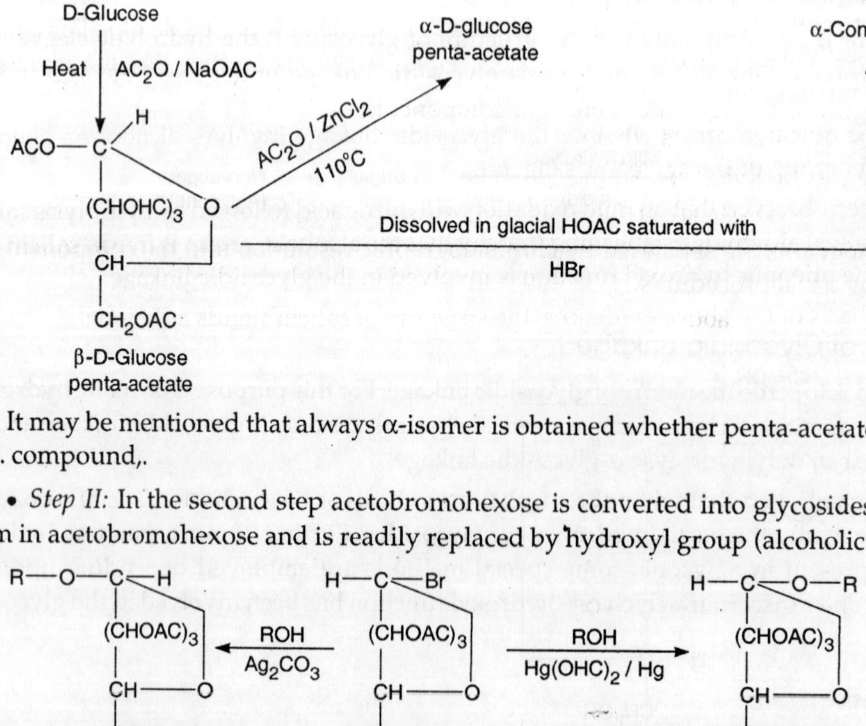

Since glycosides are stable in alkali the acetyl group is replaced by the hydrolysis in alkali to yield the desired glycoside.

2.7 Chemistry of Some Important Plant Glycosides

Chemistry of a few plant glycosides having importance are discussed below:

2.7.1 Salicin

It is a bitter glycoside and occurs in the leaves and bark of Willow plant. It is a solid, m.p. 210 °C and is optically active and laevorotatory.

- *Structure:*

1. Elemental analysis and analytical data reveals that it has molecular formula, $C_{13}H_{18}O_7$.
2. On hydrolysis with the enzyme *emulsin* it yields one molecule of salicyl alcohol and one molecule of D-glucose.

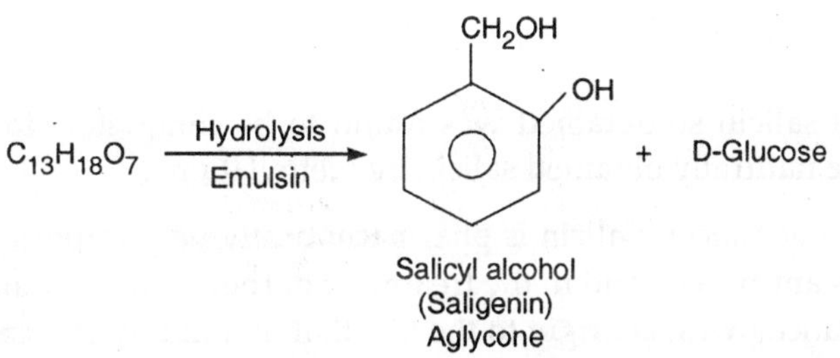

The hydrolytic cleavage clearly establishes that salicin is a glycoside of saligenin and D-glucose. Further, hydrolysis by the enzyme *emulsin* also settles that the glycosidic linkage is β in nature.

3. Now the question arises whether the glycosidic linkage involves alcohol or phenolic hydroxyl group of the aglycone, saligenin.

   It has been observed that on mild oxidation with nitric acid followed by hydrolysis salicin forms salicyl aldehyde establishing thereby that the alcoholic group is free in salicin and hence the phenolic hydroxyl function is involved in the glycosidic linkage.

   On the basis of the above evidences, the structure of salicin stands as below:

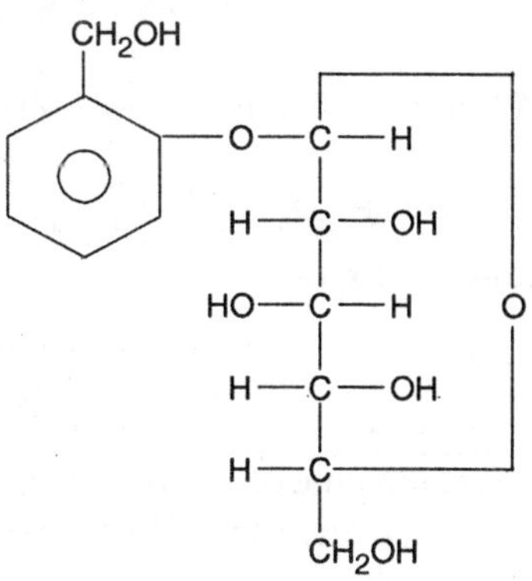

Salicin

The above structure of salicin has finally been confirmed by the synthesis of its pentamethyl derivative.

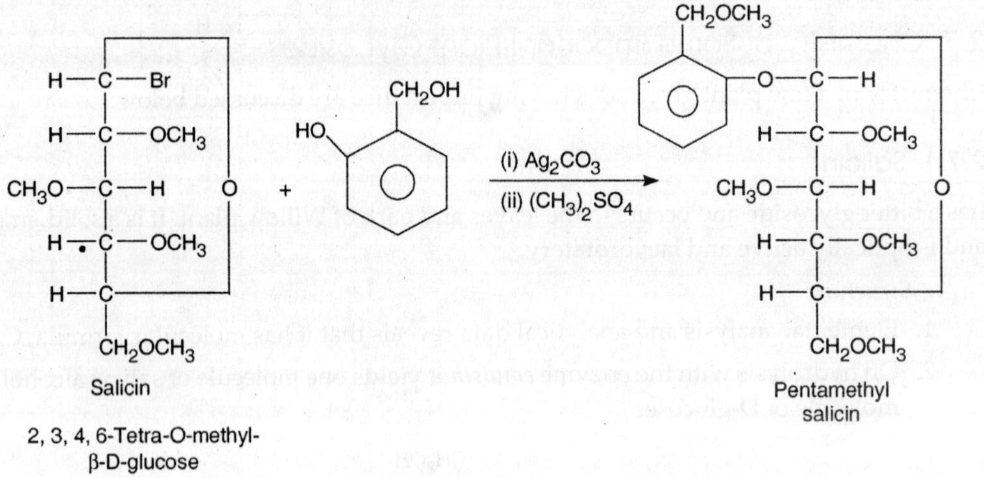

The pentamethyl salicin so obtained was found to be completely identical with that obtained from the naturally obtained salicin by methylation.

• *Importance and uses of Salicin:* Salicin is pharmaceutically very important because it has medicinal applications as antipyretic and in the treatment of rheumatism. It may be mentioned that its medicinal importance owes its origin to the fact that on mild hydrolysis it yields salicyl alcohol which on oxidation forms highly potent antipyretic and analgesic salicylic acid.

2.7.2 Ruberythric Acid

It is another important member of O-glycosides and belongs to most widely distributed plant glycosides of anthraquinone group. It occurs in the madder roots.

• *Constitution of Ruberythric Acid:* The constitution of ruberythric acid is based on the following evidences:

i. Its molecular formula has been found to be $C_{25}H_{26}O_{13}$ from analytical data.
ii. On hydrolysis with the enzyme *emulsin,* it yields one molecule of each of alizarin, D-glucose and D-xylose.

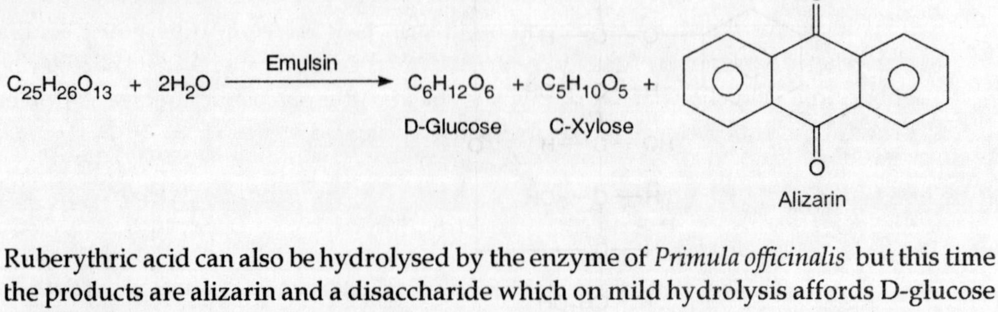

iii. Ruberythric acid can also be hydrolysed by the enzyme of *Primula officinalis* but this time the products are alizarin and a disaccharide which on mild hydrolysis affords D-glucose and D-xylose.

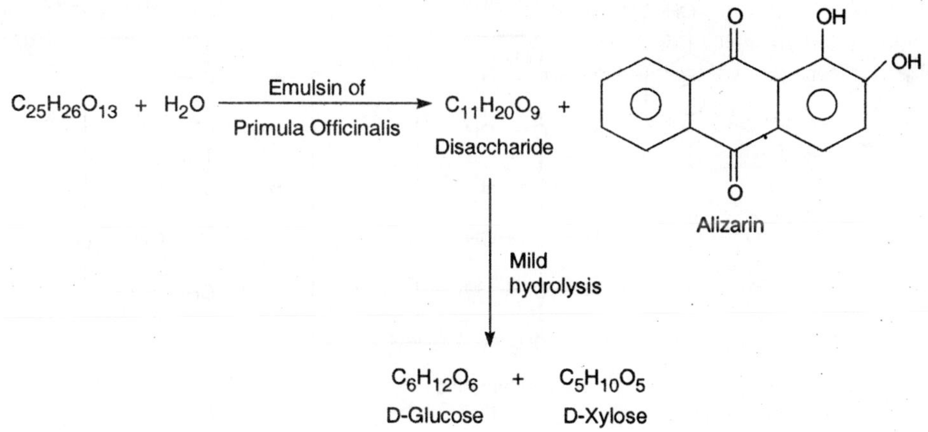

The above experiments, thus, clearly reveals that the two monosaccharides are present in the form of the disaccharide. This disaccharide has been identified as primverose as shown by its crystallographic properties. This disaccharide is 6-O-β-D-xylopyranosyl-D-Glucopyranose.

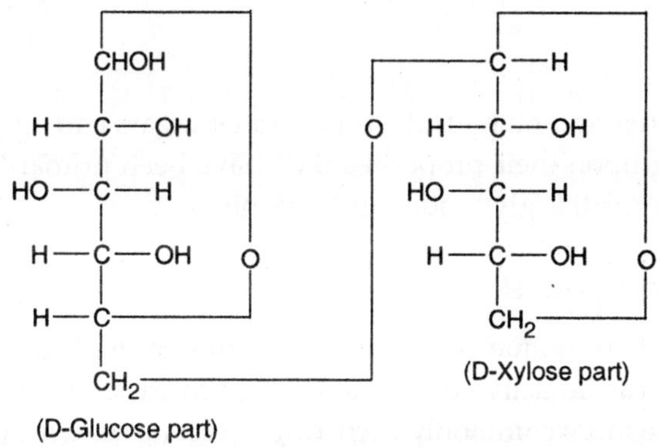

Primeverose

From the structure of primeverose it is evident that alizarin unit is linked to the glucose half of the primeverose molecule.

iv. Methylation followed by hydrolysis of ruberythric acid furnishes alizarin-I-methyl ether. This indicates that the C_1-position of alizarin unit is free in ruberythric acid, and the disaccharide primeverose is linked to hydroxyl group at C_2-position of alizarin to give ruberythic acid. Further work has shown that the glycosidic linkage is β. Hence the structure of ruberythic acid is expressed as indicated:

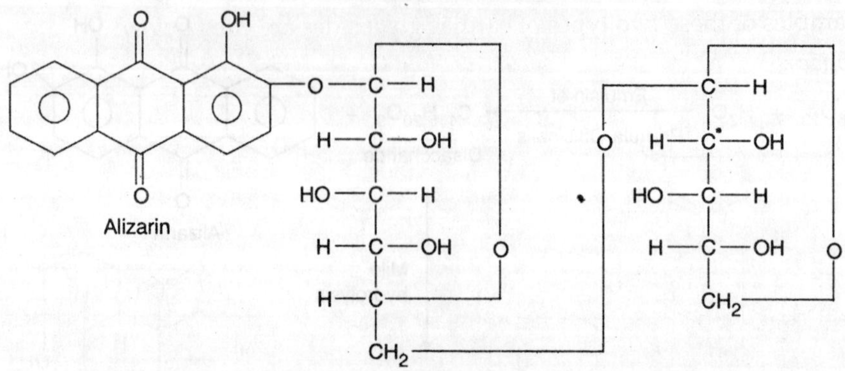

2.7.2.1 Uses of Anthraquinone Glycosides

Anthraquinone glycosides, in general, are highly potent purgatives and are frequently used in the treatment of constipation particularly for those patients who do not respond to milder dose. Besides, anthraquinone glycosides are used for the preparation of dyes. Thus ruberythric acid is employed for the manufacture of alizarin.

2.7.3 Steroidal Glycosides

These glycosides are O-glycosides and on hydrolysis generates sugars and aglycone which are steroidal in nature. Depending upon their properties they have been primarily classified into two groups, viz., cardiotonic or cardiac glycosides and saponins.

2.7.3.1 Cardiotonic or Cardiac Glycosides

These steroidal glycosides have an unique characteristic of stimulating heart muscles and for this they are referred to as the cardio-active or cardiotonic glycosides. The aglycones in these glycosides are of two types. The more commonly occurring aglycone contains α, β-unsaturated γ-lactonic ring and is known as *Cardenolides* and they show λ_{max} in the UV spectrum at 220 nm. The other aglycone is less common and contain a δ-lactonic ring with a conjugated diene system. They exhibit λ_{max} at 300 nm. These are known as *bufadienolides* or *scilladienolides*. Both these types of steroid aglycone have normal configurations at C_8, C_9, C_{10}, C_{13} and C_{17} and both contain a C_3 and a C_{14} β-hydroxyl functions. However, these two types differ in the configurations at C_3 and C_5 and in unsaturation and oxygen functions. The sugar in glycoside generally consists of several hexose residues and the glycosidic linkage to the steroid nucleus is always at C_3 and the glycosidic linkage is β-type for D-sugars and α-type for L-sugars. It may further be mentioned that in cardenolides α, β-unsaturated γ-lactone ring is present at C_{17} position in β-configuration while in butadienolides the δ-lactone with conjugated diene system is linked with C_{17} position in β-configuration. Cardenolides occur in *Digitalis purpurea, Digitalis strophanthus* and *Digitalis lanata* and butadienolides are found in some *Liliaceae* and *Ranunculaceae* plants and in toad venom.

A few examples of these two types of cardiac glycosides are cited below:

- *Cardenolides:*

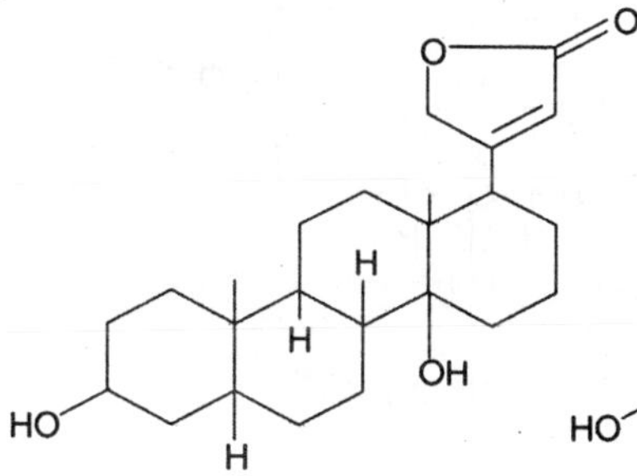

Digitoxigenin

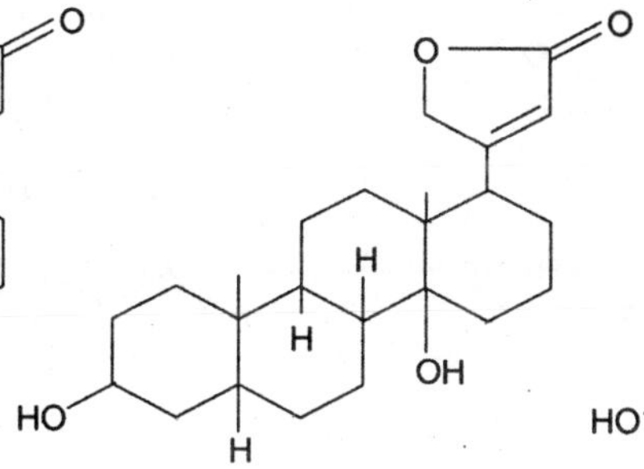

Uzarigenin

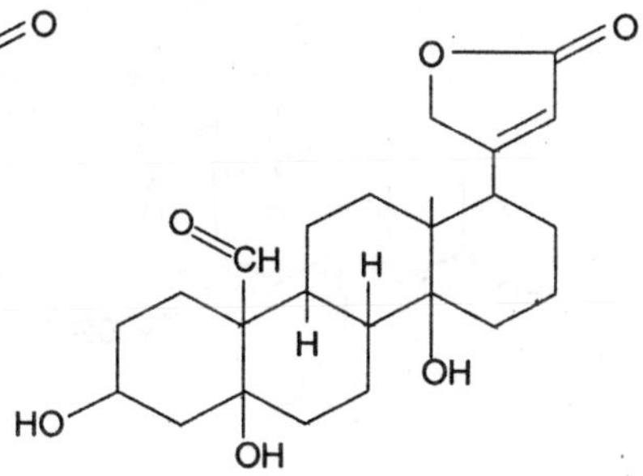

Strophanthidin

- *Bufadienolides:*

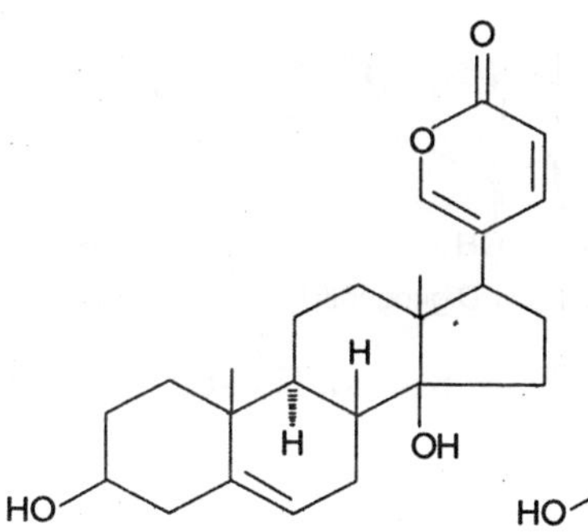

Scillaren A

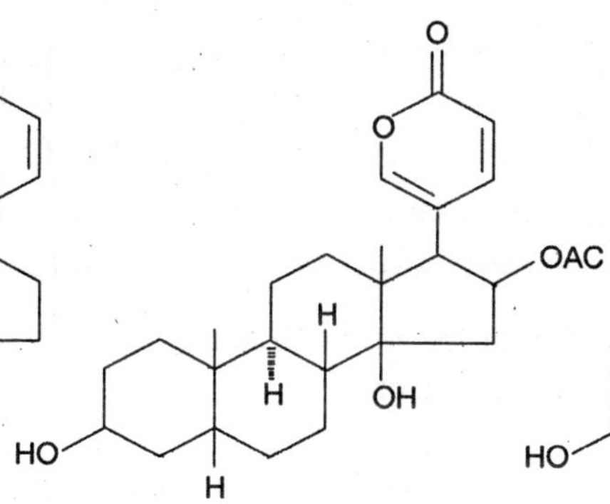

Bufatalin

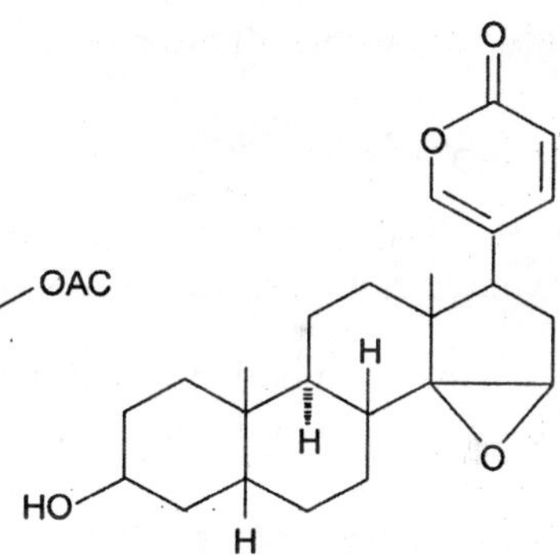

Resibutogenin

2.7.3.1.1 Uses of Cardiac Glycosides

As mentioned earlier cardiac glycosides are pharmaceutically potent organic chemicals. They are frequently used as medicines for the treatment of heart diseases. Generally they are given orally. They increase the contractions of heart and the force of heart beat. These glycosides are highly effective for the treatment of congestive heart failure and atrial fibrillation. They are also capable of increasing kidney and cardiac output.

2.7.3.2 Saponins

Saponins are plant steroid glycosides. They have a distinct property of forming foams in water like soap solution. For this reason they are mainly used as detergents. Saponins on hydrolysis yield sugars and an aglycone known as *sapogenin*. Chemically sapogenins contain a steroid nucleus with a spiroketal side-chain.

Saponins occur in many plants along with cardiotonic glycosides. The most common source of these glycosides are various species of *Digitalis*.

Some important examples of sapogenins are as noted below:

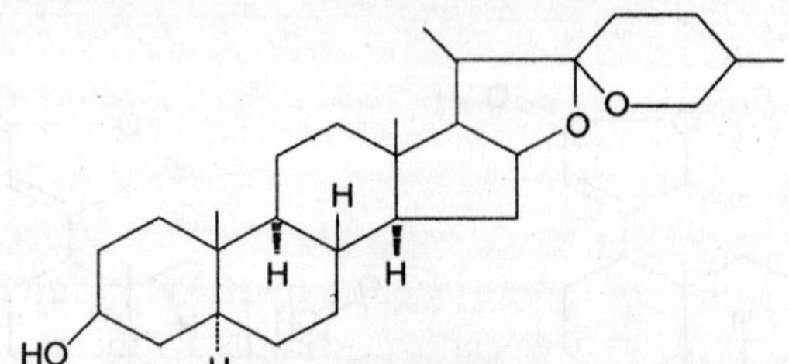

Tigogenin

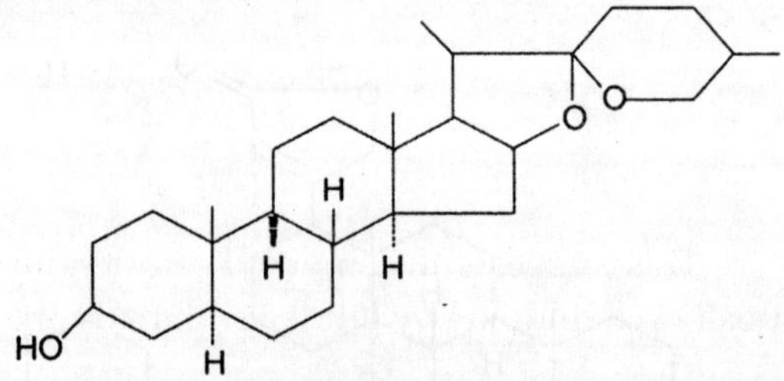

Sarsapogenin

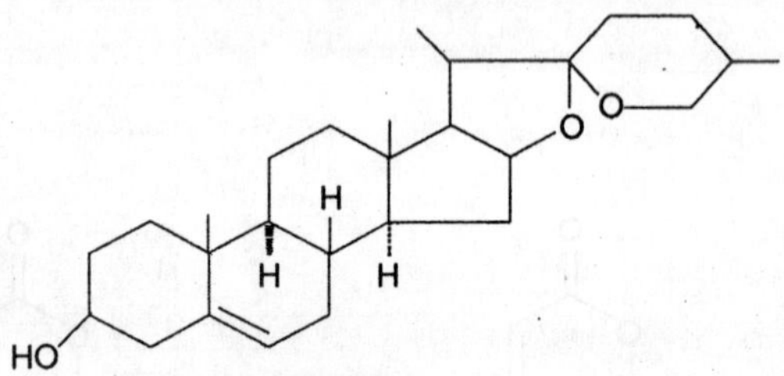

Diosgenin

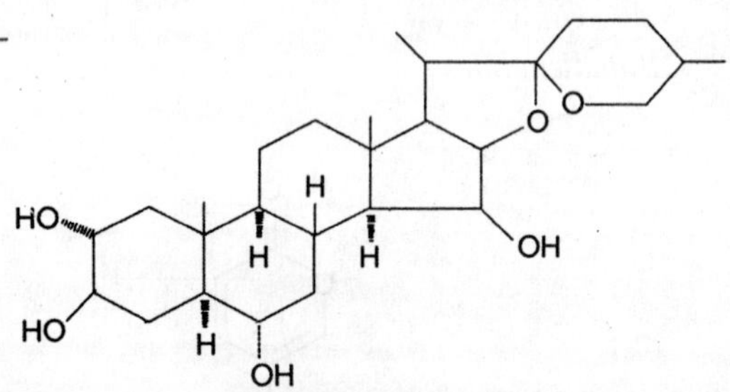

Digitogenin

It may be mentioned that sugar portion is linked with 3β-Oxygen atom. The sugars commonly present are glucose, galactose, xylose, etc.

2.7.3.2.1 Uses of Saponins

Saponins are used for variety of purposes. They are used as medicines. Saponins are not toxic to human beings if taken orally. But when used intravenously it is poisonous because under such condition haemolysis may occur. They are used as fish poisons. Fishes are killed by introducing saponins in water. They are extensively used as foaming agents in fire extinguishers and as detergents. The saponin, diosgenin, is an important starting material for the synthesis of most important sex hormone progesterone. Saponin; digitonin, is used for the estimation of 3β-hydroxy steroids because with such steroids digitonin forms complexes—digitonides.

2.7.4 Indican

Indican is another member of O-glycoside family. It occurs in indigo plant and in the wood plant. The molecular formula of indican has been found to be $C_{14}H_{17}NO_6$ and when hydrolysed with dilute hydrochloric acid or by the enzyme emulsin it affords one molecule of D-glucose and one molecule of indoxyl (3-hydroxy indole).

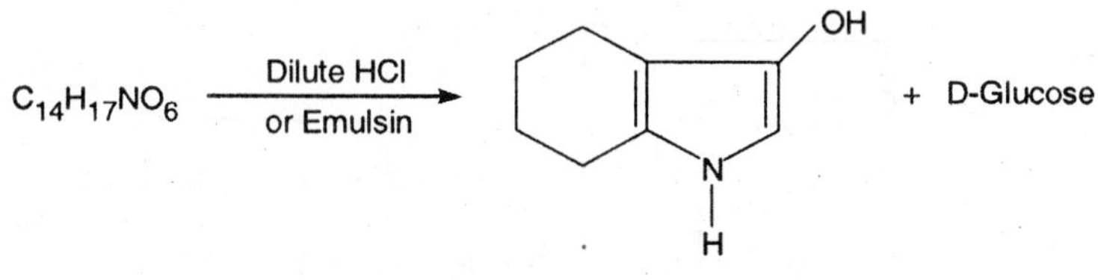

This suggests that indoxyl and D-glucose units are linked through hydroxyl group at 3 position of indoxyl by β-linkage. Finally the structure has been confirmed by its synthesis.

Thus,

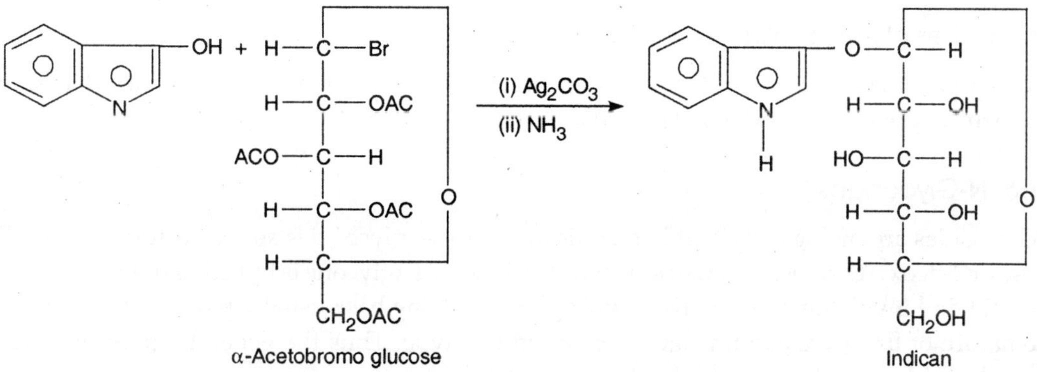

2.7.4.1 Uses of Indican

It is the main source of the natural blue dye. Indigo is the oldest known dye.

2.7.5 Amygdalin

Amygdalin is one of the earliest known glycosides and belongs to C-glycoside family. It occurs in bitter almonds. It has the molecular formula, $C_{20}H_{27}NO_{11}$ and on hydrolysis with dilute acids or enzyme emulsin gives two molecules of D-glucose, one molecule of benzaldehyde and one molecule of hydrogen cyanide.

$$C_{20}H_{27}NO_{11} \xrightarrow[\text{Acid or Emulsin}]{\text{Hydrolysis}} \underset{\text{Benzaldehyde}}{C_6H_5CHO} + \underset{\text{D-Glucose}}{2C_6H_{12}O_6} + HCN$$

Again, enzyme, *zymase* hydrolyses amygdalin into one molecule of D-glucose and one molecule of glucoside of (+) mandelonitrile which was found to be identical with naturally occurring glucoside, *prunasin*. Thus the aglycone moiety of amygdalin is mandelonitrile and sugar portion is a disaccharide. Haworth and his associates have shown that this disaccharide is gentiobiose.

On the basis of above evidences amygdalin has been represented by the following structure

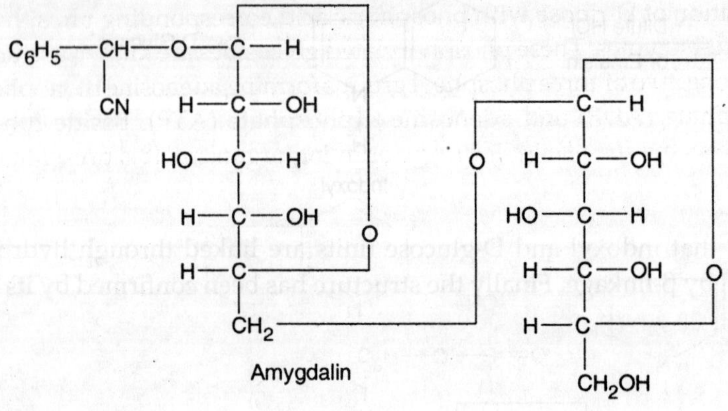

Amygdalin

2.7.5.1 Uses of Amygdalin

Amygdalin is mainly used as flavouring agent. However, it has been found that it has some therapeutic applications and may be used as sedative.

2.7.6 N-Glycosides

N-Glycosides are biologically highly significant. In these glycosides sugar portion is either D-ribose or 2-deoxy-D-ribose and the nonsugar portion—the aglycone is linked to sugar residue by a C—N bond involving a derivative of nitrogen containing base usually pyrimidine or purine. The nature of the glycoside linkage as expected is β-type. Thus the general representation of these glycosides may be expressed as below:

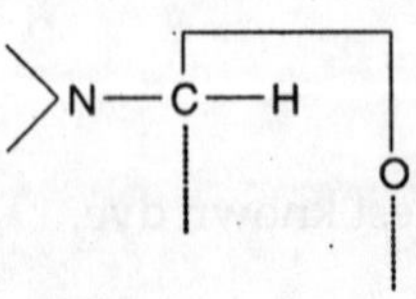

These—N-glycosides are generally known as ribonucleosides and deoxyribonucleosides. These two types of N-glycosides may be represented by the following partial structures:

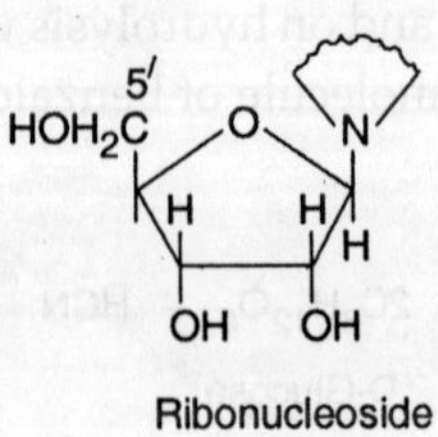

Ribonucleoside

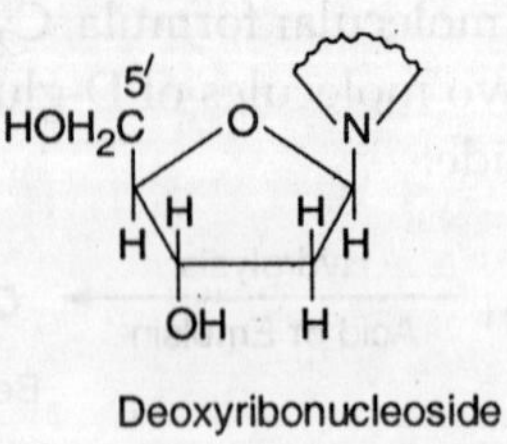

Deoxyribonucleoside

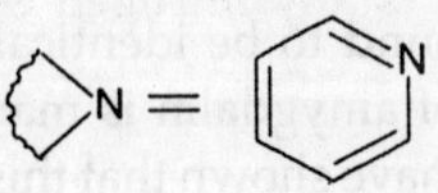

Pyrimidine

Or

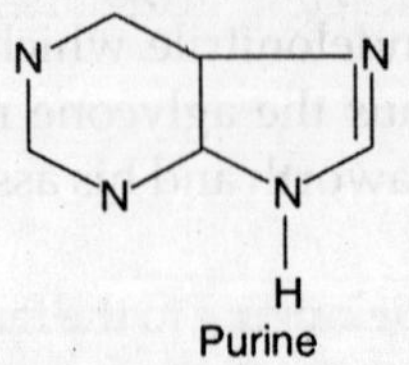

Purine

One of the important member of purine ribonucleoside is adenosine. When adenosine is esterified at 5′-position of D-ribose with phosphoric acid corresponding phosphates are formed which function as co-enzymes. These phosphorylated glycosides are known as nucleotides. These esters may contain one, two or three phosphoyl groups forming adenosine monophosphate (AMP), adenosine diphosphate (ADP) and adenosine triphosphate (ATP). Beside functioning as co-enzyme, ATP serve as the *store-house of energy* for living organism. It is present in muscle tissue.

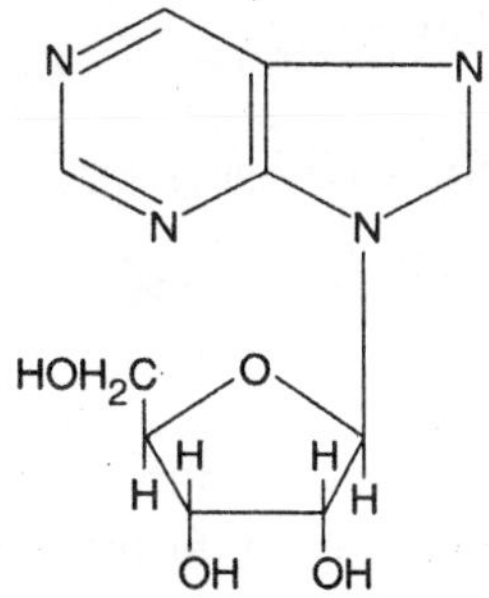

Adenosine

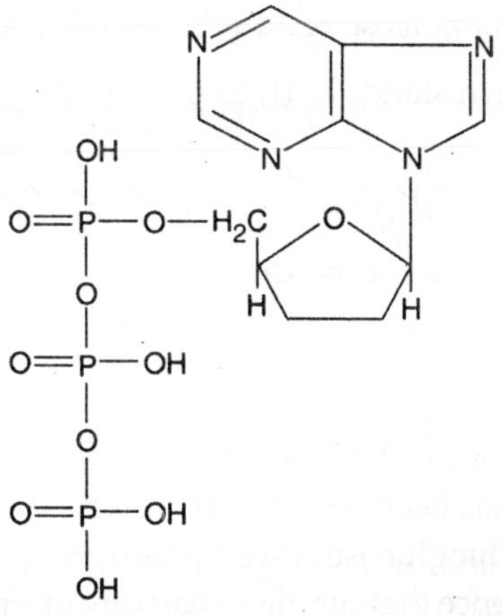

Adenosine triphosphate (ATP)

The vital nucleic acids, ribonucleic acid (RNA) and deoxyribonucleic acid (DNA) are the most essential components of every living cell. They are the polymers of a large number of nucleotides linked together through phosphate ester bonds. In DNA the sugar parts of nucleotides are joined through phosphates at 3 and 5-positions of D-ribose as shown below:

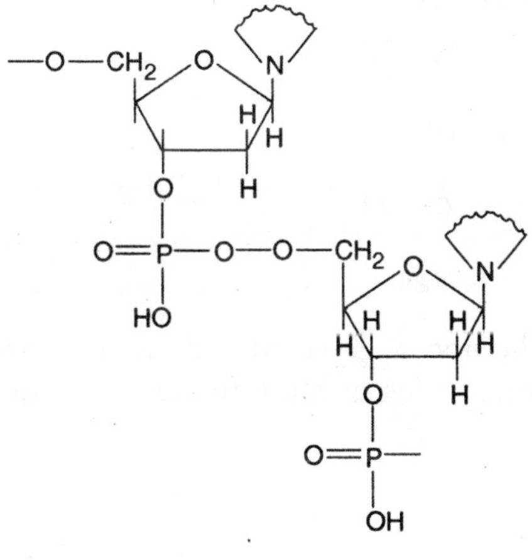

Part structure of Deoxyribonucleic acid where 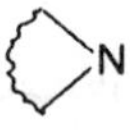 is any nitrogen containing base, pyrimidine or purine derivative.

2.7.7 Sinigrin

Sinigrin is an important glycoside belonging to the family S-glycosides. It occurs in black mustard seed. Its structure has been deduced by Gadamer on the basis of the following evidences:

i. Analytical data suggests that it has the molecular composition, $C_{10}H_{16}N_9S_2K$.

ii. On hydrolysis with the enzyme, *Myrosin* sinigrin yields D-glucose, allyl isothiocyanate and potassium hydrogen sulphate.

$$C_{10}H_{16}NO_9S_2K + H_2O \longrightarrow \underset{\text{D-Glucose}}{C_6H_{12}NO_6} + \underset{\text{Allyl isothiocyanate}}{CH_2 = CH{-}CH_2NCS} + KHSO_4$$

iii. On degradation with sodium methoxide, sinigrin forms thioglucose as one of the products indicating the fact that D-glucose residue is linked to a sulphur atom in its molecule.

Thus the structure of sinigrin stands as (I) as proposed by Gadamer.

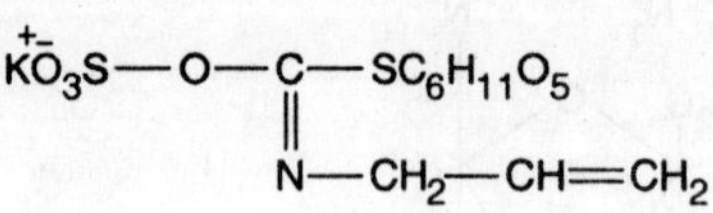

(I)

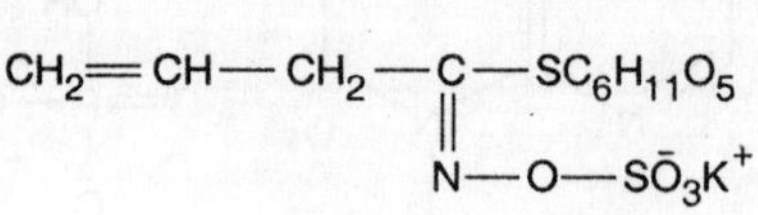

(II)

On the other hand, Ettlinger and his group suggested the structure (II) on the basis of the fact that allyl isothiocyanate is formed by lossen type of rearrangement during the hydrolysis by *myrosin*. Finally, structure (II) has been found to be correct by X-ray analysis by Waser and his associates. Thus in sinigrin the thioglucose and sulphate group are in *syn*-arrangement. Ettlinger has also synthesised sinigrin. Hence the complete structure of sinigrin may be expressed as under:

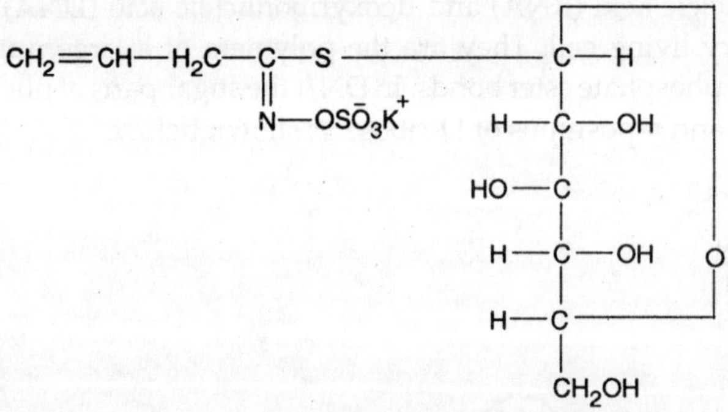

Sinigrin

It may be mentioned that besides the above glycosides there are various important compounds which are found in nature as glycosides; as for example, antibiotics erythromycin, streptomycin, anthocyanin pigments, etc.

Model Questions

1. What are glycosides? How are they classified?
2. Discuss the general method for the isolation of glycosides. What are the biological importance of glycosides?
3. Write a short note on the general method of synthesis of glycoside. How is acetobromohexose prepared?

4. What are cardiac glycosides? Why are they so named? Write the structures of some of the cardiac glycosides along with their uses.
5. What are saponins? How do they differ from cardiac glycosides. Mention a few important uses of saponins.
6. Discuss the chemisty and importance of N-glycosides.
7. Mention the name of S-glycoside and discuss its chemistry.
8. What is the natural source of amygdalin? Show that it belongs to C-glycoside family.
9. Discuss the chemistry and uses of the following:
   i. Ruberythric acid.
   ii. Salicin.
   iii. Indican.
   iv. Cardiac glycosides.

CHAPTER THREE

Amino Acids, Peptides and Proteins

INTRODUCTION

Amino acids, peptides and proteins are most vital organic compounds for living organisms. These three are interrelated with each other. Peptides are polymer of amino acids connected through ($\underset{\underset{O}{\|}}{C}$—NH—) linkage known as peptide while proteins are polypeptides. Thus amino acids can be looked upon as the structural units of proteins. In fact, a single protein molecule is made up of hundreds or even thousands of amino acid units. It may be mentioned that among the amino acids so far isolated from living organisms, about twenty odd have been found to be the components of proteins.

3.1 Amino Acids

Amino acids are those which contain both carboxylic and amino groups in their molecules. Most of the amino acids are the α-amino acids, i.e., both these functionalities are attached to the same carbon atom and so they may be represented by the following general structure:

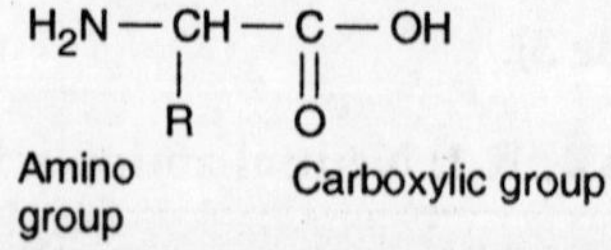

From the above general structure it is thus evident that they may be regarded as amino substituted carboxylic acid. Biologically amino acids are very significant. They are the constituents of peptides and proteins. More than hundred amino acids are known but only twenty five are obtained by the hydrolysis of typical proteins. Of these twenty five, twenty are frequently encountered in almost all the proteins. An interesting observation is that out of these twenty five, twenty three are α-amino acids and remaining two—proline and hydroxy proline contain —NH-grouping in their molecules.

3.1.1 Essential and Non-essential Amino Acids

Out of twenty five amino acids which are the constituents of proteins, ten are identified as *essential amino acids* while remaining fifteen are *non-essential* in character. *Non-essential* amino acids are those which are synthesised in the body but the *essential* amino acids cannot be synthesised in the body and so must be supplied in the form of diet. These essential amino acids also known as *indispensable amino acids* are necessary for the normal growth and development of the body. The deficiency of these acids causes serious diseases like nervous breakdown, inhibition of mental growth, etc. Sometimes continuous deficiency may even cause death in young animals.

3.1.2 Optical Activity of Amino Acids

All the naturally occurring amino acids are optically active and their absolute configuration is comparable to that of L-glyceraldehyde and thus, they may be represented by the following projection formula:

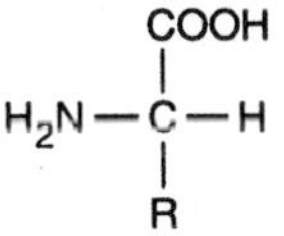

L-Amino acids

3.1.3 Nomenclature of Amino Acids

In the common system of nomenclature, they are named as the amino derivatives of the corresponding acids indicating the position of amino group by the letter α, β, γ, δ, etc.

In IUPAC system the position of amino group is indicated by number starting from 2, because carboxylic carbon atom is always 1 in this system.

3.1.4 Classification of Amino Acids

On the basis of number of carboxylic and amino groups present, amino acids have been classified into three categories.

(a) *Neutral amino acids*: In these acids there are one amino acid and one carboxylic acid (Table 1).

(b) *Basic amino acids*: These amino acids contain two amino groups and one carboxylic function in their molecule (Table 2).

(c) *Acidic amino acids*: These amino acids are those in which there are two carboxylic groups and one amino group (Table 3).

TABLE 1: Neutral amino acid

Name	Chemical name	Structure	Abbreviation
1. Glycine	Amino acetic acid	CH_2-COOH | NH_2	Gly
2. Alanine	α-amino propionic acid	$CH_3-CH-COOH$ | NH_2	Ala

Contd.

Name	Chemical name	Structure	Abbre-viation
*3. Valine	α-amino isovaleric acid	$(CH_3)_2CH-CH(NH_2)-COOH$	Val
*4. Leucine	α-amino isocaproic acid	$(CH_3)_2CH-CH(NH_2)-COOH$	Leu
*5. Isoleucine	α-amino-β-methyl *n*-valeric acid	$CH_3-CH_2-CH(CH_3)-CH(NH_2)-COOH$	Ile
*6. Phenylalanine	α-amino-β-phenyl propionic acid	$Ph-CH_2-CH(NH_2)-COOH$	Phe
7. Tyrosine	α-amino-β-(*p*-hydroxy phenyl) propionic acid	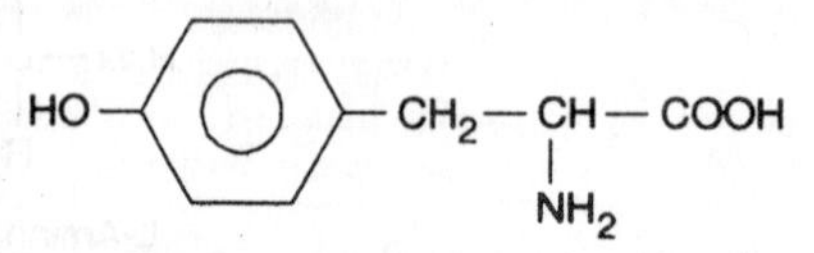	Tyr
8. Serine	α-amino-β-hydroxy propionic acid	$HO-CH_2-CH(NH_2)-COOH$	Ser
9. Cysteine	α-amino-β-mercapto propionic acid	$HS-CH_2-CH(NH_2)-COOH$	Cys
10. Cystine	Bis-(α-amino propionic acid) β-disulphide	$(-S-CH_2-CH(NH_2)-COOH)_2$	$(Cys)_2$
*11. Threonine	α-amino-β-hydroxy-*n*-butyric acid	$CH_3-CH(HO)-CH(NH_2)-COOH$	Thr
*12. Methionine	α-amino-γ-methyl thio-*n*-butyric acid	$CH_3-S-CH_2-CH_2-CH(H_2N)-COOH$	Met
13. Thyroxine	β-3, 5-Di-iodo-4(3′, 5′, di-iodo-4′-hydroxy)-phenyl-α-amino propionic acid	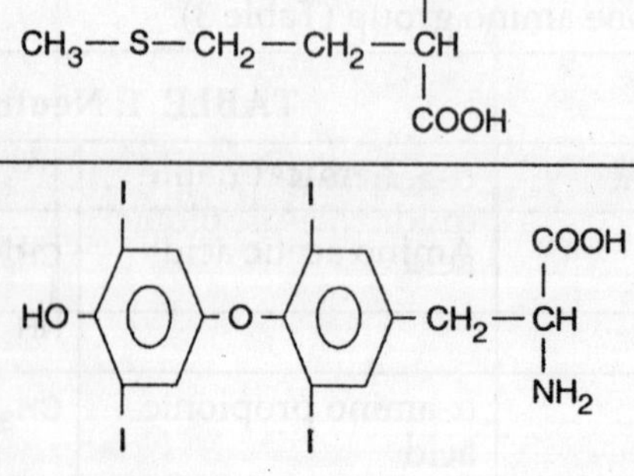	Thy

Contd

Name	Chemical name	Structure	Abbre-viation
*14. Tryptophan	α-amino-β-indole-propionic acid	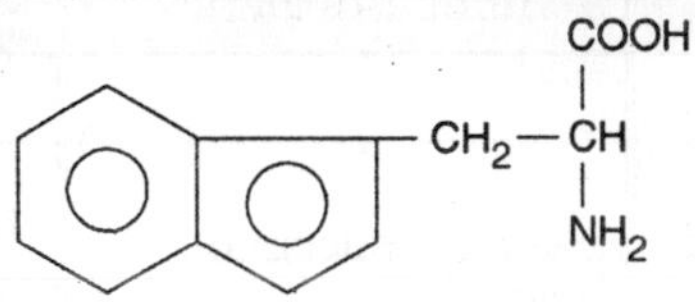	Trp
15. Proline	Pyrrolidine-α-carboxylic acid	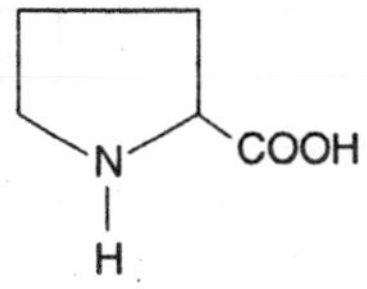	Pr
16. Hydroxy-proline	γ hydroxypyrrolidine-α-carboxylic acid	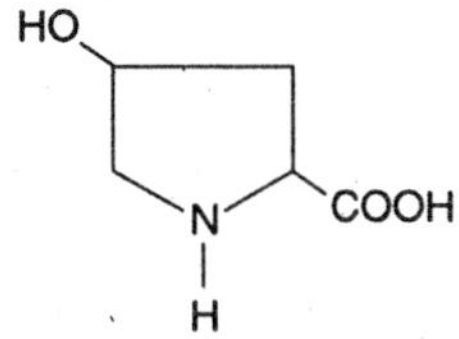	Hyp

TABLE 2: Basic amino acids

Name	Chemical name	Structure	Abbre-viation
17. Ornithine	α, δ-diamino-*n*-valeric acid	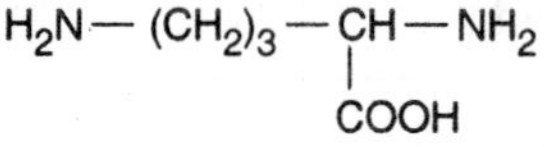	—
*18. Arginine	α-amino-δ guanidino-*n*-valeric acid	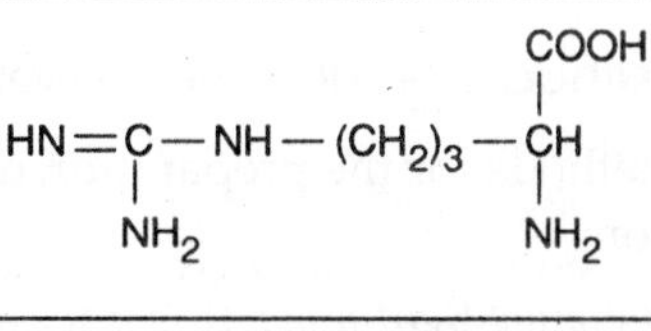	Arg
*19. Lysine	α, ε-diamino-caproic acid	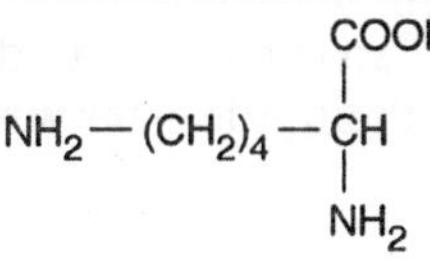	Lys
*20. Histidine	α-amino-β-imidazole-propionic acid	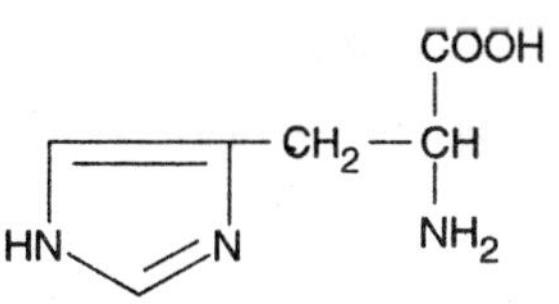	His

TABLE 3: Acidic amino acids

Name	Chemical name	Structure	Abbre-viation
21. Aspartic acid	α-amino succinic acid	$HOOC-CH_2-CH(NH_2)-COOH$	Asp
22. Aspargine	α-amino succinamic acid	$H_2N-C(=O)-CH_2-CH(NH_2)-COOH$	Aspr
23. Glutamic acid	α-amino glutaric acid	$HOOC-CH_2-CH_2-CH(NH_2)-COOH$	Glu
24. Glutamine	α-amino glutaramic acid	$H_2N-C(=O)-(CH_2)_2-CH(NH_2)-COOH$	Glu
25. β-hydroxy-glutamic acid	α-amino-β-hydroxy-glutaric acid	$HOOC-CH_2-CH(OH)-CH(NH_2)-COOH$	—

* Essential amino acids

3.1.5 General Methods for the Preparation of Amino Acids

There are several methods for the preparation of amino acids. Among these methods following are the most common:

1. *Gabriel Phthalimide Synthesis*: It is one of the best methods for the preparation of amino acids. In this method, an α-halogenated ester is treated with potassium phthalimide to form a substituted phthalimide ester which on hydrolysis under drastic condition yields α-amino acid.

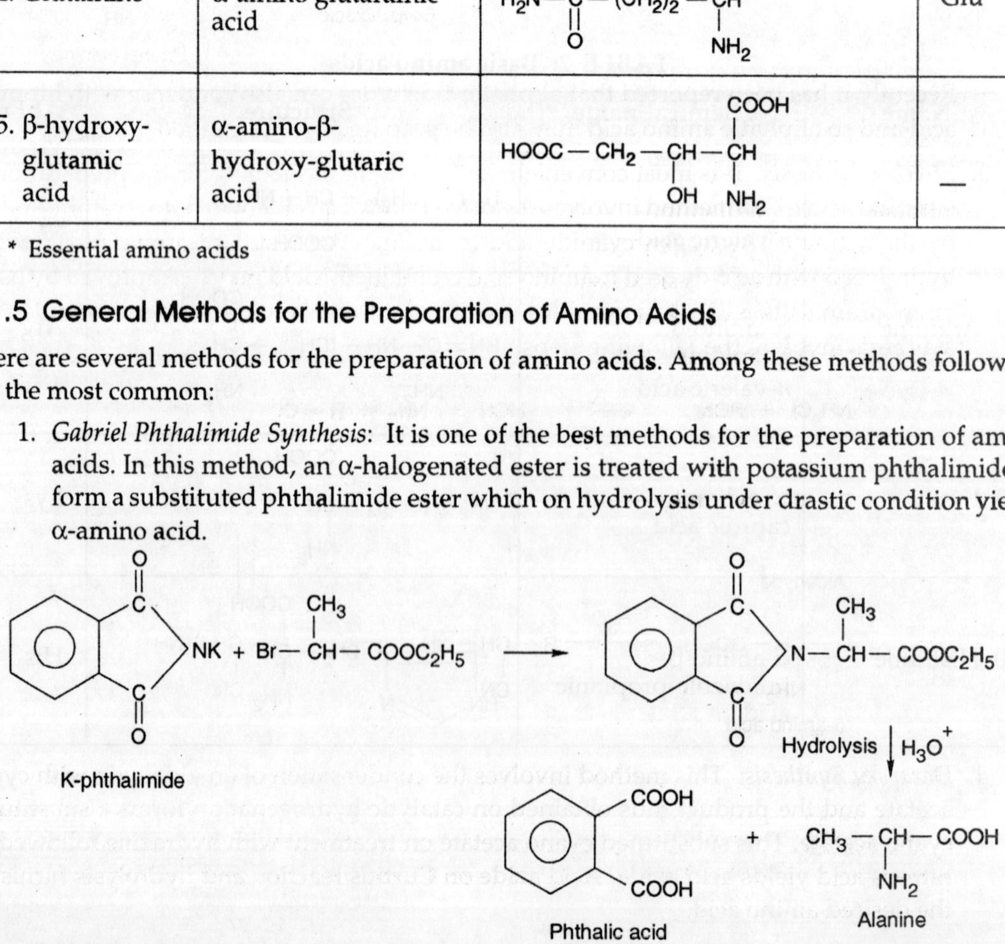

2. *Erlenmeyer Azlactone Synthesis*: This method is applicable for the synthesis of aromatic amino acids. In this method an aldehyde specially aromatic aldehyde is allowed to condense with hippuric acid (benzoyl glycine) in presence of sodium acetate in acetic anhydride solution when an azlactone is obtained. Thus,

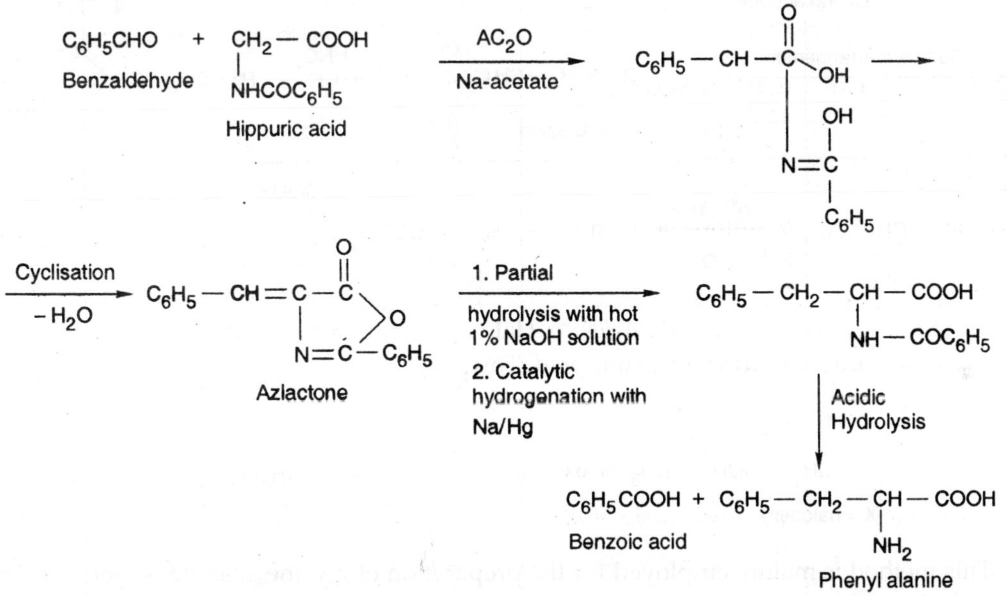

Recently it has been reported that aliphatic aldehydes can also condense with hippuric acid and so aliphatic amino acid may also be prepared by this method.

3. *Strecker Synthesis*: It is most convenient and economical method for the preparation of α-amino acids. The method involves the conversion of an aldehyde into an amino-nitrile by the action of hydrogen cyanide and ammonia. The resultant amino-nitrile when hydrolysed with acid desired α-amino acid is obtained. Yield may be improved by using ammonium salts and alkali cyanides instead of ammonia and hydrogen cyanide. The synthesis involves the following steps.

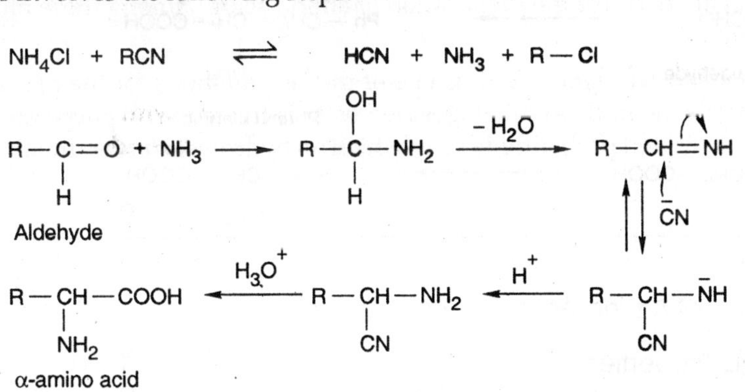

4. *Darapsky Synthesis*: This method involves the condensation of an aldehyde with cyano acetate and the product thus obtained on catalytic hydrogenation forms a substituted cyano acetate. This substituted cyano acetate on treatment with hydrazine followed by nitrous acid yields acid azide. Acid azide on Curtius reaction and hydrolysis furnishes the desired amino acid.

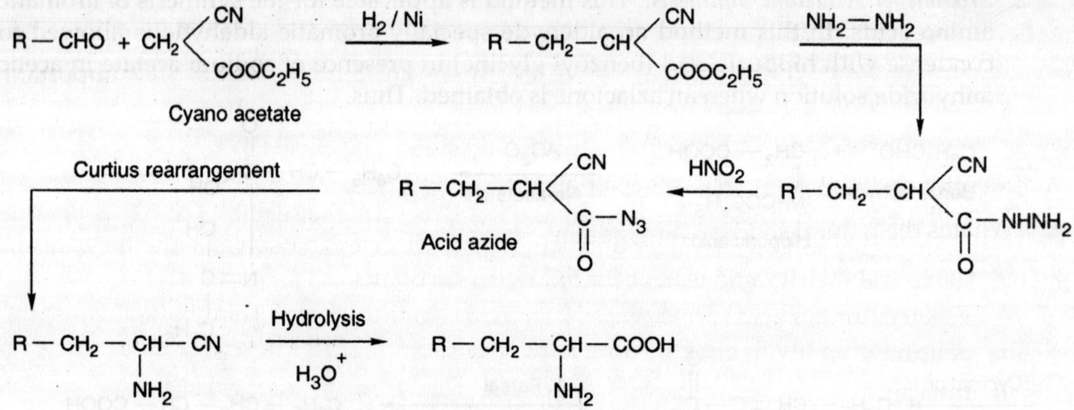

5. *Direct Amination of α-Halo Acids*: α-Halo acids on amination by alcoholic, aqueous or liquid ammonia afford α-amino acid. Thus,

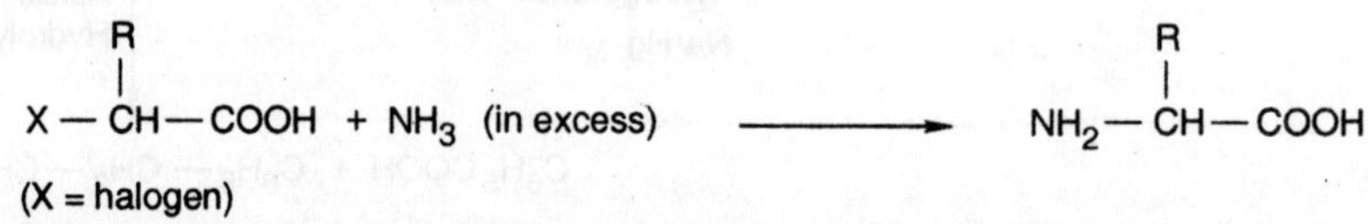

This method is mainly employed for the preparation of glycine, alanine, serine, threonine, valine and leucine.

This reaction suffers from a serious drawback that along with amino acids, secondary and tertiary amines are formed. In order to avoid the formation of these amines excess ammonia is used. In some cases use of hexamethylene tetramine in place of ammonia has been reported; however, hydrolysis of the initial product is then necessary.

PROBLEM 3.1

Prepare the following amino acids from the starting material given:

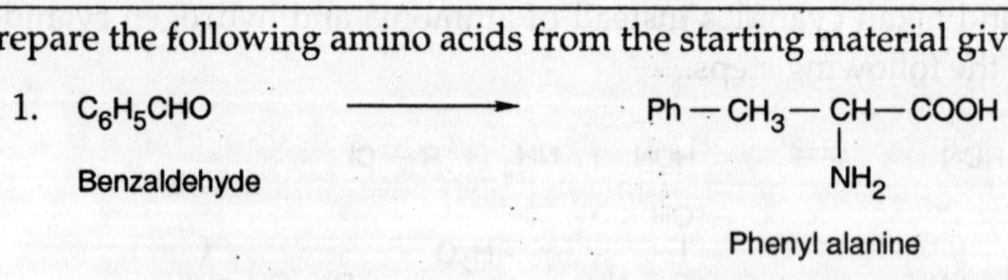

3.1.6 Properties of Amino Acids

3.1.6.1 Physical Properties

Amino acids are colourless solids. Due to the presence of both carboxylic acid function and basic amino group in the same molecule, amino acids have an unique characteristic feature. The two functionalities interact with each other internally to form a salt having both the positive and negative ions, i.e.,

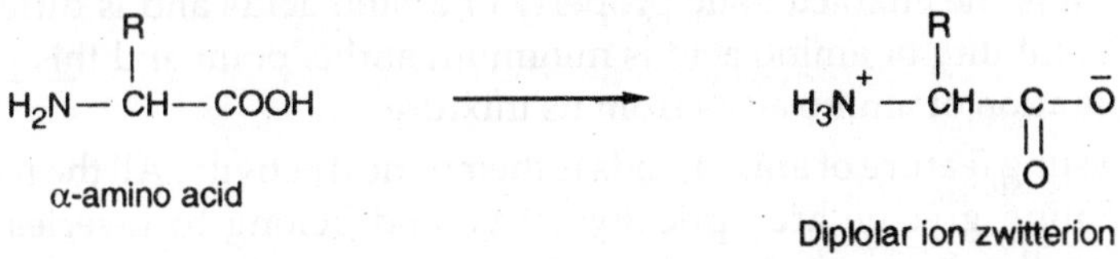

This dipolar ion is also known as internal salt or *zwitterion.*

Due to the existence of amino acids in dipolar ion structures they exhibit salt-like properties. Thus, they are highly soluble in water but sparingly soluble in organic solvents and they are high melting solids and their solutions have high dilectric constants.

As expected, amino acids are *amphoteric* in nature and in neutral solution (aqueous) they exist in an equilibriun involving following ionic species.

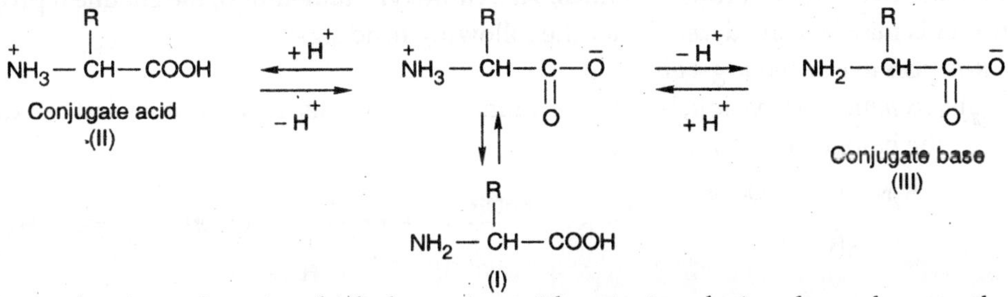

The predominant form in which the amino acids exist in solution depends upon the pH of the solution. Thus in acidic solution, i.e., at lower pH, the equilibrium shifts towards the conjugate acid form (II) but in basic solution, i.e., at higher pH, conjugate base form (III) predominates. Now if the conjugate acid is titrated against alkali and a graph of pH against alkali is plotted, it is seen that there are two equivalent points for such solution. The first equivalent point is due to the change of the conjugate acid form (II) into zwitterion (I) corresponding to pk_a of α-COOH group (pk_a 2.34) and second one indicates the change of zwitterion (I) into conjugate base (III) corresponds to pk_a of α-$\overset{+}{N}H_3$ group (pk_a 9.60). From the graph it is seen that there is a particular point at which the concentration of zwitterion is maximum and the concentrations of conjugate acid and base are minimum. The pH of this point, thus, may be considered as the pH at which the amino acid under consideration mainly exists in dipolar ion or zwitterion form. As the dipolar ion has a net charge of zero, the migration of ions under the influence of electric field is at minimum at this pH. This pH, at which the amino acid exhibits minimum migration of ions in an electric field is called *isoelectric point* (pI, point of inflection, pk_a 5.97) of the amino acid.

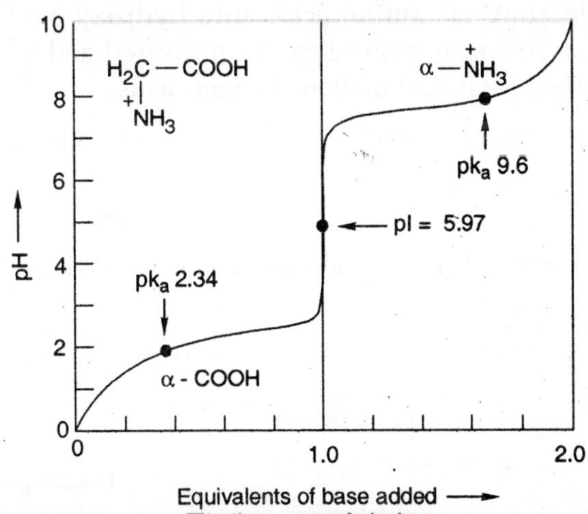

Titration curve of glycine

Isoelectric point is the characteristic property of amino acids and is different for different amino acids. The solubility of amino acid is minimum at this point and this property has been utilised in the separation of amino acids from its mixture.

Another interesting feature of amino acids is their optical activity. All the naturally occurring amino acids excepting glycine are optically active and belong to L-series and so they are represented by the following projections formula.

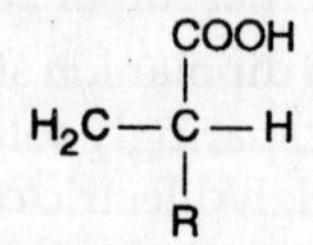

3.1.6.2 Chemical Properties

Since there are two different functionalities, viz., carboxylic and amino, the chemical properties of amino acids may be considered under the following headings:

i. *Reactions due to amino group*

(a) *Alkylation*: In basic solution, the amino group acts as a nucleophile and can displace the halogen of alkyl halides.

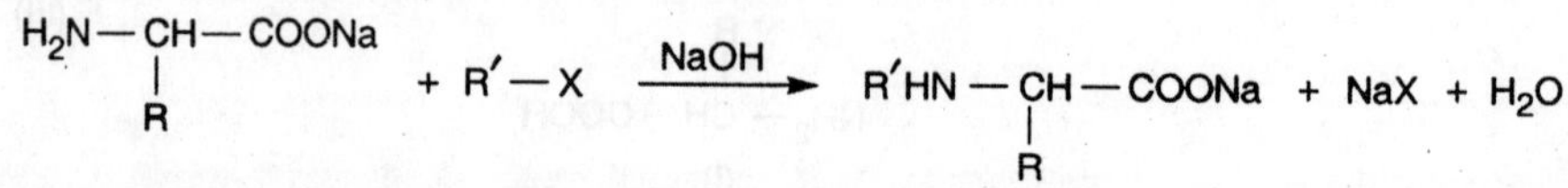

(b) On treatment with acid chlorides and acid anhydrides amino acids form acyl derivatives, i.e.,

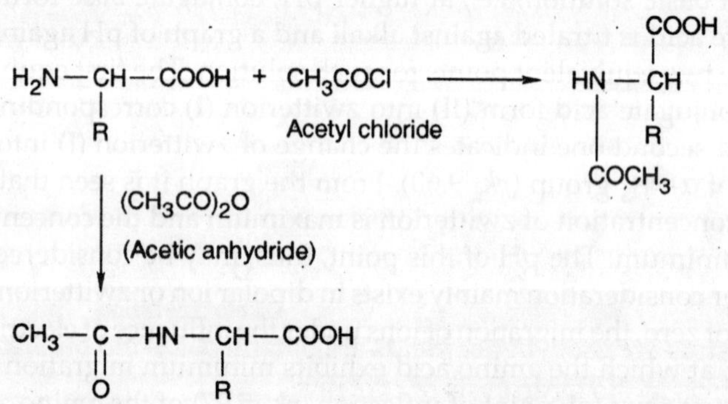

(c) Nitrous acid converts amino acids into hydroxy acid with the retention of configuration. Nitrogen evolved can be measured and in fact, this is the basis of *Vanslyke* method for the estimation of amino acids.

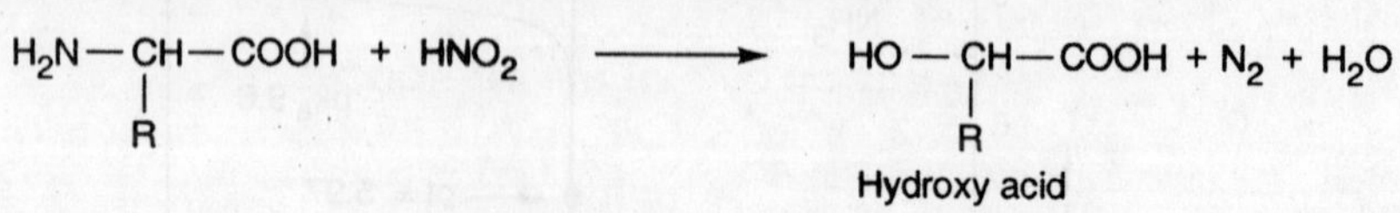

(d) *Formylation reaction*: Amino acids react with formaldehyde to form a mixture of products.

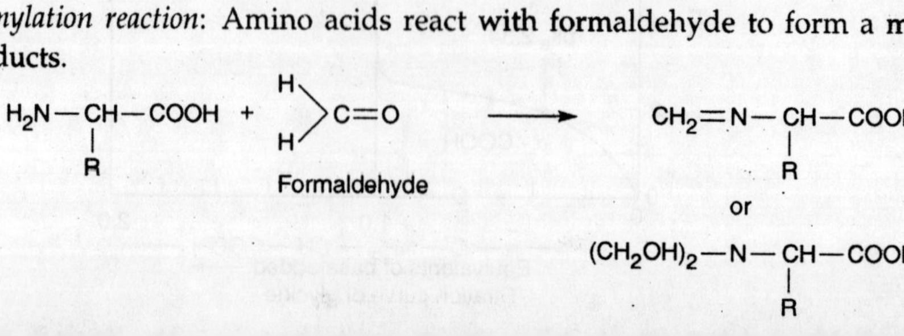

As a result amino group is totally blocked and carboxylic group of amino acid can be easily titrated with alkali. This method of titrating amino acids with alkalis is known as *Sorensen formol* titration.

ii. *Reactions due to carboxylic group*: Amino acids exhibit the typical reactions of carboxylic acids as noted below:

(a) Amino acids react with alkali to form salts.

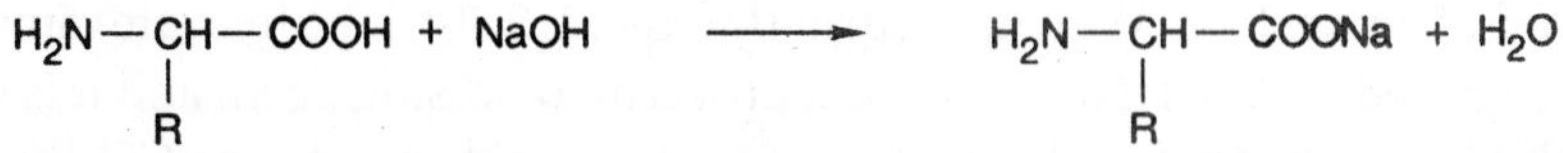

(b) Amino acids form chelate compounds with the salts of heavy metals. Thus, copper oxide forms a chelate when it is heated with the aqueous solution of an amino acid.

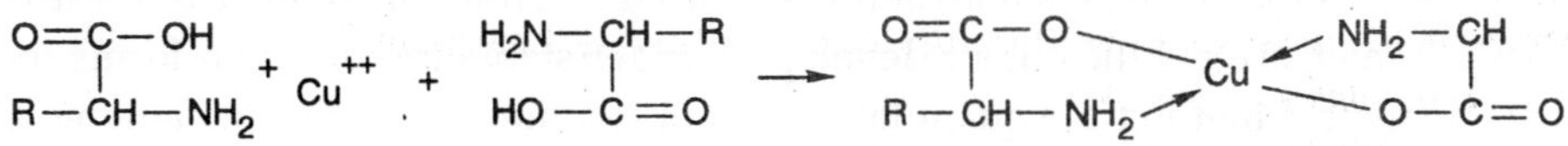

(c) *Decarboxylation*: Amino acids on heating alone or in presence of acids or bases or any specific enzyme can be decarboxylated resulting in the formation of amine.

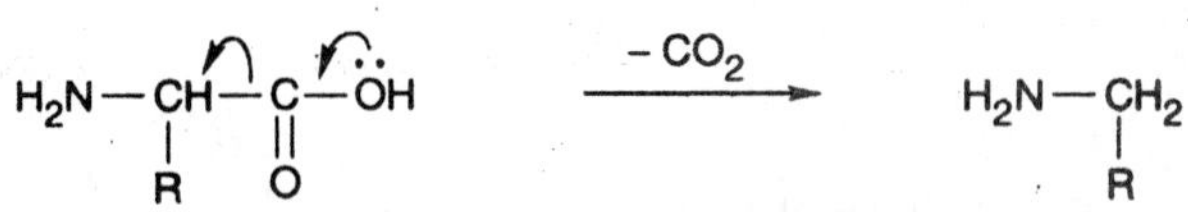

Amine

iii. *Reactions involving both the amino and carboxylic group*

(a) *Action of heat*: When amino acids are heated two molecules intereact to form 2, 5-diketo piperazines.

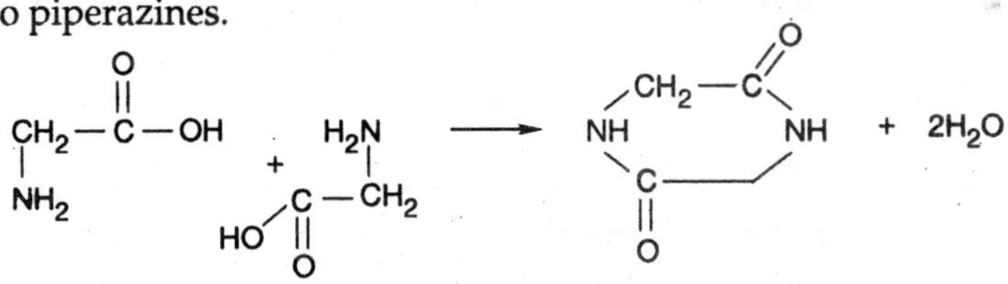

Diketo piperazine

When esters are used, better yields are obtained. Diketo piperazines are offen found as products in the hydrolysis of proteins.

(b) *Hydantoin formation*: α-amino acids react with phenyl isocyanates to form phenyl hydantoic acids which on heating in presence of acid undergo cyclisation to afford hydantoins.

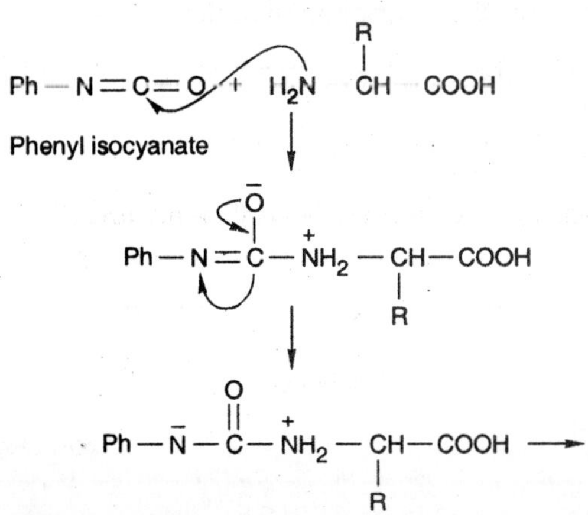

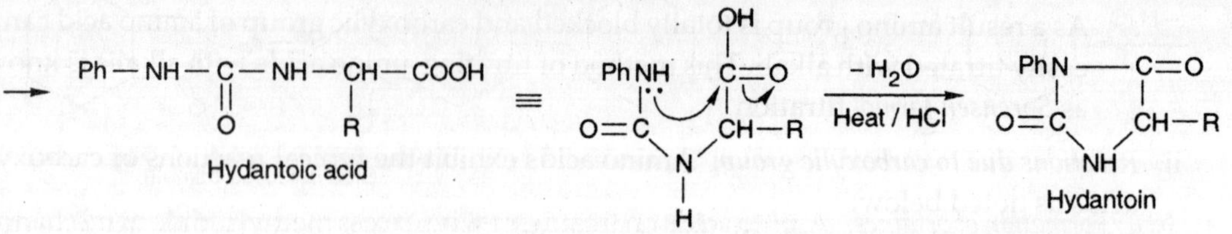

(c) *Ninhydrin reaction*: With ninhydrin (Indane, 1, 2, 3-trione hydrate) amino acids form a coloured product. Ninhydrin is a powerful oxidising agent and it is supposed that it brings oxidative decarboxylation of α-amino acids, producing CO_2, and an aldehyde having one carbon atom less than the parent amino acids. The reduced ninhydrin (A) thus formed reacts with another molecule of ninhydrin to form a blue complex. The intensity of blue colour developed under standard condition forms the basis of an useful method for quantitative test of α-amino acids. Simple amines also undergo similar reaction but without any evolution of CO_2. Evolution of CO_2 in this reaction is indicative of an α-amino acid.

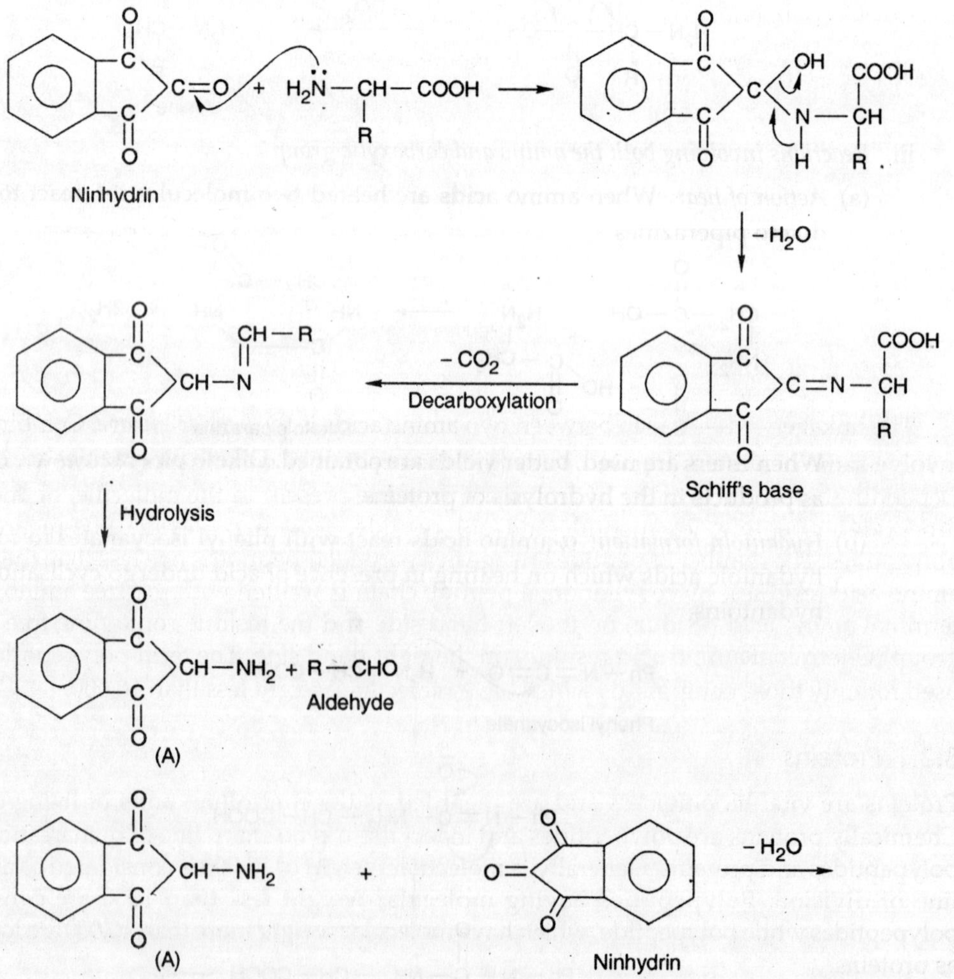

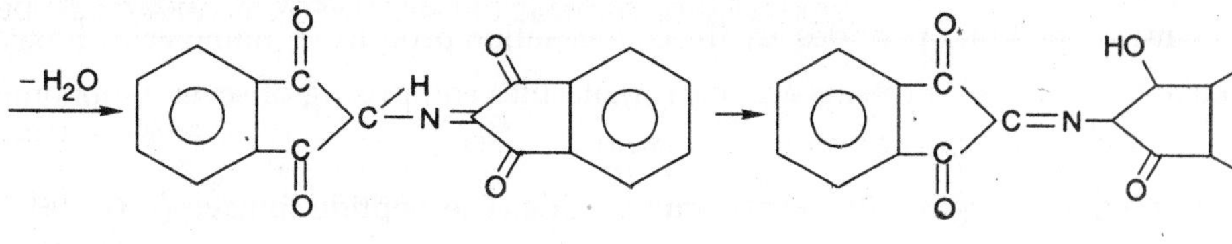

Blue coloured complex

(d) *Formation of betaines*: Amino acids on treatment with excess methyl iodide in methanolic solution yield trimethyl derivatives which are commonly known as *betaines*.

$$\overset{+}{H_3N}-\underset{\underset{R}{|}}{CH}-CO\bar{O} + 3CH_3I \longrightarrow (CH_3)_3-\overset{+}{N}-\underset{\underset{R}{|}}{CH}-CO\bar{O} + 3HI$$

Betaine

3.2 Peptides and Proteins

A peptide is composed of two or more amino acids joined together through a linkage known as *peptide linkage*. The term peptide linkage is applicable to the amide linkage between the amino and carboxylic residues of amino acids. Thus,

$$NH_2-\underset{\underset{R_1}{|}}{CH}-COOH + H_2N-\underset{\underset{R_2}{|}}{CH}-COOH$$

$$\downarrow$$

$$\text{N-terminal} \longrightarrow NH_2-\underset{\underset{R_1}{|}}{CH}-\overset{\overset{O}{||}}{C}-NH-\underset{\underset{R_2}{|}}{CH}-COOH \longleftarrow \text{C-terminal}$$

Peptide linkage

The linkage $-NH-\overset{\overset{O}{||}}{C}-$ in between two amino acids is the *peptide linkage*. Combination may involve same or different amino acids and the product of combination is known as peptide. Depending upon the number of amino acid residue present in the molecule, peptide may be dipeptide, tripeptide, tetrapeptide and polypeptide. Thus peptides may be regarded as the polyamides. The number of peptide linkage in a particular peptide is one less than the number of amino acid residues. By convention, a peptide chain is written with the free amino group (N-terminal amino acid residue) on the left-hand side and the residue containing free carboxylic group (C-terminal amino acid residue) on the right-hand side. The term polypeptide is mainly used for only those compounds which have molecular weight less than 10,000.

3.2.1 Proteins

Proteins are vital biopolymers and are regarded as the controlling units of living organisms. Chemically proteins are polypeptides and in fact there is no sharp line of demarcation between polypeptides and proteins. Generally, a molecular weight of 10,000 is considered as an arbitrary line of division. Polypeptides having molecular weight less than 1000 are considered as polypeptides while polypeptide, which have molecular weight more than 10,000 are looked upon as proteins.

It may be mentioned that peptides are the condensation product of amino acids linked by peptide linkage ($-\overset{\underset{\|}{O}}{C}-NH-$). Proteins are macromolecules comprising of several monomer of peptide. Each monomer consists of twenty amino acids. The peptide linkage ($-\overset{\underset{\|}{O}}{C}-NH-$) in proteins is identified by IR spectroscopy. In IR spectrum, proteins exhibit bands at 3300-3100 cm^{-1} for hydrogen bonded—NH—grouping and 1650 and 1550 cm^{-1} for $>C=O$ functionality.

3.2.1.1 Characteristic Features of Proteins

Proteins possess the following characteristic features:

1. Though proteins are macromolecules yet most of them are soluble in water.
2. Since proteins are the condensation product of amino acids each protein possesses a primary amino ($-NH_2$) group and primary carboxylic ($-COOH$) function in their molecule. As a result proteins exist as *Zewitter ion* and so they have *isoelectric points.*
3. Proteins are optically active due to the chiral nature of α-carbon.
4. Most of the proteins are colloidal in nature. However, some proteins are crystalline; as for example, insulin.
5. *Salting in and Salting out of proteins:* It has been observed that the solubility of proteins in water may be gradually increased by the gradual addition of proteins by the addition of neutral salt which is known as *salting in.* But if the concentration of neutral salt exceeds a particular limit precepitation of proteins occurs i.e., solubility is decreased. This decrease in solubility is termed as *salting out* of proteins. Salting out is considered as an important method for the purification of proteins.
6. *Denaturation of Proteins:* The precipitation of proteins from their solutions may be achieved by various processes such as by addition of (i) neutral salt, (ii) acids/bases, (iii) solvents (usually organic solvents such as ethanol, acetone, etc.), (iv) detergents and (v) by the application of physical means like shaking.

Since by these processes there is a change in the nature of protein (solution to solid) this phenomenon is designated as *denaturation of* proteins and the proteins thus obtained through these processes are termed as *denatured proteins.* Denatured proteins are characterised by the following characteristics:

(i) Decrease in solubility (ii) Decrease in optical activity (iii) Decrease in biological activity and increase in chemical behaviour.

On the basis of above changes in properties, particularly increase in chemical activity, it has been suggested *that denaturation is most probably due to the changes in conformation or unfolding of the protein molecule.* In general, secondary and tertiary structures of proteins are completely destroyed without any breakage in the primary structure.

It has been found that the process of denaturation in most of the cases are irreversible phenomenon, i.e., once the protein is denatured it cannot be converted to original one. The classical example of denaturation is the boiling of egg. When egg is boiled tertiary structure is destroyed and there is formation of disorganised mass of polypeptide chain as shown:

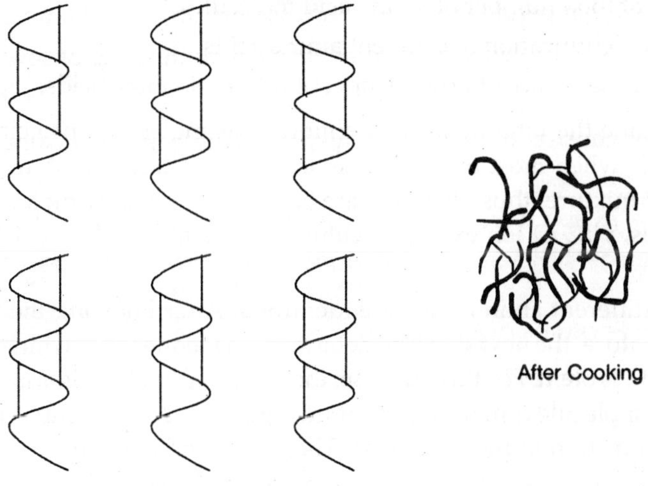

After Cooking

Before cooking Egg albumin

However, in some cases denaturation may be reversible. This reversal of denaturation is known as *renaturation* or *refolding*. The most widely illustrated example is haemoglobin which can be denatured in acid solution and the denatured haemoglobin may be converted back to original one by the treatment with alkali.

3.2.1.2 Biological Significances of Proteins

Proteins are the building units of living organisms. They serve as the basis of protoplasm. Proteins are responsible for various cellular functions as noted below:

1. Proteins, as mentioned before, serve as the building blocks of living organisms.
2. Proteins act as enzymes (catalysts) in biochemical reactions.
3. Proteins function as hormonal regulators of metabolism and control the pH of the biological system.
4. Proteins take part in necessary biological processes such as respiration, muscular contraction, active transport of cellular components, etc.
5. Proteins form antibody in living organisms which protect the different organs from the attack of external agent.

3.2.1.3 Structure of Proteins

Since proteins are highly polymeric in nature, for the convenience of elucidation, their structures have been divided into four parts, viz.,

1. Primary structure
2. Secondary structure
3. Tertiary structure and
4. Quarternary structure.

3.2.1.3.1 Determination of Primary Structure of Proteins

Primary structure of protein is primarily referred to the number, nature and sequence of amino acids along the peptide chain present. Consequently, the study of primary structure of protein involves the following steps:

(a) Determination of total number of amino acid molecules.

(b) Separation and identification of different amino acids.

(c) The settlement of sequence of arrangement of different amino acids.

In order to determine the total number of amino acids molecules, protein is subjected to hydrolysis by 6(N) HCl when most of the amino acids are hydrolysed. After hydrolysis, the solution of amino acid mixture, thus obtained, are separated by following any one of the two most common methods, viz., (i) ion exchange column chromatography or (ii) pH-dependent precipitation.

After separation, different amino acids are identified. After knowing the total number of amino acids and their nature, the next step is to determine the sequence in which different amino acids are arranged in the protein. For this purpose, the *end group* analysis is applied. Proteins are bifunctional polymeric molecule containing one amino group (—NH_2) group at one end and one carboxylic (—COOH) function at the other end. These two ends are known as *terminals*. The terminal position which contains —NH_2 group is known as *N-terminal* while terminal having —COOH group is termed as *C-terminal*. These two terminals are ascertained by the application of *tagging technique*. In this technique, protein is treated with a reagent known as tagging reagent. This reagent reacts with a particular terminal to form *tagged protein* which is subjected to partial hydrolysis either in the presence of a catalyst or an enzyme when the tagged amino acid is released and identified. The remaining protein is subjected to similar procedure and partial hydrolysis and this process is repeated till all the tagged amino acids are identified. This identification of amino acids, thus, gives an idea regarding the nature of amino acid sequence in protein. It may be mentioned that the above tagging technique has been successfully applied for the determination of N-terminal only but not for C-terminal. This is because of the lack of effective tagging reagent for C-terminal. On the other hand, many effective tagging reagents are available for N-terminal analysis. However, the most important and useful tagging agent for N-terminal analysis is 2, 4-dinitro-fluorobenzene (DNFB). DNFB reacts smoothly with a terminal α-amino group in bicarbonate-buffered aqueous ethanol to form an N-(2,4-dinitrophenyl) peptide which on hydrolysis yields DNFB-amino acid and a mixture of amino acids. As the DNP-amino acids are brilliantly coloured, they are identified by TLC and thus the amino acid residue forming N-terminal is known. Reactions taking place may be shown as below:

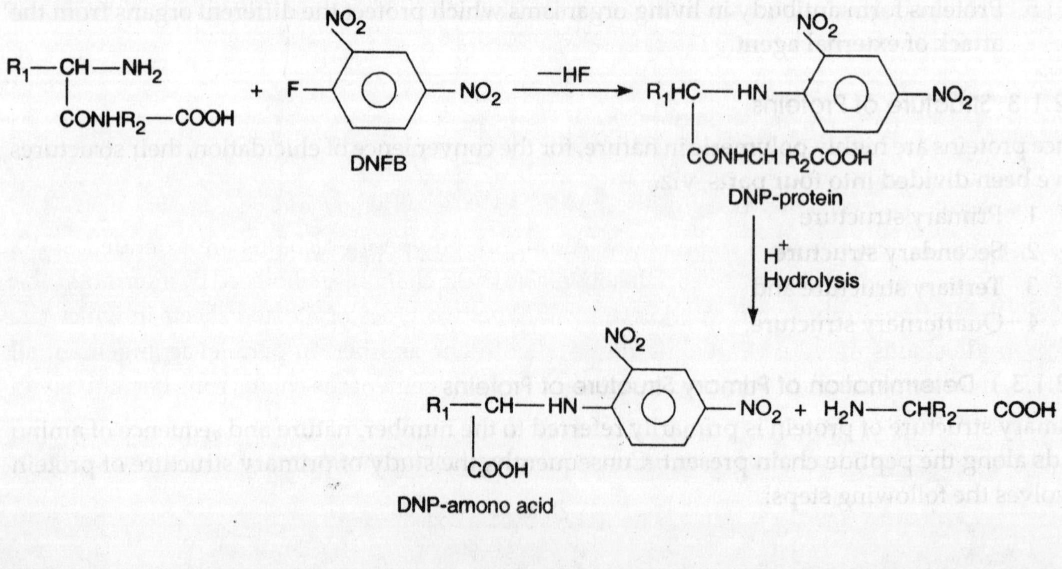

As mentioned before chemical methods for C-terminal analysis have not yet been so successful. However, C-terminal analysis may be achieved by the hydrolytic cleavage by certain enzymes such as carboxyl peptidase. A and B present in swine pancreas for peptides having free carboxylic function in the C-terminal.

3.2.1.3.2 Determination of Secondary Structure of Proteins

The secondary structure of proteins is concerned with the conformation of polypeptide chain in the protein. The conformation of peptide chain has two aspects—(i) the way in which the protein is folded and bent, and (ii) the nature of α-linkages and bonds which stabilise this structure.

Regarding the conformation of peptide chain two views have been proposed as noted below:

(a) α-helix

(b) β-helix.

α-helical conformation as shown in the figure has been proposed by Pauling and Crey. According to this view, the backbone of the polypeptide is coiled around the long axis of the protein molecule and the helix is stabilised by hydrogen bonding. Each hydrogen atom of NH_2 group of one amino acid is bonded to carbonyl oxygen of carboxylic group of another amino acid. This hydrogen bonding prevents free rotation and so helix becomes rigid. Most amino acids are accommodated as structural units in α-helix, α-helix may be either left- or right-handed and each turn of helix contains 3.7 or 5.1 amino acid residues and the diameter of a helix is about 10 A°. Wool and fibrous proteins of muscle belong to this category.

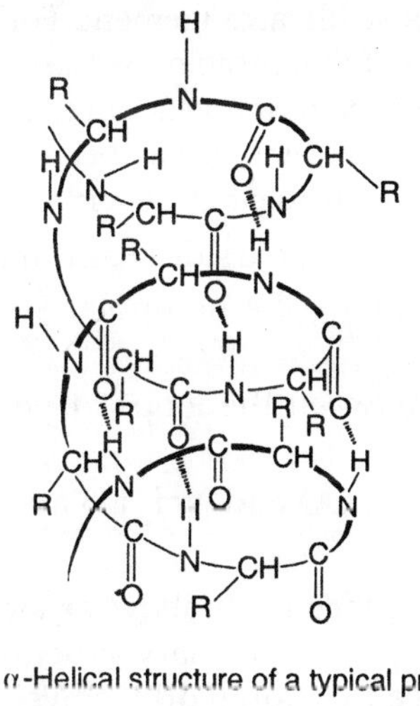

α-Helical structure of a typical protein.

In β-helical conformation as shown in the figure polypeptide chains are extended and a number of these aligned side by side in close contact. These chains are stabilised by intermolecular hydrogen binding. In this conformation there may be two types of pleated sheets in which the polypeptide chains may be parallel or antiparallel to one another. In parallel arrangement all chains run in the same directions and in antiparallel arrangement the chains run alternatively in opposite directions.

The β-helical strcutre have been found in silk and spinder-web.

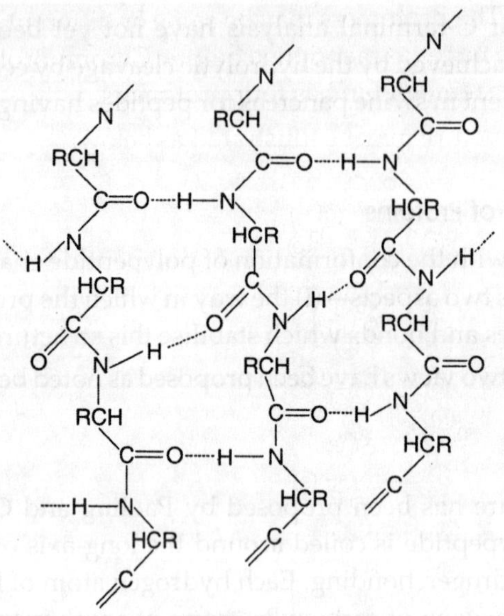

Parallel pleated sheet

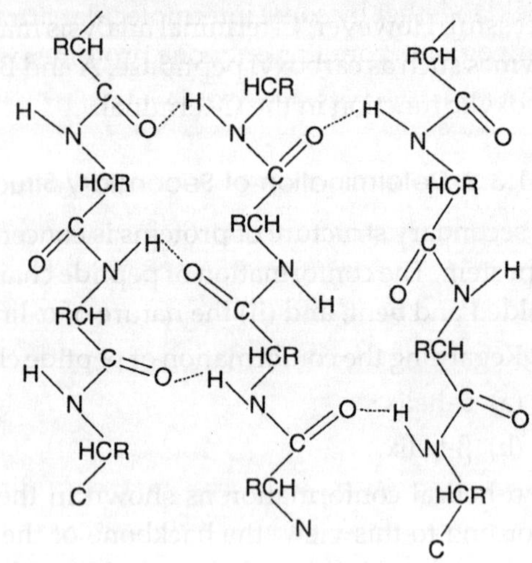

Anti-parallel sheet

3.2.1.3.3 Tertiary Structural Frame-work of Proteins

The tertiary structural frame-work of proteins refers to the orientations of the side chains in the folded molecule. The tertiary structure that a protein assumes under the normal conditions of pH and temperature is considered as its stable arrangement. For this reason this structural unit is genrally termed as *native conformation* of that protein. As the tertiary structure describes the overall spatial arrangement of polypeptide chains it reveals an exact description of molecular shape in most of the small and medium sized proteins. It has been observed that some intermolecular attractive forces as noted below are responsible for the tertiary structural unit of proteins.

i. Hydrogen bond formation between the side chain amino and carboxylic functionalities.
ii. Hydrophobic interactions among the non-polar side-chains of amino acids.
iii. Disulphide cross-linkages between the loops of poly-peptide chain.
iv. Ionic bond formation between $CO\bar{O}$ and $N\overset{+}{H}_3$ at various positions.

It has further been observed that either all the above or some of the forces may be operative in any protein. Tertiary structural frame-work has most efficiently been elaborated by physical techniques like X-ray diffraction study, ultra centrifuge, diffusion and electron microscopy. A typical diagrammatic represention of tertiary structure of protein-myoglobin is an shown below:

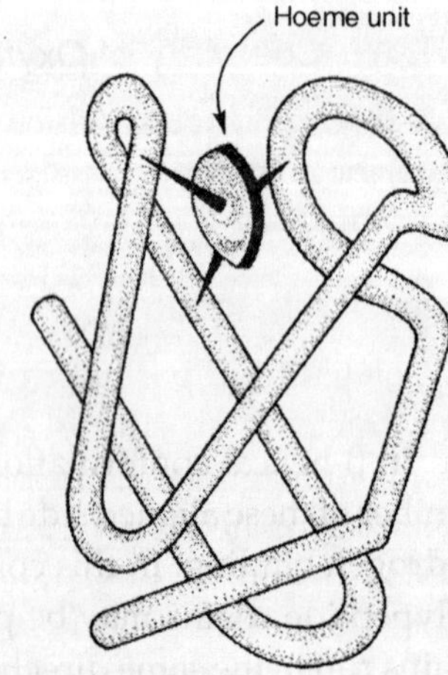

3.2.1.3.4 Quarternary Structure of Proteins

Quarternary structure of proteins involves the description of arrangements of subunits in space.

Many proteins may contain one or more polypeptide chains. In the former case, the proteins are termed as *monomeric* while in other case it is designated as *oligomeric*. The individual peptide chains in oligomeric proteins are called *protomers.* The protomers may be same or different and are held together by some intermolecular attractive forces as mentioned before. Chromoprotein, and myoglobin contains only one protomer while haemoglobin has four protomers.

The relation between four levels of protein structure may be illustrated as below:

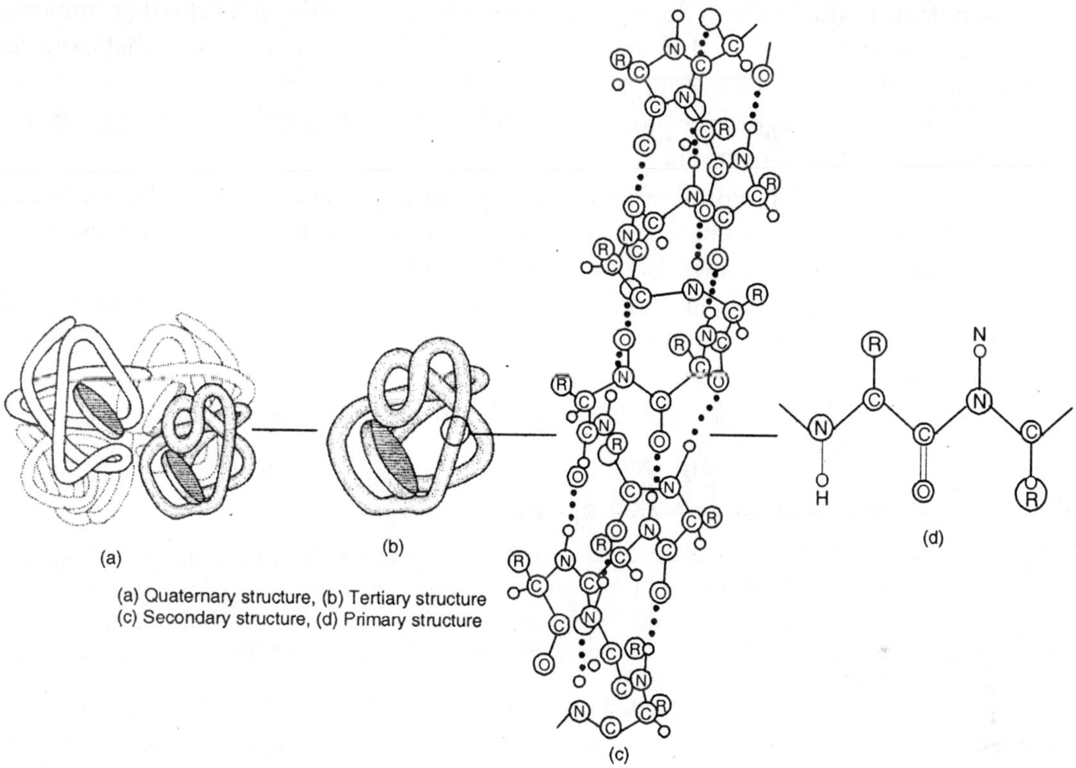

(a) Quaternary structure, (b) Tertiary structure
(c) Secondary structure, (d) Primary structure

3.2.1.4 Chemistry of Some Important Proteins

3.2.1.4.1 Chemistry of Oxytocin

Oxytocin is a hormone which occurs in posterior pituitory gland. This hormone is responsible for uterine contraction. It also excites the musculature of the intestine, gall bladder, ureter and urinary bladder. It also causes ejection of milk.

3.2.1.4.1.1 Isolation

It is isolated from posterior pituitory gland. Pituitary gland is separated from the body, dried and extracted with ethanol or acetic acid. The resulting solution is then treated with sodium chloride to coagulate all the proteins. The coagulated proteins on treatment with trichloroacetic acid are dissociated into various proteins from which by the application of paper chromatographic technique oxytocin is separated and finally it is purified by means of electrophoresis.

3.2.1.4.1.2 Constitution of Oxytocin

The constitution of oxytocin was established by Vigneaud from the following evidences:

i. Oxytocin records isoelectric point of 7.1. This value suggests the presence of free amino-group but the absence of free carboxytic group in oxytocin.

ii. When oxytocin is completely hydrolysed with acid, a mixture of eight amino acids is obtained. The identification and quantitative analysis of these amino acids reveal the presence of equimolecular mixture of eight amino acids—cystine, glycine, leucine, isoleucine, proline, aspartic acid, glutamic acid and tyrosine.

Ammonia is also obtained during hydrolysis and its estimation indicates that ammonia is present in the ratio 3 : 1 in any amino acid. This proportion suggests that oxytocin contains *three carbonamide* groups.

iii. The molecular weight of oxytocin was found to be 1000, a value which suggests the *octapeptide nature* of oxytocin.

iv. On oxidation with performic acid, oxytocin yields a disulphonic acid with a molecular weight which corresponds to oxytocin disulphonic acid. This indicates the presence of ring structure of oxytocin involving S—S linkage of cystine.

v. On controlled hydrolysis of oxidised oxytocin with hydrochloric acid, four peptides and two tripeptides along with two molecules of cysteic acid are formed. The peptides are identified by N-terminal and C-terminal analysis.

Based on the above evidences following structure has been proposed for oxytocin.

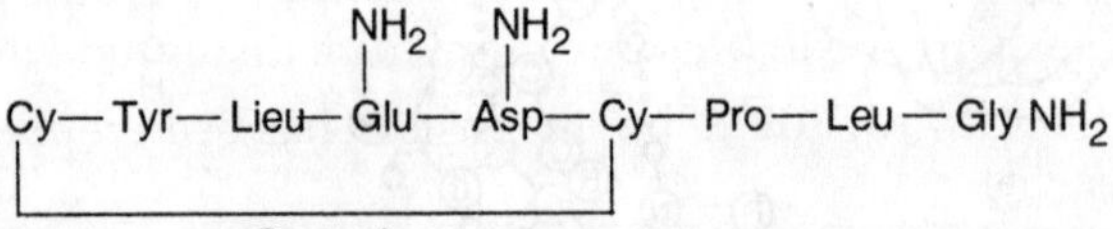

Oxytocin

3.2.1.4.2 Insulin

Insulin is a peptide hormone. It is secreted by β-cells of langerthans in the pancreas. It regulates carbohydrate metabolism in the body. Deficiency of this hormone causes a disease known as *diabetes* which is manifasted by the increase in blood glucose and excretions of sugar in urine. This disease is hereditary and can be cured by the administration of insulin. Insulin, now-a-days is prepared in large scale from the pancreas of cattle and other animals.

3.2.1.4.2.1 Isolation of Insulin

Insulin is isolated from the pancreas of shaughtered animal. As soon as the pancreas is removed from the animal it is immediately frozen and is cut into pieces. These pieces are extracted with 80% ethanol containing phosphoric acid to adjust pH at 3. At this pH level of insulin remains in solution and fats and other proteinous matter remain as suspended matters. These matters are separated from the extract by centrifugation and filtered. The filtrate which contains insulin is acidified. To this fat free solution in ethanol, picric acid is added when insulin is precipitated as picrate. The picrate is dissolved in acetone and insulin is precipitated as hydrochloride. It is further purified by chromatographic resolution.

3.2.1.4.2.2 Structure of Insulin

Insulin is a highly complex molecule and its structure has been elaborated by Frederick Sanger and for this elegant work he was awarded Nobel prize in 1958. He deduced the structure of insulin on the basis of evidences as described:

i. When insulin is hydrolysed completely, it yields 51 amino acids and six molecules of ammonia. Analysis of these amino reveals that these acids are of 17 types. From these observations it has been suggested that in insulin amino acids are repeated in the structure. The different 17 amino acids were identified and their number of molecules present has also been determined. These are: (i) leucine-6 (ii) valine-5 (iii) glycine-4 (iv) alanine-3 (v) glutamic acid-4 (vi) serine-3 (vii) phenylalanine-3 (viii) aspargine-3 (ix) glutamine-3 (x) cystine-6 (xi) histidine-2 (xii) isoleucine-1 (xiii) threonine-1 (xiv) lysine-1 (xv) proline-I (xvi) arginine-1 and tyrosine-4.

ii. When insulin is subjected to end group analysis by the use of DNFB method, two amino acids, glycine and phenylalanine are found to be present as N-terminal acid residues. This is a clear indication that insulin has two chains of *polypeptides,* one having glycine and other having phenylalanine as the terminal amino acids.

iii. Quantitative analytical experiments indicate the presence of six molecules of cystine. This suggests the presence of three disulphide S—S linkage in insulin.

iv. When insulin is oxidised by performic acids two different peptide products are obtained. These two different peptide chains are separated by preciptitation and their structures were separately elucidated.

It has been settled that one product designated as chain-A contains 21 amino acids while the other product termed as chain-B has 30 amino acid residues. These two chains are connected by two disulphide linkages and the chain-A contains one more intra disulphide linkage.

On the basis of above evidences structure of bovine insulin has been represented as under:

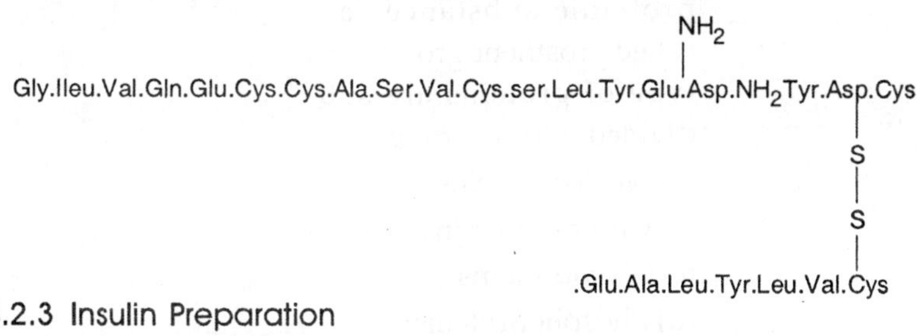

3.2.1.4.2.3 Insulin Preparation

For the treatment of diabetes different insulin preparations are used as described below:

(a) *Isophane insulin:* It is a suspension of crystalline zinc insulin with positively charged peptide mixture known as *protamine.*

(b) *Lente insulin:* It is a mixture of 30% semilente insulin and 70% ultralente insulin.

(c) *Semilente insulin:* It is a suspension of amorphons insulin. It is rapid action insulin.

(d) *Crystalline zinc insulin:* It is a purified insulin crystallised zinc salt. It is a also a rapid action insulin and lowers the blood sugar within few minutes.

(e) *Protamine zinc insulin:* It is a mixutre of zinc insulin and protamine. It is a prolonged action insulin.

(f) *Extened insulin zinc suspension:* This insulin has a delayed onset and prolonged duration of action. It is less soluble crystalline zinc insulin.

3.2.1.5 Classification of Proteins

Proteins are classified in two ways—(i) on the basis of solubility and (ii) on the basis of structure.

Classification on the basis of Solubility

Proteins

- Soluble in water and in common organic solvents (acetone, alcohol, etc). These are known as *Globular* proteins.
- Insoluble in water and in common organic solvents. These are called as *Fibrinous* proteins.

Classification based on the Structure

Proteins

- Simple
  - Albumin
  - Globulin
  - Albinoid
- Conjugated
  - In these proteins some non-proteinic substances are connected. These non-proteinic substances are called prosthetic group. This type of proteins are sub-divided into six groups—
    - (a) Nucleoproteins
    - (b) Chromoproteins
    - (c) Glycoproteins
    - (d) Phosphoproteins
    - (e) Lipoproteins
    - (f) Metalloproteins.
- Derived
  - These are denatured proteins

3.2.1.6 Synthesis of Proteins

The most popular and widely used method of synthesis of proteins is solid phase synthesis which was introduced by Merrifield in 1965. The basic feature of this synthesis is to use a synthetic insoluble resin which is a co-polymer of styrene and divinyl benzene. It is a polystyrene resin as shown below:

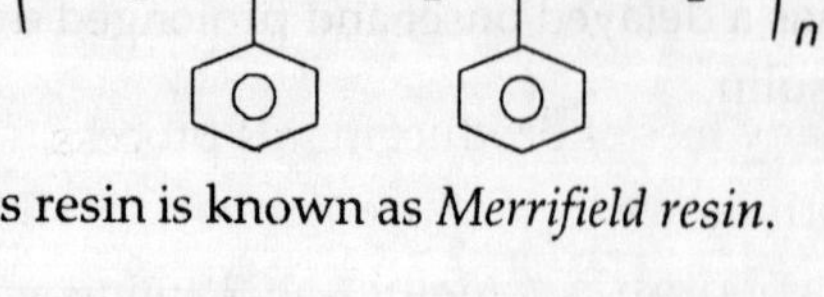

This resin is known as *Merrifield resin.*

The first step of this synthesis involves chloromethylation of polystyrene with $CH_3O—CH_2Cl$ in presence of $SnCl_4$. This chloromethylated polystyrene is now allowed to react with COOH group of N-protected amino acids in presence of dimethyl formamide (DMF) or ethyl acetate when polystyrene derivative of N-protected amino acids are formed. The product so formed is hydrolysed by HBr in presence of acetic acid to deprotect N atom of amino acids. As a result resin derivative of amino acids are obtained. This product is now allowed to condense with N-protected another amino acid in presence of dicyclohexyl carbodimide (D.C.C.) when a dipeptide is formed. The above steps are now repeated several times till the desired risin derivative of a protein is obtained. Finally, the resin is removed by hydrolysis with HBr in presence of CF_3COOH. Reactions involved may be shown as below:

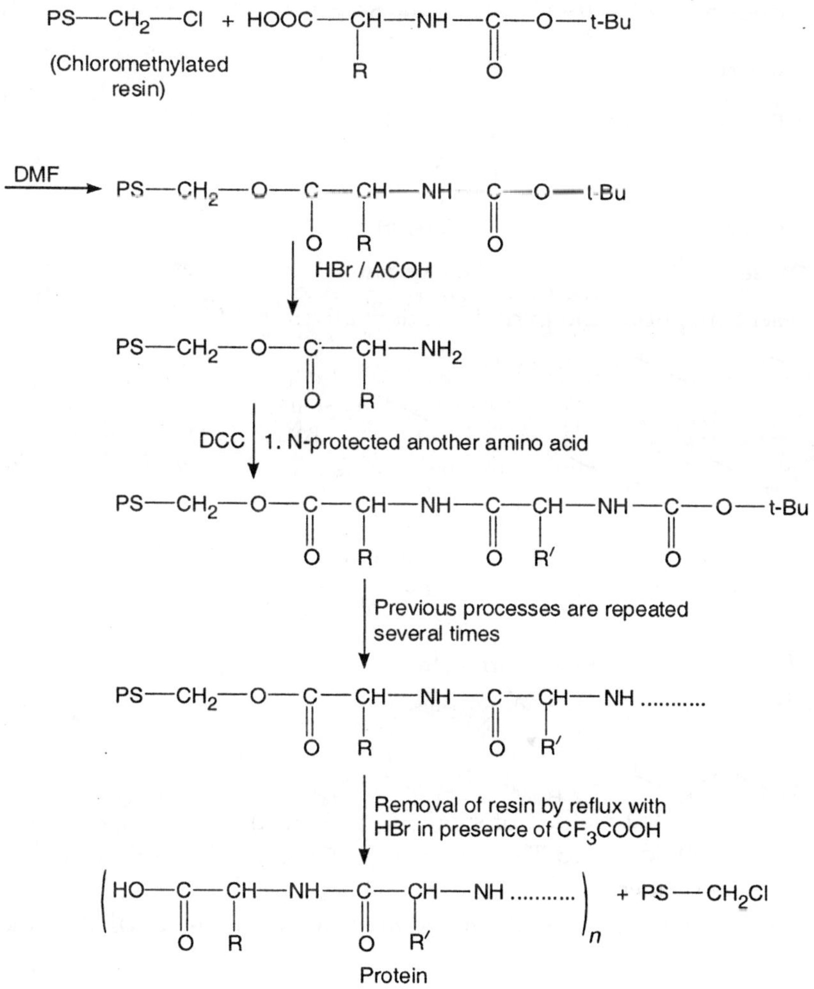

Comments:

i. Resin can be recovered unchanged without any loss of product in this process.
ii. Process is less time consuming and less laborious.
iii. This method can be applied for the synthesis of protein containing 100 amino acids.
iv. The yield of this process is very high.

v. Since the synthesis is carried out in solid phase, steps for purification is not required.

vi. The process is automatic.

3.3 Nucleic Acids

Nucleic acids are present as conjugated proteins as prosthetic group. As they occur in nuclei of the cell of living organisms they are known as *nucleic acids.* These are complex molecules and on hydrolysis form phosporic acids, sugar and some organic bases. Sugar present in nucleic acid is pentose. Among the large number of pentose only two are present in nucleic acids. These are ribose and deoxyribose.

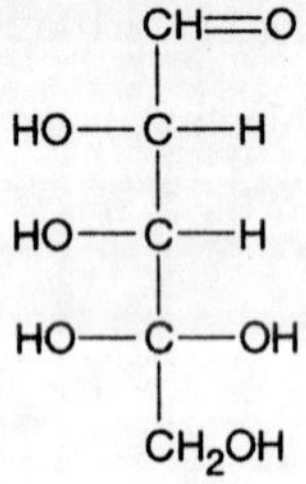

Ribose

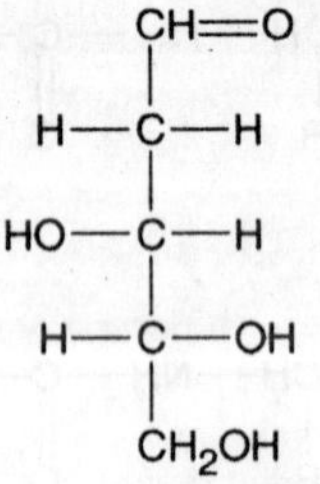

Deoxyribose

Organic bases present are purine and pyrimidine derivatives.

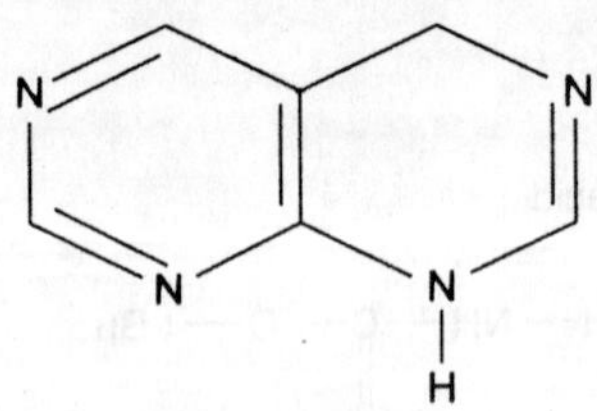

Purine

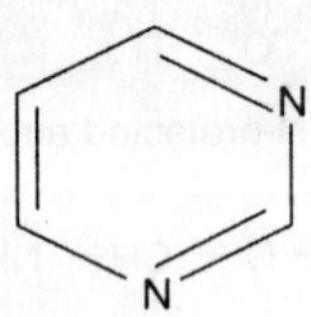

Pyrimidine

Purine derivatives that occur in nucleic acids are adenine and guanine.

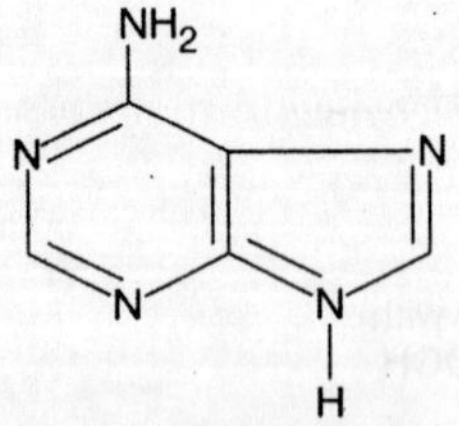

Adenine

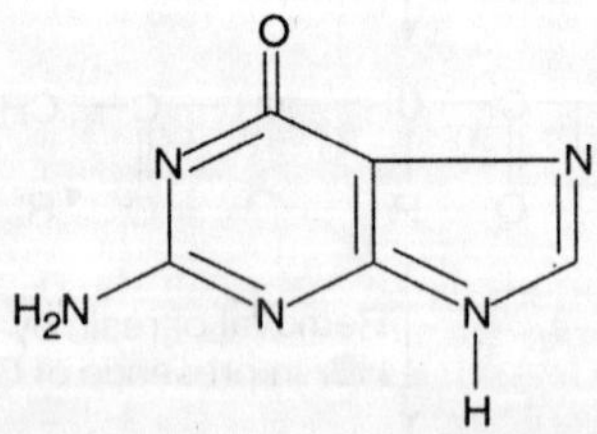

Guanine

Pyrimidine derivatives which are generally found in nucleic acids are uracil, thymine and cytosine.

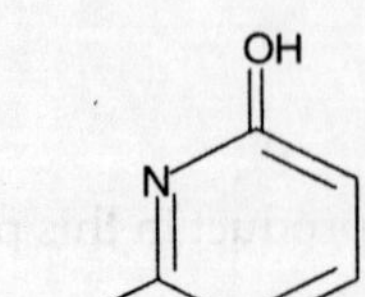

Uracil

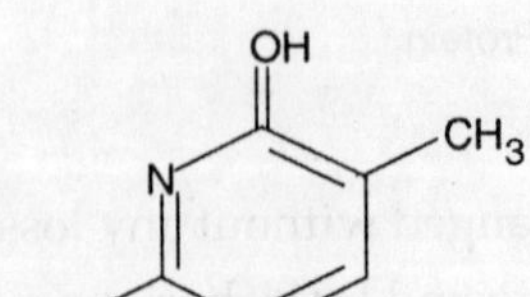

Thymine

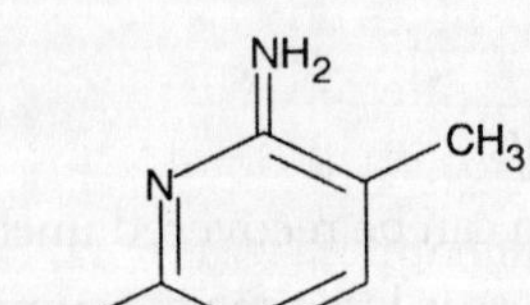

Cytosine

All these three derivatives are present in nucleic acids in keto forms.

3.3.1 Nature of Linkage (Sequence) of Different Components in Nucleic Acids

In sugar moiety phosphoric acid group is connected at C_5 and purine derivative is attached to C_1 while pyrimidine derivative in its keto form is linked to C_3 of the sugar. It may be mentioned that the sugar, pentose is present in β-form in nucleic acids. Thus a tentative structure of a nucleic acid molecule may be expressed as

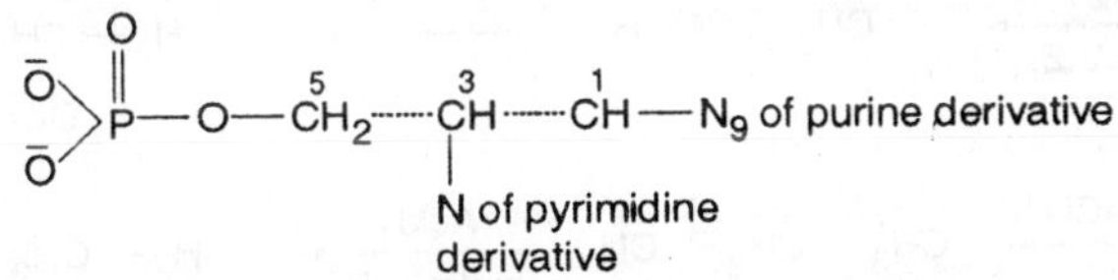

When nucleic acid is hydrolysed under mild condition phosphoric acid part is eliminated and the other part, i.e., dephosphorylated nucleic acid that is obtained is termed as *nucleotide* and nucleic acid having phosphoric acid group is known as *nucleoside.*

3.3.2 Classification of Nucleic Acids

Two types of nucleic acids are known. These are:

(i) Ribonucleic acid (RNA)

(ii) Deoxyribonucleic acid (DNA).

These two types of nucleic acids differ each other in the following respects:

(a) In RNA sugar present is ribose while in DNA it is deoxyribose.

(b) Though both contain adenine and guanine as purine derivatives but RNA has cytosine and uracil as pyrimidine derivatives while DNA contains cytosine and thymine as the correspnding derivatives.

(c) In biological system DNA controls the heredity factor and is known as store-house of genetic infomation while RNA functions as messenger.

Model Questions

1. How will you classify amino acids? Discuss some common methods of preparation of amino acids.
2. How does dipolar ion structure of amino acids influence physical properties?
3. Draw the titration curve of glycine and discuss the importance of isoelectric point.
4. How do you account for the high melting point of amino acids?
5. How are α-amino acids prepared? Describe the important reactions of α-amino acids.
6. Write notes on
   (a) Zwitterion
   (b) Isoelectric point.
7. What happens when
   (a) glycine is heated?
   (b) glycine is treated with nitrous acid?
   (c) alanine is treated with nitrous acid?

8. How will you synthesise
   (a) glycine from acetic acid?
   (b) alanine from ethyl chloride?

Hints:

(a)

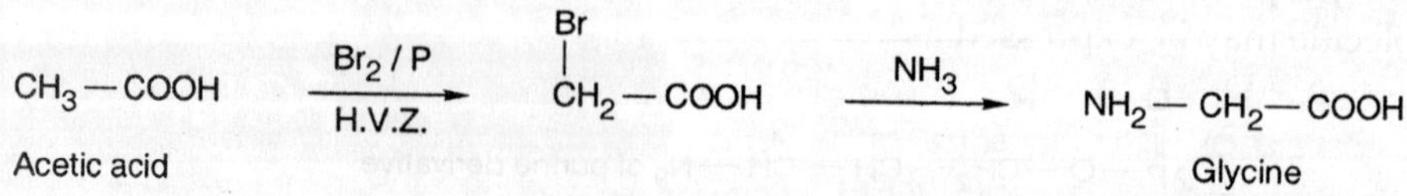

(b)

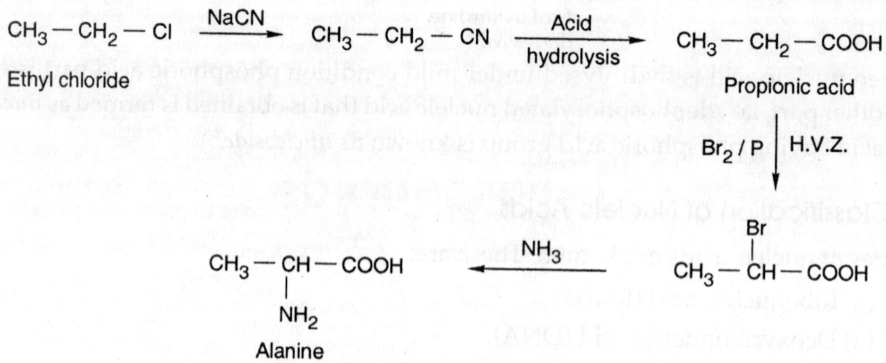

9. How will you distinguish glycine and acetamide?
   Hint: Ninhydrin test
10. What are proteins? What is the importance of protein?
11. What is peptide linkage? What is the difference between polypeptides and proteins?
12. (a) What are essential amino acids? Name a few of such acids, (b) How will you prepare glycine by Gabriel method? (c) Why the isoelectric point for aspartic acid (2.98) is much lower than that of leucine (5.98)
    Hint: Aspartic acid contains two COOH groups and one amino group but leucine has one amino group and one carboxylic group.
13. (i) Synthesise alanine by Strecker synthesis.
    (ii) Why amino acids are highly polar?
14. What are proteins? Classify them with examples.
15. Discuss in short the structure of pfotein.
16. What is meant by denaturation of proteins? Can a denatured protein be renatured?
17. What are nucleoproteins and nucleic acids? Write the names of various components present in DNA and RNA.

CHAPTER FOUR

Terpenoids

INTRODUCTION

Terpenes and terpenoids are a class of organic compounds widely distributed in plants of large number of botanical families. Originally, the term *'terpene'* was introduced for the identification of a mixture of isomeric hydrocarbons having the molecular formula $C_{10}H_{14}$, primarily occurring in terpentine and many other essential oils. But subsequently all the phytochemicals with empirical formula C_5H_8, have been brought into the same class and a new term *'terpenoids'* has been coined. Thus, the term *'terpene'* is confined only to hydrocarbons having molecular fomula, $(C_5H_8)_n$ while the term 'terpenoids' represents both the hydrocarbons and the oxygenated derivatives with $(C_5)_n$ carbon content.

4.1 Occurrence of Terpenoids

Terpenoids are widely distributed in plants belonging to different botanical families and are of frequent occurrence in fruits, leaves, stems, barks and roots of plants as pleasant smelling substances known as essential oils. Essential oils are complex mixture of hydrocarbons and their oxygenated derivatives. However, a few essential oils like oil of butter almond and oil of winter-green mainly contain only one component, viz., C_8H_5 and methyl salicylate respectively. Higher members of terpenoids, however, are found to occur in gums and resins of plants. It may be mentioned a few terpenoids have been reported to occur in animal kingdom.

4.2 Importance and Uses of Terpenoids

Pleasant smelling characteristics of this class of phytochemicals have attracted the people through-out the ages to utilise them as perfumes and food flavouring agents and, in fact, nowadays terpenoids are of immense commercial importance particularly in these two fields. Moreover, a large number of terpenoidal compounds show significant biological activities—viz., insecticidal and pesticidal activities and are being used in the field of agriculture and sericulture for protecting the loss of crop from the attack of insects and parasites. It may be mentioned in this context that these plant products are far more effective than their synthetic counterparts and at the same time they are cheap, non-toxic, non-pollutant, susceptible to easy bio-degradation and they do not leave any harmful residue neither in the fruits nor in the soil.

These phytochemicals also exhibit therapeutic activities like anthelmintic and antisecptic. Thus, terpenoids are significantly useful in pharmacy.

Besides these material aspects, terpenoids are highly interesting from chemical point of view. Structure investigation of these phytochemicals has resulted in the recognition of large variety of organic compounds having diverse skeleton pattern. The chemical studies on these phytochemicals has provided an immense fund of problems, the solution of which have afforded the stimulus for the theories that are now fundamental to organic chemisty. The descriptions of non-classical carbocation and the theories of conformational analysis have firm foundation in the chemisty of terpenoids. Again, structure investigations of terpenoids have provided a challenging source of synthetic objectives.

4.3 Properties and Structural Characteristics of Terpenoids

With a few exceptions terpenoids are colourless pleasant smelling liquids or solids, insoluble in water and readily volatile in steam. Most of them are optically active.

Almost all the members of terpenoid family have one or more double bonds and are active towards olefinic reagents and are easily oxidisable. Some of the members are very labile and are isomerised to stable forms in presence of acids. The most significant structural aspect of all the members of this class of phytochemicals is the formation of isoprene (2-methyl-1, 3-butadiene) as one of the major products on thermal decomposition.

$$\text{Terpenoids} \xrightarrow{\text{Heat}} CH_2{=}\overset{\overset{\displaystyle CH_3}{|}}{C}{-}CH{=}CH_2$$

Isoprene (C_5-unit)

The formation of this C_5-unit led to the generalisation that the carbon skeletons of terpenoids are divisible into isoprene units. This generalisation was first proposed by Wallach in 1887 under the name of *isoprene rule* which received support from the fact that isoprene may be polymerised in laboratory to yield a widely distributed terpenoid, dipentene, i.e.,

$$2C_5H_8 \longrightarrow C_{10}H_{16}$$

Dipentene

It has further been observed that the isoprene units in most of the terpenoids are joined in *"head-to-tail"* linkage, i.e., 1 : 4 linkage (branched end of the isoprene is considered as the head) as shown below:

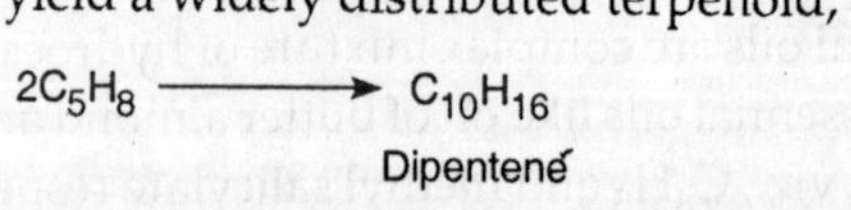

Head-to-tail Combination

This is known as *'Special isoprene rule'*. For this reason terpenoids are also known as *isoprenoids.* Some examples may be cited in favour of head-to-tail linkage.

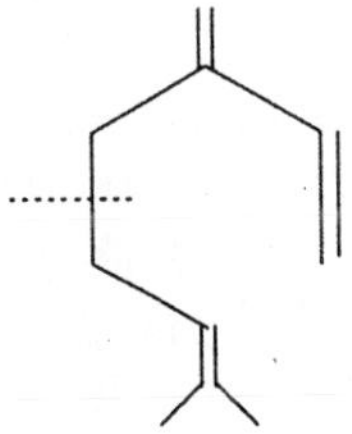

Myrcene
($2 \times C_5H_8$)

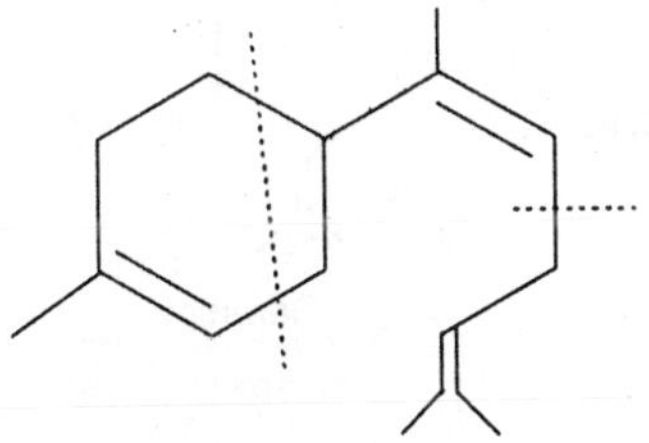

Bisabolene
($3 \times C_5H_8$)

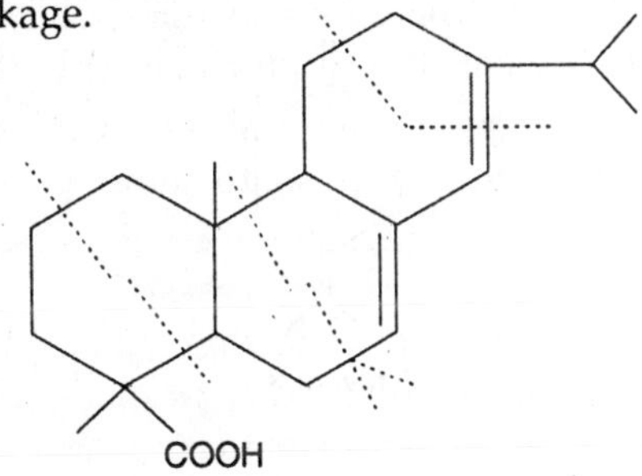

Abiectic acid
($4 \times C_5H_8$)

(Dotted lines show the head-to-tail combination)

However, there are some exceptions where there is no head-to-tail combination but the carbon skeletoms can be divided into isoprene units. Thus,

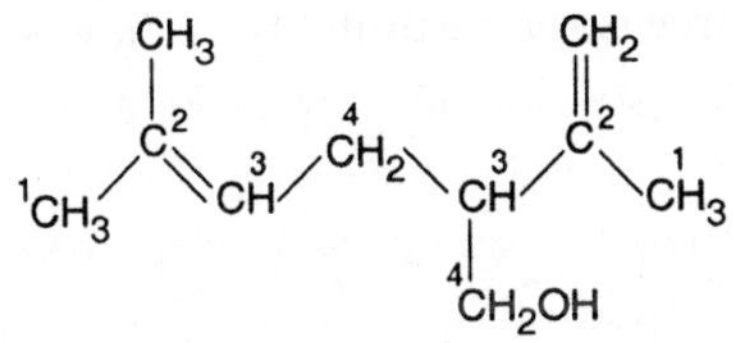

Lavandol (3, 4-combination)

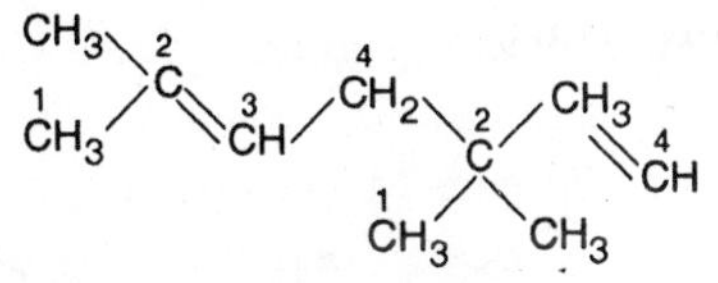

Artemisia alcohol
(3, 4-combination)

In some cases deviation from isoprene rule has been observed. Thus the structures of totarol and eremophilone cannot bė looked upon as the combination of isoprene units.

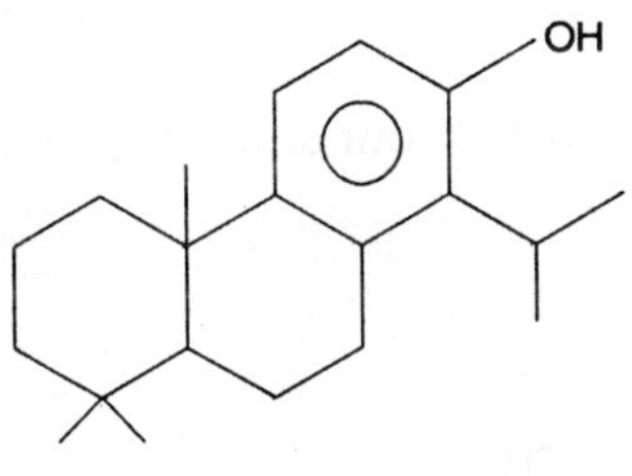

Totarol

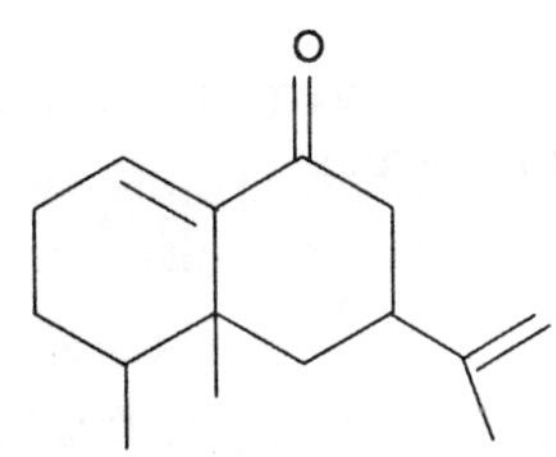

Eremophilone

4.4 Classification of Terpenoids

Terpenoids are classified primarily on the basis of number of isoprene units present in them as mentioned below:

i. *Hemiterpenes:* This category of terpenoids contains only one unit of isoprene unit in their molecule.

$$CH_2{=}\underset{|}{\overset{CH_3}{C}}{-}CH{=}CH_2$$

Isoprene

ii. *Monoterpenes*: In monoterpenes two units of isoprene molecules are linked together. They may be acyclic or cyclic in nature.

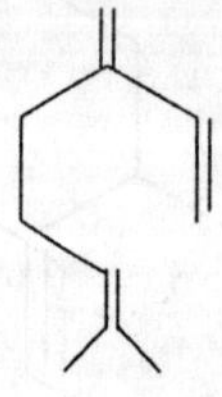

Myrcene

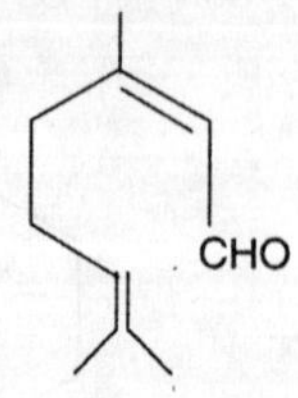

Citral

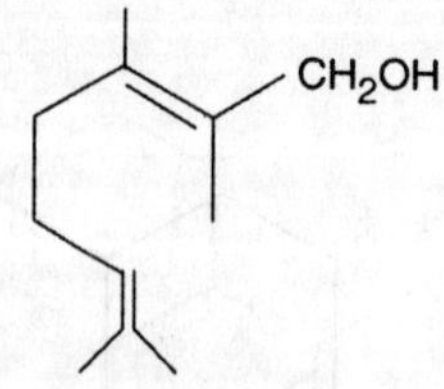

Geraniol

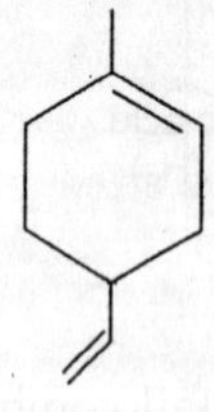

Limonene

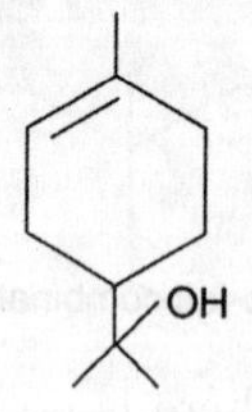

α-Terpeniol

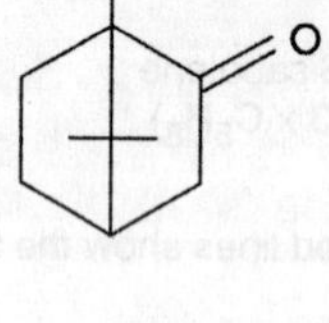

Camphor

iii. *Sesquiterpenes:* Sesquiterpenes contains three isoprene units. They may be acyclic or cylclic in nature. Thus,

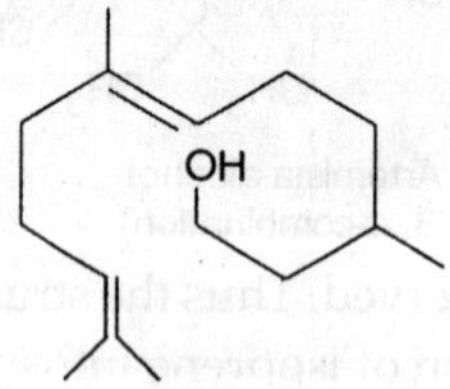

Farnesol

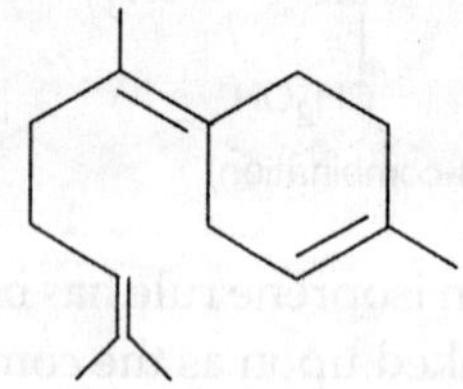

Bisabolene

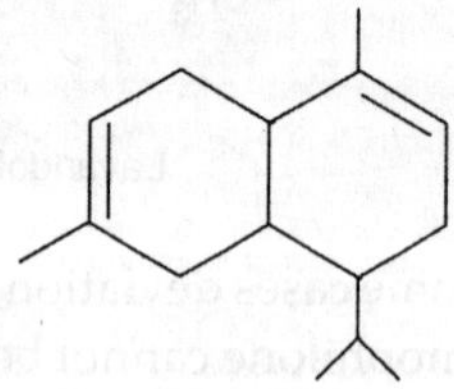

Cadinene

iv. *Diterpenes:* Diterpenes are those terpenoids in which four units of isoprene are present in their molecule.

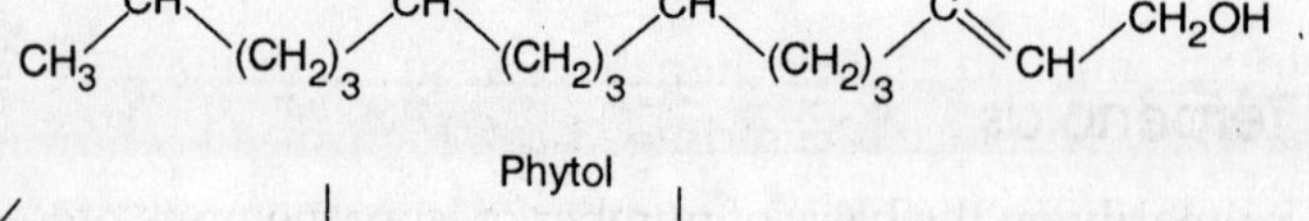

Phytol

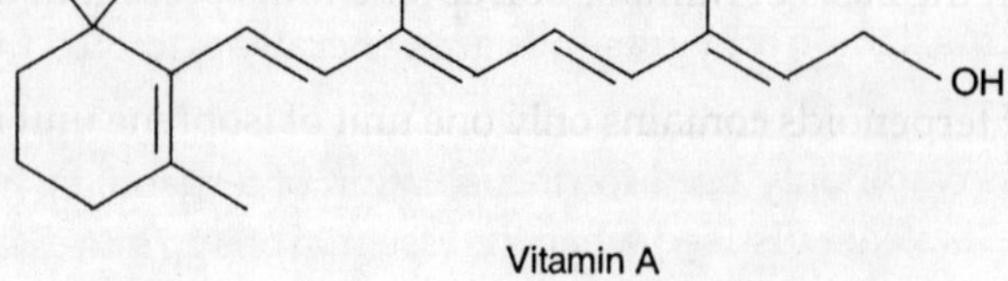

Vitamin A

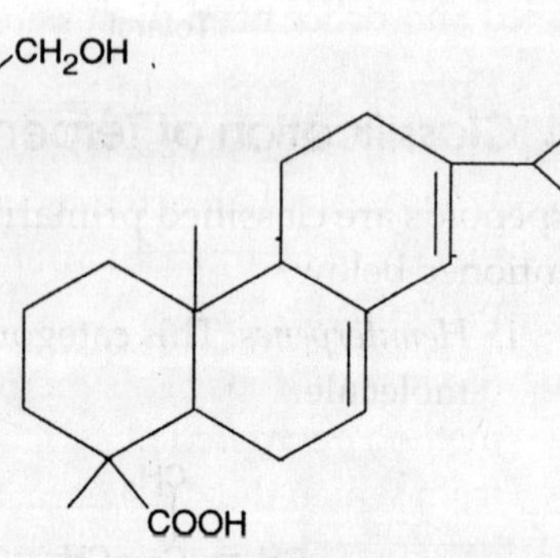

Abietic acid

v. *Triterpenes:* Terpenoids consist of six isoprene units, i.e., thirty carbon atoms. The most important members are squalene and amyrins.

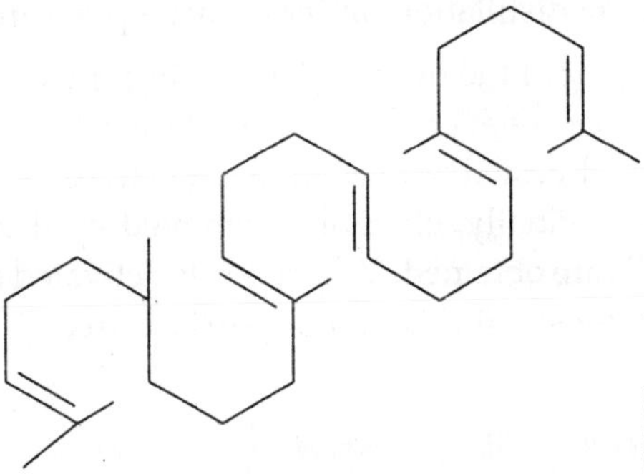

Squalene

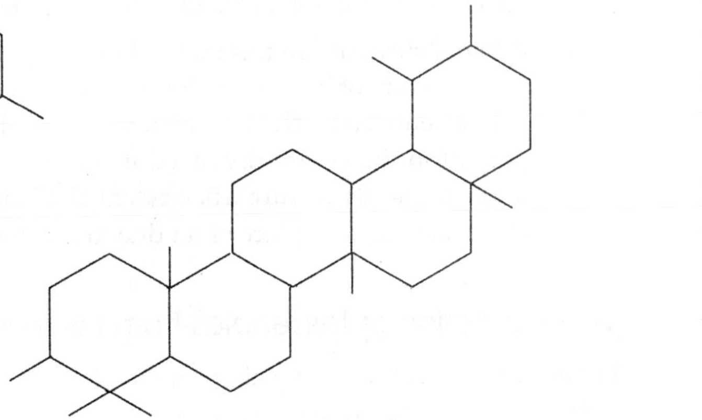

α-Amyrin

vi. *Tetraterpenes:* This category of terpenoids may be regarded as composed of eight isoprene units, i.e., forty carbon atoms. Caretenoids, the major colouring constituent of carrots, belong to this class of terpenoids.

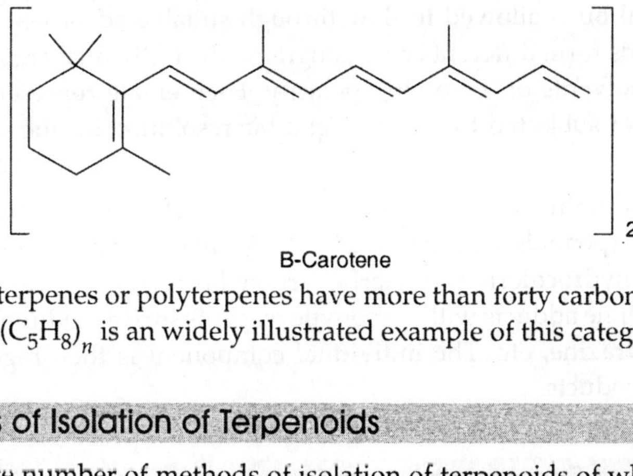

B-Carotene

vii. Higher terpenes or polyterpenes have more than forty carbon atoms in their molecules. Rubber $(C_5H_8)_n$ is an widely illustrated example of this category.

4.5 Methods of Isolation of Terpenoids

There are a large number of methods of isolation of terpenoids of which following are usually followed and hence need discussion.

i. *Expression method:* In this method plant material is crushed and the juice is filtered to remove the solid particles. The juice is centrifuged in a high speed centrifuge machine when nearly half of the essential is extracted. The remaining portion is used for the inferior quality of oil by distillation. Citrus, lemon and grass oils are generally extracted by this procedure.

ii. *Steam distillation:* This method is commonly used for the isolation of terpenoids. In this method powdered plant material is steam distilled when the essential oils go into distillate from which they are extracted by the use of low boiling organic solvents like ether and light petroleum. This method, however, suffers from a serious drawback. During steam distillation some of the constituents of essential oils such as esters may be hydrolysed and some are decomposed.

iii. *Extraction by solvents:* This method is generally employed for such essential oils which are very sensitive to heat and may be decomposed during distillation. In this method dried powdered plant material is directly treated with light petrol at a temperature of 50-60 °C and the solvent is then removed by distillation under reduced pressure.

iv. *Adsorption method:* In this method petals (part of the flower) are kept in contact with the fat (a mixture of lard and tallow) for several days at about 50 °C until the fat is saturated with essential oils. The saturated fat is then digested with ethanol when the essential oils present in the fat are dissolved in ethanol. Finally, ethanol is removed by distillation under reduced pressure when essential oils are obtained. Very recently activated coconut charcoal is used in place of fat due to greater stability and more surface area.

4.6 Separation of Terpenoids from Essential Oils

The essential oils obtained by above methods are a mixture of number of terpenoids belonging to different categories (mono-, sequi- terpenoid, etc). Chemical as well as physical methods have been employed for the separation of individual terpenoids.

(a) *Physical method:* Generally two methods, viz., fractional distillation and chromatographic resolution are used for the separation of components of essential oils. Of these two methods chromatographic method is commonly and widely used. In the chromatographic separation essential oil is allowed to flow through suitable adsorbent when different groups of terpenoids form different chromatogram. The individual chromatograms are then eluted with solvents of increasing polarity. Each eluate representing a class of terpenoids is further subjected to chromatographic resolution for the separation of its constituents.

(b) Depending upon the nature of the constituents different chemical methods are applied. Thus unsaturated terpenoids are separated by the formation of crystalline adducts with nitrosylchloride or hydrochloride. Similarly, carbonylic terpenoids are separated by the formation of crystalline adducts with carbonytic reagents such as sodiumbisulphite, 2, 4-dinotrophenyl hydrazine, etc. The individual component is then regenrated by the hydrolysis of the products.

4.7 General Methods of Determination of Structures of Terpenoids

In general similar approach is adopted as in the case of structure determination of alkaloids (vide chapter **five**) i.e., the appropriate steps for the determination of (i) molecular formula, (ii) functional nature of oxygen atom, if, present (iii) presence of unsaturation as well as the establishment of carbon skeleton and the measurement of specific rotation, etc., are undertaken. In recent years various physicochemical methods like different spectral measurements are also adopted for the determination of structures of terpenoids.

4.8 Chemistry of Some Representative Members of Terpenoids

Chemistry of some important and representative members of terpenoid family are elaborated below:

A. Monoterpenoids

4.8.1 Citral

Citral is most important member of the acyclic monoterpenoids because of the fact that the structures of other members of this group are based on that of citral. It is widely distributed in nature and occurs to the extent of 60-80 per cent in lemon grass oil. Citral is isolated as a pale yellow liquid by the fractional distillation of lemon grass oil. It is further purified by making the crystalline sodium bisulphite adduct and then decomposing it with sodium carbonate. It is optically an inactive liquid which has the smell of lemon.

4.8.1.1 Structure of Citral

The structure of citral is based on the following experimental evidences:

i. Analytical data and molecular weight determination reveals that citral has molecular formula, $C_{10}H_{16}O$.

ii. On treatment with bromine it readily forms tetra-bromo derivative indicating the presence of two double bonds in its molecule.

$$C_{10}H_{16}O \xrightarrow{Br_2} C_{10}H_{16}OBr_4$$

iii. Citral responds to carbonylic tests like formation of oxime and 2, 4-dinitrophenyl hydrazone, etc. Further it readily reduces. Fehling's solution and Tollen's reagent suggesting thereby the aldehydic nature of the oxygen atom present in it. This is further confirmed by its oxidation and reduction. On oxidation it forms geranic acid and on reduction it yields an alcohol, geraniol both having the same number of carbon atoms as citral.

$$\underset{\text{Geraniol}}{C_{10}H_{17}OH} \xleftarrow[\text{Na/Hg}]{\text{Reduction}} \underset{\text{Citral}}{C_{10}H_{16}O} \xrightarrow[Ag_2O]{[O]} \underset{\text{Geranic acid}}{C_{10}H_{15}COOH}$$

iv. Complete reduction followed by replacement of oxygen atom by two hydrogen atoms, the molecular formula of saturated hydrocarbon stands as $C_{10}H_{22}$ which can be expressed by the general formula C_nH_{2n+2}. This suggests that citral is acyclic in nature.

v. On treatment with sodium bisulphite citral forms both mono- and di-sulphite additional products indicating the presence of α, β-unsaturated aldehydic function in its molecule. This assumption is further confirmed by UV-spectral measurement which records λ_{max} at 238 nm, ∈ 13,500.

vi. The infra-red spectrum of citral exhibits a peak at 800 cm^{-1} suggesting the presence of an isopropylidene functionality ($(CH_3)_2C{=}C\langle$) in its structure.

vii. Further elaboration of the structure of citral was possible by it heating with $KHSO_4$. On such heating citral furnishes a known aromatic compound, *p*-cymene.

$$C_{10}H_{16}O \xrightarrow[\text{Heat}]{KHSO_4}$$

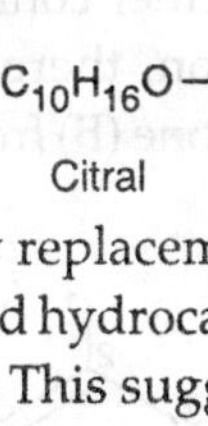

p-Cymene

Thus the relative positions of methyl group and isopropylidene functionality are settled. Based on the above evidence a tentative structure for citral may be proposed as (A) which can explain the formation of *p*-cymene.

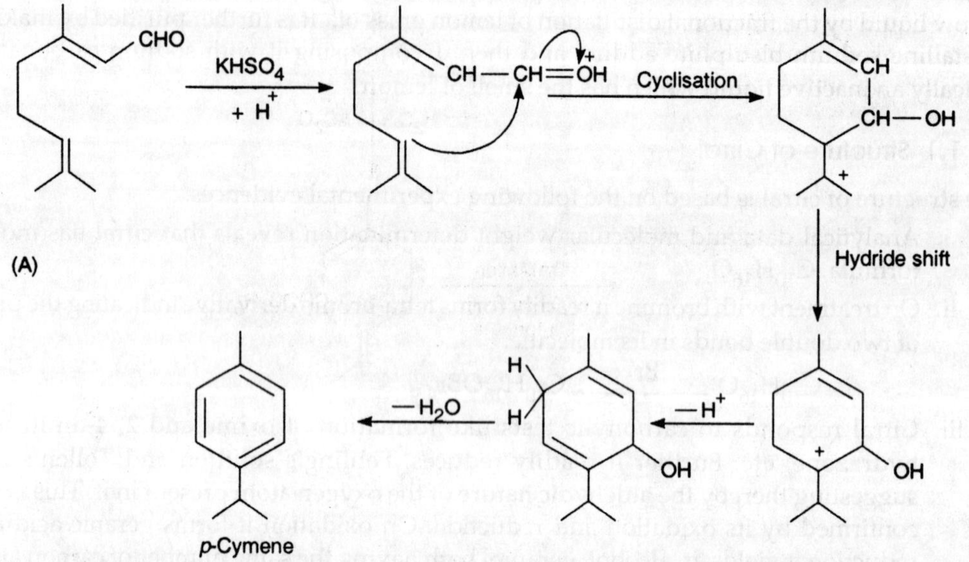

The above tentative structure (A) was further confirmed by Verley who found that when citral is treated with aqueous K_2CO_3 solution, there are formation of acetaldehyde and a compound identified as 6-methyl-hept-5-en-2-one (B) from its ozonolysis to acetone and laevulic acid (laevulinic acid).

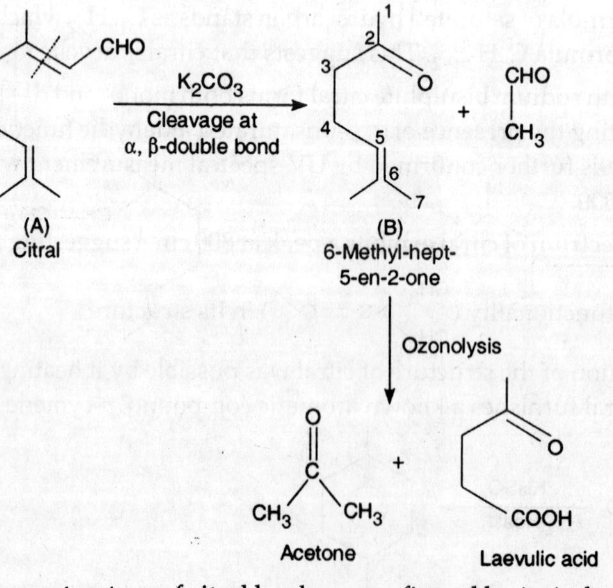

Finally, the above structure of citral has been confirmed by its independent synthesis from methyl heptenone as discussed:

(a)

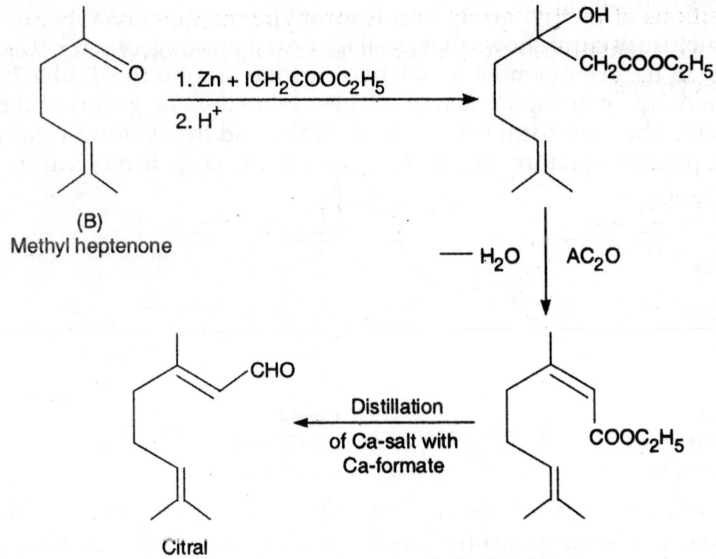
OH
CH2COOC2H5
1. Zn + ICH2COOC2H5
2. H+
(B)
Methyl heptenone
— H2O
AC2O
CHO
Distillation
of Ca-salt with
Ca-formate
COOC2H5
Citral

(b)

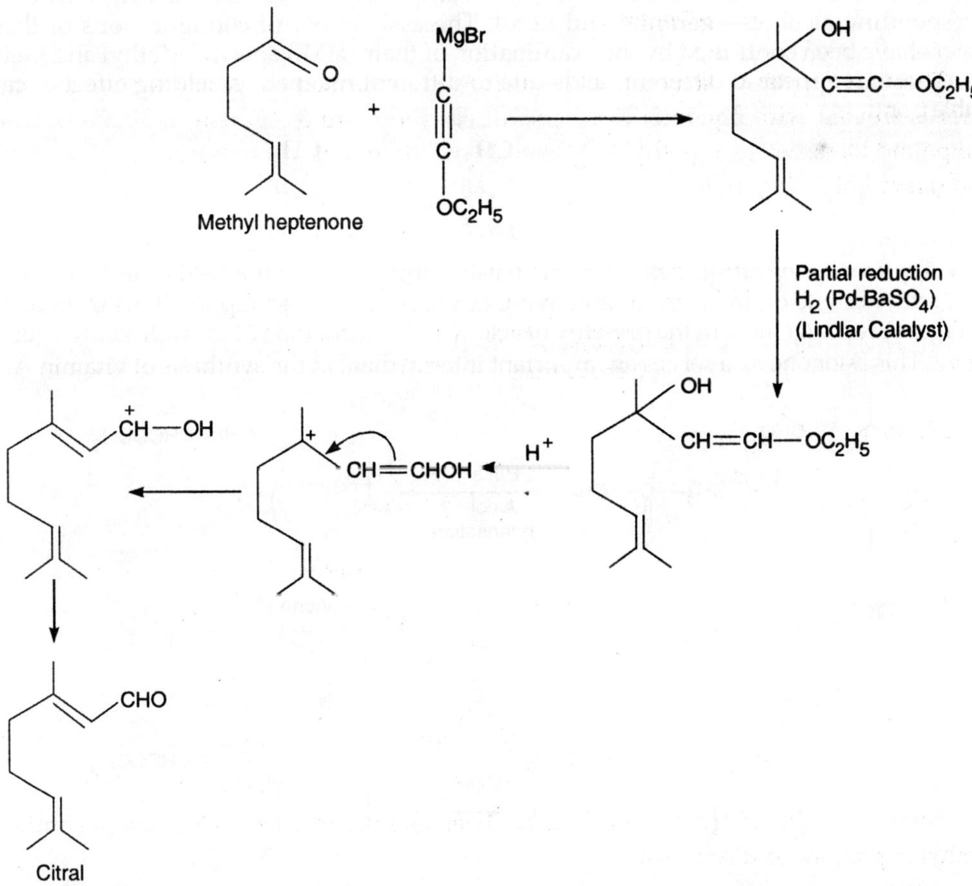
MgBr
O
C
C
OC2H5
Methyl heptenone
OH
C≡C—OC2H5
Partial reduction
H2 (Pd-BaSO4)
(Lindlar Calalyst)
OH
CH=CH—OC2H5
H+
CH=CHOH
CH—OH
CHO
Citral

4.8.1.1.1 *cis-trans* Isomerism in Citral

A careful scrutiny of the structure of citral shows that citral may exist in two geometrical isomeric forms. The two forms differ in the arrangement of aldehydic group around the double bond in 2, 3-positions—in one the aldehydic group is *cis* with respect to methylene group of the main chain while in other it is *trans*. The *trans* form is known as citral-a and the cis-form is termed as citral-b. Both the forms are present in nature and in fact, the natural citral is a mixture of both these two isomers.

Citral-a *trans*-form (E-form) (B.P. 117-119 °C/20 mm) — Citral-b *cis*-form (Z-form) (B.P. 118-119 °C/20 mm)

Due to close boiling points they cannot be separated easily by usual physical methods. However, their derivatives such as semicarbazone have to some extent different melting points. Thus semicarbazone of citral-a melts at 164 °C while that of citral-b melts at 171 °C. Citral-a on reduction with sodium amalgam forms geraniol and so it is known as *geranial*. Similarly, citral-b on such reduction yields nerol and hence is known as *neral*. The configurations of these two isomers have been settled from the consideration of relative ease of ring closure of the corresponding alcohols—geraniol and nerol. The assignment of configurations of these two isomers have been confirmed by the examination of their ^{1}HMR spectra. Methyl and methylene proton signals appear at different fields due to different magnetic shielding effect of carbonyl double bond.

	CH_3	CH_2
Citral-a	2.16δ	2.24δ
Citral-b	1.98δ	2.58δ

- ***Application of citral:*** Citral finds extensive application in the field of industry. It readily reacts with acetone or any compound having active methylene group to afford ψ-ionone which undergoes rearrangement in the presence of acid with the formation of the well-known perfume β-ionone. This β-ionone also serves an important intermediate in the synthesis of vitamin A. Thus,

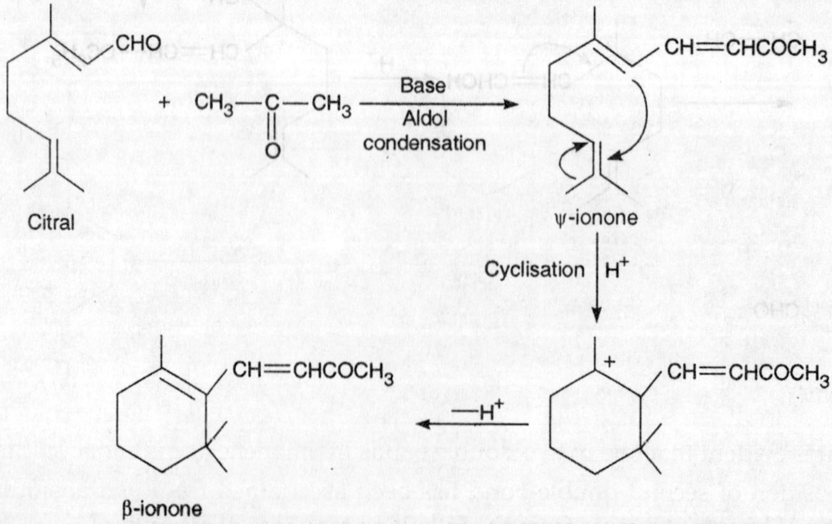

4.8.2 Limonene

It is one of the most important monocyclic monoterpene, and widely occurs in nature. It is optically active and occurs in (+), (–) and racemic forms. The (+) form generally occurs in lemon and orange oils, (–)-form in peppermint oil while racemic form is found to occur in turpentine oil. The racemic form may also be obtained by heating either of the active forms at 250 °C or by mixing equal amounts of (+)- and (–)-forms. The racemic modification is also known as *dipentene.* Limonene is extensively used in the perfume industry.

4.8.2.1 Structure of Limonene

The structure of limonene has been deduced on the basis of following evidences.

i. Limonene has molecular formula $C_{10}H_{16}$.
ii. It adds on four bromine atoms indicating the presence of *two double bonds.*
iii. Dehydrogenation of limonene with sulshur or selenium yields *p*-cymene.

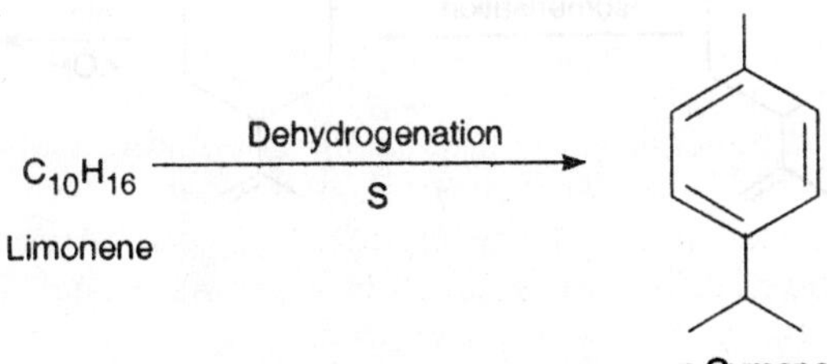

p-Cymene

This suggests the presence of six-membered carbon skeleton in limonene.

iv. The site of unsaturation in limonene has been settled from its conversion to α-terpineol. Limonene when hydrated in presence of dilute mineral acid α-terpineol is formed which on dehydration with potassium, hydrogen sulphate regenerates limonene. Thus,

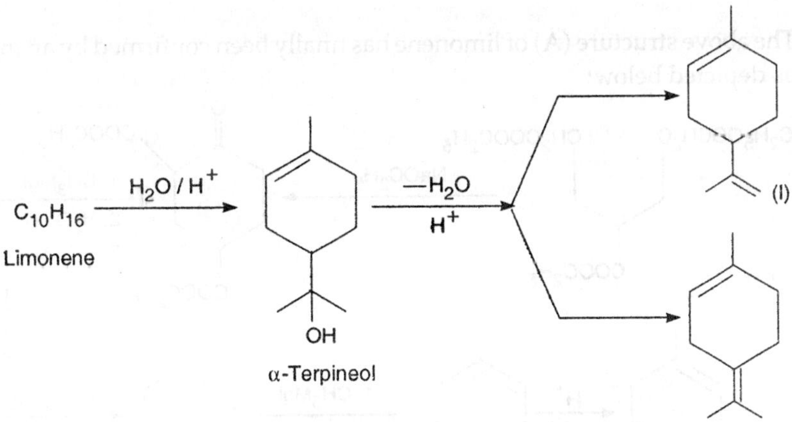

Thus it is evident that one of two double bonds in limonene one is endocyclic in nature.

v. The position of second double-bond has been ascertained from its transformation to carvone of known structure from the following sequence of reactions:

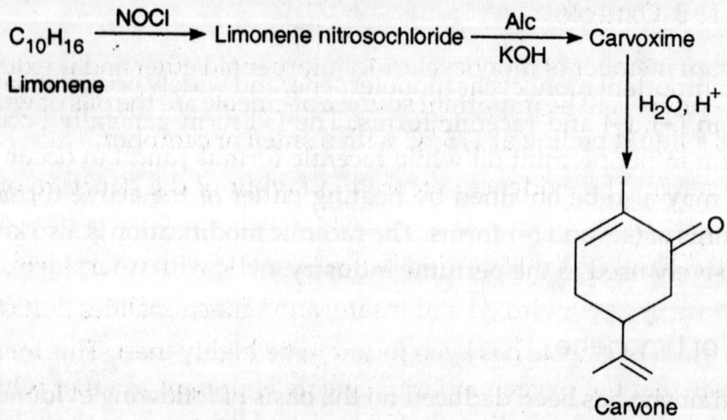

vi. **Since the structure of carvone is known, the above sequence of reactions may be written on the basis of (A) as the structure of Limonene.**

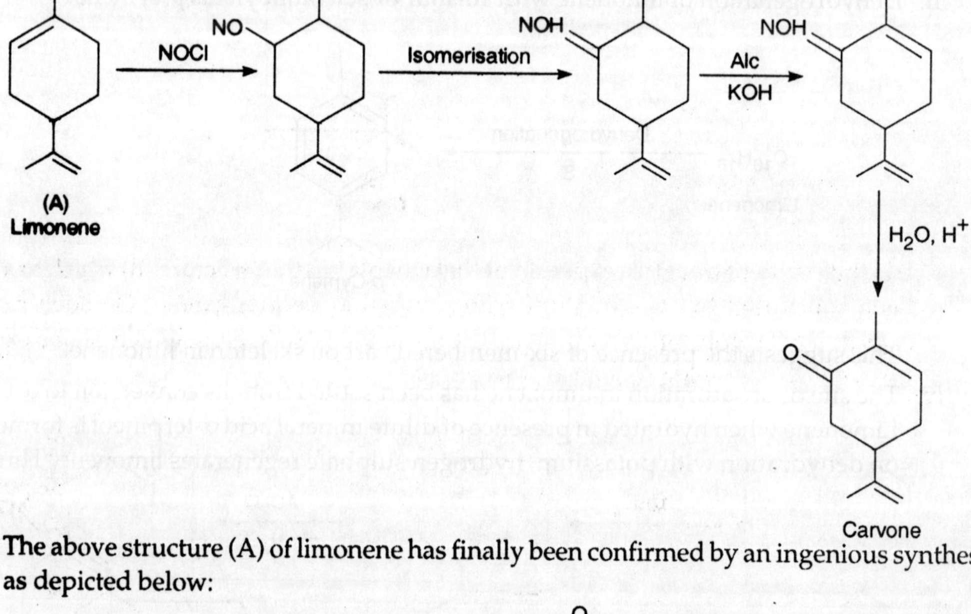

vii. **The above structure (A) of limonene has finally been confirmed by an ingenious synthesis as depicted below:**

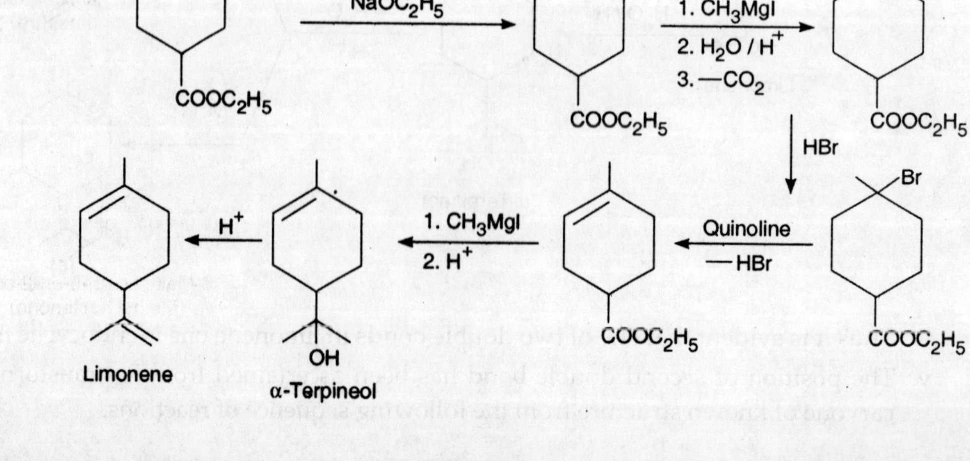

4.8.3 Cineole or 1, 8-Cineole

It is the most important member of monocyclic monoterpenoid ether and is extensively found in a large variety of essential oils. The important sources of cineole are the oils of wormseed, cajuput and eucalyptus. It is a liquid boiling at 175 °C with a smell of camphor.

- *Structure of Cineole:* The evidences secured in favour of the structure of cineole may be discussed as below:

i. Its molecular formula is $C_{10}H_{18}O$ and hence isomeric with α-terpineol.

ii. It does not possess any hydroxyl and insaturation functionalities in its molecule.

iii. The oxygen atom in cineole has been found to be highly inert. This inertness of oxygen atom suggests that the oxygen atom in cineole is present as ether which is supported from the fact that on dehydration cis-1, 8-terpin of known structure yields cineole.

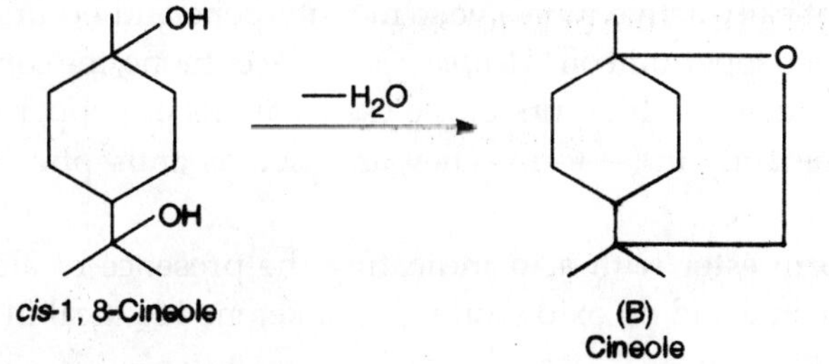

It is thus evident from this experiment that cineole has the structure (B) which has further been confirmed by its oxidation with potassium permanganate. On such oxidative experiment cineole forms methyl heptenone of known structure which can be explained through the following sequence of reactions:

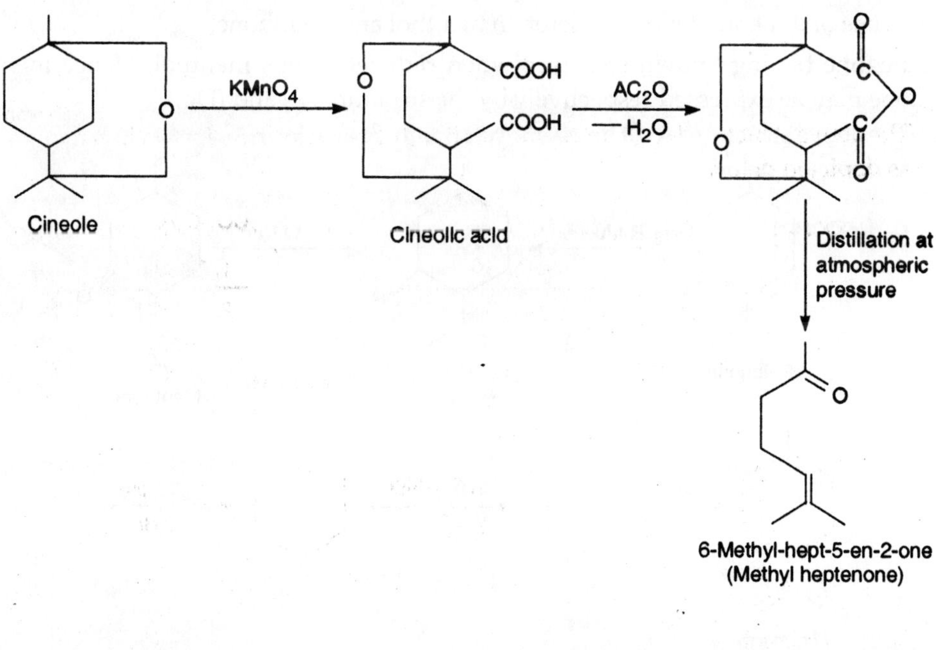

iv. It has been observed that although *cis*-1, 8-terpin has chair conformation but 1, 8-cineole possesses boat conformation, i.e.,

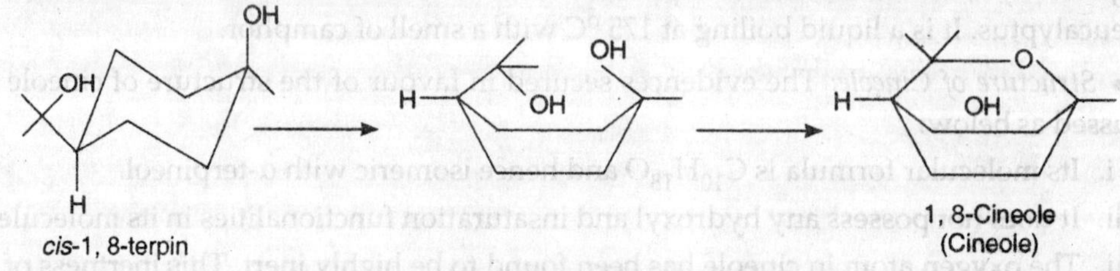

4.8.4 Menthol and Menthone

Menthol, $C_{10}H_{20}O$ is an optically active monocyclic monoterpene and occurs in nature in (–)-form. It constitutes 50-60% of peppermint oil (*Mentha piperita*) Menthone, the congener of menthol is the oxidation product of menthol. It occurs in the essential oils of peppermint (up to 35%), geranium and pennyroyal mainly in (–) form. They are used as antiseptic and as flavouring agents.

Menthol can easily form ester with acid indicating the presence of alcoholic hydroxyl (—OH) function in its molecule and on oxidation forms a ketone identical in all respects with menthone, i.e.,

$$\underset{\substack{\text{Menthone}\\\text{(Ketone)}}}{C_{10}H_{18}O} \xleftarrow{[O]} \underset{\text{Menthol}}{C_{10}H_{20}O} \xrightarrow{\text{Esterification}} \text{Acetate}$$

Menthol on dehydration followed by dehydrogenation yields *p-cymene* suggesting thereby the presence of *p*-menthane like skeleton in menthol and menthone.

Pulegone having known structure when reduced forms menthol. Hence menthol and menthone may be expressed respectively by the structure (C) and (D).

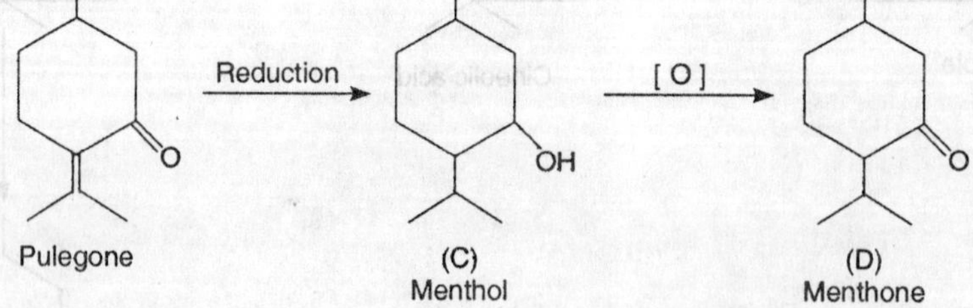

The above structures of menthol and menthone have been confirmed by their syntheses as discussed below:

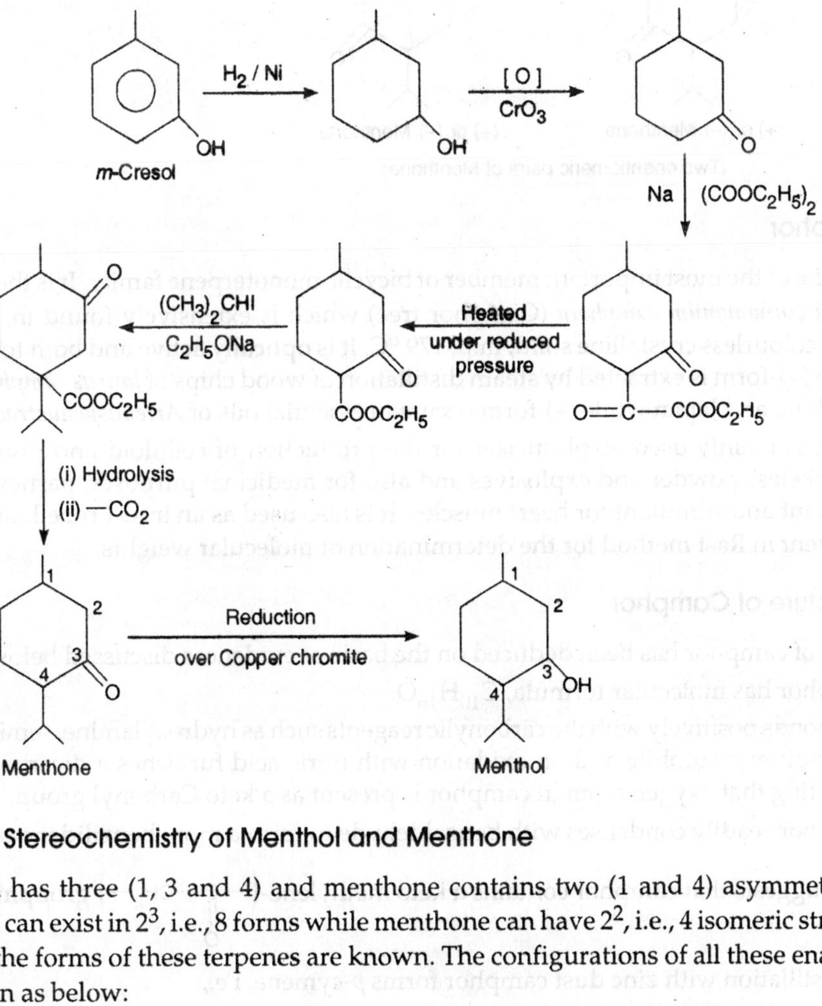

4.8.4.1 Stereochemistry of Menthol and Menthone

Menthol has three (1, 3 and 4) and menthone contains two (1 and 4) asymmetric centres. So menthol can exist in 2^3, i.e., 8 forms while menthone can have 2^2, i.e., 4 isomeric structures and in fact, all the forms of these terpenes are known. The configurations of all these enantiomers may be shown as below:

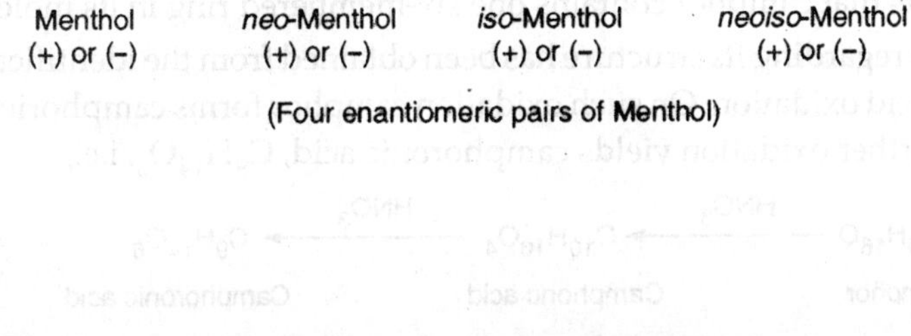

(Four enantiomeric pairs of Menthol)

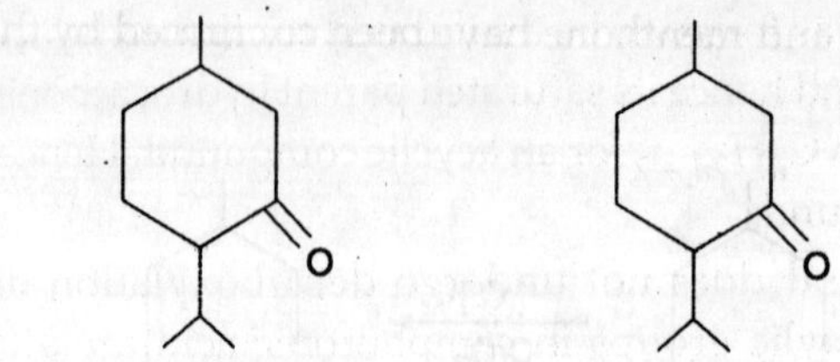

(+) or (–) Menthone (+) or (–) Menthone

(Two enantiomeric pairs of Menthone)

4.8.5 Camphor

Camphor is one of the most important member of bicyclic monoterpene family. It is the principal constituent of *cinnamonum camphora* (Camphor tree) which is extensively found in Formosa. Camphor is a colourless crystalline solid, m.p. 179 °C. It is optically active and both forms occur in nature. The (+)-form is extracted by steam distillation of wood chips of *laurus camphora* which is native of China and Japan while (–)-form occurs in essential oils of *Artemisia austrachanica.*

Camphor is mainly used as plasticiser for the production of celluloid and photographic films, for smokeless powder and explosives and also for medicinal purposes, particularly as a mild disinfectant and stimulant for heart muscles. It is also used as an insect repellent. It is also used as a solvent in Rast method for the determination of molecular weights.

4.8.5.1 Structure of Camphor

The structure of camphor has been deduced on the basis of evidences discussed below:

i. Camphor has molecular formula, $C_{10}H_{16}O$.

ii. It responds positively with the carbonylic reagents such as hydroxylamine, semicarbazide and sodium bisulphite and on oxidation with nitric acid furnishes a dicarboxylic acid indicating that oxygen atom in camphor is present as a keto Carbonyl group.

iii. Camphor readily condenses with benzaldehyde to form a monobenzilidene derivative.

This suggests that camphor contains a keto methylene-$\left(-\underset{\substack{\| \\ O}}{C}-CH_2-\right)$ grouping.

iv. On distillation with zinc dust camphor forms *p*-cymene, i.e.,

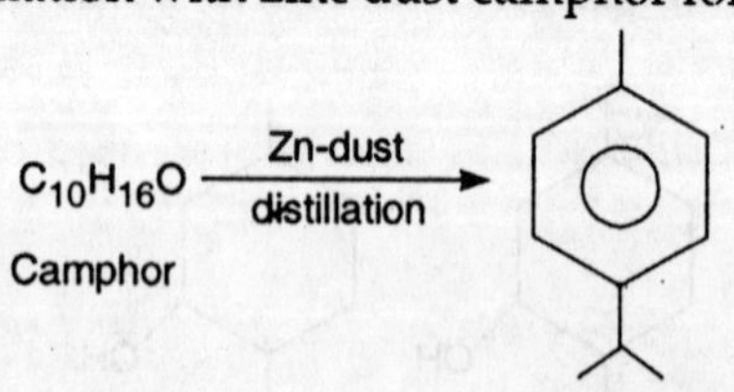

p-Cymene

This suggests that camphor contains one six-membered ring in its molecule.

v. Further clue regarding its structure has been obtained from the identification of products of its nitric acid oxidation. On such oxidation camphor forms camphoric acid ($C_{10}H_{16}O_4$) which on further oxidation yields camphoronic acid, $C_9H_{14}O_6$, i.e.,

$$\underset{\text{Camphor}}{C_{10}H_{16}O} \xrightarrow{HNO_3} \underset{\text{Camphoric acid}}{C_{10}H_{16}O_4} \xrightarrow{HNO_3} \underset{\text{Camphoronic acid}}{C_9H_{14}O_6}$$

vi. Camphoronic acid, $C_9H_{14}O_6$ was found to be a saturated tricarboxylic acid. Thus it may be written as $C_5H_{11}(COOH)_3$ and hence its saturated parent hydrocarbon is C_6H_{14} which corresponds to general formula C_nH_{2n+2} for an acyclic compound. Hence, camphoronic acid must be an acyclic compound.

vii. Camphoronic acid is stable and does not undergo decarboxylation under ordinary condition. Hence, three carboxylic groups in camphoronic acid are attached to three different carbon atoms.

viii. On distillation at atmospheric pressure it forms isobutyric acid, trimethyl succinic acid and CO_2 as the major products, i.e.,

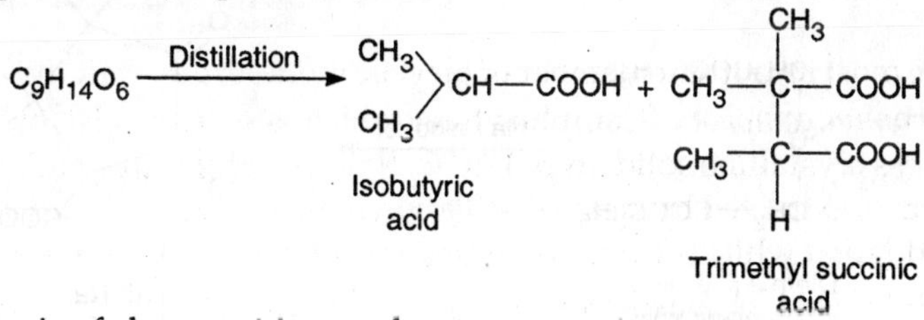

On the basis of above evidences the structure of camphoronic acid may be expressed as

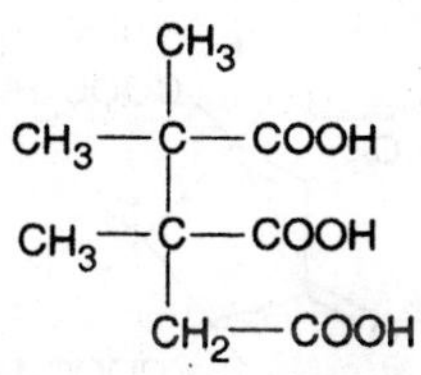

Camphoronic acid

ix. Camphoric acid, $C_{10}H_{16}O_4$, was found to be a saturated dicarboxylic acid. Since its oxidation product, camphoronic acid, has a gem dimethyl group and a separate methyl group, camphoric acid must contain three methyl groups in its molecule. Hence its molecular formula may be written as $Me_3C_5H_5(COOH)_2$ which leads to C_5H_{10} as its saturated parent hydrocarbon. This formula corresponds to C_nH_{2n} for monocyclic compound. So camphoric acid is a cyclopentane dicarboxylic acid.

x. Camphoric acid readily forms monoester but diester with some difficulty suggesting that the two carboxylic groups are different—one is primary or secondary in nature and the other is tertiary in nautre.

Based on the above evidences camphoric acid has been represented by the following structure.

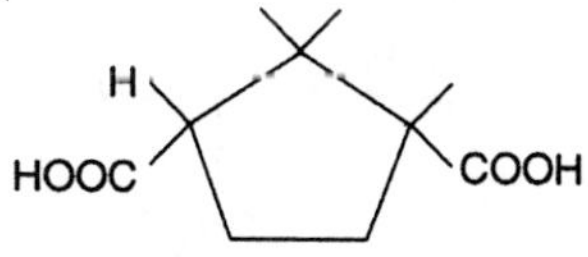

Camphoric acid

Now since camphor has a $-\overset{O}{\overset{\|}{C}}-CH_2$-grouping its structure may be written as shown:

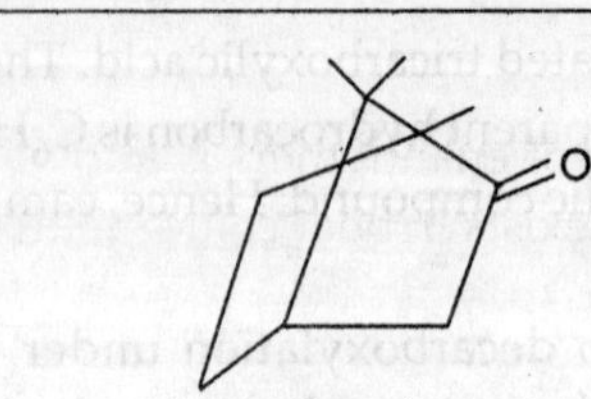

Camphor

xi. Finally the above structure of camphor has been confirmed by the following:

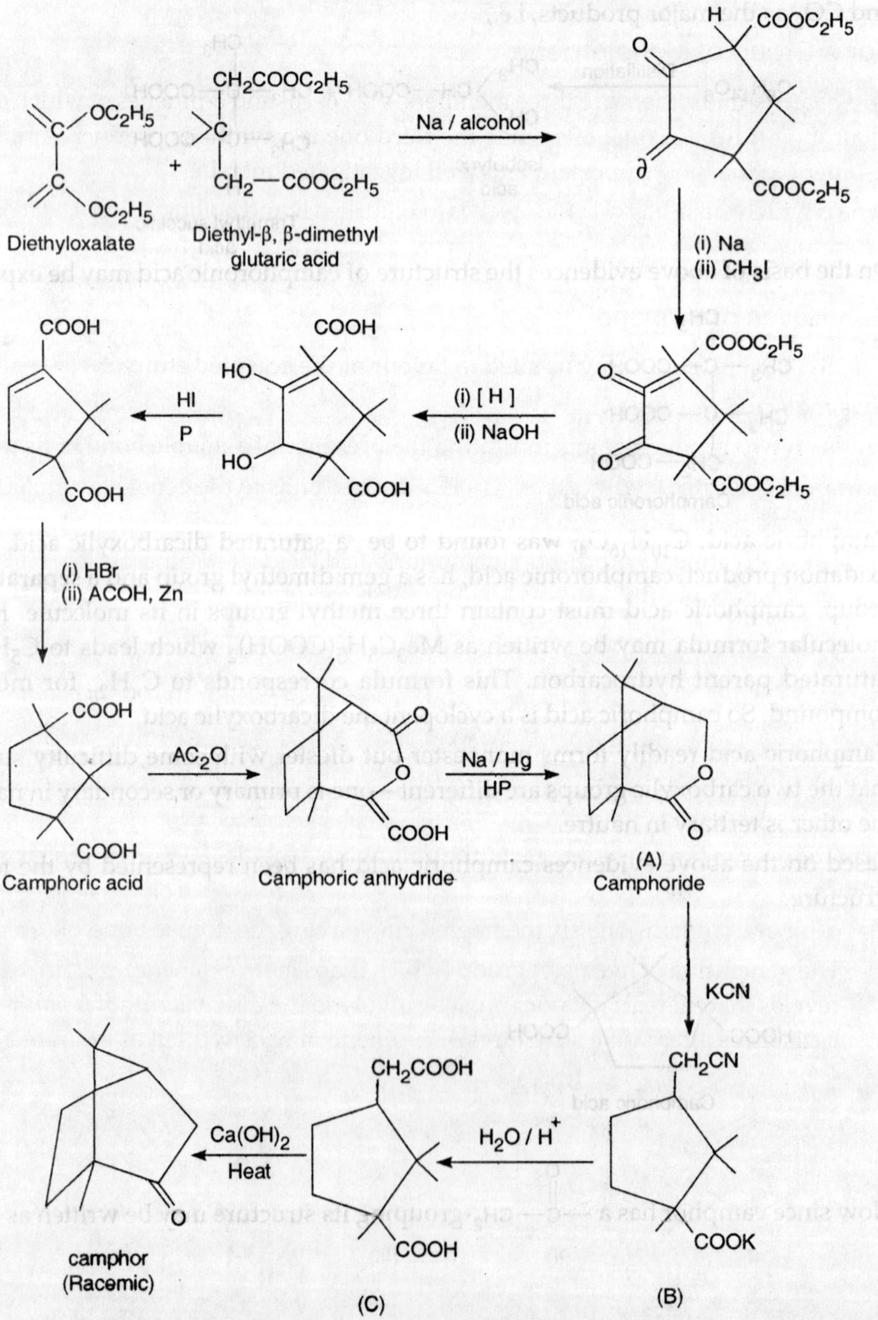

4.8.5.1.1 Stereochemistry of Camphor

Camphor has two dissimilar chiral centres but only one pair of enantiomers is known. This is because only *cis*-form is possible. It has been observed that it exists in boat conformation.

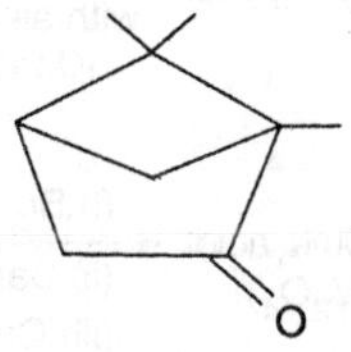

4.8.6 Pinane Group of Monoterpene

In this group of terpenoids, there are three members, viz., α-, β- and δ-pinenes of which α- and β-pinenes occur in various essential oils while the third one is a synthetic product. Among these pinenes, α-pinene is the most important and well investigated member.

α-pinene is widely distributed in nature. It is a colourless liquid boiling at 155 °C. It constitutes the major component of terpentine oil and exists in optically active forms.

4.8.6.1 Constitution of α-Pinene

Following analytical evidences may be cited in favour of the accepted sturcture of α-pinene.

i. It has molecular formula $C_{10}H_{16}$

ii. It adds on two bromine atoms indicating the presence of a double bond in its molecule.

iii. The parent saturated hydrocarbon, $C_{10}H_{10}$, corresponds to the general formula, C_nH_{2n-2} revealing a *bicyclic nature* of its structure.

iv. α-pinene on treatment with alcoholic sulphuric acid yields α-terpineol of known structure i.e.,

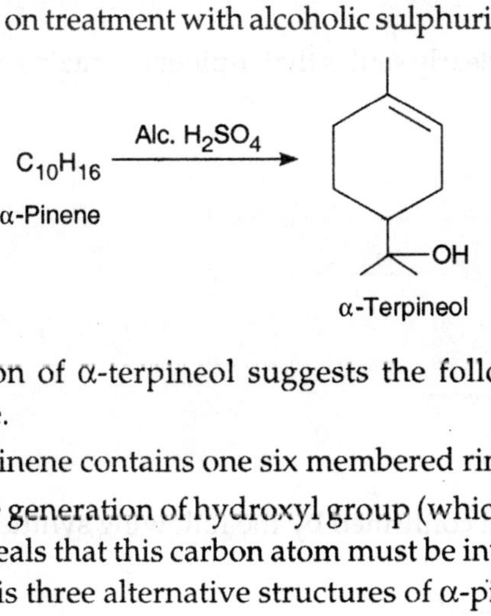

α-Terpineol

Formation of α-terpineol suggests the following facts in favour of the structure of α-pinene.

(a) α-pinene contains one six membered ring having the double bond of α-terpineol.

(b) The generation of hydroxyl group (which is absent in α-pinene) at C_8 in α terpineol reveals that this carbon atom must be involved in *the second ring of α-pinene*. On this basis three alternative structures of α-pinene may be written as indicated below:

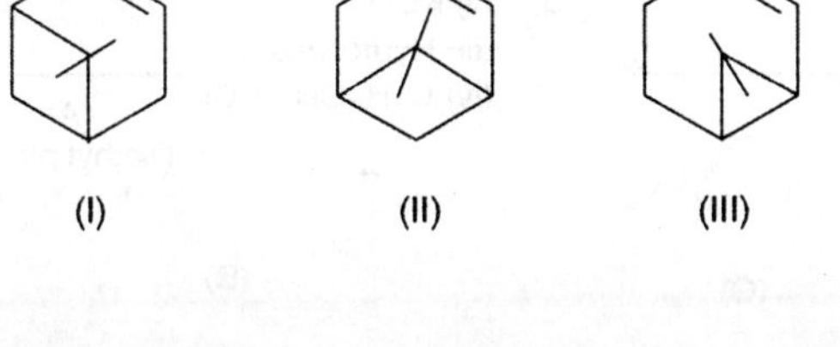

(I) (II) (III)

One of these alternatives structure (I) was found to be most probable on the basis of its oxidation to *cis*-norpinic acid.

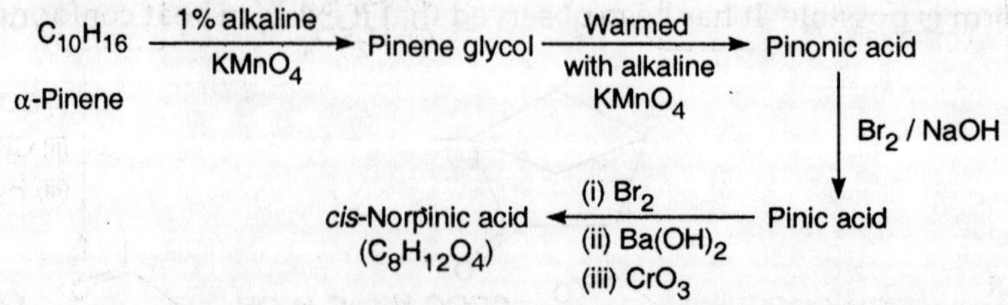

cis-Norpinic acid, $C_8H_{12}O_4$ was found to be a saturated dicarboxylic acid. So its formula may be written as $C_6H_{10}(COOH)_2$. Again, it has already been pointed out that C_8 carbon having a gem dimethyl group present in α-terpineol is not present in six-membered ring but is present in the second ring. So it may be concluded that this gem dimethyl group is present in *cis*-norpinic acid and hence its molecular formula may be written as $(CH_3)_2C_4H_4(COOH)_2$ which suggests that the saturated parent hydrocarbon of this acid is C_4H_8 corresponding to the general formula C_nH_{2n} i.e., monocyclic and four-membered ring. Thus, this *cis*-norpinic acid is a cyclobutane derivative and in fact, it has been identified as 1, 1-dimethyl-cyclobutane-2, 4-dicarboxylic acid as shown below:

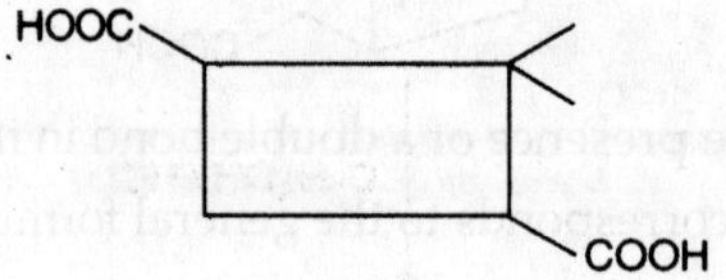

cis-Norpinic acid

The formation of *cis*-norpinic acid thus clearly settles that α-pinene contains a four membered ring as shown in the structure (I).

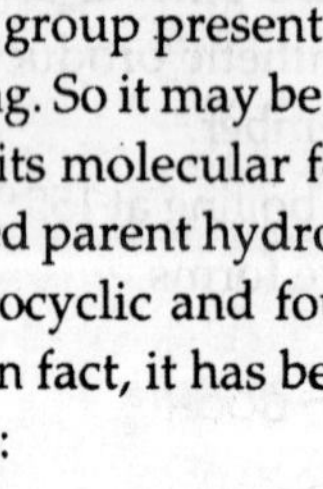

(I)
α-Pinene

Finally, the above structure (I) has been confirmed by the following synthesis:

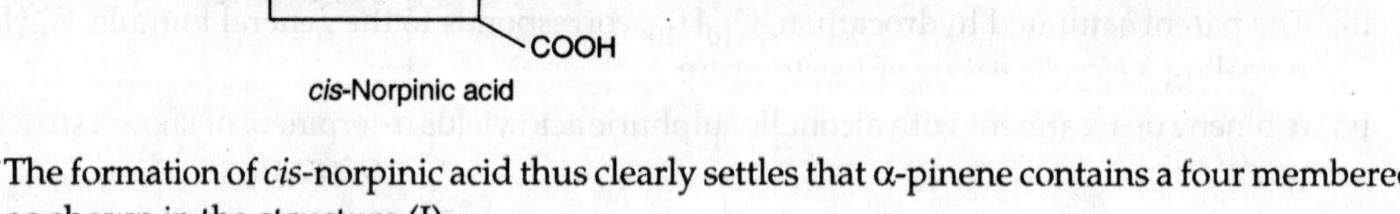

cis-Norphinic anhydride

(A)
Diethyl pinate

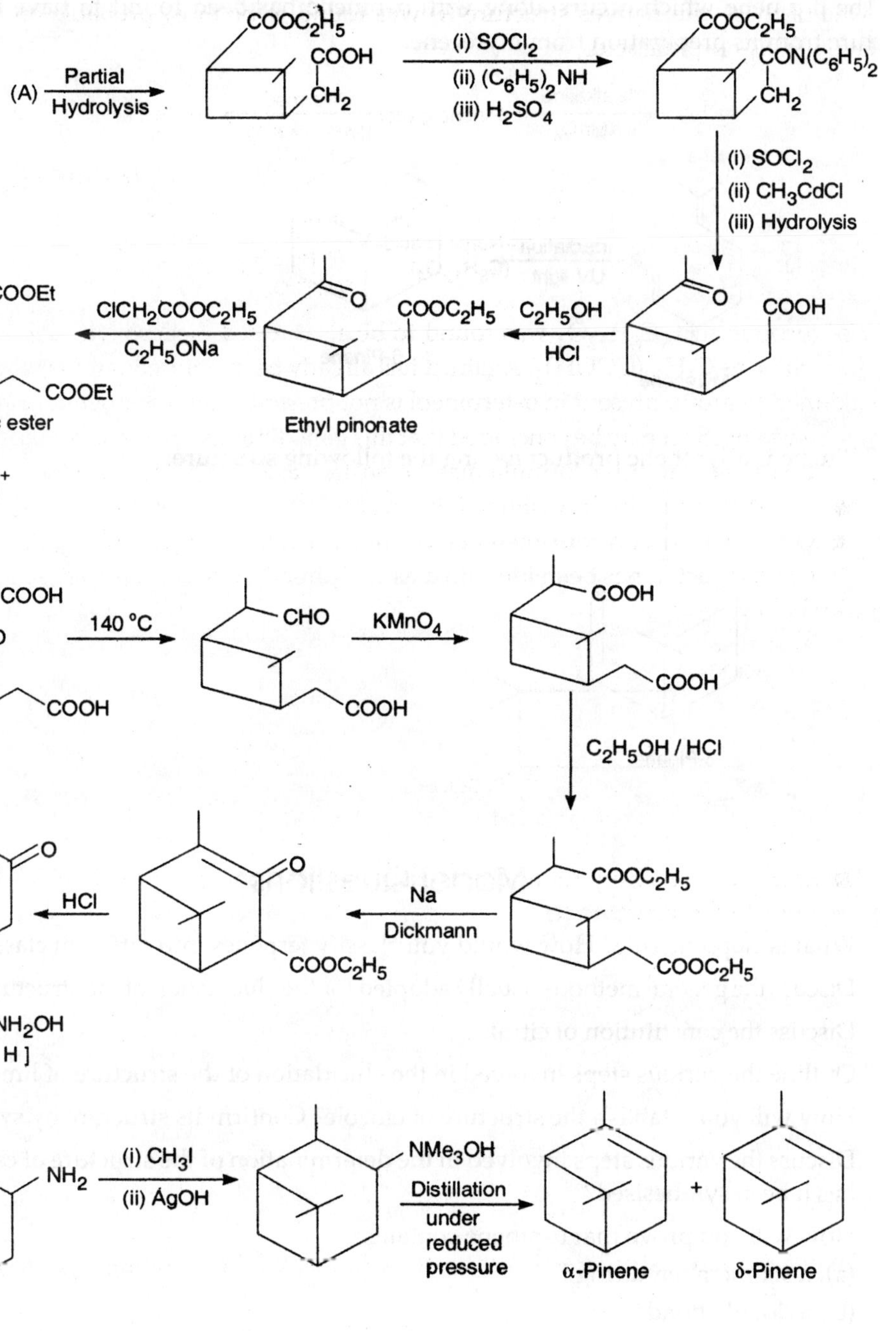

From the mixture, α-pinene was identified through the preparation of nitrosochloride derivative.

4.8.6.1.1 Stereochemistry of α-Pinene

Although α-pinene has two dissimilar chiral centres only one enantiomeric pair is known. This is due to the fact that the four-membered ring can be fused in the six-membered ring only one in the *cis*-position.

The β-pinene which occurs along with α-pinene has been found to have the following structure from its preparation from myrecene.

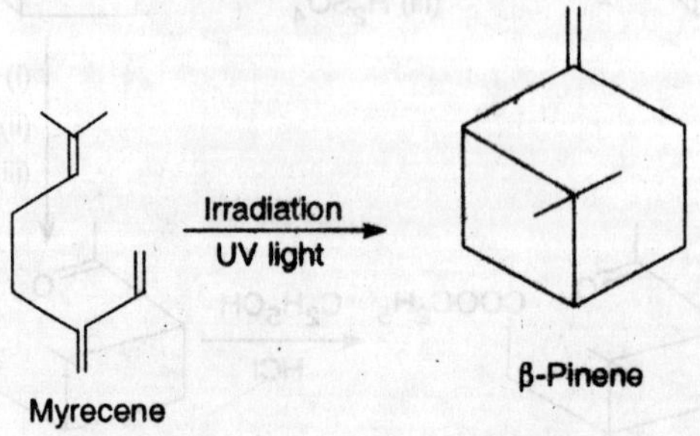

δ-Pinene is a synthetic product having the following structure:

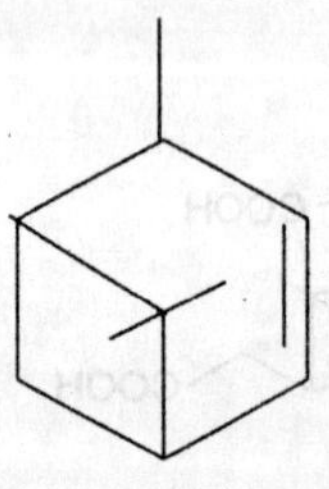

δ-Pinene

Model Questions

1. What is isoprene rule? How would you classify terpenes into different classes?
2. Discuss the general methods usually adopted for the elucidation of the structure of tarpenes.
3. Discuss the constitution of citral.
4. Outline the various steps involved in the elucidation of the structure of limonene.
5. How will you establish the structure of cineole? Confirm its structure by synthesis.
6. Discuss the various steps involved in the determination of the structure of camphor. How has it been synthesised?
7. How will you prove that α-pinene contains
   (a) a six-membered ring?
   (b) a double-bond?
   (c) a four-membered ring in its molecule?

CHAPTER FIVE

Alkaloids

INTRODUCTION

The term *'Alkaloid'* is usually applied to the members of naturally occurring chemical compounds which are basic in nature. The term *'alkaloid'* was first coined by the eminent pharmacist. W. Meissner in 1819. All the members of this class of compounds owe their basic character to nitrogen atom usually present as amino group. They occur only in certain genera and families among the large group of plants. As the investigation on the chemistry progressed, two more important characteristics of this class of phytochemicals were added to its definition. These two significant characteristics are—(i) complex structure and (ii) potential pharmocological activity. Further, in most of the members basic nitrogen atom is found in a ring. Consequently, the alkaloids are now defined as naturally occurring physiologically active nitrogen containing basic phytochemicals in which at least one nitrogen atom is present in a cyclic system.

5.1 Occurrence of Alkaloids

Thousands of alkaloids are known today, but they only occur in 10-15% of all the vascular plants. Alkaloids have not yet been isolated from lower plants like fungi, algae etc. excepting ergot alkaloids which occur in certain families of fungi, gymnosperms, or monocotyledons. They are primarily found to occur in certain dicotyledons. The alkaloids generally occur in leaves, seeds, roots and bark of plants of large number of botanical families specially in the following families:

i. Papaveraceae
ii. Rutaceae
iii. Apocynaceae
iv. Ranunculaceae
v. Solanecae
vi. Veratraceae
vii. Buxaceae
viii. Papilonaceae
ix. Euphorbeaceae, etc.

It may be mentioned that the alkaloid content of the plant varies with the season, age and locality. Closely related alkaloids generally occur in the same plant. Similarly, a particular genus or closely related genera contain the same or structurally related alkaloids. It has also been observed that simple alkaloids often occur in different unrelated plants but the very complex members generally occur in a particular species or genus of a family. It may further be mentioned that in some cases alkaloids are found to occur as salt while in other as glycosides.

5.2 Function of Alkaloids

The functions of alkaloids in plants is not yet clearly understood. Some of the views proposed by different researchers in this area may be summarised as below:

i. Alkaloids act as the reservoirs for protein synthesis.
ii. They may function as regulators in some of the activities like growth, metabolism and reproduction.
iii. Alkaloids may serve as the protective substances against insects and animals.

5.3 Isolation of Alkaloids

The general method most commonly followed for the isolation of different types of alkaloids has been proposed by Manske. This method may be described as below:

The plant material is dried, then finely powdered and first extracted with petroleum ether to remove the fatty matters. It is filtered and the filtrate is concentrated by distilling off the solvent. The concentrate is treated with dilute acetic acid where the bases, if present, are extracted as their soluble salts. The free bases are liberated by the addition of ammonia and is extracted with a suitable solvent. The solvent is evaporated and the residue thus obtained is subjected to chromatography for the separation of alkaloidal components in the usual way.

The plant material left after the extraction with petroleum ether is extracted successively with different solvents like benzene, chloroform and methanol, and in each case the basic portion is separated and is subjected to chromatographic resolution as in the case of petroleum ether extract. Finally, different basic components thus separated are processed for their purification and structure determination.

5.4 General Properties of Alkaloids

Alkaloids, in general, are crystalline, colourless and nonvolatile solid substances. But a few alkaloids like berberine is coloured. Some alkaloids are liquid. Free bases are insoluble in water but are soluble in organic solvents such as ethanol, ether, chloroform, etc. Most of the alkaloids contain tertiary nitrogen atom in a ring and may possess one or more than one nitrogen atom. They in general, have a bitter taste and exhibit optical activity. Most of them are laevorotatory although a few are dextrorotatory as for example, coniine, some of them like papaverine were found to be optically inactive. Generally, alkaloids possess significant physiological activity and have curative properties. As such they are frequently used in medicine. However, some of them are powerful poisons. Optically active alkaloids are very useful in resolving racemic acids. As mentioned earlier alkaloids in general are basic in nature and are precipitated out by some common alkaloidal reagents as mentioned below:

1. Potassium bismuth iodide (*Dragendorff's reagent*)
2. Potassium mercuric iodide (*Mayer's reagent*)

3. Iodine dissolved in potassium iodide (*Wagner's reagent*)
4. Phosphomolybdic acid (*Sonneuschein's reagent*)
5. Molybdic acid (*Frohde's reagent*)
6. Phosphotungstic acid (*Scheibler's reagent*)
7. Picric acid (*Hager's reagent*)
8. Picrolonic acid
9. Nitric acid (*Erdmann's reagent*)

Many of these reagents are used as a means of detecting alkaloids as the precipitates formed by them have characteristic colours.

5.5 General Approach for the Determination of the Molecular Structure of Alkaloids

Alkaloids as a class have attracted organic chemists partly because of their physiological activity and synthetic puzzles that they pose. Although the chemistry of alkaloids primarily is confined in the chemistry of nitrogen containing heterocyclic compounds yet the methods by which the molecular structures of individual bases have been deduced are typical of methods applied in the entire field of chemistry of natural products and are considered as the illustrations of the general and fundamental principle of organic chemistry. In general, elaboration of molecular architecture of alkaloids involves the following chemical and physical methods:

1. The crude alkaloid obtained is purified and the pure specimen, thus, obtained is subjected to elemental analysis. In general alkaloid contains carbon, nitrogen, and hydrogen and also most of them contain oxygen. This is then followed by quantitative analysis for the determination of molecular formula in the usual way. Its optical property is also measured.
2. The presence of unsaturation in the alkaloid may be ascertained by bromination or by hydroxylation with dilute alkaline permanganate.
3. The presence of unsaturation as well as the other functionalities may be ascertained from spectral particularly infrared spectral measurements.
4. *Functional Nature of Oxygen:* Oxygen atom, if present, may occur as —OH (alcoholic or phenolic), $—OCH_3$ (methoxy), $—OCOCH_3$ (acetoxy), —COOH (carboxylic), $>C=O$ (carbonyl), etc. Sometimes oxygen found to be present in lactone ring system as in the case of narcotine and hydrastine. These functionalities are detected by usual methods of organic analysis including infrared examinations. For the characterisation of different oxygen functionalities following procedures are usually adapted.
   (a) *Hydroxyl Group* (—OH): The presence of hydroxyl group in the alkaloid is usually ascertained by acetylation experiment with acetic anhydride or acetyl chloride. The exact nature (alcoholic or phenolic) of hydroxyl group is settled from (i) the solubility in caustic soda (ii) development of colour with ferric chloride solution and (iii) methylation with diazomethane. The positive response of the alkaloid with this experiments reveals the phenolic character.
   (b) *Methoxyl Group* ($—OCH_3$): The occurrence of this group in the alkaloid is confirmed by Zeisel experiment which involves the heating of the alkaloid with hydroiodic

acid at a temperature of 126 °C when methoxyl group is converted to methyl iodide. But nowadays I_{HNMR} spectral analysis is carried for the identification of methoxyl group.

(c) *Carboxylic Group* (—COOH): The presence of this functionality is carried out by usual tests, i.e., (i) solubility in aqueous sodium carbonate solution (ii) occurrence of effervescence on treatment with sodium bicarbonates and (iii) formation of ester. However, infrared spectral measurement is also used for the detection of this group.

(d) *Methylenedioxy Group* (—O—CH_2—O—): When this functional group is present in an alkaloid, formaldehyde is liberated on heating with hydroiodic acid. I_{HNMR} spectral technique is also applied.

(e) *Carbonyl Group:* The presence of this group is ascertained by the tests with carbonylic reagents particularly with 2 : 4-dinitrophenyl hydrazine. Infrared spectral analysis is highly useful in ascertaining the presence of this group.

(f) *Ester, Amide, Lactone and Lactum Groups:* These functional groups are detected by identifying the products of their hydrolysis by alkali or acid.

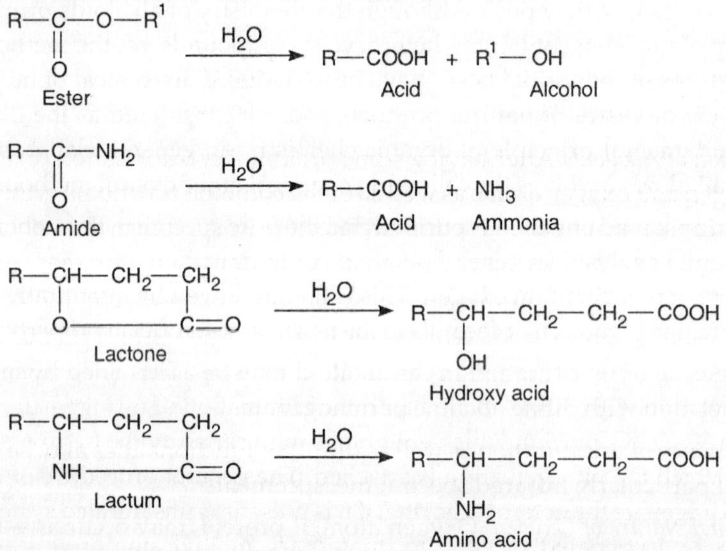

Spectroscopic technique particularly infrared spectral measurement may also be applied for identification of these functional groups.

5. *Functional Nature of Nitrogen:* Nitrogen atom is invariably present in alkaloids and in the Majority of alkaloids nitrogen forms a part of a heterocylic system. So it must be present either as a secondary amino (>N—H) or as a tertiary amino group (>N—). However, in some cases as in adrenaline, ephidrine, nitrogen is present in the form of primary amino (—NH_2) group. The functional nature of nitrogen in the alkaloid is generally determined by the following methods:

(a) The reactions of alkaloids with methyl iodide, nitrous acid and acetic anhydride are often used to ascertain the nature of nitrogen. However, it must be remembered that some alkaloids may undergo ring fission during these reactions. In general, alkaloids containing secondary nitrogen atom form N-methyl derivative while tertiary nitrogen yields quaternary salts with methyl iodide. Thus,

$$>N-H + CH_3I \longrightarrow >N-CH_3 + HI$$

$$>N + CH_3I \longrightarrow >\overset{+}{N}-CH_3\bar{I}$$

(b) Distillation of alkaloids with the aqueous solution of potassium hydroxide is used to determine the nature of nitrogen atom as well as the number of alkyl groups attached to it. Thus the formation of methyl amine, dimethyl amine and trimethyl amine reveals the attachment of one, two and three methyl groups to nitrogen atom while primary amino group, if present, forms ammonia.

(c) The reaction of alkaloid with hydroiodic acid at a temperature of 150-300 °C which is known as Herzig Meyer method, is often used to determine the presence and number of N-alkyl groups. Thus,

$$-\overset{|}{N}-CH_3 + HI \xrightarrow{150\text{-}300\,^{\circ}C} -\overset{|}{N}-H + CH_3I$$

Methyl iodide formed is estimated either volumetrically or gravimetrically. ^{1}HNMR spectroscopy can also be used for the rapid detection of these groups.

(d) Hydrolytic cleavage experiment is often used to determine the presence of amide linkage in the alkaloid.

6. *Degradation of Alkaloids:* After having some preliminary information regarding the nature of nitrogen and oxygen atoms as well as of the common functional groups, problem now remains in ascertaining the structural architecture which incorporates these functionalities. For this purpose alkaloid is subjected to degradative experiments. Some of the most frequently used such degradations are discussed in sequel.

(a) *Hofmann's Exhaustive Methylation Method:* This is one of the most important degradative experiments in alkaloid chemistry. This is because by this process heterocyclic rings are opened with the elimination of nitrogen atom and yield non-nitrogeneous portion which enlightens with certainty the nature of carbon skeleton to which the nitrogen atom is attached. The general procedure of this method is to hydrogenate the heterocyclic ring, if it is present as unsaturated system and to convert this hydrogenated product to quaternary methyl ammonium hydroxide by the treatment with excess methyl iodide followed by treatment with silver oxide. The resultant hydroxide is then heated at a temperature of 200 °C when an olefin is formed with the cleavage of C—N bond. In principle, this degradation is nothing but a β-elimination reaction and may be illustrated as below:

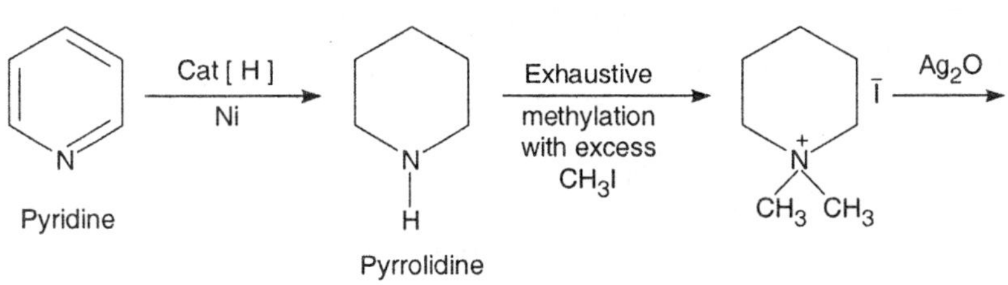

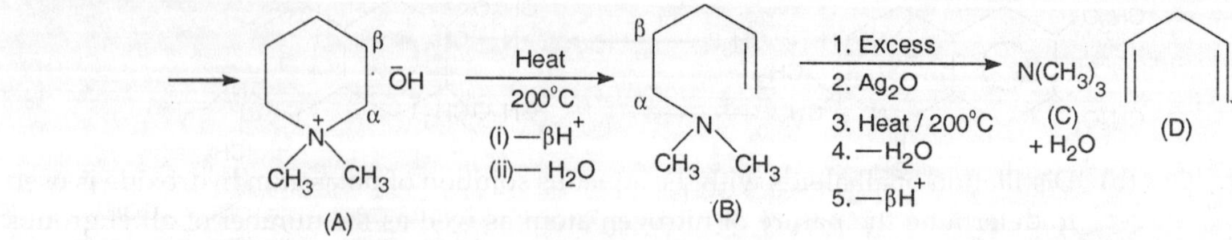

From the above sequences of reactions it is evident that if nitrogen atom is present in a ring, two complete sequences of the above reactions are to be carried out to eliminate it from the molecule. In the first set of sequences a nitrogen containing olefin (B) is formed which on further treatment of above sequences, of reactions affords a nitrogen free olefin (D) eliminating nitrogen as tertiary amine (C).

It may be remembered that since this degradation is a β-elimination reaction presence of hydrogen atom at the β-position with respect to nitrogen is an essential requirement. For this reason this degradation fails in unsaturated heterocyclic compounds and that is why such type of heterocycles are hydrogenated in the first step of this method whereby availability of β-hydrogen atoms is ensured.

Further, the quaternary ammonium hydroxide, thus, obtained should be sufficiently stable to eliminate β-hydrogen otherwise this method may not function. Thus quaternary ammonium hydroxide of tetrahedra quinoline although contains β-hydrogen atom but —C—N bond cleavage does not occur.

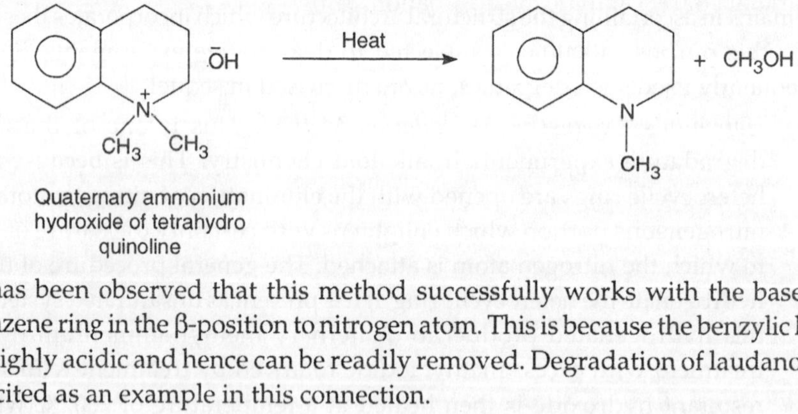

Quaternary ammonium hydroxide of tetrahydro quinoline

It has been observed that this method successfully works with the bases having benzene ring in the β-position to nitrogen atom. This is because the benzylic hydrogen is highly acidic and hence can be readily removed. Degradation of laudanosine may be cited as an example in this connection.

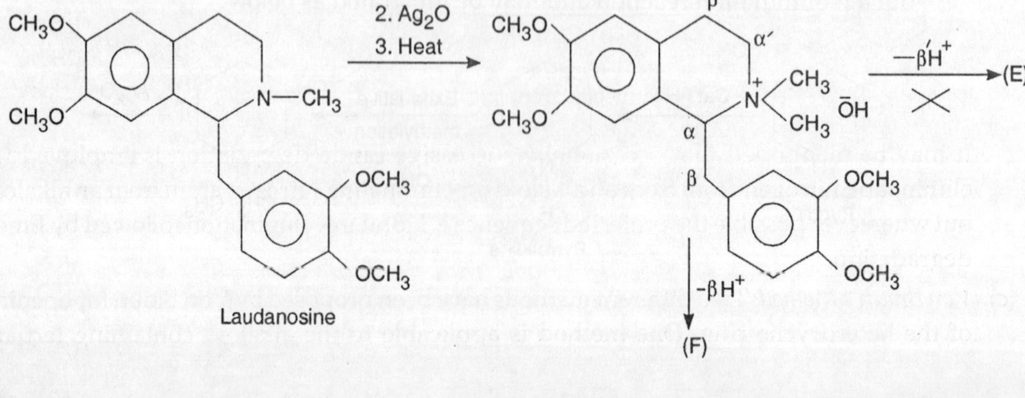

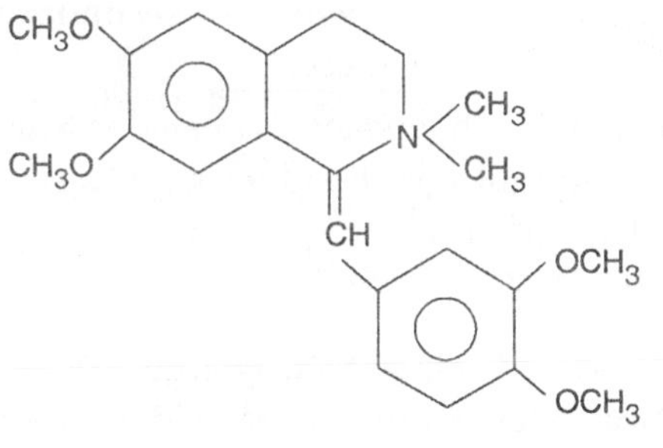

More stable due to
more extended conjugation
(F)

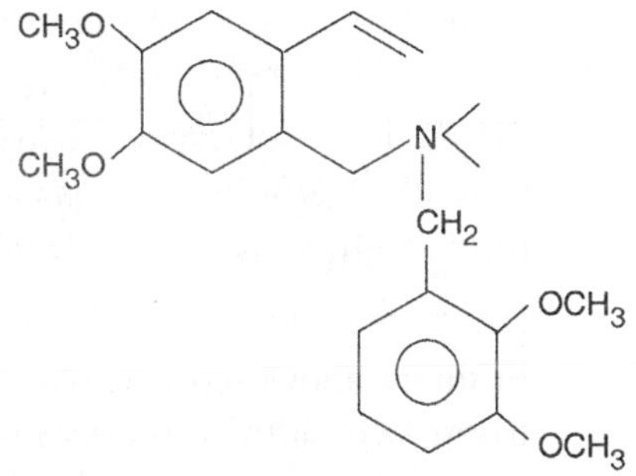

(E)

Due to the more extended conjugation styrene derivative (E) is more stable and hence is preferably formed.

The identification of non-nitrogeneous olefin (D or E) establishes the nature of carbon skeleton present in the base under consideration.

(b) *Emde's Degradation:* It has already been mentioned that the presence of β-hydrogen with respect to nitrogen is essential for Hofmann's exhaustive methylation. But there are some nitrogeneous compound where β-hydrogen is not available. In such situation Emde's degradation may be applied. In this method the final step involves the reductive cleavage of quaternary ammonium salts either with sodium amalgam or with sodium in liquid ammonia or by catalytic hydrogenation. Thus,

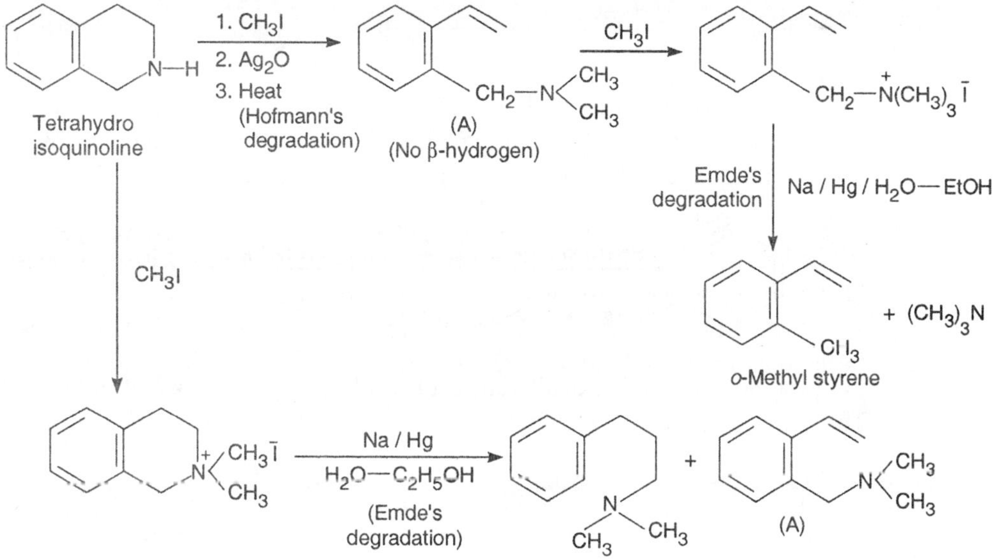

It may be mentioned that occasionally successive Emde degradation is employed for eliminating nitrogen atom from an alkaloid for eliminating nitrogen atom from an alkaloid but whereever possible the preferred sequence is Hofmann elimination followed by Emde degradation.

(c) *Von Braun's Method:* Two different methods have been proposed by Von Braun for opening of the heterocyclic ring. One method is applicable to the alkaloid containing tertiary nitrogen atom in the ring and, other is employed for opening of secondary amine containing ring compounds.

1. In the opening of tertiary nitrogen containing ring the alkaloid is treated with cyanogen bromide, CNBr as a result of which an alkyl-nitrigen bond undergoes cleavage to form an alkyl halide and a substituted cyanamide as shown below:

$$R_3N + CN—Br \longrightarrow R—Br + R_2N—CN$$

In the case of unsymmetrically substituted tertiary amine, alkyl halide is formed from the smallest alkyl substituent. Thus,

$$Et_2N—Me + CN—Br \longrightarrow CH_3Br + Et_2N—CN$$

Ring opening in the case of tertiary cyclic amines may be shown as:

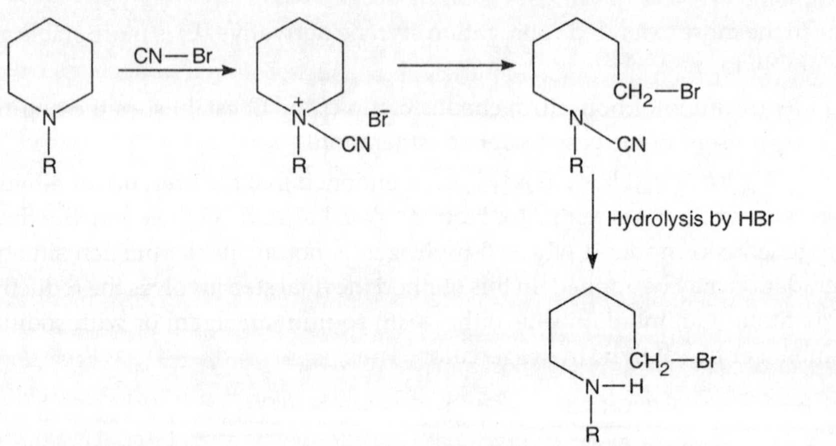

Interesting features of this method are (i) it may be successfully applied on compounds which do not respond to Hofmann method (ii) when both the methods are applicable, ring opening takes place at different points of the ring. i.e.,

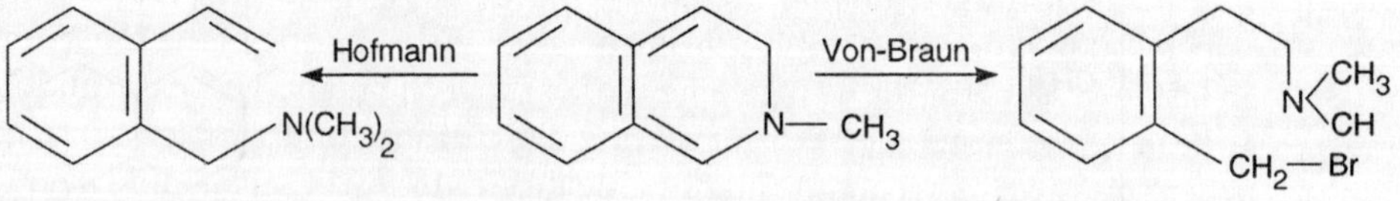

(iii) In some cases simple dealkylation of N-alkyl group occurs without ring cleavage. Thus,

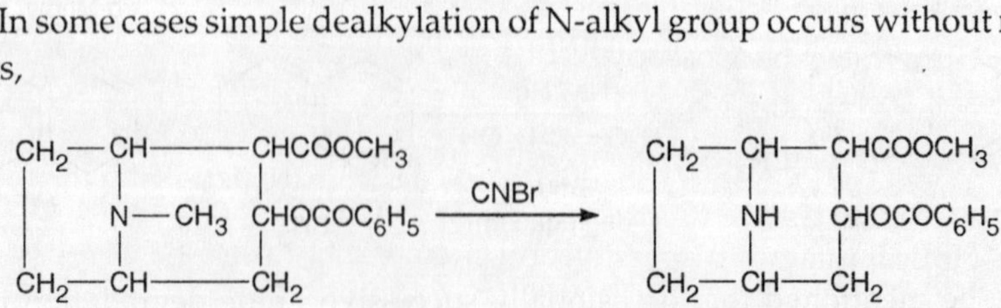

Cocaine

This method is also known as *Von Braun's Cyanogen method.*

2. In the second Von braun's method benzoyl derivative of secondary cyclic amines is treated with phosphorons halide when nitrogen is eliminated as benzonitrile with the formation of Ω-dihalo compound.

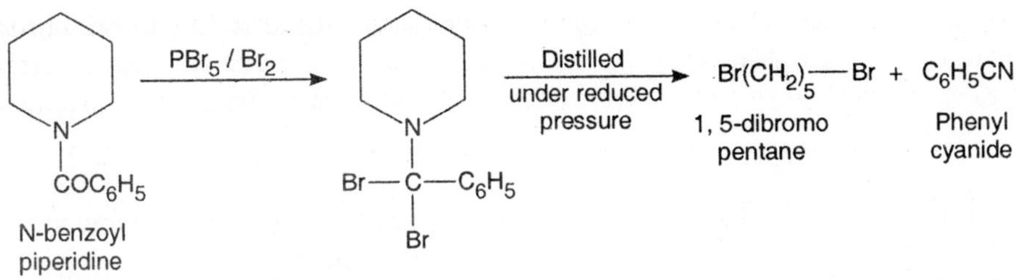

(d) *Zinc Dust Distillation:* Zinc dust distillation of alkaloid is an important method for degrading the molecule into stable smaller and easily identifiable components. Thus, morphine when subjected to zinc dust distillation furnishes phenanthrene indicating thereby the presence of phenanthrene nucleus in its molecule. Similarly cinchonine yields quinoline in such experiment revealing the presence of quinoline nucleus in its structure.

(e) *Alkali Fusion:* It is a drastic method which is normally employed to break down the molecule into simpler fragments. The identification of such simple fragments gives an insight into the nature of nucli present in the alkaloid molecule. For example, adrenaline on such fusion forms protocatechuic acid suggesting that adrenaline is a catechol derivative.

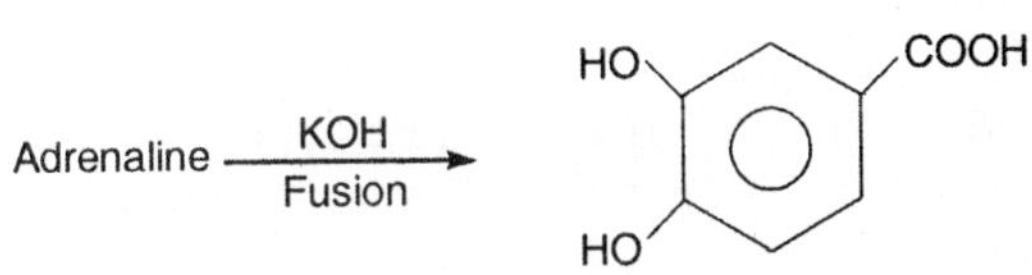

Protocatechuic acid

(f) *Dehydrogenation:* Dehydrogenation experiment with some catalysts like selenium, sulphur or palladium is one of the classical methods of degrading organic molecules and has proved very valuable in determining the structure of natural products especially alkaloids. In many cases the whole nuclear structure appears intact in the degradation products and from their proper characterisation it is possible to ascertain the nuclear structure of the compound under investigation. In general, peripheral groups such as hydroxyl and C-methyl are eliminated during such experiment.

7. *Physico chemical Techniques:* The development of some physicochemical techniques specially spectroscopic technique is now recognised as one of the most important events in last few years for the advancement of organic chemisty. These techniques have shown to be very successful methods for solving difficult structural problems in organic chemistry where classical approach could not give the final answer. In alkaloid chemistry, the most important physico-chemical methods are as under:
   (a) Ultraviolet spectroscopy
   (b) Infrared spectroscopy
   (c) Nuclear magnetic resonance spectroscopy
   (d) Mass spectrometry
   (e) Optical rotatory dispersion and circular dichroism
   (f) X-ray diffraction.

- *Ultra Violet Spectroscopy:* This spectroscopic technique has been primarily applied for the chromophoric systems present in an alkaloid and hence to establish the *structural type* to which the alkaloid belongs. For such purpose ultraviolet spectra of a large number of different types are recorded and the data are correlated with different structural pattern. From such correlation class and structural pattern such pyridine pyrolidine, quinoline, indole etc, can be easily ascertained.

- *Infrared Spectroscopy:* Infrared spectroscopy is generally used to identify the presence of various functional groups and sometimes to ascertain the absence of particular functional groups. This spectroscopic method is an important method of establishing the identify and distinction between the alkaloids.

- *Nuclear Magnetic Resonance Spectroscopy:* The development of nuclear magnetic resonance spectroscopy is now recognised as one of the most important events in the last few years for the advancement of organic chemistry. High resolution proton magnetic resonance technique has been shown to be a successful physical method for solving difficult structural problems in organic chemistry particularly in alkaloid chemistry where classical approach could not give the final answer. This epoch making technique reveals the proton environment along with the presence of C-methyl, O-methyl, N-methyl, phenolic groups, olefinic unsaturation and the nature of heterocyclic rings in alkaloid.

- *Mass Spectrometry:* In recent years mass spectrometry becomes most useful technique as it furnishes the following essential information regarding the organic molecules:
  i. Molecular weight
  ii. Molecular formula
  iii. Nature of structural architecture. It may be mentioned that this technique is although equally applicable to all types of organic molecules yet much of the success has been achieved in the case of alkaloids particularly in the field of polycyclic indole alkaloids. It is the only technique from which complete elaboration of structure is possible only with a few nanomoles of the sample.

- *X-ray Diffraction:* This instrumental technique is abundantly employed in the field of alkaloids. From this technique exact structure along with the bond angles and bond lengths can be obtained. It is also capable of furnishing information regarding the stereo-configuration of the molecule under investigation. An interesting example that may be cited in this connection is thelepogine, the complete structure of which has been settled from the X-ray analysis without the help of any other techniques.

5.6 Classification of Alakloids

There are a variety of methods in which the alkaloids are classified of which followings are significant.

5.6.1 Chemical Method

This is the most widely adopted method of classification. In this method alkaloids are classified on the basis of the nature of the ring structure present in the molecule. Thus, quinine is regarded as the quinoline type of alkaloid while morphine is considered as a phenanthrene derivative. Some of the important chemical groups of alkaloids are as under:

(a) Phenyl ethylamine group
(b) Pyrrolidine group
(c) Pyridine group
(d) Pyrrolidine-pyridine group
(e) Quinoline group
(f) Isoquinoline group
(g) Phenanthrene group
(h) Indole group.

5.6.2 Taxonomic Method

In this method of classifying alkaloids, the botanical family of the plants is taken into account. Thus alkaloids of *solanaceous group* are those which have been isolated from the *solanaceous* plants without any reference to the chemical type of alkaloids present.

5.6.3 Pharmacological Method

This method of classification lists the alkaloids according to their physiological activity. Thus analgesic alkaloids, cardioactive alkaloids, etc.

5.6.4 Biosynthetic Method

This method is the most fundamental method. It is based on the nature of building block compounds utilised by the plants in synthesizing the complex structures. Thus almost all the *indole* alkaloids are derivable from the tryptophan and mevalonic acid. Similarly, morphine, papaverine, narcotine, colchicine may be listed as phenylalanine-tyrosine derived bases. However, this method is not free from drawback. The most mentionable drawback is that the relationship which this predicts among the alkaloids is not always apparent.

It may be mentioned in this connection that among the different methods the most satisfactory method of classification of alkaloids is the chemical method which is generally followed.

5.7 Nomenclature of Alkaloids

There is no systematic method of naming the alkaloids due to the puzzling diversity in their structural architecture. In some cases names of alkaloids have been derived from the source from which they have been isolated. Thus papaverine from *Papaver somniferum*, strychnine from *Strychnos nux vomica*, etc.

In a few cases physical activity has been given importance in naming the alkaloids. Such as morphine (GK. morpheus meaning god of dream), emetine (GK. emetikos meaning to vomit). Occasionally, the names of chemists who isolated the alkaloids have also been considered. Thus, the pomegranate alkaloids were named pelletierines in the honour of the French Chemist P.J. Pelletier.

In the case of naming minor alkaloids suitable prefixes or suffixes are added to the name of the principal alkaloids, as for example, in cinchona alkaloids.

In naming isomeric alkaloids prefixes such as *iso, epi, neo, pseudo*, α, β, etc. have been used.

5.8 Chemistry of Representative Members of the Important Groups of Alkaloids

Chemistry of significant and representative members of widely occurring groups of alkaloids are furnished below to have an idea regarding their puzzling molecular architecture and pronounced pharmocological actions either curative or toxic upon the animal organisms.

5.8.1 Phenylethyl Amine Alkaloids

A large number of alkaloids of this group are known in literature. The most outstanding physiological action of these bases is to enhance the blood pressure and as such they are frequently referred to as *pressor drugs*.

5.8.1.1 Ephedrine

Ephedrine may be looked upon as a representative member of this group of alkaloid. It is one of the most important drugs of the chinese herb *Ma Huang*. It widely occurs in the genus *ephedra* along with other alkaloids. The plants belonging to the genus *ephedra* occurs in temperate and subtropical regions of Asia, America and Mediterranean countries. This alkaloid was first isolated from the ephedra by Nagai, and later Gulland and Virden obtained this base in small amount in *Taxus baccata*.

5.8.1.1.1 Isolation of Ephedrine

Ephedrine is usually isolated from the dried and powdered young stems of *Ephedra geradiana* and *Ephedra nebrodensis*, both belonging to the botanical family *gnetecae*. Nagai isolated ephedrine from *Ma Huang* by moistening the powdered young stems either with aqueous sodium carbonate or with lime water and finally extracting it with ethanol or benzene.

5.8.1.1.2 Properties and Uses of Ephedrine

It is a volatile solid with melting point of 38 °C. It is laevorotatory base having $[\alpha]_D$—6.3°. It has been in use in the treatment of variety of diseases for thousands of years. It has been successfully used in the treatment of bronchial asthma, hay fever and other allergic conditions. Recent clinical investigation reveals its usefulness as antipyretic, circulatory stimulant and sedative in cough. Ephedrine products are marketed as (i) tablet B.P. and I.P. (ii) ephedrine sulphate capsule/injection/ syrup and tablet USP (iii) ephedrine nasal drop and (iv) ephedrine hydrochloride tablet, I.P.

5.8.1.1.3 Structure of Ephedrine

The structure of ephedrine has been deduced from the following evidences:

i. From analytical data and molecular weight determination molecular formula of ephedrine stands as $C_{10}H_{15}ON$.
ii. On treatment with nitrous acid it readily forms a nitroso-compound indicating the presence of secondary amino group (—NH—) in its molecule.
iii. Ephedrine on benzoylation affords a dibenzoyl derivative. This is a clear indication that in addition to a secondary amino (—NH—) group the oxygen must be present as a hydroxyl (—OH) function.
iv. On oxidation ephedrine yields benzoic acid as the major product. This reveals the presence of a benzene ring containing a side-chain in the molecule of ephedrine.

On the basis of above evidences a part structure of ephedrine may be written as (A).

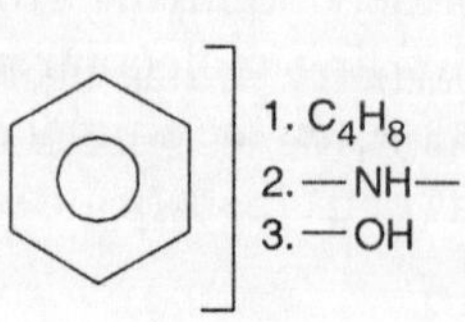

(A)

• *Nature of Side-chain in Ephedrine:* When heated with hydrochloric acid ephedrine furnishes methylamine and propiophenone, i.e.,

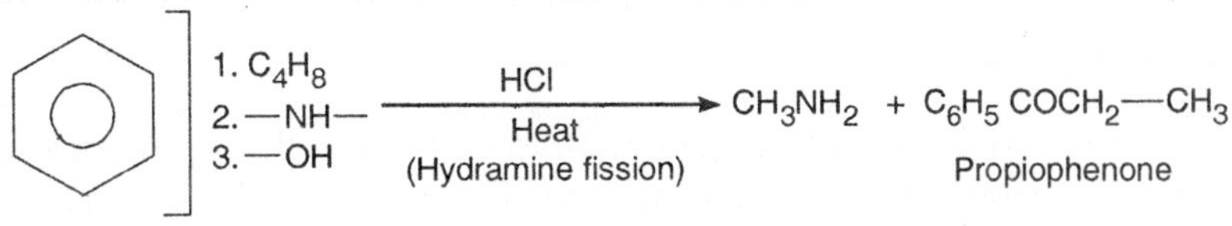

Based on the above evidences following three alternative structures (I, II and III) have been proposed for ephedrine.

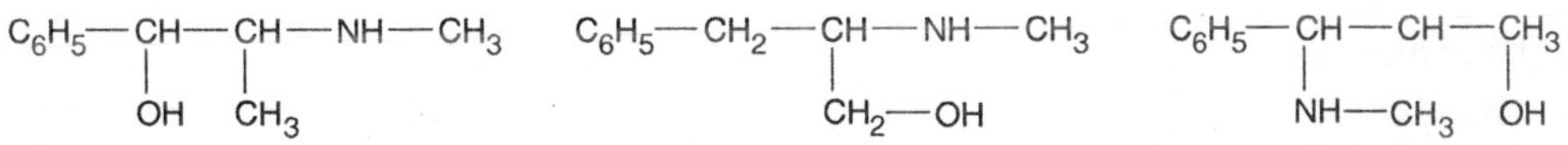

(I) (II) (III)

However, easy formation of methyl amine and propiophenone during heating ephedrine with hydrochloric acid can be best interpreted only on the basis of structure (I) through hydramine fission mechanism. Consequently, structure (I) is more likely to represent ephedrine. Thus,

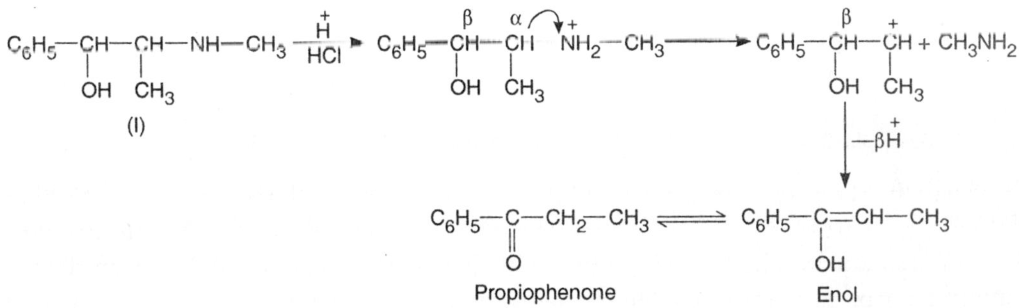

Further support in favour of structure (I) has been secured from Hofmann degradation experiment. During this experiment ephedrine yields 1, 2-methylphenyl ethyl oxide formation of which can only be explained on the basis of structure (I), i.e.,

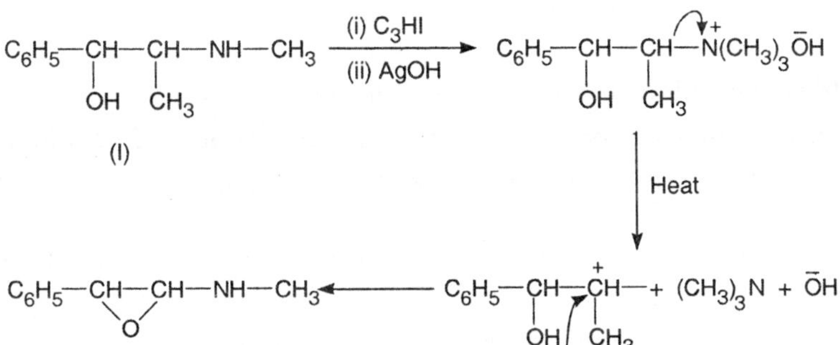

Structure (I) has also been supported by its optical activity. It has been experimentally observed that ephedrine contains two chiral centre as is evidenced from the fact that the replacement of OH group in ephedrine by hydrogen yields deoxyephedrine which is optically active. This is completely in agrement with structure (I).

5.8.1.1.4 Stereochemistry of Ephedrine

The scrutiny of the structure (I) of ephedrine reveals that it has two different chiral centres. So four optically active forms (two pairs of enantiomers) are theoretically possible and in fact, all are known as shown:

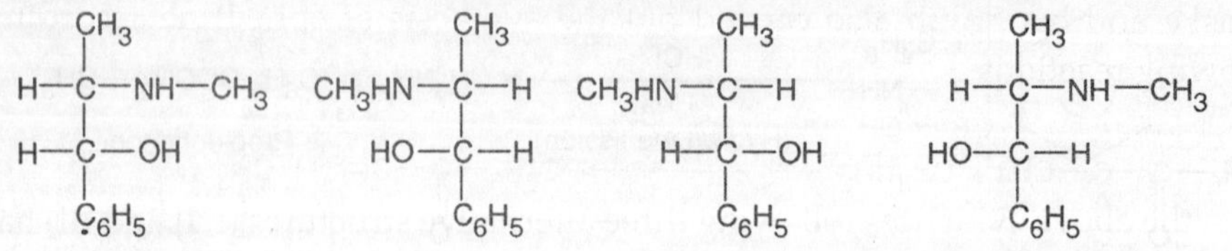

D(–) Ephedrine (A) | L(+) Ephedrine | D (+) ψ-Ephedrine | L (+) ψ-Ephedrine (B)

Out of these four forms only (–) ephedrine and L (+) pseudoephedrine are naturally occurring whereas other forms are known as synthetic compounds. The problem of the configurations of these two naturally occurring bases has been the subject of much debate.

It has been observed that both these isomers (A) and (B) can be converted to the same optically active compound (+)-desoxyephedrine by reduction with HI/P, i.e.,

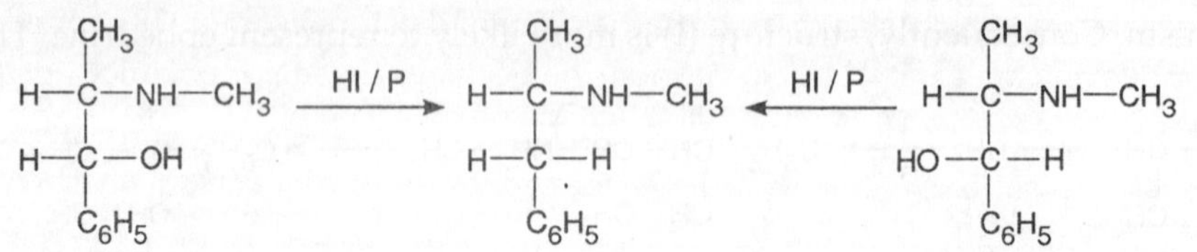

D(–) Ephedrine | (+)-Desoxy ephedrine | L (+) Ephedrine

From the above experimental evidence it is evident that both these alkaloids differ only in the configuration of carbinol carbon atom. It has been established that the absolute configuration of carbinol carbon in ephedrine is identical with that of D (–) mandelic acid whereas the absolute configuration of carbon atom containing methylamino group has been found to be identical with that of L (+) alanine.

Based on the above observation ephedrine has been given *erythro* configuration while *threo* configuration has been assigneid to pseudoephedrine. An X-ray analysis of crystalline (–) ephedrine hydrochloride has provided confirmation in this regard.

5.8.1.1.5 Synthesis of Ephedrine

Finally, the structure of ephedrine has been confirmed by various synthesis as mentioned below:

(a) *Synthesis due to Nagai and his associates:* This synthesis is of commercial interest and involves the following sequence of reactions.

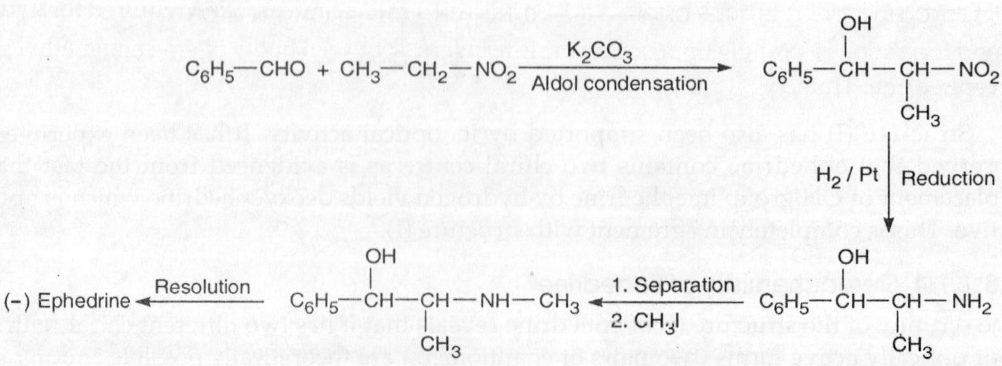

(±) Ephedrine

(b) Manske and his group also carried out the synthesis of ephedrine according to the following reactions:

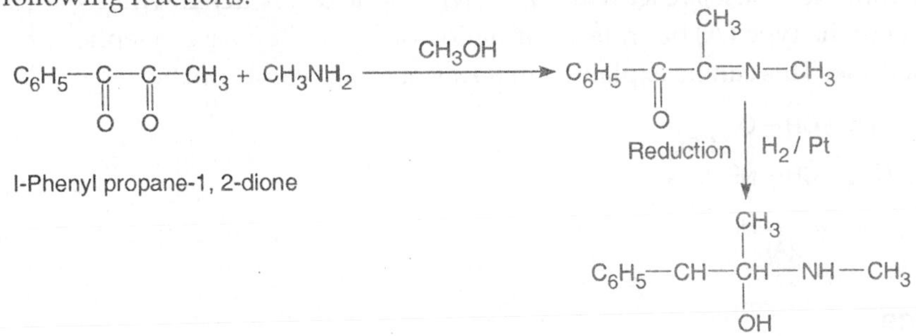

I-Phenyl propane-1, 2-dione

(±) Ephedrine

The racemic ephedrine formed is resolved by mandelic acid. Manske's synthesis is a case of stereoselective synthesis where both the pairs of diastereoisomers (±) ephedrine and (±) ψ-ephedrine are formed but (±) ephedrine becomes the major product.

(c) Synthesis carried out by Freudenberg *etal* may be looked upon as a case of stereospecific synthesis. This synthesis relates the absolute configuration of carbinol carbon atom to that of D (–) mandelic acid. Thus,

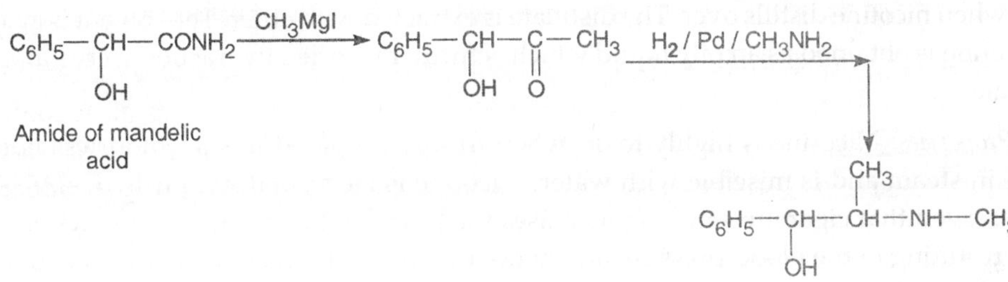

Amide of mandelic acid

D(–) Ephedrine

5.8.1.1.6 Basicity of Ephedrine

The most interesting characteristic of ephedrine is its basicity. It has been observed that D(–) ephedrine has a pk_a value of 9.14 and is an weaker base than its isomer (+) ψ-ephedrine which has pk_a value 9.22. The cause of lower basicity has been appropriately explained by Prelog on the basis of conformational analysis. According to Prelog the conformation of ψ-ephedrine is such that its conjugate acid is stabilised by internal hydrogen bonding between neighbouring OH and $\overset{+}{N}H_2—CH_3$ groups whereas appearance of similar conformation required for hydrogen bond formation is strongly opposed by the interference between bulky phenyl and methyl groups in ephedrine. Thus,

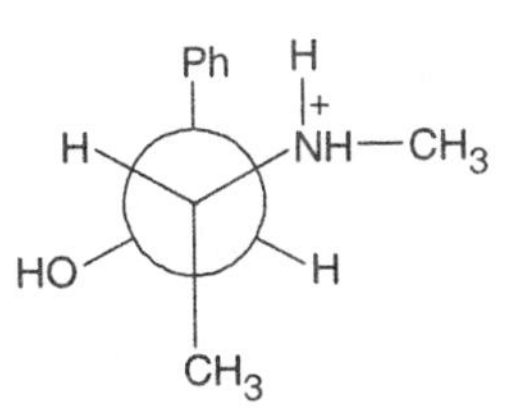

D(–)-Ephedrine
(Conjugate acid)

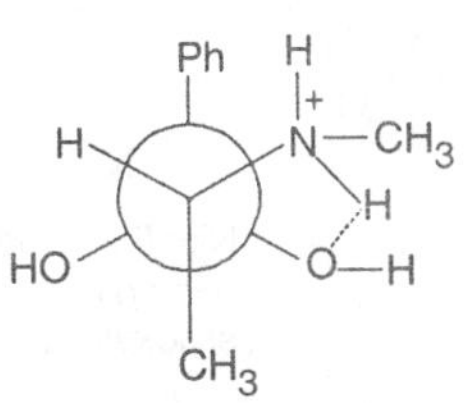

(+) ψ-Ephedrine
(Conjugate acid)

The above conformational assignments of ephedrine and ψ-ephedrine has been supported by the fact that both these bases react with diphenylboric acid (Ph_2BOH) with the formation of cyclic compound of the type (A) but rate of formation of (A) in the case of ψ-ephedrine is much faster than ephedrine. This can be explained in terms of above comformations

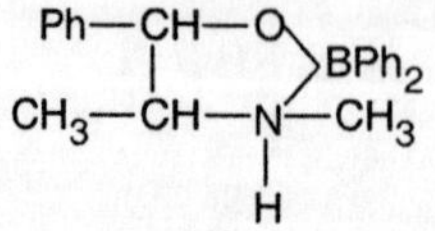

(A)

5.8.1.2 Nicotine

Nicotine belongs to pyridine-pyrrolidine group of alkaloids. It is the most important tobacco alkaloid occurring in *Nicotiana tobacum* L and other *Nicotiana* species. It usually occurs as salt with malic and citric acid. It is mainly found in the leaves. The name nicotine has been given in the honour of Sir J. Nicot, Ambassador of the king of France to Portugal.

5.8.1.2.1 Isolation

The leaves and stems of tobacco plant are dried and powdered and then distilled with the milk of lime when nicotine distills over. The distillate is extracted with ether. The solvent is evaporated and nicotine is obtained as an oily liquid which is further purified by fractional crystallisation of its oxalate.

• *Properties:* Nicotine is highly toxic, when freshly prepared it is a colourless liquid. It is volatile in steam and is miscible with water. Nicotine is laevorotatory, $[\alpha]_D = -166.50$. It has been observed that cigarette smoking increases the heart beat and causes constriction of blood vessels resulting in the blood pressure and hence disturbing blood circulation. Nicotine is used to control withdrawal symtoms of tobacco smokers.

5.8.1.2.2 Structure of Nicotine

The structure of nicotine has been deduced on the basis of following evidences:

i. It has molecular formula, $C_{10}H_{14}N_2$
ii. On treatment with CH_3I, it forms diquarternary compound indicating that both the nitrogen atoms are tertiary in nature.
iii. Nicotine when oxidised with chromic acid forms a fragment, $C_6H_5O_5N$ which has been found to be completely identical with pyridine-3-carboxylic acid which on decarbaxylation yields pyridine.

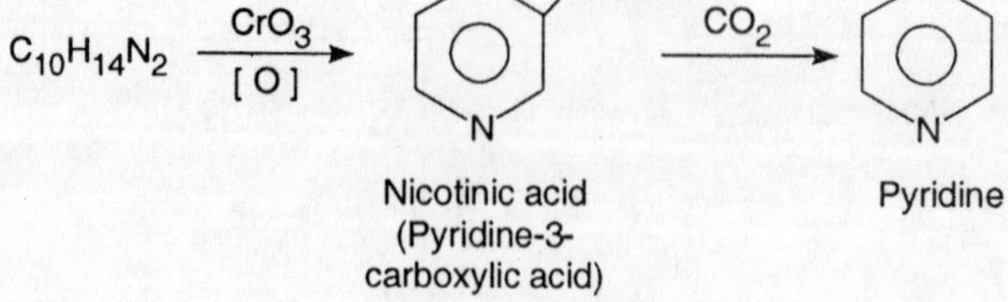

This indicates that nicotine contains a pyridine having substitution at 3-position in its ring. Thus part sturcture of pyridine may be written as

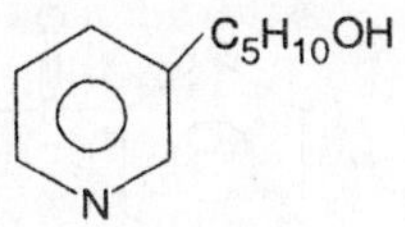

iv. Herzig-Meyer experiment suggests the presence of N-methyl group in necotine.

v. Nicotine hydroiodide when warmed with methyl iodide yields nicotine isomethoiodide which on oxdidation with potassium ferricyanide furnishes nicotone. Nictone when oxidised with chromic acids affords (–) hygrinic acid of known structure. Thus,

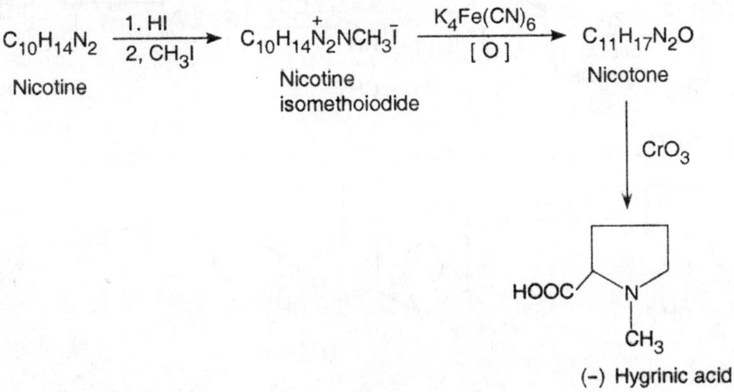

On the basis of the above observations following structure has been proposed for nicotine.

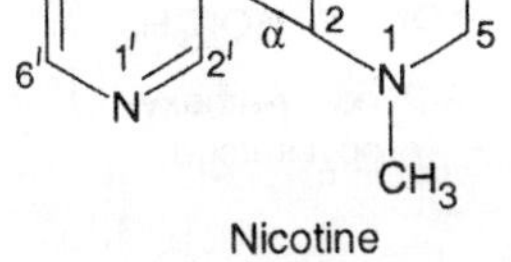

Nicotine

Thus nicotine is β-pyridil-α-pyrrole alkaloid.

vi. Above proposed structure of nicotine has been confirmed by the following syntheses.

(a) *Spath and Bretschneider's Synthesis:*

i. 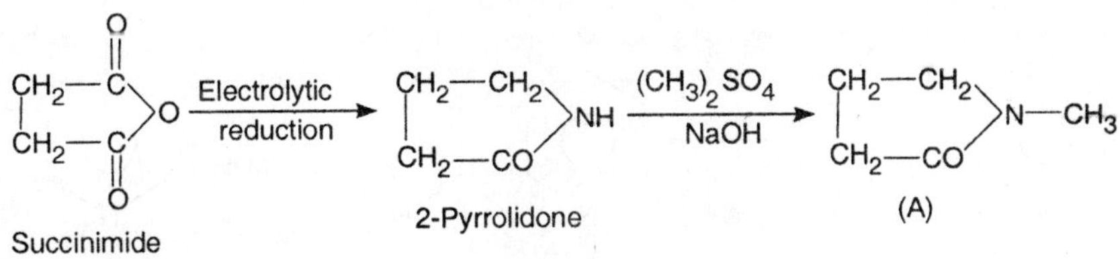

ii.

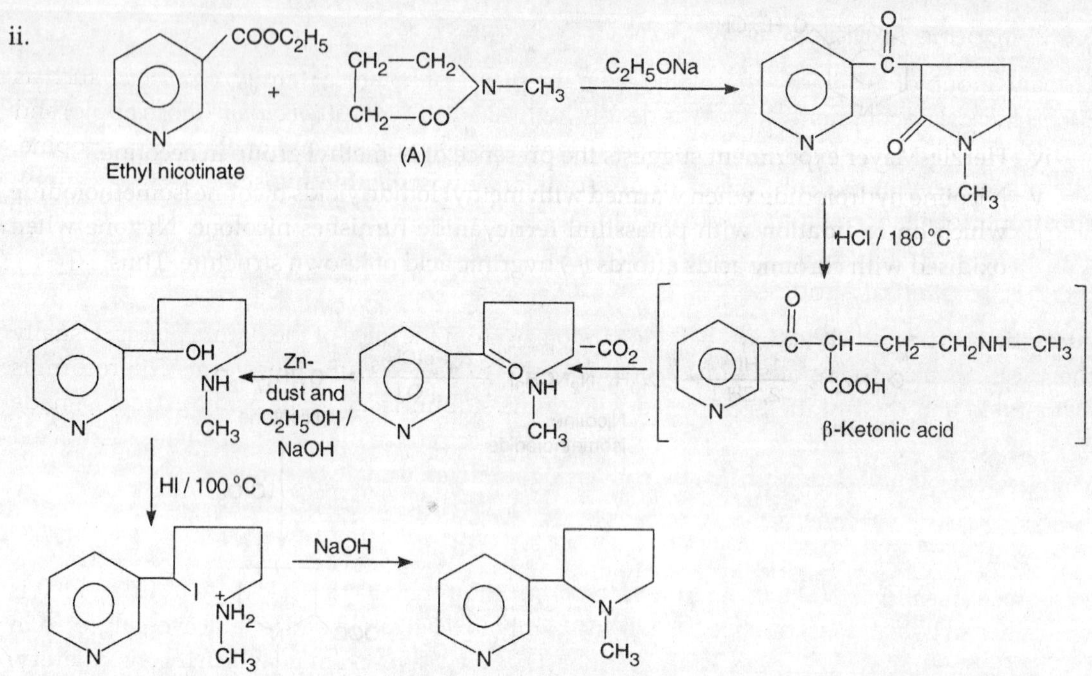

This was resolved by (+)-tartaric acid when natural (–) nicotine is obtained.

(b) *Craig's synthesis*

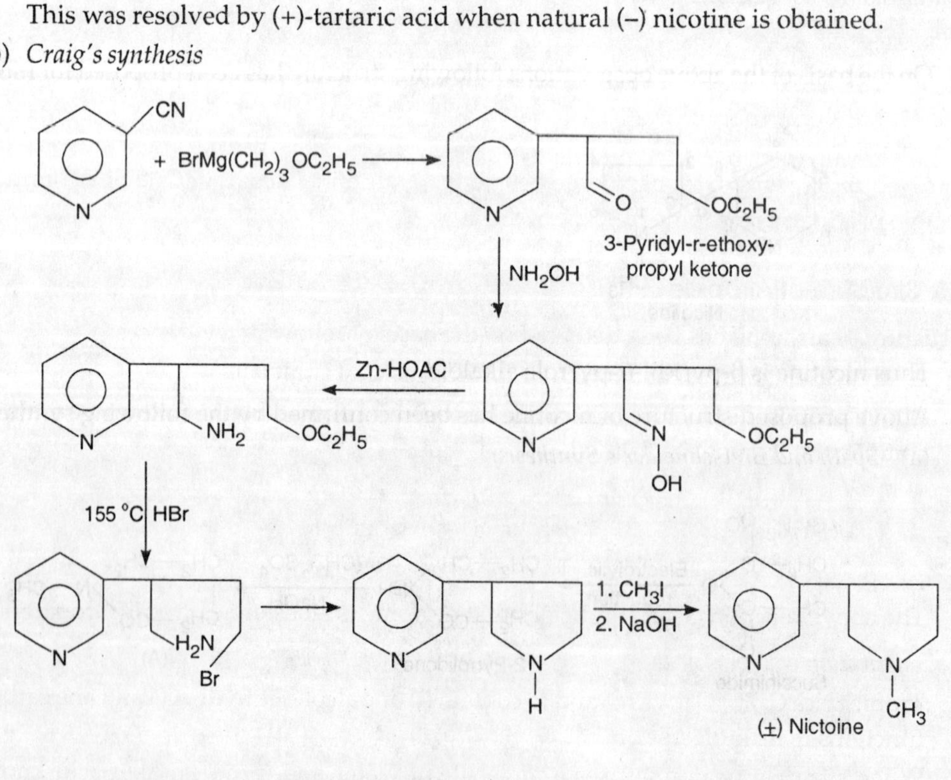

Finally, the product was resolved when (–) nicotine is obtained.

5.8.2 Tropane Alkaloids

Tropane group of alkaloids are isolated from the plants of botanical family. *Solanaceae* such as *Atropa belladonna* commonly known as deadly night shade, *Datura stramonium* (thorn apple) and *Hyoscyamus* niger (henbane). The most important member of this group of alkaloid is atropine. The other members of this group of alkaloids are hyoscyamine hyoscine, (scopolamine), apoatropine, belladomine and norhyoscyamine.

5.8.2.1 Isolation of Atropine

Atropine is extracted either from belladona roots or from the juice of the datura plants. Usually the juice is heated with potassium carbonate and is extracted with chloroform. Chloroform is evaporated and the residue is extracted with dilute sulphuric acid. The acidic extract is made alkaline with potassium carbonate when atropine is precipitated out. The precipitate is extracted with the solvent ether and purified by converting it into an oxalate or sulphate.

5.8.2.2 Properties of Atropine

Atropine is a solid crystalline compound having melting point 118 °C. It has a bitter taste. It is optically inactive and is a tertiary base. It is a highly toxic alkaloid and is fatal even ingested in moderate amount. Atropine is the racemic modification of hyoscyamine which is laevorotatory. It is beleived that atropine does not actually occur in nature. It is an artifat and is formed during the isolation of hyoscyamine.

- *Physiological activity and uses of Atropine:* Atropine dilates the pupil of the eye. A single drop of atropine solution containing 1 part of atropine in 40,000 parts of water is sufficient to dilate the pupil of the eye.

Atropine is extensively used in ophthalmology. It is also used in medicine as a muscle relaxant, and finds application as anti-spasmodic before the abdominal surgery. One of the important marketable products is atropine, BAN, USAN.

5.8.2.3 Structure of Atropine

The structure of atropine has been deduced on the basis of following evidences:

1. Analytical data reveal its molecular formula as $C_{17}H_{23}NO_3$.
2. When atropine is hydrolysed with barium hydroxide tropic acid and an alcoholic component, tropine are formed.

$$C_{17}H_{23}NO_3 \xrightarrow{Ba(OH)_2} \underset{\text{Tropic acid}}{C_9H_{10}O_3} + \underset{\text{Tropine}}{C_8H_{15}NO}$$

The above reaction clearly indicates that atropine is an ester i.e., tropine tropate.

- *Constitution of Tropic acid*

1. Tropic acid, $C_9H_{10}O_3$, was found to contain (i) one alcoholic hydroxyl and one carboxylic functions in its molecule.
2. When strongly heated it loses a molecule of water and forms another acid known as atropic acid which on oxidation yields benzoic acid. i.e.,

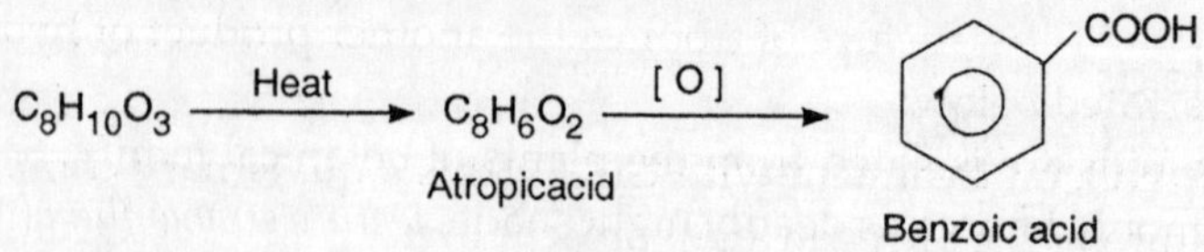

Formation of benzoic acid suggests that atropic acid, hence tropic acid, contains benzene nucleus with one side-chain on which alcoholic hydoxyl group is present. On the basis of above evidence two alternative structures have been proposed for atropic acid.

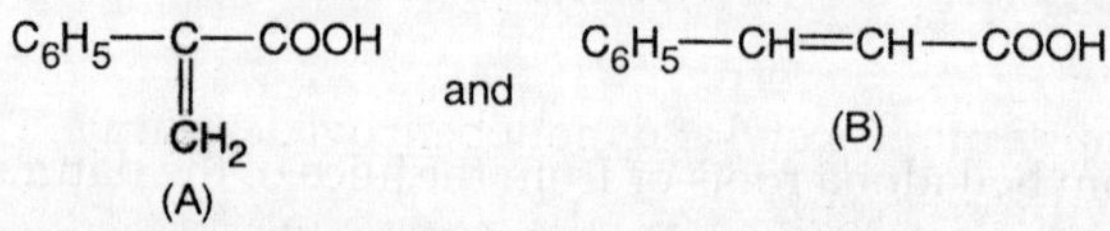

Out of these two, structure (B) is eliminated because it is an well known compound cinnamic acid. So atropic acid is (A). Again, based on the structure (A) for atropine two alternative structures (C) and (D) have been suggested for tropic acid.

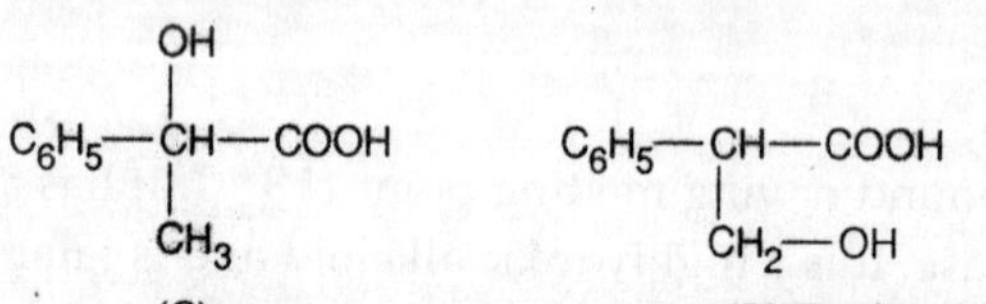

Out of these two structures tropic acid was found to be (D) from its synthesis.

(a) Synthesis due to Mackenzie and Wood:

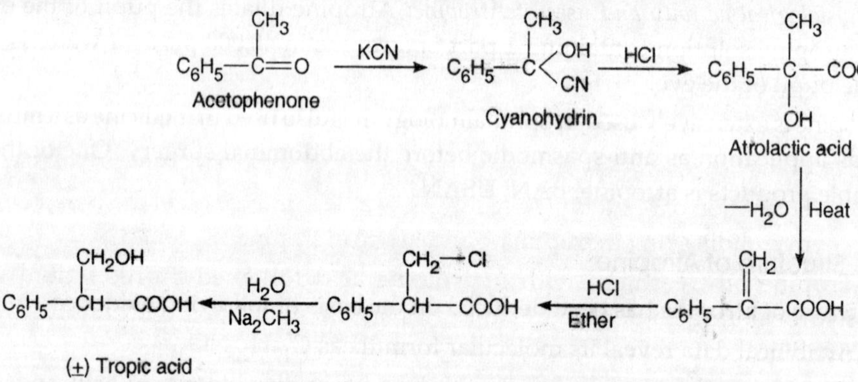

(b) Synthesis of Blicke:

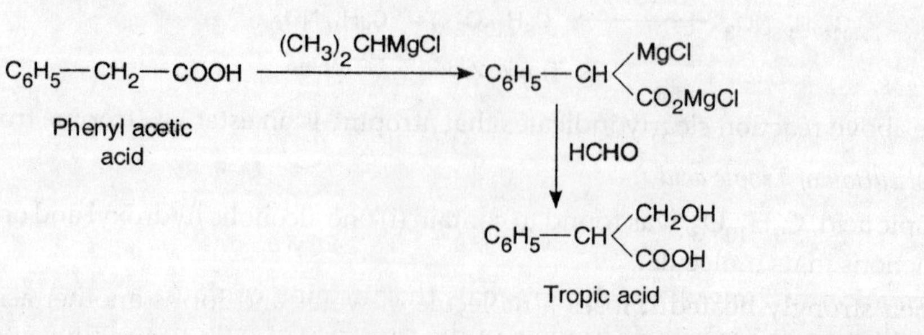

• *Structure of Tropine:* The structure of tropine, the another product of hydrolysis, is based on the evidences as narrated below:

1. Tropine, $C_8H_{15}NO$, on treatment with CH_3I forms a quaternary compound indicating the tertiary nature of the nitrogen atom present in it.
2. When fused with alkali, tropine yields methylamine suggesting the presence of $>N-CH_3$ group in its molecule. This has further been confirmed by the fact that tropine when heated with hydroiodic acid at 150 °C (Herzig Meyer method) affords one molecule of methyl iodide.
3. (a) Tropine readily forms a monoacetyl and monobenzoyl derivative. This indicates that it must contain a hydroxyl group.

   (b) Again, tropine on oxidation with chromic acid furnishes a ketone tropinone which on treatment with nitrous acid affords oximino derivative and on treatment with benzaldehyde yields dibenzylidene derivative indicating thereby (i) the secondary nature of alcoholic group and (ii) the presence of $-CH_2-CO-CH_2$-grouping in the ketone formed and hence $-CH_2-CH(OH)-CH_2-$ functionality is tropine.

   (c) Again, the ketone tropinone, on oxidation forms a dicarboxylic acid, the tropinic acid, $C_8H_{13}NO_4$ without any loss of carbon atoms. It is, therefore, logical to assume that $-CH_2-CO-CH_2-$group in the ketone, tropinone and hence $-CH_2-CH(OH)-CH_2-$ function in tropine must be in a ring.

   (d) On further oxidation with CrO_3/H_2SO_4, tropinic acid yields N-methyl succinic acid.

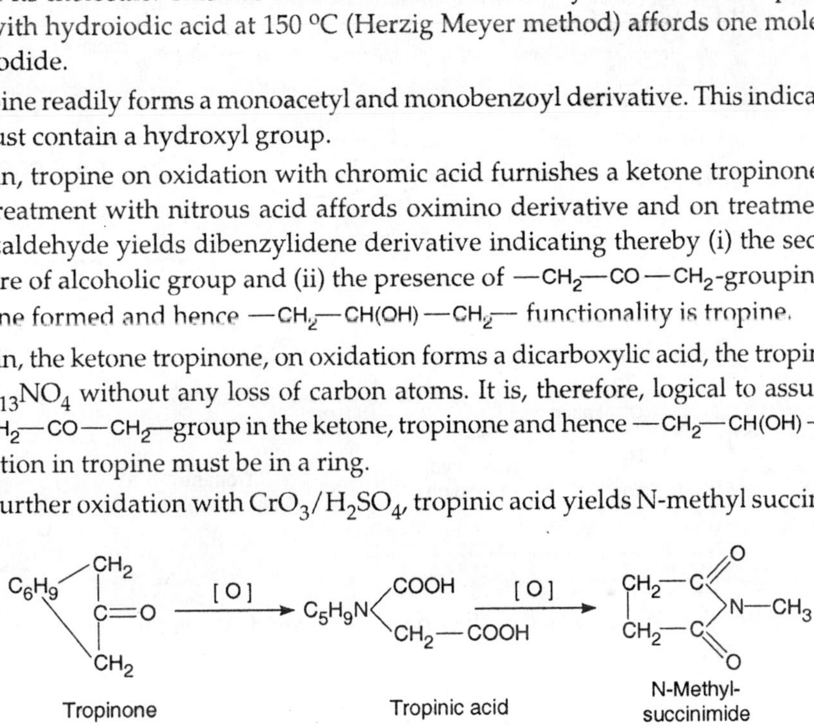

Tropinone — Tropinic acid — N-Methyl-succinimide

   Formation of N-methyl succinimide is a clear indication of the presence of N-methyl pyrrolidine ring in tropinone and hence in tropine.

4. Tropine on treatment with hydroiodic acid followed by reduction with Zn and hydrochloric acid affords tropane. Tropane on distillation with Zn-dust yields 2-ethyl pyridine.

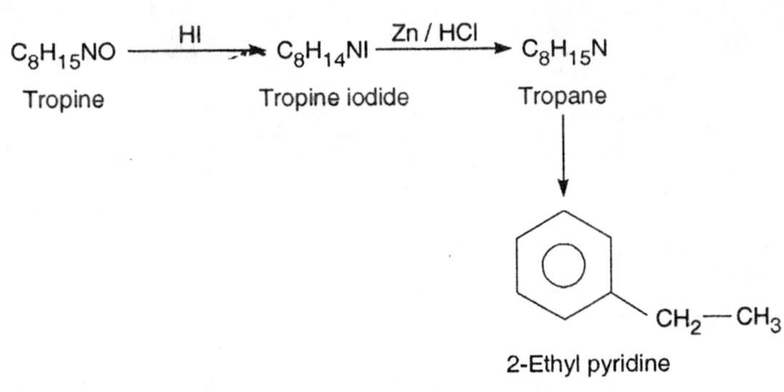

Tropine — Tropine iodide — Tropane — 2-Ethyl pyridine

Formation of 2-ethyl pyridine reveals that tropine contains a piperidine ring with substitution at 2-position. In view of the presence of both pyrrolidine and piperidine ring systems containing only one nitrogen atom it is highly rational to conclude that both the ring systems have been formed around the common nitrogen atom which is tertiary in character and contains a methyl group. Thus a probable structure of tropin has been proposed by Willstatter as below which is capable of explaining the different reactions.

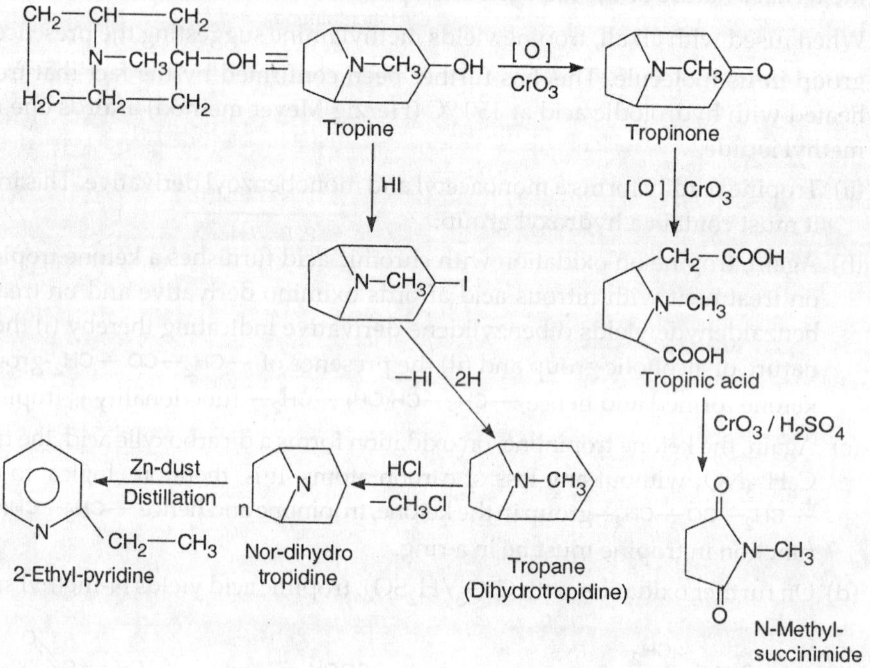

Finally, the above structure has been confirmed by its synthesis due to Willstater as depicted below:

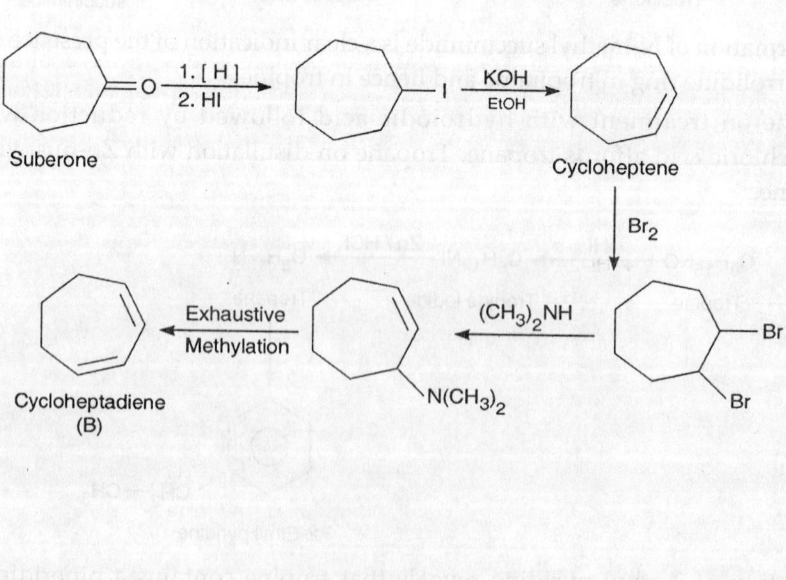

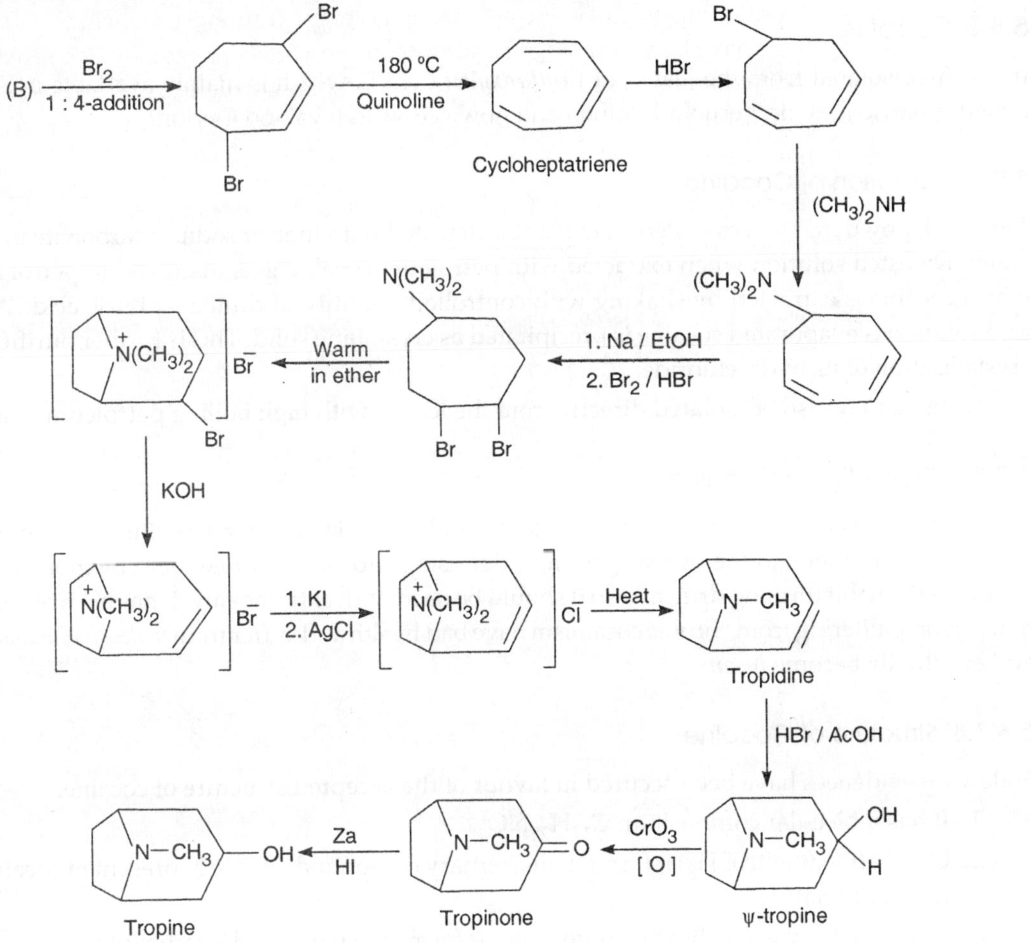

• *Structure of Atropine:* As it has been established before (vide-5.8.3-2) that atropine is an ester of tropic acid and tropine, its structure has been suggested as (A) which has been confirmed by its synthesis from tropine and tropic acid as shown below:

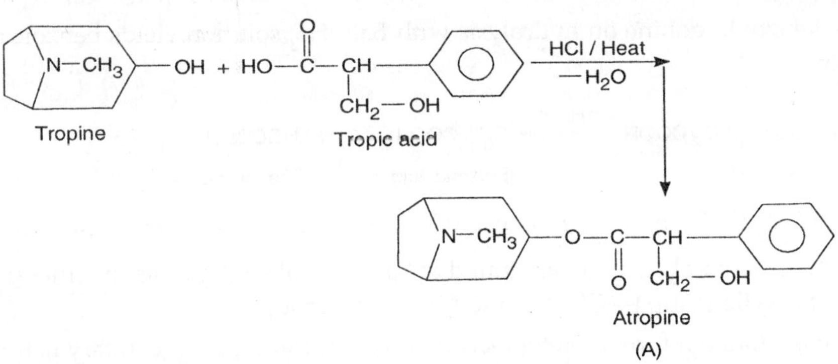

5.8.3 Cocaine

It was first isolated from the leaves of *Erythroxylon Coca* L. which is mainly available in South America particularly in Peru and Bolivia and now grows in Java and Ceylon.

5.8.3.1 Isolation of Cocaine

The dried, powdered leaves of Peruvian plant is digested with lime or sodium carbonate in little water. Digested solution when extracted with petroleum cocaine gets dissolved in petrol from which cocaine is extracted by shaking with controlled quantity of dlute sulphuric acid. When acid solution is evaporated cocaine is precipitated as crystalline solid. This is further purified by crystallisation of its hydrochloride.

Cocaine may also be isolated directly from the leaves with high boiling petroleum ether.

5.8.3.2 Properties of Cocaine

Cocaine is a crystalline solid, m.p. 98 °C. It is sparingly soluble in water. Cocaine hydrochloride is used as anaesthetic in the eye surgery and dentistry. However, it may be remembered that cocaine is the habit forming drug and so it should be used with extreme care. It has been observed that persons suffering from chronic cocainism have bad health and suffer from *widest hallucinations* and eventually become *insane.*

5.8.3.3 Structure of Cocaine

Following evidences have been secured in favour of the accepted structure of cocaine.

i. It has molecular composition $C_{17}H_{21}NO_4$.

ii. On treatment with CH_3I it forms a quarternary compound. Hence N present in cocaine is tertiary in nature.

iii. When hydrolysed by heating with water it forms methanol and a carboxylic compound, benzoyl-ecgonine, i.e.,

$$C_{17}H_{21}NO_4 \xrightarrow{H_2O} \underset{\text{Benzoyl ecgonine}}{C_{15}H_{18}NO_2\,COOH} + CH_3OH$$

This suggests the presence of carbomethoxy group (—$COOCH_3$) in cocaine.

iv. Again, benzoylecgonine on hydrolysis with $Ba(OH)_2$ solution yields benzoic acid and ecgonine.

$$C_{15}H_{18}NO_2\,COOH \xrightarrow{H_2O} \underset{\text{Benzoic acid}}{C_6H_5COOH} + \underset{\text{Ecgonine}}{C_8H_{13}NOCOOH}$$

This syggests that benzoyl ecgonine and hence cocaine contains a benzoyl group.

• *Structure of Ecgonine:* Ecgonine was found to have the following functionalities (i) tertiary N-atom (ii) a carboxylic group (—COOH) and (iii) an OH group.

Further, on oxidation it forms a ketone-ecgoninone indicating the secondary nature of OH group present. The ketone-ecgonione readily loses a molecule of CH_2 and furnishes tropinone.

Tropinone when oxidised with CrO_3 yields tropinic acid and ecgoninic acid.

$$\underset{\text{Ecgonine}}{C_8H_{12}N(OH)COOH} \xrightarrow{[O]} \underset{\text{Ecgoninone}}{C_7H_{11}NCO\ COOH} \xrightarrow{-CO_2} \underset{\text{Tropinone}}{C_8H_{13}NO}$$

$$\underset{\text{Tropinone}}{C_8H_{13}NO} \xrightarrow{[O]} \underset{\text{Ecgoninic acid}}{C_7H_{11}NO_3} + \underset{\text{Tropinic acid}}{C_8H_{13}NO_4}$$

From the above oxidative experiment it is evident that ecgonine contains a *tropane skeleton* in its molecule with hydroxyl function in the same position as in tropine.

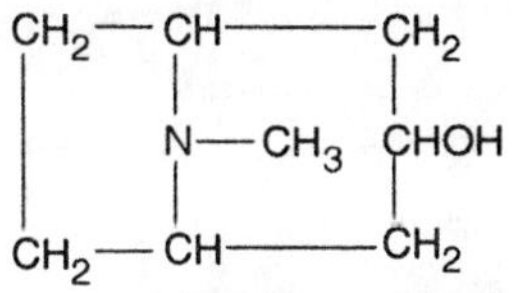

Tropine

Again, easy decarboxylation of ecgonine is a clear evidence that it is a β-keto acid. Thus the structure of ecgonine may be written as shown below:

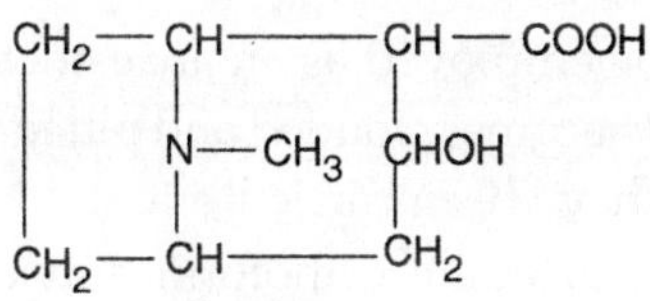

Ecgonine

The above structure of ecgonine has been confirmed by its synthesis.

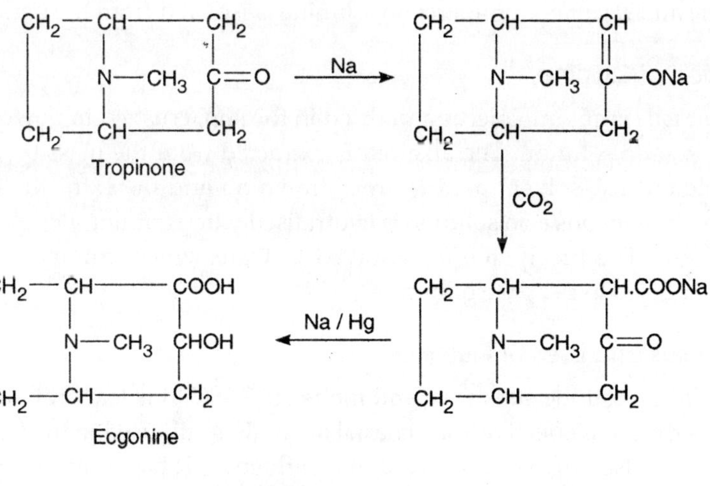

- *Structure of Cocaine:* On the basis of the structure of ecgonine, structure of cocaine logically follows as under:

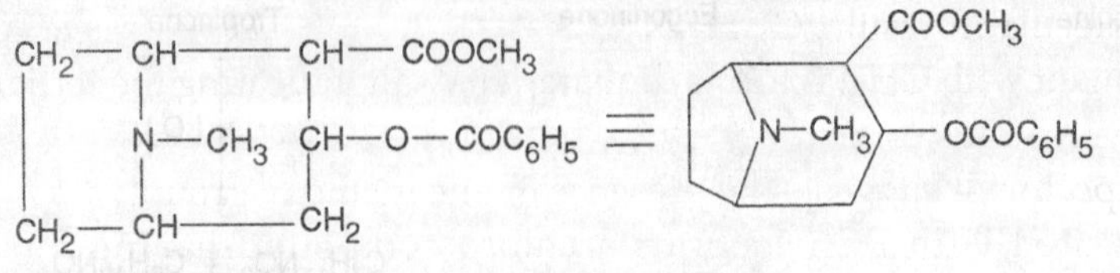

(-) Cocaine

Foddar and his collegues have established the conformation of ecgnine and cocaine as indicated below:

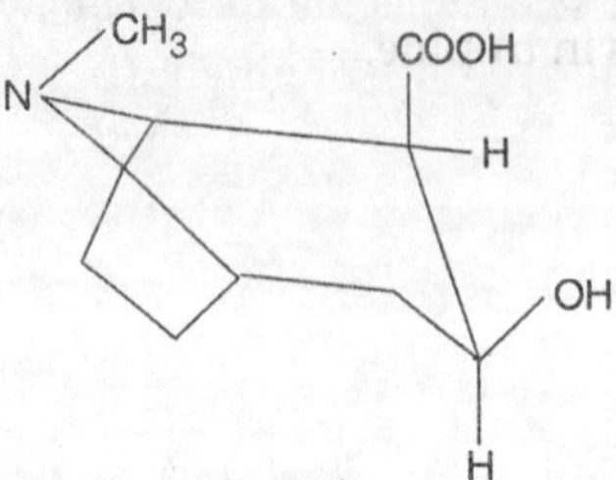

Ecgonine

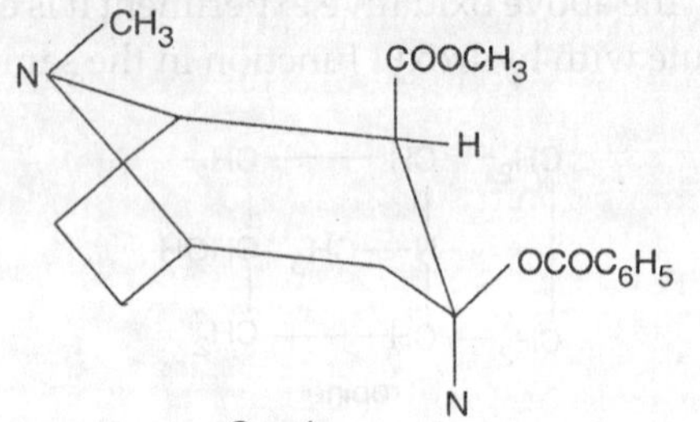

Cocaine

5.8.3.4 Some Substitutes of Cocaine

As mentioned before that although cocaine may be employed as an anaesthetic in eye surgery but its solution is highly harmful for cornea. Cornea becomes clouded and pitted following the use of this drug. For this reason, extensive researches have been carried out and a large number of substitutes of cocaine have been synthesised such as procaine, orthoform, amylcaine, eucaine etc.

5.8.4 Quinoline Alkaloid

The representative member of this group of alkaloids is quinine. It occurs in the bark of the genera *Cinchona* and *Ramifia*. Commercially quinine is isolated from the bark of *Cinchona*.

5.8.4.1 Isolation of Quinine

The bark of *Cinchona* is cut into pieces and dried in the sun, crushed to powder and mixed with lime and caustic soda solution. The alkaloid is extracted from the mass by repeated digestion with hot petroleum. The solvent petroleum is drawn off and the extract is treated with dilute sulphuric acid. The aqueous acid solution is neutralised when quinine along with other alkaloids is precipitated out. The precipitate is dissolved in water when quinine crystallises out. It is repeatedly crystallised to get pure quinine.

5.8.4.2 Properties and Uses of Quinine

Quinine is a solid crystalline substance and melts at 177 °C. It is leavorotatory and has a bitter taste. Quinine is the most effective antimalarial agent. It is still used in the treatment of malaria. In small doses it is also employed for cold and influenza. It has found to be effective as local anaesthetic, analgesic, cardiovascular stimulant and as bactericide. It is also used in the resolution of optically active enantiomers.

5.8.4.3 Constitution of Quinine

The structure of quinine has been deduced from the following evidences.

i. It has molecular formula, $C_{20}H_{24}N_2O_2$.

ii. On treatment with CH_3I it forms diquaternary salt indicating the tertiary nature of both the nitrogen atoms.

iii. Zeisel experiment suggests the presence of one methoxy group.

iv. When treated with PCl_5 it forms a chloro compound having molecular formula, $C_{20}H_{23}N_2OCl$. This suggests the presence of alcoholic hydroxyl function in quinine.

v. On careful oxidation with CrO_3 it forms a ketone. So the alcoholic OH group is secondary in nature.

vi. When oxidised with $KMnO_4$ there is formation of one molecule of formic acid and a carboxylic compound. This is a clear evidence for the presence of vinylic ($-CH{=}CH_2$) side-chain in quinine.

vii. Quinine on fusion with KOH forms two known compounds.

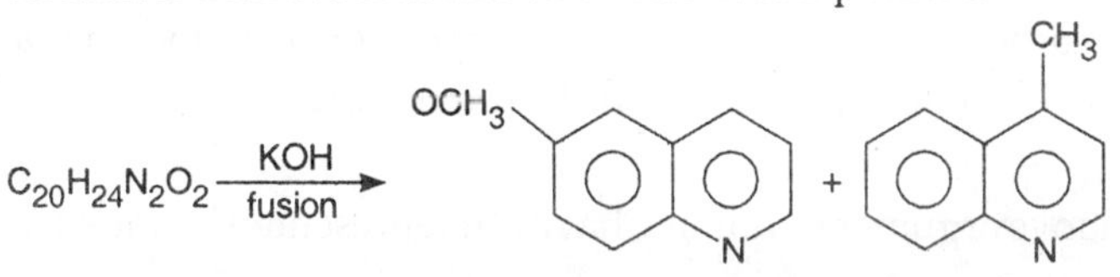

6-Methoxy quinoline 4-Methyl quinoline (Lepidine)

Formation of these two compounds suggests that out of two N-atoms in quinine one is present in quinoline ring system while second one is present in piperidine skeleton.

viii. Chloro quinine obtained by the treatment of quinine with PCl_5 is heated with alcoholic KOH when elimination of HCl occurs and an olefinic compound is formed which on hydrolytic cleavage yields 6-methoxy lepidine and meroquine. The structure of meroquinene has been deduced from chemical as well as physico-chemical evidences. Thus,

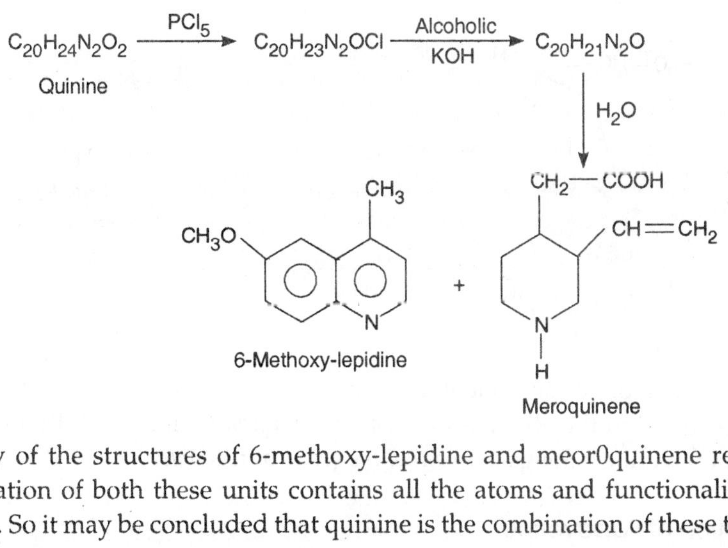

6-Methoxy-lepidine Meroquinene

Scrutiny of the structures of 6-methoxy-lepidine and meor0quinene reveals that the combination of both these units contains all the atoms and functionalities present in quinine. So it may be concluded that quinine is the combination of these two fragments.

- *Mode of attachment of 6-methoxy-lepidine and meroquinene in quinine:* In combining these two units following points are to be remembered.

i. Quinine has a secondary alcoholic OH group.
ii. Both the N atoms are tertiary in nature.
iii. Quinine has no COOH group in its molecule.

It is known that the carbon atom when present at 4-position in quinoline ring becomes very active. So it is logical to assume that he methyl carbon atom at 4-position of 6-methoxy-lepidine is most probably the point of attachment of 6-methoxy-lepidine portion with meroquinene.

Again, quinine does not contain any COOH function in its molecule. It has been generated during the hydrolytic cleavage. So it is rational to conclude that carboxylic carbon of meroquinene is the connecting point with quinoline portion.

Once again, quinine has no secondary nitrogen atom. But N-atom in meroquinene is present as secondary. So it may be logically assumed that both the carboxylic group and secondary nitrogen atom in meroquinene have been generated during the cleavage of quinine. Most probable explanation of formation of both these functionalities by a single step is that the secondary N-atom and carboxylic carbon of meroquinene portion are connected together attributing tertiary character of N-atom in quinine. Or in other words, meroquinene part exists as a bicyclic system in quinine.

On the basis of above arguments, quinine has been represented by the structure given below:

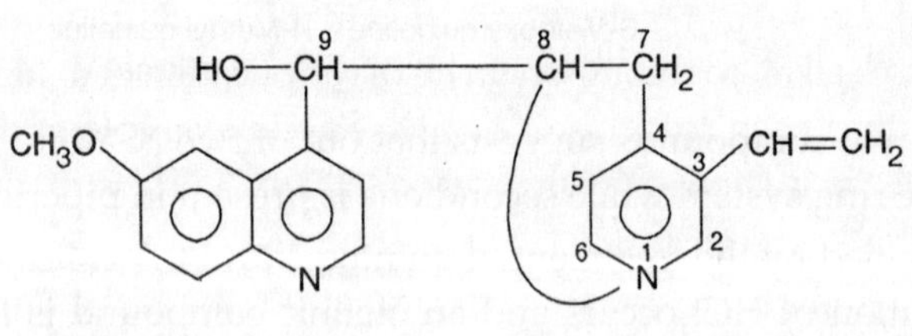

The above structure has finally been confirmed by synthesis. This structure has four chiral centres, viz., C_3, C_4, C_8 and C_9. Configuration at these centres have been settled from chemical degradations and the stereoconfigurational structure has been represented by the following expression:

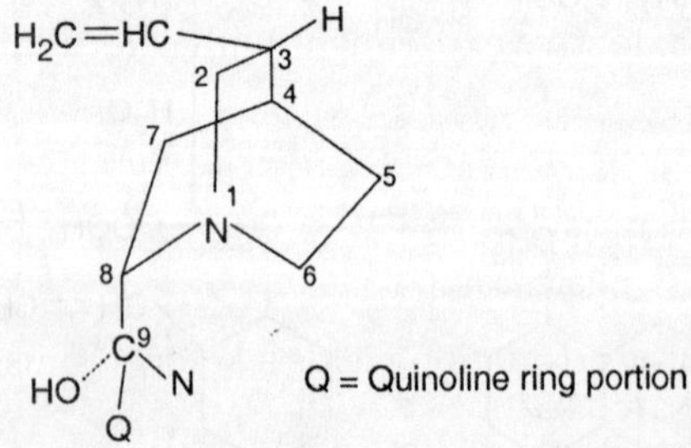

5.8.5 Papaverine

One of the major alkaloidal components of opium is papaverine. It occurs to the extent of 0.5-1% in opium. It is found in the all parts of *Papaver somniferum* Linn specially in unripe capsules. Structurally, papaverine belongs to *isoquinoline group of alkaloids.*

5.8.5.1 Isolation of Papaverine

The dried latex from unripe seed capsules of poppy is digested with lime water when morphine group of alkaloids remain in solution but the alkaloids belonging to papaverine family are precipitated. Precipitate is filtered and the residue is extracted with an organic solvent like chloroform, ether, etc. Papaverine obtained by fractional precipitation from the mixture is oxalate and is purified by crystallisation.

5.8.5.2 Properties of Papaverine

Papaverine is a colourless solid, m.p. 147 °C. It is an optically inactive tertiary base, pk_a 6.2. It forms salts and a methoiodide. It is almost insoluble in water but soluble in hot alcohol and chloroform. Physiologically it is less active than morphine. It is used as an *antispasmodic* for the relaxation of *cardiac muscles* and in the remedy of coughs. In low doses it causes light sleep but in higher doses it causes tetanus and respitatory paralysis.

5.8.5.3 Uses of Papaverine

Papaverine finds use in the following areas:

(a) It is used as a non-selective mild muscle relaxant particularly for the cardiac muscles.

(b) It is also used as mild analgesic and local anaesthetic agents.

5.8.5.4 Structure of Papaverine

Goldschmiedt and his associates during the period from 1883-1888 has been successful in elaborating the structure of this alkaloidal component by the application of oxidative degradative experiments and their work has been recognised as a very good example of the application of oxidative degradation for the elucidation of the structure of alkaloids. The structure of papaverine has been elaborated from the evidences as described in sequel.

1. Analytical data and molecular weight determination suggest that papaverine has molecular formula, $C_{20}H_{21}NO_4$.
2. On treatment with CH_3I papaverine forms a quaternary salt indicating thereby the tertiaty nature of the N-atom present in its molecule.
3. Zeisel experiment reveals the presence of four methoxyl groups in papaverine.
4. When papaverine is subjected to oxidative experiment with cold dilute permanganate an alcohol is formed, i.e.,

$$\underset{\text{Papaverine}}{C_{20}H_{21}NO_4} \xrightarrow[\text{Dil.KMnO}_4]{[O]} \underset{\text{Papaverinol}}{(C_{19}H_{19}NO_4)CHOH}$$

Papaverinol, thus, formed on vigorous oxidation yields a ketone. Thus,

$$(C_{19}H_{19}NO_4)CHOH \xrightarrow{[O]} \underset{\text{Papaveraldine}}{(C_{19}H_{19}NO_4)\!>\!C{=}O}$$

Formation of ketone from the alcohol is a clear indication that papaverinol is a secondary alcohol. It may be mentioned that both the alcohol and the ketone contain all the four methoxyl functions and the tertiary N-atom of papaverine. Formation of secondary alcohol and ketone without any loss of other functional groups during oxidative experiment with permanganate is a clear indication that papaverine contains an active methylene ($>CH_2$) group in its molecule. Thus a part structure of papaverine may be written as:

$$\left[C_{15}H_7 \right] \begin{matrix} (OCH_3)_4 \\ -CH_2 \\ \rightarrow N \end{matrix}$$

• *Nature of the Skeleton:* The nature of the skeleton present in papaverine molecule has been deduced from the following degradative experiment. Papaverine when fused with KOH it undergoes cleavage with the formation of two fragments, A, $C_{11}H_{11}O_2N$ and B, $C_9H_{12}O_2$.

$$C_{20}H_{21}O_4N \xrightarrow[\text{KOH}]{\text{Fused with}} \underset{(A)}{C_{11}H_{11}O_2N} + \underset{(B)}{C_9H_{12}O_2}$$

• *Identification of the Fragment (A)*

i. Fragment (A) was found to be basic in nature and contains a tertiary N-atom as is evidenced from the formation of quaternary salt with CH_3I.

ii. Zeisel experiment clearly establishes the presence of two methoxyl group in this fragment. Thus the part structure of (A) may be expressed as.

$$\left[C_9H_5 \right] \begin{matrix} (OCH_3)_2 \\ \rightarrow N \end{matrix}$$

Extremely low content of hydrogen in (A) reveals that this fragment is most probably cyclic and unsaturated in nature. This assumption has been corroborated by the experiments described below:

$$\underset{(A)}{\left[C_9H_5N \right] (OCH_3)_2} \xrightarrow[\text{with HI (Zeisel)}]{\text{Demethylation}} \left[C_9H_5N \right] (OH)_2 \xrightarrow{\text{Zn-dust distillation}}$$

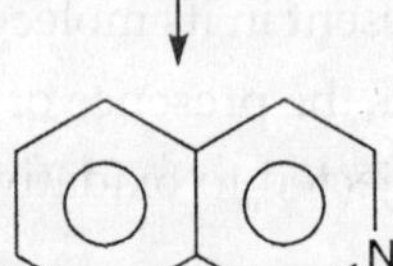

(C_9H_7N)
Isoquinoline

From the above experiments it is evident that the frequent (A), is a dimethoxy isoquinoline derivative as expreseed below:

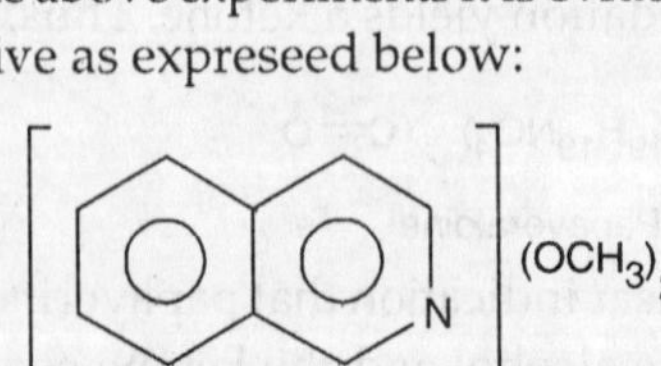

• *Location of Methoxyl Groups:* The location of two methoxyl groups in (A) has been settled from the oxidation of this fragment with permanganate solution in neutral medium. On such oxidation fragment (A) yields a dimethoxy dicarboxylic benzene derivative. This acid when heated with sodalime furnishes a known compound, veratrole, suggesting thereby the *ortho* relationship of the two methoxy groups in this portion. Again, this acid readily forms an anhydride on heating with acetic anhydride. This reveals that two carboxylic groups in this acid must be in *ortho* positions. i.e.,

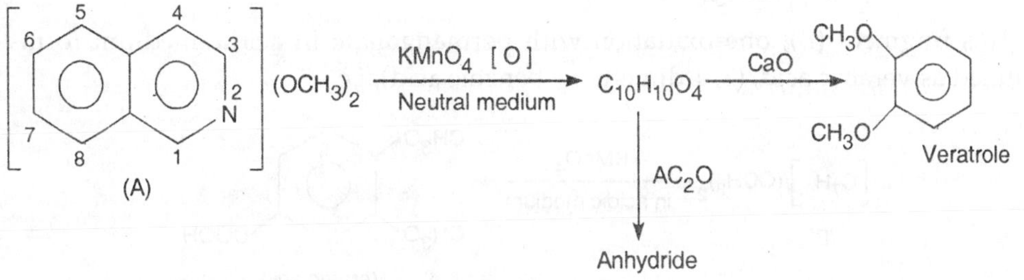

On the basis of above evidences the acid was identified as metahemipinic acid (4, 5-dimethoxy, 1, 2-dicarboxylic benzene as shown below:

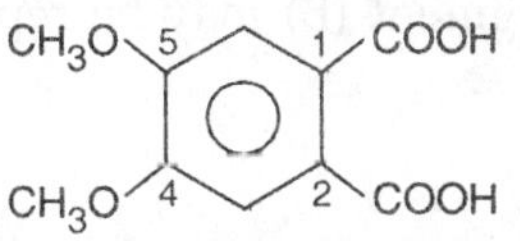

Formation of metahemipinic acid clearly indicates that the two methoxy groups in the fragment (A) are located at 6 and 7 positions of isoquinoline ring, i.e.,

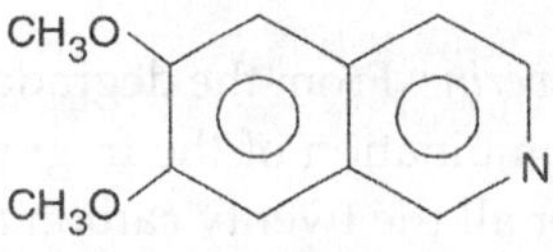
(A)

The above structure of the fragment (A) has been confirmed by its synthesis from veratraldehyde.

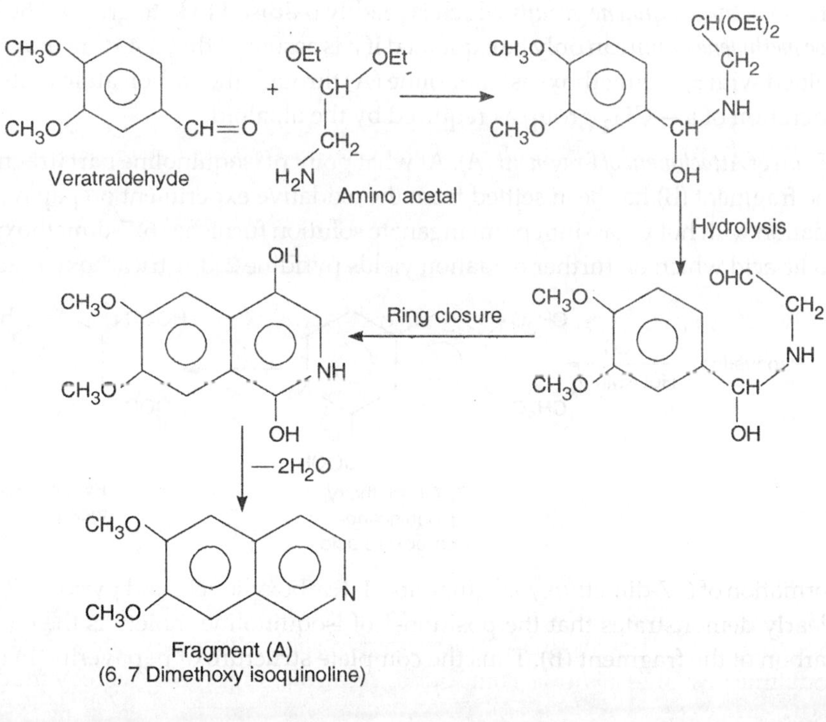

Fragment (A)
(6, 7 Dimethoxy isoquinoline)

• *Characterisation of the Fragment (B):* The fragment (B), was found to have two methoxyl groups as evidenced from Zeisel experiment and hence its part structure may be expressed as indicated below:

$$[C_7H_6](OCH_3)_2$$

This fragment (B), one oxidation with permanganate in acidic medium forms an acid identified as veratric acid, (3, 4-dimethoxy benzoic acid), i.e.,

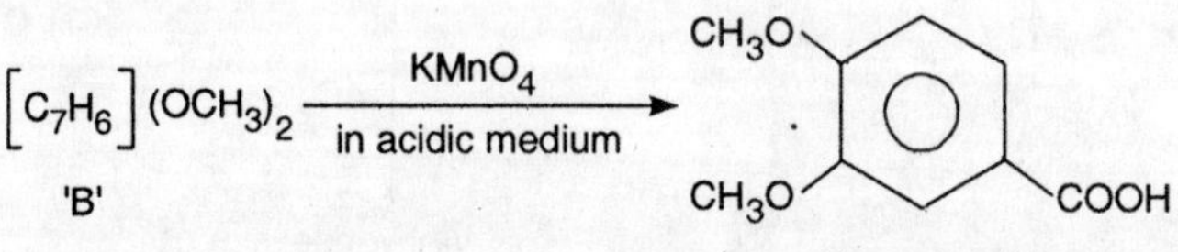

Veratric acid

A careful analysis of the product of oxidation clearly reveals that the C_7H_6 portion of this fragment contains a methylbenzene moiety. So the fragment (B) may be represented by the structure indicated below:

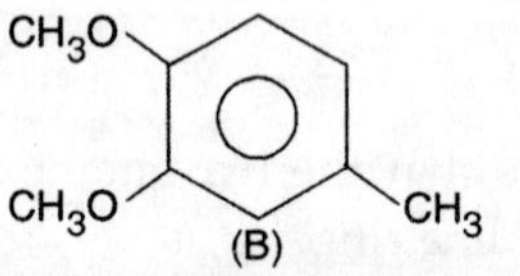

(B)
3, 4-Dimethoxy toluene

• *Mode of Linkage of the Fragments (A) and (B) in Papaverine:* From the degradative experiment discussed above it is evident that papaverine is the combination of the fragments (A) and (B) because combination of both the fragments account for all the twenty carbon atoms present in the alkaloid. Now the question arises how, these two fragments are joined to each other?

• *Point of Attachment of (B):* In answering this question it may be mentioned that papaverine: contains an *active methylene groups* which is readily oxidised to keto group. The presence of such an *active methylene group* can only be explained if it is assumed that 3, 4-dimethoxy toluene portion. (B) is joined with 6, 7-dimethoxy isoquinoline (A) through the carbon atom of its CH_3 group with the generation of a —CH_2-group as required by the alkaloid.

• *Point of Attachment of Fragment (A):* At what point of isoquinoline part (fragment (A) is linked with the fragment (B) has been settled from the oxidative experiment on papaverine. Papaverine on oxidation with hot potassium permanganate solution furnishes 6, 7-dimethoxy-isoquinoline-1-carboxylic acid which on further oxidation yields pyridine 2, 3, 4-tricarboxylic acid.

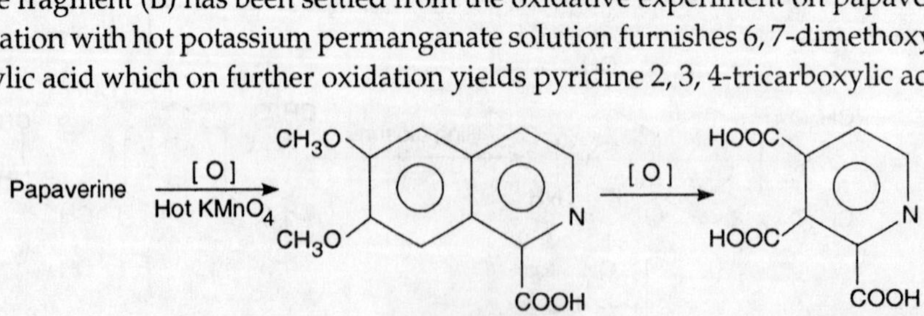

6, 7-Dimethoxy isoquinoline-1-carboxylic acid

Pyridine 2, 3, 4 tricarboxylic acid

Formation of 6, 7-dimethoxy-isoquinoline-1-1carboxylic acid and pyridine 2, 3, 4-tricarboxylic acid clearly demonstrates that the position-1 of isoquinoline moiety is the connecting point of CH_3 carbon of the fragment (B). Thus the complete structure of papaverine may be represented as:

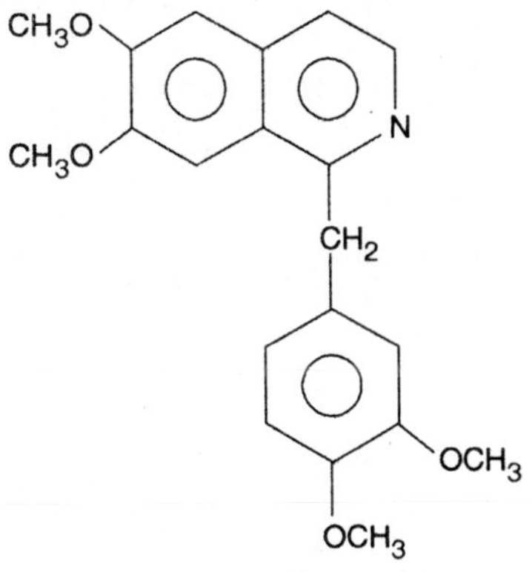

Papaverine

Finally, the above structure of papaverine has been confirmed by the following synthesis:

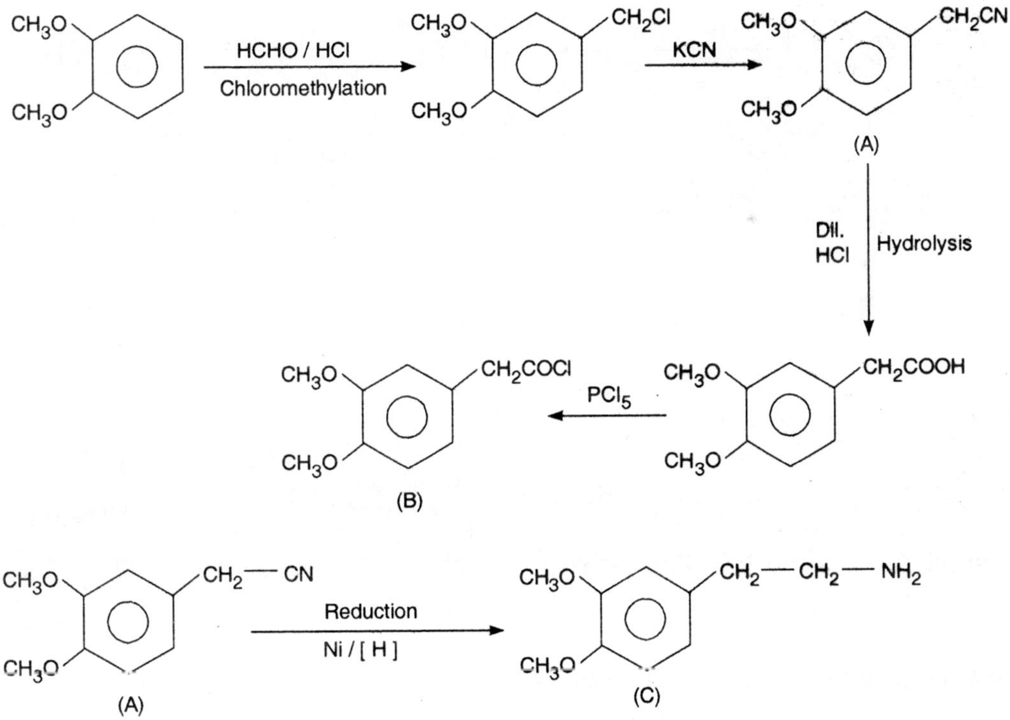

Combination of (B) and (C)

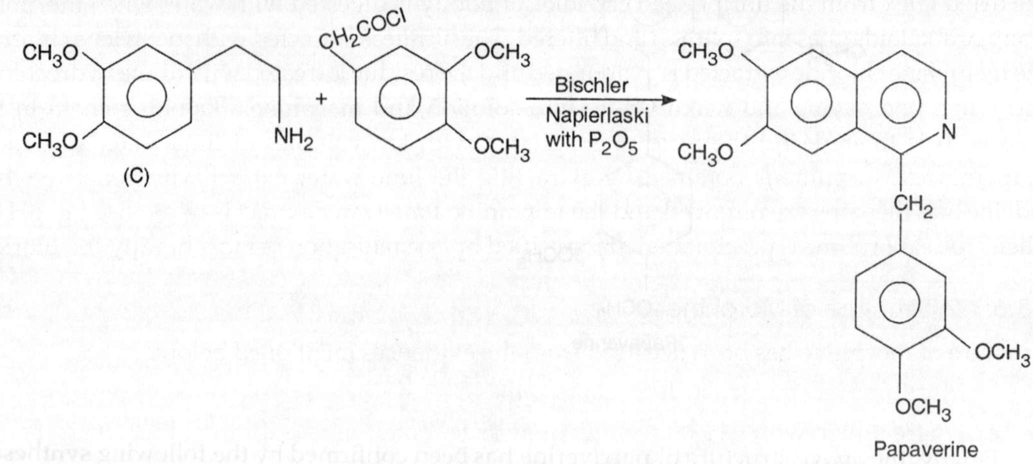

5.8.5.5 Conversion of Papaverine to Pavine

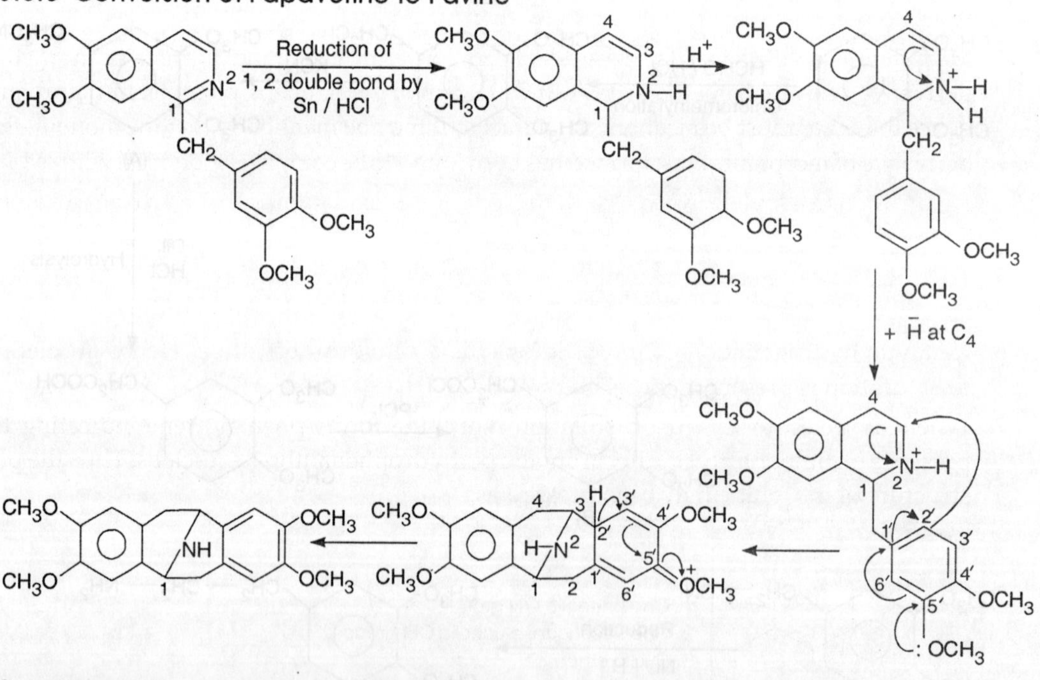

5.8.6 Phenanthrene Group of Alkaloids

5.8.6.1 Morphine

Morphine is the most important member of phenanthrene group of alkaloids. It is the chief alkaloid in opium and is present in approximately 20%. It is the first alkaloid to be isolated from opium plant, *Papaver somniferum.* Two other closely related alkaloids are codeine and thebaine. These three alkaloids are commonly known as *morphine alkaloids.* Due to the presence of phenanthrene nucleus in these alkaloids they are also known as phenanthrene alkaloids. Morphine alkaloids are extensively studied group of alkaloids.

5.8.6.1.1 Isolation of Morphine Alkaloids

The dried latex from the unripe seed capsules of poppy is digested with water when morphine group of alkaloids goes into solution and filtered. The filtrate is extracted with methylene chloride. The methylene chloride extracted is evaporated and the residue is treated with dilute hydrochloric acid when papaverine and narcotine go into solution and morphine alkaloids remain in the residue. It is filtered and the residue is agitated with ten volumes of lime water at a room temperature. Morphine is obtained by extracting the lime water extract with benzene when codeine and thebaine are removed and the remaining lime water extract is neutralised to pH 8.0 when crude morphine is precipitated. It is purified by crystallisation as morphine hydrochloride.

5.8.6.1.2 Structure of Morphine

Structure of morphine has been deduced from the evidences mentioned below:

1. Morphine has molecular formula $C_{17}H_{19}NO_3$.
2. On treatment with CH_3I it forms a quaternary compound indicating the tertiary nature of nitrogen atom.
3. On acetylation it forms a diacetate suggesting the presence of two hydroxyl functions in its molecule.
4. Morphine is soluble in alkali, gives colouration with $FeCl_3$ and forms a monomethyl derivative with diazomethane. So out of two hydroxyls, one is phenolic in nature and hence the other must be alcoholic in character. It may be mentioned that the monomethyl derivative of morphine, thus, formed has been found to be completely identical with *codeine.*
   Again, monomethyl derivative (codeine) on careful oxidation with CrO_3 forms a ketone. So the alcoholic OH group is secondary in nature.
5. The third oxygen atom was found to be extremely inert in nature and so it has been assumed that the third oxygen atom is present as a cyclic ether in morphine.
6. Catalytic hydrogenation of morphine yields a dihydro derivative. Hence an olefinic unsaturation is present in morphine.
7. When subjected to Zn-dust distillation morphine forms phenanthrene indicating the presence of either partly or fully aromatic perhydrophenanthrene nucleus. Thus the part structure of morphine may be expressed as:

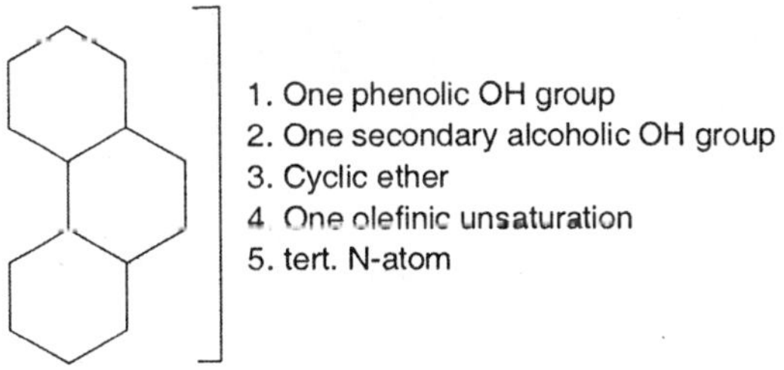

(Partly or fully aromatic)
(B)

• *Nature of* N-*Containing Chain:* Actual nature of nitrogen containing chain in morphine has been ascertained from the following sequence of experiments.

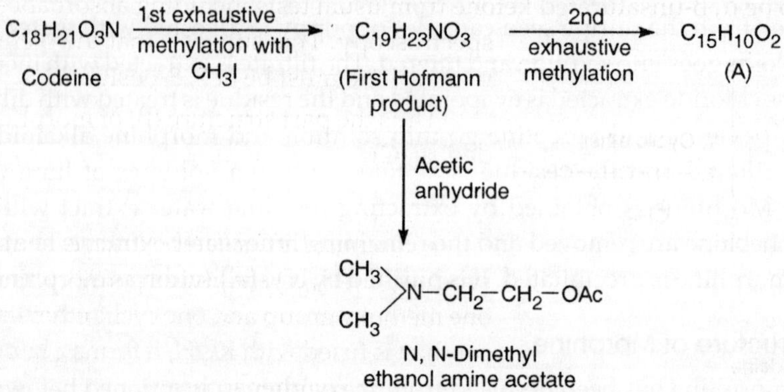

Since nitrogen atom is not eliminated during first Hofmann's exhaustive methylation experiment but requires second successive exhaustive methylation, *nitrogen in morphine is present in a ring.*

It is known that during exhaustive methylation of tertiary nitrogen atom only one methyl group is attached to nitrogen atom. So the formation of N, N-dimethyl ethanol amine acetate is a clear evidence that morphine must contain a chain $CH_3-\overset{|}{N}-CH_2-CH_2-$ (ethanamine chain) in its molecule.

- *Location of Phenolic and alcoholic hydroxyls in Morphine:* Location of these two functionalities has been settled from the following experiment:

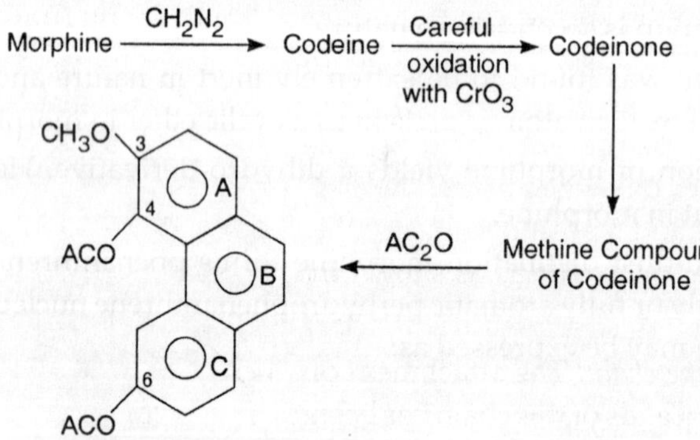

3-Methoxy, 4, 6-acetoxy phenanthrene
(A known compound)

The methoxy group at 3-position in the known phenanthrene derivative finds its origin from the methoxy group of condeinone and hence in codeine. So OCH_3 *group in codeine or phenolic-*OH group in morphine must be at 3-position of perhydrophenanthrene nucleus. Again, as phenolic-OH group is at 3-position ring (A) must be aromatic in character.

It is known that keto group on treatment with acetic anhydride generates acetoxy group. Therefore, out of two acetoxy groups, one must be from the keto group of codeinone. As the ring (A) is aromatic so keto group cannot be present in the ring (A). So acetoxy group at 6-position must be due to keto group. So alcoholic —OH group in codeine and morphine must be at 6-position.

• *Site of olefinic unsaturation in Morphine:* The oxidation product of codeine, i.e., codeinone was found to be α, β-unsaturated ketone from usual tests including absorbance maxima in UV-spectroscopy. This suggests that the olefinic unsaturation in morphine must be at 7, 8-positions.

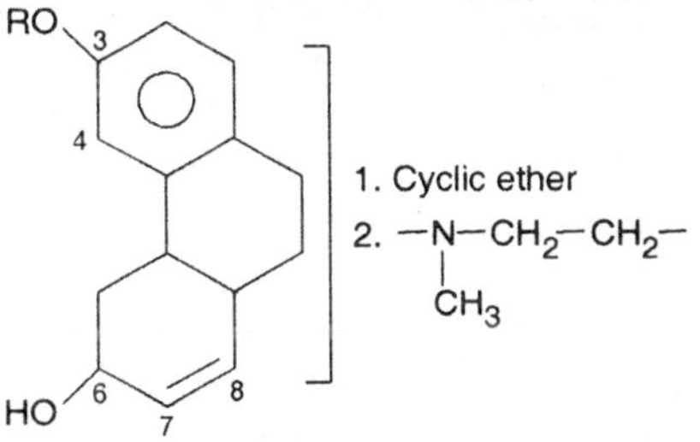

(C)
R = HO Morphine
R = CH_3, Codeine

Thus the part structure (B) of morphine may be extended as (C).

• *Placement of Cyclic ether linkage:* The second Hofmann product, $C_{15}H_{10}O_2$ (A) (vide p. 692) was found to contain one methoxy group and one cyclic ether linkage. When this product is fused with KOH, it forms a known compound 3, 4, 5-trihydroxy phenanthrene, i.e.,

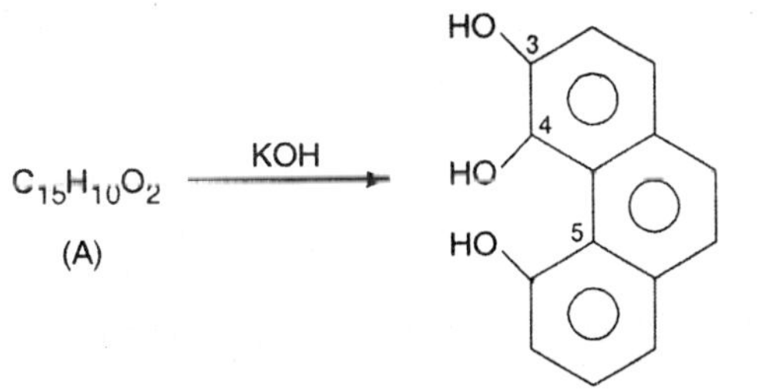

3, 4, 5-Trihydroxy phenanthrene

It is known that any ether when fused with KOH is converted to two - OH groups. Thus, of the three hydroxyl functions in the known compound one finds its origin from methoxy group and other two from cyclic ether linkage. The —OH group at 3-position is originated from —OCH_3 group and so —OH groups at 4 and 5 positions must be derived from cyclic ether linkage. Thus cyclic ether linkage in morphine and codeine must be in between 4 and 5 positions. Hence the part structure (C) may further be extended as shown in (D).

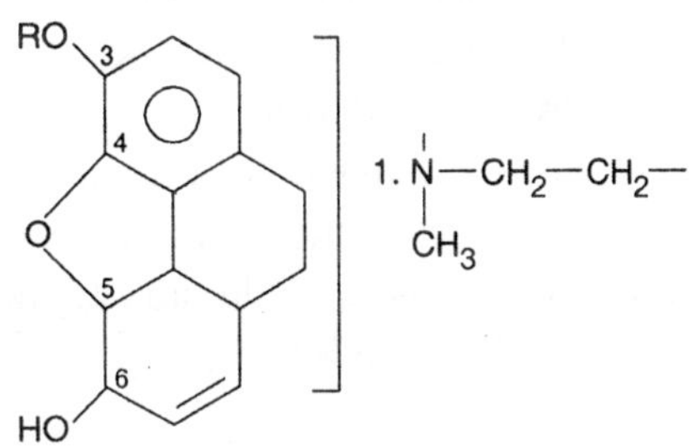

(D)
R = H, Morphine
R = CH_3, Codeine

• *Attachment of Ethanamine chain:* The attachment of two ends—nitrogen and carbon ends of this chain has been settled from the following experiments:

(a) *Connection of nitrogen end:*

Codeine on oxidation by CrO_3 forms in addition to the expected product, codeinone, an unexpected product identified as 10-Hydroxy codeine. When this newly formed 10-hydroxy codeine is subjected to exhaustive methylation (Hofmann's elimination) there is formation of a ketone with the elimination of nitrogen containing chain. This ketone was found *not to be α, β unsaturated* ketone which suggests that it is the OH group at 10 position which has been converted to keto group during Hofmann's degradation. This is only possible if N-atom of ethanamine chain is connected at the adjacent position of newly introduced OH group. Thus, N-atom of this chain is connected at 9 position and so the structure (D) may be extended to (E)

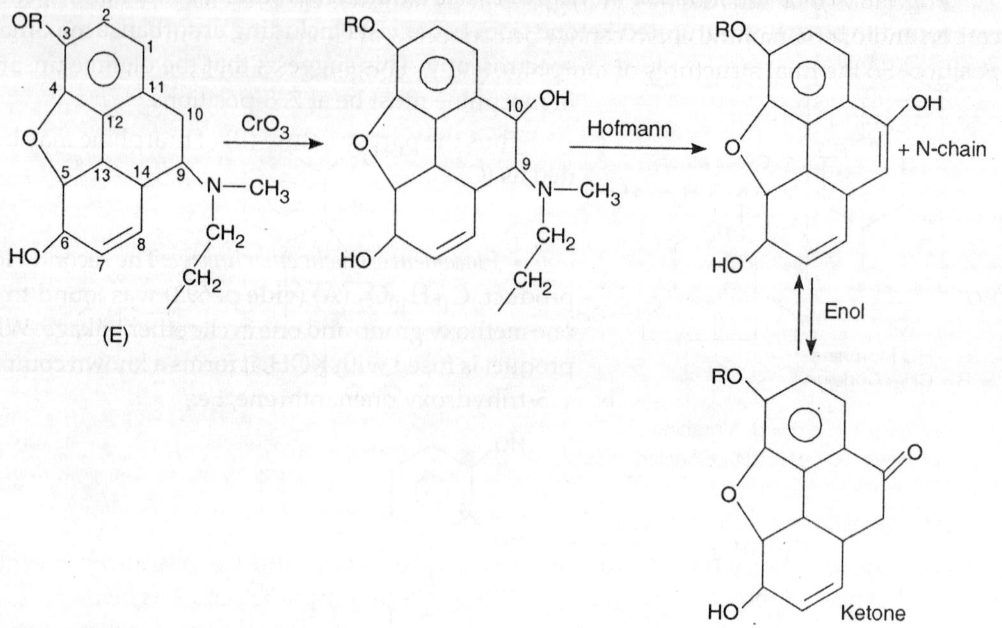

(b) *Position of Carbon end:*

Ethanamine chain in morphine cannot survive during any chemical experiment. This suggests that the carbon end is connected to any angular position. There are three such angular positions, viz., 5, 13 and 14 positions in morphine molecule. Out of these three positions, 14 has been excluded on the ground that thebaine, the very closely related congener of morphine and codeine, has a double bond and C_8—C_{14} position.

[Thebaine contains two—OCH_3 groups, and—two double bonds which are conjugated and on hydrolysis with dilute H_2SO_4 it readily forms codeinone].

The choice in between remaining two positions—5 and 13 has been decided by Beckmann transformation on the oxime of dihydrocodeinone when an aldehydic compound is formed. The formation of an aldehyde can only be explained if there are cleavages of C_5—C_6 and C_5-Oxygen bonds as shown below:

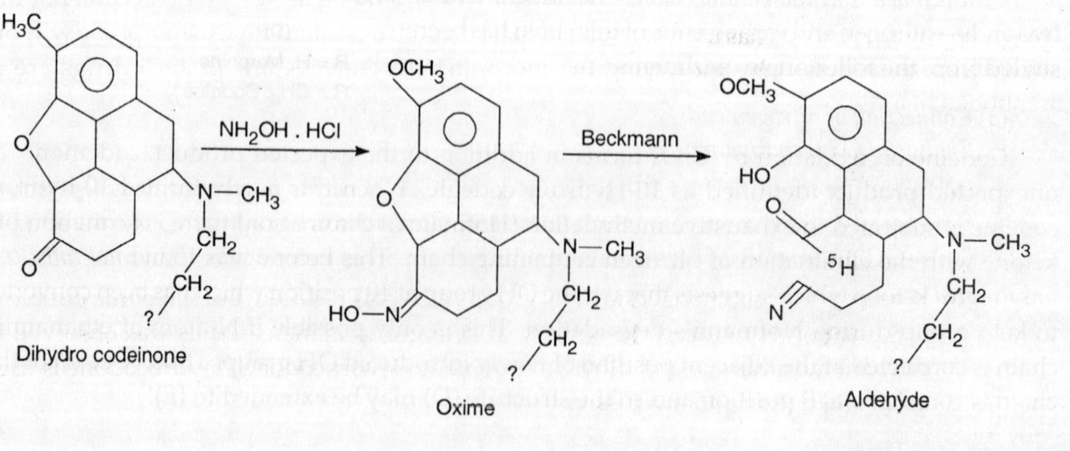

Formation of aldehydic (—CHO) group at C_5 indicates the presence of H atom at C_5. Hence carbon end of ethanamine chain cannot be connected at C_5 and thus it must be attached to C_{13} position. So the final structures of morphine and its congeners stand as below:

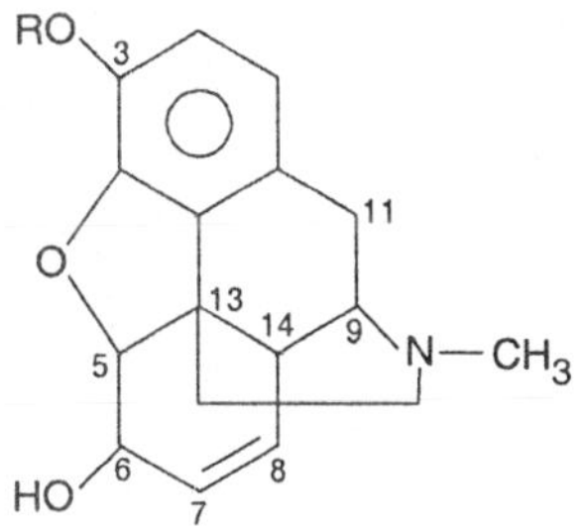

R = H, Morphine
R = CH_3, Codeine

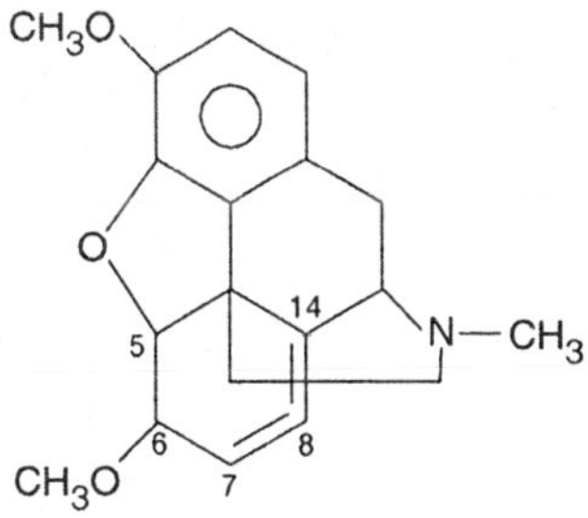

Thebaine

The above structure of morphine has finally been confirmed by its synthesis and its stereochemistry at different chiral centres (C_5, C_6, C_{13}, C_{14} and C_9) has also been settled by chemical experiments. The configurational structure of morphine stands as below:

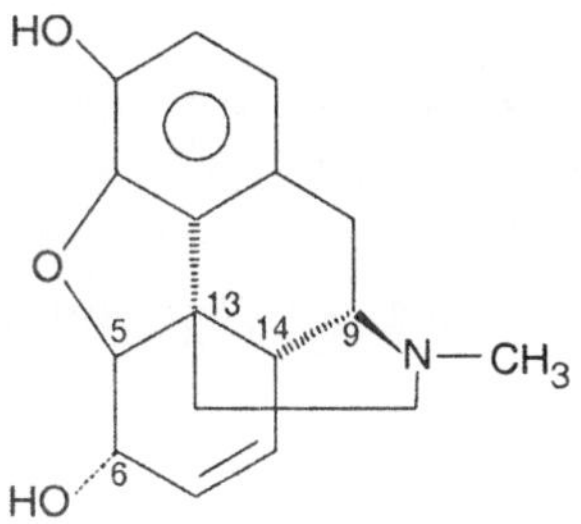

Morphine

5.8.6.1.3 Uses of Morphine Alkaloids

Morphine itself has a strong analgesic and sedative action and so is used in controlling severe pain. But it has a marked habit forming effect and so it should be used with great care. For this reason, an extensive work has been carried out to find out drugs alternative to morphine without any habit forming effect by modifying the morphine structure. A few of such drugs are as mentioned below:

1. *Change in Oxygenation pattern*
   (a) When phenolic OH at C_3 is changed to OCH_3, *Codeine* is formed. It is less active analgesic than morphine. But when alcoholic hydroxyl group at C_6 is converted to —OCH_3, *heterocodeine* is obtained which is six times more active than morphine.
   (b) When C_6—OH is changed to keto, group activity is reduced, but if olefinic double at 7, 8 position is reduced the activity of keto group is increased as was observed in dihydro morphinone and dihydro codeinone (Hydrocodonel. Hydrocodone is used as an analugesic and antitussive.

(c) Removal of alcoholic function at C_6 yields 6-desoxymorphine having ten times more activity than morphine.

(d) When both the hydroxyl functions are acetylated, *heroin* is formed. It is 2-3 times more active than morphine.

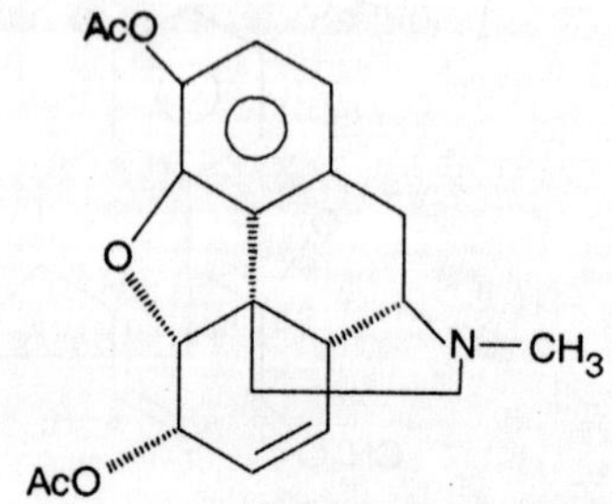

Heroin

(e) When C_{14}—H is replaced by OH function in dihydro morphinone, oxymorphone is obtained. It has ten times the potency of morphine.

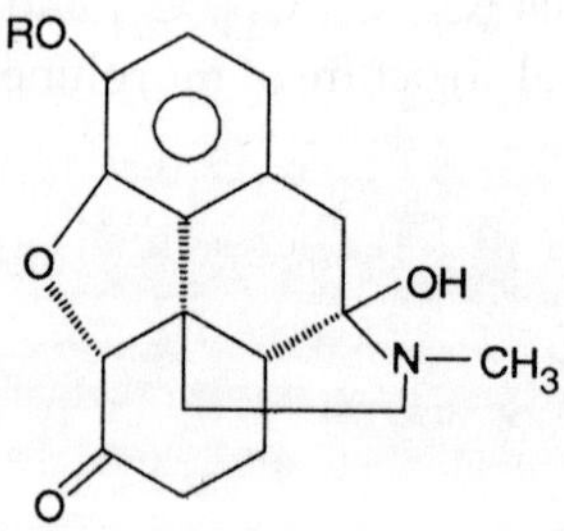

R = H, Oxymorphone, R = CH_3, Oxycodone

Similar derivative of dihydrocodeinone known as oxycodone is extensively used as oral analgesic.

2. *Change in the Substitution at nitrogen atom:* Change in the nature of substitution at nitrogen atom changes the activity remarkably. Thus, when methoyl group at N is replaced by H atom, activity is significantly (75%) reduced, but if phenethyl group is introduced in place of methyl group, there is 14-times increase in the activity over morphine. Again, if bulkier group like propyl, isobutyl, cyclopropyl methyl, allyl, etc., present on nitrogen atom, the resulting derivatives become narcotic antagonist.

5.8.7 Reserpine

It is the main component of *Rauwolfia* species particularly *Rauwolfia serpentina* and *Rauwolfia vomitoria* which are primarily indegenus to south-east Asia. The extracts of *R serpentina* are used as folk medicines in India for centuries for a variety of purposes like hypertension, epilepsy, insanity, headache, dermatological disorders.

It has been isolated as a crystalline slightly yellowish powder by following the usual procedure for the isolation of alkaloids. It is sparingly soluble in common organic solvents excepting chloroform, benzene, ethyl acetate, etc. in which it is readily soluble. It responds to various colour reactions specific to indole alkaloids.

5.8.7.1 Structure of Reserpine

Structure of reserpine is based on the evidences as laid down below:

1. It has molecular formula $C_{33}H_{40}O_9N_2$.
2. On treatment with CH_3I it forms a monoquaternary compound indicating the fact that out of two nitrogen atoms only one is basic and tertiary in nature.
3. Zeisel experiment reveals that reserpine contains six methoxy groups.
4. (a) On hydrolysis with KOH it forms methyl alcohol, reserpic acid and 3, 4, 5-trimethoxy benzoic acid, i.e.,

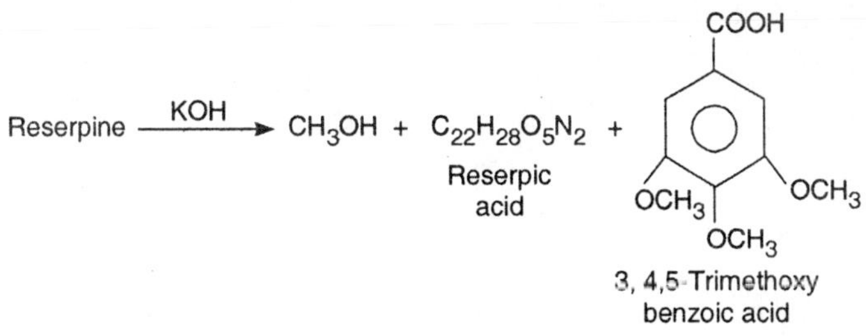

(b) Again esterification of reserpic acid with CH_2N_2 followed by benzoylation with 3, 4, 5-trimethoxy benzoyl chloride regenerates reserpine.

Reserpine, therefore, is the methyl ester as well as trimethoxy benzoate of reserpic acid.

5. (a) Reserpine responds to Adamkiwicz's colour reaction (conc. H_2SO_4 + trace of $K_2Cr_2O_7$- deep blue to green colour) which is specific for a β-Carboline system (A).

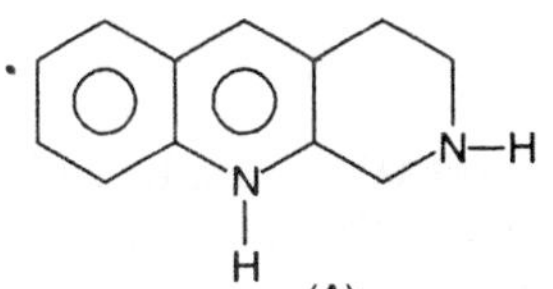

(A)

(b) Zn-dust distillation yields isoquinoline as one of the products. This is indicative of the presence of a tertrahydro-isoquinoline ring system in reserpine.

(c) Methyl reserpate obtained by the treatment of resperpic acid with diazomethane, when subjected to selenium distillation forms yobyrine and hydroxy yobyrine, i.e.,

$$\text{Methyl reserpate} \xrightarrow[\text{Se}]{\text{Dehydrogenation}} \underset{\text{Yobyrine}}{C_{19}H_{16}N_2} + \underset{\text{Hydroxy Yobyrine}}{C_{19}H_{16}N_2O}$$

The UV-spectrum of hydroxy yobyrine is similar to that of harmol (X_{max} 230, 299 nm) and it has been identified as 11-hydroxy yobyrine (B) from synthesis from harmine

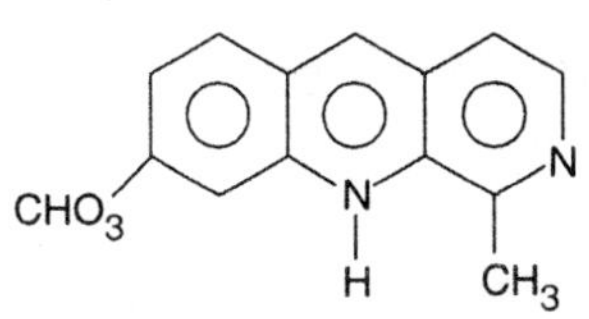

Harmine

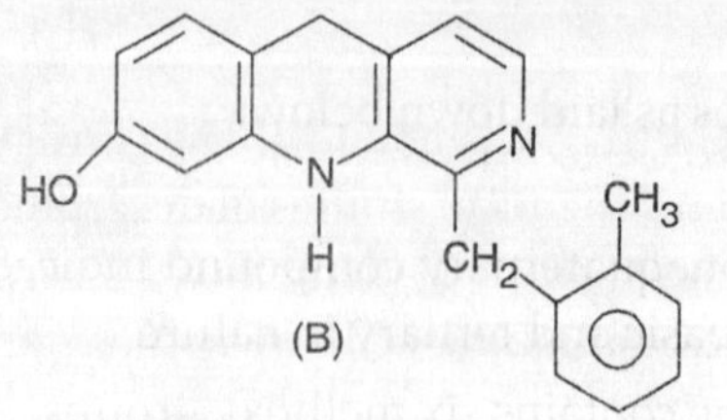

(B)

Based on the above evidences, the structure of reserpine may be expressed as below:

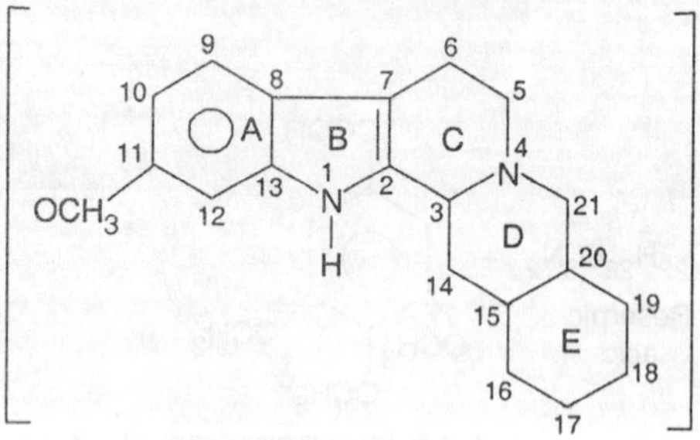

1.—COOCH$_3$
2.—3, 4, 5-trimethyoxy benzoyl group
3.—OCH$_3$

- *Locations of Different functional Groups in Reserpine:* It has been observed that in yohimbinoid indole alkaloids substituents are generally present in ring (E). When reserpic acid is fused with KOH hydroxy isophthalic acid is formed.

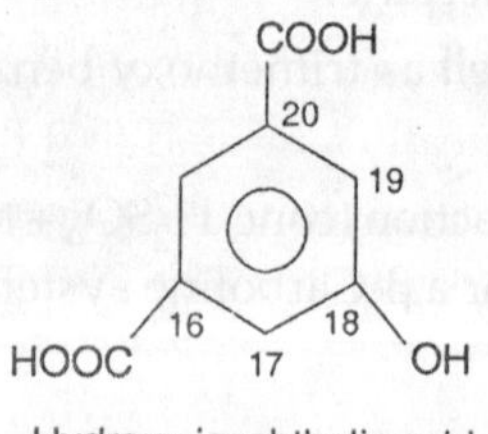

Hydroxy isophthalic acid

Formation of hydroxy isophthalic acid suggests that during KOH fusion, D-ring undergoes cleavage and benzene ring originates from the ring (E). From the analysis of the structure of hydroxy isophthalic acid it is evident that —COOH and —OH groups in reserpic acid must be located at C_{16} and C_{18} positions respectively. This is further supported by the fact that on treatment with acetic anhydride reserpic acid forms a γ-lactone indicating the fact that these two functionalities are located in 1, 3-relation in reserpic acid.

On the biogenetic ground it has been assumed that —OCH_3 group is present at C_{17} position. Thus the structure of reserpine may be represented as below:

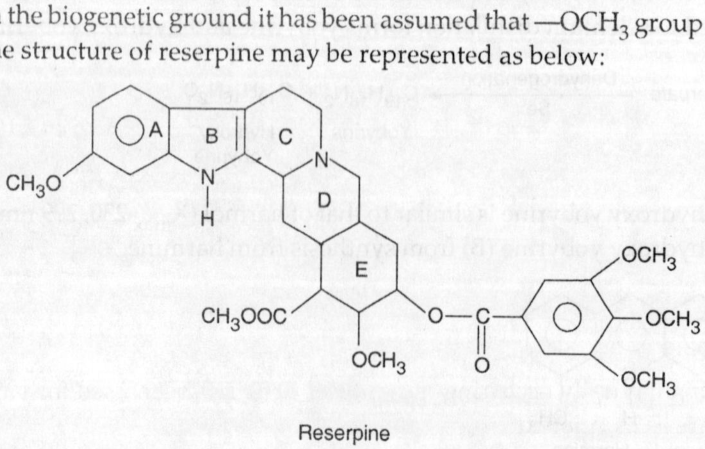

Reserpine

5.8.7.1.1 Stereochemistry of Reserpine

Reserpine has several chiral centres, viz., C_3, C_{15}, C_{16}, C_{17} and C_{20}. The configurations at these centres have been ascertained on the basis of stereochemical studies of deserpine—a congener of reserpine and structurally it is completely identical with 11-demethoxy reserpine. It has been observed that deserpine can be converted to α-yohimbine of known configuration through a series of reactions.

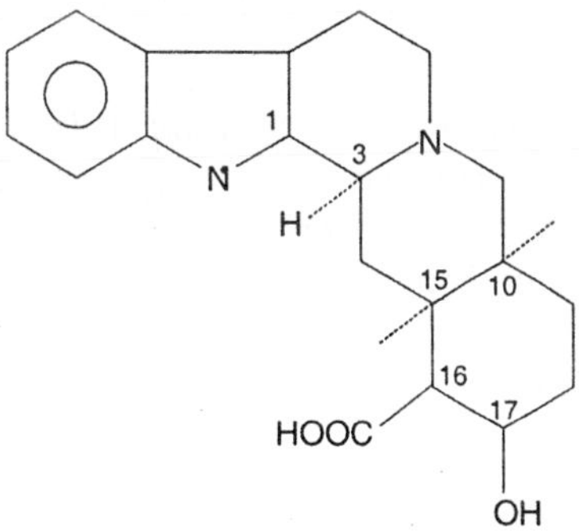

α-Yohimbine

It may be remembered that both reserpine and deserpine easily isomerise at C_3 on treatment with acid and since the sequence of reactions for the conversion of deserpine to α-yohimbine involves treatment of acid more than once, it has been logically assumed that the configuration of C_3 in deserpine and hence in reserpine should be opposite to that of α-yohimbine. Again when reserpic or deserpic acid is refluxed with acetic anhydride and sodium acetate there is ready formation of a lactone which suggests that C_{18}—OH and C_{16}—COOH must be in the same direction. As C_{16}—COOH group is β, hence C_{18}—OH must be β in these two compounds. Hence trimethoxy benzoyloxy group in reserpine must be β in nature.

Thus complete stereochemical structure of reserpine may be expressed as under which has finally been confirmed by sysnthesis.

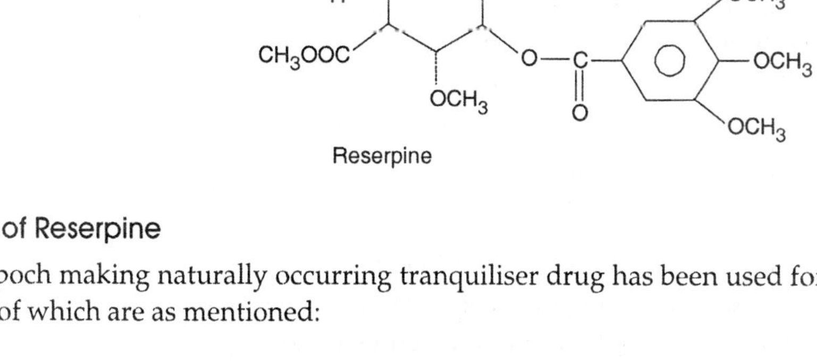

Reserpine

5.8.7.1.2 Uses of Reserpine

Reserpine, an epoch making naturally occurring tranquiliser drug has been used for variety of purposes some of which are as mentioned:

i. Reserpine is used as a sedative for mild anxiety and chronic psychoses.
ii. Reserpine has been found to be a contraceptive and radioactive agent.
iii. It is used in combination with thiazide diuretics for the management of mild hypertension.
iv. Reserpine is used as a peripheral antihypertensive, as a central depressant.
v. It may also be used in poultry feeds as a sedative and to prevent arotic rupture.
vi. It may also be used for the treatment of asthma and dermatological disorders.

5.8.8 Ergot Alkaloids

These are the alkaloids isolated from parasites *ergot* or *Secale cornutum*. This parasite originates from filamentous fungus *Claviceps purpurea*. It grows on rye and other grasses and cereals. Ergot finds extensive applications as medicines because of its action on uterus and vasomotor centre. As many as twenty one alkaloids have been isolated so far from ergot of which following four are important.

(1) Ergotamine (2) Ergotaminine (3) Ergosine and (4) Ergosinine.

5.8.8.1 Structures of Ergot Alkaloids

These four alkaloids are structurally very closely related. The first and most important member of this group of alkaloids is *ergotamine*. Its constitution has been elaborated on the basis of evidences as depicted below:

1. The molecular formula of *ergotamine* as deduced from analytical data stands as $C_{33}H_{35}N_5O_5$.
2. On hydrolysis with alkali ergotamine yields d-lysergic acid along with α-hydroxy alanine, d-proline and l-phenyl alanine. Thus,

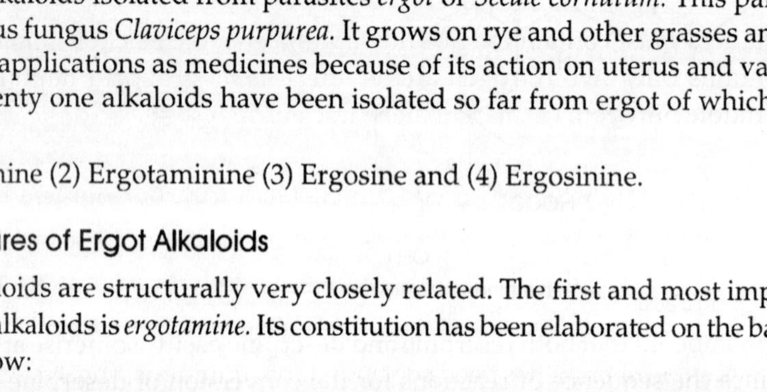

From the formation of above products during alkaline hydrolysis it is evident that the complete elaboration of the structure of ergotamine may be considered under two headings, viz., (i) structure of lysergic acid and (ii) constitution of non-lysergic acid portions along with their mode of combination with lysergic acid moiety.

A. *Structure of Lysergic Acid:*

Lysergic acid, $C_{16}H_{16}N_2O_2$, was found to contain (i) one COOH group (ii) one non-basic nitrogen present as >NH (iii) one >N—CH_3 functionality and one olefinic double bond by usual tests. When dihydro lysergic is subjected to alkaline fusion with KOH it forms 3, 4-dimethyl indole, I-methyl-5-aminonaphthalene and methylamine, i.e.,

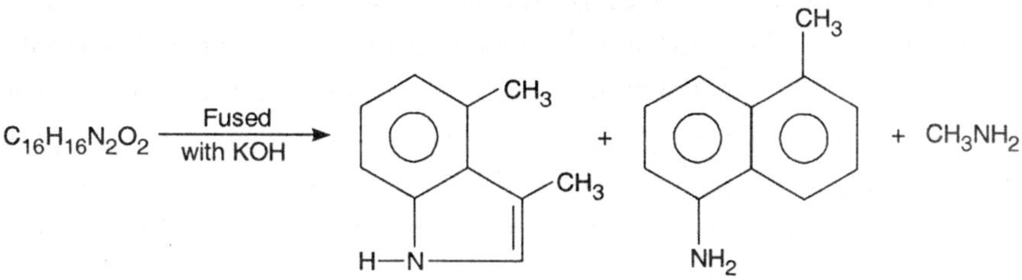

3. 4-Dimethyl indole

1-Methyl-5-amino-naphthalene

Thus lysergic acid must contain indole and naphthalene nucleus in its molecule. Again, as lysergic acid contains only two nitrogen atoms, the —NH_2 group in naphthalene must be originated from indole nitrogen, i.e., naphthalene nucleus in lysergic acid is connected with the indole N-atom.

Once again, lysergic acid when oxidised with HNO_3, a tricarboxylic acid is formed which on distillation with sodalime yields quinoline. i.e.,

$$\text{Lysergic acid} \xrightarrow[HNO_3]{[O]} \text{Tricarboxylic acid} \xrightarrow[\text{Sodalime}]{\text{Distillation}} \text{Quinoline}$$

From the above experiment it has been concluded that quinoline ring system is also present in lysergic acid molecule.

In order to explain the presence of indole, naphthalene and quinoline ring systems in lysergic acid, a tetracyclic structure as shown below has been proposed for this molecule. Thus the part structure of lysergic acid may be expressed as under:

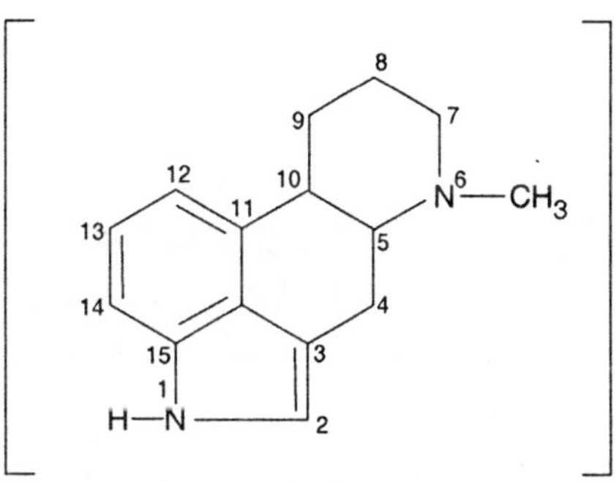

+ One COOH

+ One olefinic double bond

Lysergic acid

• *Location of Carboxylic group in lysergic acid:* Dihydrolysergic acid when heated one molecule of water is eliminated and there is formation of a compound—(A). The compound (A) responds to Keller reaction (blue colouration with conc. H_2SO_4 and glacial acetic acid containing a trace of iron chloride) which is *specific for a lactam functionality.* The compound (A) readily absorbs a mole equivalent of hydrogen suggesting the presence of an easily reducible olefinic double bond in it. Formation of a lactam having an easily reducible double bond can be explained if lysergic acid contains a β-amino acidic system in its skeleton. This is possible if carboxylic group be present either at 8 or at 4 position. However, the position 4 has been discarded on the basis of the observation that dihydrolysergic acid is thermally highly stable. Hence the part structure of lysergic acid may be extended as shown:

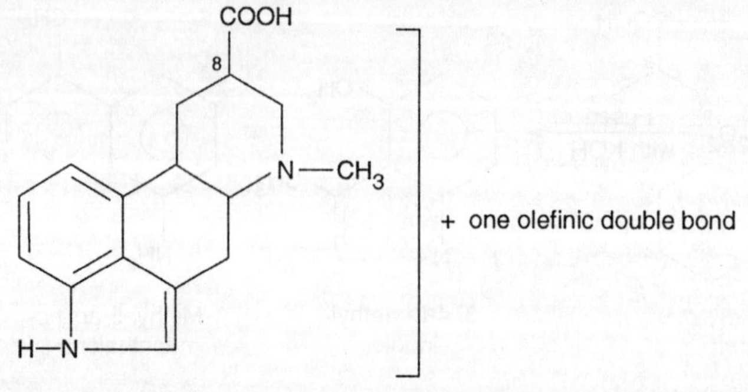

The supportive evidence in favour of location of carboxylic group at 8 has been secured from the fact that the formation of lactam (A) can be properly explained as depicted below:

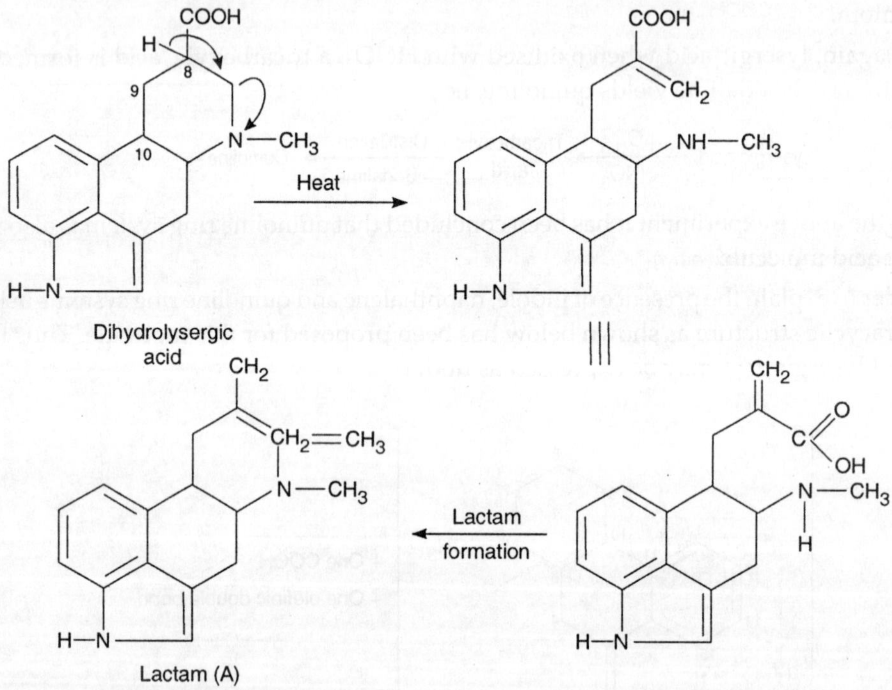

• *Site of olefinic double-bond in lysergic acid:* The site of olefinic unsaturation in lysergic acid has been settled from the fact that when lysergic acid itself is heated, once again a lactam of the type (A) is formed, but this lactam contains one additional double bond than the lactam (A). This is obvious because lysergic acid has already an olefinic double bond. Thus this lactam is a diene. UV spectral measurement clearly reveals that this diene is conjugated in nature. This is possible if lysergic acid has its olefinic unsaturation at 9 and 10 positions. Consequently the complete structure of lysergic acid may be represented as shown:

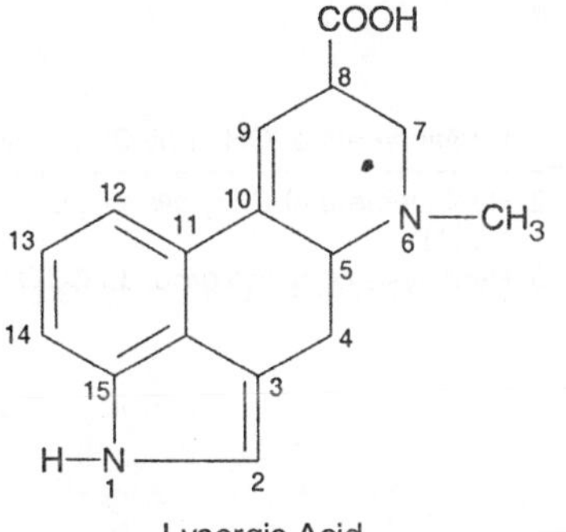

Lysergic Acid

The above structure of lysergic acid has finally been confirmed by the following synthesis.

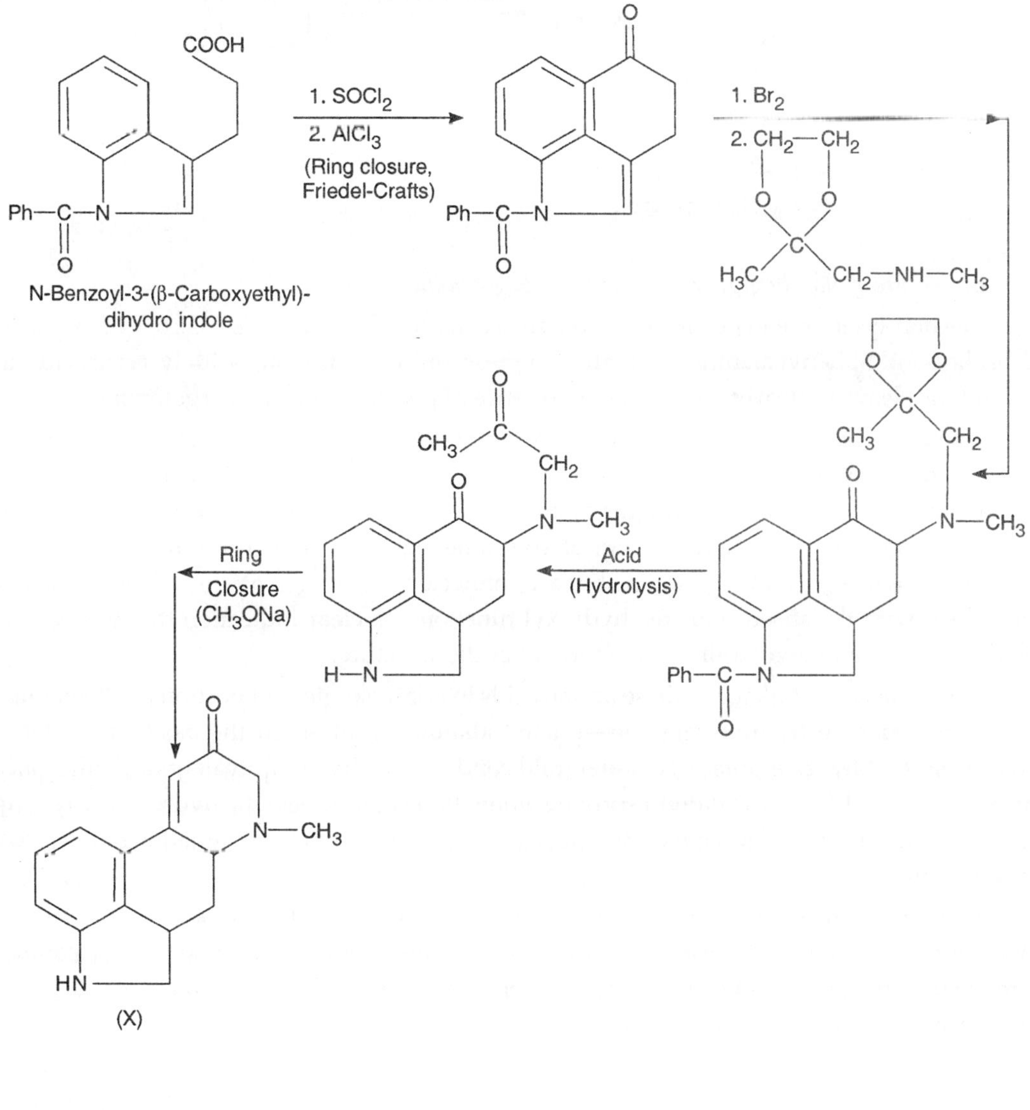

(X)

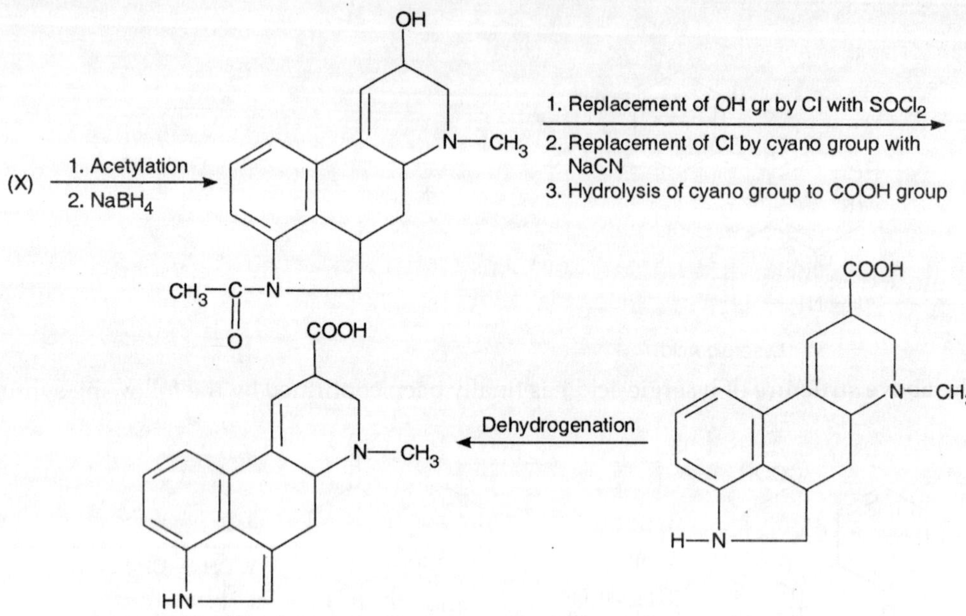

(±) Lysergic acid

B. *Nature of Non-lysergic Acid Portion in Ergotamine:*

The non-lysergic acid portion of ergotamine consists of amino acids, viz., α-hydroxy alanine, d-proline and l-phenyl alanine. Formation of these amino acids along with lysergic acid during hydrolytic cleavage clearly indicates the presence of peptide linkage in ergotamine.

Again, ergotamine itself does not contain any carboxylic function. Hence the carboxylic groups in this amino acids originate from peptide linkage during hydrolysis. Once again, ergotamine contains only two nitrogen atoms, presence of which has already been established in lysergic acid portion. It is therefore logical to assume that the amino groups in these amino acids are not present as such in ergotamine but are connected to nitrogen atoms of lysergic acid. This fact along with the absence of free hydroxyl function is a clear indication that various amino acids are present in ergotamine in the form of cyclic structure.

The sequence of linkage of these amino acids in non-lysergic acid portion has been found to be in the order—α-hydroxy alanine—phenyl alanine—proline on the basis of the fact that hydrolysis of dihydro ergotamine under mild condition with one equivalent of alkali in alcohol affords pyruvoyl-L-phenylalanyl-L-proline along with lysergic acid. [α-hydroxy alanyl portion is converted to pyruvoyl moiety under the reaction condition by the elimination of the molecule of ammonia].

Further, treatment of dihydro ergotamine with hydrazine yields diketopiperazine, i.e., lactam of phenyl alanine and proline as one of the major products. This reveals that phenyl alanine and proline moieties are linked to each other in such a way as to develop a six-membered ring along with a five-member cyclic system as shown:

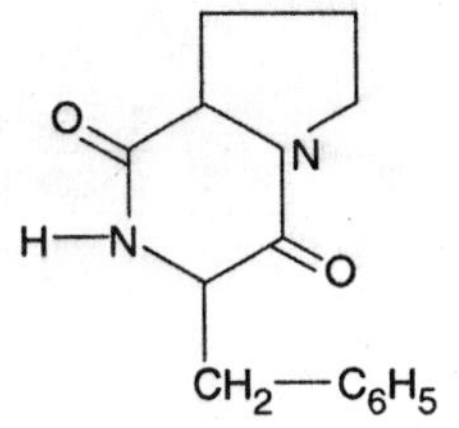

Now by combining the above diketopiperazine with α-hydroxyalanine, the structure of non-lysergic acid moiety stands as under:

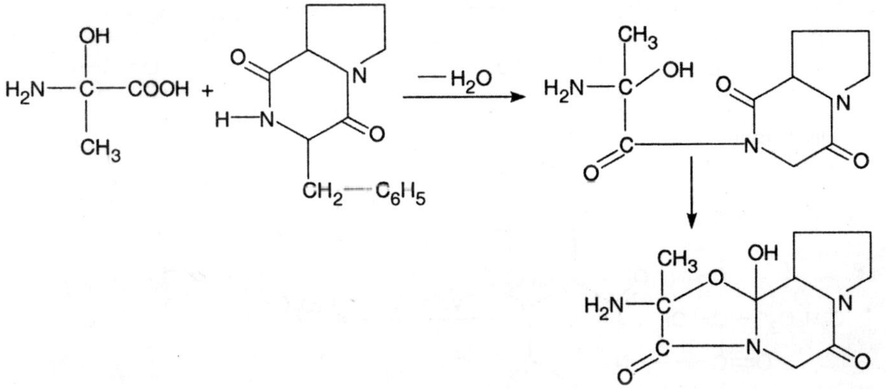

Non-lysergic acid portion

C. *Mode of Linkage between Lysergic acid and Non-lysergic Acid in Ergotamine:*

It has been observed that when ergotamine is subjected to hydrolysis under *mild condition* lysergic acid-amide, known as ergine is formed. This reveals that lysergic acid portion and non-lysergic acid moiety in ergotamine are connected by an amide linkage. This is possible if COOH group of lysergic acid and —NH_2 function of non-lysergic portion are linked to each other. Thus, the complete structure of ergotamine may be represented as below:

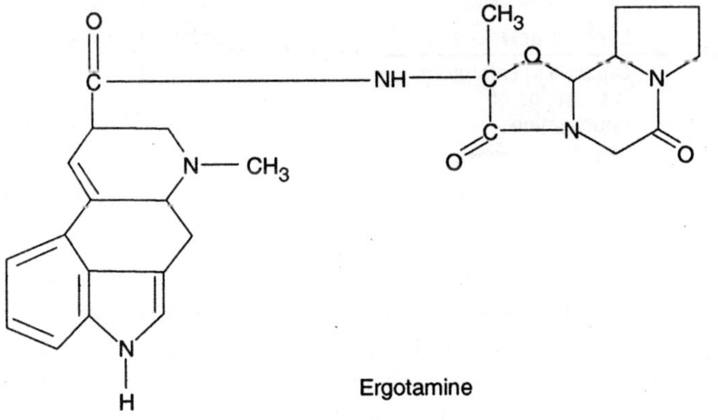

Ergotamine

The above structure of ergotamine has finally been confirmed by synthesis as discussed in sequel.

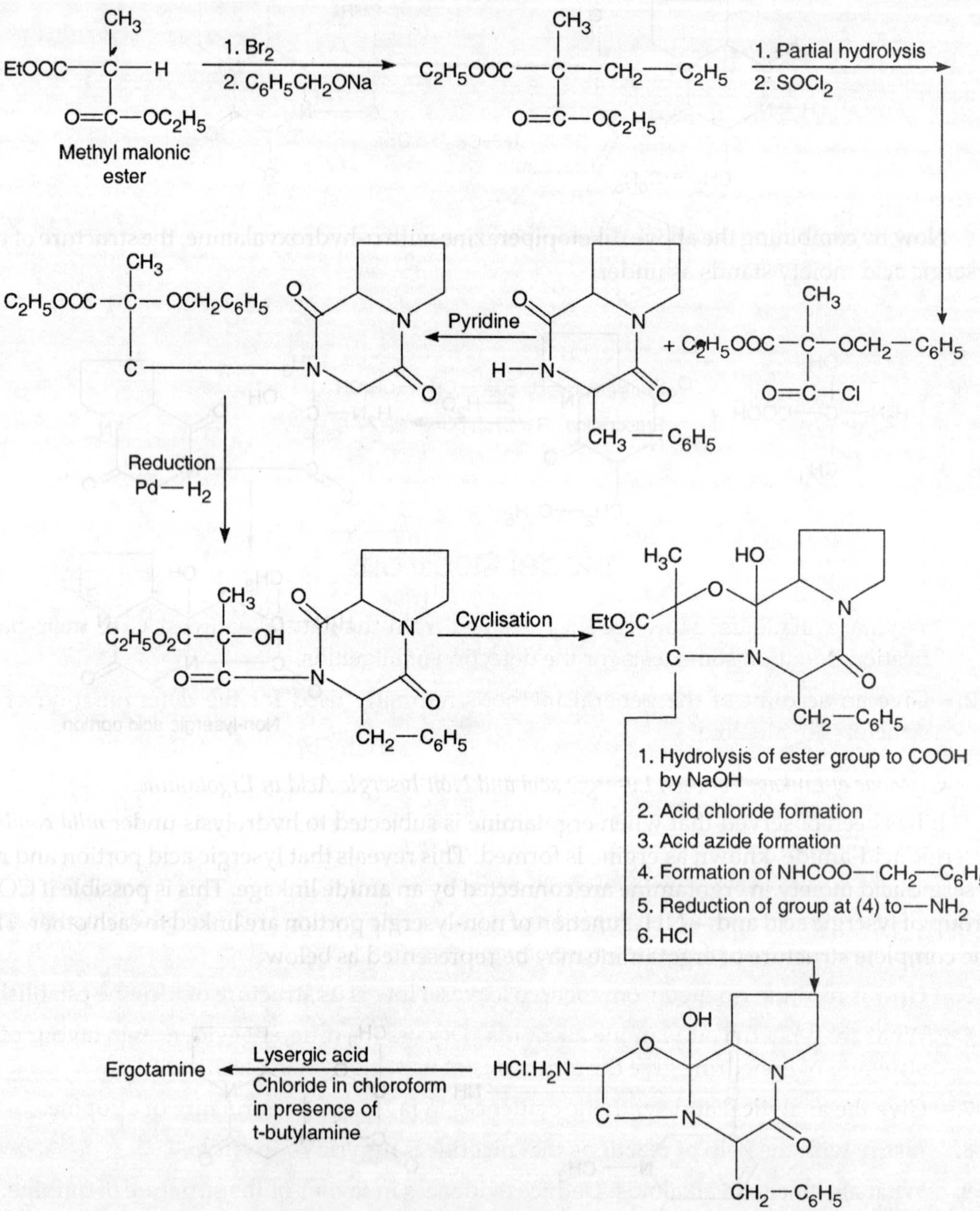

The congeners are closely related to ergotamine. Thus ergotine and ergocristine differ from ergotamine in the nature of substitution only as shown below while other three alkaloids, viz., ergotaminine ergosinine and ergocristinine have similar structure as their counter part only differing in the fact that they contain isolysergic acid instead of lysergic acid. Lysergic acid and isolysergic acid differ only in the configuration of COOH group at C_8 position. Thus,

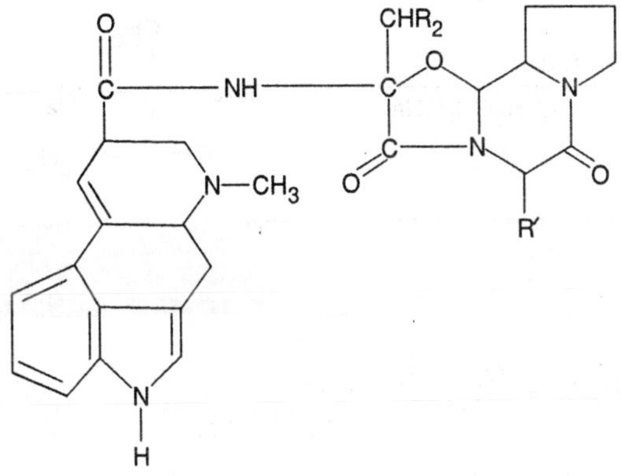

Ergosine, R = H, R′ = $-CH_2-CH(CH_3)_2$

Ergocristine, R = CH_3, R′ = $-CH_2-C_6H_5$

Model Questions

1. What are alkaloids? How are they isolated from the natural sources? Give their classification. Mention some tests for the detection of alkaloids.
2. Give an account of the general methods normally used for the determination of the structures of alkaloids.
3. How is the presence of the following found out?
   (a) Five and seven membered rings in tropine.
   (b) Two reactive methylene groups in tropinone.
   (c) β-Hydroxy acid linkage in tropic acid.
4. Give a brief account of the graded oxidation of papaverine and discuss its importance in the determination of the structure of papaverine.
5. How is nicotine isolated from tobacco leaves. How is its structure of nicotine established.
6. What are β-phenyl ethylamine alkaloids? Discuss the different evidences in favour of the structure of ephedrine give the structures of its various stereoisomers.
7. Give the analytical and synthetic evidences in favour of the structure of atropine.
8. Justify with the help of reactions that nicotine is β-pyridy-λ-pyrrole.
9. What are cinchona alkaloids. Deduce evidences in favour of the structure of quinine.
10. Describe the isolation and physiological properties of cocaine. Describe its structure. Mention the name of a few cocaine substitute.
11. What are the principal alkaloids of opium and how are they isolated? Discuss the structure of morphine.
12. Write the structures and uses of some important derivatives of morphine.
13. Discuss the various evidences for the structure of reserpine.
14. How will you prove presence of (i) indole ring in reserpine (ii) phenolic hydroxyl in morphine (iii) isoquinoline ring in papaverine?

CHAPTER SIX

Purines

6.1 Introduction

Purines are, in fact, are polyhetero cyclic compounds in which two heterocyclic rings, viz., pyrimidine and imidazole (1, 3-diazole) are fused together as shown below:

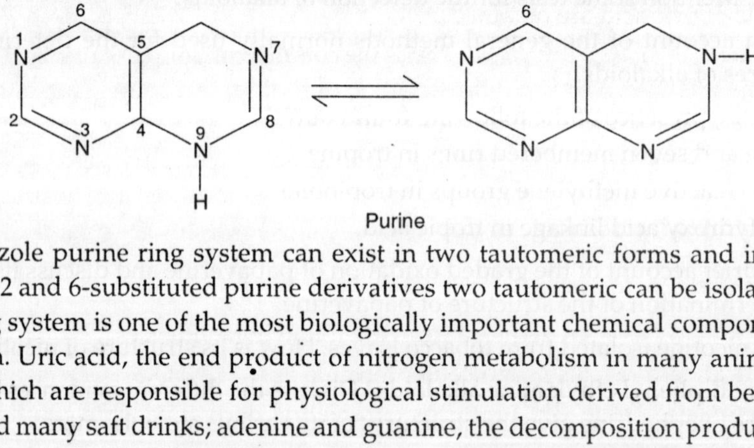

Purine

Like imidazole purine ring system can exist in two tautomeric forms and in some cases particularly for 2 and 6-substituted purine derivatives two tautomeric can be isolated.

Purine ring system is one of the most biologically important chemical components present in living system. Uric acid, the end product of nitrogen metabolism in many animals, caffeine theobromine which are responsible for physiological stimulation derived from beverages such as tea, coffee and many saft drinks; adenine and guanine, the decomposition products of nucleic acids are all purine derivatives. The different purines are named as purine derivatives. However, some of the popular trivial names such as uric acid, caffeine, etc. still exist. Though there is no rigid classification of purines but they are classified *into two categories*, viz., oxypurine i.e., uric acid, caffeine, etc. and aminopyrines such as adenine guanine, etc.

The parent compound, purine itself does not occur naturally but it can be synthesised as below:

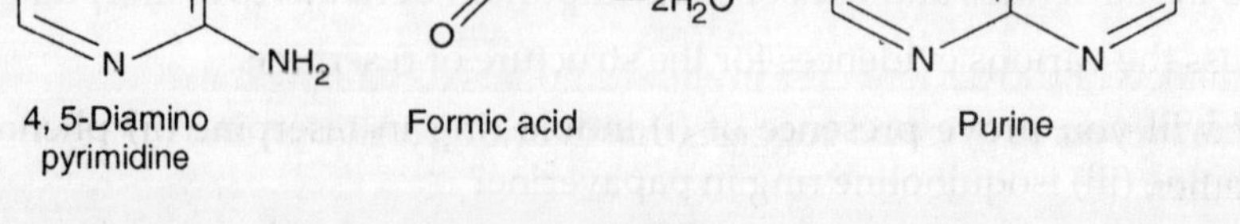

4, 5-Diamino pyrimidine   Formic acid   Purine

Purine is a solid, m.p. 212-213 °C. It behaves as a weak base but is stronger base than pyrimidine, but weaker than imidazole. It is soluble in water but sparingly soluble in organic solvents.

6.2 Chemistry of Some Purine Derivatives

6.2.1 Oxypurine

6.2.1.1 Uric Acid (2, 6, 8-Trihydroxy Purine).

6.2.1.1.1 Occurrence of Uric Acid

Uric acid was first isolated by Scheele and Bergmann in 1776 from urinary *Calculi.* However, it is present in large amount in excreta of birds and reptiles. *Gauno,* the excrement of seabirds contains up to the extent of 90 per cent in the form of ammonium nitrate. Normal blood contains only 0.2 per cent of uric acid as its sodium salt, but in patients suffering from gout, this amount may rise as much as 9 mg per cent and it gets deposited in joints and in other places. Excessive amount of uric acid sometimes is accumulated in the bladder and kidney as stones.

6.2.1.1.2 Isolation of Uric Acid

(a) *From Human Urine:* Human urine is concentrated and is treated with concentrated hydrochloric acid and is allowed to stand in cold for more than twenty four hours when crystals of uric acid are obtained.

(b) *From Guano or Snake's Excrement:* This is the commercial source of uric acid. The powdered excrement is dissolved in a dilute solution of sodium carbonate. The solution is boiled at a temperature of 80-100 °C till the evolution of ammonia ceases. The solution is filtered and is acidified with hydrochloric acid, and cooled when uric acid crystallises out. It is purified by redissolving in sodium carbonate solution and reprecipitating with concentrated hydrochloric acid.

6.2.1.1.3 Structure of Uric Acid

Structure of uric acid has been deduced from the following evidences.

i. Analytical data reveals its molecular formula as $C_5H_4N_4O_3$.

ii. On methylation with CH_3I it forms tetramethyl derivative which on hydrolysis yields four molecules of methylamine.

$$C_5H_4N_4O_3 \xrightarrow{CH_3I} \underset{\text{Tetramethyl uric acid}}{C_9H_{12}N_4O_3} \xrightarrow{H_2O} 4CH_3NH_2$$

Above experiment clearly suggests that uric acid contains four imino (—NH—) groups.

iii. On oxidation with dilute nitric acid uric acid forms alloxan and urea in equivalent amounts.

$$C_5H_4N_4O_3 \xrightarrow{HNO_3} \underset{\text{Alloxan}}{C_4H_2N_2O_4} + \underset{\text{Urea}}{CH_4N_2O}$$

Formation of alloxan and urea in equal amounts containing the requisite number of carbon atoms present in uric acid suggests that in uric acid alloxan and urea molecules are linked together.

iv. (a) When alloxan is hydrolysed with alkali it yields one molecule each of two known compounds—mesoxalic acid and urea.

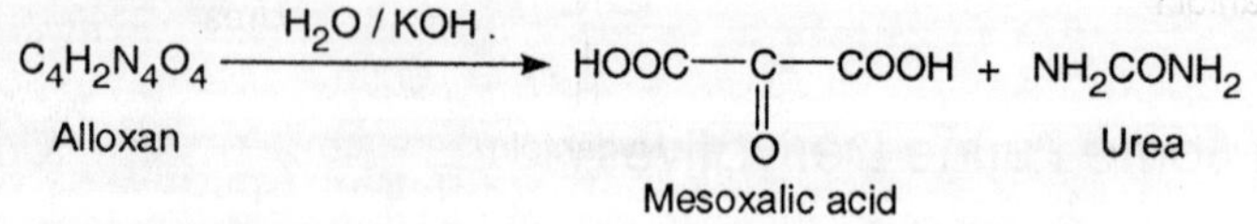

(b) When mexoxalic acid and urea are heated together alloxan is formed.

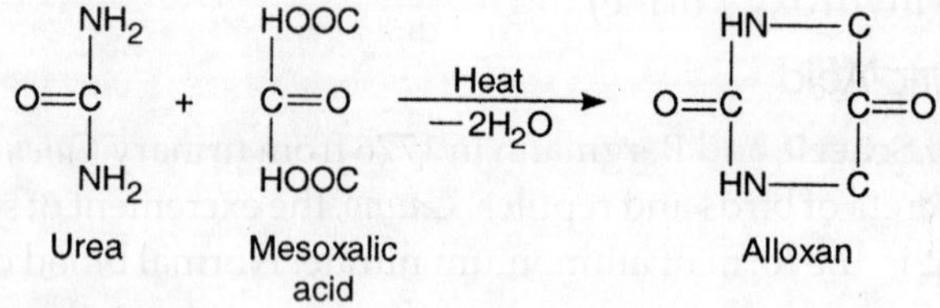

Formation of alloxan during hydrolysis is a clear indication that a pyrimidine nucleus is present in uric acid.

(v) (a) When uric acid is subjected to vigorous oxidation with neutral or alkaline $KMnO_4$ allantoin and carbon dioxide are formed.

$$\underset{\text{Uric acid}}{C_5H_4N_4O_3} \xrightarrow[KMnO_4]{[O]} \underset{\text{Allantoin}}{C_4H_6O_3N_4} + CO_2$$

(b) Again, allantoin when oxidised with nitric acid, forms parabanic acid and urea. The structure of parbanic acid has been confirmed by its synthesis from oxalyl chloride and urea, i.e.,

$$\underset{\text{Allantoin}}{C_4H_6N_4O_3} \xrightarrow[HNO_3]{[O]} \underset{\text{Parabanic acid}}{C_4H_6N_2O_3} + \underset{\text{Urea}}{NH_2CONH_2}$$

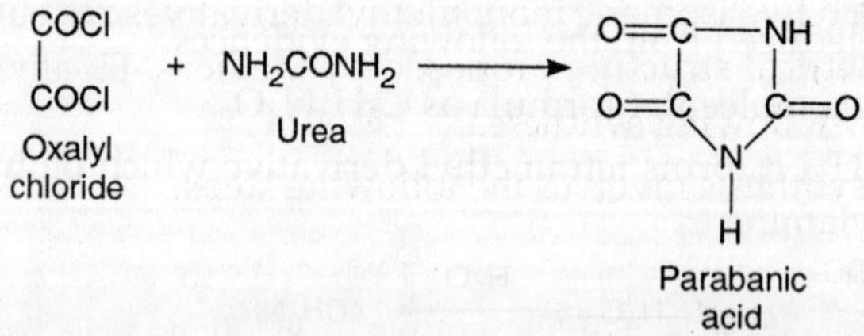

Formation of parabanic acid reveals that allantoin and hence uric acid contains an imidazole ring in their nuclei.

Further from the formation parabanic acid and urea it is obvious that in allantoin parabanic acid and urea are linked together.

But the question arises to which carbon atom urea molecule is linked? in order to get the answer allantoin has been subjected to reductive cleavage by hydroiodic acid at 100 °C when hydantoin of known structure and urea are obtained.

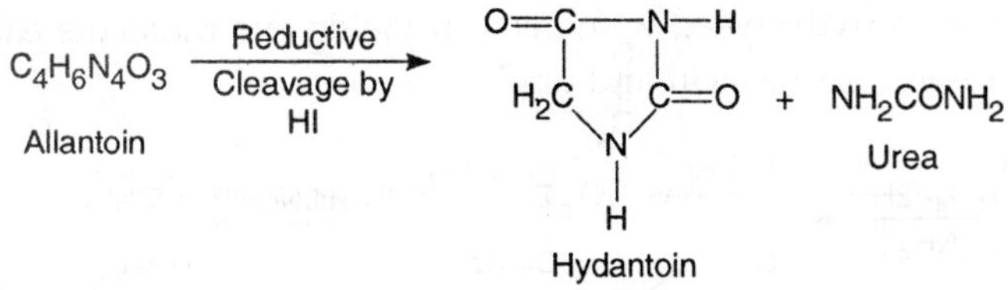

On the basis of the structure of hydantoin, the following structure has been proposed for allantoin which can clearly explain all its reaction described above.

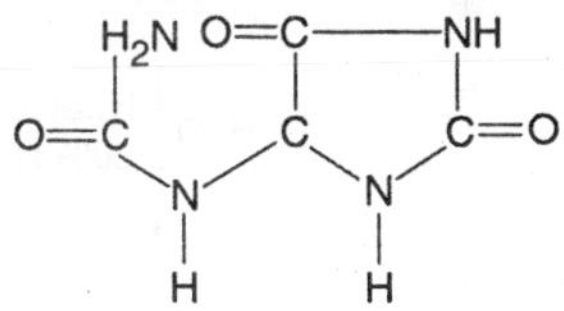

Allaintoin

Now from the evidence (Va) it is evident that one carbon atom is lost during oxidation of uric acid to allantoin. In order to fit this extra carbon atom in allantoin two alternative structures have been proposed for uric acid keeping in mind that both the pyrimidine as well as imidazole nuclei contained in it.

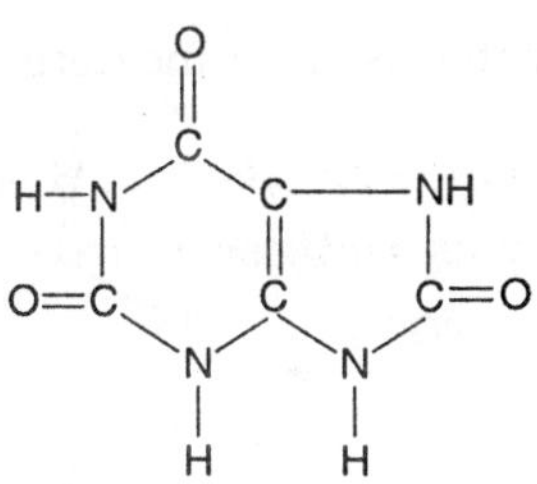

Medicus formula

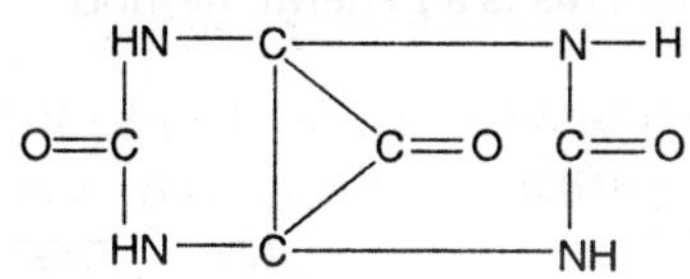

Fittig formula

Out of these two alternatives Medicus structure was found to be correct by Fischer from its methylation experiment in which two isomeric monomethyl derivatives are obtained which can only be explained by unsymmetrical structure proposed by Medicus. Finally, the structure of uric acid has been confirmed by following syntheses.

i. *Baeyer's synthesis:* This synthesis involves the following steps.

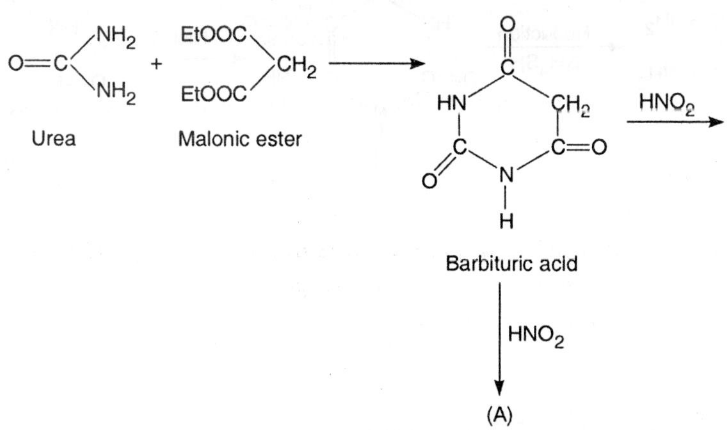

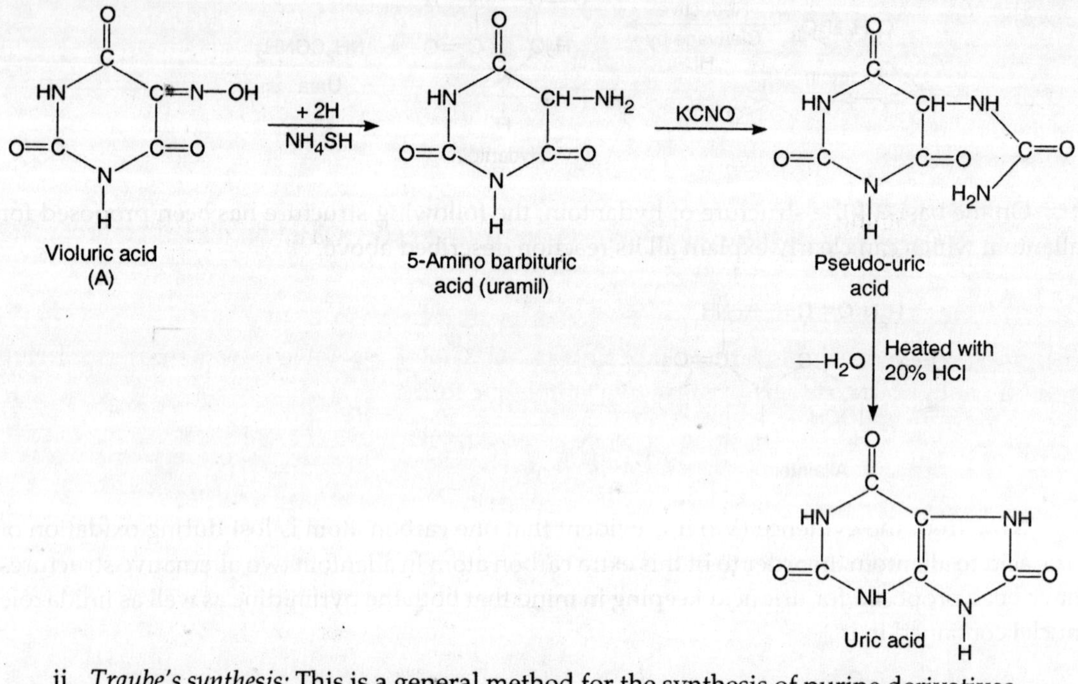

ii. *Traube's synthesis:* This is a general method for the synthesis of purine derivatives.

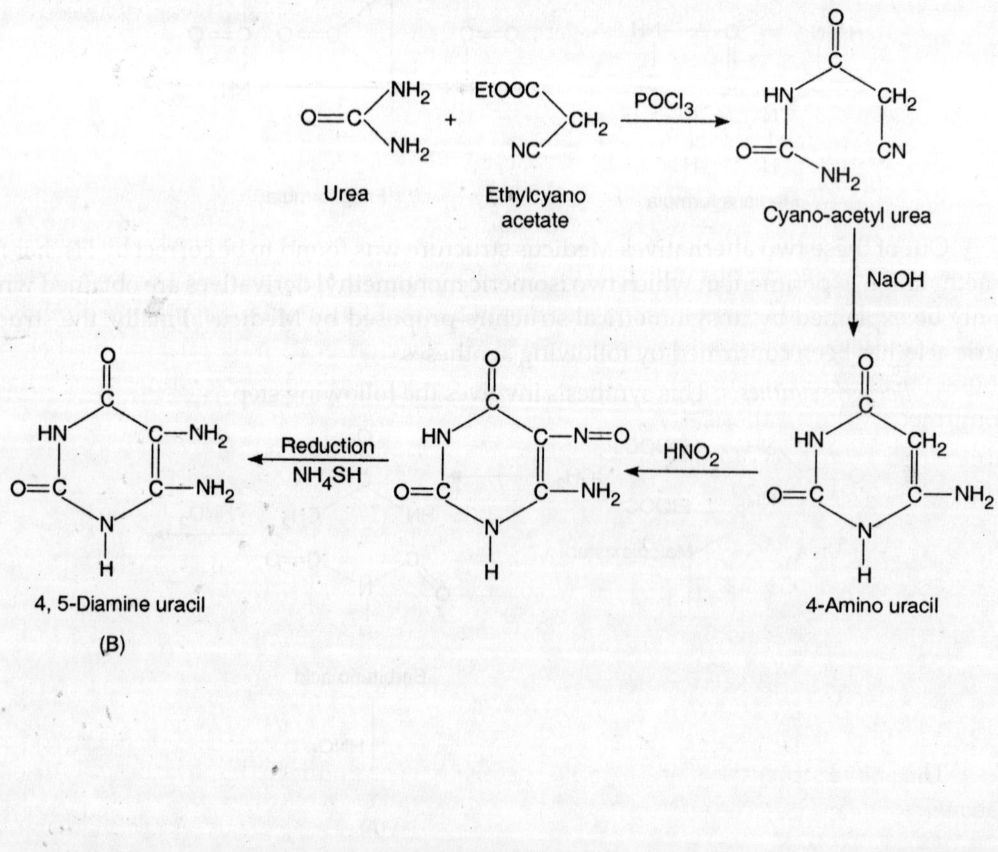

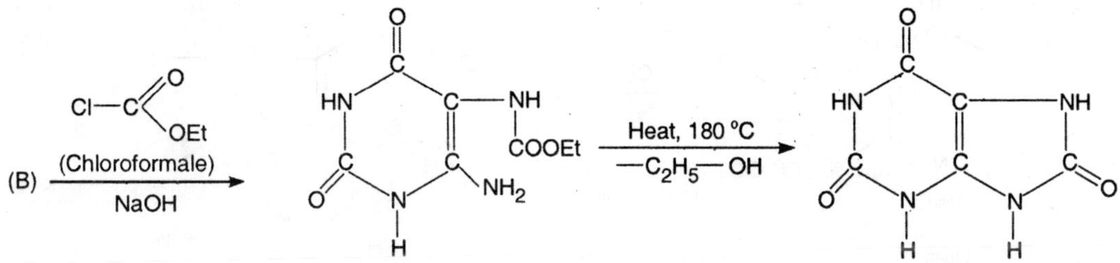

Uric Acid

6.2.1.1.4 Properties of Uric Acid

It is a crystalline white powder decomposing at 400 °C. It is insoluble in water but sparingly soluble in hot water. Uric acid exists in two tautomeric forms.

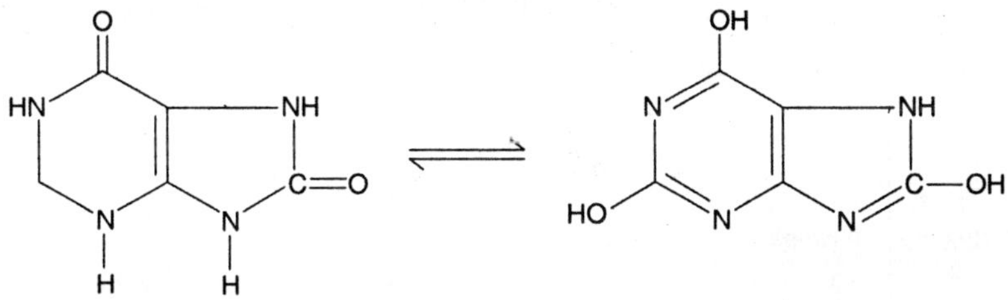

Lactam form Lactim form

Of these two forms lactam form predominates. It behaves as a weakly dibasic acid and forms two series of salts.

6.2.1.2 Xanthine Bases

6.2.1.2.1 Xanthine (2, 6-Dihydroxy Purine)

It is the parent compound of three major bases, viz., caffeine, theobromine and theophylline. It occurs widely in plants like tea, lupin seedlings etc. It also occurs in many animal tissues. Its derivatives are of great physiological importance.

When oxidised with potassium chlorate in hydrochloric acid solution it yields alloxan and urea indicating that xanthine contains uric acid skeleton in its molecule. On the basis of the above observation following structures have been proposed for xanthine which has been confirmed by the synthesis.

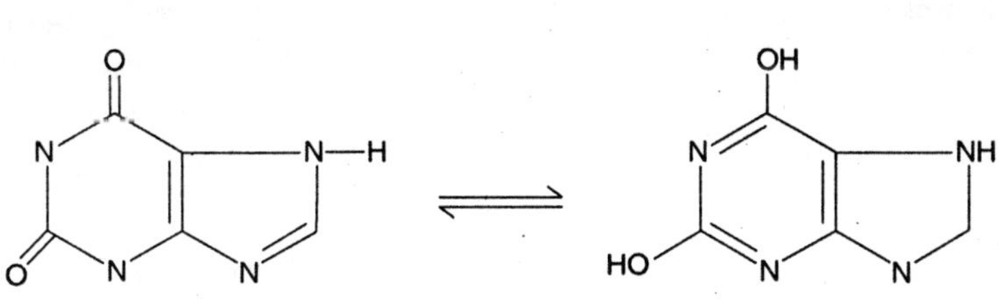

Keto form Enol form

- *Synthesis of Xanthine*

i. *Due to Traube:*

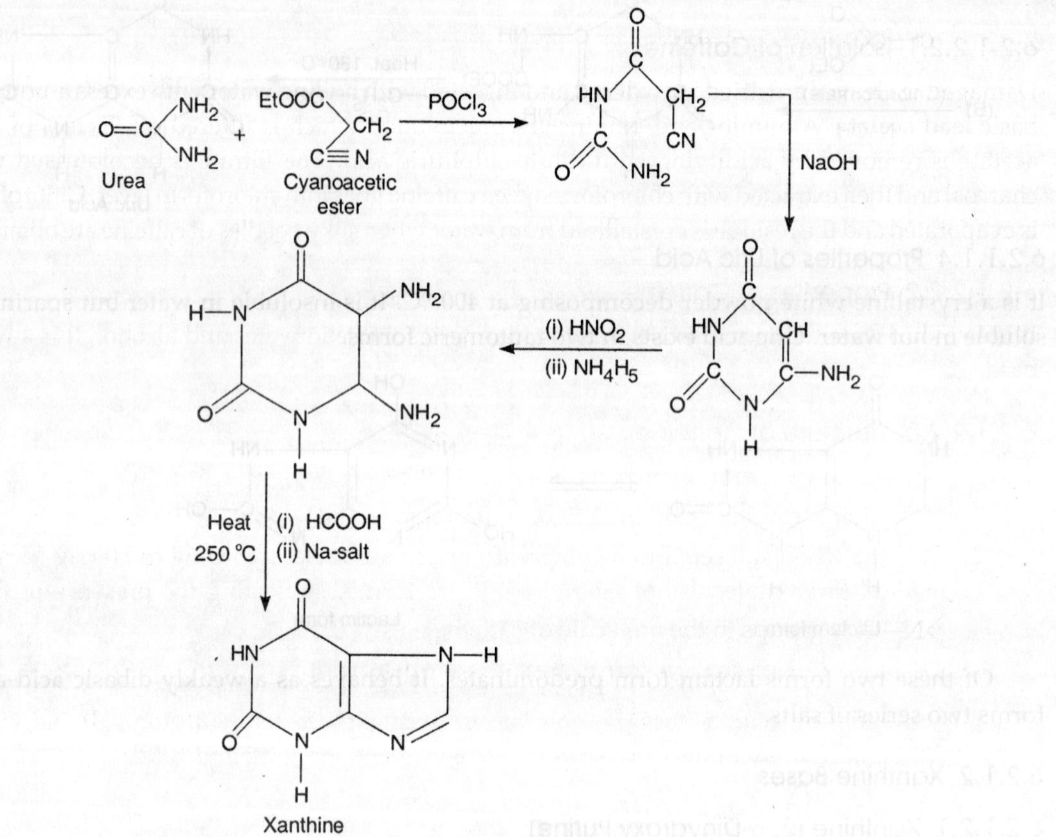

ii. *Due to Fischer:*

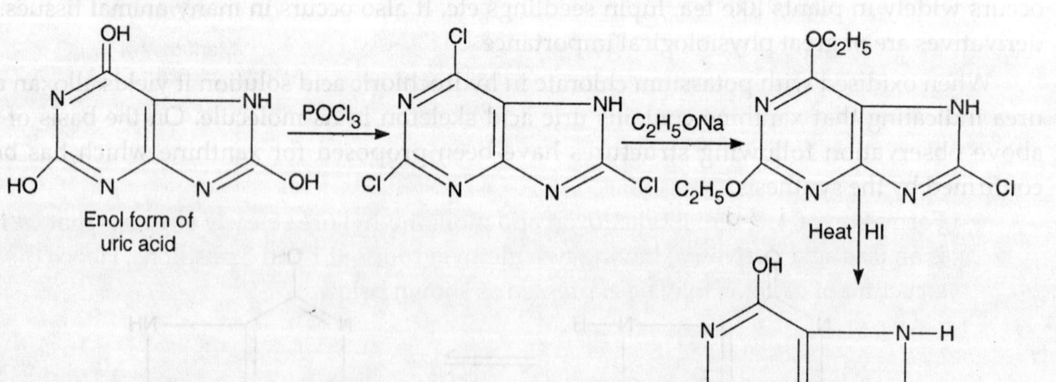

6.2.1.2.2 Caffeine or Theine

It is one of the most important member of xanthine group of purine bases. It occurs in tea *(Theu sinsis)*, coffee *(Coffea arabica)*, colanuts *(Cola acuminate)*, mate *(Ilex paraguayensis)* and many other plants. A cup of tea or coffee contains about 0.1g of caffeine. Cafeine was first isolated simultaneously by Pelletier, Runge and Robiquet in coccoa beans.

6.2.1.2.2.1 Isolation of Caffeine

Damaged tea leaves are dried, powdered and digested with boiling water with excess amount of basic lead acetate. Albumins and tannins are precipitated which is filtered off. Excess of lead acetate is removed by acidifying with dilute sulphuric acid. The filtrate is decolourised with charcoal and then extracted with chloroform when caffeine goes into chloroform layer. Chloroform is evaporated and the residue is crystallised from water when silky needles of caffeine are obtained.

6.2.1.2.2.2 Properties of Caffeine

It is a colourless solid, m.p. 235-238 °C. It is sparingly soluble in water and alcohol. It is a weak base.

6.2.1.2.2.3 Structure of Caffeine

The structure caffeine is established on the basis of following evidences.

1. Molecular formula of caffeine has been found to be $C_8H_{10}N_4O_2$.
2. Caffeine when subjected to heating with hydrolodic acid according to Herzig-Meyer's method three molecules of methyliodide are formed indicating the presence of three $>N-CH_3$ groups in the molecule of caffeine.

$$C_5HNO_2(N-CH_3)_3 + HI \longrightarrow C_5HO_2N(NH)_3 + 3CH_3I$$

3. On oxidation with potassium chlorate in hydrochloric acid solution caffeine yields equimolecular amounts of 1, 3-dimethyl alloxan and monomethyl rurea.

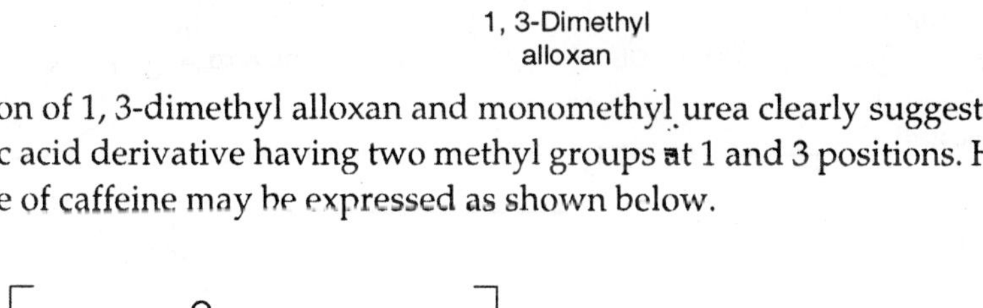

Formation of 1, 3-dimethyl alloxan and monomethyl urea clearly suggests that caffeine is an uric acid derivative having two methyl groups at 1 and 3 positions. Hence the part structure of caffeine may be expressed as shown below.

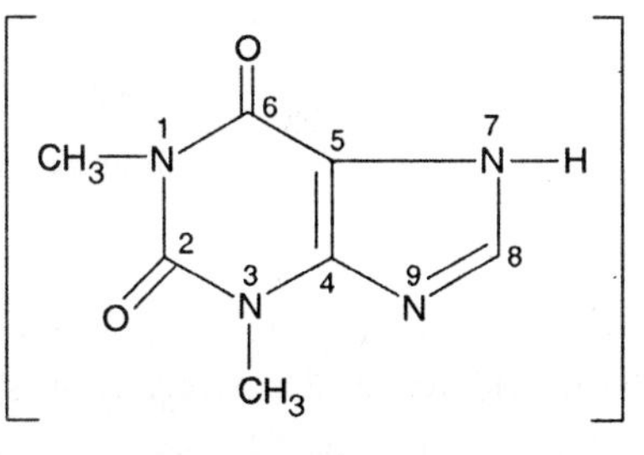

1. One $>N-CH_3$ group

• *Position of thrid* $>N-CH_3$ *group in Caffeine:* From the above part structure it is evident that the third $>N-CH_3$ may be either at 7 or at 9 position. Consequently two structures (A) and (B) have been proposed for caffeine.

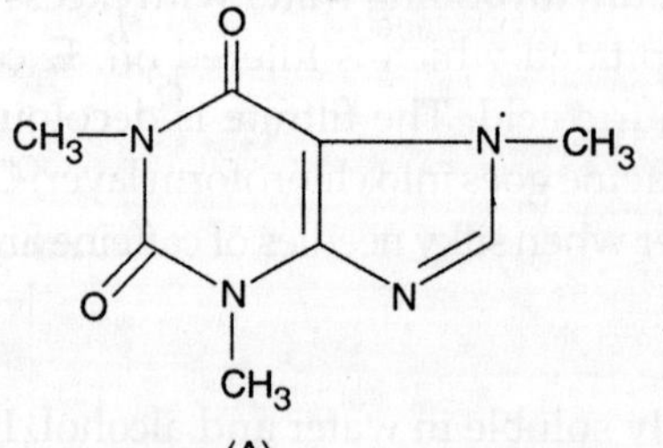

(A)

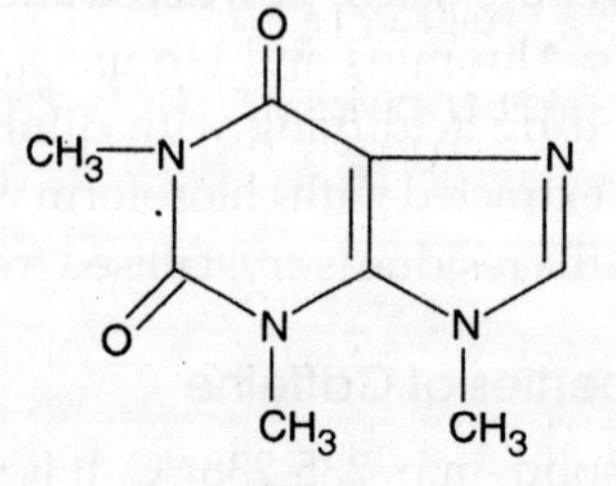

(B)

In order to decide which one (A or B) is the correct structure of Caffeine, oxidative experiment under drastic condition was employed. On such experiment caffeine yields symmetrical dimethyloxamide ($CH_3-NH-\underset{O}{\underset{\|}{C}}-\underset{O}{\underset{\|}{C}}-NH-CH_3$) formation of which is only possible from the structure (A) and hence the correct structure of caffeine stands as (A) which has been confirmed by synthesis.

6.2.1.2.2.4 Synthesis of Caffeine

i. *Fischer's synthesis:* In this synthesis the starting material is uric acid and it involves the following steps:

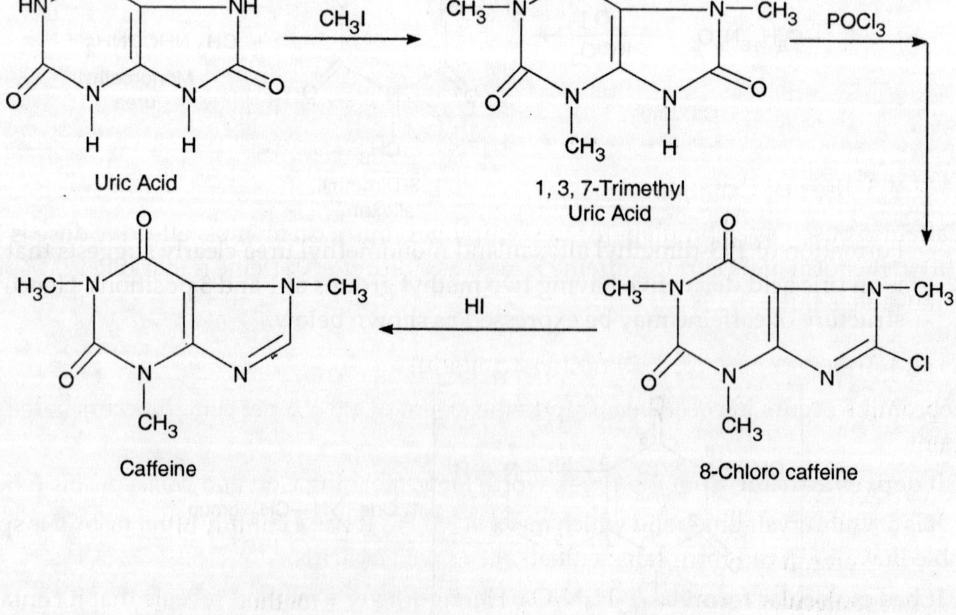

ii. *Traube's synthesis:*

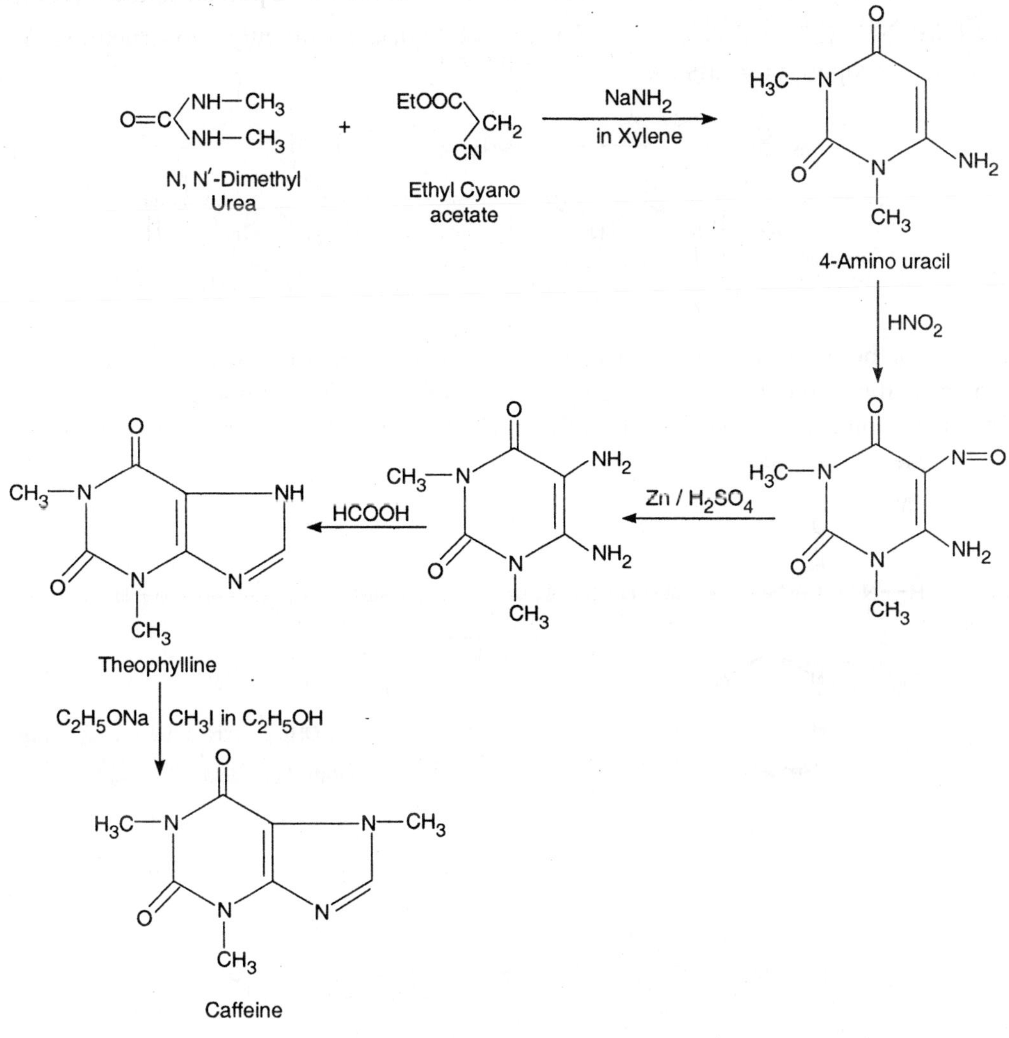

6.2.1.2.2.5 Uses of Caffeine

(i) Caffeine is used as a stimulant for the central nervous system, most effective dose is 150-250 mg (ii) In the form of its citrate, caffeine is used as a diuretic. Caffeine is marketed as aspirin and caffeine tablets B.P.

6.2.1.2.3 Theobromine (3, 7-Dimethyl Xanthine)

Theobromine occurs in cocao beans up to the extent of 1.5-2.5 per cent. It occurs in tea in trace amount.

It derives its name from the Greek word, *theos*, meaning God and *broma* means food.

It is a white crystalline solid which melts at 337 °C. It has a faintly bitter taste. It is sparingly soluble in water. It can form salts with alkalis as well as acids.

It has molecular formula, $C_7H_8N_4O_2$. Herzig-Meyer's method reveals that it contains two $>N-CH_3$ groupings. On methylation of its silver salt with methyl iodide, it forms caffeine, and

1, 3, 7-trimethyl xanthine. On the basis of the above observations two alternative structures have been suggested for theobromine.

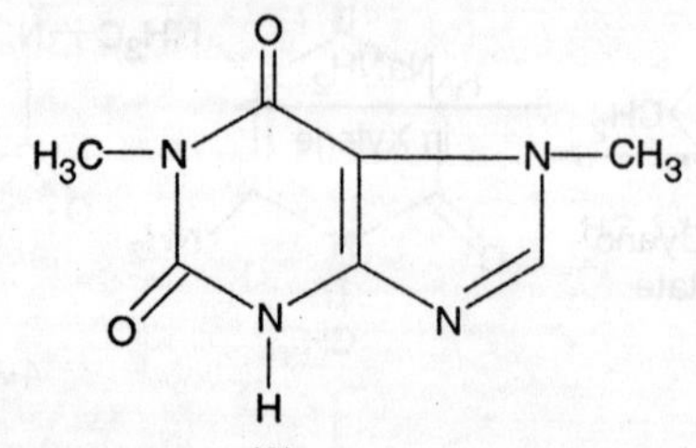

(A)

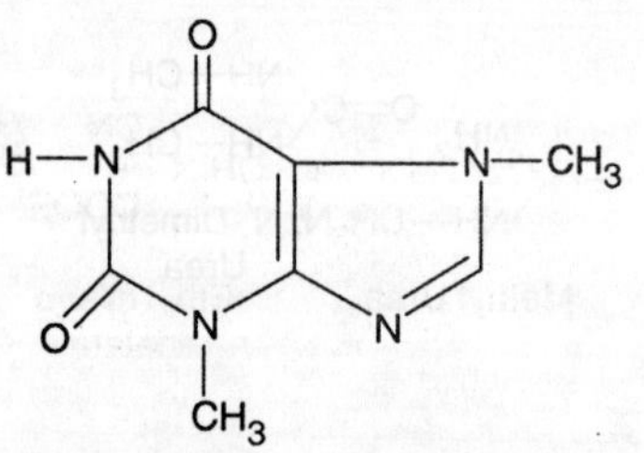

(B)

Out of these two alternatives structure (B) has been found to be correct because theobromine can be synthesised either from 3-methyl or 7-methyl uric acid but not from 1-methyl uric acid. Thus theobromine is 3, 7-dimethyl xanthine which has finally been confirmed by the synthesis.

i. *Fischer's synthesis:*

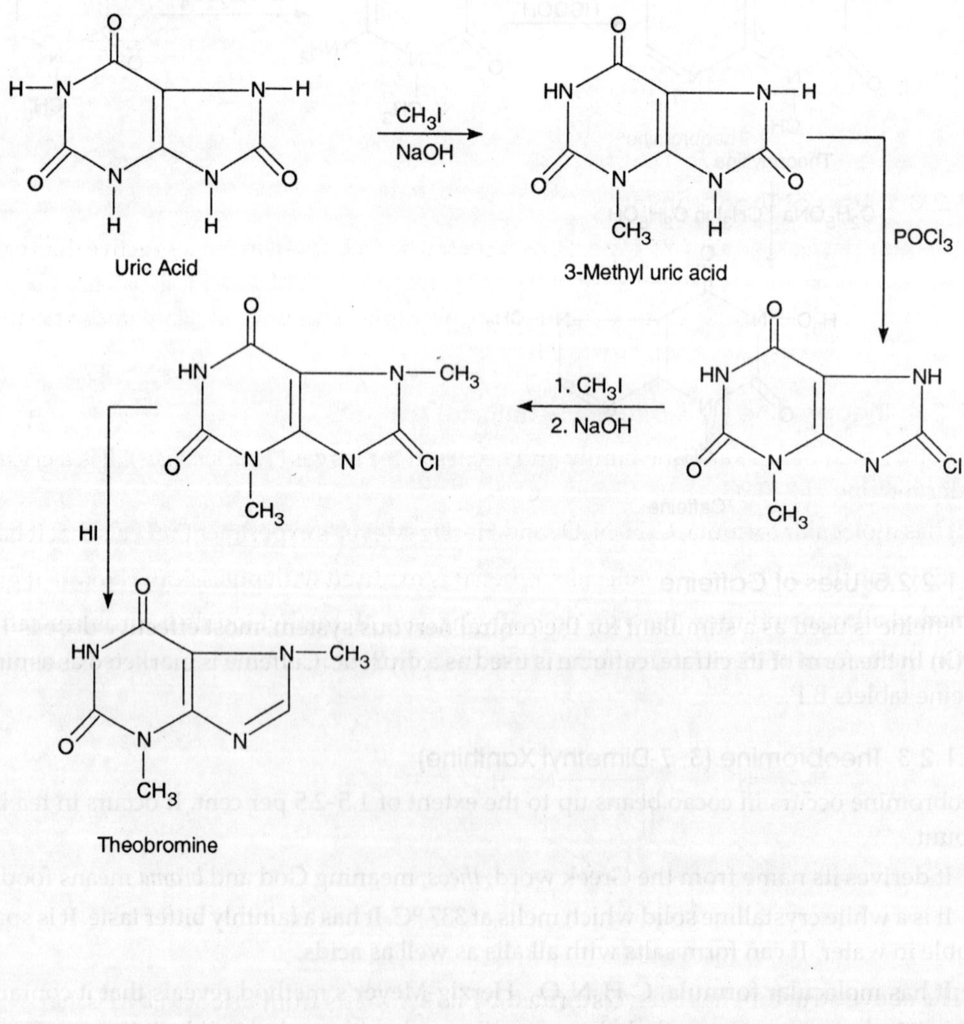

ii. *Traube's synthesis:*

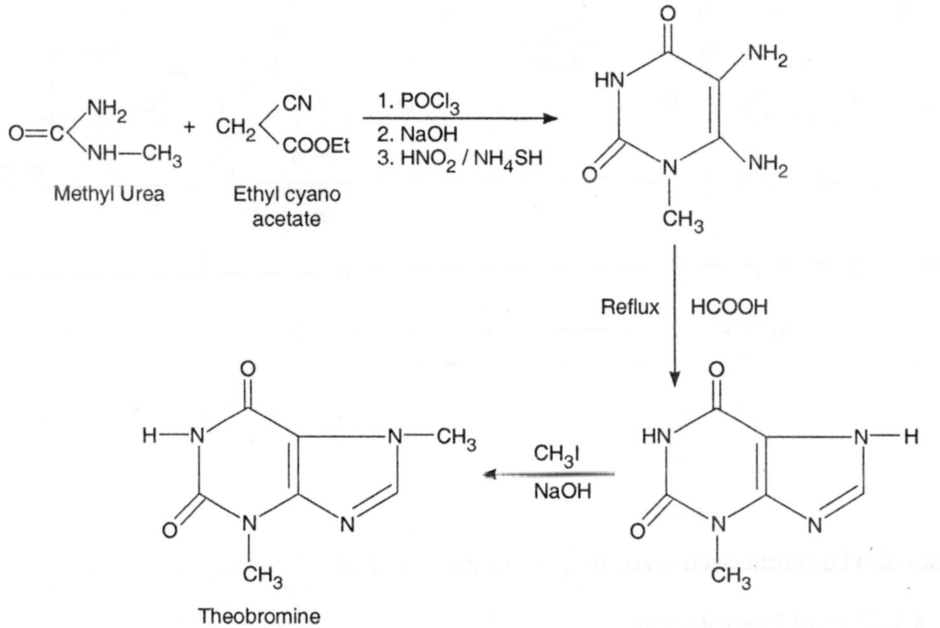

6.2.1.2.3.1 Uses of Theobromine

Theobromine possesses a stimulating action on central nervous system but less active than caffeine. It is also used as a diuretic but because of its low solubility in cold water it is usually used in the form of more soluble double salt, i.e., sodium theobromine sodium salicylate under trade name '*Diuretin*'. It is also used as a remedy for dropsy.

6.2.1.2.4 Theophylline (1, 3-Dimethyl Xanthine)

It is another member of xanthine family and occurs in tea leaves (*Thea sinensis*). It is a crystalline powder melting at 270 °C.

It has molecular formula, $C_7H_8N_4O_2$ and Herzig-Meyer's experiment reveals that it has two $>N-CH_3$ functionalities in its molecule. When it is oxidised with potassium chlorate it gives 1, 3-dimethyl alloxan and urea. Further, on methylation with methyl iodide it furnishes caffeine.

On the basis of the evidences, structure of theophylline may be represented as below.

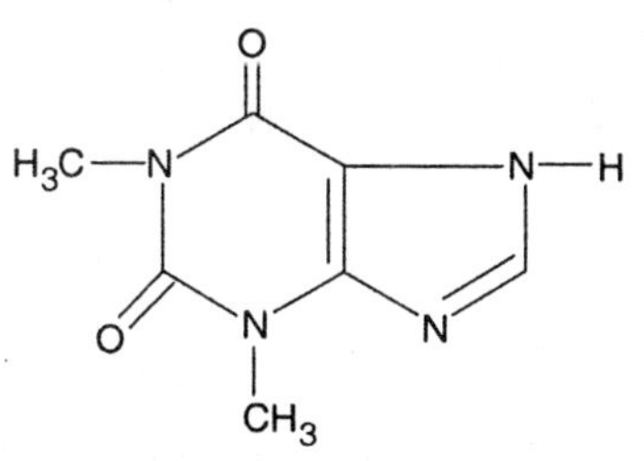

Theophylline

The above structure has been confirmed by its synthesis from uric acid by Fischer.

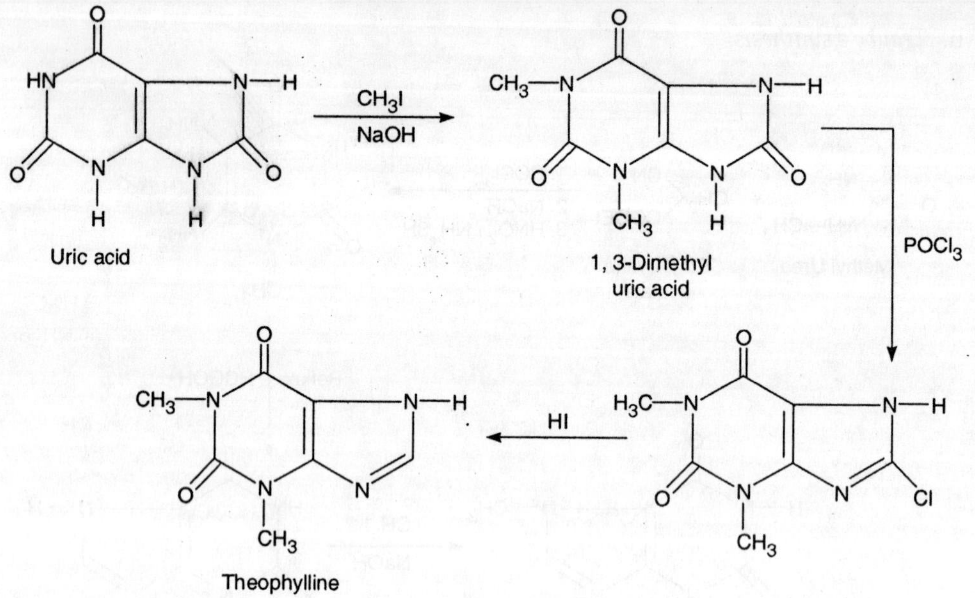

It can also be synthesised according to Traube's method.

6.2.1.2.4.1 Uses of Theophylline

It stimulates the central nervous system but is less active than caffeine.

It is used as a diuretic also and in this respect it is more powerful than caffeine and theobromine. It is marketed as aminphylline injection and tablets and also as choline theophylline tablets.

6.2.1.2.5 Hypoxanthine (6-Hydroxypurine)

Hypoxanthine occurs in tea extract and is frequently found in association with xanthine. It usually occurs in the muscles, spleen, liver and pancreas. It is a cystalline powder decomposing at 150 °C. Structurally it was found to be 6-hydroxy purine which has been confirmed by synthesis as described below:

i. *Due to Fischer:*

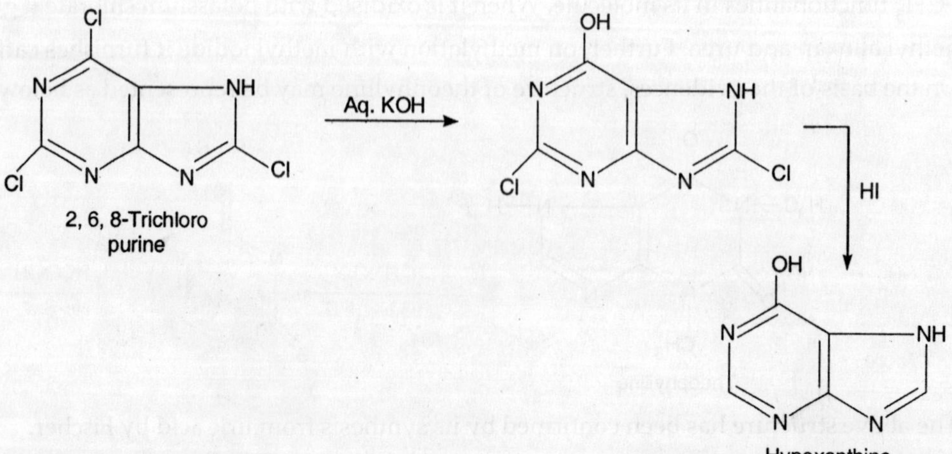

ii. *Traube's synthesis:*

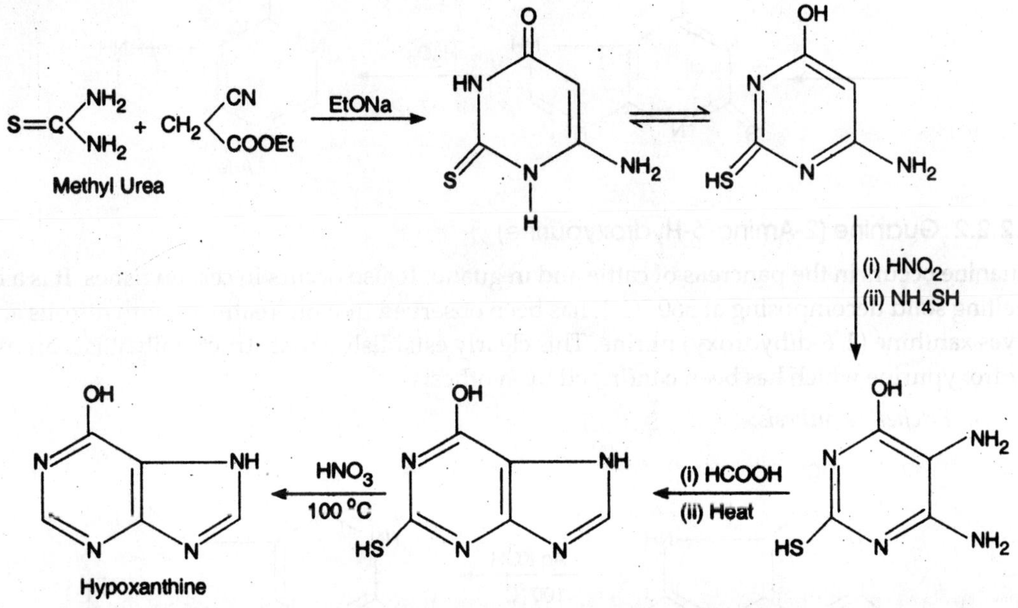

6.2.2 Aminopurine

6.2.2.1 Adenine (6-Aminopurine)

This occurs in the pancreas of cattle and in the tea extract. It is a solid and decomposes at 365 °C. Its structure has been settled on the fact that it shows similar reactions of purines and on treatment with nitrous acid forms hypoxanthine of known structure. Finally, its structure was established by synthesis.

i. *Fischer's synthesis:*

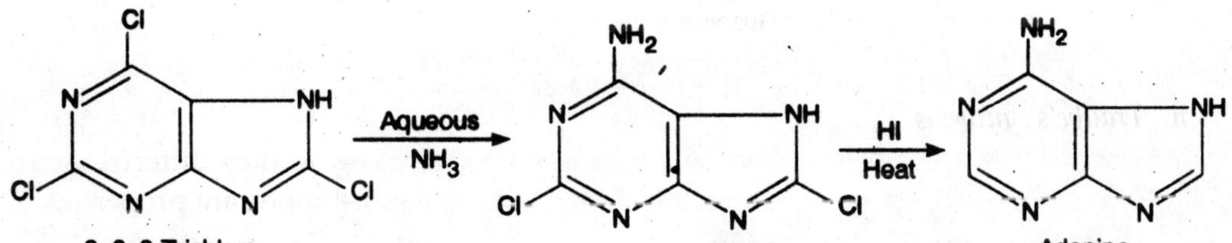

ii. *Traube's synthesis:*

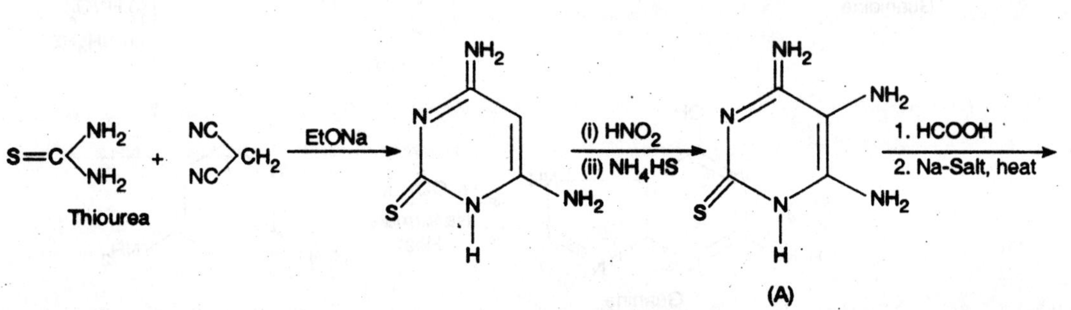

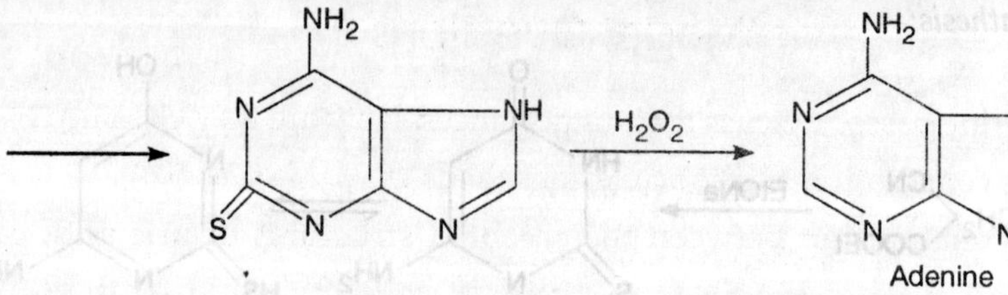

6.2.2.2 Guanine (2-Amino-6-Hydroxypurine)

Guanine occurs in the pancreas of cattle and in guano. It also occurs in certain fishes. It is a high melting solid decomposing at 360 °C. It has been observed that on treatment with nitrous acid it gives xanthine (2, 6-dihydroxy) purine. This clearly establishes that structurally it is 2-amino-6-hydroxypurine which has been confirmed by synthesis.

i. *Fischer's synthesis:*

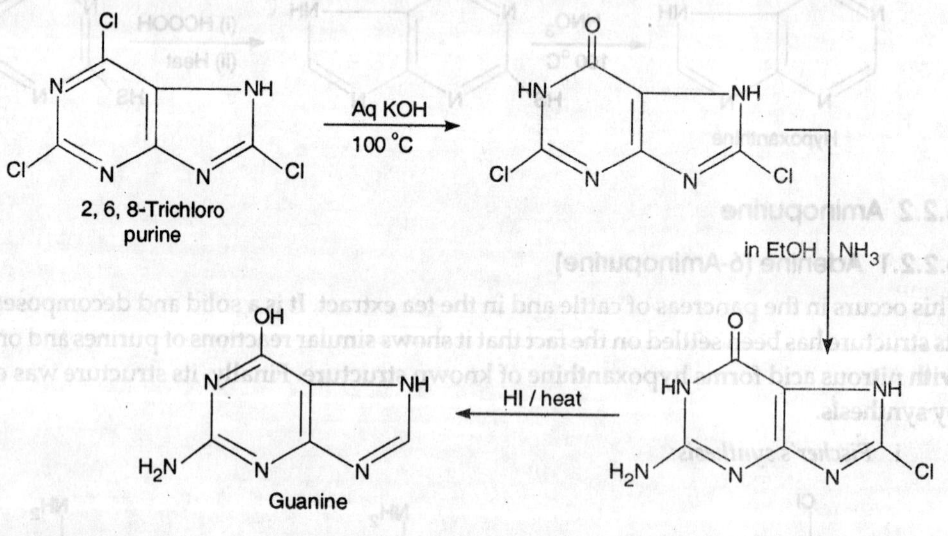

ii. *Traube's synthesis:*

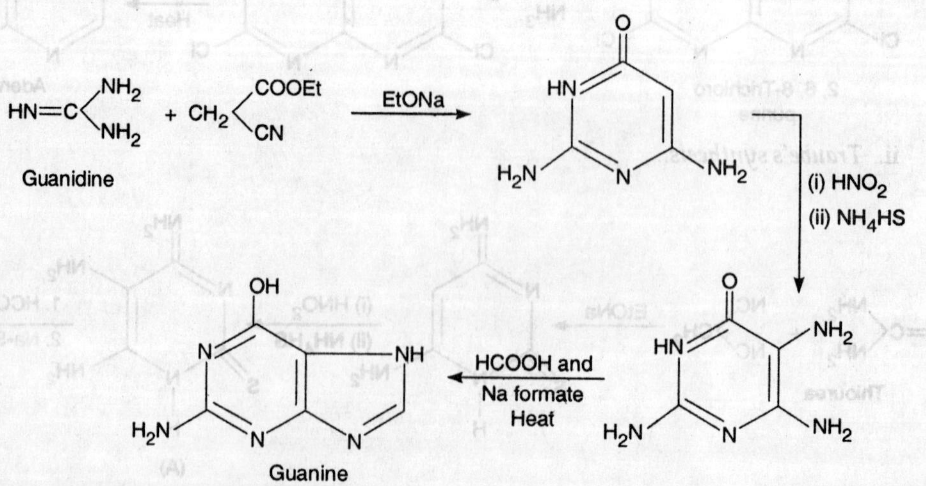

Model Questions

1. What are purine bases? Discuss their importances. How are they classified?
2. How has the constitution of uric acid established?
3. Discuss the relationship between the accepted structures of uric acid, caffeine and theobromine.
4. How is uric acid related to xanthine?
5. Discuss the structure of caffeine and give its synthesis.
6. How is caffeine isolated from tea leaves? Give its synthesis, properties and uses.
7. How would you establish the relationship between xanthine bases?
8. Discuss the synthesis of
   (a) Caffeine
   (b) Theophylline
   (c) Theobromine.

CHAPTER SEVEN

Lipids

7.1 Introduction

The term "Lipid" may be defined as a set of biomolecules which are soluble in organic solvents but insoluble in water. The set of biomolecules that forms lipids are variety of natural products occurring both in plants and animals. Chemically they belong to ester class of organic compounds and yield monocarboxylic acid (saturated and unsaturated) on hydrolysis. The lipids include oils, fats waxes and phospholipids.

7.2 Classification

Lipids are classified under following heads:

i. *Fats and Oils:* These are simplest lipids and mainly consist of triesters of glycerol and fatty acids with C_{12}-C_{22} carbon atoms chain. These esters are commonly known as *triglycerides.*

ii. *Waxes:* Waxes differ from fats and oils in the nature of ester chain. They are not the esters of glycerol but are the esters of long chain fatty acids with long chain monohydric alcohols.

iii. *Phospholipids:* These lipids differ from the simple lipids in the fact that they also contain phosphorous and nitrogen in their molecules.

7.2.1 Fats and Oils

As stated these are the simplest lipids found in nature and are triesters of long chain fatty acids and glycerol. They constitute one of the major sources of diet. These esters may be solid or liquid in nature. Fats are usually solids while oils are liquids. It has been observed that in general fats are the glycerides of long chain saturated fatty acids but in oils fatty acids are mostly unsaturated in nature. Recent scientific investigation reveals that excessive consumption of fats is injurious to health and causes coronary heart diseases. That is why it is advisable to use sunflower oil, soyabean oil, corn oil and other white oils as cooking media. This is because oils specially those mentioned, contain higher percentage of unsaturated fatty acids and they can decrease the level of cholesterol in blood, and hence risk of heart disease may be minimised.

7.2.1.1 Occurrence and Extraction of Fats and Oils

Fats and oils are widely distributed in nature—both plant and animal kingdom. In plants they mainly occur in seeds while in animals they are present under the skin and in the muscles.

From plants sources fats and oils are extracted by the following steps:

- *Step* I: *Cold pressing:* The seeds are crushed and then pressed in hydraulic press in the cold. In this way mainly high grade oils are obtained.
- *Step* II: The pressed cake obtained in step-I is heated and pressed further. This step is known as *hot pressing*. This step gives second grade oils.
- *Step* III: The pressed cake remained after hot pressing is crushed and extracted with organic solvent to obtain further quantity of oil.

7.2.1.1.1 Refining

The crude fats and oils obtained by the above processes is treated with alkali to neutralise free acids and to coagulate any colloidal impurities that may be present. After this, fats and oils are bleached by warming with animal charcoal or plaster of Paris or Fuller's earth.

7.2.1.1.2 General Physical Properties of Fats and Oils

Fats and oils are in general odourless and tasteless in pure condition. They are lighter than water and insoluble in water but are readily soluble in common organic solvents. Fats containing higher proportion of saturated fatty acids melt at relatively higher temperature but those containing higher proportion of unsaturated fatty acids melt at relatively low temperature.

7.2.1.1.2 Chemical Properties of Fats and Oils

As stated before fats and oils are chemically esters and hence they in general exhibit similar chemical behaviour as that of simple esters as mentioned below:

(a) *Hydrolysis:* Fats, like esters, undergo hydrolysis on heating with super heated steem or mineral acids or alkalies or enzyme.

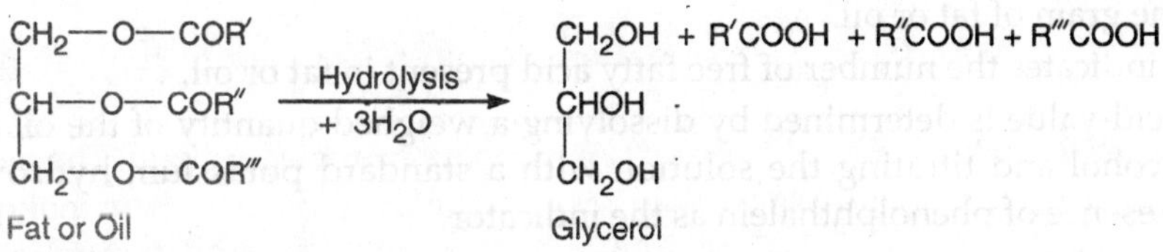

It may be mentioned that the hydrolysis is carried out with alkali when there is formation of sodium salt of fatty acids which are generally termed as soap and the process is known as *saponification*. This reaction is the basis of *soap industry*.

(b) *Hydrogenation:* Oils containing unsaturated glycerides can readily undergo hydrogenation in presence of finely divided nickel forming solid fats. Thus,

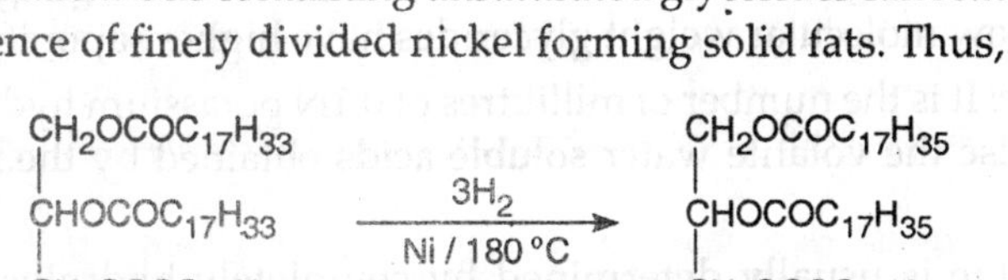

This hydrogenation process is the basis of commercial production of hydrogenated oils ('Vanaspati ghee' or margarine). This process is usually termed as *hardening of oils* because it raises the melting point of the fat. In industry, hydrogenation is not carried out to completion but is stopped as soon as the fat of desired level is obtained. The completely hydrogenated fat are too hard to be useful for kitchen purpose.

(c) *Hydrogenolysis:* Fats and oils can be cleaved into long chain aliphatic alcohols and glycerol by passing excess of hydrogen through fats and oils in presence of copper chromium catalyst at high temperature and under pressure.

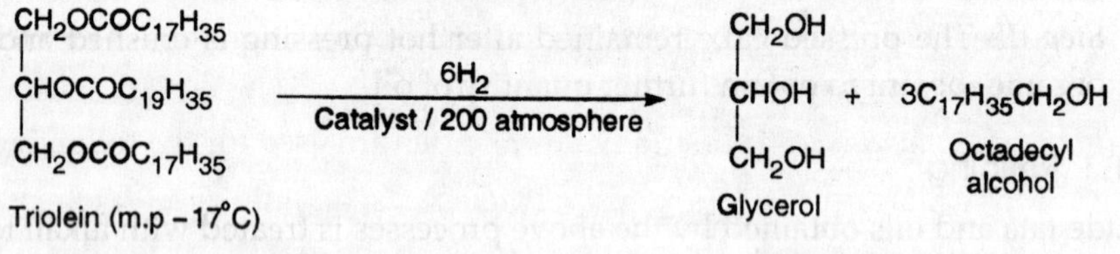

(d) *Rancidification:* On keeping fats and oils for a long storage in contact with air and moisture an unpleasant odour is developed. Such fats and oils are known as *rancid oils.* It has been suggested that some chemical changes occur for the development of rancidity such as (i) enzymatic hydrolysis in presence of micro-organisims and enzymes with the formation of bad smelling lower fatty acids (ii) air oxidation of unsaturated acid giving aldehydes and ketones having unpleasant flavour (iii) β-oxidation of saturated acids forming ketones with unpleasant odour. It is, therefore, desirable that fats and oils must be protected from air and moisture during storage.

7.2.1.1.4 Analysis of Fats and Oils

Analysis of fats and oils involves some physical tests such as determination of melting point, viscosity, specific gravity, etc. and some chemical determinations like acid-value, iodine-value, saponification value, Reichert-Meissi-value, etc. These determinations reveal the quality of a given fat and oil.

(a) *Acid-value:* It is the number of milligrams of potassium-hydroxide needed to neutralise one gram of fat or oil.
It indicates the number of free fatty acid present in fat or oil.
Acid-value is determined by dissolving a weighed quantity of the oil or fat in neutral alcohol and titrating the solution with a standard potassium hydroxide solution in presence of phenolphthalein as the indicator.

(b) *Iodine-value:* It is the measure of number of unsaturation present in fats and oils. It is defined as the number of grams of iodine required to combine with the hundred grams of fats and oils. Higher iodine value indicates greater degree of unsaturation.

(c) *Saponification-value:* It represents the number of milligrams of potassium hydroxide required to hydrolyse one gram of fat or oil. Fats and oils containing higher percentage of short chain and low molecular weight glycerides have higher saponification value.

(d) *Reichert-Meissi value:* It is the number of millilitres of 0.1N potassium hydroxide solution required to neutralise the volatite water soluble acids obtained by the hydrolysis of 5 gram of the fat.

Reichert-Meissi value is usually determined by completely hydrolysing a weighed quantity of the fat or oil with alkali. The resulting solution is acidified with sulphuric acid and then steam distjlled. The distillate is titrated with 0.1N potassium hydroxide solution. The Reichert-Meissi value is particularly important for testing purity of ghee or butter.

7.2.1.1.5 Importance of Fats and Oils

Fats and oils are important chemical components both for biological and industrial purposes.

(a) *Biological importance:* The main function of fats and oils in animal is to act as an *energy reserve.* When triglycerides are converted to carbon dioxide and water by biochemical reactions, they yield more than twice as many kilocalories per gram as do carbohydrates and proteins. Male human being normally contains 21% and females have 26% fat. This fat content is sufficient to enable us to survive starvation for 2-3 months. Thus fats and oils may be used as food.

(b) *Industrial importance:* Industrially fats and oils are used for the following purposes.

i. Many fats and oils are extensively used in soap industry.
ii. Oils, like linseed oil are frequently used in the manufacture of paints, varnishes and lacquers.
iii. They are important raw materials for the preparation of higher alcohols used in the manufacture of *synthetic detergents.*
iv. *Oil cloth* and *linoleum* require linseed oil for their manufacture.
v. Oils like castor oil and croton oil are used as purgative.
vi. Castor oil is used as lubricant.
vii. Oils are used in the preparation of hair oils, candles, polish, etc.
viii. Oils such as linseed oil and tung oil (china wood oil) form hard, elastic and water insoluble coatings when exposed to air in thin layers. This phenomenon is known as *drying* and such oils are termed as *drying oil*. Mechanistically, the process of drying involves partial oxidation, polymerisation and colloidal gel formation. Drying oils are used in the manufacture of shellac, varnish and paints.
ix. Oils like ground nut oil, are used in the manufacture of *vegetable ghee* or *margarine.*

7.2.2 Waxes

Waxes are the esters of long chain fatty acids with long chain monohydric alcohols. Waxes are low melting solids and cannot be made soluble in water by boiling. Large variety of waxes are known as mentioned below:

(a) *Bee Wax:* It is the major constituent of honeycomb of the bee. It is myricyl palmitate ($C_{15}H_{33}COOC_{16}H_{35}$). It is used in the preparation of candles, lipsticks, cosmetic creams as well as boot, floor and furniture polisher.

(b) *Carnauba Wax:* It is primarily myricyl cerotate, $C_{25}H_{31}COOC_{30}H_{61}$ and occurs in *Carnauba* plam leaves native in Brazil. It is used as coating on stencil and carbon papers.

(c) *Supernacete Wax:* It is extracted from the cavity of the sperm whale. It is cetyl palmitate, $C_{15}H_{31}COOC_{16}H_{31}$. It is used in the manufacture of soaps, skin-ointments and cosmetics.

7.2.3 Phospholipids

Phospholipids contain only two acyl groups and in place of the third, a phosphate group. The parent structure is diacetyl glycerol phosphate or phosphatidic acid as shown:

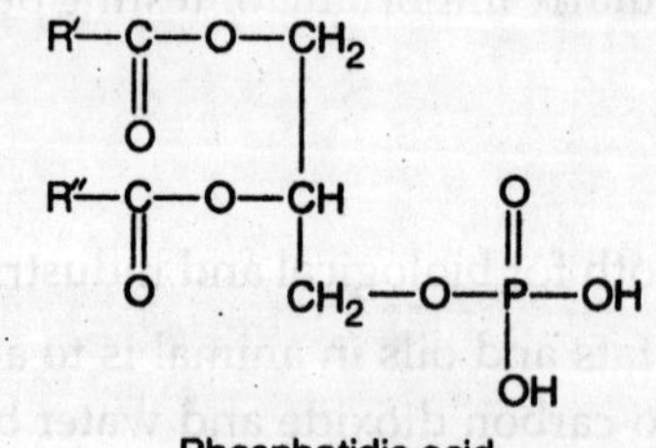

Phosphatidic acid

Usually, the phosphoric acid part a nitrogen base is connected, when the base is *cholamine,* $CH_2OH—CH_2—NH_2$, the phospholipid is known as *Kephalin* and when the base attached is *choline,* $CH_2OH-CH_2-N(CH_3)_3\}\overline{OH}$, the phospholipid is called *lecithin.* These compounds have betaine structures as indicated below:

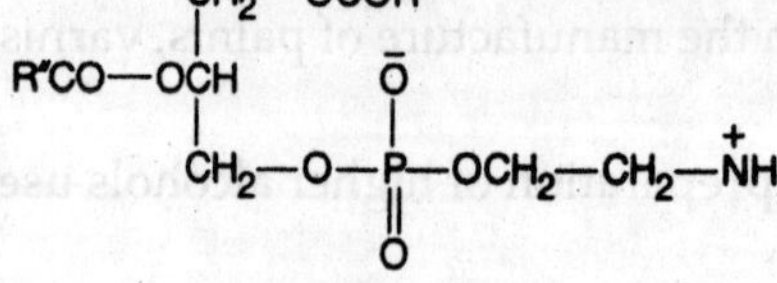

Kephalin

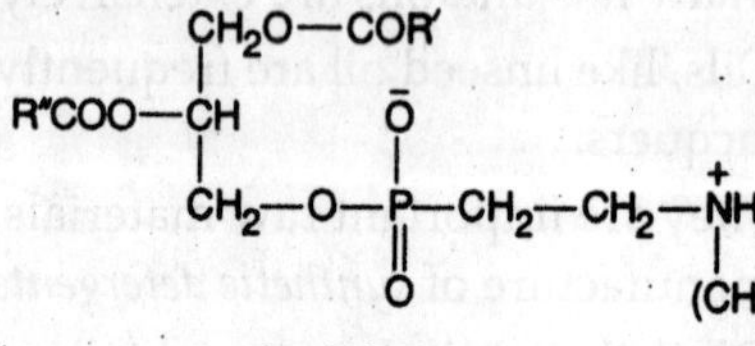

Lecithin

Sometimes kephalin may contain L-serine in place of aminoethanol. Phospholipids are also known as phosphoglycerides.

Phospholipids are found in the membranes of the cells which are the basic structural element of living organisms.

Phospholipids are amphipathic and resemble soaps and detergents. The lipophilic part in phospholipids is the long chain fatty acids and the hydrophilic part is ionic end. In cell, phospholipids exist in bilayers. They constitute the walls that not only enclose the cell but also very selectively control the passage in and out of the various substances like nutrients, waste products, hormones, etc.

Model Questions

1. What do you mean by the term fats oils, and waxes? How do they differ? Discuss the methods of isolation of fats and oils and mention their some important properties.
2. Define and give examples of
   (a) acid-value (b) iodine-value
   (c) saponification-value (d) Reichert-Meissi-value
   (e) hardening of oil (f) lipids
   (g) phospholipids (h) rancidification.
3. What are lipids? How would you classify lipids with examples?
4. Chemically what are fats and oils? Discuss various physical and chemical properties of fats and oils.
5. How the quality of an oil is determined? Mention some parameters for the assessment of the quality of an oil.

CHAPTER EIGHT

Phenolic Compounds

(Flavones, Isoflavones, Coumarins, Lignans and Tannins)

Phenolic compounds are a vast group of naturally occurring chemical compounds with diverse skeleton pattern. They contain at least one phenolic moiety in their skeletons. Among the different structural types of this group of phytochemicals only a few, viz., flavones and isoflavones, coumarin, lignans and tannins deserve special attention. Most of these compounds possess various degrees of antioxidant or free radical scavenging properties. Many of these phytochemicals possess medicinal properties and have long been used as drugs such as etoposide and teniposide, the two anticancer lignan drugs.

8.1 Flavones and Isoflavones

Flavones and isoflavones are naturally occurring pigments. Both of these two types of pigments occur in nature either in free state or as glycosides. However, isoflavones are not so widespread as flavones. Chemically these two classes are hydroxylated phenyl derivatives of *Chromene* and they differ in the position of phenyl nucleus in chromene nucleus. Thus,

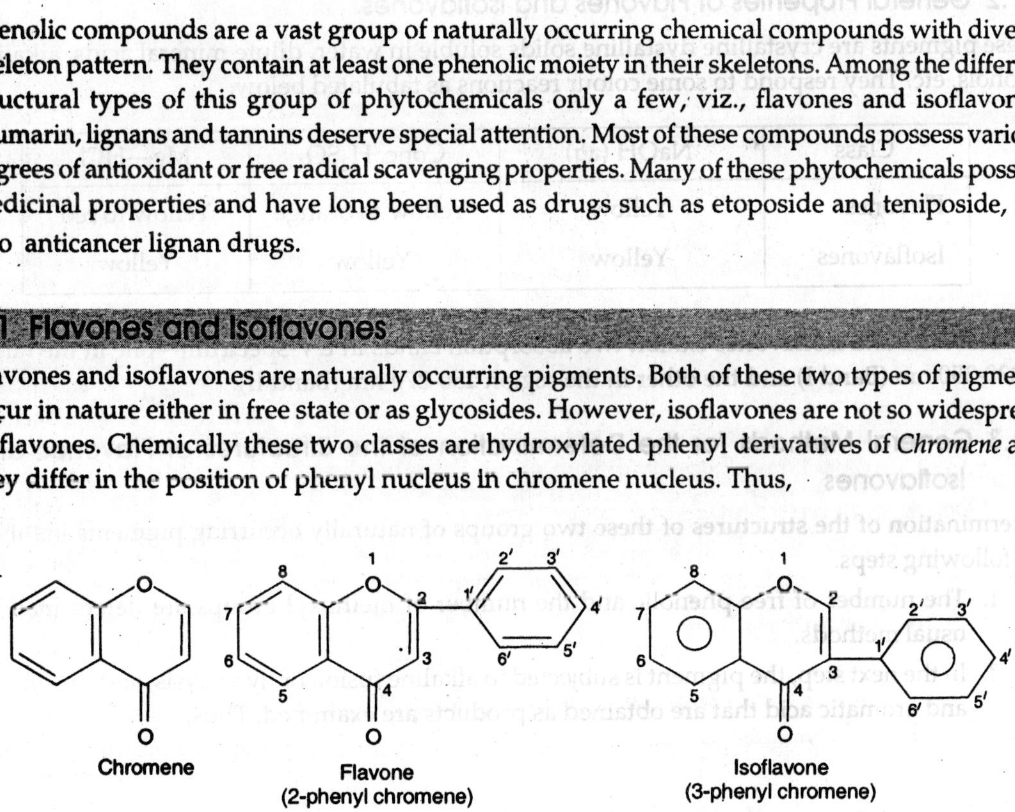

Chromene

Flavone (2-phenyl chromene)

Isoflavone (3-phenyl chromene)

In almost all the cases 5 and 7 positions are hydroxylated and frequently one or more positions (3′, 4′ and 5′) of the phenyl ring are also hydroxylated. In both classes, some of the positions may be alkylated. It has been observed that generally position 5, 7 and 4 are unmethylated but 3′ and 5′ positions are often methylated.

Most of the flavonoids have been found to be potent antioxidant agents. Many flavonoids possess anti-inflammatory, antihepatoxic, antitumour, antimicrobial and antiviral properties. Many medicines and medicinal plants contain flavonoids as the active compounds. It is believed that due to their antioxidant properties flavonoids present in fresh furits and vegetables act as preventive agents against cancer and heart diseases. Rutin, a very commonly occurring flavone glycoside is included in various multivitamin preparations. Hesperidin, another flavone glycoside of *citrus* peels has been included in a number of dietary supplement and found to have a beneficial effect for the treatment of capillary bleeding.

8.1.1 Isolation of Flavones and Isoflavones

The plant material containing these pigments is extracted with boiling water and the tannins are removed as lead salt by means of lead acetate. The filtrate is diluted with water acidified with HCl and boiled for a few hours when these sugar-free pigments are precipitated. The precipitate is extracted with alcohol and purified by fractional crystallisation of its acetate.

8.1.2 General Properties of Flavones and Isoflavones

These pigments are crystalline dystalline solids soluble in water, dilute mineral acids, alkalies, alcohols, etc. They respond to some colour reactions as tabulated below:

Class	NaOH (aq)	Conc. H_2SO_4	Mg—HCl
Flavones	Yellow	Yellow to orange	Yellow to red
Isoflavones	Yellow	Yellow	Yellow

Flavones and isoflavones exhibit two absorption bands in UV-spectrum—one in the range of 330-350 nm (Band I) and the other in the region 250-270 nm (Band II).

8.1.3 General Methods for the Determination of the Structures of Flavones and Isoflavones

Determination of the structures of these two groups of naturally occurring pigments involves the following steps.

1. The number of free phenolic and the number of methoxyl groups are determined by usual methods.
2. In the next step, the pigment is subjected to alkaline fusion or hydrolysis, and the phenol and aromatic acid that are obtained as products are examined. Thus,

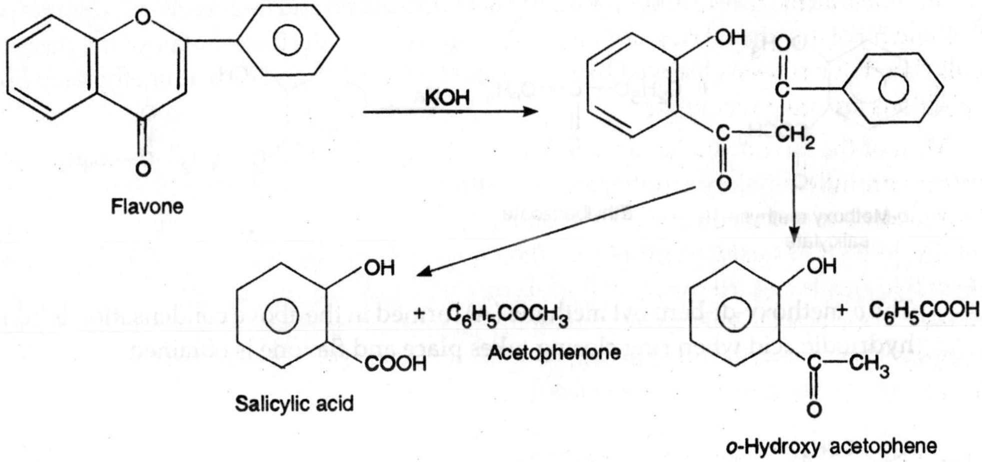

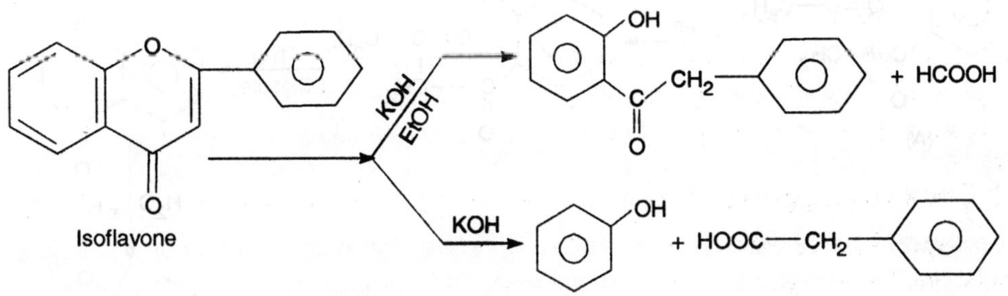

3. Finally the structure is confirmed by synthesis.

8.1.4 Some Important Methods of Synthesis of Flavones and Isoflavones

8.1.4.1 Synthesis of Flavones

Flavones are commonly prepared by the following methods.

8.1.4.1.1 Kostanecki Method

It is an important general method for the synthesis of flavones. This method involves the condensation of either an alkylated salicylic acid with acetophenone or ortho-alkylated acetophenone with the ester of an aromatic acid in presence of metallic sodium. Thus,

1. 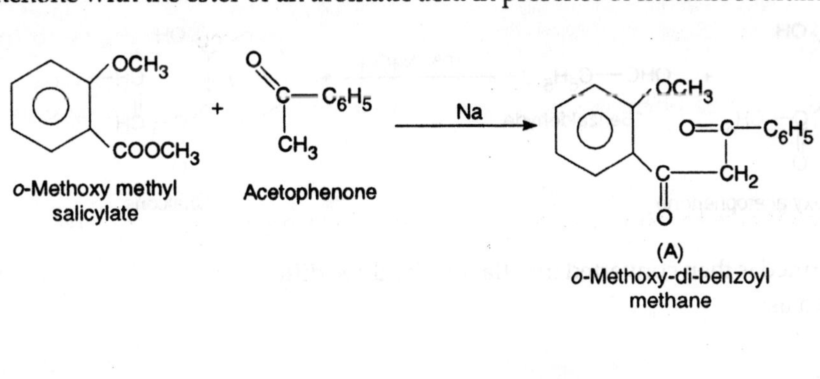

ii. 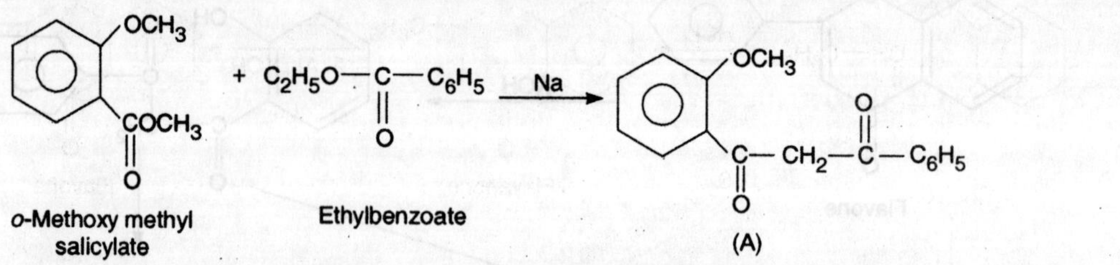

The *o*-methoxy-di-benzoyl methane (A) formed in the above condensation is boiled with hydriodic acid when ring closing takes place and flavone is obtained.

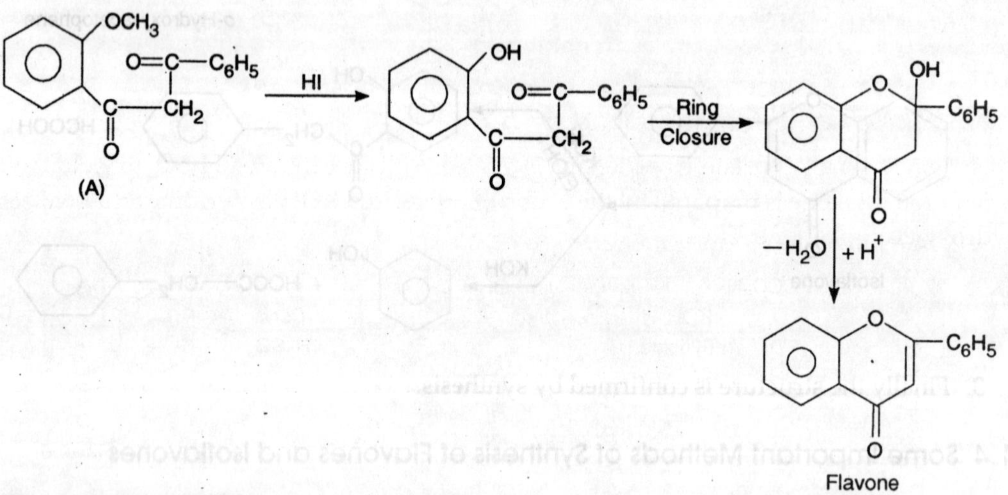

8.1.4.1.2 Chalcone Method

It is also a general method developed by Kastanecki and his associates. This method consists of the conversion of chalcone into flavone. The first step of this synthesis involves the condensation of *o*-hydroxy acetophenone with an aromatic aldehyde to form a chalcone in presence of 10% NaOH alcoholic or aqueous solution.

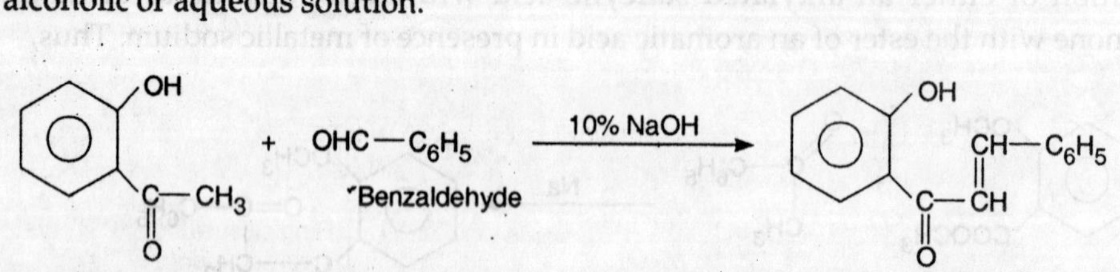

Chalcone formed is then converted into flavone by three different ways. These three methods may be illustrated as:

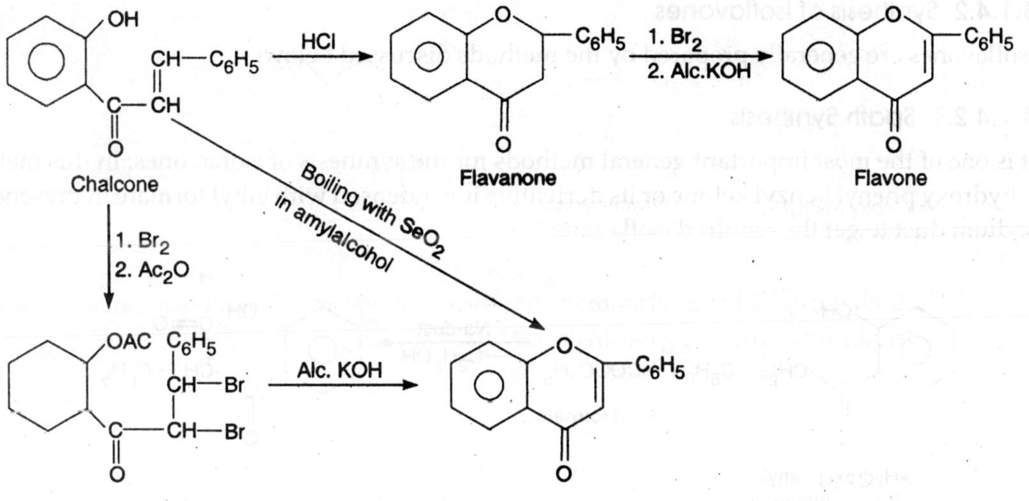

8.1.4.1.3 Baker-Venkatraman Method

In this method an appropriate 1, 3-diketone is treated with concentrated H_2SO_4 to yield flavone. The required diketone is prepared by the action of pulverised KOH in pyridine on *o*-benzoate of *o*-hydroxy-acetophenone. Thus,

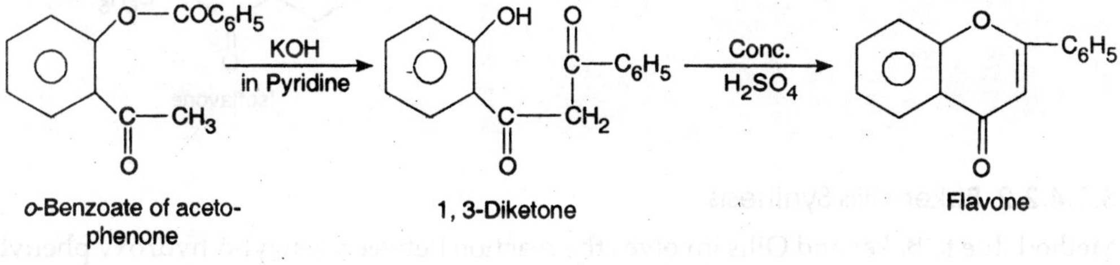

8.1.4.1.4 Robinson Method

It is the most useful general synthetic method for the prepavation of flavones. It consists of heating *o*-hydroxy acetophenone with the anhydride of benzoic acid in presence of sodium benzoate.

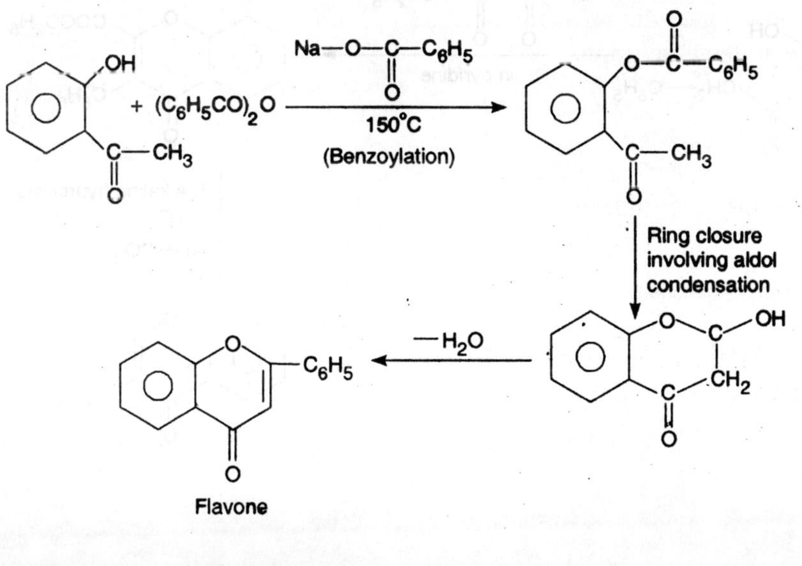

8.1.4.2 Synthesis of Isoflavones

Isoflavones are generally prepared by the methods discussed below:

8.1.4.2.1 Spath Synthesis

It is one of the most important general methods for the synthesis of isoflavones. In this method *o*-hydroxy phenyl benzyl ketone or its derivative is condensed with ethyl formate in presence of sodium dust to get the required isoflavone.

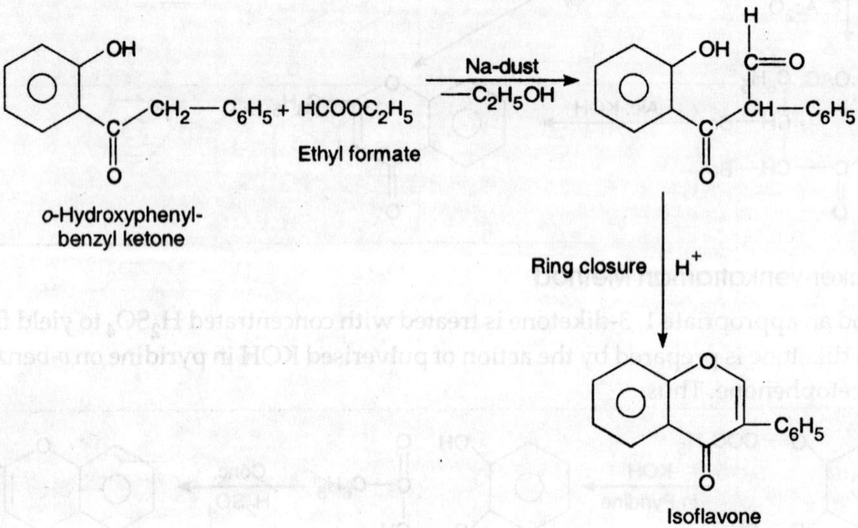

8.1.4.2.2 Baker-Ollis Synthesis

Method due to Baker and Ollis involves the reaction between benzyl-o-hydroxy phenyl ketones with ethoxalyl chloride in pyridine at room temperature. The products, on alkaline hydrolysis followed by acidification and heating yields isoflavones,

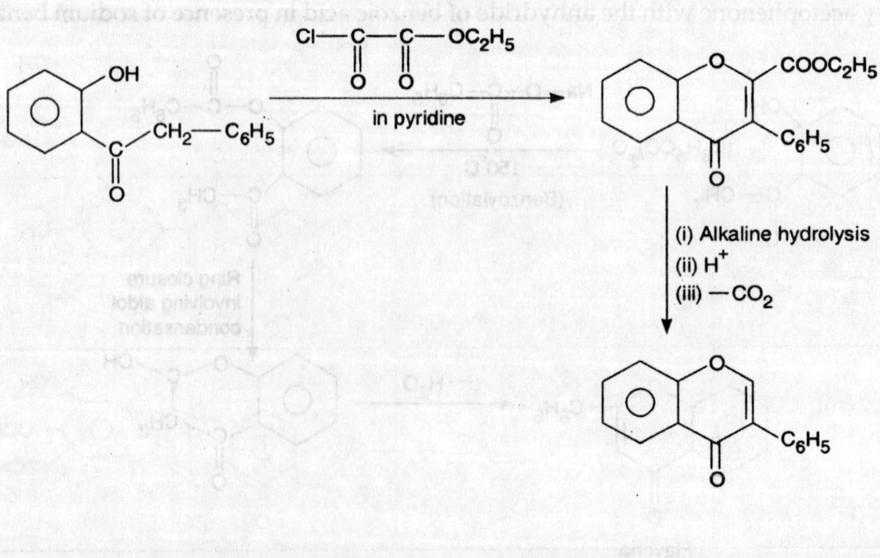

8.1.4.3 Some Common and Important Flavones and Isoflavones

Some important and extremely common flavones and isoflavones are tabulated below:

Sl. No.	Common Name	Chemical Nature	Structure
1.	Flavone	2-Phenyl-benzo-γ-pyrone	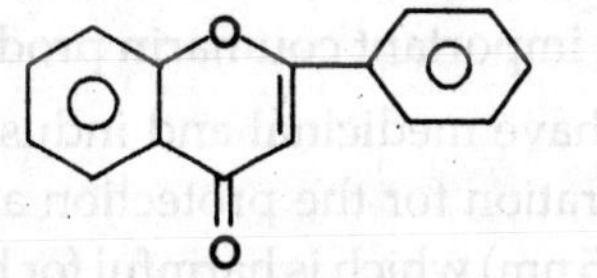
2.	Chrysin	5, 7-Dihydroxy-flavone	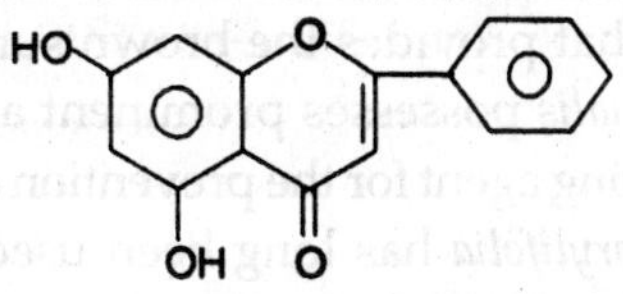
3.	Apigenin	5, 7, 4′-Trihydroxy flavone	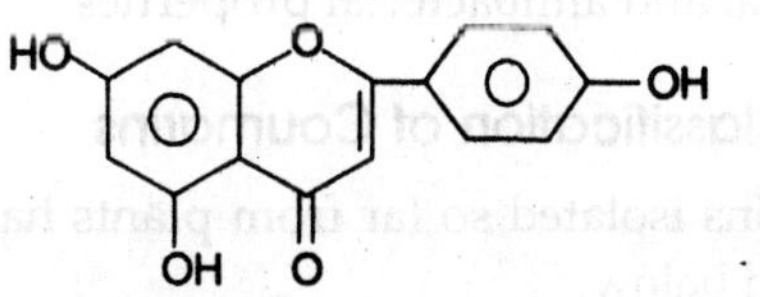
4.	Luteolin	5, 7, 3′, 4′-Tetrahydroxy flavone	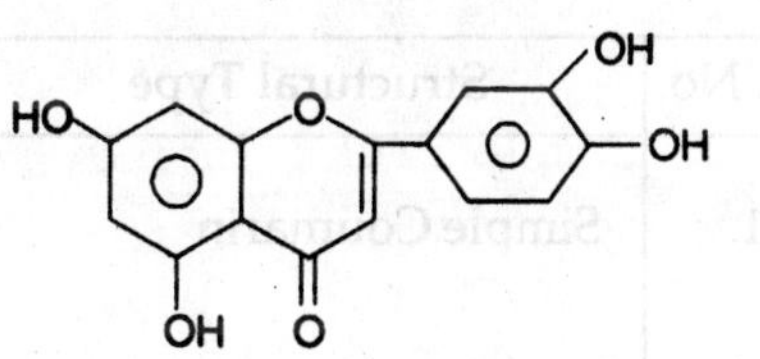
5.	Isoflavone	3-Phenyl-benzo-γ-pyrone	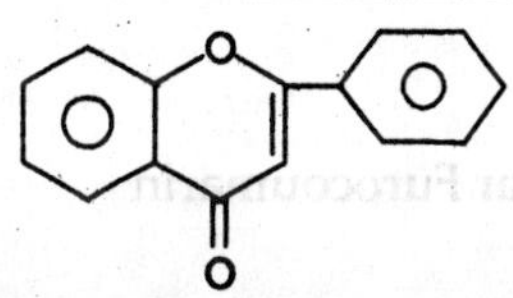
6.	Daidzein	7, 4′-Dihydroxy isoflavone	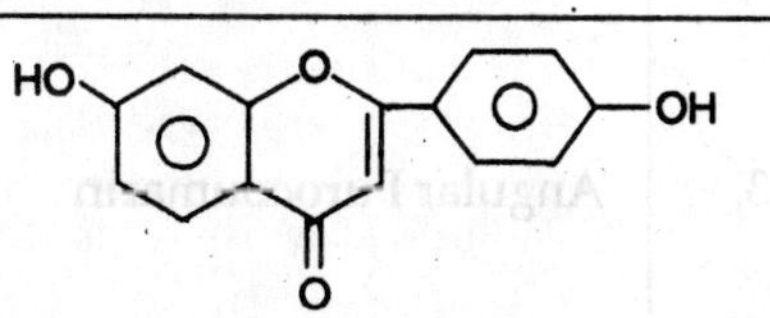
7.	Genistein	5, 7, 4′-Trihydroxy isoflavone	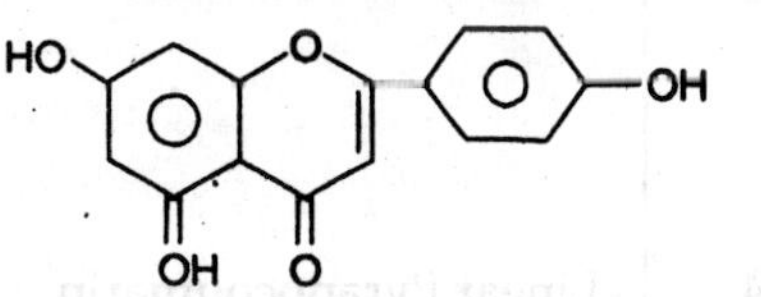
8.	Irigenin	5,7, 3′-Trihydroxy- -6, 4′, 5-trimethoxy isoflavone	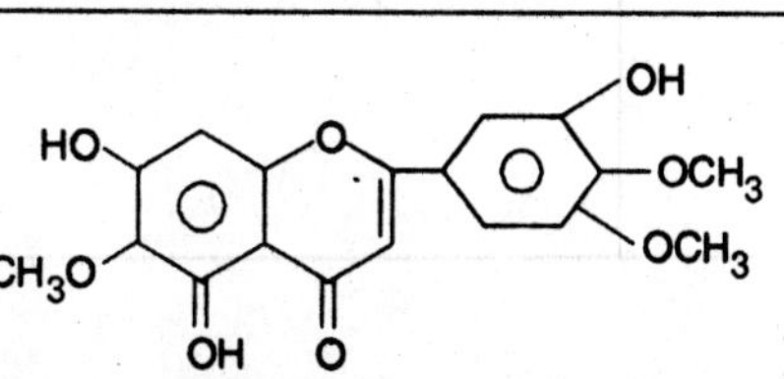

8.2 Coumarins

Coumarins are the largest group of I-benzopyran derivatives mainly occur in higher plants. Majority of coumarins have oxygen function at C-7 position as in the case of umbelliferone (7-hydroxy coumarin). Umbelliferone is considered as the structural and biological parent of the highly oxygenated coumarins. They abundantly occur in different plant families, viz, *Apiaceae, Asteraceae, Fabaceae, Lamiaceae, Moraceae, Rutaceae* and *Solanaceae*. However, *Apiaceae* and *Rutaceae* are the two most important coumarin producing plant families.

Coumarins have medicinal and industrial uses. Many members of this group are used in sunscreen preparation for the protection against sun ray because they absorb short wave UV-radiation (280-315 nm) which is harmful for human skin, but transmits the long wave UV-radiation (315-400 nm) that provides the brown sun-tan. Dicumarol, a dimeric coumarin obtained from *Melilotus officinalis* possesses prominent anticoagulant property and is used in medicine as an anti-blood clotting agent for the prevention of thrombosis. Psoralen, a linear furo coumarin isolated from *Psorlea corylifolia* has long been used in the treatment of vertigo. Many coumarins have antifungal and antibacterial properties.

8.2.1 Classification of Coumarins

Coumarins isolated so far from plants have been classified on the basis of structural types as tabulated below:

Sl. No.	Structural Type	Representative Member
1.	Simple Coumarin	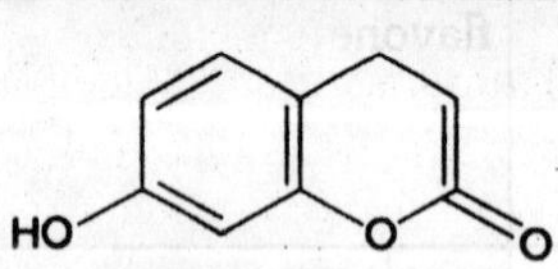 umbelliferone
2.	Linear Furocoumarin	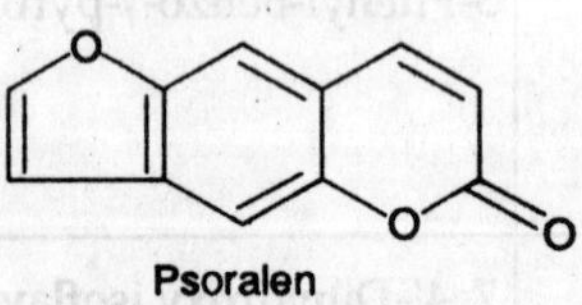 Psoralen
3.	Angular Furocoumarin	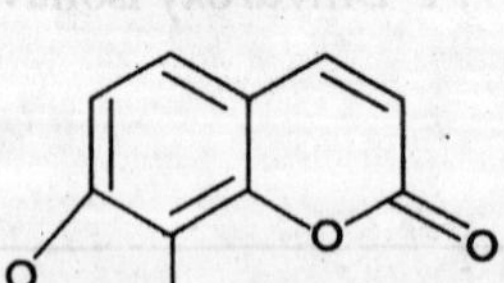 Angelicin
4.	Linear Pyranocoumarin	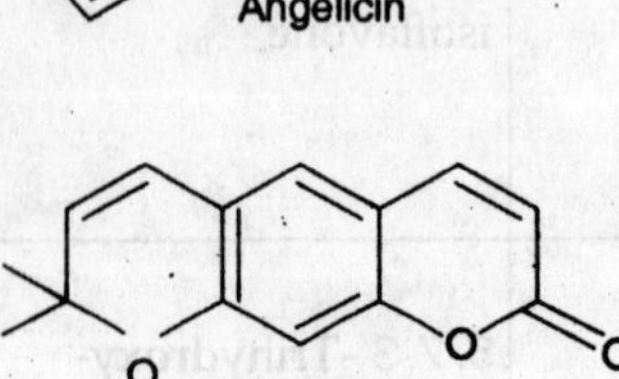 Xanthyletin

Sl. No.	Structural Type	Representative member
5.	Angular Pyrocoumarin	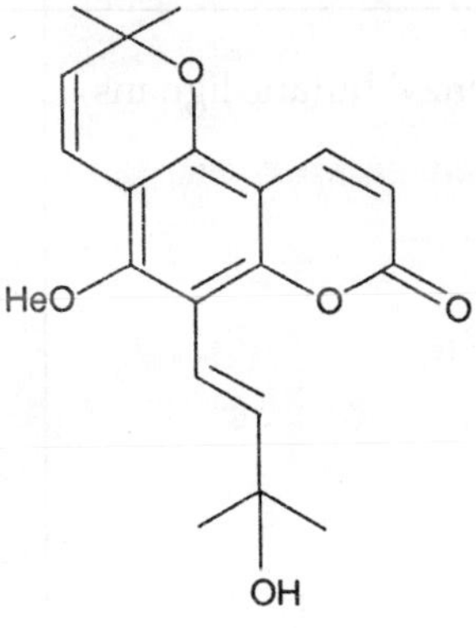 Avicennol
6.	Dimeric Coumarin	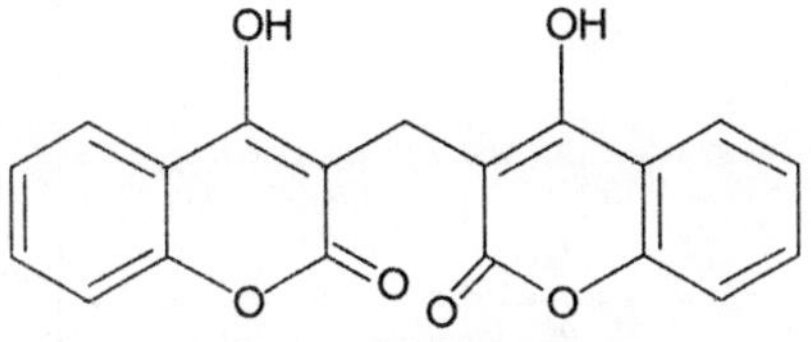 Dicoumarol
7.	Prenylated Coumarin	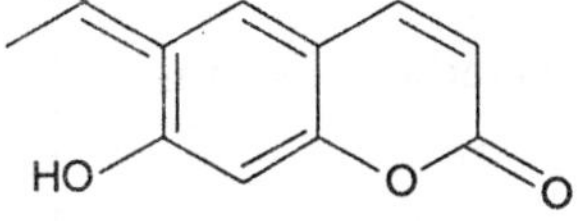 Dimethyl suberosin

8.3 Lignans

Lignans are a widely distributed plant phenolics, biosynthesised from the union of two phenylpropane molecules. They are, in general, cinnamoyl alcohol dimers, however cyclisation and other structural modifications result in various structural types. Naturally occurring lignans with a few exceptions are optically active. They exhibit significant physiological or pharmacological properties as for example podophyllotoxin which acts as antitumor agent. Lignans abundantly occur in plants of *Asteraceae, Piperaceae, Phytolaceae, Rutaceace, Pinaceae, Berberidaceae* and *Magnoliaceae* families. Some of the important structural types of lignans encountered in nature are as:

Sl. No.	Type	Representative Member
1.	Simple dibenzyl butane lignans	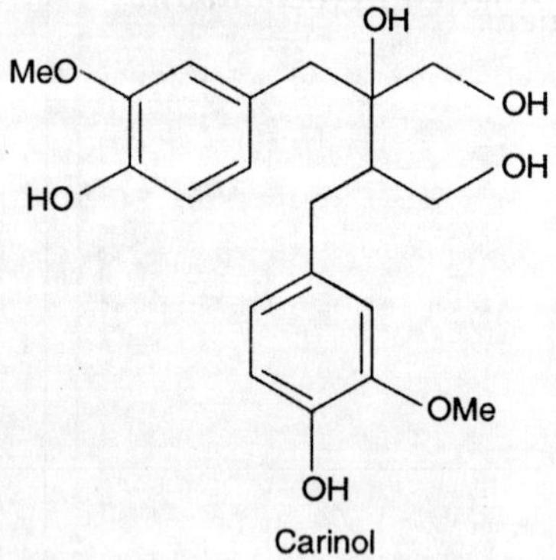Carinol
2.	Epoxylignans	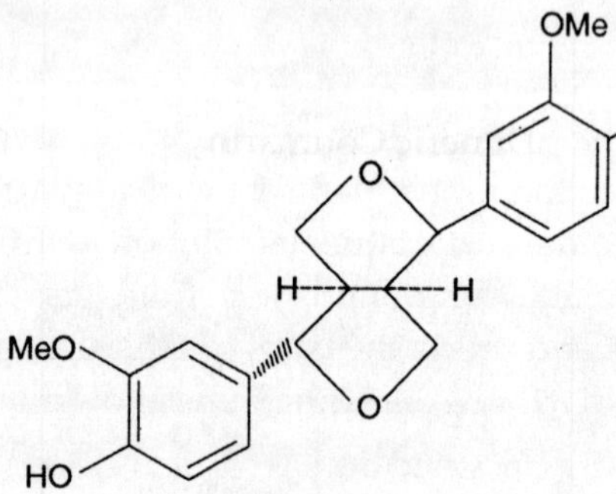Pinoresinol
3.	Dibenzocyclooctadiene lignans	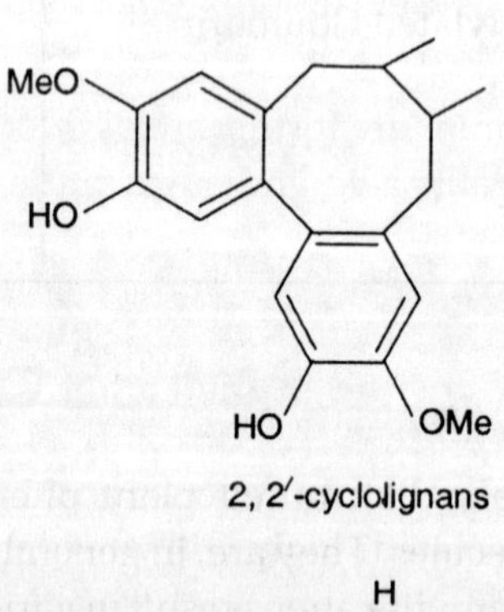2, 2′-cyclolignans
4.	Dibenzobutyrolactone lignans	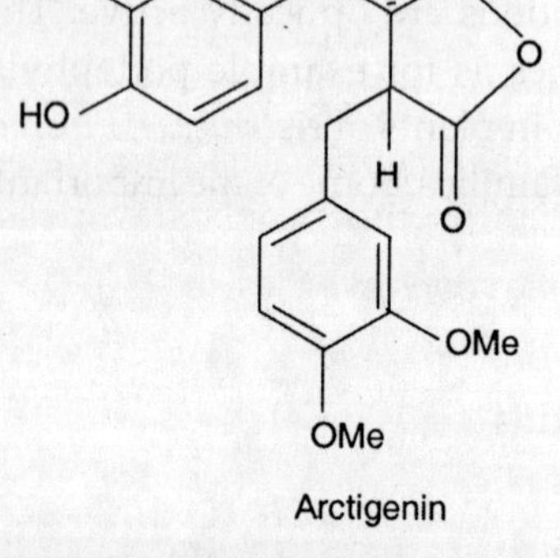Arctigenin

Sl. No.	Type	Representative Member
5.	Neolignans	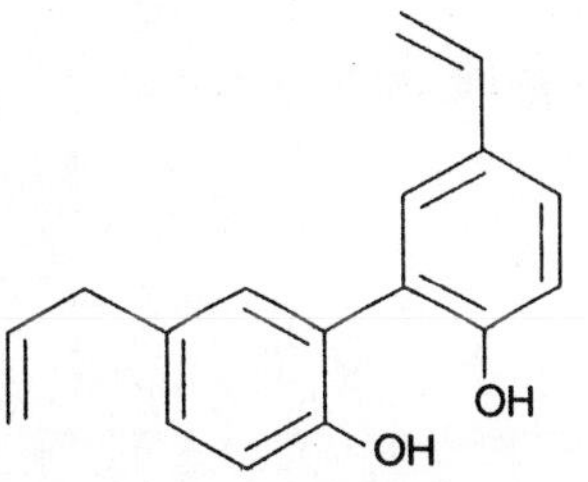 Magnolol

8.4 Tannins

Tannins are heterogeneous group of natural products and are widely distributed in plant families. They are normally found in unripe fruits but disappear during ripening. It is assumed that tannins provide protection to the plants from the microbial attack. Tannins are amorphous substances and form colloidal acidic aqueous solution with astringent taste. They form dark blue or greenish black water soluble compounds with iron salts. They form insoluble and indigestible compounds with proteins and this is the basis of their use in leather industry (tanning process) and for the treatment of diarrhoea, bleeding guns and skin injuries.

Tannins are classified into two broad classes viz., (i) condeused tannins and (ii) hydrolysable tannins. On treatment with acids or enzymes hydrolylable tannins undergo cleavage into simpler molecules while condensed tannins under similar condition form water insoluble complex molecule.

Hydrolylable tannins are further subdivided into *gallotannins* and *ellagitannins*. Gallotannins on hydrolysis form gallic acid and sugar but ellagitannins yield sugar, gallic acid and ellagic acid.

Model Questions

1. What are flavones? How flavones and isoflavones are related? How these two types of pigments are isolated? How will you identify these two kinds of pigments.
2. How are the structure of flavone determined? Illustrate your answer with a suitable example.
3. Discuss some general methods for the synthesis of flavones.
4. Discuss the general approach for the determination of the structure of isoflavones? Name some important members of isoflavone and write their structures.
5. How are isoflavones synthesised?
6. Write notes on:
   (a) Coumarins
   (b) Tannins
   (c) Lignans.

BIBLIOGRAPHY

1. "Organic Chemistry", Francis A. Carey, 3rd Edition, Tata Mcgraw-Hill, 1986.
2. "Organic Chemistry", I.L. Finar, Vol. I, ELBS, 1973.
3. "Organic Chemistry", I.L. Finar, Vol. II, ELBS, 1975.
4. "Organic Chemistry", J. Clayden, N. Greeves, S. Warren and P. Wothers, Oxford University Press, Oxford, 2001.
5. "Advanced Organic Chemistry— Reaction, Mechanism and Structure", Jerry March, 4th Edition, Wiley India, 2005.
6. "A Guide Book to Mechanism in Organic Chemistry", Peter Sykes, 6th Edition, Pearson Education, Dorling Kindersley (India) Pvt. Ltd, New Delhi, 2006.
7. "Textbook on Organic Chemisty", K.S. Mukherjee, New Central Book Agency (P) Ltd, Kolkata, 2007.
8. "Heterocyclic Chemistry— Synthesis, Reactions and Mechanisms", R.K. Bansal, Wiley Eastern Limited, New Delhi, 1990.
9. "The Principles of Heterocyclic Chemistry", A.R. Katritzky and J.M. Lagowski, Chapman and Hall Ltd, London, 1967.
10. "Natural Products, the Secondary Metabolites", J.R. Hanson, The Royal Society of Chemistry, London, 2003.
11. "Chemistry for Pharmacy Students— General, Organic and Natural Products Chemistry", S.D. Sarkar and L. Nahar, John Wiley and Sons Ltd, 2007.
12. "Pharmaceutical Organic Chemistry, Part I: Chemistry of Heterocyclic and Natural Compounds", R.R. Nadendla, Vallabh Publication, Delhi, 2005.
13. "Medicinal Chemistry", Ashutosh Kar, Wiley Eastern Ltd, New Delhi, 1992.
14. "Medicinal Chemistry", A. Burger (Ed), 2nd Edition, Interscience Publishers, Inc, NewYork, 1960.
15. "Burger's Medicinal Chemistry", M.E. Wolff, 4th Edition, John Wiley and Sons Ltd, 1981.

INDEX